To Jenny Lundberg
Best Wishes
Mark Rogers
Baltimore 1992

CURRENT PRACTICE
IN ANESTHESIOLOGY

SURGICAL TITLES IN THE CURRENT THERAPY SERIES

CURRENT PRACTICE
IN ANESTHESIOLOGY

SECOND EDITION

MARK C. ROGERS, M.D.

Professor and Chairman
Department of Anesthesiology and Critical Care Medicine
The Johns Hopkins University School of Medicine
Baltimore, Maryland

B.C. Decker
An Imprint of Mosby–Year Book

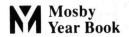

Dedicated to Publishing Excellence

Publisher: George Stamathis
Developmental Editor: Lynne Gery
Project Manager: Arofan Gregory

SECOND EDITION

Printed in the United States of America

Mosby–Year Book, Inc.
11830 Westline Industrial Drive
St. Louis, MO 63146

Library of Congress Cataloging-in-Publication Data
Current practice in anesthesiology / [edited by] Mark C. Rogers. —
　2nd ed.
　　　p.　cm. — (Current therapy series)
　Includes bibliographical references and index.
　ISBN 1-55664-269-5
　1. Anesthesiology.　I. Rogers, Mark C.　II. Series.
　[DNLM:　1. Anesthesiology.　WD 200 C976]
　RD81.C87　1992
　617.9´6—dc20
　DNLM/DLC　　　　　　　　　　　　　　　　　　　91-34676
　for Library of Congress　　　　　　　　　　　　　　CIP

92　93　94　95　96　GW/MY/MY　9　8　7　6　5　4　3　2　1

CONTRIBUTORS

ROBERT A. ABRAHAM, M.D., F.A.C.A.

Associate Professor Emeritus, Department of Anesthesiology and Critical Care Medicine, The Johns Hopkins University School of Medicine; Former Director, Division of Obstetric Anesthesia, The Johns Hopkins Hospital, Baltimore, Maryland

MAURICE S. ALBIN, M.D., M.Sc. (Anes.)

Professor, Departments of Anesthesiology and Neurosurgery, University of Texas Health Science Center, San Antonio, Texas

JAMES M. BAILEY, M.D., Ph.D.

Assistant Professor, Departments of Anesthesiology and Pediatrics, Emory University School of Medicine, Atlanta, Georgia

PAUL G. BARASH, M.D.

Professor and Chairman, Department of Anesthesiology, Yale University School of Medicine; Chief, Department of Anesthesiology, Yale-New Haven Hospital, New Haven, Connecticut

CHARLES BEATTIE, Ph.D., M.D.

Associate Professor and Director, Division of Critical Care Anesthesia, Department of Anesthesiology and Critical Care Medicine, The Johns Hopkins University School of Medicine, Baltimore, Maryland

AUDRÉE A. BENDO, M.D.

Assistant Professor, Department of Anesthesiology, State University of New York Health Sciences Center at Brooklyn, Brooklyn, New York

JONATHAN L. BENUMOF, M.D.

Professor of Anesthesiology, University of California San Diego School of Medicine, San Diego, California

IVOR D. BERKOWITZ, M.B., B.Ch.

Assistant Professor, Department of Anesthesiology and Critical Care Medicine, The Johns Hopkins University School of Medicine; Associate Director, Pediatric Intensive Care Unit, The Johns Hopkins Hospital, Baltimore, Maryland

EUGENE K. BETTS, M.D.

Associate Professor of Anesthesia, University of Pennsylvania School of Medicine; Associate Anesthesiologist-in-Chief, and Director, Division of Anesthesiology, Department of Anesthesiology and Critical Care Medicine, Children's Hospital of Philadelphia, Philadelphia, Pennsylvania

THOMAS J. J. BLANCK, M.D., Ph.D.

Associate Professor, Departments of Anesthesiology and Biomedical Engineering, The Johns Hopkins University School of Medicine, Baltimore, Maryland

CECIL O. BOREL, M.D.

Assistant Professor, Department of Anesthesiology and Critical Care Medicine, The Johns Hopkins University School of Medicine; Co-director, Neurosciences Critical Care Unit, and Medical Director, Respiratory Therapy, The Johns Hopkins Hospital, Baltimore, Maryland

LAWRENCE M. BORLAND, M.D., F.A.A.P.

Associate Professor of Anesthesiology/Critical Care Medicine and Pediatrics, University Health Center of Pittsburgh; Staff Anesthesiologist, Children's Hospital of Pittsburgh, Pittsburgh, Pennsylvania

DENIS L. BOURKE, M.D.

Associate Professor of Anesthesiology and Urology, The Johns Hopkins University School of Medicine; Director, Division of Regional Anesthesia and Pain Management, Department of Anesthesiology and Critical Care Medicine, The Johns Hopkins Hospital, Baltimore, Maryland

PHILIP G. BOYSEN, M.D.

Professor of Anesthesiology and Medicine, University of Florida College of Medicine; Associate Chief of Anesthesiology and Chief of Respiratory Care Service, Veterans Administration Medical Center, Gainesville, Florida

BARRY W. BRASFIELD, M.D.

Assistant Professor, Department of Anesthesiology, Emory University School of Medicine, Atlanta, Georgia

MICHAEL J. BRESLOW, M.D.

Assistant Professor, The Johns Hopkins University School of Medicine, Baltimore, Maryland

LINDA CAMERON, M.D.

Co-Director, Pain Management Service, Department of Anesthesiology and Critical Care Medicine, The Johns Hopkins Hospital, Baltimore, Maryland

ENRICO CAMPORESI, M.D.

Professor of Anesthesia and of Physiology, and Chairman, Department of Anesthesia, State University of New York Health Science Center at Syracuse, Syracuse, New York

EUGENIE S. CASELLA, M.D.

Assistant Professor, Departments of Anesthesiology and Critical Care Medicine and Pediatrics, The Johns Hopkins University School of Medicine; Cardiac Anesthesiologist, The Johns Hopkins Hospital, Baltimore, Maryland

ROSE CHRISTOPHERSON, M.D., Ph.D.

Assistant Professor, Departments of Anesthesiology and Critical Care Medicine, The Johns Hopkins University School of Medicine; Staff Anesthesiologist, The Johns Hopkins Hospital, Baltimore, Maryland

D. RYAN COOK, M.D.

Professor of Anesthesiology and Pharmacology, University Health Center of Pittsburgh; Director of Anesthesiology, Children's Hospital of Pittsburgh, Pittsburgh, Pennsylvania

JAMES E. COTTRELL, M.D.

Professor and Chairman, Department of Anesthesiology, State University of New York Health Sciences Center at Brooklyn, Brooklyn, New York

BENJAMIN G. COVINO, M.D., Ph.D. (deceased)

Former Professor of Anesthesia, Harvard Medical School; Former Chairman, Department of Anesthesia, Brigham and Women's Hospital, Boston, Massachusetts

ROBERT K. CRONE, M.D.

Professor of Anesthesiology and Pediatrics, University of Washington School of Medicine; Director of Anesthesiology, Children's Hospital and Medical Center, Seattle, Washington

MICHAEL N. D'AMBRA, M.D.

Assistant Professor of Anesthesia, Harvard Medical School; Assistant Anesthetist, Cardiac Anesthesia Group, Massachusetts General Hospital, Boston, Massachusetts

DONNA LYNN DARK-MEZICK, M.D.

Assistant Professor of Anesthesiology, University of South Alabama College of Medicine; Staff Anesthesiologist, University of South Alabama, Mobile, Alabama

J. KENNETH DAVISON, M.D.

Assistant Professor of Anesthesia, Harvard Medical School; Associate Anesthetist, Massachusetts General Hospital, Boston, Massachusetts

STEPHEN DERRER, M.D.

Assistant Professor, Department of Anesthesiology and Critical Care Medicine, The Johns Hopkins University School of Medicine, Baltimore, Maryland

ROSS DICKSTEIN, M.D.

Assistant Professor, Department of Anesthesiology and Critical Care Medicine, The Johns Hopkins University School of Medicine, Baltimore, Maryland

TODD DORMAN, M.D.

Fellow, Surgical Intensive Care Unit, Department of Anesthesiology and Critical Care Medicine, The Johns Hopkins University School of Medicine, Baltimore, Maryland

JEFFREY N. DORNBUSCH, M.D.

Assistant Professor of Anesthesiology, Columbia University College of Physicians and Surgeons; Assistant Anesthesiologist, Columbia-Presbyterian Medical Center, New York, New York

TOBY EAGLE, C.R.N.A.

Chief Nurse Anesthetist, The Johns Hopkins University Hospital, Baltimore, Maryland

WILLIAM F. ECKHARDT, M.D.

Instructor in Anesthesia, Harvard Medical School; Assistant in Anesthesia, Massachusetts General Hospital, Boston, Massachusetts

SCOTT M. ELEFF, M.D.

Assistant Professor, Department of Anesthesiology and Critical Care Medicine, The Johns Hopkins University School of Medicine, Baltimore, Maryland

JEFFREY C. ELMORE, M.D.

Assistant Professor, Department of Anesthesiology, University of Texas Southwestern Medical School; Attending Anesthesiologist, Division of Cardiovascular Anesthesiology, Southwestern Medical Center, Dallas, Texas

NABIL R. FAHMY, M.D., F.F.A.R.C.S., D.A.

Associate Professor of Anesthesia, Harvard Medical School; Anesthetist, Massachusetts General Hospital, Boston, Massachusetts

MARC FELDMAN, M.D.

Assistant Professor, Department of Anesthesiology and Critical Care Medicine; The Johns Hopkins University School of Medicine; Director, Division of Ophthalmic Anesthesia, The Johns Hopkins Hospital, Baltimore, Maryland

JOANNE L. FLOYD, M.D.

Assistant Professor of Anesthesiology, Indiana University School of Medicine, Indianapolis, Indiana

STEVEN M. FRANK, M.D.

Assistant Professor, Department of Anesthesiology and Critical Care Medicine, The Johns Hopkins University School of Medicine, Baltimore, Maryland

ELIZABETH A. M. FROST, M.D.

Professor of Anesthesiology, Albert Einstein College of Medicine of Yeshiva University; Director of Neuroanesthesia, Montefiore Medical Center, Bronx, New York

WILLIAM R. FURMAN, M.D.

Assistant Professor, Department of Anesthesiology and Critical Care Medicine, The Johns Hopkins University School of Medicine; Chairman, Department of Anesthesiology, Francis Scott Key Medical Center, Baltimore, Maryland

SIMON GELMAN, M.D., Ph.D.

Professor and Chairman, Department of Anesthesiology, and Professor, Department of Physiology and Biophysics, University of Alabama School of Medicine, Birmingham, Alabama

ADOLPH H. GIESECKE, Jr., M.D.

Jenkins Professor and Acting Chairman, Department of Anesthesiology, University of Texas Southwestern Medical School; Attending Anesthesiologist, Parkland Hospital, Dallas, Texas

MARK H. GILLIE, M.D.

Research Fellow in Anesthesiology, University of Utah School of Medicine, Salt Lake City, Utah

NISHAN G. GOUDSOUZIAN, M.D.

Associate Professor of Anesthesia, Harvard Medical School; Anesthetist, Massachusetts General Hospital, Boston, Massachusetts

GEORGE J. GRAF, M.D.

Clinical Assistant Professor of Anesthesiology and Medicine, University of California Los Angeles School of Medicine; Attending Anesthesiologist, Cedars-Sinai Medical Center, Los Angeles, California

CHRISTOPHER M. GRANDE, M.D.

Special Consultant and Chief, Special Project Branch, Department of Anesthesiology, Shock Trauma Center, Maryland Institute for Emergency Medical Services Systems, University of Maryland School of Medicine, Baltimore, Maryland

JEFFREY A. GRASS, M.D.

Instructor, Department of Anesthesiology and Critical Care Medicine, The Johns Hopkins University School of Medicine; Staff, Division of Obstetric Anesthesia, and Director, Acute Pain Service, The Johns Hopkins Hospital, Baltimore, Maryland

ROGER GRAYSON, M.D.

Assistant Professor, Department of Anesthesiology and Critical Care Medicine, The Johns Hopkins University School of Medicine, Baltimore, Maryland

GEORGE A. GREGORY, M.D.

Professor, Department of Anesthesia, University of California San Diego School of Medicine, San Diego, California

ALAN W. GROGONO, M.D. (Lond.), F.F.A.R.C.S

Chairman and Merryl and Sam Israel, Jr., Professor of Anesthesiology, Tulane University School of Medicine, New Orleans, Louisiana

CHARLES M. HABERKERN, M.D.

Assistant Professor of Anesthesiology and Pediatrics, University of Washington; Staff Anesthesiologist, Children's Hospital and Medical Center, Seattle, Washington

ANDREW P. HARRIS, M.D.

Assistant Professor, Department of Anesthesiology and Critical Care Medicine and Department of Gynecology and Obstetrics, The Johns Hopkins University School of Medicine; Chief, Obstetric Anesthesiology, The Johns Hopkins Hospital, Baltimore, Maryland

GREGG S. HARTMAN, M.D.

Assistant Professor, Department of Anesthesia, New York Hospital–Cornell Medical Center, New York, New York

NELSON HENDLER, M.D., M.S.

Assistant Professor of Neurosurgery, The Johns Hopkins University School of Medicine, Baltimore; Clinical Director, Mensana Clinic, Stevenson, Maryland

ROSEMARY HICKEY, M.D.

Assistant Professor, Department of Anesthesiology, University of Texas Health Science Center, San Antonio, Texas

CAROL A. HIRSHMAN, M.D.

Professor of Anesthesiology, Environmental Health Sciences, and Medicine, The Johns Hopkins University School of Medicine; Staff Anesthesiologist, The Johns Hopkins Hospital, Baltimore, Maryland

MARTIN J. HURD, M.D.

Resident, Department of Anesthesia and Critical Care Medicine, University of Chicago Division of Biological Sciences Pritzker School of Medicine, Chicago, Illinois

LUCILLE W. KING, M.D.

Chief, Division of Endocrinology, Wyman Park Medical Associates, Baltimore, Maryland

ELLIOT J. KRANE, M.D.

Associate Professor, Department of Anesthesiology, University of Washington School of Medicine; Co-Director, Pain and Stress Management Service, Children's Hospital and Medical Center, Seattle, Washington

JOHN R. LIPSEY, M.D.

Assistant Professor, Department of Psychiatry, The Johns Hopkins University School of Medicine, Baltimore, Maryland

EDWARD LOWENSTEIN, M.D.

Professor of Anesthesia, Harvard Medical School; Anesthetist-in-Chief, Department of Anesthesia and Critical Care, Beth Israel Hospital, Boston, Massachusetts

PHILIP D. LUMB, M.B.B.S.

Professor and Chairman, Department of Anesthesia, Albany Medical Center, Albany, New York

COLIN F. MACKENZIE, M.B., Ch.B., F.F.A.R.C.S.

Professor of Anesthesiology and Associate Professor of Physiology, University of Maryland School of Medicine; Attending Anesthesiologist, University of Maryland Medical System, Baltimore, Maryland

DEVANAND MANGAR, M.D.

Assistant Professor, Department of Anesthesia, University of South Florida College of Medicine, Tampa, Florida

GERTIE F. MARX, M.D.

Professor of Anesthesiology, Albert Einstein College of Medicine of Yeshiva University; Attending Anesthesiologist, Albert Einstein Affiliated Hospitals, Bronx, New York

M. JANE MATJASKO, M.D.

Martin Helrich Professor and Chairman, Department of Anesthesiology, University of Maryland School of Medicine; Chairman, Department of Anesthesiology, University of Maryland Medical System, Baltimore, Maryland

KATHRYN E. McGOLDRICK, M.D.

Associate Professor of Anesthesiology, Yale University School of Medicine; Attending Anesthesiologist, and Medical Director, One-Day Surgery, Yale-New Haven Hospital, New Haven, Connecticut

WARREN R. McKAY, M.D.

Assistant Clinical Professor of Anesthesia, and Director, Pain Management Center, University of California San Francisco School of Medicine, San Francisco, California

ROBERT W. McPHERSON, M.D.

Associate Professor, Department of Anesthesiology and Critical Care Medicine, The Johns Hopkins University School of Medicine; Director, Division of Neuroanesthesia, The Johns Hopkins Hospital, Baltimore, Maryland

ROBERT G. MERIN, M.D.

Professor of Anesthesiology, University of Texas Medical School at Houston; Attending Anesthesiologist, Hermann Hospital, Houston, Texas

WILLIAM T. MERRITT, M.D.

Assistant Professor, Department of Anesthesiology and Critical Care Medicine, The Johns Hopkins University School of Medicine, Baltimore, Maryland

CLAIR MILLER, M.D.

Associate Medical Director, Intensive Care Unit, Sinai Hospital, Baltimore, Maryland

EDWARD D. MILLER, Jr., M.D.

E. M. Papper Professor and Chairman, Department of Anesthesiology, Columbia University College of Physicians and Surgeons; Director, Anesthesiology Service, Presbyterian Hospital, New York, New York

JOHN N. MILLER, M.B., B.S.

Professor and Chairman, Department of Anesthesiology, and Chief, Anesthesia Services, University of South Alabama College of Medicine, Mobile, Alabama

RONALD D. MILLER, M.D.

Professor and Chairman, Department of Anesthesiology, and Professor of Pharmacology, University of California San Francisco School of Medicine, San Francisco, California

JOHN R. MOYERS, M.D.

Professor, University of Iowa College of Medicine; Attending, University of Iowa Hospitals and Clinics, Iowa City, Iowa

TERENCE M. MURPHY, M.B., Ch.B., F.F.A.R.C.S

Professor, Department of Anesthesiology, University of Washington School of Medicine, Seattle, Washington

JOLIE NARANG, M.D.

Assistant Professor, Department of Anesthesiology, Mount Sinai School of Medicine; Attending Physician, Mount Sinai Medical Center, New York, New York

ELIZABETH NICHOLAS, M.D.

Assistant Professor, Departments of Anesthesiology and Critical Care Medicine and Pediatrics, The Johns Hopkins University School of Medicine; Associate Director, Multi-Disciplinary Pain Service, The Children's Center, The Johns Hopkins Hospital, Baltimore, Maryland

DANIEL P. NYHAN, M.D.

Assistant Professor, Department of Anesthesiology and Critical Care Medicine, The Johns Hopkins University School of Medicine; Staff, Department of Anesthesiology and Critical Care Medicine, The Johns Hopkins Hospital, Baltimore, Maryland

CHARLES W. OTTO, M.D., F.C.C.M.

Professor of Anesthesiology and Associate Professor of Medicine, University of Arizona College of Medicine, Tucson, Arizona

L. REUVEN PASTERNAK, M.D., M.P.H.

Assistant Professor, Department of Anesthesiology and Critical Care Medicine, The Johns Hopkins University School of Medicine; Medical Director, Same Day Surgery Programs, The Johns Hopkins Hospitals, Baltimore, Maryland

LAUREN A. PLANTE, M.D.

Instructor in Anesthesiology, Albert Einstein College of Medicine of Yeshiva University; Assistant Attending Anesthesiologist, Albert Einstein Affiliated Hospitals, New York, New York

P. PRITHVI RAJ, M.B.B.S., F.F.A.R.C.S.

Professor of Anesthesiology, Medical College of Georgia; Executive Medical Director, Southeastern Institute of Pain Medicine, Georgia Baptist Medical Center, Atlanta, Georgia

SRINIVASA N. RAJA, M.D.

Associate Professor, Department of Anesthesiology and Critical Care Medicine, The Johns Hopkins University School of Medicine; Director, Pain Management Services, The Johns Hopkins Hospital, Baltimore, Maryland

SOMAYAJI RAMAMURTHY, M.D.

Professor, Department of Anesthesiology, University of Texas Medical School at San Antonio; Chief, Pain Management Clinic, University of Texas Health Science Center, San Antonio, Texas

PETER ROCK, M.D.

Assistant Professor, Department of Anesthesiology and Critical Care Medicine, The Johns Hopkins University School of Medicine; Chief, Section of General Surgery Anesthesia, Department of Anesthesiology and Critical Care Medicine, The Johns Hopkins Hospital, Baltimore, Maryland

MARK A. ROCKOFF, M.D.

Associate Professor of Anesthesia and Pediatrics, Harvard Medical School; Acting Chairman and Clinical Director, Department of Anesthesia, The Children's Hospital, Boston, Massachusetts

ELIZABETH L. ROGERS, M.D.

Associate Dean, University of Maryland School of Medicine; Chief of Staff, Baltimore Veterans Administration Medical Center, Baltimore, Maryland

MICHAEL F. ROIZEN, M.D.

Professor of Anesthesia and Critical Care Medicine and of Internal Medicine, University of Chicago Division of Biological Sciences Pritzker School of Medicine; Chairman, Department of Anesthesia and Critical Care, University of Chicago Hospitals and Clinics, Chicago, Illinois

BRIAN A. ROSENFELD, M.D.

Assistant Professor, Department of Anesthesiology and Critical Care Medicine, The Johns Hopkins University School of Medicine, Baltimore, Maryland

JACOB SAMUEL, F.F.A.R.C.S.

Assistant Professor, Albany Medical College, Albany, New York

DAVID L. SCHREIBMAN, M.D.

Assistant Professor, Department of Anesthesiology, University of Maryland School of Medicine; Attending Anesthesiologist, University of Maryland Medical System, Baltimore, Maryland

MARK S. SCHREINER, M.D.

Assistant Professor of Anesthesia and Pediatrics, University of Pennsylvania School of Medicine; Assistant Anesthesiologist, Children's Hospital of Philadelphia, Philadelphia, Pennsylvania

NANCY SETZER, M.D.

Associate Professor of Clinical Anesthesiology and Pediatrics, University of Miami School of Medicine, Miami, Florida

BARRY A. SHAPIRO, M.D.

Professor, Vice Chairman, and Chief, Section of Respiratory and Critical Care Medicine, Department of Anesthesia, Northwestern University Medical School; Medical Director, Respiratory Care Services, Northwestern Memorial Hospital, Chicago, Illinois

FREDERICK E. SIEBER, M.D.

Assistant Professor, Department of Anesthesiology and Critical Care Medicine, The Johns Hopkins University School of Medicine, Baltimore, Maryland

TOD SLOAN, M.D., Ph.D.

Associate Professor, Department of Anesthesiology, University of Texas Health Science Center, San Antonio, Texas

BRADLEY E. SMITH, M.D.

Professor and Chair, Department of Anesthesiology, Vanderbilt University School of Medicine; Chief, Anesthesiology Department, Vanderbilt University Medical Center, Nashville, Tennessee

DAVID S. SMITH, M.D., Ph.D.

Associate Professor, Department of Anesthesia, University of Pennsylvania School of Medicine; Director, Division of Neurosurgical Anesthesia, Hospital of the University of Pennsylvania, Philadelphia, Pennsylvania

DOUGLAS S. SNYDER, M.D., M.S.

Instructor, Department of Anesthesia and Critical Care Medicine, The Johns Hopkins University School of Medicine, Baltimore, Maryland

ROBERT SPRAGUE, M.D.

Community Chief, Anesthesia/Operative Services, Blanchfield Army Hospital, Fort Campbell, Kentucky

THEODORE H. STANLEY, M.D.

Professor, Department of Anesthesiology, University of Utah School of Medicine, Salt Lake City, Utah

JOHN K. STENE, Jr., M.D., Ph.D.

Assistant Professor, Department of Anesthesia, Pennsylvania State University College of Medicine; Director, Perioperative Anesthesia Trauma Services, The Milton S. Hershey Medical Center, Hershey, Pennsylvania

ROBERT L. STEVENSON, M.D.

Associate Professor, Department of Anesthesiology and Critical Care Medicine, The Johns Hopkins University School of Medicine; Director of Resident Education, Department of Anesthesiology, The Johns Hopkins Hospital, Baltimore, Maryland

JUDITH L. STIFF, M.D.

Associate Professor, Department of Anesthesiology and Critical Care Medicine, The Johns Hopkins University School of Medicine; Attending Anesthesiologist, Francis Scott Key Medical Center, Baltimore, Maryland

ROBERT K. STOELTING, M.D.

Professor of Anesthesiology, Indiana University School of Medicine, Indianapolis, Indiana

SUSAN G. STRAUSS, M.D.

Assistant Professor, Department of Anesthesiology, University of Washington School of Medicine; Anesthesiologist, Children's Hospital and Medical Center, Seattle, Washington

BRIAN K. TABATA, M.D.

Former Assistant Professor, Department of Anesthesiology and Critical Care Medicine, The Johns Hopkins University School of Medicine, Baltimore, Maryland; Presently Staff Pediatric and Obstetrical Anesthesiologist, Kapiolani Women's and Children's Medical Center, Honolulu, Hawaii

STEPHEN J. THOMAS, M.D.

Associate Professor and Vice Chairman, Department of Anesthesia, New York Hospital–Cornell Medical Center, New York, New York

DANIEL M. THYS, M.D.

Professor, Department of Anesthesiology, Columbia University College of Physicians and Surgeons; Director, Department of Anesthesiology, St. Luke's/Roosevelt Hospital Center, New York, New York

JOHN H. TINKER, M.D.

Professor and Head, Department of Anesthesia, University of Iowa College of Medicine, Iowa City, Iowa

JOSEPH D. TOBIAS, M.D.

Assistant Professor of Anesthesiology and Pediatrics, University of Tennessee, Memphis, College of Medicine; Director, Division of Pediatric Anesthesia and Critical Care Medicine, St. Jude Children's Research Hospital, Memphis, Tennessee

MITCHELL TOBIAS, M.D.

Assistant Professor, Department of Anesthesia, University of Pennsylvania School of Medicine, Philadelphia, Pennsylvania

I. DAVID TODRES, M.D.

Associate Professor in Anesthesia and Pediatrics, Harvard Medical School; Director, Neonatal and Pediatric Intensive Care Units, Massachusetts General Hospital, Boston, Massachusetts

SUSAN A. VASSALLO, M.D.

Instructor in Anesthesia, Harvard Medical School; Assistant in Anesthesia, Massachusetts General Hospital, Boston, Massachusetts

JOHN L. WALLER, M.D.

Professor and Chairman, Department of Anesthesiology, Emory University School of Medicine, Atlanta, Georgia

W. DAVID WATKINS, M.D., Ph.D.

Professor of Anesthesiology and Pharmacology, Duke University Medical Center, Durham, North Carolina

R. J. N. WATSON, M.A., M.B., B.Chir., F.F.A.R.C.S.

Assistant Professor of Anesthesia, University of Maryland School of Medicine; Director, Cardiothoracic Anesthesia, University of Maryland Hospital, Baltimore, Maryland

RANDALL C. WETZEL, M.B., B.S., F.C.C.M.

Associate Professor, Departments of Anesthesiology and Critical Care Medicine and Pediatrics, The Johns Hopkins University School of Medicine; Chief, Division of Pediatric Anesthesia, The Johns Hopkins Hospital, Baltimore, Maryland

ROGER S. WILSON, M.D.

Associate Professor of Anesthesia, Harvard Medical School; Anesthetist, Masssachusetts General Hospital, Boston, Massachusetts

MYRON YASTER, M.D.

Associate Professor, Departments of Anesthesiology and Critical Care Medicine and Pediatrics, The Johns Hopkins University School of Medicine; Director, Multi-Disciplinary Pain Service, The Children's Center, The Johns Hopkins Hospital, Baltimore, Maryland

JAMES R. ZAIDAN, M.D.

Professor, Department of Anesthesiology, Emory University School of Medicine, Atlanta, Georgia

RHONDA L. ZUCKERMAN, M.D.

Assistant Professor, Department of Anesthesiology and Critical Care Medicine, The Johns Hopkins University School of Medicine; Associate Director, Obstetric Anesthesiology, The Johns Hopkins Hospital, Baltimore, Maryland

PREFACE

The second edition of *Current Practice in Anesthesiology* represents a significant enlargement, and we hope a significant improvement, of the book. Seventeen chapters have been added in an attempt to make the material more complete and more comprehensive. Similarly, many of the contributors to the first edition were asked to write different chapters in the second edition. This provides fresh insight into the areas of anesthetic practice and keeps the book dynamic and changing.

It is our hope that these changes will result in a progressively more useful and interesting presentation of anesthesia, while retaining a clear-cut clinical focus designed to reflect how individual experts in the field conduct their practice.

Mark C. Rogers, M.D.

CONTENTS

CURRENT PRACTICE
IN ANESTHESIOLOGY

PREOPERATIVE CONSIDERATIONS

ANESTHETIC RISK

PETER ROCK, M.D.
JOHN H. TINKER, M.D.

Just a few decades ago, there was a major risk in anesthetizing patients for major surgery; both the anesthesia and the surgery were risky. For example, with diethyl ether as the anesthetic, to produce adequate abdominal muscle relaxation for the performance of major intra-abdominal surgery, it was necessary to deepen the patient's anesthesia to levels whereby cardiovascular collapse was possible. Patients with compromised cardiovascular systems often did not tolerate this much "physiologic trespass." During these times, there was real meaning when the surgeon would say to a patient's relative, "I'm sorry, but I don't think your mother would be able to tolerate the anesthesia."

Obviously, the situation is different today. Even the most moribund patient can be rendered pain-free for the performance of needed surgery, and that individual's abdominal muscles can be relaxed to the point of cadaveric neuromuscular paralysis, if necessary. To a large extent, we have succeeded in separating the various aspects of that totality we call "anesthesia," so that we provide hypnosis and obliteration of awareness with one set of drugs, neuromuscular blockade with another set, obtundation of untoward autonomic reflexes with a third, and postoperative analgesia with yet another group of drugs. This allows excellent flexibility during performance of modern anesthesia, but also adds myriad complexities. When one considers the possibilities of drug-to-drug interactions with the various possible combinations of the aforementioned drugs, plus the medications the patient may be taking, plus the patient's preoperative drug history, this should lead to understanding that today's "anesthesia risk" is still real, although it is much lower and is composed of additional elements rather than just the risk of anesthetic overdose. Added to the complexity of pharmacologic therapy today are invasive monitors whose placement may cause harm; electronic equipment with electric shock hazard; and complicated mechanical ventilators, which require the

proper functioning of alarms. Additionally, piped-in gas systems must be monitored to ensure that they contain the proper gas, and modern anesthesia machines are quite complex and include sophisticated airway disconnect alarms, which may not be turned on or may not work. Finally, major surgical procedures are now performed at the extremes of age and health. One can readily begin to contemplate the complexities of any discussion of anesthetic risk.

Despite the many changes in anesthesia practice and the complexity of modern anesthesia that render risk analysis difficult, some themes do emerge. The basics of good care have not changed over many years. Proper airway management is essential. Hypoxemia resulting from unintentional esophageal intubation or airway disconnection is still lethal. Patients can be overdosed with inhalational or intravenous anesthetic agents. Finally, the interaction between the patient's medical problems, drugs given to treat those problems, and anesthetic agents must be understood to lessen risk.

The next consideration is that of reportage. In the United States especially, but increasingly throughout the Western world, our colleagues in the legal profession would like to believe that they are making us more accountable for our actions by scrutinizing our records and results in detail. Whether this is true or not, such legal considerations probably are behind current reluctance to report critical incidents, lapses, errors in judgment, anesthetic overdoses, airway disconnects, and so on, even in a retrospective or statistical way, for fear of "discovery" or of being held accountable in other ways. Today, few physicians in the United States believe that there is really very much protection against legal assault and so have become extremely reticent about reporting the true incidence of these difficulties.

Another problem that still plagues us in this field is that of "self-flagellation." The flagellative school of thought about anesthesia risk is typified by a well-known statement attributed to Sir Robert Mcintosh: "I hold that there should be no deaths due to anesthesia." We are much more in agreement with the carefully reasoned agreements of Dr. Arthur S. Keats who, paraphrased, says, "Why shouldn't there be?" His contention is that we use dangerous potent drugs and combinations of drugs with major possibilities of drug-to-drug interactions in patients who are already sick and that it is unreasonable to believe that overall risk from anesthesia could ever be zero. The curious notion that because anesthesia does not do direct therapeutic good it must not do any harm seems nonsensical.

The contrast between this historical perspective regarding the anesthetic risk and contemporary views of other "risky" medical undertakings is often stark. For example, cardiac catheterization is well recognized to have risks associated with its performance. Perhaps because it is done in "sick" patients and is viewed as a highly invasive procedure, a risk of death of 1 to 5 per 1,000 cases seems acceptable. Risk of death from anesthesia is probably less than this. Similarly, every year several hundred patients suffer anaphylactic reactions to penicillin, a recognized rare complication of its use. Thus, a modern view of medicine holds that all treatments, including anesthesia, have some inherent risk.

Furthermore, no consideration of risk can be separated from that of a benefit. Today, every procedure, therapy, or drug treatment is carefully scrutinized for its risk-benefit ratio. The anesthesiologist, expert in considerations of perioperative risk assessment, is well suited to be an important member of the perioperative management team and its deliberations regarding benefit and risk of the proposed surgery.

This is not to say that no further improvements can be made in the level of quality of care in anesthesia. However, although some educators believe that browbeating their residents in training with the concept that all untoward outcomes are due to preventable errors can result in optimal vigilance, we believe that teaching residents to be truthful with themselves first and foremost is a better educational tool. Furthermore, the self-deprecatory approach may well produce so much self-doubt and guilt in trainees and practitioners as to affect their abilities in future cases. Thus anesthesiologists must take a balanced approach to discussions of anesthetic risk and must discuss and write about these risks as well as report them, while at the same time working toward statutory methods of protection against legal assault for so doing.

OVERALL RISK OF ANESTHETIC DEATH

Is it possible to find a modern study wherein reporting was sufficiently extensive and believable? The studies of Lunn and associates in Cardiff, Wales, come close to this ideal and are relatively recent. They comprise reportings on the performance of hundreds of thousands of anesthetics. The investigators made careful attempts to assign specific causes to each of the deaths that occurred in the operating room, in the recovery room, and to those that occurred within 6 days of operation elsewhere in the hospital. Lunn and colleagues attempted to classify these patients into risk categories similar to those used in the American Society of Anesthesiologists' risk classification. Careful analysis of the Cardiff data would indicate that there may be a set of simple fractions to which this reasonably modern

overall risk data can be reduced. If the patient is healthy and has had no added risk factors, total perioperative mortality (including deaths due to anesthesia, patient disease, surgery, and all other causes) is about one in 500. If a single risk factor is added, but the patient is still in overall good condition, then the overall incidence of in-hospital mortality is about one in 100. If, in addition to systemic disease, there is some preoperative impairment of ability to function normally, the risk jumps to approximately one in 50. If that impairment is cardiac failure, the risk is one in 25. Severe global preoperative impairment increases the risk to one in five. Finally, patients judged moribund or nearly so have total perioperative risks of approximately one in two.

How much of this information is useful to anesthesiologists—that is, how much of it can be remotely related to either selection or performance of the anesthetic? The notable efforts of Lunn and colleagues again provide the most modern set of answers. However, it must be remembered that the reporting in the Lunn studies was by no means perfect, even though the investigators had received assurances from the government that there would be no legal repercussions. Nonetheless, this is the best modern study of overall anesthesia risk. Deaths, which occurred either in the operating room or within a few days after surgery, were analyzed by a "blinded assessor." In one of the Lunn reports, 197 such deaths were studied. Of these, 43 percent were believed to have nothing to do with anesthesia, whereas 41 percent were believed to be partly caused by anesthesia, and an additional 16 percent were believed to be totally caused by anesthesia. The authors separately queried both the anesthesiologist and surgeon involved in each case to assess who should be "blamed" for these deaths. Needless to say, there was not much agreement. The independent "blinded assessor" agreed with the anesthesiologist alone in 33 percent of the cases, with the surgeon alone in 29 percent of the cases, with neither in 19 percent, and with both in only 18 percent of the cases.

Perhaps a sample case taken from the Cardiff study might serve to point out the difficulties inherent in any study of anesthetic risk.

A 6-month-old infant was to have had a pyloromyotomy. No vagolytic drug was given. Two percent halothane was administered after succinylcholine, 1.5 mg, was given intravenously. There was manual intermittent positive-pressure ventilation of the lungs. Although both anesthesiologist and surgeon believed that anesthesia played some part in the death, which occurred during the use of this anesthetic, the assessors considered anesthesia to be totally responsible.

This death was considered preventable and points out another major problem in any consideration of anesthetic risk. Of the deaths adjudicated by the Cardiff group to be attributable to anesthesia, five of 32 were described as unavoidable—that is, not attributable to detectable errors in judgment, wrong drug, lapses in vigilance, or departures from standards of care. This supports the contention above that by no means are all "anesthesia deaths" necessarily preventable. In the remaining 27 deaths in the Cardiff study, there were no avoidable features; even in these cases the investigators could not always find convincing evidence that, without the errors or lapses that did occur, the individuals would not have died anyway.

To summarize the Cardiff data, it was found that anesthesia was partly or totally the cause of death in about one to two cases in 10,000. This figure of one anesthetic death per 10,000 cases is probably the most modern anesthesia risk statistic currently available. Without mandatory critical incident reporting, coupled with real protection against legal assault, this statistic derived from voluntary questionnaire reprospective studies done in the late 1970s is likely to be the standard for quite some time.

Are we making any progress? Is there evidence that the current anesthesia risk statistic is better than that of the past? The answers to both of these questions are clearly *yes*. Major studies of anesthesia risk have been published since 1954, when the famous Beecher and Todd study of the performance of 599,584 anesthetics was published. As a cause of death, anesthesia was thought to be either "primary" or "contributory" in one case per 1,560 anesthetics performed. The report of the greatest anesthesia risk was made in 1961 by Dripps and colleagues, wherein a study of 33,224 cases produced an overall anesthesia "primary plus contributory" death rate of one per 115 cases.

In 1968, a larger study of 177,928 anesthetic procedures by Harrison and co-workers reported an anesthesia-related death rate of one per 3,000 cases. Thus, there does seem to be a trend toward improvement in the overall anesthesia death rate statistics. However, there is great variation as would be expected given the problems with such studies as previously noted.

How meaningful is this figure of one death due to anesthesia per 10,000 cases. First, it means that for the "average" anesthesiologist, who supervises 1,000 cases per year, there may be possibly three or more anesthetic-related deaths in the course of his or her career. For some, this may be frightening to contemplate. However, it is crucial to remember that all such statistics must be fractions; in other words, there must be a denominator to go along with this numerator. Each conscientious and competent anesthesiologist must remember that the denominator consists of the number of patients who were specifically helped, or even whose lives were saved during that anesthesiologist's career.

SPECIFIC STUDIES OF ANESTHESIA RISK

Prior Myocardial Infarction

In order to discuss the specifics of anesthesia risk, the concept of "events" must be understood. Compare, for example, estimates of anesthesia risk in patients with prior myocardial infarctions (MIs) (i.e., events) versus estimates of anesthesia risk in patients with congestive heart failure. In the former case, there has been an

event. The event tells us of the existence of a disease. Although this does not necessarily tell us much about the extent of that disease, we know that there is at least one critical coronary stenosis that has produced an infarction. By contrast, congestive heart failure is a continuum (not necessarily linear), and it is obviously much more difficult to tell where a specific patient is on that continuum. This is why most studies of perioperative risk have focused on patients who have suffered one or more particular events. Specifically, most studies have focused on the event of a previous MI. There are over 30 such studies, the first of which was produced in the late 1950s. With one recent exception, to be subsequently discussed, these studies have had a remarkable consistency through the past 2.5 decades.

A patient who has suffered a remote MI has approximately a 6 percent chance of suffering another MI during or within the 7 days following any kind of noncardiac surgery. A patient with a recent MI is at much greater risk. If that prior MI occurred 3 months previously or less, the risk of a perioperative MI is approximately 30 percent; if the prior MI occurred 3 to 6 months earlier, the risk is still high, namely 15 percent or so. Beyond 6 months after an infarction, the risk levels off at about 6 percent. The mortality from these perioperative reinfarctions is high, ranging between 50 to 70 percent in the literature.

Is there any evidence that we are getting any better? In 1983, Rao and El-Etr reported two groups of patients: the group studied prior to 1977 showed perioperative infarction rates that were almost exactly as previously described; the second group of patients studied between 1977 and 1981 had a much lower overall perioperative reinfarction rate—namely 1.9 percent. The risk for their patients with recent MIs was also much lower: less than 6 percent for infarcts within the previous 3 months and less than 3 percent for patients with infarcts within the previous 3 to 6 months. This excellent result has not been repeated to date. The authors attributed their results to the aggressive use of invasive monitors and drug therapy decisions based thereon. Whether this actually explains their results remains in some dispute, but these authors did demonstrate that improvements may be possible.

Those physicians who specialize in the perioperative management of such high-risk patients in the operating room and intensive care units believe that our specialty has made advances in the perioperative care of patients with recent MI. There is better recognition and treatment of hemodynamic factors related to myocardial ischemia (tachycardia, hypertension, congestive heart failure, pain); and improved modalities to assess myocardial performance (pulmonary artery catheters, on-line ST segment analysis, two-dimensional echocardiography, esophageal echocardiography) are available intraoperatively and postoperatively to help guide therapy. Furthermore, there is emerging thought that not all infarctions are the same and that the functional status of a patient may be important. Thus, low-level exercise stress tests, echocardiography, and nuclear imaging techniques may help identify subsets of recent MI patients at low risk for surgery. This idea, while attractive, remains to be verified.

Patients who have undergone prior successful coronary artery bypass surgery and who then undergo subsequent noncardiac surgery seem to have a remarkably low risk of perioperative MI. Maybe this is because the coronary artery bypass graft (CABG) protects the patient against a perioperative MI around the subsequent noncardiac surgery, or maybe it is because the perioperative MI that was "available to happen" occurred around the CABG itself. Whichever is operative, the fact is that the patient who has had a relatively recent (within 5 years or so) successful CABG is probably at much lower risk of a perioperative MI than a patient who has suffered a preoperative MI and has not had a CABG.

There is some evidence that the magnitude of surgery plays a role here. Ophthalmic operations performed with the patient either under local and/or regional block or general anesthesia seem to pose relatively low risks of perioperative MIs, even in patients with well-documented prior MI. Whether this is true for other relatively minor operations (minor in terms of physiologic trespass) is not known for sure. Just how much of this risk, as discussed, is on account of anesthesia is not known. Congestive heart failure (CHF) is known to be a major risk factor for the performance of anesthesia and surgery. In 1977, Goldman and associates listed it in first place—that is, most predictive of major cardiac morbidity and/or mortality after noncardiac surgery. In that study, patients with either S3 gallop rhythm or distended neck veins were noted to be at high risk for cardiac morbidity and/or mortality. Other risk factors that were predictive of morbidity in that study included greater than five premature ventricular contractions per minute, recent MI, hemodynamically significant aortic stenosis with or without coronary artery disease, and "poor general medical condition." Subsequent similar studies have indicated that operations on the great vessels, especially abdominal aortic aneurysm repair, are associated with high risk. Again, all these are studies of overall risks and are not specifically indicative of anesthesia risk. Nonetheless, they are helpful in the preoperative assessment of affected patients. It is clear from these studies that the anesthesiologist must concentrate heavily on the heart in the preoperative assessment of anesthesia risk.

Carotid Endarterectomy

An example of this risk evaluation is the attempt to assess risk in a patient who needs a carotid endarterectomy. Studies indicate that these patients have little chance of death unless they have concomitant heart or coronary artery disease. If they do have significant heart disease and undergo carotid endarterectomy, probably 3 percent will either die or suffer a postoperative stroke. More may suffer a perioperative myocardial infarction. There are numerous other studies in the literature that point to the fact that if the heart is compromised in any

way, anesthetic risk is significantly increased. Thus, there is extensive documentation in the literature leading one to contend that preoperatively great attention should be placed on the evaluation of the patient's cardiac status.

Unfortunately, what is missing is the evidence of risk reduction by preoperative testing and intervention prior to surgery. Examples of this include patients with abnormal electrocardiograms, stable exertional angina, or a history of CHF. Further cardiac evaluation might reveal significant coronary artery disease or myocardial dysfunction. Another example of this would be the question of how extensive the cardiac workup should be in a patient scheduled for major vascular surgery, such as abdominal aortic aneurysmectomy. A recent study indicated that when coronary angiography was performed in these patients, a high yield (>30 percent) of major coronary disease was discovered. Some of these patients benefitted from coronary bypass prior to their elective abdominal aneurysmectomies. However, there is no consensus in either the medical or anesthesiology communities as to how to proceed. Data do not exist to evaluate the perioperative risk reduction that could be achieved from medical treatment of coronary ischemia or heart failure. Since both angioplasty and operative myocardial revascularization procedures carry risk of infarction and death, it is by no means clear that these should be performed prior to other sorts of surgery.

Recent recognition of "silent" ischemia has further complicated these perioperative management issues. Whether affected patients require further cardiologic evaluation and treatment is unknown. Adding to this dilemma is the ability of the modern anesthesiologist to monitor safely and care for such patients in the operating room. For many patients and types of surgery, even "high-risk" patients can now have surgery.

A reasonable approach to risk assessment in such patients would involve consideration of the patient's functional status and proposed surgery. Asymptomatic patients may not require further evaluation for many types of surgery that involve minor physiologic trespass. Symptomatic patients or those with a suggestion of heart disease who are undergoing major procedures involving blood loss, large fluid fluxes, or aortic cross-clamping may require cardiologic consultation to assess the degree, if any, of coronary artery disease and/or significant myocardial dysfunction. Such an assessment may then indicate the need for further preoperative medical therapy or myocardial revascularization. Such an assessment may also allow a better "guess" as to perioperative risk and the risk-benefit ratio of the proposed surgery.

For many patients, such an evaluation may actually reveal that, in fact, the proposed surgery can proceed safely. For example, exercise stress testing may confirm the presence of coronary artery disease but also reveal that the patient develops symptoms or electrocardiographic changes only at work, heart rates, and blood pressure unlikely to be observed (or allowed to occur) in the operating room.

Finally, the anesthesiologist does not require a cardiology consultant to "clear" the patient for surgery or to make an assessment of *anesthetic* risk. Rather, we hope to learn that the patient's status is "good" for that patient, that the patient is on appropriate therapy (if needed), and that no further diagnostic or therapeutic maneuvers are necessary.

CRITICAL INCIDENTS

Every anesthesiologist knows that numerous critical incidents occur in the operating room and intensive care unit (ICU). The extensive studies of Cooper are relevant for discussion here. Cooper defines critical incident as "a human error or equipment failure that could have led (if not discovered or corrected in time) or did lead to an undesirable outcome, ranging from increased length of hospital, recovery room, or ICU stay to death." Cooper has collected many reports of these "critical incidents." They were obtained originally from volunteer anesthesiologists in the Boston community. The manner in which they were collected is relevant. First, the incidents were reported voluntarily. Cooper's 1984 report contained a total of 616 such events reported voluntarily by the physicians involved in the studies. Next, trained nonphysician interviewers contacted the same volunteer anesthesiologists and were able to elicit reports of 234 additional critical incidents, all of which met the original criteria. Next, Cooper tried a third round of reporting and, interestingly, another 239 such incidents came to light. Thus, although only receiving 616 initial reports from an enthusiastic group of physicians who were legally protected, after two rounds of close questioning a total of 1,089 such incidents were collected. Also, there were 798 "occurrences" that fell somewhat short of being critical incidents by the above definition.

By far the largest percentage of these critical incidents (70 percent) were due to human error, including disconnections related to airways or intravenous or arterial catheters; improper use of anesthesia machines; and instances wherein the wrong drug or dosage was given. The studies of Cooper and colleagues were not designed to determine an absolute critical incident rate per hour of anesthesia or per case. Their purposes were instead to understand why such errors occur and to prevent them by both better machine design and better personnel education. One of the interesting sidelights that emerged was that relieving an anesthesiologist on a long case, i.e., allowing a "break," seemed to aid the discovery of potential critical incidents. There were approximately three times as many critical incidents discovered by the relief person as were apparently caused by the relief process. Cooper and co-workers estimated that about one-half of the overall anesthesia-related mortality and morbidity they discovered would fall into "preventable" categories.

Studies such as those of Cooper and co-workers have had other effects. Quality assurance activities are very important in hospitals today and are emphasized by various accrediting bodies. Establishment of a critical incident reporting system in a department of anesthesia is reasonable in order to understand what kinds of incidents are occurring in one's own hospital and to attempt to educate the members of a department of anesthesia as to their prevention. Knowledge of what might have prevented reported incidents is a first step toward establishing reasonable standards of care.

CARDIAC ARREST IN THE OPERATING ROOM

A recent comprehensive study of anesthesia-related risk is that of Keenan and Boyan. They studied approximately 150,000 anesthetics performed at the Medical College of Virginia. There were 27 cardiac arrests that occurred in the operating room, and of these, nearly all were classified as preventable. A majority were caused by failures in airway management. Airway management catastrophes are well known to every anesthesiologist, and this result came as no surprise. Almost as many deaths were related to absolute or relative anesthetic overdose. This should not be surprising either because the therapeutic to toxic ratios for volatile anesthetics are very poor, the best being that of isoflurane, which is only about 1:5 based on animal studies. Halothane's therapeutic to toxic ratio is as poor as that of digitalis, namely 1:2. Anesthesiologists should keep in mind the fact that absolute or relative volatile agent overdose is an important cause of cardiac arrest in the operating room. An extremely important finding of this study was the importance of bradycardia as a marker of impending cardiac arrest due to either hypoxemia or volatile agent overdose. Anesthesiologists at all levels should not fail to heed the warning of significant bradycardia developing during surgery; hypoxemia and anesthetic overdose should be looked for and immediately treated.

It is likely that the overall anesthesia death rate is somewhere around one per 10,000 cases, although these figures are extremely difficult to verify because of the vicissitudes of our opportunistic adversarial legal system. Study of critical incidents and establishment of individual in-hospital reporting systems would seem proper. Specific studies of cardiac and other risks are also of use and are extensively found in the literature.

Resuscitation Attempts

One final point we wish to make is based on a review of numerous medicolegal cases that have involved anesthesia. Many of these cases do indeed involve a cardiac arrest in the operating room. Most striking have been the paltry and inadequate attempts at resuscitation that often occur. These are witnessed cardiac arrests, often with considerable monitoring, but always with an electrocardiographic monitor attached and working. Even though these cardiac arrests occur in operating rooms with fully qualified surgeons present, there are rarely instances in which the chest is opened and careful manual cardiac compression is done. There are few instances in which patients are actually put on cardiopulmonary bypass until diagnosis can be made. Blood gas control is often poor. Most importantly is the delay in recognition and prompt treatment of hypoperfusion in outright cardiac arrest. With current monitoring modalities, including pulse oximetry, end-tidal capnography, continuous noninvasive blood pressure monitoring, and electrocardiography, coupled with the most important monitor, the vigilant anesthesiologist, cardiac arrest should be recognized promptly. Effective cardiopulmonary resuscitation should be started promptly, with attention to control of the airway. Current evidence suggests that the prompt use of epinephrine is effective, particularly in those cases of cardiac arrest involving regional anesthesia. The multiple resources of the modern hospital are not always called on. Anesthesiologists and surgeons should be among the most competent cardiac resuscitators. Attention to skills in this area might also help this problem of anesthetic risk.

Dr. Arthur Keats, one of our specialty's wisest practitioners, has provided a remark that seems suitable for the close to this chapter: "To every benefit, there is a risk. The only way to guarantee immunity from risk is to do nothing at all."

SUGGESTED READING

Backer CL, Tinker JH, Robertson DM, et al. Myocardial reinfarction following local anesthesia for ophthalmic surgery. Anesth Analg 1980; 59:257–262.

Caplan RA, Ward RJ, Posner K, et al. Unexpected cardiac arrest during spinal anesthesia: a closed claims analysis of predisposing factors. Anesthesiology 1988; 68:5–11.

Cohen MM, Duncan PG, Tate RB. Does anesthesia contribute to operative mortality? JAMA 1988; 260:2859–2863.

Cooper JB, Newhower RS, Long CD, et al. Preventable anesthesia mishaps—a study of human factors. Anesthesiology 1978; 49: 399–406.

Goldman C, Caldera DL, Nussbaum SR, et al. Multifactional index of cardiac risk in non-cardiac surgical procedures. N Engl J Med 1977; 297:845–850.

Keenan RL, Boyan CP. Cardiac arrest due to anesthesia. A study of incidence and causes. JAMA 1985; 253:2373–2377.

Lunn JN, Hunter AR, Scott DB. Anaesthesia related surgical mortality. Anaesthesia 1983; 38:1090–1096.

Mahar LJ, Steen PA, Tinker JH, et al. Perioperative myocardial infarction in patients with coronary artery disease with and without aorta coronary artery bypass grafts. J Thorac Cardiovasc Surg 1978; 76:533–537.

Mangano DT, Browner WS, Hollenberg M, et al. Association of perioperative myocardial ischemia with cardiac morbidity and mortality in men undergoing noncardiac surgery. N Engl J Med 1990; 323:1781–1788.

Rao TL, Jacobs KH, El-Etr AA. Reinfarction following anesthesia in patients with myocardial infarction. Anesthesiology 1983; 59: 499–505.

Rosenfeld B, Rogers MC. Risk stratification in postmyocardial infarction patients: is six months too long to wait? J Clin Anesthesiol 1991; 3:85–87.

Steen PA, Tinker JH, Tarhan S. Myocardial reinfarction after anesthesia and surgery. JAMA 1978; 239:2566–2570.

PREOPERATIVE MEDICATION

DOUGLAS S. SNYDER, M.D., M.S.

Premedication has been defined as "preliminary medication, particularly internal medication to produce narcosis prior to inhalation anesthesia" (*Dorland's Medical Dictionary*, ed 27, 1988). This brief review focuses on limitations implicit to this definition, on the expanding role (and responsibility) of the anesthesiologist, and on the changing goals of therapy. Historically, induction of anesthesia by inhalation posed serious dangers. The major focus of premedication was to temper the storm, i.e., to minimize the risk of using "irritant vapors." This task was primarily accomplished by employing opiates, sedatives, and anticholinergics to avoid excessive salivation, coughing and laryngospasm that frequently accompanied administration of ether by open-mask. Fortunately, the practice of anesthesia has progressed, and these problems have been largely overcome by the application of new drugs and techniques. We currently face a new set of challenges, and the role(s) premedication should play in patient management is largely redefined. Premedication should be viewed in the larger sense as perioperative preparation of the patient for anesthesia and surgery. Our objectives fall into two major categories: minimizing emotional and physical stress and ensuring optimal treatment of pre-existing medical conditions. Because the latter is discussed in other chapters, this chapter focuses on general issues. Some of the data is controversial, forcing the practitioner to simply use good clinical judgment. Often it is the art as well as the science of medicine that achieves an optimal result.

A primary emphasis of preoperative preparation is to allay anxiety and to "smooth the induction of anesthesia." Despite our general successes, patients remain fearful, and this fear may not peak until the second postoperative day. An informative and reassuring preoperative visit may do much to relieve anxiety. This personal touch, even when performed briefly, is more effective than simply providing literature. In one study, premedication with intramuscular pentobarbital alone did not relieve anxiety but did produce drowsiness. Drowsiness or the appearance of calmness by the patient does not necessarily translate into patient-perceived anxiolysis. Coupling the preoperative visit with appropriate premedication is the most effective technique. Of course, any benefits derived from sedation must be balanced against the patient's general condition, previous response to drugs, and surgical procedure. Frequently, conflicting objectives must be prioritized. For example, we generally omit sedative premedication for patients with intracranial mass lesions and rely on preoperative discussion to allay apprehension. In this manner we avoid the risks of excessive sedation (hypoxia, hypercarbia, intracranial pressure elevation, airway compromise) in an unmonitored setting but often face anxious patients in the operating room. Findings supporting improved outcome following nonpharmacologic and pharmacologic control of anxiety are inconclusive, whereas serious sequelae following premedication are well documented. Sedation can be easily administered or supplemented intravenously with the patient under observation in the operating room.

BENZODIAZEPINES

There is no ideal drug, but benzodiazepines have achieved widespread popularity as premedicants. They are effective in producing sedation, anxiolysis, and amnesia. They generally cause minimal cardiovascular and respiratory depression, and there are few side effects. Diazepam is very useful in its oral form with greater than 90 percent absorption and a peak effect in 30 to 60 minutes. An average dose is 10 mg for the typical 70-kg patient. The elimination half-life is 20 to 40 hours. It is metabolized by hepatic microsomal enzymes with some active metabolites; its effects may be prolonged in the elderly and in patients with cirrhosis. As it is highly protein-bound, its effects may be increased in patients with low serum albumin levels, such as those with renal failure or cirrhosis. Administered intravenously, it is frequently associated with pain and phlebitis; $Paco_2$ has been found to increase after administration of 0.2 mg per kg, yet respiratory arrest has been reported after only 2.5 mg. It is an effective and relatively benign agent for routine oral premedication. It also offers a theoretical advantage of increasing seizure threshold for patients undergoing regional anesthesia. Two other drugs in this class are also particularly useful. Lorazepam offers a more profound amnesia than diazepam and a longer duration of action, making it particularly suitable for stressful, long procedures such as coronary artery bypass. The usual oral dose is 2 to 4 mg. It is reliably absorbed orally, but peak plasma concentrations are not achieved for 2 to 4 hours. Despite an elimination half-life of 10 to 20 hours, sedation and amnesia are prolonged as compared with diazepam (which may dissociate more rapidly from central nervous system [CNS] receptors). There are no active metabolites. Respiratory depression has been observed in patients with lung disease. A third agent, midazolam, may be administered intramuscularly or intravenously. The usual intramuscular dose is 0.05 to 0.1 mg per kg with onset in 5 to 10 minutes and a peak effect in 30 to 60 minutes. Unlike diazepam, it rarely causes pain on injection, and there is no delayed absorption. It also possesses more potent amnestic qualities than diazepam. The elimination half-life is 1 to 4 hours, which is attributed to lipid solubility, rapid redistribution to peripheral tissues, and metabolic biotransformation. Hepatic microsomal enzymes are responsible for its metabolism to essentially inactive metabolites. Rapid onset and relatively rapid recovery with minimal pain on injection make this agent particularly useful for the ambulatory setting. Profound respiratory depression has been associated with the use of midazolam, particularly in patients with chronic obstructive pulmonary disease. Deaths have been associated with the use of midazolam in elderly and debilitated patients. The manufacturer recommends administering initially no more than 2.5 mg intravenously in less than 2 minutes in a *healthy* adult. Subsequent doses should be titrated over an additional 2 minutes. All of the benzodiazepines, especially when used in conjunction with narcotics, may cause hypotension. Although benzodiazepines have been implicated in general in delaying recovery of psychomotor function, it is not clear that they prolong the overall hospital stay.

NARCOTICS

Narcotics were routinely used in the past for premedication, but their continued use for routine procedures has fallen into some disfavor. The argument that narcotics "decrease the requirement for inhaled anesthetics" probably holds little clinical significance. Several reasons favoring their use include on-going pain or anticipated painful procedures and chronic narcotic use prior to surgery. Combinations of sedatives-narcotics (with or without scopolamine) are very effective for selected procedures for which heavy premedication is desired, such as major cancer surgery or coronary artery bypass. The use of different classes of agents for heavy premedication may limit the amount of respiratory depression that would otherwise be associated with an equianalgesic dose of narcotic, but combinations commonly potentiate respiratory depression by the narcotics. The increasing use of specialized techniques such as postoperative epidural analgesia also modifies the use of narcotics as premedicants.

Morphine, a phenanthrene-derivative opioid agonist, is the standard against which all narcotics are compared. Morphine typically produces analgesia, drowsiness, and possibly euphoria. Morphine given alone may also produce dysphoria, and side effects such as nausea, vomiting, dizziness, and chest tightness are not uncommon. For patients in pain, the pain is generally reported to be less intense and/or less discomforting. Morphine depresses respiration (including rate, minute volume, and tidal volume) in patients within 5 to 10 minutes after intravenous administration or 30 to 90 minutes following intramuscular or subcutaneous administration, respectively; this depression may persist for 4 to 5 hours. Maximal analgesia occurs within 1 hour and persists for approximately 4 hours. When equianalgesic doses of narcotics are used, the degree of respiratory depression (believed to be mediated by the mu_2 receptor) is not significantly different. Morphine is particularly effective in suppressing the cough reflex, which appears to involve opioid receptors in the medulla that are activated at doses that may not depress respiration or achieve significant analgesia. Nausea and vomiting are relatively infrequent in supine patients, but 40 percent of ambulatory patients develop nausea and 15 percent develop vomiting after subcutaneous administration. The typical premedicant dose of morphine is 0.1 to 0.15 mg per kg given intramuscularly 1 hour before surgery. Onset of action is delayed owing to its relatively limited lipid solubility. It is metabolized by the liver and eliminated primarily as morphine-3-glucuronide by glomerular filtration; the elimination half-life is 2.9 ± 0.5 hours. Dosage should be reduced in the elderly and debilitated patients. As with all narcotics, it is generally contraindicated with respiratory depression or decreased respiratory reserve (emphysema, kyphoscoliosis, severe obesity) and conditions associated with elevated intracranial pressure. It may cause a marked increase in pressure in the biliary tract and spasm of the sphincter of Oddi, which might rarely produce epigastric distress; fentanyl and possibly meperidine are believed to cause lesser increases in biliary pressure. The significant histamine-releasing aspect of the drug can contribute to hypotension in the hypovolemic patient and could exacerbate or provoke an acute asthmatic attack.

Meperidine, a phenylpiperidine derivative, is a synthetic opioid chemically dissimilar from morphine. Central nervous system effects are, however, comparable to those of morphine. Although it is one-eighth as potent as morphine, it is more lipid soluble. The usual adult preoperative dose is 50 to 100 mg given intramuscularly or subcutaneously 30 to 90 minutes before surgery. Maximal analgesic affect is 30 to 50 minutes after intramuscular administration with a duration of action of 2 to 4 hours. Meperidine is chiefly metabolized in the liver, undergoing N-demethylation to normeperidine or conjugation with glucuronic acid. The elimination half-life is 3.6 hours. Prolonged administration can lead to an accumulation of normeperidine, which causes excitatory phenomena, including twitches, tremors, multifocal myoclonus, and grand mal seizures. Normeperidine has a half-life of 14 to 21 hours, increasing to 35 hours in patients with renal failure. Administered with monoamine oxidase inhibitors, patients have manifested excitation, hyperpyrexia, rigidity, convulsions, severe respiratory depression, hypotension, coma, and death. The mechanism is unknown, but the association is strong enough to contraindicate its use in patients who have received the drugs within the past 14 days. Meperidine administered in larger intravenous doses may increase heart rate (possibly owing to a structural similarity to atropine) and should be used with caution in patients with supraventricular tachycardia or coronary insuffi-

ciency. Unlike other opioids even low doses (2.0 to 2.5 mg per kg) may cause myocardial depression. Meperidine may be superior to morphine for procedures involving the biliary tract, but it also increases biliary pressure via direct (as opposed to opioid receptor-mediated) smooth muscle stimulation. Meperidine has been reported to have a higher incidence of histamine-release than morphine. It is associated with less urinary retention and constipation than morphine but lacks its antitussive properties.

Fentanyl is a synthetic opioid related to the phenylpiperidines and a congener of meperidine. It is 80 times as potent as morphine; however, analgesia by morphine lasts 2 to 3 times longer. Although fentanyl may be administered intramuscularly for premedication, it is popularly given intravenously as 50 to 100 µg for a typical 70-kg adult immediately prior to induction of anesthesia. Its lipophilic nature provides for a rapid onset and a more rapid redistribution. Peak analgesia occurs within several minutes with a duration of 30 to 60 minutes, whereas multiple and/or large doses may have prolonged effects. Fentanyl undergoes biotransformation in the liver to a more polar compound, which is excreted by the kidneys. The elimination half-life is about 3.5 hours, which is longer than the half-life for morphine. Although rapidly administered (large) doses of fentanyl may be associated with muscle rigidity and bradycardia, these findings are generally not observed with premedicant doses. Unlike morphine and meperidine, fentanyl causes minimal histamine-release, and hemodynamic variables are typically unchanged. Therefore, it is often the preferred agent in adjusted dosages for elderly or debilitated patients. In equivalent analgesic doses, fentanyl is similar to morphine and meperidine with regard to respiratory depression except that duration is shorter. Respiratory effects may persist longer than analgesia. Fentanyl may cause less nausea and vomiting than morphine and meperidine. Manufacturers now state that when fentanyl is administered to patients who have received monoamine oxidase inhibitors within 14 days, appropriate monitoring and treatment for hypertension should be readily available.

BARBITURATES AND BUTYROPHENONES

Barbiturates have been shown to be effective for both anxiolysis and sedation-hypnosis. Antianalgetic properties limit its usefulness as a premedicant for patients in pain that may lead to disorientation. Prolonged effects make these agents unsuitable for shorter procedures. The benzodiazepines have in large part replaced the barbiturates. Butyrophenones (e.g., droperidol) are useful in combination with sedatives and narcotics for unpleasant procedures that require patient cooperation, such as an awake intubation. Patients who receive droperidol alone may appear placid but may actually be dysphoric; one may be quite chagrined to discover this discrepancy on the "routine" postoperative visit. Small doses up to 2.5 mg may be used to prevent or treat nausea and vomiting. Duration of action is 3 to 6 hours. About 1 percent of patients develop extrapyramidal signs due to dopamine antagonism.

CARDIOVASCULAR THERAPY

Part of the expanded role of preoperative preparation, particularly in dealing with sicker patients, involves the maintenance of hemodynamic stability. It is generally recommended that antihypertensive, antianginal, and antiarrhythmic therapy be continued throughout the perioperative period. Hypertensive patients with atherosclerotic disease are particularly prone to develop intraoperative lability of blood pressure. Good control of blood pressure preoperatively improves perioperative control and may reduce overall risk. In addition to continuing antihypertensive medications (many prefer to withhold diuretics owing to a free water deficit that occurs with NPO status) through the morning of surgery, alpha$_2$-agonists are also being administered preoperatively to reduce hemodynamic lability. Clonidine, the best-studied example of this type, decreases the release of central catecholamines and thereby minimizes blood pressure variability. It has also been associated with reduced anesthetic requirements. One study found a lower incidence of bigeminy and a smaller increase in heart rate after intubation and another reported reduced cardiovascular responses to intubation. This preliminary work is exciting and offers new avenues for future therapies. As one might expect, side effects have been noted and include dry mouth, marked sedation, and severe bradycardia and hypotension. If it is considered important for the patient to receive medications, I recommend ordering these agents specifically as to dose, route, and time of administration. Orders such as "continue meds" are subject to interpretation and may lead to the omission of essential drugs; for example, the patient would not receive morning medication on a b.i.d. regimen (10:00 AM and 10:00 PM in our hospital) if scheduled for 8:00 AM surgery. Propranolol and clonidine have been associated with "rebound phenomena" with abrupt discontinuation. For propranolol, this can be manifested by ischemia, myocardial infarction, ventricular tachycardia, and sudden death. Severe hypertension has followed withdrawal of clonidine. Incidentally, medication taken orally at least 1 hour before surgery with less than 30 ml of water has not been associated with any increased incidence of aspiration.

ASPIRATION PROPHYLAXIS

Another area of active investigation involves minimizing the risk of aspiration. The time-honored standard of NPO after midnight for adult patients is now being questioned. Patients receiving diazepam orally with 50 ml of water have been found to have a lower gastric volume and higher pH than those patients receiving diazepam intramuscularly. (Anxiety and stress are be-

lieved to delay gastric emptying and increase gastric acid production; therefore, anxiolysis itself may reduce the risk of aspiration.) Surprisingly, patients who were fasted versus those fed orange juice or coffee 2 to 3 hours before surgery did not differ with respect to gastric volume or pH. Another study found that patients who received 150 ml of water in addition to 10 ml of water with bromsulfothalein (an indicator administered to both groups) had a significantly lower gastric volume, whereas pH did not differ. The jury is still out, but these studies certainly raise doubts about current standards. By extrapolation from animal studies, the lungs are considered "at risk" if gastric volume is greater than 25 ml, pH is less than or equal to 2.5, or if the stomach contains particulate material. Certain patients are at greater risk; for example, those with reflux from an incompetent gastroesophageal sphincter or the morbidly obese with increased gastric volume. The emergency trauma victim who has just eaten a full dinner typifies the patient with a "full stomach" who is at high risk for aspiration. To offset this risk, this patient could receive 30 ml of a nonparticulate antacid (0.3M sodium citrate). Although effective in increasing pH above a critically low level, this increase may be achieved at the expense of gastric volume. Barring other extenuating circumstances (such as active myocardial ischemia), sedative or analgesic premedication for this same patient could increase risk from aspiration. In the elective setting, prophylaxis with an H$_2$-receptor antagonist administered the evening prior to and the morning of surgery is very effective in increasing gastric pH. This treatment does not change the pH of contents already present in the stomach. This therapy can be coupled with a gastrokinetic agent such as metoclopramide to stimulate gastric emptying and reduce gastric volume on the morning of surgery. This drug also increases lower esophageal sphincter tone and is an effective antiemetic. These agents do not guarantee that the stomach is empty, however, and standard measures to protect the airway must still be used diligently. Please refer to standard references for agents, dosages, and side effects.

ANTICHOLINERGICS

Anticholinergic agents, once widely used to prevent copious secretions associated with inhalation anesthetics, are no longer needed routinely. They are specifically indicated as an antisialagogue in preparation for fiberoptic bronchoscopy; glycopyrrolate is probably more potent and longer-acting than atropine and is less likely to increase heart rate. It is most effective if administered intramuscularly (0.2 to 0.3 mg) at least 30 minutes prior to the procedure. Scopolamine (0.3 to 0.6 mg given intramuscularly or intravenously) offers more sedative, amnestic, and antisialagogue effects than atropine, but is less likely to increase the heart rate. Scopolamine and atropine both cross the blood–brain barrier. Atropine (0.3 to 0.6 mg given intramuscularly or intravenously) possesses the most potent vagolytic action of the anticholinergic drugs and is most reliable in preventing or treating bradycardia if given intravenously just before anesthesia and surgery. The anticholinergics do relax the lower esophageal sphincter, potentially increasing risk of aspiration, which may not be counteracted effectively by metoclopramide.

SELECTED CIRCUMSTANCES

Antibiotic therapy is beyond the scope of this chapter, but it is included for completeness. Antibiotics may be useful in decreasing the incidence of wound infection (e.g., compromised blood supply, large tissue destruction, remote infections) or for patients at risk (e.g., obese, elderly, diabetic, immunocompromised). Antibiotics also may prevent endocarditis in susceptible patients undergoing surgeries associated with bacteremia, but there are no prospective trials of this use. The reader is referred to appropriate texts for further information. Patients at risk for severe allergic reactions or anaphylaxis should be evaluated preoperatively. Prophylaxis may include H_1 and H_2 blockers and steroid therapy. Patients who may have adrenal insufficiency should undergo provocative testing before surgery. If this is not an option, glucocorticoid coverage may be indicated. Finally, (protracted) nausea and vomiting is not uncommon. Women, and particularly pregnant women, are predisposed. Nausea and vomiting are also associated with certain types of surgery, especially strabismus surgery, laparoscopy, and therapeutic abortions. Narcotics, nitrous oxide, isoflurane, and etomidate have been associated with an increased incidence of postoperative nausea. If controlling pain and anxiety (while avoiding offending agents) is not sufficient, droperidol, metoclopramide, and/or transdermal scopolamine are generally helpful. Phenothiazine derivatives or antihistamines also may offer effective alternative therapy.

DISCUSSION

Current trends in anesthesiology are driven both by rapid progress in medicine and changing modes of practice. The burgeoning role of outpatient surgery has focused attention on early recovery with minimal pain and nausea. We are challenged in outpatient and inpatient settings with sicker patients undergoing increasingly complex surgeries. Appropriate, thorough preoperative preparation is essential and should achieve: (1) an informed, prepared patient; (2) sedation/amnesia/analgesia; (3) hemodynamic stability; (4) respiratory stability; (5) minimal aspiration risk; and (6) optimization of selected conditions, for example, antibiosis, allergy/anaphylaxis, steroid dependence, predisposition for nausea and vomiting. This approach establishes a foundation for successful perioperative management that assumes even greater importance with current emphasis on ambulatory care and cost containment.

SUGGESTED READING

Fee JPH. Premedication. Acta Anaesthesiol Scand 1988; 87:1–5.
Hutchinson A, Maltby JR, Reid CRG. Gastric fluid volume and pH in elective inpatients. Part I: coffee or orange juice versus overnight fast. Can J Anaesthesiol 1988; 35:12–15.
Lindhal SGE. The use of midazolam in premedication. Acta Anaesthesiol Scand 1990; 34(Suppl 92):79–83.
Madej TH, Paasuke RT. Anaesthetic premedication: aims, assessment and methods. Can J Anaesthesiol 1987; 34:259–273.
White PF. Pharmacologic and clinical aspects of preoperative medication. Anesth Analg 1986; 65:963–974.

PULMONARY FUNCTION TESTING

BARRY A. SHAPIRO, M.D.

Anesthesia and surgery may pose significant challenges to the maintenance of cardiopulmonary homeostasis during the early postoperative period. In the broadest sense, pulmonary function includes the movement of gases in and out of the pulmonary tree (ventilation), exchange of oxygen across the alveolar capillary membrane (arterial oxygenation), removal of blood carbon dioxide (alveolar ventilation), and the muscular energy required for ventilation (work of breathing). Figure 1 illustrates the classic lung volumes and capacities used to quantitate pulmonary function. Determination of the total lung capacity (TLC) necessitates measurement of functional residual capacity (FRC), requiring an inert gas study or the body plethysmograph. More sophisticated pulmonary function studies such as exercise testing, diffusing capacities, and differential lung function testing are available to help ascertain whether contemplated lung excision will leave adequate pulmonary function to support life. This type of evaluation demands diagnostic testing beyond the expertise of the anesthesiologist. Although the importance of the history and physical examination, chest x-ray examination, and arterial blood gas measurements cannot be overemphasized, only *spirometric* pul-

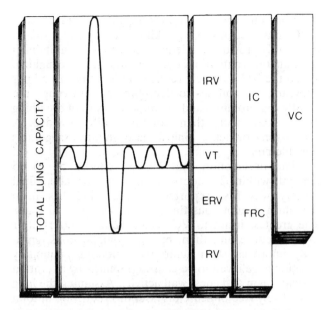

Figure 1 The divisions of total lung capcity. Total lung capacity (TLC) is the maximum amount of air the lungs can hold. The total lung capacity is divided into four primary volumes: inspiratory reserve volume (IRV); tidal volume (VT); expiratory reserve volume (ERV); and residual volume (RV). Capacities are combinations of two or more lung volumes. They are inspiratory capacity (IC), functional residual capacity (FRC), and vital capacity (VC). (Republished with permission from Shapiro BA, Harrison RA, Walton JR. Clinical application of blood gases. 3rd ed. Chicago: Year Book Medical Publishers, 1982.)

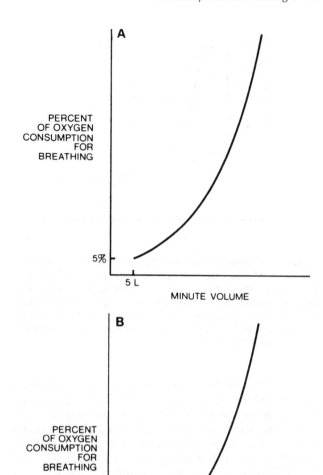

Figure 2 *A*, The work of breathing in relation to vital capacity. *B*, Point *a* represents a tidal volume of 500 ml with a VC to 5 L; point *b* represents a tidal volume of 500 ml with a VC of 1 L. (Republished with permission from Shapiro BA, Harrison RA, Walton JR. Clinical application of blood gases. 3rd ed. Chicago: Year Book Medical Publishers, 1982.)

monary function tests provide cost-effective quantitative data to help the anesthesiologist evaluate preoperative pulmonary function in terms of reserves available to meet the anticipated insults of specific anesthetic and surgical interventions.

VENTILATORY RESERVE

The work of breathing is best quantified as that portion of the total oxygen consumption that is being utilized by the ventilatory muscles ($\dot{V}O_{2VENT}/\dot{V}O_{2TOT}$). A healthy adult at rest has a $\dot{V}O_2$ of 250 ml per minute, less than 5 percent of which is utilized for breathing. However, this energy is utilized inefficiently because the pulmonary system is a to-and-fro valveless pump. As shown in Figure 2A, increasing minute ventilation causes an exponential increase in ventilatory oxygen consumption in healthy individuals. When pulmonary disease is present (dashed line, Fig. 2A), the net result of an increasing minute ventilation can be the ventilatory muscles demanding such a large portion of the $\dot{V}O_2$ and cardiac output that oxygen delivery to the rest of the body becomes insufficient.

If the respiratory rate remains constant, increases in minute ventilation can be accomplished only by increases in tidal volume. Since tidal volume can be expressed as a portion of the vital capacity (VC), Figure

2B shows the relationship between the work of breathing and that portion of the VC being used for tidal volume. Although this is a greatly simplified schema, it is a reliable clinical reflection of ventilatory reserves, since the greater the portion of the VC required for a tidal volume, the less the ability to increase tidal volume to meet stress.

SPIROMETRY

Although flow volume loops are preferred, the most readily available, least expensive, and most useful

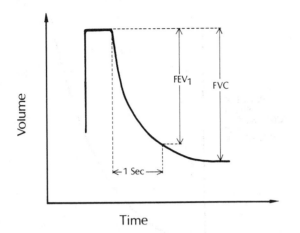

Figure 3 Schematic representation of a forced expiratory spirogram. Moving from left to right, a maximum inspiration is depicted by the rapid increase in volume (this represents inspiratory capacity). The patient holds his breath at maximum inspiration and then forces the air out as fast as possible. The total air expelled is the FVC; the volume expelled during the first second is the FEV_1.

spirometric test for routine preoperative evaluation remains the forced vital capacity (FVC). The FVC (Fig. 3) represents the maximum ventilatory volume available under stress and can be compared with predicted normals, based on sex, height, and age. The FVC expressed as a percentage of the predicted VC (%FVC) reflects restriction of ventilatory capacity and is often used to reflect ventilatory reserve. In general terms, the greater the %FVC, the greater the capability to increase ventilation without unduly taxing the cardiopulmonary system. A %FVC greater than 80 percent is normal; 70 to 80 percent, border-line normal; 60 to 70 percent reflects identifiable disease; and less than 60 percent reflects significant restriction of pulmonary function.

The forced expiratory volume in 1 second (FEV_1) is the volume of air forcefully expired during the first second of an FVC maneuver (see Fig. 3). Normally at least 70 percent of the VC can be expired during the first second. The FEV_1 is not the most sensitive or reliable index of small airway disease but because it has been used for many years and is relatively simple to derive, it remains the most widely used calculation from the forced expiratory spirogram for purposes of preoperative evaluation. The FEV_1 can be compared with the actual FVC and referred to as %FEV_1. A %FEV_1 less than 70 percent reflects airway resistance that increases the work of breathing during stress and reflects a diminishment of ventilatory reserves.

VITAL CAPACITY AND OPERATIVE INTERVENTION

In adults, the VC ranges from 55 to 85 ml per kilogram of normal body weight. An acute decrease of up to 75 percent would leave most normal individuals with a VC greater than 15 ml per kilogram, a VC that should transiently provide an adequate reserve for maintaining spontaneous ventilation, deep breathing, and coughing. When the VC is acutely reduced to less than 10 ml per kilogram, the abilities to deep-breathe and cough are greatly compromised and the required work of breathing may become more than can be readily provided. A pre-existing or acute lung disease greatly exaggerates this dilemma.

The observation that VC is reduced 50 to 75 percent within 24 hours of thoracic or abdominal surgery was first reported in 1927 and has been reconfirmed numerous times during the past 60 years. The greatest insult to VC occurs 12 to 18 hours after the procedure and then, barring complications, gradually improves. This acute restriction of pulmonary function is believed to be caused primarily by alteration of diaphragm and chest wall activity. Assuming the lung is relatively free of acute disease, this reduction in total lung capacity would occur primarily at the expense of VC, since airway closure mechanisms and surfactant activity would tend to maintain residual volume in the basilar areas. The resultant hypoxemia at room air would be caused by open, low V/Q alveoli in the dependent lung. Thus, ventilatory reserves are limited (diminished VC), and the hypoxemia is responsive to moderate levels of oxygen therapy (30 to 40 percent). Persistent hypoxemia despite 40 percent oxygen cannot be attributed to the predicted transient pulmonary restriction anticipated after abdominal or thoracic surgery.

FACTORS INFLUENCING POSTOPERATIVE PULMONARY COMPLICATIONS

Pulmonary complications range from acute ventilatory failure (acute respiratory acidosis) requiring mechanical ventilation, to pneumonia requiring antibiotic and oxygen therapy, to segmental atelectasis, which may require no more than deep breathing. The incidence of pulmonary complications after abdominal or thoracic surgery has been reported to be from 12 to 80 percent. This wide range is attributable to various definitions and criteria for identifying pulmonary complications. Studies utilizing broad criteria such as combinations of fever, sputum, and hypoxemia show relatively high rates of pulmonary complications; studies utilizing x-ray evidence of atelectasis/pneumonia reveal relatively low pulmonary complication rates.

The incidence of atelectasis/pneumonia remains controversial, and its pathogenesis has been debated since the turn of the century. Pre-existing pulmonary disease is universally accepted as a factor that increases the incidence of atelectasis/pneumonia. Retained pulmonary secretions secondary to inadequate coughing and limited ambulation is another well-accepted factor contributing to the incidence of postoperative atelectasis/pneumonia.

ANTICIPATING POSTOPERATIVE PULMONARY COMPLICATIONS

Although the limitations of any system used to predict postoperative pulmonary risk must be recognized, a practical system to guide preoperative evaluation is shown in Table 1. Because the expiratory spirogram is the most reliable means of quantitating patients at high risk for pulmonary complications, its findings are given the greatest emphasis (3 points). The %FVC grossly reflects ventilatory reserve; the %FEV$_1$ after bronchodilator grossly reflects the degree to which airway resistance will affect the work of breathing during stress. The sum of these two factors can be used to predict the degree to which the pre-existing obstructive and restrictive components of pulmonary function may compromise the ability to ventilate adequately and maintain clear lungs after abdominal and thoracic surgery.

Cardiopulmonary reserves are given 2 points (1 point for the cardiovascular system and 1 point for arterial blood gases), and 2 points are given to the postoperative capability of maintaining clear lungs (1 point for ambulation potential and 1 point for the nervous system). Each of the five categories is evaluated and the patient ascribed a total score ranging from 0 to 7 (only one score is assigned for each variable), making 7 the highest score possible.

The Low-Risk Patient

A thoracoabdominal surgical patient whose preoperative evaluation yields a score of zero has little expectation of demonstrating a postoperative pulmonary complication. The patient must be encouraged to cough and deep-breathe frequently. Ambulation should be accomplished as quickly and frequently as is reasonable. Oxygen therapy is usually not necessary after discharge from the recovery room.

The Moderate-Risk Patient

A thoracoabdominal surgical patient whose preoperative evaluation yields a score of 1 or 2 has a low incidence of postoperative pulmonary complications, and these are not life threatening and seldom prolong hospitalization. Incentive spirometry is indicated as a prophylactic measure, with therapeutic bronchial hygiene therapy instituted when indicated. Oxygen therapy is often indicated for several postoperative days.

The High-Risk Patient

A thoracoabdominal surgical patient whose preoperative evaluation yields a score of 3 or more should remain in an intensive care area for 18 to 24 hours so that serial evaluation of cardiopulmonary reserves can be accomplished and interventions readily instituted. Many of these patients may benefit from continued tracheal intubation to facilitate suctioning and deep breathing, and some may benefit from ventilator assistance. These

Table 1 Classification of Risk of Pulmonary Complications of Thoracic and Abdominal Procedures

Category	Points
Expiratory spirogram (maximum of 3 points)	
Normal (%FVC + %FEV$_1$/FVC > 150)	0
%FVC + %FEV$_1$/FVC = 100 to 150	1
%FVC + %FEV$_1$/FVC < 100	2
Preoperative FVC < 20 ml/kg	3
Postbronchodilator FEV$_1$/FVC <50%	3
Cardiopulmonary reserves (maximum of 2 points)	
Uncontrolled symptoms (dyspnea on exertion, orthopnea, paroxysmal nocturnal dyspnea, dependent edema, congestive heart failure, angina)	1
Abnormal blood gas values	1
Bronchial hygiene capability (maximum of 2 points)	
Expected ambulation within 36 hours; at least sitting up in bed	0
Bed confinement for more than 36 hours	1
Nervous system ability to maintain BH confusion, obtunded sensorium, discoordination muscular	1
weakness	1

patients most likely benefit from epidural pain control techniques and/or patient-controlled analgesia.

A preoperative FVC of less than 20 ml per kilogram signals that a patient is at high risk for postoperative acute ventilatory failure. Significant preoperative irreversible airway obstruction significantly increases the postoperative work of breathing and diminishes bronchial hygiene capability. A patient free of pulmonary infection who manifests a postbronchodilator %FEV$_1$/FVC of less than 50 percent should be considered at high risk for postoperative pulmonary complications.

BRONCHIAL HYGIENE THERAPY

No known therapy completely eliminates postoperative pulmonary complications. However, it was common practice 25 years ago to treat postoperative patients with costly bronchial hygiene therapies such as intermittent positive-pressure breathing (IPPB), aerosol therapy with and without a bronchodilator, and chest physical therapy techniques in the hope of minimizing the incidence of pulmonary complications. The findings of more than 20 years of scientific investigation are summarized in the following paragraphs.

Preoperative Therapy

Patients with significant chronic pulmonary disease or retained secretions often demonstrate significant increases in VC or FEV$_1$ with 48 hours of appropriate bronchial hygiene therapy. Preoperative instruction in breathing exercises, cough methods, and techniques planned for postoperative bronchial therapy have been shown to diminish the incidence and severity of pulmonary complications postoperatively. Preoperative instruction and psychologic reassurance appear to decrease anxiety and pain. These advantages must be weighed against the increased costs of preoperative hospitalization.

Prophylactic Therapy

It has been well established that *prevention* of postoperative pulmonary complications in patients free of lung pathology can be effectively accomplished with simple stir-up regimens such as encouraging cough, ambulation, and the frequent use of incentive spirometry. The effectiveness of more costly therapy to prevent pulmonary complications in postoperative patients with pre- existing lung disease remains controversial. However, no data suggest that thoracoabdominal surgical patients without diseased lungs postoperatively require more than frequent stir-up regimens to prevent pulmonary complications.

Therapeutic Bronchial Hygiene Therapy

Therapeutic bronchial hygiene therapy is defined as the application of techniques for the *reversal* of sequelae

attributable to inadequate bronchial hygiene mechanisms. These sequelae most commonly include retained secretions with or without absorption atelectasis documented by (1) copious, thick, or retained pulmonary secretions; (2) an inadequate cough mechanism; (3) wheezing; and/or (4) absorptive atelectasis. The need for therapy is primarily based on the patient's ability or inability to mobilize secretions—not primarily on the severity of the pulmonary disease.

SUGGESTED READING

Ford GT, Guenter CA. Toward prevention of postoperative pulmonary complications. Am Rev Resp Dis 1984; 130:4–5.

Shapiro BA, Cane RD, Peterson J, Weber D. Authoritative medical direction can assure cost-beneficial bronchial hygiene therapy. Chest 1988; 93:1038–1042.

Shapiro A, Kacmarek R, Cane RD, et al. Clinical application of respiratory care. 4th ed. St. Louis: Mosby-Year Book, 1991: 426–432.

Tisi GM. Preoperative evaluation of pulmonary function. Am Rev Respir Dis 1979; 119:293–310.

PREOPERATIVE PATIENT EVALUATION

MICHAEL F. ROIZEN, M.D.
MARTIN J. HURD, M.D.

This chapter has emerged in response to the question, What routine preoperative laboratory tests are beneficial to patients and best enable physicians to make medical assessments that improve perioperative management? These medical assessments provide an important opportunity for physicians to reduce perioperative morbidity by optimizing preoperative status and planning perioperative management. Because perioperative mortality and morbidity increase with the severity of pre-existing disease, careful evaluation and treatment should reduce their occurrence. Consequently, physicians would benefit from a reliable, efficient method of assessing patients preoperatively and then ordering laboratory tests based on that assessment.

PREOPERATIVE EVALUATION: THE CURRENT SYSTEM

The primary problem with the current system of preoperative evaluation is that many tests are ordered and obtained that do not contribute beneficially to patient care. Most studies estimate that approximately 60 percent of preoperative testing could be eliminated without adversely affecting patient care. It has been further documented that unnecessary testing tends to cause extra risk to the patient, inefficient operating room schedules, and unnecessary costs. Unnecessary testing may be hazardous to patients because of the pursuit and treatment of borderline positive or false-positive results. In addition, because newly discovered abnormalities are not noted in the patient's medical record by the physician caring for the patient, extra testing may increase the medicolegal risk for the physician.

From the 1940s to the 1960s, preoperative medical assessment relied primarily on accurate history-taking and physical examination. Then, in the late 1960s, Kaiser and Technicon introduced multiphasic screening laboratory tests. The ease and low cost of ordering and obtaining many tests made this new mode of preoperative testing seem logical and desirable. As a result, many hospitals, anesthesia departments, and outpatient surgery centers made rather arbitrary rules — recommendations that became requirements — regarding the tests that should be performed before elective surgery. When, with good intentions, anesthesiologists and surgeons tried to follow those rules, problems arose. Physicians believed that they could order inexpensive batteries of tests and thus efficiently screen for disease. Instead, because physicians were often still trying to determine which tests to order before surgery, what to do about an unexpected abnormal result on the morning of surgery, or how abnormal a result had to be before a consultant should be called in, Kaiser found that the system of preoperative multiphasic screening with multiple nonselective tests was not practical. The system produced so many false-positive and false- negative results that the subsequent harm vastly outweighed any possible benefit. In this chapter, we evaluate the goals of preoperative medical assessment and the relative importance of history-taking, the physical examination, and laboratory testing for perioperative outcome.

Routine laboratory testing is not the most effective way to evaluate patients preoperatively. Leonard and co-workers reported that biochemical screening tests had no significant value in the preoperative screening of pediatric patients who were expected to be hospitalized for less than 1 week. In another study, Korvin and associates reviewed biochemical tests given routinely to 1,000 patients on hospital admission. None of the tests produced a new diagnosis that was unequivocally beneficial to the patient. In an ambitious, controlled trial of multiphasic screening in 1,500 patients, Olsen and co-workers found no difference in morbidity between control groups and groups having screening tests. Durbridge and colleagues compared 1,500 patients who were randomly assigned to undergo or not to undergo screening tests on admission. No benefit resulted from the 8,363 tests that were performed with respect to duration of hospital stay or patient outcome.

Although laboratory screening tests can aid in optimizing a patient's preoperative condition once a disease is suspected or diagnosed, they have several shortcomings: they frequently fail to uncover pathologic conditions; their detection of abnormalities does not necessarily improve patient care or outcome; and they are inefficient in screening for asymptomatic diseases. Finally, most abnormalities discovered on preoperative screening, or even on admission screening for nonsurgical purposes, are not recorded (other than in the laboratory report) or appropriately pursued.

Domoto et al examined the yield and effectiveness of a battery of 19 screening laboratory tests performed routinely in 70 functionally intact elderly patients (average age of 82.6 years) who resided at a chronic care facility. The 70 patients underwent 3,903 screening tests. "New abnormal" results primarily occurred in five of the 19 screening tests; most of these "new abnormalities" were only minimally outside the normal range. Only four

(0.1 of all tests ordered) led to change in patient management, none of which, Domoto and colleagues concluded, benefited any patient in an important way.

Wolf-Klein and colleagues retrospectively studied the results of annual laboratory screening on a population of 500 institutionalized and ambulatory elderly patients (average age, 80 years). From the 15,000 tests performed, 756 new abnormalities were discovered, 690 of which were ignored. Sixty-six of the new abnormalities were evaluated; 20 new diagnoses resulted, 12 of which were treated. Two patients of the 500 may have ultimately benefited from eradication of asymptomatic bacteriuria (although eradication of asymptomatic bacteriuria has not been shown to improve the quality of life or extend the life-span).

Studies show that the history and physical examination are the best measures for screening for disease. Delahunt and Turnbull evaluated patients who were assessed preoperatively for varicose vein stripping or inguinal herniorrhaphy. For 803 patients who underwent 1,972 tests, only 63 abnormalities were uncovered in those patients whose history or physical findings had not indicated the need for tests; however, in no instance did the discovery of these abnormalities influence patient management. Rossello and associates retrospectively evaluated 690 admissions for elective pediatric surgical procedures. The history and physical examination indicated the probability of abnormalities in all 12 patients in whom an abnormality was found through laboratory testing. Clinical diagnosis, and not laboratory testing, was the apparent basis for any change in operative plans.

Several studies have compared outcome for groups of hospitalized patients who had routine laboratory screening tests performed to supplement the history and physical examination with that of patients who did not have routine screening tests. Wood and Hoekelman found that 28 of 1,924 children examined had changes in preoperative clinical courses (all had surgery postponed) because of abnormal history, physical examination, or laboratory examination results. Three of those 28 patients whose surgery was postponed had abnormal laboratory tests that were not indicated by history or physical examination. Thus, history or physical examination dictated appropriate laboratory testing for all but three of 1,924 patients. The abnormalities discovered for these three patients pertained to their chest radiographs. (These children were part of a study comparing perioperative outcome at two hospitals — one of which required chest radiographs as a screening test for elective surgery in children, and one of which did not.) There were no differences noted in anesthetic or perioperative complications between the two groups. Wood and Hoekelman therefore recommended that chest radiographs not be obtained routinely for apparently healthy children.

Even in a referral population, history and physical examination determine more than 90 percent of the clinical course when a patient is referred for consultation about cardiovascular, neurologic, or respiratory diseases. Other studies also have demonstrated that the history and physical examination accurately indicate all areas in which subsequent laboratory testing proves beneficial to patients. For example, Rabkin and Horne examined the records of 165 patients having "new" (i.e., a change from a previous tracing) abnormalities on the electrocardiogram (ECG) that were potentially "surgically significant" (i.e., that might affect perioperative management or outcome). In only two instances were the anesthetic or surgical plans altered by the discovery of new abnormalities on an ECG that were not indicated by history. Thus, for these 165 patients, for whom the benefits of a laboratory test should have been maximal (because a new abnormality was detected during the course of preoperative assessments), the history or physical examination determined case management most of the time. Even in one of the two instances of altered case management—a patient having atrial fibrillation—the physical examination should have indicated that an ECG needed to be performed. A history or physical examination was not available for the other patient.

In summary, the studies cited above point to the inadequacy of routine laboratory tests as an independent means of assessing patients preoperatively. It has been shown that many of these laboratory tests are considered superfluous to patient care management. History and physical examination are considered the most effective ways to screen for disease; laboratory tests can be used to screen for disease when such tests have proven effective but are better used to confirm clinical diagnoses or to optimize a patient's condition before surgery.

Random testing may not be beneficial and may even present extra risk to the patient. Unnecessary testing may lead physicians to pursue and treat abnormalities based on borderline positive and false-positive results. Few studies examine whether increased tests and the follow-up of false-positive tests adversely affect patients. Roizen retrospectively examined the adverse effects of chest x-ray examinations on patients. In this study population of 606 patients, 386 extra chest radiographs were ordered without being indicated. In those 386 patients, one elevated hemidiaphragm and probable phrenic nerve palsy was found that may have resulted in improved care for that patient. In addition, three lung shadows were found that resulted in three sets of invasive tests, including one thoracotomy, without discovery of any disease. These procedures caused considerable morbidity for those patients, including one pneumothorax and 4 months of disability.

In another study, Turnbull and Buck examined the charts of 2,570 patients undergoing cholecystectomy to determine the value of preoperative tests. The history and physical examinations successfully indicated all tests that ultimately benefited the patients, with four possible exceptions. But again, in those four patients it is doubtful if any benefit actually occurred. Among them was one patient whose emphysema was detected only by chest x-ray examination; he underwent preoperative physiotherapy without subsequent postoperative complications. Two patients had unsuspected hypokalemia (3.2 and 3.4 mEq per liter, respectively) and received

potassium treatment before surgery. Data in the literature now indicate that no harm occurs to patients undergoing an operation with this degree of hypokalemia, and severe potential harm may be caused by treating such patients with oral or intravenous potassium. The fourth patient in whom possible benefit occurred received a blood transfusion before cholecystectomy for an asymptomatic hemoglobin concentration of 9.9 g per deciliter. Since cholecystectomy is not normally associated with major blood loss, it is concluded that this patient also received no benefit and only the risk of transfusion from that preoperative laboratory test. Thus, it is not clear that any patient in this study benefited from preoperative screening tests that were not indicated.

In another study, only two patients at most (who had eradication of asymptomatic bacteriuria) benefited from the 9,270 screening tests that were obtained. At least one patient was seriously harmed from the pursuit of abnormalities on screening tests and their treatment; this woman developed atrial fibrillation and congestive heart failure after thyroid therapy was instituted for borderline low thyroxine and free thyroxine index (FTI) tests. It is unclear if these investigators examined other patients for potential harm arising similarly from the pursuit and treatment of abnormalities.

When batteries of laboratory tests yield abnormal results that are neither pursued nor noted, medicolegal risk for physicians increases. Extra testing—testing that is not warranted by findings on a medical history—does not serve as medicolegal protection against liability. A series of studies (Roizen reviews these) shows that 30 to 95 percent of all unexpected abnormalities found on preoperative laboratory tests are not noted on the chart preoperatively. Many reports of preoperative radiographs, for example, are not on the chart before anesthesia is administered. This lack of notation occurs not only at university medical centers, but in community hospitals also. Data show that failing to pursue an abnormality that has been detected poses a greater risk to medicolegal liability than does failing to detect that abnormality. In this way, extra testing results in extra medicolegal risk to physicians.

Random preoperative testing is inefficient for operating room schedules. According to hospital administrators in the United States, surgeons say that they order preoperative tests to satisfy the anesthesiologist: they find it easier just to order all the tests and let the anesthesiologist sort them out. Surgeons also believe that it is much more efficient to order batteries of tests than to have the anesthesiologist, who sees the patient the night before or the morning of surgery, try to get the tests on an emergency basis. These surgeons apparently do not realize that abnormalities detected by tests done in this battery fashion are not discovered until the night before or the morning of surgery, if at all. Then abnormal results on these tests delay or postpone schedules, as extra effort and time are wasted in obtaining consultant reviews of false-positive or slightly abnormal results.

IMPLEMENTATION
OF PREOPERATIVE EVALUATION

There are at least three methods of determining the laboratory tests to be ordered for a patient. The surgeon or anesthesiologist who sees the patient prior to the scheduled procedure can obtain the history and perform the physical examination. Second, a clinic can be set up in the outpatient facility to perform these two tasks early enough to ensure that the appropriate laboratory tests or consultations can be obtained without delaying schedules. Third, a questionnaire answered by the patient can be used to indicate appropriate laboratory tests.

Of the first method one might ask, Can the appropriate testing be easily generated from the surgeon's preoperative visit? One study found that it could. At the University of California, San Francisco, Kaplan et al found that even a partial history conveyed enough information to indicate correctly all but 22 abnormalities (none of which affected patient outcome) in more than 2,785 preoperative blood tests obtained (counting the complete blood count and simultaneous multichannel analysis of six variables [SMA 6] as one test). Knowing only the admission diagnosis, previous discharge diagnoses, and scheduled operation and using previously determined indications for laboratory testing enabled detection of virtually all abnormalities that would have been detected by routine screening.

As regards the patient questionnaire, several groups have tested the effects and sensitivity of orally administered or written questionnaires as a means of linking the selection of laboratory tests with a patient's medical history. In 1987, McKee and Scott used an orally administered set of 17 questions and patient demographics to select preoperative tests for 400 patients. They found that age was the best predictor of abnormalities on preoperative tests. Complications occurred most commonly in patients who reported positive symptoms on the questionnaire and who were older.

A recent study determined that the responses of patients to written questions can be used to predict which laboratory tests will yield abnormal results for those patients. After the patient answers the questionnaire, a plastic overlay reveals what tests are indicated. If the patient cannot answer the questions, a standard group of tests is ordered. Even in a tertiary care hospital that admits very sick patients, more than 60 percent of these laboratory tests now routinely obtained could be eliminated. The elimination of such tests could result in a 93 to 97 percent reduction in patient charges and hospital costs.

The protocols outlined in Tables 1 and 2 are guidelines for using clinical judgment in ordering laboratory tests. A careful history and physical examination of the patient are required, with special attention to testing whenever indicators of disease entities listed in the tables are discovered. The protocol clearly places the burden on whoever takes the history to do so accurately.

We do not say that all standard screening tests should be discontinued. Some are beneficial—the fecal

Table 1 Current (1990) Minimal (? Maximal) Laboratory Test Recommendations Based on Benefit Exceeding Risk in Asymptomatic Patients Scheduled for Peripheral Surgical Procedures

Age (years)	Male	Female
≤ 40	–	? pregnancy test*
40–49	Hct ECG	Hct ? pregnancy test*
50–64	Hct ECG	Hct ECG
65–74	Hct BUN ECG ? CXR†	Hct BUN ECG ? CXR†
≥ 75	Hct BUN, glucose ECG CXR†	Hct BUN, glucose ECG CXR†

*If patient cannot rule out pregnancy definitely.
†Benefit-risk ratio of chest x-ray examination for asymptomatic individuals older than 60 years of age is not clear, but it appears that risk exceeds benefit until the patient is older than 74 years.
BUN = blood urea nitrogen; CXR = chest x-ray examination; ECG = electrocardiography; Hct = hematocrit.

occult blood test for individuals older than 40 years of age (every 2 years or every year in high-risk groups), the pap smear (every 3 years for women who are sexually active, or every year for women at high risk), and the mammogram (every year for women older than 50 years of age or for those older than 40 years in high-risk groups). That is the point of the screening history—to identify individuals likely to benefit from testing. Although the rationale for the choice of tests is beyond the scope of this chapter, some specific tests deserve comment.

Hemoglobin, Hematocrit,
and White Blood Cell Counts

How many asymptomatic patients have a degree of abnormality on hematocrit or the white blood cell (WBC) count that alters perioperative management? I would define the following values as not meriting intervention perioperatively: a hematocrit of 27 to 54 for patients undergoing operations during which major blood loss is unlikely, and a WBC of 2,400 to 16,000 per cubic millimeter for individuals not undergoing insertion of a prosthesis. When values fall outside these ranges, we recommend seeking alternative diagnoses before the institution of anesthesia or surgery. The data available in the literature indicate that either preoperative hematocrit or hemoglobin levels should be determined for all surgical patients older than 60 years of age. Hematocrit and red blood cell antigen screening is warranted for all patients undergoing procedures involving possible loss

Table 2 Simplified Strategy for Preoperative Testing*

Preoperative conditions suspected	HGB		WBC	PT/PTT	PLT/BT	Elect	Creat/BUN	Blood glucose	SGOT/ALK PTASE	X-ray examination	ECG	Pregnancy	T/S
	M	F											
Surgical procedure with blood loss	X	X											X
without blood loss													
Neonates	X	X											
Age <40 yr		X											
Age 40–59 yr		X									•		
Age ≥60 yr	X	X								X	X		
Cardiovascular disease							X			X	X		
Pulmonary disease										X	X		
Malignancy	X	X	○		○					X			
Radiation therapy			X							X	X		
Hepatic disease				X					X				
Exposure to hepatitis									X				
Renal disease	X	X				X	X						
Bleeding disorder				X	X								
Diabetes						X	X	X			X		
Smoking ≥20 pk yrs	X	X								X			
Possible pregnancy												X	
Diuretic use						X	X						
Digoxin use						X	X				X		
Steroid use						X		X					
Anticoagulant use	X	X		X									

*Not all diseases are included in this table. Please use your judgment for patients with diseases not included.

• = maybe; ○ = leukemias only; X = obtain; BT = bleeding time; Creat/BUN = creatinine or blood urea nitrogen; ECG = electrocardiography; Elect = Na$^+$, K$^+$, Cl$^-$, CO_2, proteins; HGB = hemoglobin; PLT = platelet count; PT = prothrombin time; PTT = partial thromboplastin time; SGOT/ALK PTase = serum glutamic oxaloacetic transaminase phosphatase; T/S = blood typing and screen for unexpected antibodies; WBC = white blood cell count.

Modified from: Roizen MF. Preoperative evaluation. In: Miller RD, ed. Anesthesia. 3rd ed. Vol. 1. New York: Churchill Livingstone, 1990: 743; and Kaplan EB, Sheiner LB, Boeckmann AJ, et al. The usefulness of preoperative laboratory screening. JAMA 1985; 253: 3576–3581; Blery C, Fourgeaux B, et al. Evaluation of a protocol for selective ordering of preoperative tests. Lancet 1986; 1:139–141.

of more than 2 U per 70 kg of body weight. WBCs appear to be rarely indicated in asymptomatic individuals but might be considered when a prosthesis is to be inserted.

Blood Chemistries and Urinalysis

What blood chemistries would have to be abnormal, and how abnormal would they have to be, to justify changing the perioperative management? Abnormal hepatic or renal function might change the choice and dose of anesthetic or adjuvant drugs. About one in 700 supposedly healthy patients is actually harboring hepatitis, and one in three of those will become jaundiced. However, in a prospective study of the HealthQuiz (see below) involving 3,500 patients, our group found no asymptomatic patient who denied exposure to hepatitis who then became jaundiced after uneventful surgery. These data imply that either the screening history suffices or the incidence of asymptomatic hepatitis is decreasing. Unexpected abnormalities are reported for 2 to 10 percent of patients with multiphasic screening, and these abnormalities lead to many additional tests that usually (in approximately 80 percent of cases) have no significance for the patient. Unexpected abnormalities that are significant arise in 2 to 5 percent of patients studied. Of these abnormalities, approximately 70 percent are related to blood glucose and blood urea nitrogen (BUN) levels. The 2 to 20 additional tests on the

screening SMAs 6-21 panels lead to very few important discoveries affecting anesthesia. In fact, the false-positive rate is so high (96.5 percent for the test for calcium) that the value representing cost versus benefit for most of these tests (even when the initial tests are free) is negative, as is the value representing benefit versus risk.

If a screening test for hepatitis is desired, because the incidence of hepatitis is 0.14 percent and/or because one wishes to avoid the potential legal problems of postanesthetic jaundice, only three tests appear to be justified: serum glutamic-oxaloacetic transaminase (SGOT), blood glucose, and BUN. Even then, the last two are indicated only for patients older than 64 years of age. In fact, if the data from our group on asymptomatic liver disease can be generalized, no blood chemistry tests are warranted for patients younger than 64 years of age. Furthermore, if the antibody test that detects non-A, non-B hepatitis (now called hepatitis C) proves as useful after infection has occurred, the medicolegal risk posed by postanesthetic jaundice will be even less.

Abnormalities are commonly found on urinalysis. The quality of urinalysis results obtained by dipstick technique has been variable at best. In addition, these abnormal results do not usually lead to beneficial changes in management. Most of the results that do lead to beneficial changes could have been obtained by history or determination of BUN and glucose levels, tests that are already recommended for all patients older than 64 years of age. Thus, urinalysis, although initially inexpensive, becomes an expensive test to justify on a cost-benefit or benefit-risk basis.

Chest X-Ray Examination

What abnormalities on chest radiographs would influence management of anesthesia? Certainly, it may be important to know about the existence of tracheal deviation; mediastinal masses; pulmonary nodules; a solitary lung mass; aortic aneurysm; pulmonary edema; pneumonia; atelectasis; new fractures of the vertebrae, ribs, or clavicles, dextrocardia; or cardiomegaly before proceeding to anesthesia and surgery. However, a chest radiograph probably would not detect the degree of chronic lung disease requiring a change in anesthetic technique any better than would the history and physical examination. The data reviewed by Roizen show that abnormalities are rare in the asymptomatic individual. In fact, if the patient is asymptomatic and younger than 74 years of age, the risks of chest x-ray examination probably exceed the possible benefits. This analysis is, of course, predicated on maximizing benefit to society in general, as one cannot predict in advance which patients will benefit or which will be harmed.

Electrocardiography and Screening for Cardiac Disease

Although individual episodes of myocardial ischemia may not produce symptoms, almost all patients without diabetes or autonomic insufficiency have symptoms that lead one to screen for myocardial disease. We present an algorithm in Figure 1 for pursuing laboratory testing for cardiovascular disease.

Pulmonary Function Testing

These expensive tests are rarely needed but are useful for determining those who may benefit from bronchodilator therapy and to predict risk for thoracic operations before obtaining informed consent. The indications for pulmonary function tests in Table 3 seem justified by the data.

Clotting Function Studies

Virtually no asymptomatic patient in the literature has had unequivocal benefit from clotting function studies preoperatively. Most patients show symptoms or have a medication history suggesting that clotting function tests may be necessary. Aspirin at 60 mg per 70 kg of body weight per day does not seem to pose a risk for bleeding, but the data are not available for 300 mg or more administered within 12 hours of surgery. Since the pharmacology of aspirin changes when more than 2 g per 70 kg is consumed per day, patients should be evaluated if they cannot stop aspirin early enough to have no appreciable acetylsalicylic acid (ASA) level for 24 hours before surgery (the period without ASA necessary to

generate the approximately 50,000 new platelets per cubic millimeter needed for normal platelet aggregation) or if surgical hemostasis cannot be assured or a regional procedure into a closed space is planned. Figure 2 presents an algorithm for determining whether coagulation tests are indicated.

Other Tests: Pregnancy and AIDS Screening

Tests for acquired immunodeficiency syndrome (AIDS) and pregnancy, and screening for hemoglobinopathy and malignant hyperthermia raise ethical issues that may require close attention to institutional policy and the immediate availability of counseling services. Moreover, all of these tests have associated risks. The physician may therefore decide to limit testing to only at-risk populations (e.g., for pregnancy testing, only female patients who believe they may possibly be pregnant).

Testing of the asymptomatic population for AIDS is not likely to be the most effective way of uncovering the disease. Of the more than 135,000 people in the United States who have had AIDS, only one person has not been gay, had sex with a prostitute, used intravenously administered drugs and shared needles, been stuck with a needle, cared for a family member with AIDS, been born of a woman with AIDS, or received a blood transfusion after 1979. One program screening for human immunodeficiency virus in asymptomatic individuals was able to produce an "acceptably low false-positive rate" by diagnosing HIV infection only after one sample of blood produced positive results on four different tests and after a second sample of blood had been used for verification. Thus, for pregnancy, hemoglobinopathies, and AIDS, the history is still best at identifying those at risk for the condition.

We believe that because we biased the analysis to favor laboratory testing, the tests listed in Table 1 may be more than is needed but certainly are not less than indicated. Just as good an argument could be made for no testing of asymptomatic individuals in low-risk groups.

THE "SMART TECHNOLOGY"* SOLUTION TO EFFICIENT, LESS EXPENSIVE QUALITY CARE

However, even when physicians attempt to choose tests selectively based on the history and/or physical

*"Smart technology" is the use of new configurations of chips, microprocessors, circuit boards, memory banks, and software to allow us to inexpensively practice more efficient, less costly, and higher quality medicine. As the hardware becomes smaller and more powerful and the software becomes more versatile, the age of "high-tech" is being replaced by the age of "smart tech" just as the relatively expensive "horseless carriages" were replaced by today's cars. We can embrace smart-tech solutions such as this as we have embraced oximeters to reduce costs and improve quality.

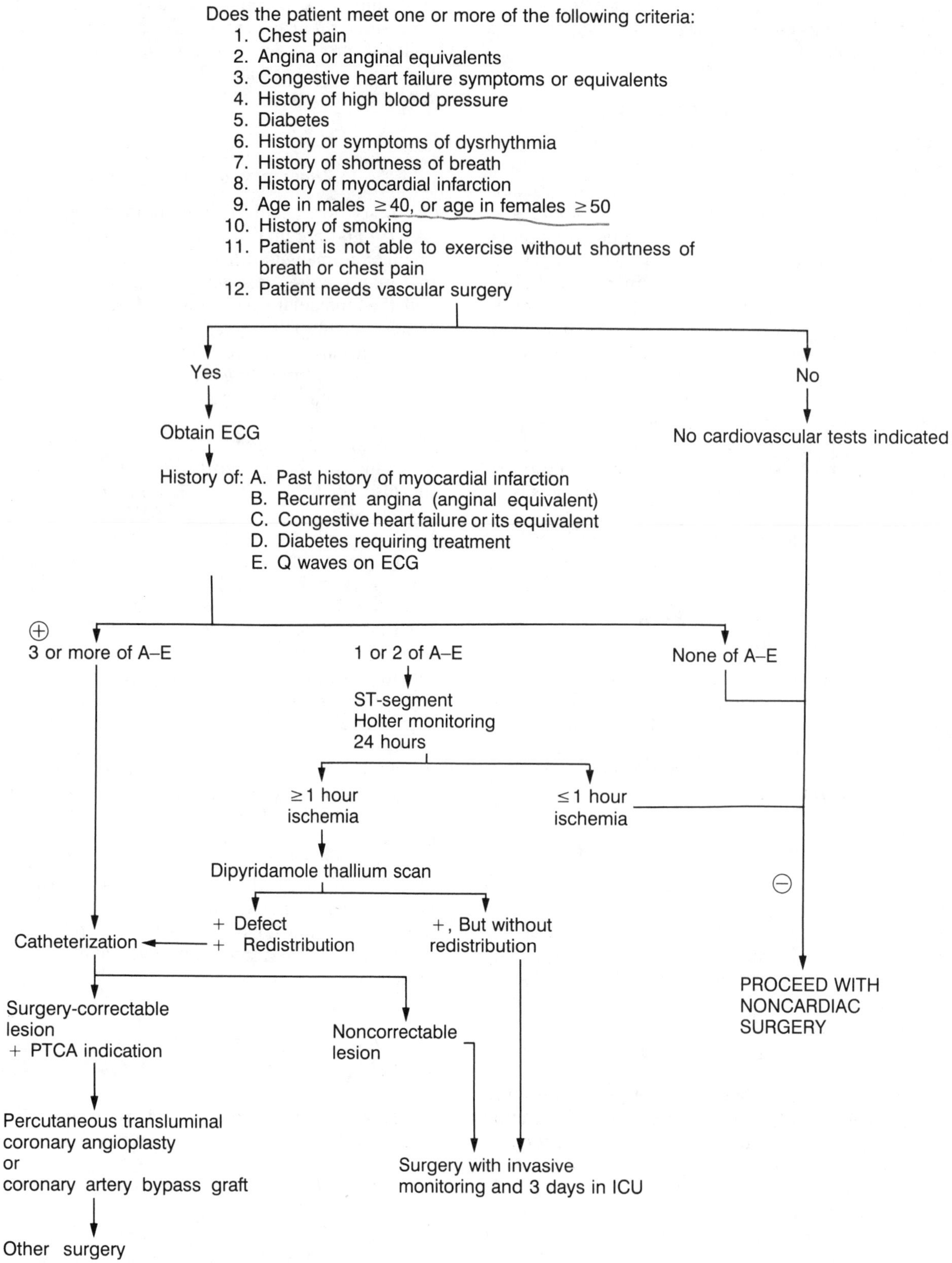

Does the patient meet one or more of the following criteria:
1. Chest pain
2. Angina or anginal equivalents
3. Congestive heart failure symptoms or equivalents
4. History of high blood pressure
5. Diabetes
6. History or symptoms of dysrhythmia
7. History of shortness of breath
8. History of myocardial infarction
9. Age in males ≥40, or age in females ≥50
10. History of smoking
11. Patient is not able to exercise without shortness of breath or chest pain
12. Patient needs vascular surgery

Yes

No

Obtain ECG

No cardiovascular tests indicated

History of: A. Past history of myocardial infarction
B. Recurrent angina (anginal equivalent)
C. Congestive heart failure or its equivalent
D. Diabetes requiring treatment
E. Q waves on ECG

⊕
3 or more of A–E

1 or 2 of A–E

None of A–E

ST-segment
Holter monitoring
24 hours

≥1 hour ischemia

≤1 hour ischemia

Dipyridamole thallium scan

Catheterization ◄── + Defect
+ Redistribution

+, But without redistribution

⊖

Surgery-correctable lesion
+ PTCA indication

Noncorrectable lesion

PROCEED WITH NONCARDIAC SURGERY

Percutaneous transluminal coronary angioplasty
or
coronary artery bypass graft

Surgery with invasive monitoring and 3 days in ICU

Other surgery

Figure 1 How to decide which cardiovascular laboratory tests to obtain: Use history to segregate patients into groups to test and/or monitor invasively.

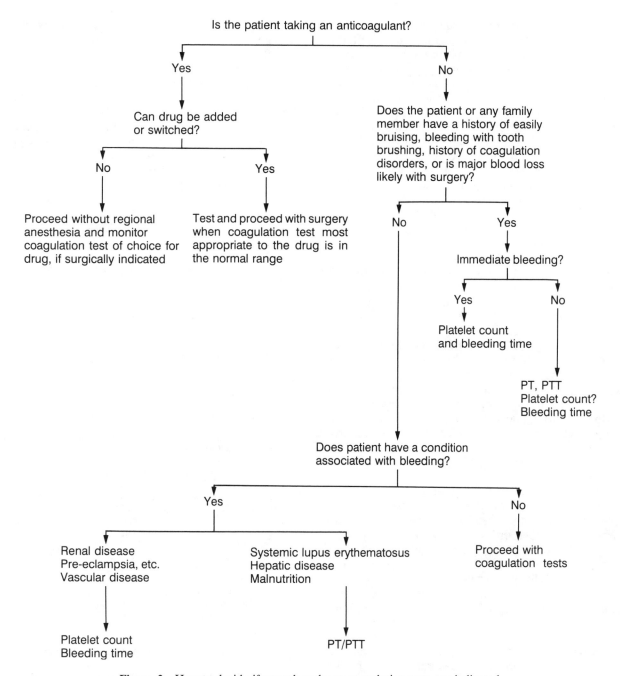

Figure 2 How to decide if coagulopathy or coagulation tests are indicated.

examination of a patient, errors are made in ordering tests. When surgeons and anesthesiologists agreed on indications for testing, 30 to 40 percent of patients who should have had tests did not get them, and 20 to 40 percent of patients who should not have had tests got them. For instance, Blery and co-workers used a protocol based on suspected disease to order preoperative tests selectively for 3,866 surgical patients in France and found that even after clinicians had been educated with regard to indications, 30 percent of tests ordered were not indicated and another 22 percent of tests that were indicated were not obtained. Thus by ordering tests in the usual way, surgeons and anesthesiologists both increased costs and failed to obtain possibly valuable

Table 3 Indications for Pulmonary Function Tests

History of at least one of the following:

1. Chronic obstructive pulmonary disease
2. Shortness of breath
3. Orthopnea

Also at least one of the following needs to be determined:

1. Reversibility of bronchospasm
2. Baseline condition if intubation is expected preoperatively
3. Risk for lung resection (maximal midexpiratory flow rate, maximum breathing capacity, diffusing capacity for carbon monoxide)

information. Blery subsequently questioned anesthetists to assess whether management of the patient suffered from omission of one or more preoperative tests. Only 0.2 percent of omitted tests would have possibly been useful. Blery did not examine how many times such data might have led to pursuits that harmed patients.

Charpak et al examined the value of preoperative screening chest radiographs in 3,849 patients. Surgeons and anesthesiologists agreed that any lung or cardiovascular disease, malignant disease, current smoking history in patients older than 50 years of age, major surgical emergencies, immunodepression, or lack of prior health examination in immigrants were indications for ordering a chest radiograph. The surgeons ordered or did not order the chest radiograph after seeing the patient. Even with this agreement with regard to indications, however, of a total of 1,426 chest radiographs that should have been ordered in this group of 3,849 patients, 271 radiographs were ordered although they were not recommended, and 596 were not ordered although they were recommended. While clinical judgments may account for some of these recommendations, it is presumed that many extra chest radiographs ordered or not ordered were simply errors. If there are this many errors in a single test trial, more laboratory tests are likely to generate more errors. Preliminary data from studies of ours attest to this error rate. The problem is how to order tests that are appropriate to each patient without decreasing efficiency. We believe that selective ordering strategies are better than previous nonselective methods of ordering tests, but an even easier, more efficient method exists.

At the University of Chicago and at least 13 other institutions, a health quiz is given to patients on a four-button computer machine similar to the child's game "Donkey-Kong, Jr." Improvements in technology, graphics, and voice properties make it relatively inexpensive to display clearly (or read clearly) questions about a patient's health on a portable 8 inch × 6 inch × 1 inch hand-held box.* The surgeon or anesthesiologist can have this box in his/her office and, after both have agreed upon indications, it can be used by the patient to suggest the tests needed. The "smart-tech" box simply asks patients yes/no questions. It then generates a printout of the answers to the questions and a symptom summary, as well as suggested laboratory tests based on

the agreed upon indications and the patient's answers. It also gives reminders about items in history important to anesthesia care, such as allergies and capped teeth. It does not save me much time when I see patients, but it improves the quality of time I spend with them. And it suggests tests that would be appropriate for each patient based on that patient's medical history and accepted indications for testing. The physician, surgeon, or anesthesiologist can then override or add to suggested tests before ordering preoperative tests. The "Health-Quiz" and its printout take less than 10 minutes for the patient to complete.

SUGGESTED READING

Blery C, Szatan M, Fourgeaux B, et al. Evaluation of a protocol for selective ordering of preoperative tests. Lancet 1986; 1:139–141.
Charpak Y, Blery C, Chastang C, et al. Prospective assessment of a protocol for selective ordering or preoperative chest x-rays. Can J Anaesth 1988; 35:259–264.
Delahunt B, Turnbull PRG. How cost-effective are routine preoperative investigations? NZ Med J 1980; 92:431–432.
Domoto K, Ben R, Wei JY, et al. Yield of routine annual laboratory screening in the institutionalized elderly. Am J Public Health 1985; 75:243–245.
Durbridge TC, Edwards F, Edwards RG, et al. Evaluation of benefits of screening tests done immediately on admission to hospital. Clin Chem 1976; 22:968–971.
Kaplan EB, Sheiner LB, Boeckmann AJ, et al. The usefulness of preoperative laboratory screening. JAMA 1985; 253:3576–3581.
Korvin CC, Pearce RH, Stanley J. Admission screening: clinical benefits. Ann Intern Med 1975; 83:197–203.
Leonard JV, Clayton BE, Colley JRT. Use of biochemical profile in Children's Hospital: results of two controlled trials. Br Med J 1975; 2:662–665.
Olsen DM, Kane RL, Proctor PH. A controlled trial of multiphasic screening. N Engl J Med 1976; 294:925–930.
Rabkin SW, Horne JM. Preoperative electrocardiography: its cost-effectiveness in detecting abnormalities when a previous tracing exists. Can Med Assoc J 1979; 121:301–306.
Rabkin SW, Horne JM. Preoperative electrocardiography: effect of new abnormalities on clinical decisions. Can Med Assoc J 1983; 128:146–147.
Roizen MF. Preoperative evaluation. In: Miller RD, ed. Anesthesia. 3rd ed. Vol. 1. New York: Churchill Livingstone, 1990:743.
Roizen MF, Kaplan EB, Schreider BD, et al. The relative roles of the history and physical examination and laboratory testing in preoperative evaluation for outpatient surgery: the "Starling Curve" of preoperative laboratory testing. Anesthesiol Clin North Am 1987; 5:1, 15–34.
Rossello PJ, Cruz AR, Mayol PM. Routine laboratory tests for elective surgery in pediatric patients. Bull Assoc Med Puerto Rico 1980; 72:614–623.
Turnbull JM, Buck C. The value of preoperative screening investigations in otherwise healthy individuals. Arch Int Med 1987; 147:1101–1105.
Wolf-Klein GP, Holt T, Silverstone FA, et al. Efficacy of routine annual studies in the care of elderly patients. J Am Geriatr Soc 1985; 33:325–329.
Wood RA, Hoekelman RA. Value of the chest x-ray as a screening test for elective surgery in children. Pediatrics 1981; 67:447–452.

---

*Dr. Roizen has been involved in the development of three systems designed to facilitate preoperative ordering of indicated tests. The University of Chicago is developing one of these methods, a lap-top video preoperative health questionnaire, into a commercial product. If the product is successful, Dr. Roizen will benefit financially, as the University distributes a royalty and/or partial ownership right in such commercialized inventions to its faculty.

ASTHMA

JOSEPH D. TOBIAS, M.D.
CAROL A. HIRSHMAN, M.D.

Asthma is generally defined as a clinical syndrome of wheezing and dyspnea characterized by reversible airway narrowing, mucosal edema, and increased secretions. Since it affects roughly 2 to 5 percent of the general population, anesthesiologists are frequently faced with the problem of providing a safe anesthetic for this group of patients.

Although several new medications for the treatment of asthma have been introduced over the past 5 years, these have had little impact on the overall course of the disease. In fact, deaths due to asthma have been increasing. Aside from its impact on daily life, asthma significantly increases the risk of anesthetic morbidity.

PREOPERATIVE EVALUATION

A thorough preoperative history and physical examination are essential. The aim of the preoperative evaluation is to detect the presence of clinically significant respiratory dysfunction and to assess the effectiveness of therapy in order to maximize preoperative therapy. Furthermore, the patient should be encouraged to stop smoking for as long as possible before the anesthetic is administered, in the hope of decreasing airway reactivity.

LABORATORY INVESTIGATION

Because there is no specific laboratory test to identify asthma, the diagnosis is generally made on clinical grounds. Pulmonary function testing (PFT) (discussed in detail in another chapter of this text) is indicated in cases where the diagnosis is in doubt and may help in the evaluation of the effectiveness of the current treatment regimen. If PFT reveals obstructive disease, testing is repeated after the administration of aerosolized bronchodilators to assess the reversibility of bronchoconstriction.

Degree of reversibility =

$$\frac{\text{postbronchodilator PFT} - \text{prebronchodilator PFT}}{\text{prebronchdilator PFT}}$$

A value greater than 15 percent for the forced expiratory volume in 1 second (FEV_1) indicates the presence of significant reversible airway disease and demonstrates that the patient is not in optimum condition for anesthesia. In such cases, additional medical therapy is appropriate. Further laboratory tests such as arterial blood gas analysis and chest films are not routinely indicated.

TREATMENT

Drug Therapy

To understand the mechanisms of action of the therapeutic agents used in the treatment of asthma, a brief review of the physiology of the control of airway caliber is necessary. Airway caliber is regulated by a balance between the parasympathetic and sympathetic nervous systems. The parasympathetic nervous system promotes constriction of airway smooth muscle and mediates the rapid reflex changes in airway caliber initiated by endotracheal tubes and other irritating substances. This effect is mediated through vagal afferents and efferents after stimulation of subepithelial irritant receptors. This reflex arc can be interrupted by several pharmacologic agents, including muscarinic antagonists, local anesthetics such as lidocaine (with serum levels of 1 to 4 μg per milliliter), potent inhalational agents, and ketamine.

The bronchoconstrictive effects of the parasympathetic nervous system are balanced by the sympathetic nervous system. Although there is very little direct sympathetic innervation of the lung, bronchodilatation is mediated through the effects of circulating endogenous catecholamines (epinephrine) or exogenous agents on airway receptors. Two types of airway receptors have been described: alpha and beta$_2$. While stimulation of beta$_2$ receptors leads to bronchodilatation, the role of the alpha receptor is controversial. Some studies suggest that alpha stimulation induces bronchoconstriction, while other studies have found alpha stimulation to have little or no effect.

In addition to the two limbs of the autonomic nervous system, recent attention has focused on the nonadrenergic, noncholinergic nervous system. The mediators of this system include neuropeptides such as substance *P*, which is released from sensory nerves by an axon reflex. These peptides increase vascular permeability and mucus secretion as well as induce bronchoconstriction. These mediators are degraded by the neutral endopeptidase enzymes in the airway epithelium. Inhibition of these enzymes by influenza and other viruses has been proposed as one of the factors accounting for airway hyperreactivity associated with upper respiratory infections.

The therapeutic agents currently used in the treatment of asthma include methylxanthines, sympathomimetics, anticholinergics, steroids, and cromolyn sodium.

Sympathomimetics

Sympathomimetics are the most effective bronchodilators currently available. They lead to bronchodilatation through interaction with beta$_2$ adrenergic receptors. This interaction leads to adenylate cyclase activation, which produces increased intracellular levels of cyclic adenosine monophosphate (AMP). Cyclic AMP activates protein kinase A, which inhibits myosin phosphorylation and results in bronchodilatation.

All beta-agonists have a basic catecholamine structure with specific substitutions to the molecule, which enhance beta$_2$ selectivity or prolong the duration of action. Isoproterenol is the standard agent in the group. Other agents such as metaproterenol, terbutaline, and albuterol differ in the functional groups substituted on the benzene ring and on the ethylamine side-chain.

Because several beta$_2$ selective agents are available, the use of nonselective agents is no longer recommended except when intravenous administration is necessary. Isoproterenol is the only agent approved for intravenous use in the United States. Selective beta$_2$ agents can be administered orally, subcutaneously (terbutaline), and by inhalation. Aerosol delivery offers several advantages, including a much higher concentration at the target organ (lungs), lower systemic concentrations and therefore lower systemic effects, and a prolonged duration of action. No true advantage exists among the currently available agents, since the duration or action (3 to 6 hours) and beta$_2$ selectivity are relatively equal. Newer agents with longer durations of action (salmeterol and formoterol) are currently being evaluated.

Unwanted cardiovascular effects occur with the use of any of the beta-adrenergic agonists. Although less severe with selective beta$_2$ agents, at the doses used some degree of beta$_1$ stimulation occurs leading to tachycardia, palpitations, and tremor. Other side effects include hypokalemia, urinary retention, and central nervous system stimulation. All of these side effects tend to decrease in severity with time.

Theophylline

Theophylline is a methylxanthine derivative which has been used for 50 years in the treatment of asthma. Although less effective than beta-adrenergic agonists, it is still frequently used in the United States to treat asthma.

Although this agent has been in clinical use for several years, the exact mechanism of action remains unknown. Proposed mechanisms have included phosphodiesterase (PDE) inhibition, adenosine antagonism, anti-inflammatory effects, and the release of endogenous catecholamines. The time-honored theory of action has been through PDE inhibition. However, the concentration needed to inhibit PDE in vitro far exceeds those levels obtained in clinical use (10 to 20 µg per milliliter). Although theophylline does exhibit adenosine antagonism in clinically achievable concentrations, enprophylline (a closely related xanthine compound available in Europe) has superior bronchodilatory properties and is not an adenosine antagonist. We have recently evaluated the role of endogenous catecholamines in the effects of athiophylline preparation. In the basenji-greyhound dog model of asthma, we found that during thiopental-fentanyl anesthesia, aminophylline increased endoge-

nous catecholamine (epinephrine and norepinephrine) levels and attenuated histamine-induced bronchoconstriction. This attenuation was blocked by pretreatment with propranolol without affecting catecholamine levels. Furthermore, during 1.5 minimum alveolar concentration (MAC) halothane anesthesia (an agent known to block the release of endogenous catecholamines), no increase in endogenous catecholamines was noted and no attenuation of histamine-induced bronchoconstriction was achieved. Although the acute in vivo action may relate to the release of endogenous catecholamines, this mechanism is unlikely to explain its chronic beneficial effects. Studies in humans have shown that endogenous catecholamine levels, although initially elevated after aminophylline infusion, return to baseline after 12 to 24 hours. Therefore its chronic actions on airways may be derived from a secondary effect. These chronic effects may result from its anti-inflammatory actions. Theophylline inhibits the late response to allergens and may thereby inhibit submucosal edema formation.

The bronchodilatory properties of theophylline increase linearly from serum levels of 5 to 20 µg per milliliter. At levels greater than 20 µg per milliliter, toxic side effects become more frequent, with 75 percent of patients exhibiting side effects when levels reach 25 µg per milliliter. Rapid, reliable techniques are available for monitoring serum theophylline levels, thus helping to avoid toxic levels.

Theophylline is generally administered orally two to three times per day (as a sustained-release preparation) on a regular basis to prevent recurrent attacks of asthma. In the acute treatment of bronchospasm, theophylline is administered intravenously. As theophylline is poorly soluble in water, concentrated solutions for intravenous use are compounded with a pharmacologically inactive base (ethylenediamine). Aminophylline consists of 2 molecules of theophylline compounded with one molecule of ethylenediamine. Therefore, when the dosage is estimated based on weight, 75 to 80 percent of the dose is theophylline itself, while the rest is the inactive base.

The apparent volume of distribution is approximately 50 percent of lean body weight. Therefore, for each milligram per kilogram of theophylline, serum levels increase by 2 µg per milliliter. For example, a loading dose of 6 mg per kilogram of aminophylline (4.8 mg per kilogram of theophylline) would result in a serum concentration of 9.6 µg per milliliter. This loading dose is then followed by a continuous maintenance infusion of 0.2 to 1.0 mg per kilogram per hour (Table 1). Dosing is based on lean (not actual) body weight, and levels should be checked 30 to 60 minutes after a loading dose and 3 to 4 hours after a change in the continuous infusion rate.

Theophylline is eliminated from the body by the hepatic microsomal enzyme P450 system. Several factors, including underlying disease processes, age, and the use of other medications, can alter theophylline clearance (Table 2). Decreased clearance (leading to increased levels) can occur with hepatic dysfunction, congestive heart failure, cor pulmonale, and viral infections, and in patients who are either very young (younger

Table 1 Guidelines for Maintenance Infusion Rates of Aminophylline

Age	Aminophylline Dose (mg/kg/hr)
0–4 weeks	0.2
4 weeks–1 year	0.2–0.5
1–9 years	1.0
10–55 years	0.4–0.6
Over 55 years	0.2–0.3

Table 2 Theophylline Clearance

Decreased Clearance	Increased Clearance
Congestive heart failure	Pregnancy
Cor pulmonale	Cigarette smoking
Liver disease	Phenobarbital
Acute hypoxemia	Phenytoin
Old age	Carbamazepine
Age < 1 year	Rifampin
Cimetidine (not ranitidine)	Isoproterenol
Erythromycin	
Troleandomycin	
Allopurinol	
Oral contraceptives	

than 1 year) or very old (older than 60 years). Clearance can also be decreased by several medications. Theophylline clearance may be increased by any one of several factors, and therefore frequent monitoring of serum levels is mandatory, especially when one of these conditions is present.

Although relatively effective in controlling asthmatic symptoms, theophylline has fallen out of favor with many physicians because of its relatively high incidence of side effects. These adverse effects, which can occur in the presence of therapeutic serum levels, include tremor, restlessness, nausea and vomiting from direct central stimulation, tachycardia, and tachydysrhythmias from myocardial stimulation as well as from catecholamine release. Furthermore, the incidence of dysrhythmias is increased during inhalational anesthesia with halothane, but not enflurane or isoflurane. Central nervous stimulation and seizures can occur at levels of 30 μg per milliliter. Recent concern has centered on the occurrence of electroencephalographic abnormalities and learning disabilities in children receiving long-term theophylline therapy.

Anticholinergics

Anticholinergics represent one of the oldest remedies for asthma, outdating even the use of epinephrine. Stramonium has been used for hundreds of years in herbal teas and by inhalation to treat asthma. The currently available anticholinergics are either tertiary compounds (atropine, scopolamine) or quaternary compounds (glycopyrrolate, ipratropium). These agents block airway muscarinic receptors, leading to broncho-

dilatation. Although several different types of muscarinic receptors have been identified, currently available preparations are nonselective. This nonselective blockade may also block inhibitory receptors on cholinergic nerves which control acetylcholine release. This blockade leads to the increased release of acetylcholine, which can antagonize the effects of the anticholinergics. Selective blockade of M_3 receptors may overcome this problem.

Quaternary compounds are generally favored over tertiary compounds; since they do not cross the blood-brain barrier, there is less systemic absorption and no central nervous system effects. These agents are particularly effective in patients with a reactive component of chronic obstructive pulmonary disease.

Although atropine effectively attenuates bronchoconstriction, its use by aerosol and certainly its intravenous use may be accompanied by significant systemic effects. These effects include tachycardia, blurred vision from mydriasis, dry mouth, urinary retention, and drying of secretions. These effects are uncommon with the aerosolized use of quaternary compounds such as glycopyrrolate or ipratropium. However, because both of these agents can precipitate bronchospasm, they should be administered with a beta-adrenergic agent. This effect has been attributed to the additives in the solution.

Cromolyn

Cromolyn is the prototype of a new series of drugs capable of controlling asthmatic symptoms. Although it has no role in the acute treatment of bronchospasm, it is generally effective in preventing recurrent attacks. It is administered as an aerosol and is particularly effective in preventing exercise-induced bronchospasm. Although initially thought to act by stabilizing mast cells and thereby preventing mediator release, recent studies suggest that it also affects inflammatory cells (macrophages and eosinophils). It is relatively free of adverse side effects and no interactions with other medications have been reported.

Corticosteroids

The use of corticosteroids is a potent weapon in the treatment of chronic asthma as well as status asthmaticus. Like many of the other drugs used to treat asthma, their mode of action remains poorly understood. They most likely act by either altering the beta-adrenergic limb or by modulating inflammation. Corticosteroids increase beta-receptor density and function, thereby improving the response to endogenous or exogenous catecholamines. Steroids also modulate various components of the inflammatory response and through this action may modulate asthmatic symptoms.

Various corticosteroid preparations exist which can be administered orally, intravenously, and by aerosol. For daily maintenance therapy, aerosol delivery by metered dose inhaler is currently the preferred method. As with other inhaled agents, this route increases delivery to the target organ while minimizing systemic effects. To treat acute attacks and during the perioperative period, the intravenous route is preferred. As long as equipotent doses are used, no real advantage exists for any of the intravenous preparations, except that methylprednisolone has fewer mineralocorticoid effects. It may offer some advantage by avoiding the undesirable side effects affecting salt and water balance.

The short-term use of corticosteroids is relatively safe and free of adverse side effects. However, prolonged use of these agents can have significant adverse effects. These effects can be minimized by alternate-day dosing and by aerosol administration. Side effects of long-term steroid use include osteoporosis, weight gain, hypertension, cataracts, glucose intolerance, central nervous system disturbances, and hypokalemia.

Other Therapies

Since the control of asthma remains quite difficult, the search for the "magic bullet" continues. As these "additional therapies" are used more frequently, the anesthesiologist is likely to be confronted by such patients.

As stated previously, the role of the alpha-adrenergic nervous system in asthma remains controversial. Manipulation of the alpha limb has been met with mixed results. However, reports exist on the successful treatment of asthma with alpha-blockers such as phenoxybenzamine. Moreover, Prezant and Aldrich presented two patients in whom the use of droperidol decreased airway pressures and improved compliance, presumably from alpha-adrenergic blockade.

More recently, Okayama et al reported the beneficial effects of magnesium sulfate on forced vital capacity and FEV_1 in ten asthmatic patients. Lindeman et al have shown that, in dogs, the effects of magnesium result from its actions as a voltage-sensitive calcium channel blocker.

Other "additional therapies" include the antihistamine ketotifen fumarate and the macrolide antibiotic troleandomycin. Troleandomycin has steroid-sparing effects, but only with methylprednisolone. This effect is related to its inhibition of the cytochrome P450 system, thereby prolonging the serum half-life. Other attempts to decrease steroid doses by modulating the inflammatory response have included therapy with gold and methotrexate.

Perioperative Care

Because airway instrumentation is the event most likely to precipitate acute bronchospasm, any measure to avoid it is useful. In asthmatics, intraoperative wheezing occurs more commonly after intubation (6.4 percent) than during either general anesthesia by mask or regional anesthesia (2 percent). Therefore, when appropriate, regional anesthesia or general anesthesia by mask is preferred.

As always, careful preoperative evaluation is mandatory. Preoperative drug regimens should be maxi-mized and elective cases should be postponed in patients with recent upper respiratory tract infections or recent bouts of wheezing. Emergency anesthesia in patients with asthma is occasionally necessary, and there exists a certain subpopulation of patients with asthma who are never asymptomatic. In such cases, therapy should be maximized as time permits.

There are no controlled studies showing the superiority of any preanesthetic medication. Anxiety should be alleviated as it can exacerbate asthma. Although no controlled studies exist, one or two preoperative doses of corticosteroids may be beneficial and are mandatory in patients receiving chronic steroid therapy. The use of all other routine asthma medications should be continued. Although the acute administration of aminophylline during deep inhalational anesthesia (1.5 MAC) may be ineffective (because of inhibition of endogenous catecholamine release by halothane), it may offer protection during induction and emergence. Furthermore, its chronic mode of action may not involve catecholamine release.

As mentioned previously, the event most likely to induce bronchospasm is tracheal intubation. Therefore, when intubation is required, a deep level of anesthesia should be obtained before airway manipulation. Thiopental was previously believed to cause bronchospasm through histamine release; however, it does not in itself induce bronchoconstriction but rather provides a light anesthesia during which airway manipulation can lead to bronchoconstriction.

Ketamine hydrochloride is the induction agent of choice in the severe asthmatic and the actively wheezing patient. It produces bronchodilatation through both a direct effect on airway smooth muscle and through catecholamine release. Intravenous lidocaine (1 to 1.5 mg per kilogram) given 1 to 2 minutes before intubation is a useful adjunct.

After induction, deep inhalational anesthesia should be obtained before airway manipulation. Although we have shown that the three commonly used agents provide equal protection, halothane is preferred since it is less pungent and therefore less likely to cause coughing.

Although no drugs are absolutely contraindicated, it is best to avoid those known to cause histamine release such as curare, atracurium besylate, and perhaps morphine. Maintenance anesthesia is best maintained with nitrous oxide and one of the inhalational agents. Because a light plane of anesthesia can lead to bronchospasm, it is best to keep these patients deeply anesthetized.

Many asthmatics require ENT procedures, and ENT surgeons frequently use topical epinephrine and cocaine. The combination of these two agents with aminophylline and halothane can be lethal. In such patients, it may be wise to change to either enflurane or isoflurane after induction and encourage the surgeon to use other vasoconstrictors.

Even with the most meticulous care, intraoperative bronchospasm can still occur. When severe bronchospasm occurs (assuming that other causes for wheezing and increased airway pressures have been ruled out), it is generally best to ventilate by hand with 100 percent oxygen. Treatment involves deepening the level of anesthesia by increasing the concentration of the inhalational agent. Beta-adrenergic agonists should be administered through the endotracheal tube by means of a t-adapter. Terbutaline can be administered subcutaneously. Other strategies include incremental doses of ketamine and/or lidocaine. Most importantly, in severe cases, a servo ventilator such as the Siemens 900C can be used in the operating room, since its capabilities are greater than those of ventilators on the anesthesia machine.

SUGGESTED READING

Barnes PJ. A new approach to the treatment of asthma. N Engl J Med 1989; 321:1517–1527.

Hirshman CA. Airway reactivity in humans: anesthetic implications. Anesthesiology 1983; 58:170–177.

Kingston HCG, Downes H, Hirshman CA. Antibronchospastic drugs. In: Smith NT, Miller RD, Corbasci AN, eds. Drug interactions in anesthesia. Philadelphia: Lea and Febiger, 1985:100.

Kingston HCG, Hirshman CA. Perioperative management of the patient with asthma. Anesth Analg 1984; 63:844–855.

Lindeman KS, Hirshman CA, Freed AN. Effect of magnesium sulfate on bronchoconstriction in the lung periphery. J Appl Physiol 1989; 66:2527–2532.

Okayama H, Aikawa T, Okayama M, et al. Bronchodilating effect of intravenous magnesium sulfate in bronchial asthma. JAMA 1987; 257:1076–1078.

Prezant DJ, Aldrich TK. Intravenous droperidol for the treatment of status asthmaticus. Crit Care Med 1988; 16:96–97.

Tobias JD, Kubos KL, Hirshman CA. Aminophylline does not attenuate histamine-induced bronchoconstriction during halothane anesthesia. Anesthesiology 1989; 71:723–729.

CHRONIC OBSTRUCTIVE PULMONARY DISEASE

PHILIP G. BOYSEN, M.D.

Chronic obstructive lung disease (COPD) is most often the result of a long history of cigarette use. The diagnosis and assessment of COPD is of particular importance to the practicing anesthesiologist for a number of reasons. Surgical procedures that involve the upper abdomen or thorax cause impairment of lung function in the immediate postoperative period. This is usually associated with a loss of lung volume, atelectasis, and development of infection. In order to improve function and outcome, it is essential to realize the degree of impairment and maximization of function. During the immediate postoperative period, a given patient with COPD may not be able to tolerate the superimposed restrictive ventilatory defect, even though this is transient. Further, resection of lung tissue may leave the impaired patient in a functional status incompatible with survival. COPD and lung cancer often share the same etiology (i.e., tobacco use), so that a candidate for resectional cure of a lung cancer must be carefully evaluated from a physiologic standpoint.

HISTORY AND PHYSICAL EXAMINATION

Assessment of the COPD patient begins with a directed history and physical examination. A long history of smoking may interfere with the ability to clear secretions and to develop an effective cough. Patients with established COPD can be divided into emphysema, or type A COPD, and chronic bronchitis, or type B COPD. Differences are detailed in Table 1.

The classic history obtained from the COPD patient with chronic bronchitis confirms the diagnosis. These patients produce sputum for a period of at least 2 months during consecutive calendar years. As the disease progresses, they begin to develop the atypical "blue-bloater" habitus: they are fat, edematous, and cyanotic. Cyanosis is compatible with the tendency toward chronic hypoxemia and arterial oxygen desaturation. In addition, progression of disease results in hypercarbia, through mechanisms not completely understood. The process develops slowly so as to allow compensation by renal mechanisms, resulting in metabolic alkalosis and a near-normal hydrogen ion concentration. Since hypoxemia, and to a lesser extent, hypercarbia are potent stimuli to the pulmonary vascular bed, pulmonary vascular resistance will eventually be sustained. Right heart failure and cor pulmonale are the inevitable result. Alteration in right heart hemodynamics result in jugular venous distention, increased hepatojugular reflux, and peripheral edema. When hepatic perfusion is impaired, metabolism of many drugs is altered. In the chronically hypoxic patient with coronary artery disease, left heart failure may also result. Productive cough and purulent sputum are evidence of colonization and often result in parenchymal infection. Repeated episodes of respiratory failure are characteristic and can usually be managed conservatively without tracheal intubation or mechanical ventilation.

The emphysematous patient is rarely hypoxic despite severe alterations in lung and chest wall mechanics.

Table 1 Classification of COPD Patients

	Type A Emphysema "Pink Puffer"	Type B Chronic Bronchitis "Blue Bloater"
Body weight	Thin/emaciated	Overweight/edematous
Hypoxia	No	Yes
Hypercarbia	No	Yes
Cyanosis	No	Yes
Cor pulmonale	No	Yes
Erythrocytosis	No	Yes
Cough/sputum	Minimal	Significant
Colonization/infection	Minimal	Significant
Repeated episodes of respiratory failure	Few	Many
Bronchospasm	Minimal	Often significant
Hyperinflation/gas trapping	Significant	Minimal
Bullous disease	Yes	Unusual

There is little tendency toward carbon dioxide retention, and thus increased pulmonary vascular resistance and right heart failure are both uncommon. Sputum is scanty, usually nonpurulent, and there is little tendency toward colonization and infection. Lack of hypoxia and cyanosis results in a "pink" patient, and altered mechanics result in the "puffer" appearance. Whereas the bronchitic patient has near-normal lung volumes and a chest radiograph showing increased vascular and parenchymal markings, the emphysematous patient has flat diaphragms, hyperlucent lung fields with decreased pulmonary and vascular markings, and a slim cardiac silhouette. Loss of lung parenchyma is due to the destructive influence of tobacco, which destroys the alveolocapillary membranes. When lung parenchyma is destroyed, the tethering effect of the lung parenchyma is also lost, increasing the tendency toward airway collapse. The patient "puffs"—i.e., adapts a breathing pattern to minimize airway collapse. Typically the patient leans forward, breathes slowly through pursed lips, and maintains a quiet demeanor to maintain his or her respiratory mechanics. Hyperinflation is another mechanism used to maintain peripheral airways. Episodic respiratory failure is infrequent. It has been said that the emphysematous patient has only one episode of respiratory failure: the last.

PULMONARY FUNCTION TESTING

The diagnosis of COPD is made by history and physical examination. Corroborative data and documentation of physiologic dysfunction are obtained from pulmonary function testing. Spirometry and arterial blood gas analysis are of particular interest. In order to generate useful data, three forced vital capacity maneuvers are performed and a time versus volume tracing is recorded. Forcing the vital capacity maneuver accentuates airway collapse. Since volume (L) per unit time (sec) ensures exhaled flow (4 sec), an arbitrary point is used to assess exhaled flow. Thus, the forced expiratory

volume at one second ($FEV_{1.0}$) assesses exhaled flow and the forced vital capacity (FVC) measures total exhaled volume. The ratio of $FEV_{1.0}$/FVC is the hallmark of expiratory flow obstruction. Reduction of the FEV is characteristic of restrictive physiology, and the FVC is well preserved until late in the course of COPD. At that time, reduction in FVC is accompanied by severe hyperinflation and gas trapping. For this reason, lung volume determinations are often performed. Emphysema usually shows increased functional residual capacity (FRC) and residual volume (RV), with little change in total lung capacity (TLC). The FRC/TLC and RV/TLC ratios are thus increased. Chronic bronchitis shows relatively little change in lung volumes unless there is significant bronchospasm. Diffusing capacity changes little if at all; emphysema is characterized by loss of effective surface available for gas transfer; therefore, diffusing capacity is often increased.

The response to bronchodilators is usually assessed during spirometry. A nebulized bronchodilator is administered, and three spirograms are repeated. Improvement in FVC, $FEV_{1.0}$, or midflow measurements suggest an improved outcome with adequate perioperative therapy.

TREATMENT

A suggested approach to perioperative therapy is outlined in Table 2. For noncardiac thoracic surgery and upper abdominal surgery, such therapy is particularly important. This regimen should be implemented as soon as possible before surgery, continued intraoperatively, and maintained through the postoperative period. As a general rule, 80 percent of preoperative function is recovered by the third postoperative day, the radius occurring within 24 hours.

Additional measures are helpful to reverse the superimposed restrictive ventilatory defect, recruit alveolar volume, and improve arterial oxygenation. These therapeutic maneuvers are all designed to achieve a

Table 2 Therapeutic Regimen to Maximize Function*

Metered dose (inhaler) atropine analogue
Metered dose (inhaler) beta$_2$ agonist
Metered dose (inhaler) nonabsorbable steroid
Phosphodiesterase inhibitor, e.g., aminophylline
   Orally
   intravenously
Parenteral steroids†
Short-course broad-spectrum antibiotics‡

*Mainly for chronic bronchitis
†If evidence of adrenal suppression or parenteral dosing past 6 months.
‡With evidence of purulent sputum.

deep, sustained inspiration. They include coached deep breathing exercises, sustained maximal inspiration using incentive spirometric devices, and passive lung inflation with an intermittent positive pressure breathing device. The latter is especially helpful in selected COPD patients who use such a device at home to nebulize bronchodilators.

Anesthetic management may also be altered in the COPD patient. Since ventilation-perfusion abnormalities are characteristic of the pathophysiologic syndrome, anesthetic uptake may be impaired owing to a prolonged time constant. In the emphysematous patient, hyperinflation and gas trapping may further interfere with the movement of anesthetic gas. For the patient with chronic bronchitis and a tendency to retain carbon dioxide, the administration of narcotics, sedatives, and volatile anesthetic agents may accentuate a known or anticipated tendency to cause significant alveolar hypoventilation. Circulatory abnormalities may be present, including pulmonary vascular hypertension, cor pulmonale, and impaired liver perfusion. For drugs that depend on hepatic mechanisms for metabolism and elimination, altered pharmacokinetics will result. Therapy for underlying abnormalities may result in side effects, such as catecholamine sensitivity and arrhythmias, and fluid-electrolyte and/or acid-base disorders complicated by diuretic therapy.

During anesthetic emergency, additional time may be required to remove alveolar gas, again because of ventilation-perfusion abnormalities. The tendency to hypoventilate may be accentuated by residual volatile anesthetic, sedatives, or narcotics or residual neuromuscular paralysis.

Because of the blunted response to an elevated or rising carbon dioxide tension, pain management techniques should be optimized for the surgical COPD patient. Patient-controlled analgesia (PCA) is a technique utilizing small intravenous narcotic doses, limited to specific intervals that can be self-administered by the patient. The intent is to avoid both subtherapeutic and toxic blood levels of analgesics. The psychological impact of control over the pain management system has the putative advantage of resulting in lower total dosing per unit time.

Intrathecal or epidural analgesia and narcotics should be considered for all thoracotomy patients. For the COPD patient with upper abdominal surgery, epidural analgesia may be of particular benefit, since there is some evidence that in addition to superior pain relief, there is a further benefit in improved pulmonary function. To maintain adequate pain relief without causing respiratory depression, naloxone can be administered as necessary or by continuous infusion. Naloxone is also useful for urinary retention and pruritus. For the latter, diphenhydramine hydrochloride (Benadryl) can be added if necessary.

SUGGESTED READING

American Review of Respiratory Disease. Supplement: the rise in chronic obstructive pulmonary disease mortality. Am Rev Respir Dis 140(3 Part 2).

Bone RC. Managing acute respiratory failure in COPD patients. J Respir Dis 1979; 1:60–77.

Bone RC. Treatment of respiratory failure in advanced chronic obstructive pulmonary disease. Med Clin North Am 1981; 65: 563–578.

Derenne J-P, Fleury B, Pariente R. State of the art: acute respiratory failure of chronic obstructive pulmonary disease. Am Rev Respir Dis 1988; 138:1006–1033.

Powell JR, Vozeh S, Hopewell P, et al. Theophylline disposition in acutely ill hospitalized patients: the effect of smoking, heart failure, severe airway obstruction, and pneumonia. Am Rev Respir Dis 1978; 118:229.

Rosen RL. Acute respiratory failure and chronic obstructive lung disease. Med Clin North Am 1986; 70:895–907.

Silver MR, Bone RC. Acute respiratory failure and chronic obstructive pulmonary disease. In: Ledingham McA, ed. Recent advances in critical care medicine. Vol 3. 1987:31.

HYPERTENSION

EDWARD D. MILLER, Jr., M.D.

The elevation in systemic blood pressure may be the only sign that a patient about to undergo a surgical procedure is at risk for developing complications during the perioperative period. The decision either to proceed with or to delay the procedure on a single measurement of blood pressure is not justified. To proceed, however, in the face of significantly elevated blood pressure is also unwise. What then are the guidelines for making this decision? To appreciate the problem more fully, one must understand the underlying condition that an elevation in blood pressure represents. Thus, a broad classification of hypertension is necessary.

Blood pressure greater than 160/90 mm Hg on three consecutive readings is all that is required to label a patient as hypertensive. However, since that label may result in a medical work-up, treatment with various drugs, and increased premiums for life insurance, the diagnosis must be made accurately. It is now appreciated, for example, that some patients have an elevation in blood pressure secondary to the "white-coat syndrome." By this we mean that blood pressure is elevated when a physician first takes the patient's blood pressure. This reading can often be corrected on subsequent measurements by allowing the patient to rest comfortably in a quiet room while leaving the blood pressure apparatus in place, and by having nonthreatening discussions with the patient.

Once an elevation in blood pressure has been established, one must determine the type of hypertension. When only systolic blood pressure is elevated, the patient is often elderly and has stiff arteries. This is because aging results in a progressive decrease in the elasticity of the arteries, which produces an increase in systolic pressure only. Currently, systolic hypertension alone is not treated in the vast majority of patients.

The patient whose systolic and diastolic blood pressure values are both elevated is the one commonly thought to be hypertensive. Diastolic blood pressures greater than 115 mm Hg indicate that the patient has severe hypertension. Surgery should be postponed until the patient has been properly evaluated. Patients whose blood pressure ranges from 140/90 mm Hg to 160/95 mm Hg are borderline hypertensives. The increased rate of heart disease for these borderline hypertensive patients is similar to the rate for those with true hypertension. Therefore, they are at risk for perioperative complications. Patients whose diastolic pressure ranges from 95 to 115 mm Hg are labelled mild to moderate hypertensives; they are often being treated medically.

Hypertensive patients have elevated blood pressure for a variety of reasons. Therefore, it is important to determine as well as possible whether the patient has primary (essential) hypertension or secondary hyperten-sion (hypertension due to an underlying cause). Since 95 percent of hypertension is primary, chances are that no underlying cause will be noted. However, if, for example, the patient has underlying renal disease, then secondary hypertension is likely.

SECONDARY HYPERTENSION

Forms of secondary hypertension include renal, endocrine, and neurologic problems as well as pregnancy.

Renal forms of secondary hypertension include hypertension in patients in renal failure and in patients whose blood pressure is elevated secondary to stenosis of the renal artery. Renal failure can be diagnosed by measuring blood urea nitrogen (BUN), creatinine, and potassium. Renovascular hypertension is more difficult to diagnose. A younger patient with recently diagnosed hypertension becomes a prime candidate for intravenous pyelography to evaluate the rapidity with which the dye is excreted from the kidneys. A delayed excretion from one kidney would require further evaluation.

Endocrine forms of hypertension are rare but deserve special attention. Patients with primary aldosteronism have an increase in plasma aldosterone, which results in retention of sodium and therefore an increase in blood pressure. Concomitantly, there is a loss of potassium through the kidneys. The serum potassium is therefore markedly decreased. A serum potassium level of less than 2 mEq per liter is not unknown in patients with primary aldosteronism. Patients with Cushing's syndrome also have elevated blood pressure. Excess amounts of cortisol result in sodium retention as well. Because other stigmata of Cushing's disease are present, diagnosing the cause of hypertension is more easily done.

Pheochromocytoma, although a rare cause of hypertension, deserves special attention, because patients who are not diagnosed preoperatively have a very high mortality rate intraoperatively. How can one be assured that the hypertensive patient does not have a pheochromocytoma? One cannot; but one can have a high index of suspicion. For example, a clue is provided when the patient is young and has significant hypertension. If the patient's symptoms include palpitations, periods of extreme nervousness, weight loss, constipation, or other signs of sympathetic overdrive, then the patient should be referred for work-up. One must remember that pheochromocytoma is the great mimicker and that it can take many forms. One should also remember that not all patients with pheochromocytoma have an elevation in blood pressure. Preoperative treatment of patients with pheochromocytoma consists of alpha- and beta-blockade for 1 to 2 weeks before surgery.

Hypertension secondary to neurologic causes and pregnancy is diagnosed more easily and will not be discussed in further detail here. Suffice it to say that the treatment of these two disorders is not based on the same principles that apply to other forms of hypertension. For example, an elevation of blood pressure in the patient with a neural injury is not treated, because blood flow in the brain stem depends on this high pressure. Similarly, therapy during pregnancy is aimed at treatment of the hypersensitive sympathetic nervous system and the decreased fluid volume present in the pregnant patient.

ESSENTIAL HYPERTENSION

The cause of essential hypertension is multifactorial; no one mechanism is clearly the cause. It would appear that heredity, membrane defects, sodium intake, the sympathetic nervous system, and circulating hormones all play important roles in blood pressure control. Drug therapy and diet to control blood pressure work on a variety of these factors and are discussed further in this chapter.

Although the underlying cause of hypertension is unknown, some important physiologic changes occur. First, in hypertension, cardiac output is normal and peripheral resistance is elevated. Second, the vasculature is more reactive than in the normotensive patient. Third, plasma volume is decreased in hypertension.

The fact that peripheral resistance is increased and that cardiac output is normal directs the course of the antihypertensive therapy. To decrease cardiac output to lower blood pressure would not be the proper approach. Therefore, the therapies that are currently available work on the peripheral resistance side of the equation.

The increased vascular reactivity that occurs in hypertension is thought to be caused by the increased mass of vascular smooth muscle in the arterioles. Because the arterioles are the controllers of resistance in the body, small increases in smooth muscle have a profound influence on vascular tone. It is thus easy to see why a stimulus such as an intubation causes blood pressure to increase more in the hypertensive patient than in the normotensive patient. The resistance, already disproportionately increased in hypertension, is increased even more when painful stimuli occur.

The decrease in plasma volume that is seen in hypertension has consequences for the intraoperative management of the patient. Because the induction of anesthesia is often associated with changes in vascular resistance, the volume status of the patient before anesthesia is important. For patients with a decreased plasma volume, hypovolemia occurring before induction may result in significant hypotension. This is accentuated in the patient with hypertension and may be further exaggerated by therapy with diuretics. Rehydration of the hypertensive patient is therefore essential before induction.

DRUG THERAPY

The initial step in treating hypertension has generally been to advise the patient to lose weight, increase exercise, and decrease sodium intake. Often, these relatively simple steps are all that are necessary to bring blood pressure to more normal values.

Until recently, the next step in therapy was to introduce a thiazide diuretic. Seventy percent of hypertensive patients have had effective blood pressure control with this therapy alone. How the diuretic decreases blood pressure is not exactly clear. Since the plasma volume in the hypertensive patient is already reduced, further reduction in volume does not seem to be the likely mechanism. However, because diuretics cause the loss of sodium from cells, they may exert their influence by this mechanism. Since sodium and calcium are so intimately linked, it is likely that the loss of sodium induced by the diuretic causes a loss of sodium and, potentially, calcium from vascular smooth muscle, thus resulting in less contractility. It is also possible that sodium is lost from sympathetic nerve terminals, thereby influencing the amount of catecholamines that are released secondary to sympathetic stimulation. Whatever the mechanism, there is a negative aspect to the treatment of hypertension with diuretics: total body potassium may be depleted, thus causing low serum potassium levels. This may present a problem during the preoperative period when the laboratory values are noted. This will be discussed in more detail later.

One of the consequences of treating hypertension with diuretics is that plasma renin activity is elevated. With the increase in plasma renin activity, there is also an increase in angiotensin IIa potent vasoconstrictor. To offset this increase in angiotensin II, low-dose beta-blockade has been used in combination with diuretics to manage the hypertensive patient effectively.

There is some evidence to suggest that treating hypertensive patients with diuretics has resulted in a small but significant increase in sudden death. Whether this suggestion will be substantiated by larger clinical studies awaits the passage of time. However, concern over this issue has led to new approaches for the treatment of mild hypertension. Two main categories of drugs have been used, the converting enzyme inhibitors and the calcium channel blockers.

The effective treatment of the patient with essential hypertension by converting enzyme inhibitors was not initially anticipated. Most patients with hypertension have normal or low plasma renin activity. Therefore, the possibility of blocking the conversion of angiotensin I (no pressor properties) to angiotensin II was not foreseen as helpful. However, studies showed no correlation between plasma renin activity and the ultimate decrease in blood pressure seen in patients with essential hypertension when they were treated with a converting enzyme inhibitor. The implication is that the measurement of plasma renin activity is not a good indicator of the importance of the renin-angiotensin system in blood pressure support. The use of converting enzyme inhibitors has increased in popularity because of the few side effects associated with these compounds. Current therapy is aimed at administering agents that cause enzyme inhibition for 24 hours with once-daily therapy.

More recently, calcium channel blockers have been used to treat hypertension. We know that some agents have more influence on coronary or cerebral beds, while others influence conduction in the heart. Calcium channel blocks that work primarily on the peripheral circulation have been used to treat hypertension effectively. Whether these agents can cause regression of left-ventricular hypertrophy (to be discussed later) has not been studied. Certainly, however, patients with coronary artery disease are being treated with calcium channel blockers. Some of these patients, who are also hypertensive, have had their hypertension controlled with only one agent.

A variety of other classes of antihypertensive agents are currently available. Central acting alpha$_2$ agonist agents, alpha-blockers, smooth muscle relaxants, and sympatholytic agents have all been employed (for details of those agents, see a standard pharmacology text). For the anesthesiologist, understanding how these drugs work can influence the intraoperative management of the patient. For example, knowing that a patient had been treated with a beta-blocker, the anesthesiologist would not be alarmed by a slower than normal heart rate. The anesthesiologist would also know that the normal signs of light anesthesia could be masked by such therapy.

What does one do about the use of antihypertensive agents before anesthesia and surgery? Antihypertensive agents should be continued up to the time of surgery and restarted as soon as possible during the postoperative period. With proper control preoperatively, the intraoperative course is much more smooth.

It has even been suggested that the mild hypertensive patient might derive significant benefit from a single oral administration of a beta-blocking agent before surgery. One study showed that the incidence of ischemia was markedly less when this therapy was used. Further studies are needed to validate this.

ADDITIONAL CONCERNS

What additional concerns should one have when evaluating the hypertensive patient who is scheduled for surgery? Since hypertension affects three main organs—the heart, the kidneys, and the brain—it behooves the anesthesiologist to ask the appropriate questions and order the appropriate tests.

The most important concern with hypertension is its deleterious effects on the heart. Whatever mechanism is responsible for the elevation in blood pressure, the result is the same. The heart needs to work against an increased pressure load. Just as the heart hypertrophies in a patient with aortic stenosis, the same occurs in a patient with hypertension. The hypertrophy in the left ventricle is the major concern. Routine tests (electrocardiography, chest x-ray examination) may not provide evidence of left-ventricular hypertrophy. However, echocardiography has conclusively demonstrated that hypertrophy does occur and is something that we need to be concerned about.

Why the concern with left-ventricular hypertrophy? First, there is increased muscle mass. Because of the increased mass, more blood flow is needed. Secondly, it is estimated that 50 to 60 percent of patients with hypertension have some coronary artery disease. If there is an increase in mass and the potential for a decrease in supply, then ischemia may occur. Furthermore, the increased intracavitary pressure that occurs in hypertension creates the potential for subendocardial myocardial ischemia. Under what condition does this occur? It does not occur in all hypertensive patients. It appears that in hypertension, the most important factor is *heart rate*, not elevation in blood pressure. The elevation in blood pressure, I believe, is a predisposing factor for the hypertensive patient. The fact that the patient has hypertension is why he may have perioperative problems. With long-standing hypertension, he has a reactive vasculature, he has increased myocardial mass; and he may have coronary artery disease. When one superimposes tachycardia on this, the stage is set for myocardial ischemia.

The data supporting the theory that hypertension is a factor in intraoperative myocardial ischemia and or infarction is not strong. This is because blood pressure, not heart rate, has been the focus of most studies. However, in studies that examine the influence of heart rate on ST segment depression, results show that alteration in heart rate is more important than alteration in blood pressure. As has been shown in patients with mild hypertension, periods of myocardial ischemia are best correlated with increases in heart rate, not increases in blood pressure. It is known that the hypertensive patient has a greater output of catecholamines during periods of stress than does the normotensive patient. Therefore, it is imperative that maneuvers that stimulate the patient be blunted adequately in the hypertensive patient. Blunting such responses in the normotensive patient would be commendable. In the hypertensive patient, it is mandatory. Tachycardia, because of its deleterious effect on diastolic time, causes a decrease in coronary blood flow. Because of the hypertrophy and associated increased oxygen consumption of the left ventricle, which is working against an increased pressure head, the potential for myocardial ischemia is intensified. Hypertensive patients that present for surgical procedures with increased heart rates are at risk for myocardial ischemia. The cause for the increased heart rate should be sought and treated appropriately (e.g., volume, pain). The anesthesiologist must pay strict attention to the patient intraoperatively to prevent increases in heart rate. A variety of drugs are now available to accomplish this task, including narcotics, propranolol, and esmolol.

The second organ that is at risk in patients with hypertension is the kidney. Several studies have shown that with hypertension, there is a progressive loss of nephron function. Long-standing blood pressure elevation results in a loss of nephrons and blood flow through the kidney that is not as brisk as in the normotensive patient. Similarly, autoregulation of blood flow through the hypertensive kidney is shifted to the right. This means that short periods of hypotension result in decreased blood flow throughout the kidney. Unfortunately, this margin of safety cannot be ascertained with routine tests. Blood urea nitrogen and creatinine are normal in most hypertensive patients. However, if either of these values is elevated in the hypertensive patient, one must determine the underlying cause. Does the patient have underlying renal disease with hypertension, or does the patient have long-standing hypertension with renal involvement? The determination should be made preoperatively.

The third organ affected by hypertension is the brain. The elevation in blood pressure causes a shift in the autoregulatory curve. The higher the pressure, the greater the shift to the right. As is seen in kidney involvement, periods of hypotension may result in decreased blood flow to the brain. This again shows that the margin of safety for the hypertensive patient is not as great as it is for the normotensive patient. How does this alter our work-up of the hypertensive patient? First, one should delve into more detail in the patient's history. A history of light-headedness, blurry vision, fainting, or collapse should alert the anesthesiologist to potential problems with the central circulation. An examination of the carotid vessels by palpation and auscultation should also be done. Positive findings in any of these areas mean that the patient should be more fully evaluated to see whether additional medical or surgical therapy should be instituted. It must be remembered that hypertension is the forerunner of coronary, renal, and cerebral vascular disease.

PREOPERATIVE TESTS

What does the physician then order before surgery for the hypertensive subject? Although most normotensive patients need minimal laboratory work, this is not true for the hypertensive patient. A patient with true hypertension requires the following baseline tests: hematocrit, blood urea nitrogen (BUN), creatinine, and potassium. If the hematocrit is low and the BUN and creatinine levels are elevated, then renal failure exists and further work-up is necessary. If the potassium is abnormally low, one must consider an aldosterone-producing tumor. If the serum potassium is moderately

low (2 to 3 mg per liter), the patient should be questioned about diuretic therapy and potassium supplements that are used.

A great deal of controversy exists concerning serum potassium levels. It is my opinion that if the patient has a serum potassium level of 2.5 or greater, shows no arrhythmias, and is not taking digoxin-like preparations, then surgery should proceed. The risks of rapid potassium replacement outweigh the potential benefits.

Other laboratory examinations are necessary for the hypertensive patient. A chest radiograph may or may not show an increase in the size of the left ventricle. Even if there is no increase in heart size, one cannot assume that left-ventricular hypertrophy has not occurred. An electrocardiogram may also be normal despite an increase in left-ventricular mass. However, a normal electrocardiogram is reassurance that the disease has not progressed too far.

What additional tests might be ordered and when should they be ordered? I believe that if any of the routine studies show an abnormal result, then additional studies should be done. For example, if a hypertensive patient reports vague symptoms of chest pain, coronary artery disease should be the presumed diagnosis until it has been otherwise proven. Echocardiography, stress test, and a thalium scan would all be appropriate. We know that the risk of coronary artery disease is high in the hypertensive patient. We should therefore document its existence if it is present. Our goal should be to identify the patients who are at risk and do what we can in the operating room to prevent unfortunate consequences.

SUGGESTED READING

DeSimone G, Lorenzo L, Moccia D, et al. Hemodynamic hypertrophied left ventricular patterns in systemic hypertension. Am J Cardiol 1987; 60:1317–1321.

Goldman L. Cardiac risks and complications of noncardiac surgery. Ann Intern Med 1983; 98:504–513.

Prisant M, Frank M, Carr A, et al. How can we diagnose coronary heart disease in hypertensive patients? Hypertension 1987; 10:467–472.

Prys-Roberts C, Foex P, Greene LT. Studies of anesthesia in relation to hypertension IV: the effect of artificial ventilation on the circulation and pulmonary gas exchange. Br J Anaesth 1972; 44:335–348.

Wikstrand J. Left ventricular function in early primary hypertension: functional consequences of cardiovascular structural changes. Hypertension 1984; 6(suppl III):108–116.

CORONARY ARTERY DISEASE

BRIAN A. ROSENFELD, M.D.

Many patients presenting for anesthesia and surgery in the United States have some degree of coronary artery disease (CAD). During the perioperative period, this CAD poses a significant risk for morbidity and mortality (Table 1). In this discussion, I concentrate on patients who are being anesthetized for noncardiac surgery but who have concurrent coronary heart disease, and I examine (1) preoperative assessment of the patient; (2) the determinants of perioperative ischemia and infarction; (3) monitoring modalities; and (4) therapy that can minimize risk.

PREOPERATIVE ASSESSMENT

The initial assessment of patients with possible CAD involves a good history, physical examination, and basic laboratory studies.

History

When taking a history from someone with possible CAD, it is important to ask specific questions. The classic symptoms of angina (substernal chest pain with exercise) can be obtained from some patients. However, many patients will describe atypical complaints, shortness of breath without pain, or no symptoms at all. Many elderly or debilitated patients will be unable to exercise at all, and other patients will have subconsciously decreased their level of activity below their anginal threshold. In these patients, questions about risk factors (e.g., family history, diabetes, smoking, peripheral vascular disease) and medications can be helpful. If information is available, questions about the patient's exercise tolerance are extremely beneficial.

Any history of prior angina, positive work-up for CAD, or myocardial infarction (MI) will identify patients with known CAD. In these patients, determining the severity of their disease and associated risk factors for perioperative morbidity and mortality are important. Evidence of the severity of CAD can be gleaned from the patient's exercise tolerance, results of exercise stress tests, stress thallium tests, and coronary angiography. The type and amount of anti-anginal medications they require can also be helpful in assessing disease severity.

Associated risk factors for perioperative ischemia and infarction in patients with CAD include (1) recent MI, (2) congestive heart failure, and (3) unstable angina. Patients with congestive heart failure and unstable angina should have surgery delayed, unless the procedure is an extreme emergency. In patients with a recent

Table 1 Risk of Anesthesia and Surgery in the Patient with Coronary Artery Disease

Factors	Risk
Stable effort related angina easily controlled by rest or medication. Good exercise tolerance. No arrhythmia or signs of heart failure.* No myocardial infarction within 1 year prior to surgery.	Low: Routine monitoring and post-operative care
Symptoms controlled by significant medication. No arrhythmia or signs of heart failure.* No myocardial infarction within 6 months prior to surgery.	Moderate: Monitoring and postoperative care should depend upon the magnitude of the procedure
Symptoms usually controlled by medication. There may be history of arrhythmia or heart failure.* No myocardial infarction within 6 months prior to surgery.	Moderate–High: Need to treat any symptoms of CHF prior to surgery. Will usually require invasive monitoring.
Unstable angina or congestive heart failure with or without arrhythmias	High: Only emergency surgery should be scheduled. Full monitoring is mandatory.
Myocardial infarction less than 6 months prior to surgery	If negative symptom-limited exercise stress test (4–6 weeks post-MI), probably in low-risk group. If positive test, high-risk group and should receive further work-up.

*Ejection fraction <40%, cardiomegaly and/or congestion on chest roentgenogram, moderate-severe wall motion abnormality.

MI (less than 6 months), delaying surgery for 6 months has recently been questioned and should be evaluated on an individual basis.

Physical Examination

The physical examination will rarely provide much additional information about patients with suspected CAD. It will, however, provide evidence of concomitant myocardial disease, which may influence perioperative risk. On physical examination, evidence of ventricular failure should be particularly noted. A finding of basilar rales, an S_3 murmur, or both suggests left ventricular failure. Neck vein distention, hepatomegaly, and peripheral edema are additional findings that suggest either left and/or right heart decompensation. The other major physical findings of interest would be evidence of aortic stenosis and arrhythmias. Aortic stenosis is important because of its association with chest pain that may or may not be due to concomitant CAD, and its effect on cardiac performance. Arrhythmias (particularly ventricular) may be a manifestation of underlying left ventricular dysfunction. During the preoperative evaluation, it is important to assess the adequacy of peripheral pulses for monitoring purposes. Of course, blood pressure and heart rate should also be noted. In particular, if the patient is being treated with a beta-adrenergic–blocking drug, basal heart rate is one index of the adequacy of the therapy.

Laboratory Examination

The more complete the laboratory examination, the better able the physician will be to assess the risk and type of monitoring necessary for perioperative management. However, cost effectiveness must always be considered when making decisions about preoperative testing. This was demonstrated by Hertzer at the Cleveland Clinic, who did coronary angiography on all patients presenting for peripheral vascular disease (PVD) surgery.

Minimum laboratory examinations for every patient with a history of CAD should include measurement of hemoglobin, serum creatinine (for assessment of renal function), electrolytes for patients taking any type of diuretic drug, electrocardiography (ECG), and chest roentgenography. The ECG can confirm a past myocardial infarction, present ischemic changes, and any baseline abnormalities that will make perioperative ECG monitoring problematic. The chest roentgenogram is important for assessing signs of congestive failure (dilated left ventricle, pulmonary edema). More formal noninvasive cardiovascular diagnostic methods are frequently required to document CAD and assess the perioperative risk.

The goal of further preoperative testing is to identify patients who would benefit from (1) myocardial revascularization surgery or angioplasty prior to their noncardiac surgery, (2) intensive intraoperative and postoperative measures to reduce the operative risk, (3) a more limited surgical approach, or (4) canceling surgery altogether.

These tests include the exercise stress test (EST), stress thallium, dipyridamole thallium, and continuous Holter monitoring. Both the EST and stress thallium test require patients to increase their heart rate by exercising. Ischemia is then documented by the appearance of ST segment changes on the ECG or by decreased thallium uptake (representing coronary hypoperfusion). The dipyridamole thallium scan and continuous Holter monitoring have recently shown promise for preoperatively predicting postoperative cardiac events in patients with PVD. Neither test requires the patient to exercise, which is frequently necessary in this high-risk group. Continuous Holter monitoring is easily performed and relatively inexpensive but is limited by baseline ECG abnormalities. Dipyridamole thallium testing is expensive and requires specialized testing facilities but is not limited by baseline ECG changes. At the present time, no single test has the sensitivity and specificity to be considered the ideal screening procedure.

Results of these tests may prompt increasing medications, more aggressive perioperative monitoring and management, or coronary angiography.

Risk Assessment

The risk of suffering a perioperative myocardial infarction is 0.15 to 0.55 percent in the general population. Patients who have recently suffered a MI have a greater risk. Historically, this risk was between 4 and 8 percent and increased substantially if the MI was within 6 months. Recent studies have demonstrated a much lower risk in patients with a recent MI, whether it was longer than or less than 6 months previously. These improved results no doubt are due to increased awareness and improved perioperative management techniques. These include the addition of invasive monitoring, close postoperative observation, and controlling myocardial oxygen supply-demand imbalances.

When assessing patients with a recent MI, it is important to remember they represent a very diverse group. We know from the cardiology literature that post-MI symptom-limited exercise stress testing stratifies patients into low, moderate, and high-risk groups for subsequent cardiac events based on the presence of ischemia and left ventricular (LV) dysfunction. In the anesthesia literature, affected patients are lumped together chronologically on the basis of time since MI (i.e., 0–3, 3–6, and >6 months) and not physiologically. There is good reason to believe that their perioperative risk can also be stratified using similar testing. Table 1 includes a generalized risk schema for patients with CAD, based on the literature and personal experience.

DETERMINANTS OF PERIOPERATIVE MYOCARDIAL ISCHEMIA AND INFARCTION

The determinants of perioperative myocardial ischemia and infarction have expanded during recent years.

It was previously believed that imbalances of myocardial oxygen supply and demand were determined exclusively by changes in hemodynamics, hematocrit, and arterial oxygenation. It is now believed that changes in plasma viscosity, coagulation, fibrinolysis, and platelet activation are factors in the development of perioperative ischemia and infarction.

Hemodynamic changes continue to be the major cause of perioperative myocardial ischemia. Hemodynamics are also what anesthesiologists can control most with pharmacologic and fluid manipulations. The single hemodynamic parameter that has been consistently demonstrated to correlate with perioperative ischemia is tachycardia. Tachycardia not only increases myocardial oxygen demand, but also decreases myocardial oxygen supply by decreasing diastolic filling time. Any physiologic perturbation that causes tachycardia may lead to myocardial ischemia. These include pain, fever, anemia, hypovolemia, hypercarbia, and hypoxemia. Other hemodynamic causes of ischemia are hypotension (particularly in patients with pre-existing hypertension and left ventricular hypertrophy), increased preload, increased afterload, and changes in contractility. Some authors have suggested that the heart rate should never be higher than the systolic blood pressure. This may sound simplistic, but in patients with CAD this is good advice. Increases in preload, afterload and contractility have their most detrimental effect in patients with LV dysfunction. Because of this, patients with concomitant CAD and LV dysfunction are extremely difficult to manage perioperatively.

Anemia and hypoxemia are well-established causes of myocardial ischemia. Anemia causes ischemia by decreasing myocardial oxygen supply. It may also cause ischemia by increasing myocardial oxygen demand from the tachycardia that ensues. It is not known what the ideal hematocrit is. It is probably patient specific, based on the patient's systemic oxygen consumption and coronary microcirculatory flow. A good rule of thumb is to maintain the hematocrit at a level at which peripheral oxygen demands are met without causing tachycardia. If there is evidence of ischemia, raising the hematocrit can be helpful.

Changes in plasma viscosity, coagulation, fibrinolysis, and platelet activation have been demonstrated in patients with CAD compared with normal controls. These changes are especially increased during episodes of unstable angina and infarction. Many of these same changes can be seen in postoperative patients, which may predispose those with stenotic coronary lesions to worsening of their ischemia and infarction.

Increases in plasma viscosity correlate with elevated serum fibrinogen levels. Fibrinogen levels (acute phase reactant) increase at 48 to 72 hours postoperatively. The associated increase in plasma viscosity can alter the rheologic properties of the coronary microcirculation, decreasing perfusion and predisposing to thrombosis.

The postoperative changes in coagulation (increased procoagulant) involve elevated levels of coagulation factor proteins and decreased levels of antithrombin III. Additionally, there is decreased fibrinolytic activity in many postoperative patients. This has been demonstrated by elevated levels of plasminogen activator inhibitor.

Platelet activation has not been well studied in the postoperative period. What is known is that general anesthetics depress platelet function in vitro, whereas catecholamines and the "stress response" increase aggregation. Regional anesthesia, which attenuates the stress response of surgery, may similarly decrease platelet activation.

Teleologically, this hypercoagulable state makes sense for most postoperative patients. However, for patients with CAD, this situation may put them at increased risk for myocardial ischemia and infarction.

MONITORING FOR MYOCARDIAL ISCHEMIA

Modalities for monitoring myocardial ischemia include the standard surface ECG, computer-assisted ST segment scanning, pulmonary artery catheter (SGC), and two-dimensional transesophageal echocardiography (2D-TE).

Electrocardiography

The surface ECG is the most commonly used modality for detecting myocardial ischemia. This is because of its proven sensitivity and specificity, ease of application, and minimal expense. The most commonly used leads for intraoperative monitoring are leads II and V_5. Precordial lead V_5 is the most informative lead for diagnosing ischemia, and lead II is most useful for diagnosing arrhythmias (prominent P waves). When one is using a standard limb lead ECG, a modified V_5 lead can be obtained by moving lead I to the V_5 position and monitoring lead I.

Computer-Assisted ST Segment Scanning

A recent modification to improve the surface ECG involves micropressor scanning of ST segments. This can include visual observation of a trend recorder (which is now included on many new ECG monitors), or a sound alarm from a continuous Holter monitor. The sound alarm, currently used exclusively for research, offers promise for future 24-hour ischemia monitoring.

For some patients, any monitoring tool using ECG ST segments is of limited value. Baseline ECG abnormalities, which include bundle branch block, pacemaker-induced depolarizations, digoxin effect, and nonspecific ST segment changes, render interpretation difficult to impossible. If these abnormalities are present, other monitoring tools should be employed.

Pulmonary Artery Catheter

Use of the SGC for diagnosing ischemia comes from observations during cardiac catheterization that patients with ischemia frequently had elevations in their pulmonary capillary wedge pressure. This elevation is caused by a reduction in diastolic relaxation that occurs during early ischemia. When the left ventricle becomes ischemic, it becomes less compliant and pressures increase. The problem is that most focal ischemic changes (unless associated with a papillary muscle) do not lead to significant increases in wedge pressure.

In 1981, Kaplan and Wells demonstrated the effectiveness of SGC monitoring for intraoperative ischemia. In their study involving 40 patients undergoing coronary bypass surgery, more ischemia was detected by SGC than by ECG. The combination of SGC and ECG together was better than either technique alone. Subsequent studies have not supported these findings. Although relatively insensitive to focal ischemia, SGC monitoring represents an additional method for detecting ischemia. Its use should be considered when baseline changes preclude ECG techniques. It should definitely be considered for patients with CAD and LV dysfunction who are undergoing surgeries involving large volume shifts.

Two-Dimensional Transesophageal Echocardiography

Limitations in the sensitivity of the ECG and SGC monitoring have led to the intraoperative use of 2D-TE. This method reveals focal changes in systolic wall motion thought to be representative of the ischemia that precedes ECG changes. The problems with this technique are that (1) it lacks specificity (i.e., all focal systolic wall motion abnormalities may not be caused by ischemia); (2) it is very operator-dependent; and (3) it is expensive. The present use of 2D-TE appears to be at critical points during surgery—for instance, coming off of cardiac bypass or during aortic cross-clamping.

Monitoring for myocardial ischemia has taken on greater importance with the observation that hemodynamic control alone will not abolish ischemia. For this reason, close observation of monitors intraoperatively and postoperatively is advocated.

PERIOPERATIVE THERAPY

The perioperative period is associated with elevated catecholamine levels and the potential for major hemodynamic fluctuations. This requires therapy directed toward maintaining a good myocardial oxygen supply-demand balance. To do this, anesthesiologists must employ analgesics, anxiolytics, beta-blockers, nitrates, calcium channel blockers, and on the rare occasion, mechanical devices. How much and what type of drug to use will depend on the clinical situation and the severity of the patient's disease.

Analgesics and Anxiolytics

Analgesics and anxiolytics are beneficial throughout the perioperative period. Used preoperatively, these drugs serve to decrease patient anxiety. Because anxiety

situations have been shown to be a potent factor for exacerbating ischemia, it is incumbent on anesthesiologists to begin treatment prior to the morning of surgery. Intraoperatively and postoperatively, analgesics attenuate the stress response and thereby decrease tachycardia and hypertension.

Beta-Blockers

Beta-blockers have been demonstrated in perioperative studies to decrease heart rate, blood pressure, ischemia, and arrhythmias. Their membrane-stabilizing properties also decrease platelet aggregability. Most beta-blockers come in intravenous form, and the decision to use one over another is dictated by the clinical situation and the potential for adverse effects.

Patients who are chronically taking beta-blockers need to have them maintained perioperatively, because of the rebound hyperadrenergic state that will occur with beta-blocker withdrawal. This hyperadrenergic state normally occurs 24 to 48 hours after withdrawal, but will occur much earlier in the perioperative period because of the elevated catecholamine levels.

Specific events in the perioperative period have been shown to be associated with the development of tachycardia and ischemia in patients with CAD. These include line placement, laryngoscopy and intubation, surgical incision, and emergence from anesthesia. For attempting to block a short-lived tachycardiac response (i.e., intubation), a short-acting beta-blocker like esmolol is ideal. When more long-term heart rate control is indicated, atenolol, labetalol, or esmolol infusions can be used. Patients with reactive airway disease and LV dysfunction are at risk for decompensation when beta-blockers are administered. In these patients, a trial of esmolol (elimination half-life of 9 minutes) is indicated.

Nitrates

Nitrates are an important part of therapy for CAD. In the heart, nitroglycerin enhances myocardial flow to ischemic areas, improves the ratio of endocardial to epicardial perfusion, and increases collateral flow. The mechanism of the antianginal effect of nitroglycerin probably involves a combination of systemic venodilation and coronary vasodilation. Determining the specific site of action in a patient is difficult, and the site may vary depending on the clinical situation.

When nitrates are used, it is important to establish a therapeutic endpoint. The resolution of pain, normalization of ECG changes, or preload reduction are some examples of desired endpoints. Prophylactic nitroglycerin has not been shown to be efficacious when begun preoperatively. Furthermore, the development of tolerance to intravenous nitroglycerin can limit its usefulness when used prophylactically.

The systemic hemodynamic properties of nitroglycerin limit its effectiveness as an antihypertensive agent. Very high doses of nitroglycerin are required to affect the arteriolar resistance vessels. Therefore, at lower doses, blood pressure changes are probably caused by reduced preload (decreased cardiac output). Any reflex tachycardia from lower cardiac output also will be detrimental to the patient with CAD. When using nitroglycerin for blood pressure control, invasive hemodynamic monitoring is warranted.

Calcium Channel Blockers

Perioperative gastrointestinal absorption problems limit the use of calcium channel blockers to intravenous verapamil and sublingual nifedipine. Nifedipine is the preferred agent because its antihypertensive and coronary vasodilating properties are better. In the near future, intravenous formulations of second-generation calcium channel blockers will be available.

Nifedipine given sublingually has an onset of action within minutes. The vasodilation that occurs is limited to the arterial vessels, and the hypotensive effect is directly related to the pretreatment blood pressure. The vasodilating action of nifedipine in non–beta-blocked patients causes a reflex tachycardia. This limits its usefulness as a single agent, but makes it the drug of choice for hypertensive bradycardic patients.

Intra-Aortic Balloon Pump

In certain situations in which surgery is necessary and patients have severe, inoperable CAD or refuse coronary artery bypass graft surgery, the intra-aortic balloon can be used. This provides excellent temporary antianginal therapy, which can be placed in the operating room. The major contraindication to this treatment involves vascular access, and the complication rate can run as high as 25 percent.

SUGGESTED READING

DeBusk RF. Specialized testing after recent acute myocardial infarction. Ann Intern Med 1989; 110:470–481.

Eagle KA, Coley CM, Newell JB, et al. Combining clinical and thallium data optimizes preoperative assessment of cardiac risk before major vascular surgery. Ann Intern Med 1989; 110:859–866.

Gallagher JD, Moore RA, Jose AB, et al. Prophylactic nitroglycerin infusions during coronary artery bypass surgery. Anesthesiology 1986; 64:785–789.

Hertzer NR, Beven EG, Young JR, et al. Coronary artery disease in peripheral vascular patients. Ann Surg 1984; 199:223–233.

Kaplan JA, Wells PH. Early diagnosis of myocardial ischemia using the pulmonary arterial catheter. Anesth Analg 1981; 60:780–793.

London MJ, Hollenberg M, Wong MG. Intraoperative myocardial ischemia: localization by continuous 12-lead electrocardiography. Anesthesiology 1989; 69:232–241.

Mangano DT. Perioperative cardiac morbidity. Anesthesiology 1990; 72:153–184.

Mangano DT, Browner WS, Hollenberg M, et al. Association of perioperative myocardial ischemia with cardiac morbidity and mortality in men undergoing noncardiac surgery. N Engl J Med 1990; 323:1781–1788.

Rosenfeld BA, Rogers MC. Risk stratification in post-myocardial infarction patients: is six months too long to wait? J Clin Anesth 1991; 3:85–87.

Rozanski A, Bairey CN, Krantz DS, et al. Mental stress and the induction of silent myocardial ischemia in patients with coronary artery disease. N Engl J Med 1988; 318:1005–1012.

LIVER DISEASE

ELIZABETH L. ROGERS, M.D.

Mortality from surgery in patients with pre-existing liver disease is highest in those with acute hepatitis, those with poorly compensated chronic hepatitis, and those with unsuspected liver problems. Reduction of perioperative risk involves preoperative assessment of the severity and acuity of the liver process, optimization of hepatic function and correction of associated co-morbid problems, and attempts to avoid precipitation of further liver deterioration.

Not all patients with liver disease are jaundiced, and not all patients with jaundice have liver disease. Frequently patients in early stages of acute viral or acute obstructive liver disease have symptoms that occur before jaundice. Similarly, patients with inactive cirrhosis may be marginally compensated and therefore not clinically jaundiced before the stress of surgery. Failure to consider liver disease in these patients can lead to unnecessary surgery, or surgery without the precautions necessary in a patient with liver disease. On the other hand, jaundice can occur without disease of the liver in patients with acute hemolysis, large hematomas, and in people with congenital conjugating deficiencies as occur in Gilbert's syndrome. Neither of the later two groups of patients are at increased risk from surgery because of their jaundice.

Jaundice may be classified as prehepatic, acute disease, and chronic disease. Common causes of jaundice are listed in Table 1. Prehepatic causes of liver disease usually can be recognized by the lack of hepatic symptomatology or physical findings and the presence of normal liver enzymes, albumin, and prothrombin time. This is an important category, for as many as 7 percent of the population of the United States have Gilbert's syndrome and become clinically jaundiced with stresses such as fasting, loss of sleep, trauma, or vigorous exercise.

Acute parenchymal liver disease is the category most

Table 1 Common Causes of Jaundice

Prehepatic
  Hemolysis

Acute Disease
  Viral hepatitis
  Drug-induced hepatitis
  Acute extrahepatic obstruction

Chronic Disease
  Alcoholic liver disease
  Chronic active hepatitis
  Primary biliary cirrhosis
  Metabolic disorders
  Cirrhosis
  Malignancy

likely to be missed by physicians, and the one most likely to be responsible for unexpected surgical deaths. Reasons for acute parenchymal disease include viral hepatitis, drug-induced hepatitis, veno-occlusive disease, and trauma. Acute viral hepatitis is most frequently caused by viruses such as hepatitis A, hepatitis B, hepatitis C, other forms of non-A, non-B hepatitis, and cytomegalovirus in adults. Cytomegalovirus, Epstein-Barr virus, coxsackievirus, measles, and herpes virus infections are common in children. In the presence of acquired immunodeficiency syndrome, toxoplasmosis and tuberculosis have become important causes of infectious hepatitis. Veno-occlusive disease of the hepatic veins, or Budd-Chiari syndrome, was once found as a rare complication of cirrhosis; more frequently now, it is seen as an acute complication in patients who are bone marrow transplant recipients. Acute extrahepatic obstruction, which is frequently a reason for surgery, may be due to choledocholithiasis, sclerosing cholangitis, or tumor of the common duct of the head of the pancreas.

Chronic liver disease may be symptomatic, as in patients with chronic active hepatitis or primary biliary cirrhosis, or asymptomatic and occult as in cryptogenic cirrhosis, hepatoma, or hemochromatosis. Chronic active hepatitis is a progressive disorder caused by a virus, drugs, or idiopathic causes. More frequent in women, symptoms of amenorrhea, fatigue, arthralgias, and fever may accompany the abnormality of hepatic function. Primary biliary cirrhosis is suspected when 40- to 60-year-old women present with intense itching, very high concentration of alkaline phosphatase, and a positive reaction for antimitochondrial antibody. Metabolic disorders such as hemochromatosis, porphyria, and Wilson's disease also cause chronic liver disease. Iron deposition in the skin, pancreas, heart, and liver is responsible for the so-called bronzed diabetic with hemochromatosis and cirrhosis. On the other hand, the findings of chronic liver disease, hemolytic anemia, and ataxia with absent serum ceruloplasmim and deposition of copper in the liver occurs with Wilson's disease.

Alcohol abuse is one of the most frequently cited reasons for chronic liver disease in the United States. Ingestion of more than four drinks per day on average can be associated with chronic progressive liver disease, regardless of the socioeconomic or nutritional status of the patient.

Numerous drugs can cause liver disease. The most common drugs that cause liver disease or alteration of hepatic function include methyldopa (Aldomet), isoniazide, halothane, phenothiazines, oral hypoglycemics methyltestosterone, antithyroids, sulfonamides, azathioprine, and oral contraceptives.

RECOGNITION OF THE PATIENT WITH LIVER DISEASE

A carefully taken clinical history and physical examination, combined with attention to the results of commonly ordered chemistry studies is unlikely to miss significant liver disease. A disturbing study by Powell-Jackson, however, showed that 31 patients who underwent unnecessary laparotomy with unsuspected liver disease did so because insufficient attention was paid to the history and physical examination. An additional five patients underwent exploratory surgery because liver function testing was either omitted or ignored.

Preoperative evaluation of patients should include careful questioning and chart review to determine if a history of jaundice exists. With a history of jaundice, evaluation to rule out chronic active hepatitis, cirrhosis, or anesthetic-related jaundice should be accomplished.

One should try to elicit a report of symptoms commonly associated with liver disease such as malaise, fatigue, anorexia, nausea and vomiting, or pruritus in addition to jaundice. Review of previous operations (including biliary tract surgery) and anesthetics, blood transfusions, allergies, alcohol intake, and drug history is important. References to drugs known to be associated with liver disease should be evaluated. Presence of right upper quadrant pain, fever with rigors, nausea, or pruritus is suggestive of cholecystitis or cholangitis.

Jaundice with scleral icterus is usually discernible when the serum bilirubin concentration is greater than 3 mg per deciliter. Asterixis, ascites, and petechiae or bruises as well as jaundice are evidence of hepatic failure. Spider telangiectasias, Dupuytren's contractures, palmar erythema, and gynecomastia are evidence of chronic liver disease. Portal hypertension may be manifested by ascites, splenomegaly, caput medusa (prominent veins on the anterior abdominal wall), and esophageal varices. The liver is usually enlarged if active hepatic disease is in process. Extreme tenderness should alert the physician to the presence of inflammation or infection.

Patients with well-compensated inactive cirrhosis may not have the usual signs of chronic liver disease, and as many as 50 percent of such patients may have a normal physical examination. Absence of physical findings, therefore, does not rule out liver disease.

The depth of encephalopathy is one of the most clinically useful ways of following the severity of hepatic failure. Encephalopathy is frequently classified on a scale of one through five. Grade I encephalopathy is usually noticed only if attention is paid to detail; the patient may have altered sleep habits or altered effect. The most commonly recognized depth of encephalopathy is Grade II, in which slurred speech may be present, the patient may be drowsy but easily responsive, and asterixis is present. By Grade III, the patient is stuporous and may respond primarily to noxious stimuli. By Grade IV, the patient is unresponsive to normal stimuli and may exhibit decorticate or decerebrate posturing. Complete recovery from Grade IV encephalopathy is rare once cerebral edema has developed.

The usual battery of tests commonly ordered to evaluate for the presence of liver disease includes those tests that indicate liver functioning and those that indicate an active process. The tests most likely to have abnormal results when hepatic function declines are bilirubin and albumin concentrations and prothrombin time. The tests most frequently used to screen for active liver disease include alkaline phosphatase, SGOT, and SGPT. Aspartate aminotransferase, or SGOT, is elevated in alcoholic, obstructive, and hepatitic processes, whereas alanine aminotransferase, or SGPT, is most frequently elevated in viral or drug-induced hepatitis. The highest levels of SGOT are seen in toxic hepatitis or fulminant hepatic failure due to viral hepatitis. Alcoholic hepatitis can be associated with severe acute damage, or with only moderate increases of SGOT and sometimes no elevation of SGPT, and it is the third most likely process to be discovered in otherwise asymptomatic people, only behind diabetes mellitus and hypercholesterolemia.

The most frequently uncovered processes in these people with previously unsuspected disease are acute viral hepatitis and alcoholism. Screening for liver disease by ordering a panel of tests including bilirubin, albumin, prothrombin time, alkaline phosphatase, SGOT, and SGPT is therefore recommended by this author. The combination of a careful history and physical examination with the above-listed screening tests can rule out serious hepatic disease or point to a likely diagnosis in most cases. Use of more expensive, high technology testing is recommended only after the above-mentioned test results have been analyzed.

Once obstructive jaundice is suspected, ultrasonography followed by visualization by endoscopic retrograde cholangiopancreatography (ERCP) or percutaneous transhepatic cholangiography (PTC) is recommended. Ultrasonography and computed tomography (CT) scans have revolutionized the ability of physicians to noninvasively identify obstruction of the biliary tree, neoplastic lesions within the liver, major alteration of hepatic architecture, and iron deposition. Ultrasonography is especially useful in identifying gallstones and extrahepatic obstruction, and is sometimes preferred because its use avoids radiation exposure. It is, however, less reliable than a CT scan for stones lodged in the distal bile duct, and may yield insufficient information in patients with acute abdominal processes caused by increased bowel gas, which interferes with the study. The CT scan, on the other hand, is somewhat less sensitive to operator expertise, and is sensitive in detecting mass lesions within the liver, hemochromatosis, and cirrhosis in addition to dilated intrahepatic ducts and vascular lesions greater than 1 cm. Once extrahepatic obstruction has been determined, the cause can usually be determined by either ERCP or PTC.

Patients with symptoms, physical findings, or laboratory evidence of a hepatic process should have the diagnosis more firmly established before surgery if delay is possible. An algorithm for the care of the jaundiced patient is shown in Figure 1.

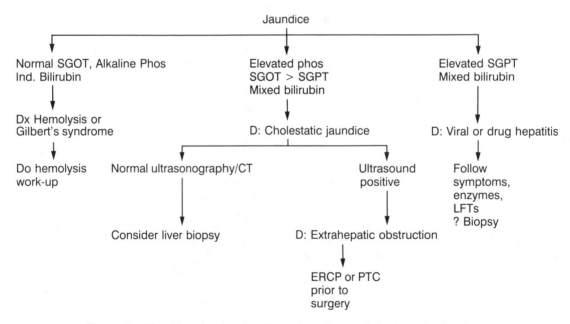

Figure 1 Algorithm showing the diagnosis and care of the jaundiced patient.

Patients with parenchymal liver disease, especially those with acute hepatitis of viral or drug etiology, those with alcoholic hepatitis, and those with uncompensated chronic liver disease, are at risk of increased morbidity and mortality from surgery. Patients with unexplained liver disease who are contemplating elective surgery are therefore frequently advised to undergo liver biopsy to assess the type and degree of active liver disease. Delay of surgery for patients with confirmed alcoholic hepatitis, acute viral hepatitis, and acute drug-associated hepatitis may result in considerable reduction in surgical morbidity.

Liver biopsy using ultrasound or CT scan guidance is used to make the diagnosis in mass lesions of the liver, thus frequently avoiding the need for purely exploratory surgery in these cases.

RISK FACTORS FOR SURGERY

In general, for patients with obvious liver disease, the risk of anesthesia and surgery increases with the degree of preoperative liver disease, the development of hepatic hypoxia or hypotension during the procedure, and the development of extrahepatic complications during the perioperative period.

There is some evidence that the mortality risk from surgery may be higher when liver disease is present but not suspected. In a series of patients studied by Powell Jackson, patients undergoing exploratory laparotomy experienced a 31 percent mortality rate and 61 percent morbidity rate when liver disease was present but ignored or not suspected prior to surgery. Patients with preoperative liver biochemical abnormalities have been advised to delay elective surgery until a thorough evaluation of their liver problem has been accomplished and the course of their liver disease observed.

Patients with acute viral hepatitis have been shown to experience a 9.5 percent mortality rate and 11.9 percent morbidity rate when undergoing elective surgery. For this reason, elective surgery is usually postponed for at least 3 to 4 weeks after the development of suspected acute viral hepatitis. As liver function may not completely return to normal for up to 1 year following acute viral hepatitis, and as there is a 30 percent loss of liver function in at least half of the patients with even mild preoperative abnormality of liver function, the decision to undergo the elective procedure at all should be carefully reviewed. Sifkin has recommended that patients not undergo surgery after acute viral hepatitis until the results of their liver function tests return completely to normal. Certainly the risks of operating on a patient before their liver function returns completely to normal must be balanced against the risk of further delaying surgery.

Acute drug hepatitis in patients undergoing hip repair likewise carries an increased risk of surgery, with mortality rates reported from 10 to 80 percent.

The risk of surgery in patients with alcoholic hepatitis in whom Mallory hyaline bodies are found on biopsy specimen is significantly higher than the biochemical abnormalities would suggest, and may approach 40 to 60 percent. Molitch recommends that patients with evidence of alcoholic hepatitis present on the biopsy specimen should have surgery delayed 6 to 12 weeks until abstention from alcohol and nutritional repletion allow body temperature, leukocytosis, and hyperbilirubinemia to return to normal.

In patients with chronic liver disease, the development of postoperative complications is usually related to the degree of preoperative derangement of hepatic function. Patients with known stable chronic liver disease, who undergo anesthesia where care is taken to minimize hepatic ischemia and hepatotoxicity, may well have nearly normal morbidity rates. The risk of developing complications increased from 16 percent to 35 percent when there was increased BSP retention or a low serum albumin concentration. Cirrhotic patients with poorly compensated liver function may experience morbidity and mortality rates of higher than 90 percent. Even in reasonably well-compensated patients with cirrhosis, the risk of mortality increases sixfold when emergency surgery is performed.

By the time jaundice is clinically detectable, the mortality rate may be as high as 40 percent. Factors associated with increased postoperative mortality in patients with chronic liver disease include bilirubin greater than 3.5 mg per deciliter, prothrombin time prolonged for more than 2 seconds, increase in partial thromboplastin time longer than 2 seconds, hypoalbuminemia, poor nutritional state, presence of encephalopathy, ascites, and infection. The risk of surgery increases as the number of adverse factors present increases.

Despite all of the new studies available and new techniques of assessing patients, Child's classification system remains the most useful rapid way to estimate the liver disease's contribution to risk from surgery. The modification of Child's assessment shown in Table 2 can be used for initial risk assessment in patients with chronic liver disease undergoing a major surgical procedure.

Surgical mortality increases from 1 to 15 percent for patients who are Child's Class A, and up to 80 to 100 percent for those who are Class C. Most physicians do not recommend elective surgery for those patients who are Child's Class C.

MODIFIABLE RISK FACTORS IN LIVER DISEASE

Survival of the patient with liver disease depends on attention to detail, gentle but timely correction of modifiable risk factors, and avoidance of iatrogenic complications. When time permits, it may pay to delay elective surgery until hepatic function returns to normal, nutrition is improved, ascites are controlled, renal function is maximized, encephalopathy is cleared, coagulopathy has improved, and fluid and electrolyte abnormalities have improved. This delay may improve the

Table 2 Modification of Child's Classification: Risk From Surgery
Due to Liver Disease

| | Risk to Patient | | |
Factors	Minimum	Moderate	Severe
Bilirubin	< 2 mg/dl	2–3 mg/dl	> 3 mg/dl
Albumin	> 3.5 mg/dl	3–3.5 mg/dl	< 3 mg/dl
Prothrombin time prolongation	<2 sec	2–3 sec	> 3 sec
Ascites	None	Controlled	Uncontrolled
Encephalopathy	None	Provoked	Grade II–IV
Nutrition	Excellent	Good	Wasting

survival even in patients with moderately severe cirrhosis. Even with urgent surgery, survival will improve as the above-mentioned factors are improved or normalized. Only truly emergent surgery should occur without stabilization of the hepatic parameters.

Malnutrition is common in patients with liver disease, and is a known source of increased morbidity and mortality from surgical procedures in patients with and without liver disease. Although the prognostic nutrition index (PNI) has been shown to correlate with surgical morbidity in patients with liver disease, liver disease itself may affect the albumin concentration and thus the PNI, making it less predictive in patients with liver disease. Preoperative nutritional repletion is important if time allows. Induction of a positive nitrogen balance is primary. Lactulose administration may help avoid encephalopathy with mild protein loads. The use of low-protein diets, with and without branched-chain amino acids, remains the mainstay of therapy. For the short term, branched chain amino acids may be better tolerated and serve to normalize the serum's amino acid profile. Although perioperative albumin may be necessary for tissue oncotic pressure reasons, long-term use of albumin is not advantageous from a nutritional perspective.

Patients with new-onset ascites or ascites associated with new-onset renal failure or encephalopathy should undergo diagnostic paracentesis to exclude spontaneous bacterial peritonitis which may occur in the absence of symptoms. Restriction of sodium intake to less than 1 g per day, discontinuation of nonsteroidal anti-inflammatory agents that increase fluid accumulation, and administration of spironolactone are all recommended. Lasix should be used only in low doses, and only after it has been shown that the above-stressed measures did not prompt diuresis. Overaggressive diuresis of the patient with liver disease may initiate hepatorenal syndrome. Large-volume paracenteses accompanied by albumin infusion and central venous pressure monitoring has been suggested when there is insufficient time for slow diuresis to occur.

Serum creatinine is one of the strongest risk factors for predicting death in patients undergoing liver transplantation. Iatrogenic reasons for development of renal failure in hospitalized liver patients are the overaggressive use of potent diuretics or the administration of nonsteroidal anti-inflammatory agents or aminoglycosides. Treatment consists first and foremost in discontinuation of the offending agents. Administration of a rapid fluid challenge to raise the central venous pressure to 3 to 8 mm H_2O is a useful way to see if renal flow and function have been affected by hypovolemia.

Control of hepatic encephalopathy revolves around the use of lactulose orally or rectally plus the correction of potentially precipitating factors such as gastrointestinal bleeding, use of sedatives, infection, infection, and electrolyte abnormalities.

Coagulopathy is related to insufficient synthesis of factors in the thrombin cascade, splenic sequestration of platelets, fibrinolysis, diffuse intravascular coagulopathy, and capillary fragility. Correction of prothombin time by administration of vitamin K is seen in patients with obstructive liver disease but rarely in patients with severe hepatocellular disease. Although administration of fresh-frozen plasma and platelets immediately before and during surgery may help to reduce the risk of bleeding; the mortality of surgery may be as high as 45 percent in patients with elevated fibrin degradation products preoperatively.

Correction of dilutional hyponatremia or hypokalemia preoperatively is important. Dilutional hyponatremia most frequently is iatrogenic and occurs in association with excess free water administration in an effort to avoid exacerbation of ascites in a patient who already has inappropriate secretion of antidiuretic hormone. Hypokalemia occurs from a combination of secondary hyperaldosteronism associated with diuretics, diarrhea, and poor dietary intake.

Although hyperbilirubinemia has been shown to be a risk factor for surgery, correction of the hyperbilirubinemia by percutaneous stint placement has not been associated with decreased morbidity.

ANESTHETIC CONSIDERATIONS

A history of jaundice following previous anesthetic use should be ascertained. If the jaundice occurred after halothane anesthesia, without other obvious explanation, then an alternative anesthetic should be used in following anesthetic experiences. For patients with liver disease who do not have a demonstrated sensitivity to halothane, halothane does not need to be avoided and may well be an agent of choice.

The most important consideration in choice of agents will depend on the surgery contemplated and the ability of the anesthesiologist to maintain blood pressure and oxygenation during the procedure. Few agents are available that are clearly hepatotoxic; however, most agents will reduce hepatic blood flow associated with decreased splanchnic flow. This is true for agents administered by the epidural and spinal routes. The agents that have the least effect on hepatic blood flow are halothane, enflurane, and nitrous oxide.

In addition to the necessity to minimize hepatic flow diminution, maintenance of adequate oxygen supply to the liver is crucial in avoiding deterioration of hepatic function during the perioperative period. Attention to detail, monitoring of arterial oxygen saturation, control of blood pressure, and control of bleeding during surgery will then be the major factors promoting survival in the perioperative period.

SUGGESTED READING

Aranha GV, Greenlee HB. Intra-abdominal surgery in patients with advanced cirrhosis. Arch Surg 1986; 121:275–277.

Arroyo V, Gines P, Planas R, et al. Management of patients with cirrhosis and ascites. Semin Liver Dis 1986; 6(4):353–369.
Child CG, III. The liver and portal hypertension. In: Dunphy JE, ed. Major problems in clinical surgery. Philadelphia: WB Saunders., 1964:15.
DiCecco SR, Wieners EJ, Wiesner RH, et al. Assessment of nutritional status of patients with end-stage liver disease undergoing liver transplantation. Mayo Clin Proc 1989; 64:95–102.
Doberneck RC, Sterling WA, Allison DC. Morbidity and mortality after operation in nonbleeding cirrhotic patients. Am J Surg 1983; 146:306–309.
Friedman LS, Maddrey WC. Surgery in the patient with liver disease. Med Clin North Am 1987; 71(3):453–476.
Harville DD, Summerskill WHJ. Surgery in acute hepatitis. JAMA 1963; 184(4):257–261.
Jackson FC, Christopherson EB, Peternel WW, et al. Preoperative management of patients with liver disease. Surg Clin North Am 1968; 48(4):907–928.
Lindenmuth WW, Eisenberg MM. The surgical risk in cirrhosis of the liver. Arch Surg 1963; 86:235–242.
Molitch ME, ed. Management of medical problems in surgical patients. Philadelphia: FA Davis, 1982: 219–252.
Powell-Jackson P, Greenway B, Williams R. Adverse effects of exploratory laparotomy in patients with unsuspected liver disease. Br J Surg 1982; 69:449–451.
Rogers EL, Rogers MC. Fulminant hepatic failure and hepatic encephalopathy. Ped Clin North Am 1980; 27(3):701–713.
Siefkin AD, Bolt RJ. Preoperative evaluation of the patient with gastrointestinal or liver disease. Med Clin North Am 1979; 63(6):1309–1320.

DIABETES MELLITUS

FREDERICK E. SIEBER, M.D.

Diabetes mellitus is a disease commonly encountered by the anesthesiologist. The vast majority of patients with diabetes have either type I, juvenile-onset, insulin-dependent diabetes or type II, adult-onset, non-insulin–dependent diabetes. More than 90 percent of all diabetic patients have type II diabetes and are not prone to ketoacidosis. In the United States, type II diabetes has a 1 to 5 percent incidence and type I diabetes a 0.5 percent incidence, with perhaps an equal percentage of undiagnosed patients of both types. In addition, more than 200,000 new cases of diabetes are diagnosed each year in the United States. It is estimated that 50 percent of all diabetic patients require an operation during their lifetime. Because of the frequency with which the diabetic patient presents to surgery, it is important for the anesthesiologist to be familiar with the perioperative management of this disease.

It is debatable which is the major risk factor for surgery and anesthesia: diabetes mellitus or its related end organ disease. The controversy is illustrated by the studies concerning screening for gallstones in the dia-betic population. Older studies showed an increase in postoperative mortality in diabetics with acute cholecystitis. These results lead to recommendations for gallstone screening in asymptomatic diabetic patients. A study at the University of North Carolina showed an increased incidence of postoperative complications associated with biliary tract surgery and diabetes, but when the long-term complications of diabetes are accounted for, diabetes does not appear to present a greater risk to patients undergoing surgery. Several investigators have found that morbidity and mortality associated with acute cholecystitis were independent of diabetes and were determined primarily by the presence of vascular or renal disease. To date, I am unaware of any study that has definitively shown that diabetes under reasonable control contributes significantly to morbidity and mortality as compared with the patient's underlying complications or metabolic problems. This point is worth emphasizing because the anesthesiologist presented with a diabetic patient must remember to pay close attention not only to the intraoperative management of blood glucose, but also to the complications of diabetes.

Nonetheless, it is important to recognize that in certain surgical populations, intraoperative management of diabetes may assume critical importance in influencing surgical outcome. For instance, there is an increasing body of evidence that hyperglycemia occurring before and during a neurologic event may contribute to a poor neurologic outcome. Although the evidence from animal studies is convincing, human data are less definitive. Studies by Longstreth et al at the University of Washington showed a correlation between hyperglycemia and poor neurologic outcome after out-of-hospital cardiac arrest. However, the authors subsequently refuted this study, showing that the hyperglycemia exhibited in patients with a poor neurologic outcome was secondary to the duration and difficulty of resuscitation. Therefore, poor neurologic outcome was better predicted by the difficulty of the resuscitation rather than the hyperglycemia per se. At Cornell, Pulsinelli et al have found a correlation between hyperglycemia and poor stroke outcome in patients with moderately elevated initial blood glucoses following stroke. In addition, hyperglycemia has been correlated with greater cerebral edema on head computed axial tomography (CAT) scan following stroke. However, the question remains whether the hyperglycemia is a stress response to a large stroke or whether hyperglycemia contributes to the poor stroke outcome. Within the surgical setting, the author has shown that patients who incur strokes as a result of carotid endarterectomy have an elevated blood glucose in association with a poor neurologic outcome. Whether or not hyperglycemia in the diabetic has similar detrimental effects on neurologic outcome is controversial. However, most authorities believe that diabetes presents a similar scenario and that higher blood glucose levels in the diabetic may influence neurologic outcome. It may therefore be prudent to control blood glucose tightly in situations where neurologic insults may occur.

In the diabetic mother, blood glucose is important in determining neonatal outcome during labor and delivery. Neonatal hypoglycemia (defined as a blood glucose less than 40 mg during the first 12 hours of life), may be influenced by both maternal glucose control during the latter half of pregnancy and maternal glycemic control during labor and delivery. Maternal glucose levels greater than 90 mg during delivery significantly increase the frequency of neonatal hypoglycemia. Therefore, glucose boluses should be avoided in the peripartum period, and strict blood glucose control should be initiated. Additionally, episodes of hypotension in the diabetic mother during regional anesthesia may be associated with lower pH and base excess in the neonate.

Recent animal studies have shown that moderate hypoglycemia not associated with electroencephalogram (EEG) changes may cause profound changes in cerebral blood flow and metabolism. This becomes particularly important during hyperventilation or hypotension. Nuclear magnetic resonance (NMR) studies have demonstrated that hypoglycemia in combination with hyperventilation may lead to rapid depletion of high energy phosphates in the brain, which in turn leads to a flat EEG and inability of the brain to vasoconstrict. Additionally, moderate hypoglycemia interferes with brain autoregulation at lower blood pressures. It becomes imperative for the anesthesiologist dealing with "brittle" diabetics to avoid hypoglycemia, as even moderate levels may have neurologic consequences in the proper setting.

Poorly controlled diabetes may cause severe metabolic abnormalities, and patients can present with diabetic ketoacidosis or hyperglycemic hyperosmolar nonketotic coma. With these patients, perioperative management strongly influences outcome.

Other theoretical risks of diabetes in the surgical setting are based on diabetic animal models that show defects in wound healing which were partially corrected by the administration of insulin even without the restoration of euglycemia. However, the importance of these findings in humans has not been determined. In addition, the diabetic may be prone to infections during the perioperative period.

PHYSIOLOGY

The alterations that occur in glucose physiology in diabetic patients are associated with the stresses of fasting and surgery.

Normal Fasting Physiology

During fasting, adaptive changes occur that cause the mobilization of endogenous energy sources to maintain the metabolic rate. During a 24-hour fast, certain organs such as the brain preferentially oxidize glucose at a rate of 110 to 200 g per day, and in the absence of exogenous glucose, glycogenolysis and gluconeogenesis helps in meeting this need. During the initial 24 hours of starvation, liver glycogenolysis occurs at high rates to produce this glucose. Other tissues such as the heart, skeletal muscle, and renal cortex utilize free fatty acids or ketone bodies as their primary fuel source, accounting for some of the triglyceride mobilized.

Perioperative Changes in Glucose Metabolism

The major influence causing the immediate postoperative catabolic state is the stress response. The surgical stress response is characterized by increases in sympathetic tone, glucagon levels, pituitary hormone levels (notably adrenocorticotropic hormone [ACTH] and growth hormone) and interleukin-1. During the perioperative period, elevations of plasma norepinephrine and epinephrine occur. Epinephrine and norepinephrine stimulate liver glycogenolysis and gluconeogenesis and inhibit glucose uptake by insulin-dependent tissues. Both the alpha and beta effects of the catecholamines may influence glucose metabolism. For instance, through its beta effects, epinephrine increases metabolic rate. At the same time, the alpha and beta effects have profound influences on pancreatic function. Beta-receptor stimulation enhances insulin and glucagon release, whereas alpha-receptor stimulation inhibits the release of insulin. During the intraoperative and immediate postoperative course, alpha effects predominate to cause suppression of insulin secretion. Decreased insulin levels coupled with increased gluconeogenesis and insulin resistance cause hyperglycemia and glucose intolerance, prompting the term "diabetes of injury." During the following convalescent stage, the hormonal milieu maintains the elevated levels of gluconeogenesis while glucose uptake by the peripheral tissues is normalized and insulin secretion increases. The pancreas is also able to respond normally to excess glucose loads. One of the contributing factors to this change in glucose kinetics is the hormonal shift from alpha to beta catecholamine effects. Plasma glucagon levels rise after surgery and promote hepatic amino acid uptake, gluconeogenesis, and glycogenolysis. However, the increase in splanchnic glucose production with glucagon is a transient phenomenon, and it is only with the combined effects of all the stress hormones that the level of hepatic gluconeogenesis is maintained. Increased pituitary release of ACTH leads to elevated glucocorticoid levels, which can produce a moderate glycemic response as well as a sustained nitrogen loss. Postoperative elevations in growth hormone have an anabolic effect, causing nitrogen retention, protein synthesis, lipolysis, and decreased peripheral glucose uptake. The net effects of the neuroendocrine response on metabolism during the convalescent stage of tissue injury include elevation of blood sugar levels, stimulation of lipolysis, and an increased rate of gluconeogenesis, resulting in increased protein breakdown and nitrogen excretion.

During surgery, blood glucose concentrations in nondiabetic patients may increase to as high as 60 mg% above preoperative levels. The amount of surgical stress is the primary determinant of the absolute increase in glucose values. Inadequate insulin secretion, the stress hormone milieu, and the preoperative fasting state make the diabetic patient more susceptible to hyperglycemia, hypovolemia, osmotic diuresis, ketosis, and possible changes in acid-base balance. Hyperglycemia may have detrimental effects if allowed to go untreated. Osmotic diuresis secondary to the osmotic activity of glucose occurs when the patient's blood glucose exceeds the renal glucose threshold (approximately 180 to 250 mg%). This osmotic diuresis can result in dehydration and electrolyte abnormalities. Although hyperglycemia per se does not have direct effects on the patient's acid-base status, the ketone bodies that result from inadequate insulin therapy can elicit such effects. Acetoacetic acid and beta-hydroxybutyric acid may alter pH status by the accumulated dissociation of hydrogen ions.

Pharmacology

Several pharmacologic issues are important in the perioperative management of the diabetic.

Steroids

During procedures in which high doses of glucocorticoids are given, steroid-induced diabetes may occur. If hyperglycemia could cause problems in this setting, the approach to these patients can be modified by avoiding intraoperative glucose administration. Should the anesthesiologist elect to use insulin in this setting, there are

no good studies showing that steroid-induced hyperglycemia increases surgical morbidity.

Beta-Blockers

Beta-blockers inhibit the beta-catecholamine effects on carbohydrate and fat metabolism. Propranolol can prevent the increase in plasma free fatty acids as well as selectively inhibit the lipolytic action of catecholamines. In addition, the hyperglycemic response to epinephrine is reduced by beta-adrenergic blockers. In normal individuals, propranolol does not effect the rate or magnitude of the decrease in plasma glucose after administration insulin. However, it does slow the recovery from hypoglycemia. Because of the interference with the hypoglycemic response, diabetics who receive beta-blockers and are undergoing surgery must have their blood glucose concentrations carefully monitored whenever insulin is administered.

Insulin

The onset of action of intravenous regular insulin takes place within 10 minutes, with the maximum effect occurring within 1 hour. When discontinued, the effects dissipate within 60 to 90 minutes. The intravenous administration of 2 to 3 U of regular insulin per hour during surgery provides circulating insulin levels in the midphysiologic range and promotes the consumption of 12 to 15 g of glucose per hour.

Oral Hypoglycemic Agents

Oral hypoglycemic agents may have effects lasting for as long as 36 hours (chlorpropramide). These agents should be withheld before surgery.

PREOPERATIVE EVALUATION

In the preoperative evaluation of the diabetic surgical patient, one should assess for end organ disease.

Cardiac Disease

The most common cause of death in patients with diabetes mellitus is coronary artery disease, which accounts for one-third of all deaths in diabetics older than 40 years of age. In addition, compared with the general population, diabetics are more than twice as prone to have heart disease. It is controversial whether diabetics are more likely to have coronary artery disease than the general population. However, when compared with age-matched controls, diabetics have more incidents of atherosclerotic vessel involvement, more myocardial infarctions, and greater coronary collateralization. The severity and extent of coronary artery lesions are not related to the severity of the diabetes. Therefore, some common factor among diabetics (e.g., hyperglycemia) and not the duration or severity of diabetes may be the underlying factor causing accelerated atherosclerosis. This emphasizes that coronary artery disease should be sought for and expected even in mild, easily controlled diabetes.

Myocardial infarction is more common in the diabetic population. Because of the autonomic neuropathy that occurs with long-standing diabetes, it has been assumed that there is an increased incidence of silent myocardial infarctions in diabetics. Electrocardiographic studies of diabetic patients show multiple abnormalities despite a lack of symptoms. Exercise stress testing has shown that while 26 percent of a control population will exhibit ST-segment abnormalities, greater than 50 percent of diabetics may show ST-segment abnormalities during stress testing, with the incidence increasing with long-standing diabetes.

The diabetic population has a greater incidence of congestive heart failure. In the Framingham study, a 20-year follow-up demonstrated that diabetic males were twice as likely and diabetic females were five times as likely to have congestive heart failure. When coronary artery disease, hypertension, age, and other risk factors were taken into account, diabetics — especially females — were still at increased risk for congestive heart failure. Diabetics exhibit a range of cardiac abnormalities. The young asymptomatic diabetic may have subclinical abnormalities of left ventricular function, the incidence of which is unknown. During early diabetes, a noncompliant ventricle may be observed where the patient has an abnormal exercise tolerance and dyspnea secondary to elevated filling pressures and diastolic dysfunction. With progression of diabetes, patients gradually develop systolic dysfunction as well as elevated filling pressures and decreased ejection fraction. It is important to note that congestive heart failure can exist in the absence of hypertension or coronary artery disease.

In diabetics, hypertension is more prevalent than in the general population. From the Framingham study we know that hypertension compounds the risk of cardiovascular events. For example, hypertensive diabetic patients are at increased risk for stroke and transient ischemic attacks when compared with nonhypertensive diabetics.

There is a greater incidence of sudden cardiac death in diabetic patients than in the general population, although the exact cause of these events is not clearly delineated at this time.

Urologic Disorders

Voiding dysfunction has an estimated incidence of 25 to 87 percent in diabetics. The incidence correlates with the duration and severity of illness. Voiding dysfunction may lead to urosepsis and subsequent postoperative complications.

Renal Disorders

Kidney disease with or without hypertension is common in the diabetic population, with close to half of insulin-dependent diabetics eventually developing renal insufficiency. In addition, renal failure contributes significantly to the cause of death in type I diabetics. It is important that adequate hydration and good urine output be maintained during surgical procedures in diabetic patients. This point should be emphasized during radiologic procedures, when injected contrast agents may contribute to renal insufficiency.

Diabetic Neuropathy

Because of the increased frequency of peripheral neuropathy, a careful neurologic evaluation should be performed preoperatively, especially if regional anesthesia is considered. Attention must be paid to intraoperative positioning and padding of all pressure points to prevent ulceration and postoperative infection.

The autonomic neuropathies may involve one of several organ systems (e.g., the cardiovascular, gastrointestinal, and genitourinary systems). The genitourinary problems have been described previously. Within the cardiovascular system, subclinical autonomic dysfunction is probably quite common in the diabetic. Although the patient is often asymptomatic, the earliest signs are impaired vagal innervation of the heart, as demonstrated by the absence of heart rate variation during respiration. With progression of autonomic dysfunction, a fixed resting tachycardia and abnormal cardiac response to postural changes or exercise may be evident. The presenting clinical symptoms may include decreased exercise tolerance, orthostatic hypotension, and palpitations, syncope, or weakness on assuming an upright posture. The decrease in exercise tolerance has been attributed to a blunted increase in heart rate at low exercise secondary to an impaired ability to withdraw vagal tone. Similarly, an increase in heart rate may be blunted at high exercise levels secondary to impaired sympathetic tone. Orthostatic symptoms in diabetics may be secondary to a blunted increase in norepinephrine that occurs with assuming the upright posture. However, before ascribing any postural hypotension to diabetes, it is important to rule out other causes. The occurrence of autonomic cardiovascular dysfunction in the diabetic may be important in light of reports of unexplained cardiac arrest occurring in young patients with severe autonomic neuropathies.

Gastroparesis (gastroparesis diabeticorum) and impaired esophageal motility are common diabetic autonomic neuropathies. Although overt symptoms of esophageal dysfunction are rare, studies have shown a 56 percent incidence of abnormal esophageal motility in diabetic patients. There is a 20 to 30 percent incidence of delayed gastric emptying in the diabetic patient. These patients are usually asymptomatic or intermittently symptomatic with a clinical presentation consisting of gastric reflux, nausea, vomiting, and anorexia. Poor control of diabetes or hyperglycemia can contribute to poor gastric emptying. In these patients, metaclopramide may be useful in doses of 10 mg IV administered approximately 30 minutes before induction. In addition, aspiration precautions must be taken when anesthetizing these patients.

During hypoglycemic episodes, glucagon and epinephrine are released to increase the blood glucose level. The release of these hormones may be impaired, however, in diabetics secondary to impaired epinephrine secretion and blunted hypoglycemic symptomatology.

Laryngoscopy and Intubation

Diabetes may be associated with a higher incidence of difficult laryngoscopy and intubation. In patients with Type 1 diabetes, stiff joint syndrome may occur ultimately affecting all joints including those of the cervical and thoracic spine. Often these patients are of short stature and do not present prior to puberty. Several investigators have described up to a 40 percent incidence of difficult laryngoscopy in severe diabetics.

INTRAOPERATIVE MANAGEMENT

Diabetes encompasses a spectrum of diseases. However, each type of diabetes has specific insulin requirements for metabolic control during the perioperative period. In general, perioperative management of the diabetic can be divided into three strategies. With type II diabetes controlled with diet alone, no specific insulin or oral hypoglycemic regimen is indicated, especially if the surgery is of a minor nature. With the type I diabetic, most experts agree that perioperative management should include either subcutaneous or intravenous insulin. With regard to the type II patient requiring either oral hypoglycemic agents or insulin therapy, there is no consensus on the approach to perioperative glycemic control. This controversy stems from the large range of insulin requirements in this population coupled with the lack of data showing differences in outcome between various perioperative regimens. Perioperative care of diabetics involves managing the metabolic problems of catabolism, ketoacidosis, and hyperglycemia, and follows several principles:

1. Insulin requirements may differ dramatically with the type of operation and stress of the procedure.
2. Diabetic patients are a heterogeneous group, and their management must be adjusted on an individual basis.
3. In these days of cost containment, financial constraints may dictate the type of therapy diabetic patients receive. The shortest duration of hospitalization may be an important consideration.
4. A team approach is best in managing these complicated cases. Their overall care should be coordinated by the internist or endocrinologist most familiar with the patient. It is essential that close communication exist between the surgeon, anesthesiologist, and internist.
5. Morbidity and mortality in diabetic surgical patients is primarily from cardiovascular events and infection. It is unlikely that perioperative glucose control has much effect on these outcomes, although a theoretic argument can be made for an association between hyperglycemia and infection. Therefore, unless tight control is indicated, the anesthesiologist should concentrate on good sterile technique and cardiovascular physiology. The author does not wish to downplay metabolic considerations, but the evidence suggests that cardiovascular events are more important in determining surgical outcome.

With these principles in mind, the first decision which the clinician must make is whether or not insulin is required perioperatively. Diabetics as a group have a relative insulin deficiency. As previously alluded to, there are increased insulin requirements during anesthesia and surgery. At present, there is no proven method for predicting the need for insulin during surgery. In general, most authorities agree that it is safest to give insulin to every diabetic patient during the perioperative period, except for those who are diet controlled, type II, and undergoing minor surgery. The amount of insulin given is determined on an individual basis by the daily insulin requirements, the preoperative condition, the desired blood glucose control, and the extent of the surgery. For type II diabetic patients, subcutaneous or intravenous insulin administration is equally feasible. For the brittle type I juvenile onset diabetic patient, however, intravenous insulin provides the most reliable route. Whenever insulin is administered perioperatively, blood glucose monitoring is mandatory. Capillary glucose monitoring with glucose oxidase strips is adequate, and the frequency of blood glucose monitoring depends on the severity of the patient's illness and the desired range in which the physician wishes to maintain the blood glucose. Most diabetologists advocate maintenance of the blood glucose within the range of 80 to 200 mg%. For the patient undergoing elective surgery, preoperative admission is helpful to allow time for medical evaluation as well as obtaining fine metabolic control.

Fine or loose control can be obtained using either glucose, insulin, K^+ infusions, or subcutaneous insulin injections in conjunction with glucose infusions. Protocols that are helpful in my practice are shown in Tables 1 and 2.

The physician should have a low threshold for hospital admission in diabetic outpatients. It is best if diabetic patients are earliest on the operating room schedule. Patients with implantable insulin pumps should be managed under the direction of a diabetologist.

It is not always possible to optimize diabetic care, especially in emergency situations. In these cases, the urgency of the situation is dictated by the nature of the surgery. I believe, however, that there are few surgical situations which dictate immediately anesthetizing a

Table 1 Protocol for Tight Metabolic Control

Indications:
  Labor and delivery
  Neurosurgical procedures
  Brittle diabetes

Rationale:
  The amounts of insulin and glucose given should be related.
    Investigators have shown that an infusion of 0.25 to 0.33 U
    per gram of glucose provides good glycemic control.

Regimen:
  Preoperatively:
    (1) Discontinue subcutaneous insulin
    (2) Obtain baseline blood glucose
    (3) NPO after midnight
    (4) Add 5 U regular insulin to 500 ml of 5% dextrose solution
        and run at 100 ml/hr
    (5) Check blood glucose every 2 to 4 hours
    (6) Add K^+ to solution as needed as determined by
        electrolytes
  Intraoperatively and postoperatively:
    The infusion is continued until the patient is taking well PO
      and preoperative insulin therapy can be reinstituted. Glucose
      determinations are made every 2 to 4 hours.

Adjustments:
  If blood glucose is less than 100 mg, decrease the infusion to
    3 U insulin per 500 ml. A blood glucose >200 mg% is treated
    with an increase in insulin of 8 to 10 U per 500 ml 5% dextrose
    solution.
  Conditions that increase insulin requirements include patients
    receiving >1.5 U insulin/kg/day, obesity, steroids, infection,
    liver disease, and cardiopulmonary bypass.*

---

*For precise insulin adjustments in these cases, refer to the following article: Alberti MM, Gill GV, Elliot MJ. Insulin delivery during surgery in the diabetic patient. Diabetes Care 1982; 5:65–77.

Table 2 Protocol for Loose Metabolic Control

Indications:
  Most surgical cases involving diabetic patients, especially when
    lack of personnel or outpatient surgery is a concern

Rationale:
  Principle 5 (see text)

Regimen:
  Preoperative:
    NPO after midnight
  Intraoperatively and postoperatively:
  On the morning of surgery start intravenous solution containing
    5% dextrose at a maintenance rate; give ½ to ⅔ of AM dose
    of insulin as subcutaneous NPH early in the morning; continue
    glucose infusion intraoperatively and postoperatively; continue
    blood glucose monitoring every 2 to 4 hours intraoperatively
    and postoperatively using sliding scale coverage with regular
    insulin; reinstitute preoperative insulin regimen when patient
    taking PO adequately.

At the very minimum, I prefer to see a blood pH greater than 7.25 and a blood glucose less than 400 mg% before administering anesthesia. Diabetic ketoacidosis can present with symptoms that mimic the acute abdomen; therefore it is imperative that ketoacidosis be treated first, as in many cases these symptoms may resolve.

The choice of anesthesia is not greatly influenced by the presence of diabetes. No particular anesthetic agent or technique has been shown to decrease perioperative morbidity and mortality in these patients.

SUGGESTED READING

Alberti MM, Gill GV, Elliot MJ. Insulin delivery during surgery in the diabetic patient. Diabetes Care 1982; 5:65–77.
King LW, Snyder DS. Diabetes and other endocrine disorders. In: Breslow MJ, Miller CF, Rogers MC, eds. Perioperative management. St. Louis: CV Mosby, 1990: 292–313.
Schade DS. Surgery and diabetes. Med Clin North Am 1988; 72:1531–1544.
Sussman KE, Draznin B, James WE, eds. Clinical guide to diabetes mellitus. New York: Alan R. Liss, Inc., 1987.

patient in diabetic ketoacidosis. In these cases, even a 4- to 6-hour period to treat the patient's underlying metabolic abnormalities will significantly enhance postoperative outcome. Treatment of diabetic ketoacidosis is complicated and beyond the scope of this chapter. For discussions on the management of this disorder, the reader is referred to some excellent texts on this subject.

KIDNEY DISEASE

CLAIR MILLER, M.D.

Preoperative considerations for patients with kidney disease fall into two distinctly different categories: (1) assessment of patients with less than normal (but not end-stage) renal function and (2) assessment of patients with end-stage renal disease who require dialysis for survival. Goals for anesthetic management of these two categories of patients vary markedly. Preservation of existing renal function is the primary perioperative goal for normal patients and for patients with less than normal kidney function. In contrast, supportive management of the physiologic abnormalities of end-stage renal disease is the major goal for dialysis patients who require anesthesia and surgery. Because of these differences, in this chapter preoperative considerations for patients with decreased renal function are discussed separately from preoperative considerations for patients with end-stage renal disease.

PREOPERATIVE ASSESSMENT OF RENAL IMPAIRMENT NOT REQUIRING DIALYSIS

Preservation of existing renal function is a challenging perioperative goal. Of all the physicians involved in the care of surgical patients, the anesthesiologist is in the best position to oversee and to begin effective management that is likely to achieve this goal. The following discussion first presents an overview of the problem of renal deterioration in the perioperative time and then discusses specific preoperative strategies that are aimed at preserving renal function.

Overview

Careful preoperative assessment and management of patients with functional kidneys is important because prognosis for patients who develop any degree of acute renal impairment in the perioperative time is worse than for patients who maintain stable indices of renal function during and after anesthesia and surgery. Furthermore, perioperative mortality appears to increase in parallel with the level to which kidney function deteriorates. In a large series of cardiac surgical patients, for example, perioperative mortality was approximately 1 percent in patients who maintained normal serum creatinine concentrations throughout the perioperative time. The mortality rate increased to 11 percent in patients in whom postoperative creatinine concentrations increased from normal values to 1.5 to 2.5 mg per deciliter, and mortality further increased to 24 percent in patients in whom serum creatinine levels exceeded 2.5 mg per deciliter at any time in the postoperative period. Table 1 summarizes mortality rates that are reported for

Table 1 Mortality Rates in Acute Postoperative Renal Failure Requiring Dialysis

Procedure	Mortality (%)
General surgery/trauma	50–79
Major vascular surgery	50–100
Cardiac surgery	50–100

patients who develop acute renal failure severe enough to require dialysis after a variety of surgical procedures. Acute postoperative renal failure severe enough to require dialysis develops in 0.5 to 1.5 percent of trauma patients, in 1.5 to 2.5 percent of patients after cardiac surgery, and in 2.0 to 2.5 percent of patients after abdominal aortic reconstruction.

The overall incidence of developing renal dysfunction after anesthesia and surgery is not known. However, some level of renal deterioration (assessed by serial creatinine determinations) develops in 2 to 5 percent of all adult hospital admissions. Patients in whom serum creatinine levels increase during hospitalization have a much higher mortality rate than patients with stable creatinine concentrations throughout their hospital course. Patients with pre-existing renal insufficiency appear to have a greater tendency for acute perioperative renal deterioration.

The two major causes of acute perioperative renal deterioration are (1) decreased renal perfusion and (2) nephrotoxin exposure (Table 2). In surgical patients, renal perfusion deficits are probably more common and more important mediators of renal dysfunction than are nephrotoxic exposures. Although the renal ischemic effects of poor left ventricular function, cardiopulmonary bypass, and aortic cross-clamping undoubtedly contribute to development of acute renal failure in some patients, renal deterioration in most surgical patients appears to be due to inadequate intravascular volume repletion. Intravascular dehydration enhances the nephrotoxic effects of aminoglycosides and radiocontrast agents. Diabetic patients have a tenfold greater risk for renal deterioration during hypovolemic episodes than nondiabetic control patients.

Thus, the major risk factors for acute perioperative renal dysfunction include (1) intravascular dehydration; (2) procedures that require interruption of renal blood flow, such as cardiopulmonary bypass and aortic cross-clamping; (3) presence of poor left ventricular function; (4) pre-existing renal insufficiency; (5) diabetes; and (6) perioperative exposure to aminoglycosides or radiocontrast agents.

Perioperative renal deterioration is a more common and more lethal complication than is generally appreciated. Failure of modern dialysis therapy to decrease substantially the excessive mortality rates suggest that acute perioperative renal failure is mediated by processes that result in widespread systemic injury that is often irreversible. Postoperative renal failure, then, appears to be a marker for the severity of the initiating insult rather than an unfortunate complication that requires treatment.

Preoperative Recommendations

Preoperative assessment and perioperative monitoring of renal function is largely limited to serial determinations of blood urea nitrogen (BUN) values, serum creatinine concentrations, and timed measurements of urine volume. Sophisticated monitoring modalities that are available to monitor and guide therapy for the cardiovascular and respiratory systems are not available for renal monitoring. Despite these limitations, there are important aspects of preoperative assessment and planning that will help to prevent renal deterioration in the perioperative time.

Serum BUN and creatinine concentrations should be measured within 24 hours prior to surgery, and these values should be compared to previous determinations. Acute elevations of BUN and creatinine that are discovered preoperatively should prompt an immediate search for reversible causes of acute renal deterioration such as volume contraction, acute left ventricular failure, or nephrotoxin exposures. Surgery should be postponed until BUN and creatinine concentrations return to baseline values in elective cases. It is unreasonable and dangerous to expose a patient with acute renal injury to the many additional risk factors for renal deterioration that are known to exist in the perioperative time.

Every effort must be made to maintain effective left ventricular preload throughout the perioperative time. Preoperative fluid deficits from NPO status, dehydrating effects of bowel preparations, nausea and vomiting, and the osmotic consequences of radiocontrast agents must be replaced prior to anesthetic administration. Intraoperative blood loss, evaporative losses, and extravascular sequestration of fluid must also be replaced to maintain adequate intravascular volume. Intravascular pressure measurements with central venous or pulmonary artery catheters may be needed to judge the adequacy of intravascular volume repletion in some cases. If any doubt exists, it is generally preferable to overhydrate rather than to restrict fluids in surgical patients. The consequences of fluid overload can be easily and reversibly treated, but ischemic postoperative renal failure is associated with high mortality.

Table 2 Causes of Perioperative Acute Renal Failure

Decreased renal perfusion
  Intravascular volume contraction
  Impaired left ventricular function
  Cardiopulmonary bypass
  Aortic cross-clamping

Nephrotoxin exposure
  Aminoglycosides
  Radiocontrast agents
  Anesthetic agents

Continuous assessment of urine flow should be made in all cases in which either large blood losses, large fluid shifts, or deliberate interruptions of renal blood flow are anticipated. Although urine output is not a very sensitive indicator of renal blood flow, maintenance of normal urine output intraoperatively provides reassurance that intravascular volume is adequate. Complete cessation of urine flow is often associated with reversible mechanical obstruction of the urinary collecting system. Oliguria during anesthesia and surgery often occurs despite normal renal blood flow and normal renal function. "Surgical oliguria" is caused by salt and water retention that is mediated by stress-induced sympathetic nervous system hyperactivity, activation of the renin-angiotensin-aldosterone system, and release of antidiuretic hormone. Nevertheless, a search for occult intravascular dehydration must be made if urine flow rate decreases markedly during the course of an anesthetic.

Anesthetic management of patients with less than normal renal function is guided by the physiologic requirements of the patient rather than by avoidance of one or another anesthetic drug or technique that may have adverse effects on the kidney. Renal function is adversely affected during spinal or epidural anesthesia only to the extent that sympathetic nervous system blockade produces arterial hypotension and renal hypoperfusion. Halogenated anesthetic agents do not appear to be important mediators of renal injury. Because occasional case reports describe fluoride nephrotoxicity after administration of enflurane, enflurane is probably best avoided, especially in patients with preoperative renal insufficiency. Of the halogenated agents in common use today, only enflurane is metabolically defluorinated and likely to cause direct nephrotoxicity. Renal blood flow is normally autoregulated at clinically important concentrations of all halogenated anesthetic agents. Renal tubular cells are not damaged on exposure to halothane or isoflurane. Thus, preservation of renal function is largely independent of the anesthetic agent or techniques used.

PREOPERATIVE ASSESSMENT OF END-STAGE RENAL FAILURE REQUIRING DIALYSIS

There is probably no other group of patients who undergo as many surgical procedures in their lifetimes as do dialysis patients. Although most of the procedures performed are required to establish vascular access for dialysis, other surgical procedures are being performed more and more commonly. When planning anesthetic management for dialysis patients, the anesthesiologist is confronted not only with the disease that caused the kidneys to fail in the first place (these problems are discussed elsewhere in this book), but also with the physiologic complications of renal failure itself. This section presents an overview of the problem of anesthetic management of dialysis patients and then discusses specific preoperative recommendations for management that are aimed at decreasing the incidence and severity of complications related to the physiologic abnormalities of end-stage renal disease.

Overview

Although vascular access procedures are performed safely with the patient under regional, local, or general anesthesia, major invasive procedures with the dialysis patient under either general or regional anesthesia are associated with higher mortality rates than similar procedures in patients with normal renal function. Overall mortality after major procedures is 5 to 6 percent. Of patients who die, approximately 10 percent die of hyperkalemia within the first 24 hours after operation, approximately 20 percent die of excessive postoperative bleeding within the first few days after operation, and approximately 40 percent die of septic complications at 1 to 2 weeks postoperatively. Severe cardiovascular dysfunction accounts for about 20 percent of the remaining deaths.

Nonlethal complications occur regularly after anesthesia and surgery in dialysis patients. These complications also reflect the physiologic abnormalities of end-stage renal failure. Thus, 36 percent of patients require emergency dialysis within the first 24 hours after operation to treat hyperkalemia. Hypotension and hypertension occur in approximately 20 percent of patients over the first day postoperatively; these problems appear to reflect changes in intravascular volume status. Shunt or fistula thrombosis develops in about 10 percent of patients over the first postoperative week. Septic complications, including pneumonia, wound infections, and septicemia develop in about 25 percent of patients over the first and second postoperative weeks. Most of these complications can either be eliminated or their effects blunted by careful preoperative assessment and management. The following section offers recommendations for preoperative management for each of the expected physiologic abnormalities encountered in end-stage renal failure (Table 3).

Preoperative Recommendations

Anemia

Serum hematocrit and red blood cell indices should be measured preoperatively and compared with previous values from dialysis records. Acutely decreased hematocrit values and/or indices that reveal other than the

Table 3 Abnormalities of End-Stage Renal Failure That Alter Anesthetic Management

Anemia
Bleeding abnormalities
Cardiovascular and blood volume abnormalities
Electrolyte and metabolic abnormalities
Infectious complications
Pharmacologic alterations

expected normochromic normocytic anemia of renal failure should prompt an immediate investigation into other causes of anemia before surgery proceeds. Before human recombinant erythropoietin was available for widespread use, hematocrit values of less than 30 percent were commonly encountered in functionally anephric patients. This level of anemia is generally well-tolerated even at levels of hemodynamic stress that are common in the perioperative time. However, red blood cell transfusions should be given as needed throughout the perioperative time as in any other surgical patient.

Bleeding Abnormalities

Laboratory assessment of coagulation parameters is unlikely to alter clinical management because a bleeding tendency from abnormal platelet function is assumed to be present. If measured, the bleeding time may be slightly prolonged and the platelet count mildly depressed. Prothrombin and partial thromboplastin times should be normal. Dialysis partially corrects platelet dysfunction in uremia, and dialysis within 24 hours prior to anesthesia and surgery remains the hemostatic therapy of choice in dialysis patients. If excessive bleeding is encountered perioperatively, or if the planned surgical procedure is normally associated with large blood losses, desmopressin (deamino-8-D-arginine vasopressin) administration may shorten the bleeding time, increase circulating levels of Factor VIII/von Willebrand antigen, and decrease perioperative blood loss in uremia. Dialysis patients are at high risk for stress-induced gastrointestinal bleeding in the perioperative time and should be routinely treated prophylactically with either histamine-2 receptor blockers, antacids, or sucralfate.

Cardiovascular and Blood Volume Abnormalities

Assume that clinically important coronary artery disease is present. Multiple risk factors for ischemic heart disease including hypertension, hyperlipedemia, and abnormal carbohydrate metabolism are almost uniformly present in dialysis patients, especially elderly patients. The presence of myocardial ischemia and myocardial dysfunction carry the same perioperative prognostic significance in dialysis patients as in other patients with ischemic heart disease and must be treated accordingly.

As with any other surgical patient, intravascular volume must be adequately maintained throughout the perioperative time. Potassium-free saline solutions should be used to replete fluid losses and maintain left ventricular preload. Blood volume repletion and cardiovascular management may be difficult in uremic patients because of myocardial dysfunction; presence of arteriovenous shunts, and the unpredictable effects of uremia, acidosis, and adrenergic stimuli on the cardiovascular system. Invasive intravascular monitoring may be required to guide fluid therapy in some cases. Because many dialysis patients are anuric, mobilization of "third-space" fluid in the postoperative time may be accompanied by rapid development of pulmonary edema and respiratory failure. Careful postoperative observation for fluid overload and regular well-timed dialysis therapy will avoid these complications. Care must be taken to protect the fistula site from injury during positioning prior to anesthesia and surgery.

Electrolyte and Metabolic Abnormalities

Serum electrolytes should be measured within 12 to 24 hours before the operation. An "anion gap" acidosis is normal. However, a serum bicarbonate concentration below 12 to 15 mEq per liter should prompt an immediate investigation for other causes of metabolic acidosis. Serum potassium concentrations will be on the high side; the measured level should be compared with those recorded on dialysis records to get an idea of what level of hyperkalemia is normally tolerated without untoward sequelae. Further laboratory investigation is unlikely to alter anesthetic plans.

All dialysis-dependent patients should receive dialysis therapy within 12 to 24 hours prior to anesthesia and surgery. Such therapy will abruptly decrease serum potassium concentrations and will largely eliminate the need for emergency dialysis in the immediate postoperative time to treat life-threatening hyperkalemia. Preoperative hemodialysis may be difficult to achieve in patients who require vascular access procedures. However, peritoneal dialysis and hemodialysis through specialized venous catheters should be used even in these difficult patients in order to manage hyperkalemia, advanced uremia, and severe metabolic acidosis preoperatively. There is no need to subject any patient with uncontrolled complications of end-stage renal failure to the risks of anesthesia and surgery for an elective procedure.

Infectious Complications

Strict adherence to aseptic techniques during all intravascular cannulations is mandatory in dialysis pa-tients. Dialysis patients are more susceptible to infectious innoculations than are patients with normal renal function, and septic complications are a leading cause of death in dialysis patients who undergo anesthesia and surgery. Hepatitis B and C virus infections are common in dialysis patients, and care must be taken to avoid self-innoculation of these infectious agents by anesthesiologists who care for these patients.

Pharmacologic Alterations

Standard dosages of barbiturates, benzodiazepams, and narcotic analgesics may cause excessive and prolonged sedation and respiratory depression in functionally anephric patients. These drugs should be titrated in small incremental dosages to the desired effects only under the direct observation of the anesthesiologist. Anesthetic drugs and techniques should be chosen to meet the physiologic requirements of the patients rather than to avoid one or another drug or technique. Local, regional, and general anesthetic techniques can all be safely and effectively administered to dialysis patients. All nondepolarizing neuromuscular blocking drugs can be safely used with careful neuromuscular monitoring in uremic patients, but atacurium and vecuronium may be the preferred agents because they are eliminated virtually independently of renal mechanisms. Succinylcholine increases serum potassium concentration by 0.5 mEq per liter in patients with or without renal failure and should probably not be used in patients with end-stage renal failure.

SUGGESTED READING

Myers BD, Moran SM. Hemodynamically mediated acute renal failure. N Engl J Med 1986; 314:97–105.
Shusterman N, Strom BL, Murray TG, et al. Risk factors and outcome of hospital-acquired acute renal failure: clinical epidemiologic study. Am J Med 1987; 83:65–71.
Spurney RF, Fulkerson WJ, Schwab SJ. Acute renal failure in critically ill patients: prognosis for recovery of kidney function after prolonged dialysis support. Crit Care Med 1991; 19:8–11.
Zaloga GP, Hughes SS. Oliguria in patients with normal renal function. Anesthesiology 1990; 72:598–602.

HEMATOLOGIC DISORDERS

BARRY W. BRASFIELD, M.D.

Hematologic problems in the patient presenting for elective or emergency surgery have a direct impact on the outcome of a procedure. Such problems, however, influence the timing and the extent of an operative procedure. For example, although recent aspirin ingestion may be inconsequential to the patient undergoing an elective inguinal hernia repair, it may be of paramount importance for the patient presenting for emergency cerebral aneurysm repair. In addition, the controversy over the infectious and immunologic effects of blood transfusions demands the pursuit of a rational approach to the management of perioperative anemia, based not only on long-standing traditions but on a constantly refined understanding of the physiology of the consequences of anemia.

Although much research is being conducted concerning the effects of anesthesia, stress, and surgery on immune function, it is premature to draw firm conclusions about the function of white blood cells during the perioperative period. Therefore, this chapter focuses on conditions associated with red blood cells, platelets, and serum factors related to hemostasis and thrombosis.

PERIOPERATIVE MANAGEMENT OF ANEMIA

While the definition of anemia with regard to its morphology may seem straightforward, with regard to its physiology, it is much more difficult to grasp (Table 1). As our understanding of the effects of blood loss and anemia on wound healing, cardiopulmonary physiology, and patient tolerance has increased, so have the recognition and incidence of the hazards of transfusion. At a time when the possibility of life-threatening, even fatal, infection is a constant concern of physicians and patients alike, several recent symposia and publications have emphasized the importance of basing transfusion practices on rational scientific principles, not anecdotal experience. These principles begin with an understanding of the consequences of anemia.

A recent National Institutes of Health (NIH) conference on the consequences of anemia failed to reach a consensus on the level of hemoglobin that would automatically demand red blood cell transfusion. Attempts to define a minimal acceptable hemoglobin level have focused on the primary nutritive function of blood, that of providing oxygen to the tissues. The maintenance of an adequate oxygen-carrying capacity requires a thorough understanding of oxyhemoglobin saturation and cardiac output as well as the impact of anesthetics, coexisting disease, and surgical stress on the various components of the equation. In general, chronic anemia (to a hemoglobin level of 8 g per deciliter) in an otherwise healthy patient has not been associated with increased perioperative morbidity and mortality (Table 2). On the other hand, patients who have decreased compensatory tissue perfusion (e.g., coronary artery disease), increased tissue oxygen needs (e.g., burns or sepsis), or an inability to increase cardiac output (e.g., congestive heart failure) may require hemoglobin concentrations in excess of 10 g per deciliter. Although techniques such as oxygen delivery–oxygen consumption curves and Svo_2 monitoring have been used in attempts to maximize the oxygen supply/demand ratio, the utility of these remains controversial.

PERIOPERATIVE TRANSFUSION

Despite the absence of scientific data supporting a minimal acceptable hemoglobin level or hematocrit (MAH), it is still common to expose patients to the risks of homologous blood transfusion to maintain a fixed MAH of 10 g per deciliter or 30 percent. As surgical and anesthetic techniques have improved and transmissible diseases such as human immunodeficiency virus (HIV) and non-A, non-B hepatitis have become more widespread, the need to define and institute rational perioperative transfusion strategies has become mandatory.

Table 1 Classifications of Anemia

I. Relative
  A. Pregnancy-related
  B. Volume overload
  C. Age-related
II. Absolute
  A. Morphologic class
    1. Macrocytic (vitamin B_{12}, folate)
    2. Normocytic (blood loss, "chronic disease")
    3. Microcytic (iron, thalassemia)
  B. Pathophysiology
    1. Increased destruction (hemolytic anemia)
    2. Decreased production (nutrition related, age related)
    3. Sequestration/loss of platelets
    4. Combination of B1–3
  C. Association with certain diseases/conditions
    1. Pregnancy
    2. Renal failure
    3. Liver disease
    4. Alcoholism
    5. Nutritional deficiencies
    6. Infection (HIV, SBE, sepsis)
    7. Age related (prematurity, elderly)
    8. Blood loss

Table 2 Conditions That May Require Hemoglobin > 8 g per Deciliter

Coronary artery disease
Congestive heart failure
Sepsis
Burns
Carbon monoxide poisoning
Adult respiratory distress syndrome
Pregnancy

Consideration of the possible need for perioperative transfusion should be initiated, when possible, weeks before the planned procedure. The safest technique available to the patient presenting for an elective procedure is predeposit autologous blood donation. Liberal criteria for selecting patients for autologous donation have allowed patients with coronary disease and extremes of age, and those who are pregnant to donate without significant morbidity. Limitations based on the ability to replenish red blood cell mass allow donation only every 7 to 10 days. In the near future, use of recombinant human erythropoietin (r-HUEPO) may stimulate red blood cell production sufficiently to allow more frequent donation. Many patients donate up to 48 hours before the planned procedure, which allows sufficient time for re-equilibration of intravascular volume.

If a patient needs more units than can be collected within the shelf life of the first collected unit, autologous blood can be frozen. This can be especially important to the individual with a rare blood type or with unusual antibodies. Although new adenosine-based additive solutions have made liquid storage possible for up to 42 days, the Food and Drug Administration allows frozen red blood cell storage for up to 3 years. If this time is extended (some believe 10 to 11 years may be possible), private citizens could conceivably store their blood in a community blood center to be used if the need were to arise. The availability of both autologous blood and frozen red blood cell storage is currently limited, depending on the geographic area and the willingness of the local blood center to participate in such programs.

Other blood components—namely, plasma and platelets—have been collected for autologous use. Patients having cardiopulmonary bypass, for example, may benefit from such collections in the maintenance of postbypass hemostasis.

Perioperative Hemodilution

For surgical patients expected to require blood replacement but temporally constrained from autologous donation, hemodilution may be an alternative. Replacement of fresh whole blood with cell-free substitutes (lactated Ringer's at 3 ml per milliliter of whole blood or hetastarch at 1 ml per milliliter of whole blood) can be performed in the operating room before induction of anesthesia. This technique may require careful monitoring of arterial and central venous pressures, especially when a target hematocrit of less than 26 to 28 percent is used. The collected whole blood can then be used to replace blood lost during the procedure, usually starting with the lowest hematocrit unit and preserving the highest hematocrit (i.e., the first collected unit[s]) blood for reinfusion after the major blood loss. Concomitant diuresis may be necessary, because red blood cell mass is increased at the end of the procedure. Studies in patients undergoing spinal fusion have shown that hemodilution dramatically decreases the need for homologous transfusions; other studies have reported similar results in pediatric cases and in cardiac surgery, in which hemodilution is used routinely during cardiopulmonary bypass. In these patients, hemodilution has been shown to improve the patency of bypass grafts. In a study of free flap survival, lower hematocrits were found to correlate with increased flap survival. Other studies have reported increased platelet counts and improved hemostasis in patients who undergo preoperative hemodilution. Despite concerns over tissue hypoxia, complications have been minimal.

Intraoperative Blood Salvage

Several devices designed to salvage autologous red blood cells from a surgical field have recently been developed. The semicontinuous-flow cell-washing centrifuge has now reached a stage of automation that makes it practical and cost effective if 2 to 3 U of red blood cells are recovered. Widespread use of autotransfusion without significant incidence of complications has been reported for patients undergoing cardiac, vascular, and orthopedic surgery and liver transplants. Theoretic contraindications to its use include surgery for malignant tumors and bowel surgery or surgery in the area of other contaminated fields. Washing the cells in 0.9 percent normal saline before transfusion effectively removes fat, bone chips, and other particulate matter but may also remove significant amounts of platelets and plasma. These products may therefore need to be given to effect hemostasis when more than 6 to 8 U have been reinfused. Careful monitoring of coagulation status and appropriate replacement of indicated factors have generally been effective in the adjunctive management of patients receiving salvaged blood.

Anesthetic Technique

Once decisions concerning the need for and methods of blood replacement have been addressed, the question of whether the type of anesthesia influences blood loss should be considered.

Deliberate hypotension as an adjunct to general anesthesia has been reported to reduce intraoperative blood loss during surgery for scoliosis, hip arthroplasty, major head and neck surgery, and thoracoabdominal dissections. Studies of benefit have been published for radical cystectomy, middle ear surgery, and pediatric surgery. Although definitions of hypotension vary, most define it as reduction in systolic pressure to 80 to 90 mm Hg or a mean blood pressure of 50 to 75 mm Hg. Total hip replacement best illustrates the benefits of hypotension, with blood loss reduced by approximately 50 percent and transfusions reduced by 20 to 83 percent. Many different methods have been used, including administration of trimethaphan, sodium nitroprusside, inhalational agents, beta-blockers, labetalol (combined alpha- and beta-blocker), nitroglycerin, and various combinations. As for which technique is most effective, studies demonstrate no difference in blood loss between a method that decreases cardiac output (trimethaphan) versus one that increases cardiac output (sodium nitroprusside) when the same target blood pressure is achieved. Complications associated with deliberate hypotension have been surprisingly low, probably because the technique is avoided in patients with vascular disease or hypertension, conditions that may increase the risk of hypotensive organ ischemia. Careful monitoring with intra-arterial and central venous pressures is generally indicated when a deliberate hypotensive technique is used. In some centers, somatosensory-evoked potential monitoring or electroencephalographic monitoring is used, especially during scoliosis surgery, when spinal manipulation may precipitate neurologic injury.

Regional anesthesia (usually epidural or spinal anesthesia) has a beneficial effect on intraoperative blood loss in patients undergoing prostatectomy and other pelvic or lower extremity surgery. Several randomized prospective controlled studies in patients undergoing total hip replacement demonstrated a reduction of 30 to 40 percent in blood loss. Studies comparing epidural anesthesia, general anesthesia with spontaneous ventilation, and general anesthesia with positive-pressure ventilation found a strong correlation between central and peripheral venous pressures and blood loss. Regional anesthesia, associated with the maintenance of lower venous pressures, results in less perioperative blood loss and decreased postoperative thromboembolism. Therefore, these methods should be used as often as procedures and patient cooperation will allow.

Directed Donations

More frequently, patients are requesting that they not be given homologous blood transfusions from "strangers." In such cases, it may be possible to use direct, or recipient-designated, donations. Such donations are frequently received from family members or close friends whose blood group is compatible with the patient's. The method may also be helpful for a child whose need of platelets can be satisfied by a parent who possesses at least one haplotype human lymphocyte antigen (HLA) match. Nevertheless, as pressure to allow directed donations increased in 1983 with the advent of the acquired immunodeficiency syndrome (AIDS) scare, the American Red Cross, the American Association of Blood Banks, and the Council of Community Blood Centers issued a joint statement on directed donations that strongly recommended that such programs not be conducted. Their reluctance was based not only on an absence of scientific evidence that directed donations were safer than volunteer donations but also with concerns for the increased burden placed on blood collection centers by directed donor programs. While not preventing the risk of homologous transfusions entirely, directed donations may nevertheless reduce the anxiety associated with perioperative transfusion.

Figure 1 suggests a rational algorithmic approach to the perioperative maintenance of an MAH. This scheme obviously depends on careful cooperation between anesthesiologist and surgeon, with considerations, when

possible, weeks before the planned surgical procedure. As autologous and directed donation programs continue to expand and intraoperative hemodilution and blood salvage increase, the use of homologous blood transfusion with its associated risk should significantly decline.

DISEASES OF RED BLOOD CELLS

Sickle Cell Anemia

Disorders of red blood cells include those conditions associated with too few and dysfunctional cells (sickle cell anemia) and conditions associated with too many cells (polycythemia). Hemoglobin S is the most important hemoglobin variant in regard to perioperative implications. Perioperative vaso-occlusive crises resulting in pulmonary or coronary emboli, renal failure, and strokes usually occur in patients with greater than 50 percent hemoglobin S. Sickle cell anemia, in which 85 to 95 percent of native hemoglobin is the S form, presents in approximately 15 in 10,000 American blacks. Sickling is exacerbated by hypoxemia, hypothermia, dehydration, acidosis, and low-flow states.

Preoperative management of the patient with sickle cell disease should include evaluation for significant end-organ dysfunction as well as consultation with a hematologist for the conduct of partial exchange transfusion. Many clinicians recommend a target hemoglobin S of 40 to 50 percent before all but the most emergent operative procedures are performed. Maintenance of adequate oxygenation, hydration, normothermia, and acid-base balance is crucial to good outcome. Pain management may be difficult in the patient who has been using high-dose narcotics to control sickle pain; regional techniques should be used for pain control when feasible.

Polycythemia

Polycythemia is defined as the presence of a spun hematocrit of greater than 40 percent in women or greater than 52 percent in men. Relative polycythemia is characterized by normal or decreased total red blood cell mass accompanied by a low plasma volume. It is associated with chronic fluid loss, hypertension, obesity, smoking, and stress. Absolute erythrocytosis may result from one of many hemoglobinopathies, but more commonly it is caused by excessive erythropoietin production, or so-called secondary polycythemia. Secondary polycythemia can be further divided into cases in which there is a reasonable physiologic cause for the increase in red blood cell mass and into those in which there is autonomous production of excessive erythropoietin. The most commonly reported causes of polycythemia are listed in Table 3.

The preoperative evaluation and management of polycythemia must include a consideration of the physiologic effects of the erythrocytosis. In hypoxemic patients with limited cardiac output, the elevated

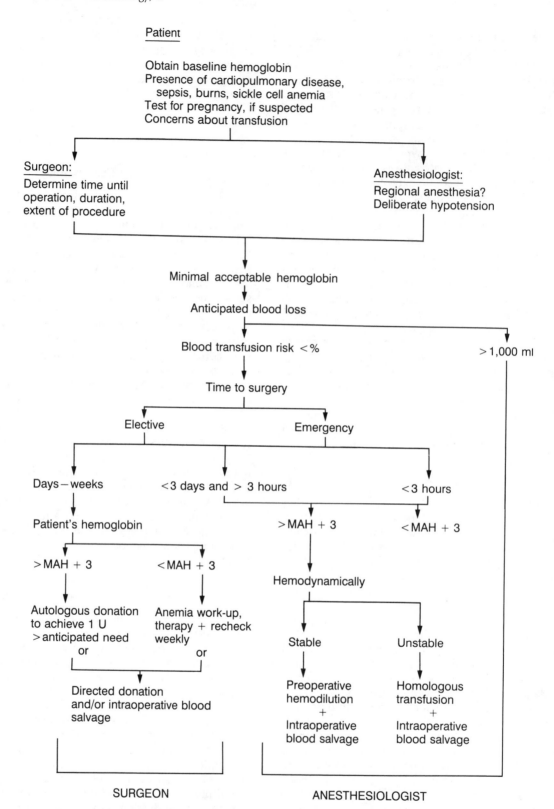

Figure 1 Perioperative management of anemia.

hematocrit may represent an important physiologic adaptation for the preservation of oxygen delivery to the tissues. On the other hand, the patient with an erythropoietin-producing tumor who is experiencing headache, tinnitus, and hypertension may benefit from preoperative phlebotomy. The target hematocrit should be in the range of 40 to 44 percent. If significant blood loss is anticipated, these patients make excellent candidates for preoperative hemodilution. Limited physiologic reserve during phlebotomy may demand judicious

Table 3 Causes of Absolute Polycythemia

Physiologic responses
  Chronic carbon monoxide poisoning
  High altitude
  Chronic hypoxemia (e.g,. right-to-left shunts, severe chronic
    obstructive pulmonary disease)

Pathologic states
  Polycythemia vera
  Renovascular disease
  Renal tumors, cysts
  Uterine myomas
  Cerebellar hemangiomas
  Hepatomas

Table 4 Drugs Implicated in Thrombocytopenia

Decreased production of platelets
  Ethanol
  Thiazides
  Estrogens

Increased destruction of platelets
  Quinine/quinidine
  Penicillin
  Cephalothin
  Thiazides
  Gold
  Heparin
  Ranitidine
  Methyldopa

replacement of lost blood volume with crystalloid or colloid solutions in appropriate quantities. If factors such as smoking, hypertension, or obesity are prevalent, elective surgery may be postponed until appropriate corrective therapy has been undertaken. Patients with polycythemia are known to have a high incidence of postoperative thromboembolic events. Appropriate measures for deep venous thrombosis prophylaxis, such as intermittent compression stockings, thromboembolic device (TED) hose, or subcutaneous heparin, should be instituted whenever feasible.

PLATELET ABNORMALITIES

Platelet abnormalities fall into one of three broad categories: a paucity of platelets (thrombocytopenia), an overabundance of platelets (thrombocytosis), and dysfunctional platelet syndromes (thrombocytopathia). During the perioperative period, the vast majority of clinical platelet problems involve the first and last of these abnormalities, generally manifested as a coagulopathy.

Thrombocytopenia

Most commonly, the presence of a reduced platelet count during the perioperative period (< 100,000 per cubic millimeter) is secondary to blood loss and subsequent hemodilution. A recent study in which the transfusions consisted of adenosine-based packed red blood cells demonstrated that clinical bleeding was most closely associated with decreases in platelet counts to less than 70,000 per cubic millimeter after transfusions consisting of 0.6 to 1.0 patient blood volumes.

On occasion, patients may present either preoperatively or perioperatively with thrombocytopenia. In these cases, the causes may be secondary to the decreased production of platelets, increased platelet destruction, platelet sequestration, platelet loss, or a combination of these factors. Alcohol abuse is well known for its ability to depress megacaryotic production by bone marrow; it may also increase the incidence of sequestration, especially in the chronic alcoholic with cirrhosis and hypersplenism. Thrombocytopenia is also caused by the use of certain drugs. Table 4 lists those most commonly associated with thrombocytopenia.

The only significant consequence of thrombocytopenia is bleeding, which tends to be variable and intermittent; spontaneous bleeding rarely occurs until the platelet count decreases to less than 50,000 per cubic millimeter. While more serious bleeding occurs at counts of less than 10,000 to 20,000 per cubic millimeter, the severity of bleeding correlates poorly with platelet count, especially in chronic thrombocytopenia. Initial manifestations of thrombocytopenia are petechiae in skin or oral mucosa, along with cutaneous ecchymoses (purpura). More serious manifestations include epistaxis, gingival bleeding, hemorrhagic vesicles in mucus membranes, hematuria, menometrorrhagia, and gastrointestinal bleeding. Intracranial hemorrhage, that most dreaded of complications of thrombocytopenia, rarely occurs in the absence of other hemorrhagic manifestations.

Thrombocytopathia

When bleeding occurs in the presence of a normal prothrombin time, activated partial thromboplastin time, and quantitative platelet count (> 100,000 per cubic millimeter), the most common cause is a qualitative platelet abnormality. Qualitative platelet abnormalities are often not detected preoperatively because routine preoperative screening tests (prothrombin time, activated partial thromboplastin time, platelet count) of hemostasis are normal. Although there are reported cases of inherited qualitative platelet abnormalities, acquired abnormalities are much more routinely encountered. During the perioperative period, these are caused by drugs, uremia, liver disease, and cardiopulmonary bypass.

An increasingly large number of drugs, both over-the-counter and prescription, have been demonstrated to have both in vitro and in vivo platelet inhibitory activity. Aspirin ingestion, for example, is a common cause of dysfunctional platelets. In one survey, 52 percent of the patients presenting for emergency surgery had ingested some aspirin-containing compound within the previous 8 to 10 days. Ingestion of aspirin during pregnancy has been associated with significantly greater peripartum bleeding in both the mother and neonate. Preoperative ingestion of aspirin in patients undergoing cardiac surgery is clearly associated with greater blood loss. The effect of aspirin on platelets, because it is irreversible, may necessitate delaying an operative procedure with significant risk (e.g., craniotomy) for 7 to 10 days (the life span of the circulating platelets) from the time of last ingestion. When it is not possible to postpone a procedure, the use of platelet transfusions or the antidiuretic hormone analogue desmopressin acetate (DDAVP) may be indicated to control the bleeding tendency. The use of nonsteroidal anti-inflammatory drugs is somewhat controversial. Several studies of these agents during the perioperative period have shown no significant effect on bleeding time or perioperative blood loss. However, many investigators recommend discontinuing these agents 2 to 4 weeks before major operations. Other drugs that affect platelet function either in vivo or in vitro are listed in Table 5.

Another commonly encountered cause of acquired platelet dysfunction is uremia. The clinical manifestations of uremic bleeding include petechiae, epistaxis, and gastrointestinal bleeding. It is now commonplace to dialyze uremic patients just before the surgical procedure to correct volume status, hyperkalemia, and acidosis, and also to help reduce the risk of perioperative bleeding. Dialysis clearly reduces the risk of bleeding in approximately half of uremic patients, but there is no clear association between the degree of uremia and the bleeding tendency. Because platelet dysfunction with impaired platelet–blood vessel wall interaction appears to be the major cause of bleeding in uremia, increasing the circulating quantity of von Willebrand factor has been postulated to be beneficial. The increase in the bleeding time has been corrected by the use of cryoprecipitate and, most recently, DDAVP. The use of these agents during the perioperative period, in conjunction with dialysis, should significantly reduce surgical risk in patients with uremia.

Hypothermia, long believed subjectively to be associated with increased bleeding, has been recently shown in animal studies to cause a decrease in thromboxane production, which correlated with an increase in bleeding time. Warming the skin to normal temperature restored the bleeding time to normal. These data suggest that the effects of cardiopulmonary bypass on platelet function are at least partially mediated by the accompanying hypothermia. Depletion of von Willebrand factor may also have a role in this condition, as DDAVP has been used successfully to correct the bleeding diathesis in postbypass patients.

Platelet Transfusions

When platelets are administered to a patient with a quantitative or qualitative platelet defect, it is important to measure the increment in the measured platelet count and to evaluate the function as well as the survival time of the transfused cells. Survival measurements determine the required frequency of transfusion, while the initial platelet increment correlates most closely with the immediate clinical response. In recipients with thrombocytopenia, the platelet increment can be expected to be approximately 50 to 60 percent of the transfused num-

Table 5 Drugs That May Affect Platelet Function

Aspirin
Cephalosporins (especially moxalactam)
Dextrans
Dipyridamole
Ethanol
Methylxanthines (caffeine, aminophylline, theophylline)
Nitrofurantoin
Nitroglycerin
Nitroprusside
Nonsteroidal anti-inflammatory drugs (NSAIDs)
Penicillins (penicillin G, carbenicillin, ticarcillin, ampicillin)
Phenothiazines (chlorpromazine, promethazine, trifluoperazine)
Propranolol
Tricyclic antidepressants (amitryptiline, nortryptiline, imipramine)

ber, usually resulting in an increase in the measured platelet count of 5,000 to 10,000 per cubic millimeter per transfused unit in the average adult. Causes of reduced increments include hypersplenism, alloimmunization, fever and infection, and consumptive coagulopathy. Evaluation of function in vivo may be more difficult and is most simply done by repeated measures of the template bleeding time. Further research is needed to confirm the value of newer tests of primary hemostasis, such as the sonoclot and thromboelastography.

Controversy exists concerning the use of regional anesthesia in the patient with thrombocytopenia or thrombocytopathia. Although studies have shown safe administration of anesthetics to a few patients with HELLP (hemolysis, elevated liver [enzymes], low platelets) syndrome (counts of 40,000 to 70,000 platelets per cubic millimeter), most clinicians would defer spinal or epidural anesthesia if the platelet count is less than 100,000 per cubic millmeter. This number was cited as the minimum acceptable platelet count in a group of 61 parturients with peripartum thrombocytopenia who underwent epidural anesthesia without neurologic sequelae. Likewise, the presence of thrombocytopathia, which prolongs the template bleeding time beyond 12 minutes, may be considered a contraindication to major conduction blockade.

Thrombocytosis

Thrombocytosis, defined as a platelet count greater than 350,000 per cubic millimeter, is most frequently associated with heavy smoking, iron deficiency anemia, malignancy, postsplenectomy, and chronic inflammatory diseases such as rheumatoid arthritis. In these conditions, isolated thrombocytosis is not associated with an increased morbidity or mortality during the perioperative period. When platelet counts of 1,000,000 per cubic millimeter or more accompany a myeloproliferative disorder, thrombotic events may not only precipitate the surgery but may make the postoperative period more risky as well. Treatment of thrombocytosis associated with such disorders as polycythemia vera, primary thrombocythemia, agnogenic myeloid metaplasia, and others may involve phlebotomy, plateletpheresis, or chemotherapy. Thrombosis in these disorders tends to involve the large vessels, such as the splenic artery or vein, hepatic vein, or mesenteric artery. Plateletpheresis may result in rebound thrombocytosis within 24 to 72 hours, requiring repeated use until the perioperative period has passed or chemotherapy is effective.

PROBLEMS OF HEMOSTASIS

Hemostasis is a complicated process involving blood cells (primarily platelets), blood vessels, and blood factors derived from different tissues. One attempt to simplify problems in hemostasis has been to divide it into categories (Fig. 2). Surgical bleeding, the most common type of postoperative bleeding, is the simplest to deal with. With this type of bleeding, suture, cautery, ligature, and adjuncts such as fibrin glue, topical thrombin, gelatin foam, oxidase cellulose, and absorbable collagen hemostat provide surgical control of hemostasis, the discussion of which is beyond the scope of this chapter. Nonsurgical bleeding can be broken down into two broad categories: disorders of primary hemostasis (local vasoconstriction and formation of platelet plug) and

disorders of secondary hemostasis, which reaches its pinnacle in the formation of cross-linked fibrin. Disorders of primary hemostasis almost always involve platelet defects, which are discussed above. The bulk of this section focuses on disorders of secondary hemostasis, their evaluation, and their treatment.

Secondary hemostasis is a process best described as a cascade of biochemical interactions among a number of primarily hepatic and endothelial cell-derived factors. The interactions culminate in the production and eventual degradation or lysis of a fibrin clot. The balance between clot production and lysis is a process that is constantly being refined—not only within the body, but in our understanding of its intricacies. As biochemical and immunologic techniques have improved, the characterization of abnormalities in the coagulation cascade has likewise improved sufficiently to provide some understanding of the consequences of the inherited or acquired deficiencies of some of the components of this process. There are only three commonly encountered inherited coagulopathies: hemophilia A and B, and von Wille-

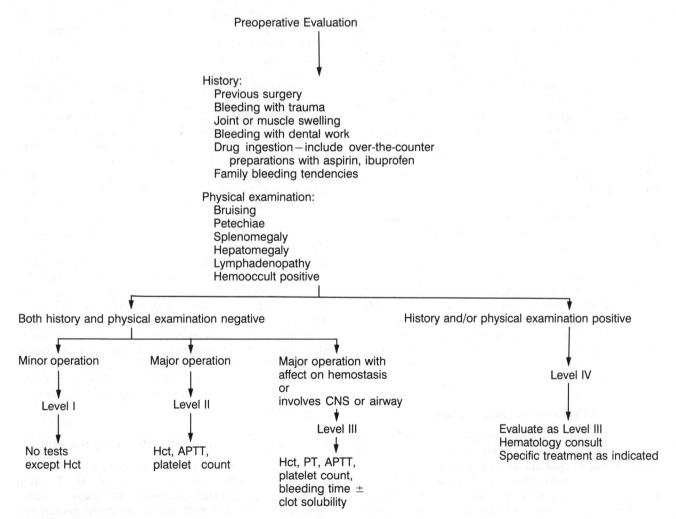

Figure 2 Hemostasis during the perioperative period. APTT = activated partial thromboplastin time; PT = prothrombin time. Modified from Rappaport.

brand disease. Although these patients deserve the expertise of a hematologist during the perioperative period, it is important for the anesthesiologist to appreciate the basics of managing these disorders.

Hemophilia A and B

Hemophilia A, or factor VIII deficiency, is a sex-linked hereditary disorder with a frequency of approximately one in 10,000 American men. Hemophilia B, or factor IX deficiency, has a reported incidence of 0.25 per 10,000 men. Approximately 30 percent of hemophilia A cases arise spontaneously. The frequency and severity of bleeding in most hemophiliacs corresponds with the biologic assay of the missing plasma factor.

Correction of the bleeding diathesis in the hemophiliac presenting for surgery should be achieved using a combination of factor-containing materials, assays for factor activity, coagulation profiles (prothrombin time/partial thromboplastin time/template bleeding time), and evaluation for circulating inhibitors. In severe factor VIII deficient patients, circulating inhibitors may make elective surgical procedures impossible. Inhibitors have been reported in 4 to 6 percent of factor VIII deficient patients, with the incidence reportedly as high as 20 percent in those with activity less than 1 percent of normal. Replacement therapy for hemophilia may be achieved with fresh frozen plasma (FFP), cryoprecipitate, or specific factor concentrates. FFP carries the risk of volume overload with amounts sufficient to achieve the desired 50 percent of normal activity. Cryoprecipitate has the disadvantage of possessing variable amounts of factor VIII activity. At the same time, it carries the relatively low risk of infectious agent transmission of FFP, because it is from a single donor. Lyophilized antihemophilic factor, while providing the most reliable and lowest volume titer of factor activity, carries the highest risk of infectious disease transmission because of its pooled origin. In a study of 42 hemophiliacs in Ohio, 31 had lymph node enlargement and/or splenomegaly; four died of opportunistic infections; three died of chronic hepatitis; one died of Burkitt's lymphoma; one died of non-Hodgkins lymphoma; and one died of primary pulmonary hypertension. While screening tests for HIV has minimized the risk of HIV infection in hemophiliacs, it is prudent to remain cautious in recommending administration of blood and body fluids during the perioperative period for the routine management of the patient with hemophilia.

von Willebrand Factor Deficiency

An autosomal dominant disorder, von Willebrand factor (vWF) deficiency usually presents as a prolonged bleeding time in a patient with a history of epistaxis, easy bruising, or excessive bleeding after tooth extraction. The incidence is estimated at seven in 100,000; however, mild forms of the disorder often escape clinical detection. It is one of few coagulation factors that is not

derived primarily from the liver; rather, it is derived from vascular endothelium.

The role of vWF in hemostasis is twofold. Its first role is to bind with factor VIII and maintain its presence in the circulation; the other is to facilitate the binding of platelets to collagen. Failure of the endothelium to secrete adequate quantities of vWF thus impairs primary as well as secondary hemostasis. There can be considerable variability in the amount of clinical bleeding with vWF deficiency, not only among patients, but at varying times in the same patient. Several types of vWF deficiency have been identified: type I, with a vWF antigen of 15 to 60 percent of normal; type III, with undetectable levels of antigen; and types IIa and IIb, in which there is a selective deficiency of the larger (bioactive) multimers of plasma vWF. There is also a pseudo–von Willebrand's disease, in which there is an abnormal affinity of platelets for vWF.

Preoperative evaluation and preparation of the patient with von Willebrand's disease should include a routine bleeding time (preferably Duke), prothrombin time, activated partial thromboplastin time, and determination of the specific type of deficiency. The risks of the operative procedure should also be evaluated. Platelet-active substances such as aspirin should be strictly avoided for 10 to 14 days before elective procedures. Management of prolonged bleeding times may include the use of cryoprecipitate (one to three bags per 10 kg of body weight per day) to reduce the Duke bleeding time to 5 minutes for large surgical procedures. For small procedures (e.g., dental extractions or hernia repair) in type I patients, the use of vWF-stimulating agent DDAVP may be adequate, especially when combined with a fibrinolysis inhibitor such as epsilon-aminocaproic acid (EACA). In a report of five patients given a single dose of DDAVP (0.3 µg per kilogram) along with EACA, excellent dental hemostasis was achieved. In another report, four patients underwent surgery (tonsillectomy, cystectomy, carpal tunnel release, and salpingo-oophorectomy) with DDAVP alone. These drugs provide the advantage of avoiding the infectious and immunologic risks of cryoprecipitate transfusion. It should be pointed out, however, that this therapy is reportedly useful only for type I patients; type II patients may not have enough endogenous vWF factor production to stimulate, and the vWF produced by type II patients may not be effective. One author also points out that DDAVP administration has been associated with mild thrombocytopenia in some instances; this may theoretically cause patients with pseudo–von Willebrand's disease to experience worsening bleeding if given DDAVP.

Other Causes of Perioperative Coagulopathy

The most common cause of perioperative coagulopathy in the face of normal platelet counts and function is hemodilution, usually secondary to massive transfusion. A recent study with adenosine-based packed red blood cells found that replacement of more than 1.5

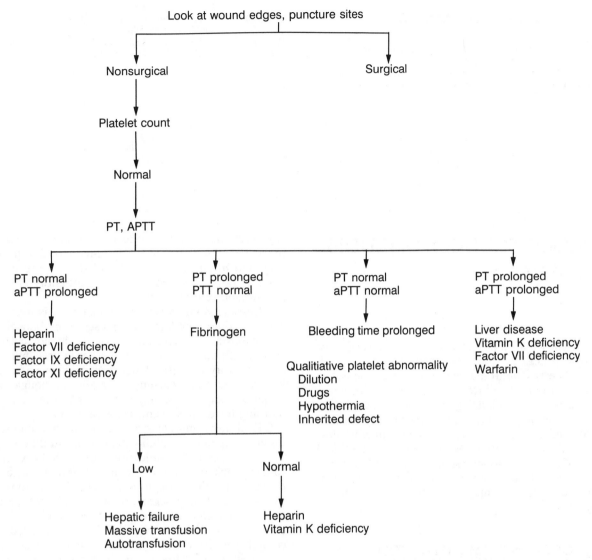

Figure 3 Intraoperative bleeding. aPTT = activated partial thromboplastin time; PT = prothrombin time; PTT = partial thromboplastin time.

blood volumes may be required before hemodilution is manifested as a nonsurgical coagulopathy. While the prothrombin time and activated partial thromboplastin time remain the most commonly used standard tests, it should be noted that these tests may exceed control values by 1.5 times without clinical evidence of coagulopathy. It is important in the massively transfused patient to consider the interaction of hypothermia, thrombocytopenia, and hemodilution before initiating factor replacement with fresh frozen plasma. As noted in Figure 3, measurement of the fibrinogen level may be indicated if both the activated partial thromboplastin time and prothrombin time are prolonged. If it is low, the best source of fibrinogen is cryoprecipitate.

Other commonly encountered causes of coagulopathy are liver disease and the administration of sodium warfarin (Coumadin). In these instances, patients clas-

sically present with an elevated prothrombin time with a normal activated partial thromboplastin time. FFP and/or vitamin K may be indicated for these conditions, depending on how urgently normal clotting parameters must be established. Heparin therapy results in a prolonged activated partial thromboplastin time; if urgent correction is needed, administration of protamine may be necessary, with the dosage being approximately 1 U of protamine per unit of heparin activity present. The dosage can be determined empirically or by using the activated clotting time. The significant incidence of anaphylactoid reactions to protamine should temper enthusiasm for its use. Heparin's effect is 2 to 4 hours without reversal.

As with red blood cell product administration, the rational approach to the bleeding patient can result in definitive therapy while minimizing risk.

SUGGESTED READING

Homi J, Reynolds J, Skinner A, et al. General anesthesia in sickle cell disease. Br Med J 1979; 1:1599–1601.
Sandler SG, Naiman JL, Fletcher JL. Alternative approaches to transfusion: autologous blood and directed blood donations. Prog Hematol 1987; 15:183–219.

Symposium: Current concepts in transfusion practice. Acta Anaesthesiol Scand 1988; 32(suppl):1–80.
Watson-Williams EJ. Hematologic and hemostatic considerations before surgery. Med Clin North Am 1979; 63:1165–1189.

NEUROMUSCULAR DISORDERS

CECIL O. BOREL, M.D.

Neuromuscular illnesses result from a variety of pathologic processes that can affect the spinal cord, peripheral nerves, neuromuscular junctions, or muscles. Thus, the perioperative care of patients with neuromuscular diseases is challenging, because these disease processes may all adversely affect respiratory, cardiovascular, and nutritional balance. Acute illness, anesthesia, and surgery often overwhelm the functional capacity of disturbed organ systems to respond to stress, and they unmask the severity of the underlying neuromuscular disorder that may have been underestimated preoperatively.

ORGAN SYSTEM DYSFUNCTION IN NEUROMUSCULAR DISEASE

Respiratory System Involvement

Breathing depends on effective skeletal muscle activity. While the extent of respiratory system involvement relies on the type, distribution, and duration of neuromuscular disease, ventilatory disability is often disproportionate to general muscle weakness. Thus, essential respiratory functions, such as inspiratory ventilatory effort, forced expiratory effort (cough), and maintenance of airway patency can be impaired even in a relatively strong patient.

The insidious loss of ventilatory reserve and inability to increase minute ventilation on demand are often the initial effects of impaired respiratory function in neuromuscular disease. Perioperative changes in lung function and increased metabolic rate frequently increase the work of breathing and result in respiratory muscle fatigue and ventilatory insufficiency. Early responses to increased inspiratory work include: (1) frequent changes in respiratory pattern in order to alternate work between primary muscles and accessory respiratory muscles and

(2) increasing respiratory rate to allow more efficient use of weakened muscles, resulting in increased inspiratory time and in an increased ratio of dead space to tidal volume. Both responses decrease ventilatory efficiency and worsen ventilatory failure.

Chronic ventilatory muscle weakness is associated with impaired ventilatory responses to carbon dioxide and hypoxia. The altered responses do not correlate closely with static pressures and other indirect measures of respiratory strength. Patients usually have a baseline hypercapnia that worsens at night. Although some patients complain of daytime somnolence and early morning headaches, many are asymptomatic.

Expiratory muscle dysfunction in neuromuscular disease impairs the ability to cough. Additionally, it further exacerbates reductions in forced expiratory capacity observed after abdominal and thoracic procedures. Impaired cough and retained secretions lead to collapse of lung segments and predispose patients to bacterial contamination and pneumonia. Microatelectasis has been implicated in the reduced lung compliance, decreased functional residual capacity, and increased work of breathing observed in patients with respiratory muscle dysfunction related to neuromuscular disease.

Impaired laryngeal and glottic muscle function occurs in patients with neuromuscular disease and, when severe, results in recurrent aspiration and airflow obstruction. Airway muscles, including those of the tongue, jaw, retropharynx, glottis, and larynx, can be affected by any neuromuscular disease process that affects respiratory muscles. Also, cranial nerves can be affected by neuromuscular disease processes specific to the brain stem or lower cranial nerves. The gag reflex results in constriction and elevation of the pharynx. It is mediated by the sensory fibers of the glossopharyngeal nerve synapsing in the nucleus ambiguus, which sends efferent fibers to the striated muscles of the pharynx. A decrease in the gag reflex because of a decreased sensation in the retropharynx or incompetent motor response leads to recurrent aspiration of pharyngeal contents. Residual anesthesia and persistent effects of muscle relaxants administered intraoperatively, which can result in postoperative aspiration and positional airway obstruction in normal patients, exacerbate upper airway muscle dysfunction in patients with neuromuscular disease.

Cardiovascular System Involvement

Cardiovascular involvement ranges from autonomic dysfunction with neuropathic diseases to myocardial failure with myopathic diseases. During the perioperative period, the cardiovascular response to anesthetics, blood loss, dehydration, and infection is hindered if the cardiovascular system is impaired by neuromuscular disease. Because of the broad dependence of the cardiovascular system on nerve and muscle function, patients with neuromuscular illness commonly have low cardiac reserve.

The autonomic nervous system regulates the heart rate, inotropic state, venous tone, and systemic vascular resistance. Heart rhythm is balanced by sympathetic and parasympathetic influences; cardiac arrhythmias ranging from sinus tachycardia to bradycardia and asystole occur when either system is impaired. Resting tachycardia and postural hypotension have been associated with intraoperative hemodynamic instability and the need for vasopressor therapy, and unexplained cardiorespiratory arrest during anesthesia has been reported to occur in patients with dysautonomia. Vasomotor dysfunction causes postural hypotension as a result of decreased vasoconstriction, or it may cause hypertension as a result of a hypersensitivity response to peripheral vasomotor paresis. Volume and electrolyte disorders frequently occur in dysautonomic diseases because the autonomic nervous system controls distribution of systemic blood flow, modulates blood volume by sodium retention through aldosterone release, and limits insensible loss of fluids from the sweat glands. Hypovolemia may be relative, the result of venous pooling, or it may be absolute, the result of increased insensible volume losses. Hypovolemia is a potent stimulus for the release of arginine vasopressin from the pituitary gland, which results in water retention and an increase in venous tone. Patients with dysautonomia frequently become hyponatremic during the perioperative period because of the combination of hypovolemia, arginine vasopressin release, stress, and volume replacement with hyponatremic solutions.

Myopathic diseases may involve cardiac muscle, resulting in congestive heart failure, complex cardiac arrhythmias, or the formation of a mural thrombus in the heart.

Nutritional Involvement

Appetite, deglutition, gastric emptying, intestinal motility, defecation, and metabolic requirements are affected to some degree in most patients with chronic neuromuscular diseases. Patients avoid eating or drinking when swallowing function is impaired. Paralytic ileus results in the loss of nutrient absorption from the intestine when the autonomic enervation to the gut is impaired. Protein energy malnutrition aggravates ventilatory dysfunction and probably increases the risk of wound dehiscence and infection. The role of preoperative nutritional support is controversial, but repletion therapy is probably beneficial since postoperative return to normal dietary intake is prolonged in patients with neuromuscular disease. Vagal damage during generalized demyelinating neural disorders may lead to delayed gastric emptying and disordered gastric acid secretion during times of perioperative stress.

PREOPERATIVE ASSESSMENT

Respiratory Function

Preoperative assessment of respiratory dysfunction in patients with neuromuscular disease requires assessment of oxygenation, ventilatory muscle function, and airway integrity (Table 1). Paradoxic inspiratory movement of the abdomen and rib cage (Fig. 1) and the use of the accessory ventilatory muscles suggest involvement of the diaphragm by neuromuscular disease. Forced vital capacity and inspiratory force measurements are useful in assessing overall ventilatory muscle strength. An increased carbon dioxide partial pressure (Pco_2) on baseline arterial blood gases implies a decreased ventilatory drive. A history of aspiration or positional airway obstruction suggests neuromuscular involvement of bulbar musculature. The patient's reaction to a small sip of

Table 1 Criteria for Preoperative Ventilatory Assessment

	Normal	*Borderline*	*Failure*
Oxygenation			
Saturation	>97% on room air	>95% on O_2	<95% on O_2
PO_2	>75 on room air	>75 on O_2	<75 on O_2
Chest x-ray atelectasis	None	Subsegmental	Lobar
Ventilation			
Blood gases	Normal Pco_2	$Pco_2 < 50$	$Pco_2 > 50$
	Normal pH	Normal pH	pH <7.37
Inspiratory force (cm H_2O)	<50	<30	>30
Vital capacity (ml)	>15/kg	10–15/kg	<10/kg
Airway			
Swallowing	Liquids and solids	Solids only	Aspirates
Breathing	Unobstructed	Positional	Obstruct

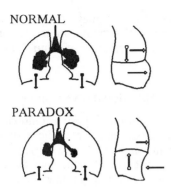

Figure 1 Inspiratory paradoxic motion of the diaphragm occurs when the abdomen moves inward during inspiration.

water may be used as a bedside assessment of swallowing capability.

Preoperative Plasma Exchange Therapy

The removal of circulating toxic substances is effected by physical separation of plasma from formed elements of the blood and subsequent reinfusion of the formed elements with a plasma replacement. Preoperative plasma exchange in patients with severe myasthenia gravis who are undergoing thymectomy reduces the need for postoperative mechanical ventilation, decreases time to extubation, and decreases the duration of the stay in the intensive care unit. Plasma exchange improves ventilatory function when used early in the course of the disease in patients with Guillain-Barré syndrome.

Cardiovascular Function

The extent and severity of autonomic dysfunction is difficult to assess noninvasively. Orthostatic hypotension, resting tachycardia, paralytic ileus, anhydrosis, and constricted pupils are all clinical signs of generalized autonomic dysfunction. The loss of beat-to-beat variability in the heart rate is probably the most sensitive indicator of autonomic cardiac involvement. The presence of clinical signs of dysautonomia may indicate profound hemodynamic instability from adrenergically active anesthetics or blocking drugs.

Cardiomyopathy from myopathic illness is relatively common, and preoperative history and assessment of the electrocardiogram, echocardiogram, and chest radiograph will identify most individuals with serious involvement. The standard electrocardiogram is the most reliable tool for diagnosing suspected cardiac involvement. Tall right precordial R waves and Q waves in leads I, aVL, and V5–6 are most characteristic. Conduction system abnormalities and arrhythmias are also frequent findings. Left ventricular dysfunction and mitral valve prolapse are frequently found on echocardiography. Determination of creatine phosphokinase (CPK) has long been used to identify active systemic myopathy, but it may not accurately detect myocardial dystrophy.

Nutritional Assessment

A history of weight loss, poor appetite, or difficulty swallowing should be sought during the preoperative period. Laboratory confirmation of hypoalbuminemia, anemia, hypocalcemia, and decreased transferrin levels suggest serious preoperative malnutrition that requires repletion therapy to prevent infection and improve wound healing.

NEUROMUSCULAR EFFECTS OF ANESTHETIC AGENTS

General Anesthesia

Inhalational anesthetics (halothane, enflurane, and isoflurane) suppress neuromuscular transmission and, at high concentrations, reduce the force of muscle contraction by as much as 50 percent. Because blood anesthetic levels decrease in normal patients, clinically important muscle weakness on emergence from anesthesia is not apparent. However, even low concentrations of residual inhalational anesthetics in patients with neuromuscular disease may prolong the return of baseline neuromuscular function postoperatively.

Muscle Relaxants

The perioperative effects of depolarizing and nondepolarizing muscle relaxants depend on the type of neuromuscular disease, and each class of drugs must be used cautiously (Table 2). Depolarizing relaxants, such as succinylcholine chloride, may cause pathologic muscle contracture and lethal hyperkalemia in patients with neuropathic muscle denervation. Succinylcholine increases serum potassium concentrations in normal patients, and the exaggerated release of intracellular potassium may produce lethal hyperkalemia in patients with denervated muscle. Pretreatment with nondepolarizing relaxants does not prevent succinylcholine-induced hyperkalemia, which develops approximately 3 weeks after an acute denervation injury. Consequently, depolarizing relaxants should be avoided in all patients with chronic motor neuropathy. Nondepolarizing muscle relaxants have normal effects in patients with denervated muscle, but the clinical response may be prolonged.

The intensity and duration of nondepolarizing relaxants is enhanced in patients with myasthenia gravis. While some anesthesiologists avoid administering nondepolarizing agents in these patients, other practitioners use small doses while carefully monitoring the extent of relaxation with train-of-four electrical stimulation. The effect of depolarizing relaxants in patients with defects of neuromuscular transmission is variable. Some patients are resistant to succinylcholine chloride, but others develop prolonged noncompetitive block. It is probably wise to avoid muscle relaxants in patients with myasthenia gravis.

Muscle relaxants have variable and unpredictable effects in patients with primary muscle diseases. Relax-

Table 2 Response to Muscle Relaxants in Neuromuscular Disease

Neuromuscular Dx	Nondepolarizing	Depolarizing
Muscular denervation	Normal	Hyperkalemia
Myasthenia gravis	Increased	Resistant
Myasthenic syndrome	Increased	Increased
Myotonia	Normal to increased	Spasticity
Muscular dystrophy	Normal to increased	Cardiac arrhythmia

ants have little effect on the muscle tone of diseased fibers, since the site of disease is distal to the neuromuscular junction. However, the response of normal muscle fibers may be exaggerated, and smaller doses of both depolarizing and nondepolarizing agents may be required. Abnormal contracture of facial and respiratory musculature in response to depolarizing agents in myotonic patients may both make orotracheal intubation impossible and impair mechanical ventilatory efforts.

Regional Anesthesia

Successful administration of major conduction anesthetics has been reported for a variety of neuromuscular diseases. No data exists to indicate that regional techniques combined with local anesthetics adversely affect the progression of neuromuscular diseases. Major conduction blockade also produces sympathectomy, which can exacerbate hypotension in patients with pre-existing autonomic dysfunction.

PREOPERATIVE ASSESSMENT OF SPECIFIC NEUROMUSCULAR DISEASE

Myelopathy

Amyotrophic Lateral Sclerosis

Amyotrophic lateral sclerosis (ALS) is characterized by degeneration of the lower motor neuron, motor nuclei of the brain stem, and the descending pathway of the upper motor neurons. Progressive muscular atrophy and bulbar muscle weakness with fasciculations are its clinical manifestations.

Atrophy and weakness of respiratory muscles eventually lead to ventilatory failure and death. The impairment of ventilatory musculature, especially airway muscles, affects anesthetic management. Aspiration is a clear danger during the perioperative period, when muscular deficits are exaggerated. Although respiratory reserve is reduced as a result of muscle weakness and skeletal deformity, the ventilatory drive is not impaired. The response to muscle relaxants, either depolarizing or nondepolarizing, is altered in ALS. Therefore, whenever possible, administration of muscle relaxants should be avoided. Epidural anesthesia has been safely conducted in several patients.

Multiple Sclerosis

Multiple sclerosis (MS) is a demyelinating disease of the brain and spinal cord. Various stressful situations, particularly those associated with elevated body temperature, exacerbate the symptoms of MS. Demyelinization of neural tissue can predispose patients to local anesthetic neurotoxicity. MS patients may have increased autonomic lability. For these reasons, spinal anesthesia is generally contraindicated. General anesthesia does not appear to pose an additional hazard to patients with MS.

Peripheral Neuropathy

Guillain Barré Syndrome

Guillain Barré is an inflammatory polyneuropathy that can affect all motor, sensory, autonomic, and cranial nerves. Ascending muscle weakness and the loss of deep tendon reflexes are the major clinical manifestations. Motor involvement may include ventilatory and facial musculature. Nerve conduction studies differentiate polyneuropathy from high cervical spinal cord lesions or transverse myelitis. Other causes of acute polyneuropathy, such as acute intermittent porphyria and heavy metal poisoning, must be excluded.

Respiratory failure in Guillain-Barré syndrome often begins with weakness of forced exhalation and impaired cough. Atelectasis leading to hypoxia may develop rapidly. Inspiratory muscle weakness usually develops later. Elevation of carbon dioxide tension portends rapidly progressive ventilatory failure. Abnormal swallowing and glottic dysfunction may occur at any time in the course of the disease.

Autonomic dysfunction frequently accompanies motor weakness in patients who progress to ventilatory failure. Sinus tachycardia and repolarization abnormalities are commonly observed on electrocardiogram. Intermittent bradyarrhythmias have resulted in death in some patients. Episodic hypertension and profound hypotension regularly occur in patients with severe disease. Continuous arterial blood pressure monitoring may be indicated, and pulmonary artery catheterization may assist fluid and pressor management.

Acute Intermittent Porphyria

Acute intermittent porphyria (AIP), an inherited disorder of porphyrin metabolism, is characterized by painful abdominal crises that mimic the acute abdomen. The ventilatory musculature and autonomic nervous system are often involved by the neuropathic process.

Barbiturates have been associated with enzyme induction that worsens the syndrome. Although it is rare for any anesthetic to induce symptoms during latent porphyria, both anesthesia and surgery appear to worsen an acute attack. Numerous anesthetics, including barbiturates, etomidate, enflurane, and methoxyflurane, have been shown to induce porphyrin synthesis. Ketamine and propofol have been used without adverse sequelae, and no harmful effects are expected to occur with the use of opiates, local anesthetics, nitrous oxide, or isoflurane. Adverse reactions to muscle relaxants, however, are associated with denervation sensitivity. Regional anesthetic techniques may be appropriate during an acute attack, although major conduction techniques risk interaction with the autonomic neuropathy commonly seen in porphyria.

Neuromuscular Junction Disease

Myasthenia Gravis

Myasthenia gravis is characterized by weakness and fatigability of skeletal muscles. Autoimmune-mediated reduction of the number of acetylcholine receptors at the neuromuscular junction results in the inability to sustain or repeat muscular contractions. Electromyographically, this abnormality corresponds to "fade" of muscle contraction observed during repetitive nerve stimulation after neuromuscular blockade with nondepolarizing muscle relaxants. Muscle strength improves similarly in both myasthenia gravis and nondepolarizing blockade after administration of anticholinesterase drugs. Glucocorticoids and regular plasma exchange are effective in patients with severe disease and ventilatory impairment. Thymectomy reduces symptoms in most patients with severe disease and causes total remission in some.

Preoperative preparation of patients with myasthenia gravis includes assessment of pulmonary mechanical functions such as forced vital capacity and negative inspiratory force, arterial blood gases, chest x-ray, and determination of upper airway competence. If severe abnormalities are encountered, surgery should be postponed to allow upward adjustment of anticholinesterase medication or plasma exchange therapy unless the patient is already receiving maximal medical therapy. Preoperative plasma exchange decreases the patient's time on mechanical ventilation and shortens the stay in the intensive care unit following thymectomy. Anticholinesterase medications should be continued until the morning of surgery.

The use of muscle relaxants should be avoided when possible because myasthenic patients are 10 to 100 times more sensitive to their effects than normal patients. If muscle relaxation is required, succinylcholine chloride may be the drug of choice for short-term management, but the onset of "phase II" block occurs at very low doses in these patients. The patient's return to preoperative

neuromuscular function is facilitated by resuming anticholinesterase medication before emergence from anesthesia. Intravenous infusion of neostigmine (Prostigmin) ($\frac{1}{60}$ of the usual daily oral dose of pyridostigmine bromide over 24 hours) should begin during wound closure. Mechanical ventilatory support should continue postoperatively until all criteria for adequate ventilatory function and airway patency are met. Postoperatively, patients with severe disease may improve muscle strength and ventilatory capacity after plasma exchange, and this therapy may shorten the time to tracheal extubation.

Myasthenic Syndrome (Eaton-Lambert Syndrome)

Unlike myasthenia gravis, myasthenic syndrome is characterized by muscles that may temporarily increase power during the first few contractions. Bulbar musculature is less likely to be involved. The response to anticholinesterase drugs is variable, but these patients are extremely sensitive to both depolarizing and nondepolarizing muscle relaxants.

Muscular Dystrophy

Muscular dystrophies, a group of primary muscular disorders of unknown cause, begin in childhood and pursue a rapid and progressive course to death. The incidence of serious perioperative complications in patients with muscular dystrophy is relatively low, because most surgical procedures are performed early in the course of these diseases.

Duchenne Muscular Dystrophy

Duchenne muscular dystrophy is the most common and severe syndrome. Cardiac muscle and the diaphragm are involved in the dystrophic process. Nondepolarizing muscle relaxants may result in either a normal or prolonged response. The response to depolarizing neuromuscular blockade may be normal, but cardiac arrest, possibly caused by hyperkalemia, has been reported after administration of succinylcholine chloride. Other arrhythmias, unrelated to drug therapy, have precipitated cardiac arrests during the immediate postoperative period.

Myotonic Dystrophy

Myotonia implies an abnormal persistence of induced or voluntary muscle contractions. The increased muscle tone may be caused by a generalized membrane defect in which muscle membranes have normal resting potentials but increased resistance to electrical conduction.

Respiratory and cardiac involvement complicate anesthetic management. Ventilatory dysfunction is characterized by swallowing difficulties and an altered ventilatory drive that elevate resting PCO_2. The degree of cardiac involvement does not correlate with the severity of skeletal muscle involvement. Death from cardiac arrhythmia is common in this group of patients; the electrocardiogram may reveal bradycardia and delayed intraventricular conduction. Hyperglycemia may result from a membrane-mediated resistance to insulin.

Anesthetic management can be complicated by the sensitivity of the patient to respiratory depressants and to the difficulty in assisting ventilation because of rigidity of the jaw and chest caused by respiratory muscle myotonic spasm. Succinylcholine chloride may induce rigidity. Although general anesthesia, spinal anesthesia, and depolarizing relaxant drugs cannot break a myotonic contracture, the response to nondepolarizing relaxants may be normal.

Myopathy

Central Core Disease

The importance of recognizing this myopathic disease is its association with malignant hyperthermia. It is essential to take all precautions to avoid malignant hyperthermia when anesthetizing patients with central core disease.

Proximal muscle weakness is a common feature of this disease and may be associated with secondary skeletal changes, such as hip dislocation, kyphoscoliosis, funnel chest, mandibular hypoplasia, and short neck. Bulbar and respiratory musculature is spared. The electrocardiogram is normal.

Glycogen Storage Diseases

This group of related illnesses is notable for the build-up of glycogen in muscle. This build-up results in a diffuse pattern of muscle weakness in which proximal muscles are often more involved than peripheral muscles. The muscles of ventilation may be severely involved, resulting in profound diaphragmatic weakness and ventilatory failure. Cardiomyopathy, which may also be present, can limit cardiac reserve. Anesthetic management should be planned to support ventilation in the perioperative period so that cardiac reserves are not stressed.

Familial Periodic Paralysis

The two forms of familial periodic paralysis are defined by serum potassium levels. In the hypokalemic form, weakness is exacerbated by carbohydrate or salt loading or from rest following strenuous exercise. Flaccid paralysis of voluntary muscle may last for as long as 36 hours, but bulbar and ventilatory musculature are spared. The severity of skeletal muscle weakness does not correlate well with serum potassium levels. Anesthesia and surgery may initiate an episode of weakness. Consequently, prolonged postoperative monitoring is indicated even after a benign intraoperative course. Since hypothermia or glucose and salt loading can precipitate an attack, careful intraoperative monitoring

of temperature and levels of glucose and electrolytes is important.

Attacks from hyperkalemic periodic paralysis tend to be of shorter duration and are often related to exercise and cold temperatures. The elevation of serum potassium may be mild and short-lived and may represent hypersensitivity of the muscle membrane to acetylcholine or mechanical stimulation. Glucose/insulin or calcium infusions can be used to treat the acute attack. Electrocardiographic monitoring and temperature monitoring are essential. Muscle relaxants should be avoided, since succinylcholine chloride can induce hyperkalemia, and neostigmine reversal of nondepolarizing muscle relaxants can induce myotonia from excessive acetylcholine elevation.

Malignant Hyperthermia

Malignant hyperthermia is the most feared and often lethal syndrome related to anesthetic drug administration. Inciting anesthetics trigger a hypermetabolic state that results in elevated temperature and diffuse rhabdomyolysis that is often associated with muscle rigidity. Rhabdomyolysis follows prolonged muscle rigidity and results in gross elevations in the levels of serum creatinine kinase and myoglobin. Disseminated intravascular coagulation and renal failure may occur during this time.

Other neurologic and myopathic illnesses have been associated with malignant hyperthermia. Except for central core myopathy, however, the association may be coincidental. Nevertheless, myopathic and neuropathic disorders appear to share pathogenic mechanisms with malignant hyperthermia, resulting in positive muscle contracture tests, and can result in clinical reactions during anesthesia. Caution should therefore be exercised during anesthesia with this group of patients.

Halogenated volatile anesthetics and succinylcholine chloride trigger the malignant hyperthermic response in susceptible individuals. Even so, a susceptible patient may have been previously anesthetized with triggering anesthetic drugs without a clinically apparent reaction. Any patient who appears to be at an increased risk for developing malignant hyperthermia must be managed carefully and with heightened awareness during anesthesia. Because of the effectiveness of nontriggering anesthetic techniques in avoiding malignant hyperthermic crisis, pretreatment with dantrolene is often unnecessary. A carefully administered nontriggering anesthetic will not induce the clinical syndrome, even in a patient with a history of a full-blown crisis. This approach depends on the expectation that prompt diagnosis and effective treatment with dantrolene are available whenever necessary.

SUGGESTED READING

Duncan PG. Neuromuscular diseases. In: Katz J, Steward DJ, eds. Anesthesia and uncommon pediatric diseases. Philadelphia: WB Saunders, 1987:509.

Azar I. The response of patients with neuromuscular disorders to muscle relaxants: a review. Anesthesiology 1984; 61:173–187.

Perloff JK. The heart in neuromuscular disease. Curr Prob Cardiol 1986; 11:509–557.

Vincken W, Elleker MG, Cosio MG. Determinants of respiratory muscle weakness in stable chronic neuromuscular disorders. Am J Med 1987; 82:53–58.

Gronert GA, Mott J, Lee J. Aetiology of malignant hyperthermia. Br J Anaesth 1988; 60:253–267.

THYROID, PARATHYROID, AND ADRENAL DISORDERS

DOUGLAS S. SNYDER, M.D., M.S.
LUCILLE W. KING, M.D.
MICHAEL J. BRESLOW, M.D.

HYPERTHYROIDISM

Hyperthyroidism, characterized by the increased production of triiodothyronine (T_3) and/or tetraiodothyronine (T_4), is generally manifested by signs and symptoms of excess thyroid hormone. The findings may be subtle or profound; one may observe anything from listlessness, apathy, or weight loss, to obvious sweating, vasodilation, and tachycardia. Successful management is predicated on establishing the diagnosis, which can be particularly difficult to make in the elderly with apathetic hyperthyroidism. Patients are typically women between the ages of 20 and 40 years. Hyperthyroidism most often causes a hyperdynamic state, manifested by increased cardiac output, tachycardia, or arrhythmia. These changes appear to be caused by thyroid hormone alone; serum catecholamines are not increased, and the cardiovascular response to catecholamines is unaltered.

The most dangerous complication of hyperthyroidism in surgical patients is thyroid storm, which usually develops 6 to 18 hours postoperatively and may last for several days. In older studies, thyroid storm occurred in 10 to 32 percent of unprepared hyperthyroid surgical patients and was associated with a high mortality rate. Historically, treatment of thyroid storm with iodine alone resulted in a mortality rate of 60 to 70 percent; the addition of steroids and beta-adrenergic–blocking agents has reduced mortality to 25 percent. Although propranolol is effective in controlling heart rate, it does not reliably prevent thyroid storm. Manifestations of thyroid storm include hyperpyrexia, tachycardia, and severe hypotension. In addition to reducing thyroid hormone levels and blocking their systemic effects, emergency supportive strategies include fluid therapy, administration of oxygen, and mechanical cooling devices. Because aspirin displaces T_4 from binding proteins, it should be avoided.

Many regimens are available for preoperative preparation of the hyperthyroid patient; if at all possible, the patient should be euthyroid before any elective surgical procedure is performed. Propylthiouracil (PTU), iodine, hydrocortisone, and beta-adrenergic–blockers decrease thyroid hormone levels or block peripheral effects. One hundred to 300 mg of PTU orally every 8 hours blocks oxidation, organification, and coupling of thyroid hormone and also blocks the peripheral conversion of T_4 to T_3. PTU generally produces clinical improvement within 1 to 2 weeks and a euthyroid state within 6 to 7 weeks. After PTU is started, saturated solutions of potassium iodide (SSKI, 40 mg per drop), five drops orally three times daily, can be added to block thyroid hormone release and inhibit organification. Sodium iodide, 1 g intravenously every 8 to 12 hours, can be substituted for SSKI. Hydrocortisone, 100 mg intravenously every 8 hours, decreases extrathyroidal T_3 production and protects against possible decreased adrenal reserve. Propranolol or other beta-blockers (such as esmolol) can be administered orally or intravenously and titrated against heart rate. While beta-adrenergic blockade can be hazardous in patients with congestive heart failure, cardiac function can actually improve in the profoundly tachycardic patient. If beta-blockade is not tolerated, reserpine or guanethidine may be substituted. Preoperative examination of the hyperthyroid patient must include a careful evaluation of the airway for tracheal compression or deviation by a large goiter, which could make intubation difficult. Indirect laryngoscopy, both preoperatively and postoperatively, is useful to document normal vocal cord movement.

Anesthetic management is based on theoretic considerations; preoperative and intraoperative drugs that exacerbate the effects of elevated thyroid hormones should be avoided. Atropine, for example, may prevent sweating, and both cyclopropane and ether increase serum catecholamines that could worsen a baseline hyperdynamic state. Drugs that undergo extensive biotransformation into toxic substances, such as methoxyflurane, are best avoided. Controversy exists as to whether hyperthyroid patients are at increased risk for developing volatile anesthetic-induced hepatotoxicity. Rats pretreated with T_3 and anesthetized with enflurane or halothane in 21 percent oxygen develop centrilobular hepatic necrosis. Hyperthyroid patients have been found to have a higher incidence of postoperative elevation of lactate dehydrogenase (LDH) levels but do not appear to have an increased incidence of postoperative hepatic dysfunction. However, large, well-controlled, prospective trials are lacking. Special attention to eye care intraoperatively is important to prevent corneal ulceration, since 5 percent of hyperthyroid patients have proptosis.

HYPOTHYROIDISM

Hypothyroidism, characterized by a deficiency of thyroid hormone, is often an insidious disease and requires a high index of suspicion. Among the adult population, 0.5 to 0.8 percent have documented hypothyroidism, but undiagnosed or untreated disease probably occurs more frequently. Forty to 50 percent of cases are caused by previous thyroid resection or radioactive iodine treatment. Symptoms include lethargy, intolerance to cold, constipation, and apathy; the physical examination may reveal periorbital edema, lateral thinning of eyebrows, brittle hair, goiter, hypothermia, and bradycardia. Among the various manifestations of hypothyroidism, only prolongation of the relaxation phase of deep tendon reflexes, husky voice, and dry skin have been found to be statistically predictive. Cardiomegaly, pleural effusion, ascites, and peripheral edema can mimic congestive heart failure. The association of spontaneous hypothermia, hypoventilation, congestive heart failure, and decreased consciousness suggests the presence of myxedema coma. Diagnosis is confirmed by appropriate laboratory testing; patients with subclinical disease often have normal T_4 levels and mildly elevated thyroid-stimulating hormone (TSH) levels, whereas patients with overt disease usually have markedly reduced T_4 levels and elevated TSH levels.

Depressed myocardial function can be seen with hypothyroidism. Decreases in cardiac output are caused by both bradycardia and reduced stroke volume. Myxedematous infiltration of the myocardium, alterations in sarcoplasmic reticulum function, and reduced myosin ATPase activity may all contribute to decreased contractility. Although reversible conversion of beta-adrenergic receptors to alpha-adrenergic receptors occurs in hypothyroidism, there is no direct evidence for reduced cardiac responsiveness to exogenous catecholamines. Despite evidence of subnormal cardiac function, hypothyroidism is rarely responsible for overt heart failure and its presence is suggestive of underlying heart disease. Sixty percent of patients with overt hypothyroidism develop protein and mucin-rich pericardial effusions; however, tamponade is rare because of the gradual rate of fluid accumulation. Electrocardiographic changes in hypothyroidism include sinus bradycardia, flattening or inversion of T waves in lead II, and low amplitude P, QRS, and T waves. Careful preoperative assessment of cardiovascular function and reserve is required in hypothyroid patients.

Pulmonary function is also impaired in hypothyroid patients. Hypoxic and hypercapnic ventilatory drives are often markedly depressed. Mechanical strength is usually normal, although reversible reduction of maximal breathing capacity and diffusing capacity occurs in some overtly hypothyroid patients. Respiratory failure associated with myxedema is usually associated with obesity, unrelated intrinsic lung disease, or coma.

Other abnormalities seen in hypothyroid patients include (1) increased sensitivity to drugs that depend on metabolic transformation for their elimination (e.g., narcotics); (2) hyponatremia caused by impaired free water clearance; (3) adynamic ileus; and (4) delayed gastric emptying. Hypothyroid patients are also prone to develop hypoglycemia, anemia, and hypothermia. Finally, concomitant adrenal insufficiency occurs in some hypothyroid patients. If unrecognized, this can result in perioperative cardiovascular instability. Although plasma levels of T_3, T_4, and TSH are corrected fairly quickly following institution of thyroid hormone replacement, reversal of organ-specific abnormalities can be surprisingly slow. Abnormal muscle biopsies have been noted 7 to 15 months after initiation of replacement therapy. Recovery of hypoxic ventilatory drive is variable and depends on the severity of the initial disease process. In one study, mildly hypothyroid patients demonstrated normal responsiveness to hypoxia in 3 weeks, whereas this required 3 to 6 months in myxedematous patients; hypercapnic ventilatory response did not improve with hormonal replacement. A single, intravenous bolus of T_4 produces peak increases in the basal metabolic rate within 10 to 12 days. An intravenous bolus of T_3 increases the basal metabolic rate more quickly, usually within 36 to 72 hours. A large intravenous dose of T_3, however, can exceed tissue storage capacities and transiently elevate plasma levels sufficiently to cause cardiovascular complications, including angina, arrythmias, and sudden death. When thyroid hormone must be given intravenously, as for the treatment of myxedema, small doses of T_4 should be used.

Untoward events associated with anesthesia and surgery in the hypothyroid patient include hypotension, cardiac arrest, and increased sensitivity to drugs, with prolonged unconsciousness and coma. Establishing a euthyroid state in patients before elective surgery is therefore generally recommended. In a retrospective study of hypothyroid patients undergoing surgery, there was a higher prevalence of risk factors such as hypertension and anemia, but because there was no difference in the incidence of intraoperative or postoperative complications, the authors concluded it was safe to proceed with surgery in mild-to-moderate hypothyroidism. The advisability of performing an operation in patients with severe hypothyroidism could not be addressed due to their limited number. By contrast, a prospective analysis of perioperative outcome reported an increased incidence of intraoperative hypotension and heart failure in hypothyroid patients. Postoperatively, these patients were found to have a higher incidence of gastrointestinal and neuropsychiatric problems and a lower incidence of fever despite comparable rates of infection.

The hypothyroid patient with symptomatic coronary artery disease who is scheduled to undergo coronary artery bypass presents a unique challenge, since establishing euthyroidism can exacerbate ischemia. Medical management of patients with coexisting hypothyroidism and coronary artery disease has proven ineffectual in controlling ischemic symptoms or hypothyroidism, suggesting that perhaps coronary artery bypass should assume a dominant role in management. In a small study of patients with incapacitating angina and severe hypothyroidism, uneventful perioperative courses were noted when limited thyroid replacement was administered before coronary revascularization, and full replacement was achieved after surgery. Similarly, no perioperative morbidity or mortality was observed in a small study of untreated hypothyroid patients undergoing coronary artery bypass surgery, whereas almost 50 percent of patients who received thyroid replacement preoperatively suffered myocardial infarctions.

Based on the above data, careful management of patients with mild-to-moderate hypothyroidism should result in a safe and uneventful perioperative course. Preoperative neutralization of gastric acid with H_2 antagonists or the use of agents that increase gastric emptying may reduce the risk associated with pulmonary aspiration of gastric contents. Slow induction of anesthesia with cricoid pressure may be safer than a rapid-sequence induction, because the former technique may result in less hypotension and provide some protection of the airway. Care should be taken to avoid inadvertent hypocarbia during controlled ventilation, since carbon dioxide production is reduced at low metabolic rates. While prospective studies are lacking, no anesthetic agent or technique has been shown to be superior in the management of the hypothyroid patient. Dosages of sedatives and narcotic drugs need to be titrated to desired clinical effects to minimize prolonged postoperative depression. Despite the general clinical impression that intraoperative anesthetic requirements are reduced, hypothyroidism does not appear to affect the dose of potent inhalation anesthetics necessary to prevent skeletal muscle responses to noxious stimuli. However, volatile agents may cause excessive hypotension as a result of underlying myocardial depression, attenuated baroreceptor function, and hypovolemia. Careful observation of hemodynamic parameters and early recognition of congestive heart failure are therefore very important. Defective thermogenic mechanisms increase susceptibility to hypothermia; since hypothermia has been associated with increased mortality in hypothyroid patients, every effort should be made to prevent the loss of body heat intraoperatively.

In summary, hypothyroid patients are probably more sensitive than normal individuals to the adverse effects of anesthetic agents. Careful management of patients with mild-to-moderate hypothyroidism should result in a good outcome if preoperative replacement therapy is not possible or advisable. Existing data concerning outcome in severely hypothyroid patients are inadequate. These patients should be considered to be at high risk, and only truly emergent procedures should be performed before correction of thyroid insufficiency is undertaken.

HYPERPARATHYROIDISM

Hyperparathyroidism is characterized by the increased secretion of parathyroid hormone (PTH). Primary hyperparathyroidism usually causes hypercalcemia and hypophosphatemia. It may be detected in asymptomatic patients because of elevated serum calcium levels on routine screening tests or can present with findings such as mental status changes, bone pain, or recurrent nephrolithiasis. Incidence approaches two per 1,000 individuals per year in the older (age >60 years) female population; in the older male population, the incidence is half that of this female population, and it is even lower in younger populations. Eighty-five percent of cases involve a single gland (81 percent adenoma, 4 percent carcinoma), while 15 percent involve hyperplasia of all glands (usually chief-cell hyperplasia). Six to 10 percent of patients have ectopic parathyroid adenomas located in the thymus, thyroid, and pericardium, or behind the esophagus. Hyperparathyroidism may be a component of Multiple Endocrine Neoplasia type I or II.

Signs and symptoms of hyperparathyroidism are secondary to hypercalcemia. Renal complications are most common, due to either calcium deposition in renal parenchyma or recurrent nephrolithiasis, which may lead to urinary tract obstruction and repeated bouts of infection. Polyuria, reversible acute renal insufficiency, interstitial nephritis, and nephrosclerosis have all been reported. Changes in glomerular filtration and tubular function can lead to loss of sodium, dehydration, and hyperuricemia. Hyperchloremic acidosis may also develop. Chronic hypercalcemia may cause hypertension, particularly in the setting of advanced renal failure. Hypercalcemia is associated with increased myocardial contractility and shortening of the QT interval. Decreased myocardial automaticity, atrioventricular block, atrial fibrillation, ventricular extrasystoles, and ventricular tachycardia have also been described, and the effects of digitalis preparations are potentiated. Despite these reports, several studies have found no significant perioperative ventricular arrhythmias in surgical patients with mild hypercalcemia. Classic skeletal abnormalities of hyperparathyroidism include osteitis fibrosa cystica and severe osteopenia, although these are uncommon. Pseudogout and chondrocalcinosis are also associated with primary hyperparathyroidism. Central nervous system manifestations may range from mild personality disturbances to psychiatric disorders, mental obtundation, or coma. Reversible proximal muscle weakness, easy fatigability, and atrophy are also seen. Abdominal pain, nausea, and anorexia are common, and peptic ulcer (with Multiple Endocrine Neoplasia type I and associated Zollinger-Ellison syndrome) and pancreatitis may occur.

Because of the range and subtlety of manifestations of hypercalcemia, a high index of suspicion is often required to make the diagnosis of hyperparathyroidism. Immunoassay of PTH is increasingly useful, but may detect inert fragments. The differential diagnosis of hypercalcemia is large, and malignancies and other serious illnesses must be excluded. The reader is referred to standard endocrine texts for further discussion of the topic.

Secondary hyperparathyroidism, characterized by a compensatory increase in PTH, can develop in any illness associated with hypocalcemia. Secondary hyperparathyroidism occurs in patients with some forms of osteomalacia, pseudohypoparathyroidism (a hereditary disorder caused by deficient end-organ response to PTH), and chronic renal disease, as well as with malabsorption and decreased vitamin D metabolism. Tertiary hyperparathyroidism refers to hypercalcemia that follows correction of the stimulus for PTH secretion in patients with secondary hyperparathyroidism (e.g., renal transplantation); this hypercalcemia is mild and transient, reflecting a lack of adaptation of hyperactive parathyroid glands.

Preoperative preparation includes correction of intravascular volume depletion and electrolyte problems, and attention to potential renal, cardiac, and central nervous system involvement. Volume depletion is to be expected because of pre-existent anorexia, vomiting, and urinary concentrating defects associated with hypercalcemia. Patients may also have potassium and magnesium depletion. The choice of therapy depends on the underlying disease, the severity of the hypercalcemia, the serum inorganic phosphate level, and renal, hepatic, and bone marrow function. Mild hypercalcemia (serum calcium level of < 12 mg per deciliter) can usually be managed by hydration with normal saline and small doses of furosemide. Sodium infusion inhibits the absorption of calcium in the proximal tubule and increases its delivery to the loop of Henle, and diuretics such as furosemide prevent its reabsorption and promote calciuresis. Rehydration alone may lower serum calcium by 2 mg per deciliter. Severe hypercalcemia (>15 mg per deciliter) requires rapid correction. Aggressive hydration and diuresis (e.g., up to 6 L of saline per day, with up to 100 mg of intravenous furosemide every 1 to 2 hours) are effective but should be undertaken only with careful monitoring and when cardiac function is adequate. Correction of hypophosphatemia is also important; hypophosphatemia increases gastrointestinal absorption of calcium, stimulates the breakdown of bone, and impairs uptake of calcium by bone. Low serum phosphate impairs cardiac contractility and may cause skeletal muscle weakness, hemolysis, and platelet dysfunction. Oral phosphate therapy (recommended dosage of 1 g of phosphate phosphorus per day in four divided doses) is preferred over intravenous therapy except in extreme emergencies, because of the risk of causing hypocalcemia and metastatic calcification. Glucocorticoids (recommended dosage of 40 to 100 mg of predisone daily in divided doses) inhibit intestinal absorption of calcium and increase urinary calcium excretion. Calcitonin reduces osteoclast activity and number, thereby inhibiting bone resorption. Calcitonin is administered either by intravenous, intramuscular, or subcutaneous injection, in a dose of 25 to 50 U every 6 to 8 hours. Calcium is usually reduced

within 1 to 2 hours; 25 to 50 percent of patients develop resistance with prolonged use. Mithramycin inhibits osteoclast activity. Its onset of action is 6 to 12 hours, with a duration of up to 6 days, and the usual dose is 25 μg per kilogram administered intravenously over 4 to 24 hours. Because this drug has toxic side effects, including bone marrow suppression, nephrotoxicity, and hepatic necrosis, its use is usually limited to patients with hypercalcemia secondary to malignancy.

Surgery is considered the treatment of choice for primary hyperparathyroidism since it prevents subsequent osteoporosis. However, in elderly, high-risk patients with cardiovascular or pulmonary disease, medical management may be preferable, particularly if serum calcium levels are less than 11 mg per deciliter. There are several reports of parathyroid surgery being performed with the patient under local or regional anesthesia; obviously, positive localization with ultrasonography, radionuclide scanning, computed tomography, or parathyroid venous sampling is important. With surgery, hypercalcemia resolves in 95 percent of cases; permanent hypocalcemia develops in less than 5 percent. Re-exploration has a success rate of up to 72 percent, and the risk of postoperative hypoparathyroidism approaches 30 percent.

Serum calcium declines within 24 to 48 hours after successful surgery, generally stabilizing in the low-to-normal range for 4 to 5 days, until remaining parathyroid tissue resumes hormone secretion. Increased phosphorus clearance usually occurs 3 days postoperatively. Fifty percent of patients develop postoperative hypocalcemia which may, in part, be related to hemodilution. Severe postoperative hypocalcemia is more common in patients with severe preoperative bone resorption, high serum alkaline phosphatase levels, renal impairment, and vitamin D deficiency ("hungry bone syndrome"). For mild asymptomatic hypocalcemia, oral calcium supplements should suffice; for severe hypocalcemia, intravenous calcium is required. The rate and duration of supplementation is determined by the severity of symptoms and the patient's response to therapy. Patients can rarely develop stridor resulting from hypocalcemia-induced laryngospasm.

No evidence exists that any specific anesthetic technique is preferable in these patients. Although inorganic fluoride ion derived from enflurane metabolism can cause a transitory hyperparathyroidism, the clinical significance of this finding has not been established. Monitoring neuromuscular function is important; increased sensitivity to succinylcholine has been reported, as has a reduced response to atracurium. Careful positioning of the patient during surgery is recommended to avoid pathologic bone fractures in osteopenic patients. Since the head and neck are generally elevated during parathyroid surgery, a risk of venous air embolism exists. Pneumothorax, hemodynamic disturbances caused by carotid sinus manipulation, and phrenic nerve and lymphatic duct injury can occur.

As in other surgeries involving the neck, bleeding can lead to airway compromise. The recurrent laryngeal nerve is also subject to injury. Unilateral nerve injury may present as hoarseness; recovery usually occurs within several weeks and, frequently, no intervention is required. By contrast, bilateral recurrent laryngeal nerve injury, which is rare, often requires immediate intubation to stabilize the airway. Routine preoperative and postoperative indirect laryngoscopic examination is recommended to rule out nerve injury, especially if the patient has undergone prior neck surgery.

HYPOPARATHYROIDISM AND OTHER HYPOCALCEMIC STATES

Hypoparathyroidism, a deficiency of PTH production, is characterized by hypocalcemia and resultant neuromuscular symptoms. Postoperative hypoparathyroidism is probably the most common form, resulting from excision of the parathyroid glands or damage to their vascular supply during surgery for thyroid disorders, hyperparathyroidism, or radical neck dissection for cancer. Symptoms may develop at any point from several days to months and even to years after surgery. Other causes include neck trauma, granulomatous diseases, infiltrating processes (malignancy, amyloidosis), and treatment with radioactive iodine for thyroid disease. Hypocalcemia also occurs with pseudohypoparathyroidism, a hereditary disorder characterized by end-organ resistance to PTH. These patients have characteristic skeletal and developmental defects, may be mentally retarded, and have an increased incidence of diabetes and hypothyroidism. Patients with pseudopseudohypoparathyroidism have these same abnormalities but are not hypocalcemic. Hypomagnesemia (magnesium level <0.8 mEq per liter) occasionally causes hypocalcemia by suppressing secretion and impairing peripheral responsivity to PTH. In patients with renal insufficiency, hypocalcemia is usually caused by phosphate retention and impaired synthesis of 1,25-dihydroxycholecalciferol. The etiology of hypocalcemia associated with burns and pancreatitis is less clear; suppression of PTH secretion has been described.

Symptoms of hypocalcemia are primarily related to increased neuromuscular irritability. Tetany and convulsions are the most serious complications. Latent tetany can often be demonstrated by tapping the facial nerve and producing a contraction of the facial muscles (Chvostek's sign) or by eliciting carpopedal spasm by inflating an arm tourniquet for approximately 3 minutes (Trousseau's sign). Patients may exhibit fatigue, depression, paraesthesias, or skeletal muscle cramps. Acute hypocalcemia can present with stridor or apnea. Hypotension and congestive heart failure have been associated with hypocalcemia; a relative insensitivity to the effects of beta-adrenergic agonists has also been reported. Delayed ventricular repolarization contributes to a prolongation of the QT interval on the electrocardiogram. Although this may be a reliable sign for serial assessment in an individual patient, it is relatively insensitive for the detection of hypocalcemia.

The general objective of treatment is to restore calcium levels toward normal preoperatively by using supplemental dietary calcium and vitamin D. To treat chronic hypoparathyroidism, the recommended dose of oral elemental calcium is 1.5 to 2 g (as lactate, gluconate, or carbonate salts) with 50,000 IU of vitamin D per day (range 25,000 to 200,000 IU per day). For maximal response to therapy to be achieved, 2 to 4 weeks or longer may be required. (By contrast, simple vitamin D deficiency can be treated with as little as 100 IU of vitamin D per day.) Severe symptoms often require treatment with calcium gluconate (10 to 20 ml of a 10 percent solution administered intravenously over several minutes, followed by a continuous infusion of 1 to 2 mg per kilogram per hour of elemental calcium). These patients require close monitoring of serum calcium concentrations and clinical status. Few data exist concerning anesthetic management. Hypocalcemia can cause neuromuscular blockade, probably secondary to reduced acetylcholine release from the neuromuscular junction and decreased sensitivity of the motor end-plate to depolarization. Alkalosis reduces ionized calcium and may cause tetany, especially with underlying hypocalcemia. Several cases of tetany occurring with the patient under general anesthesia have been reported; the diagnosis is commonly inadvertent, with Trousseau's sign being observed after the blood pressure has been taken repetitively by cuff. Respiratory alkalosis (hyperventilation) and intravenous hydration (dilutional hypocalcemia) are often contributory. Neonatal tetany has a peak incidence during the first 2 weeks of life, and is associated with gastrointestinal conditions. As a latent condition in patients that may necessitate surgery, it has been reported to contribute to the development of frank tetany during general anesthesia. Occlusion of the endotracheal tube due to tetany-induced masseteric spasm has been reported. In such cases, intravenous succinylcholine effected immediate relaxation of the jaws. Other effective treatments include intravenous calcium gluconate and, theoretically, reversing hyperventilation; administering an acidifying agent or increasing the inspired concentration of carbon dioxide has also been recommended. Muscle relaxants should be administered conservatively under the guidance of neuromuscular blockade monitoring. Because severe hypocalcemia may cause heart failure or render the heart insensitive to digoxin, the patient's myocardial status must be closely monitored throughout anesthesia.

ADRENAL INSUFFICIENCY SECONDARY TO STEROID THERAPY

It is standard dogma that patients receiving long-term steroid therapy are at risk for acute adrenal insufficiency during the perioperative period unless appropriate steroid coverage is provided. This section addresses the following issues: (1) the duration of steroid therapy that produces suppression of the hypothalamic-pituitary-adrenal (HPA) axis; (2) the time course of recovery of the HPA axis after withdrawal of steroid therapy; (3) the evaluation of the HPA axis; and (4) the guidelines for perioperative glucocorticoid coverage.

Although it is impossible to define precisely the shortest duration or the smallest dose of steroids that will produce HPA suppression, suppression clearly can develop early after exogenous steroid administration. One study found that the cortisol response to insulin-induced hypoglycemia and adrenocorticotropic hormone (ACTH) administration was significantly reduced in healthy male volunteers who had received prednisone, 25 mg twice daily, for only 2 days. It is generally recommended that patients taking the equivalent of 20 to 30 mg of prednisone daily for more than 1 week should be considered to be at risk for having HPA suppression and for developing adrenal insufficiency during the perioperative period.

The duration of HPA axis suppression after steroid therapy is variable, but may persist for 12 months. Hypothalamic-pituitary function is the first component of the HPA axis to return to normal after chronic suppression; this is followed by the return of adrenocortical function. Therefore, the demonstration of normal adrenocortical responsiveness indicates HPA axis recovery. The intravenous ACTH stimulation test is a safe, simple, and reliable means of evaluating adrenocortical function preoperatively in patients who have received prior glucocorticoid therapy. Cortisol responses to 250 μg of exogenous ACTH correlate well with maximal cortisol levels during anesthesia and surgery; perioperative cortisol secretion will likely be normal if a normal adrenal response to ACTH stimulation is demonstrated preoperatively.

If such preoperative testing cannot be done, it must be assumed that the patient who received high-dose glucocorticoid treatment for 2 to 3 weeks during the preceding year is at risk for developing adrenocortical insufficiency during surgical stress. The current recommended schedule for corticosteroid supplementation is outlined in Table 1. The recommended dose of 300 mg of hydrocortisone daily is based on approximations of the maximal daily glucocorticoid output of the adrenal glands rather than on studies that critically assess actual requirements during stress. Recent studies suggest that

Table 1 Glucocorticoid Coverage Schedule for Surgery

1. Hydrocortisone phosphate or hemisuccinate, 100 mg IM, on call to the operating room.
2. Hydrocortisone phosphate or hemisuccinate 50 mg IM or IV in recovery room and every 6 hours for the next three doses.
3. Decrease to 25 mg every 6 hours for 24 hours if postoperative recovery is satisfactory.
4. Taper to maintenance dosage over next 3 to 5 days.
5. Increase cortisol dosage to 200 to 400 mg over 24 hours if fever, hypotension, or other complications occur.

Republished with permission from Baxter JD, Tyrell JB. The adrenal cortex. In: Felig P, Baxter JD, Broadus AE, et al, eds. Endocrinology and metabolism. McGraw-Hill: New York, 1981:462.

less hydrocortisone, perhaps only normal replacement doses (equivalent to 25 mg of hydrocortisone per day), may be adequate to prevent Addisonian crisis during the perioperative period.

In summary, patients may have suppression of the HPA axis if they have received supraphysiologic dosages of glucocorticoids for 2 to 3 weeks within the past 12 months. The ACTH stimulation test accurately and reliably assesses the integrity of the HPA axis since responsiveness of the adrenal gland is the last component of the HPA axis to recover. Patients who are shown to be or who are suspected of being adrenally insufficient should receive glucocorticoid coverage during the perioperative period.

SUGGESTED READING

Axelrod L. Glucocorticoid therapy. Medicine 1976; 55:39–65.

Edis AJ. Prevention and management of complications associated with thyroid and parathyroid surgery. Surg Clin North Am 1979; 59:83–92.

Goldmann DR. Surgery in patients with endocrine dysfunction. Med Clin North Am 1987; 71:499–509.

Graber AL, Ney RL, Nicholson WE, et al. Natural history of pituitary-adrenal recovery following long-term suppression with corticosteroids. J Clin Endocrinol 1965; 25:11–16.

Mackin JF, Canary JJ, Pittman CS. Thyroid storm and its management. N Engl J Med 1974; 291:1396–1398.

Murkin JM. Anesthesia and hypothyroidism: a review of thyroxine physiology, pharmacology, and anesthetic implications. Anesth Analg 1982; 61:371–383.

ACQUIRED IMMUNODEFICIENCY SYNDROME

IVOR D. BERKOWITZ, M.B., B.Ch.

Acquired immunodeficiency syndrome (AIDS) is a "new" disease that was first described in 1981. Since that time, hundred of thousands of cases have been diagnosed and reported in this country and throughout the world. The disease is now in a rapid growth phase, and because of its widespread prevalence, it is essential that the anesthesiologist understand its etiology, modes of spread, protean manifestations, and the implications of the disease with regard to anesthetic care.

AIDS is an acquired, virus-induced disease characterized primarily by cell-mediated immunodeficiency. The etiologic agent, a retrovirus, has been variously termed the human immunodeficiency virus (HIV), the human T-cell lymphotropic virus type III (HTLV-III), the lymphadenopathy-associated virus (LAV), or the AIDS-associated retrovirus (ARV). HIV isolates are not genetically identical, rather, they comprise a closely related family of antigenically different strains. The virus is composed of a core that is surrounded by a protein core shell. The core consists of viral RNA, reverse transcriptase, and viral proteins. A lipid bilayer viral envelope containing various glycoproteins surrounds the viral core. These various proteins and glycoproteins are the antigens against which host antibodies are made and detected in the Western blot test. Cellular infection is initiated by the attachment of the envelope protein to CD4 receptors on the membrane of a specific CD4+ subset of T lymphocytes with subsequent cell damage and death. The HIV virus also infects other CD4+ cells, such as macrophages, glial cells, chromaffin cells of the gut, and rectal mucosal cells to initiate infection. Death of CD4+ cells (T-helper lymphocytes and some macrophages) leads to immunodeficiency with resultant recurrent bacterial, viral, fungal, and protozoal infections that are characteristic of the severely ill patient with AIDS (Table 1). The failure of immune tumor surveillance, together with other unknown factors, permits the development of otherwise uncommon neoplasms, particularly Kaposi's sarcoma and lymphoreticular malignancies.

When first described, AIDS appeared to be confined to particular high-risk groups. These included male homosexuals, intravenous drug abusers, recent Haitian immigrants, and hemophiliacs. Soon thereafter, recipients of multiple blood transfusions, infants of high-risk mothers (e.g., intravenous drug abusers, prostitutes, and heterosexual mothers with bisexual husbands) were added to these high-risk groups. HIV can also be transmitted between heterosexuals, and it is this mode of transmission that accounts for a growing number of AIDS cases in the United States.

CLASSIFICATION OF HIV INFECTION

Not all patients with HIV infection demonstrate the classic, initially described, clinical picture of AIDS, which is characterized by constitutional symptoms of weight loss, fever, chronic diarrhea, lymphadenopathy, severe immunodeficiency with life-threatening opportunistic infections (see Table 1), and secondary neoplasms. Long-term follow-up of patients with HIV infection has demonstrated that there is, indeed, a wide spectrum of clinical manifestations of HIV-related disease. Many patients are either asymptomatic or have generalized lymphadenopathy, whereas others present the severe full-blown progressive disease. Table 2 describes the recent Centers for Disease Control (CDC) classification of HIV-related infection. Other nomenclatures and classifications schemes (e.g., "lymphadenopathy syndrome" [LAS] or "AIDS-related complex" [ARC]) are in use. Equivalents can be found in the new CDC classification.

DIAGNOSTIC TECHNIQUES

The presence of HIV infection can be determined by laboratory techniques that include viral culture and the

Table 1 Opportunistic Infections in Patients with AIDS

Viral	*Protozoal*
Cytomegalovirus	*Pneumocystis carinii*
Pneumonia	Pneumonia
Chorioretinitis	*Toxoplasma gondii*
Encephalitis	Encephalitis
Colitis	Brain abscess
Disseminated	Myocarditis, pericarditis
Herpes simplex	*Cryptosporidium muris*
Encephalitis	Enteritis
Mucocutaneous	*Isospora belli*
Disseminated	Enteritis
Varicella zoster	
Primary	
Disseminated	*Bacterial*
Epstein-Barr	*Mycobacterium*
Oral hairy leukoplakia	*avium-intracellulare*
Lymphoid interstitial	Enteritis
pneumonitis	Pneumonia
	Disseminated
Fungal	Legionella
Candida albicans	Pneumonia
Oropharyngitis	Infections with "non-
Vaginitis	opportunistic" bacteria
Esophagitis	(e.g,. *Mycobacteria tuberculosis*,
Disseminated	*Streptococcus pneumoniae*,
Cryptococcus neoformans	*Haemophilus influenzae*,
Meningitis	salmonellae)
Pneumonia	
Disseminated	
Histoplasma	
Disseminated	
Aspergillus	
Pneumonia	

Adapted from Groopman JE. Clinical symptomatology of the acquired immunodeficiency syndrome (AIDS) and related disorders. Prog Allergy 1986; 37:188, by permission of S. Karger AG, Basel.

detection of antibodies to HIV virus and its protein components. The most specific technique for diagnosing HIV infection is virus isolation. However, this technique is relatively insensitive, technically difficult, and not widely available. HIV infection is usually indirectly identified by determining the presence of antibody to the virus. The enzyme-linked immunosorbent assay (ELISA) determines the presence of antibody reacting with inactivated virus. It is the primary screening test for HIV infection because of its high degree of sensitivity (greater than 99 percent), its reproducibility and low cost. False-positive results do occur, however, and the Western blot immunofluorescence assay or similar assays that identify specific antibodies to the protein and glycoprotein components of the viral core and envelope are now the primary confirmatory tests. Other laboratory immunologic abnormalities in patients with AIDS include polyclonal elevation of immunoglobulins, decreased number of CD4-positive lymphocytes (reflected by a reduction in the ratio of T-helper/T-suppressor lymphocytes), and functional abnormalities in T lymphocytes, natural killer cells, B lymphocytes, monocytes, and macrophages.

PREOPERATIVE EVALUATION

The widespread, multiple-organ dysfunction characteristic of this disease is caused either by the direct cytopathic effects of the virus, by opportunistic infections, or by secondary tumor development. This necessitates a thorough preoperative evaluation of the patient by the anesthesiologist before surgery. This evaluation can be achieved only with a detailed knowledge of the HIV disease and its complications. The intravenous drug abuser who is at high risk for acquiring HIV infection may have additional problems. He or she may already be severely compromised from an anesthetic point of view by cardiac valve damage secondary to endocarditis, pulmonary disease from septic emboli, talc granulomata, or pulmonary hypertension, as well as by renal disease, especially the nephrotic syndrome.

Pulmonary System

The pulmonary system is often compromised in patients with AIDS, either by opportunistic infections caused by a wide array of viral, bacterial, and fungal pathogens, or by lymphocytic interstitial pneumonia (LIP), which is a common complication, particularly in the pediatric AIDS patient. Opportunistic pneumonia is most frequently caused by *Pneumocystis carinii*, but cytomegalovirus and atypical mycobacteria are also common pulmonary pathogens. In addition, the pulmonary function of the intravenous drug abuser with AIDS may be compromised by pulmonary fibrosis (from talc granulomata) and pulmonary hypertension. Appropriate preoperative evaluation should therefore include a chest x-ray examination and arterial blood gas analysis. Pulmonary function tests should also be included if

respiratory symptoms are present and if general anesthesia is planned. Usually *Pneumocystis carinii* pneumonia in the AIDS patient is manifested radiologically by diffuse, bilateral, interstitial infiltrates. However, patients may be symptomatic, with tachypnea, fever, and hypoxia, and still have a normal chest film. Postoperative ventilation may be required for the AIDS patient with severely compromised lung function who is to undergo major surgery.

Cardiovascular System

In patients with HIV infection, involvement of the cardiovascular system is becoming recognized more frequently. Cardiac complications include myocarditis, pericarditis with effusion, and dilated cardiomyopathy. Myocarditis, a relatively infrequent complication, can be caused by the HIV virus or by opportunistic cytomegalovirus, *Toxoplasma*, and mycobacteria infections. AIDS patients with pericardial disease usually have concomitant myocardial disease (e.g., Kaposi's sarcoma) or opportunistic myocarditis. Dilated cardiomyopathy, the most common cardiac dysfunction in AIDS patients, is characterized by congestive heart failure with four-

Table 2 Classification of HIV Infection

1. Acute infection. Mononucleosis-like syndrome associated with seroconversion.
2. Asymptomatic infection. Patient is asymptomatic, but with serologic or culture evidence of infection.
3. Persistent generalized lymphadenopathy. Palpable lymphadenopathy (>1 cm) at two or more extrainguinal sites for more than 3 months, in absence of concurrent illness rather than HIV infection to explain findings.
4. Other HTLV-III disease.
   Subgroup A: Constitutional disease.
   One or more of the following: fever or diarrhea for more than 1 month or 10 percent baseline weight loss, in absence of concurrent illness other than HIV infection to explain findings.
   Subgroup B: Neurologic disease.
   One or more of the following: Dementia, myelopathy, or peripheral neuropathy, in absence of concurrent illness other than HIV.
   Subgroup C: Secondary infectious disease.
   Infectious disease associated with HIV infection or at least moderately indicative of a defect of cell-mediated immunity (see Table 1).
   Subgroup D: Secondary cancers.
   Diagnosis of one or more cancers known to be associated with HIV infection and at least moderately indicative of a defect in cell-mediated immunity (Kaposi's sarcoma, non-Hodgkin's lymphoma, or primary lymphoma of brain).
   Subgroup E: Other conditions in HIV infection.
   Clinical findings or diseases that cannot be assigned to the classifications above that may be attributable to HIV infection and are indicative of a defect in cell-mediated immunity. These include chronic lymphoid interstitial pneumonitis, other infectious diseases, and neoplasma not listed above.

From Centers for Disease Control. Classification system for human T-lymphotropic virus type III/lymphadenopathy-associated virus infections. MMWR 1986; 35:334.

chamber enlargement, ST wave changes, and echocardiographic evidence of generalized hypokinesis. If cardiac symptomatology exists, the preoperative cardiac work-up should include electrocardiography and echocardiography.

Gastrointestinal System

AIDS patients with chronic diarrhea (which characterizes the AIDS syndrome), gastroenteritis, complicating opportunistic gastrointestinal infections (e.g., cryptosporidiosis), and dysphagia from candida esophagitis can develop dehydration and electrolyte disturbances. If undiagnosed, these complications, particularly hypokalemia, place the patient with AIDS at risk for general anesthesia.

Central Nervous System

Soon after its discovery, HIV was noted to be not only lymphotropic but also neurotropic. Neurologic diseases that influence anesthetic management affect more than 50 percent of patients with AIDS. The central nervous system involvement is caused not only by direct infection of neurons and glia with HIV, but also by opportunistic central nervous system infections and central nervous system tumors, such as primary central nervous system lymphoma and metastatic Kaposi's sarcoma. Subacute encephalopathy, which causes AIDS-related dementia or the AIDS dementia complex (ADC), is the most common central nervous system disease in patients with AIDS. These syndromes present as a subacute encephalitis with dementia and progressive motor disturbances accompanied by tremors, gait disturbances, and even paraplegia. Ten to 20 percent of HIV-infected patients may present with neurologic symptoms of AIDS-related dementia before other signs of HIV infection appear. Other neurologic complications of HIV nervous system involvement include atypical aseptic meningitis with cranial nerve neuropathies, and spinal vacuolar myelopathy with a Guillain-Barré–like syndrome. Opportunistic infections, such as toxoplasma and herpes simplex encephalitis, and cryptococcal, listerial, and mycobacterial meningitis are common. Central nervous system involvement with metastatic Kaposi's sarcoma and primary central nervous system lymphomas, as well as AIDS-related cerebrovascular disease, produce serious neurologic disease. Patients with such central nervous system involvement can demonstrate intracranial hypertension, seizures, dementia, coma, and peripheral nerve damage. These are important clinical features that must be carefully considered in planning a safe and rational anesthetic. A preoperative cranial computed tomographic or magnetic resonance imaging scan of patients with neurologic signs and symptoms will alert the anesthesiologist to the presence of a space-occupying lesion or to evidence of elevated intracranial pressure.

Hematopoietic System

Hematopoietic abnormalities are almost a sine qua non of HIV infection. Lymphopenia, neutropenia, anemia, and thrombocytopenia are common. A characteristic form of immune thrombocytopenia can develop in patients with AIDS, and this responds in varying fashion to steroids, danazol, and splenectomy. Serious bleeding complications are uncommon despite often severe thrombocytopenia. Radiation treatment for lymphoma and antimicrobial chemotherapy—for example, ganciclovir (dihyroxopropoxymethyl guanine, or DHPG), pentamidine, amphotericin B, and trimethoprim-sulfamethoxazole for opportunistic infections may aggravate the hemopoietic disturbances. Judicious administration of packed red blood cells and platelet transfusions must be part of the preoperative preparation of the patient with AIDS, particularly when major surgery is contemplated.

Renal System

Renal involvement and electrolyte disturbances, which frequently complicate the course of patients with HIV infection, have important implications for the anesthesiologist. Hyponatremia, the most common electrolyte disturbance, occurs in approximately 60 percent of hospitalized AIDS patients. Gastrointestinal fluid loss from diarrhea is the most frequent cause of hyponatremia, but other etiologies include AIDS-related adrenal insufficiency and inappropriate antidiuretic hormone secretion secondary to *Pneumocystis* pneumonia or pulmonary lymphoma.

Renal parenchymal disease, which includes acute tubular necrosis, miscellaneous tubular-interstitial and vascular diseases, and a distinct, recently described HIV-associated nephropathy that causes irreversible renal failure, frequently complicates the course of patients with HIV infection. This mandates the preoperative evaluation of renal function with urinalysis and blood urea nitrogen, creatinine, and electrolyte determination.

ANESTHETIC MANAGEMENT

The choice of anesthetic techniques for patients is wide and is determined largely by underlying organ involvement and the planned surgical procedure. Local anesthesia, supplemented by sedation with intravenous narcotics such as fentanyl combined with an intravenous benzodiazepine such as midazolam, provides safe and effective amnesia and relief of pain for many minor procedures. These include fiberoptic bronchoscopy with bronchial brushings, alveolar lavage, transbronchial lung biopsy, Hickman catheter placement, sigmoidoscopy, and superficial lymph node and skin biopsies. Droperidol and other drugs with pryamidal side effects should be avoided in patients with ADC who display parkinsonian-like symptoms, because of their potential for exacerbating the movement disorder. General anesthesia is required for other diagnostic and therapeutic procedures, including brain biopsy in patients with suspected herpetic or *Toxoplasma* encephalitis, splenectomy for patients with AIDS-associated immune thrombocytopenia, and colectomy for patients with perforated cytomegalovirus colitis. Special precautions must be taken during induction of anesthesia if myocardial dysfunction or intracranial hypertension are present. The selection of muscle relaxants should be based on a thorough knowledge of the extent of the neurologic involvement and the state of renal function. Administration of succinylcholine should be avoided in patients with myelopathy, hemiparesis, and peripheral neuropathy because of the risk of life-threatening hyperkalemia. Atracurium besylate is the muscle relaxant of choice in patients with renal failure. Because of its epileptogenic potential, enflurane should be avoided in patients who have neurologic involvement characterized by seizures.

TRANSMISSION PRECAUTIONS

An important and certainly emotionally charged issue in caring for patients with HIV infection is the potential for transmission of a uniformly fatal disease to health care workers. A rational approach to this problem must be based on an understanding of the epidemiology and possible modes of transmission of AIDS in the hospital setting. Although the virus has been detected in many body fluids, including blood, semen, vaginal secretions, saliva, urine, tears, cerebrospinal fluid, and breast milk, epidemiologic evidence has implicated only blood, semen, and vaginal secretions as important in transmitting the HIV infection. HIV infection is not acquired by casual contact. The most likely potential sources of infection for the anesthesiologist are either direct parenteral inoculation of blood or exposure of mucous membranes to blood-contaminated body fluids. The risk of acquiring HIV infection after needle-stick exposure is approximately 1 percent. This relatively low degree of infectivity can be contrasted with a 6 to 30 percent risk of infection with hepatitis B after a needle-stick exposure to a carrier of that virus. The risk to the health care worker of acquiring HIV infection from exposure of mucous membranes is rare indeed. Nevertheless, because of the lethal nature of AIDS, measures must be taken to protect the operating room staff. Because of the increasing incidence of HIV infection and the fact that the infectivity of patients is unknown, the blood and body fluids of every patient must be regarded as infectious. Universal precautions should therefore be adopted to avoid exposure to blood and other body fluids.

The CDC have provided guidelines for the protection of health care workers. These resemble the guidelines set forth for those working with patients with hepatitis B (Table 3). Patients may be transported from their rooms to the operating suite by the usual patient

Table 3 Guidelines for Protecting Operating
Room Personnel

Contaminants	Precautions
Avoid contact with blood and body fluids of patients	"Universal precautions." Wear gloves when direct contact with blood or mucous membranes is likely. Wash hands thoroughly if contamination occurs. Wear masks, gowns, and glasses if more extensive exposure is likely.
Take extreme care when handling sharp instruments and needles	Do not recap, bend, or remove needles from disposable syringes. Discard into puncture-resistant containers.
Sterilize contaminated nondisposable equipment (e.g,. laryngoscope blades, temperature probes)	Use "high-level disinfectant" (e.g., 1:10–1:100 sodium hypochlorite solution or commercial "sterilants").

escort service. They need to wear masks only if reverse isolation is necessary or if they are infected with a contagious opportunistic agent. To prevent skin contact with contaminated blood, gloves should be worn, particularly when performing invasive procedures such as intravenous or arterial line placement and when there is exposure to mucous membranes and their secretions, such as during endotracheal intubation and the insertion of nasogastric tubes and other catheters. Gowns should be worn when clothes are likely to be contaminated with blood or blood-contaminated secretions. Other precautions, such as wearing masks and glasses, are indicated if aerosolization is likely to occur. Although oral and airway secretions may contain virus, epidemiologic evidence suggests that exposure to these secretions is rarely, if ever, the mode of acquisition of HIV infection by health care workers. Contamination with blood, however, may render these secretions more infectious. Hands should be thoroughly washed after gown and gloves have been removed and before one leaves the operating room. Extraordinary care must be taken to prevent injury to hands from needles, scalpels, and other sharp instruments. Placing stopcocks in intravenous lines minimizes the use of needles for intravenous injection. After use, needles and scalpel blades must be placed in puncture-resistant containers for disposal. To reduce the hazard of injury, needles must not be recapped, manipulated, or removed from disposal syringes before being discarded.

Disposable anesthesia circuits and disposable soda lime and ventilator filters can be used. Disposable laryngoscope blades are convenient. After a soap and water scrub to remove secretions and blood, metal laryngoscope blades should be sterilized or disinfected with a commercial germicide or a disinfectant such as a dilute (1:10) solution of household bleach.

Resuscitation equipment such as Ambu bags and

face masks should be readily available in all areas where cardiopulmonary resuscitation might be required. Such availability protects the personnel performing cardiopulmonary resuscitation and mouth-to-mouth resuscitation from potential exposure to infectious oral secretions.

SUGGESTED READING

Berry AJ. Infection control in anesthesia. Anesth Clin North Am 1989; 7:967–981.

Centers for Disease Control. CDC recommendations for prevention of HIV transmission in health-care settings. MMWR 1987; 36:35–185.
Conte JE. Infection with human immunodeficiency virus in hospitals: epidemiology, infection control, and biosafety considerations. Ann Intern Med 1986; 105:730–736.
Green ER. Acquired immunodeficiency syndrome: an overview for anesthesiologists. Anesthesiology 1986; 65:1054–1058.
Warner MA, Kunkel SE. Human immunodeficiency virus infection. Anesth Clin North Am 1989; 7:795–811.

THE GERIATRIC PATIENT

WILLIAM T. MERRITT, M.D.

In chronologic terms, a definition of aging seems clear. Persons 65 to 79 years of age have been called "elderly," those 80 to 90 years "aged," and those older than 90 years the "very old" (Muravchick). From a physiologic viewpoint, however, there is wide variation within each of these age groups, ranging from those who are incapacitated because of disease to those who engage in athletic competition. This physiologic variation, as reflected in the American Society of Anesthesiologists Physical Status classification, affects perioperative morbidity and mortality (Djokovic and Hosking). It has been estimated that more than 100,000 persons older than 65 years of age die perioperatively each year. As anesthesiologists, our goals are to discern a reasonable amount of preoperative information regarding a patient's health and to attempt to manipulate appropriate physiologic, pharmacologic, and environmental variables in an effort to improve outcome.

The elderly represent the most rapidly growing segment of our population. In 1981, 11.4 percent (approximately 22 million) of Americans were older than 65 years of age (Stephen). Persons older than 85 years of age use twice the Medicare dollars as those 20 years younger. Persons older than 90 years old will number nearly 2 million by the year 2000. By design or default, surgeons and anesthesiologists will be caring for these people in increasing numbers. It is important to review periodically the important variables of direct and indirect concern to the anesthesiologist in the perioperative care of elderly patients.

GENERAL CHANGES

Because of changes (Kenney) in body composition during the aging process, there is a redistribution of cellular and extracellular water. Approximately 55 percent of the body weight of a young adult represents water, whereas in the elderly individual this decreases to about 50 percent. In younger patients, roughly one-third of this water is extracellular. Normal aging does not alter the absolute volume of extracellular water; it increases in proportion to intracellular water. Lean body mass decreases more or less in proportion to a loss of muscle mass; however, because body fat is not lost with aging, it increases in proportion to the other compartments. There is only a slight decline in blood volume past the age of 80 years. These changes, taken together, indicate a relative dehydration during the aging process. Such changes can have significant effects on pharmacodynamics (discussed below). Electrolyte composition changes little with aging, but many elderly patients do take diuretics, which can greatly alter homeostatic balance. Basal metabolic rate has fallen by one-quarter in the 80-year-old compared with the young adult, partially because of a decrease in metabolically active cells (Lonergan).

THERMOREGULATION

Thermoregulation in the elderly can be altered at all levels: input (afferent), processing (hypothalamic), and output (efferent). Temperature discrimination in the skin is certainly decreased. In the young, a change of 1°C is discernable, but an elderly patient may not be able to discriminate changes of 2°C or more. Although the majority of elderly persons have normal hypothalamic central thermoregulation, some have lower set points and are at risk for clinical hypothermia when exposed to cold environments.

Most problems with loss of temperature occur because of changes in efferent pathways of temperature conservation or heat generation. In the setting of a decrease in the density of cutaneous vessels, there is decreased autonomic control of cutaneous vasculature and impaired ability to close skin arteriovenous shunts. Internal warmth is constantly being dissipated. Thermogenesis is altered as well. Onset is delayed, and the intensity of shivering is decreased. Moreover, anesthetic agents alter thermoregulation. Halogenated agents appear to lower set points. Regional anesthesia paralyzes autonomic control of cutaneous vessels; those vessels not blocked are not able to compensate as well as in the younger patient.

In the face of all these changes, we place patients in operating rooms with cold temperatures, induce high convective loss as a result of multiple air exchanges per hour, high evaporative losses from surface preparation solutions, and exposed visceral surfaces, and risk conductive loss due to cold or inadequately warmed fluids and blood. It is no wonder that patients older than 60 years average temperatures one-third of a degree lower than those in younger adults. Since they have normal set points but lower temperatures, the gradient to be restored is greater. Unfortunately, shivering can increase oxygen consumption by three to eight times and overwhelm limited cardiopulmonary reserves. It is incumbent upon both anesthesiologists and surgeons to worry about these problems and seek common ground solutions. In addition, severe hypothermia alters glomerular and tubular function and decreases both renal excretion and hepatic metabolism of drugs.

THE BRAIN

Evidence for neurologic dysfunction is common in the elderly population. Deterioration in memory and intellectual activity; gait and mobility impairment; changes in sleep patterns; and altered sensory function, including impaired vision, hearing, taste, and smell are common accompaniments of the aging process. The human brain diminishes in both weight and volume with aging. Thirty percent of cerebral cortical neurons are lost between the ages of 20 and 90 years. Betz cells are lost from the cortex, and Purkinje cells are lost from the cerebellum. Numerous changes including development of lipofuscin pigment granules; loss of dendrites; and creation of neurofibrillary tangles, neuritic plaques, and neuraxonal spheroids are described in the aging brain (Everitt). In general, these changes are worse in patients with Alzheimer's disease, which is much more prevalent than previously believed (Evans).

Biochemical explanations for these neurologic changes that occur with aging are not complete. It is known that there are changes in protein synthesis. DNA levels in the brain do not appear to decrease with age, but RNA is greatly decreased in certain areas of the brain. Ganglioside content decreases as well. Glycolytic metabolism decreases in both normal individuals and those with dementia.

Cholinergic (acetylcholine), catecholaminergic (dopamine, norepinephrine, serotonin), and GABA-ergic neurotransmitters decrease with age. There is a significant decrease in the brain of dopamine and the enzyme tyrosine hydroxylase, which is important for the synthesis of both dopamine and norepinephrine. Such changes are marked in patients with Parkinson's disease. The defect in the cholinergic system, which is part of normal aging, is much more evident in those with Alzheimer's disease.

Anesthetic agents and sedatives are administered in the setting of these age-altered changes of central nervous system (CNS) function. There is a distinct decrement in minimal alveolar concentration (MAC) with aging. This term refers to a measure of the amount of inhalational anesthetic required to suppress reaction to the stimulus of surgery. Unfortunately, cardiovascular depression with anesthetics may be increased in the elderly as well. Because there is not a direct relationship between the amount of anesthesia required to suppress recall, movement, or autonomic stimuli and that associated with cardiovascular depression, one may have difficulty achieving appropriate levels of anesthesia without undue loss of myocardial function. In the elderly, the half-life is increased for virtually all of the sedative-hypnotic classes of drugs (Larson). Mental function will very likely be impaired beyond the standard period for which patients remain in the postanesthesia care unit. Hypothermia and hypercapnia may potentially slow recovery. Premedication may not have "worn off." Drugs used to treat gastric acidity (e.g., cimetidine) can prolong the metabolism of benzodiazepines, leading to prolonged sedation. Disorientation can actually persist for several days; up to 3 percent of patients over 90 years of age will experience this (Woodrow). Delirium is a particular risk in the hospitalized elderly. It is associated with abnormal sodium values, illness severity, preexisting dementia, fever or hypothermia, psychoactive drug use, and azotemia. Death is more common in this group (Francis).

THE INTEGUMENT

The skin is often not thought of as an organ system, but actually serves a number of important complimentary functions. It has numerous sensory functions, serves as a barrier to water loss and against invasion by microorganisms, and because of its vascularity, is the major organ of thermoregulation. With aging, the mechanical strength of the skin weakens, which may account for the ease of blister formation in the elderly. Loss of water content and elasticity leads to the loose, wrinkled appearance of skin in the aged. As a barrier to body water loss, the skin seems to function effectively as it ages. But as subcutaneous fat loss occurs, the insulating capacity of the skin diminishes. Loss of reticuloendothelial cells in the epidermis contributes to a loss of effectiveness as a barrier to infection. In addition, wound healing is retarded. Most of our problems with the integument of the aged have to do with adhesive tape injury, blistering associated with infiltrated intravenous lines, and pressure necrosis from prolonged immobility with insufficient padding on an operating room table, and are largely preventable.

THE CARDIOVASCULAR SYSTEM

In 1968, Cole pointed out that one-half of postoperative deaths are directly related to myocardial disease (Cole). The state of the cardiovascular system often presents the most perplexing questions prior to an operation. Short of a clearly defined history of daily jogging or vigorous walking, or anginal pain, congestive heart failure, a distinctive electrocardiogram (ECG) or arrythmia, or the results of invasive or noninvasive cardiovascular testing, it is often difficult to be reasonably sure what the functional capacity of the cardiovascular system is. How will a given patient tolerate the administration of anesthesia and the subsequent emergence period when anesthetics disappear and some form of pain treatment takes over? Will the asymptomatic, sedentary 70-year-old man develop ischemia with tachycardia, and what is tachycardia (i.e., "too fast") for him—60, 80, 100, or 120 beats per minute? Will a short period (e.g., several minutes) of relative hypotension (systolic pressure of 80 mm Hg in a patient who normally has a pressure of 190 mm Hg) have effects on the heart, brain, kidneys, and other organ systems? Conversely, what will be the effects of brief hypertension, especially if it occurs with tachycardia, during intraoperative events such as intubation, incision, nerve stimulation, or topical epinephrine administration? Is there any way to be certain how much of a medication is enough to achieve the desired effect? What about sustained hypertension and tachycardia in the anxious preoperative patient or in the postoperative patient who is uncomfortable with pain? These are questions the anesthesiologist ponders when dealing with the older patient, whether for a limited procedure or for major surgery. Unfortunately and all too often, there are few immediate answers. Common sense dictates that anesthetic and pharmacologic prudence are in order. Not infrequently an anesthesiologist will request that a patient be evaluated by a cardiologist. This should be done *not as clearance for anesthesia,* but to obtain assistance from a potentially more experienced source in getting an answer to a specific question: Is this chest pain angina, is it unstable angina, is medical management essentially optimal, what is the significance of the murmur heard, what is the cardiovascular status of this bedridden patient? Answers to these questions may help quantify risks for discussions with the patient, may dictate further preoperative treatment or evaluation, and should help in the choice of intraoperative and postoperative monitoring.

As the cardiovascular system ages, many changes are considered normal. The arterial tree stiffens, resulting in a modest increase in blood pressure. Compensatory, modest left ventricular hypertrophy occurs. During this same period, systolic pressure increases by approximately 25 mm Hg in normal men and 35 mm Hg in normal women, with a diastolic pressure peaking in the sixth decade of life and declining slightly over the next 20 years or so. Autonomic receptors are much less sensitive to stimulation as a person ages, and plasma levels of norepinephrine rise, reflecting altered autonomic modulation. In contrast to earlier studies conducted primarily in hospitalized patients that showed a progressive age-associated decrease in cardiac output (Brandfonbrener and co-workers), more recent studies that carefully *excluded* patients with cardiovascular disease (by extensive noninvasive testing such as radionuclide scanning) demonstrate that there is no significant age-associated decrease in cardiac output. With stress, the normal aging heart cannot increase heart rate as well, but maintains output by an appropriate increase in stroke volume from an increased end-diastolic volume (Rodeheffer). There are changes in the heart's conduction system as well. Fatty deposits envelop the sinoarterial (SA) node and may eventually so isolate the node from atrial muscle that the sick sinus syndrome may result. SA pacemaker cells decrease in number after about 60 years of age, so that by the age of 75 years only 10 percent remain. Changes in the bundle of His include increased fibrous, adipose, and amyloid deposits and loss of cells. Variable fibrosis of the cardiac "skeleton" occurs. The prevalence of first-degree atrioventricular block increases but there should be little effect on conduction within the ventricle. The ECG will demonstrate progressive leftward shift of the QRS axis, evidence of increased left atrial size, and may occasionally (2 percent) even show right bundle branch block in apparently healthy persons. Although isolated supraventricular and ventricular ectopic beats are more frequent in elderly patients, bradycardia, high-grade atrioventricular blocks, and atrial flutter or fibrillation are uncommon in the healthy heart.

The average elderly patient, however, does not climb mountains or jog, and does not come for surgery fresh from a spotless cardiac evaluation. Ten to twenty percent of patients over the age of 60 years have distinct historical evidence of coronary artery disease (angina, history of myocardial infarction, an abnormal ECG). Stress evaluation of heart function uncovers previously unrecognized ischemia and doubles this number (Lakatta). Thus half of those at risk for perioperative myocardial ischemia may be unrecognized prior to operation. Such data force us to treat the elderly patient expectantly and gingerly.

THE RESPIRATORY SYSTEM

Physiologic respiratory reserve is lost with aging, but in healthy elderly persons, daily activities should not be limited. These changes are steady, but are most marked after 60 years of age. In youth, the chemosensitive cells of the respiratory center of the brainstem and the peripheral chemoreceptors in the carotid and aortic bodies monitor the effectiveness of breathing. Respiration is controlled around specific levels of carbon dioxide and oxygen. In the elderly, this may not be so. Elderly patients experience increasing periods of apnea and hypoxemia during sleep; some investigators say that two-thirds of the elderly have this problem. There is a marked reduction in response to hypercapnia, and the arterial Po_2 must fall farther before there is an increase in minute ventilation. The relative bradycardia with stress seen in the elderly may impair oxygen delivery as well. This change in ventilation seems to be caused by a reduced responsiveness of ventilatory drive or neural output from the respiratory center rather than by altered function of the chemoreceptors themselves.

The strength of muscle contraction decreases by 15 to 35 percent by 80 years of age, and for the respiratory system, much less force is likely to be generated. This is contributed to by stiffening of the chest wall, loss of muscle mass, decrease in energy-rich phosphate compounds, and atrophy of type two fibers. Functional residual capacity increases with age, creating a flattened diaphragm which is less efficient (LaPlace's law). Airway protective reflexes are lost with aging as well, presumably a factor in the increasing incidence of aspiration pneumonia seen in the elderly (Pontoppidan).

At rest, the elderly do fairly well in spite of these changes, and the diaphragm is able to handle ventilatory requirements. As reserve functions are called into play for additional demands, however, problems may arise. A good cough, for example, requires high air flow and coordination of both diaphragm and chest wall musculature. Measurements of maximal expiratory flow decrease by about 30 percent with aging; for example, FEV_1 decreases by about 30 ml per year in the nonsmoker. In the presence of decreased strength, as well as pain, an adequate cough may not be possible. Increased work load on respiratory musculature (e.g., mild airway obstruction) or spontaneous breathing through a small endotracheal tube may lead to fatigue and failure of respiration. In addition, cilia decrease in number and effectiveness, resulting in less than optimal removal of debris.

Elastic recoil of the lung parenchyma decreases, which lessens the force that holds open small airways. If closing volume exceeds functional residual capacity, airway closure with tidal breathing may occur, altering the distribution of ventilation. In addition, vital capacity decreases by approximately 20 ml per year, coincident with a residual volume increase of the same magnitude. As this ventilation and perfusion mismatching develops, there is a widening of the alveolar to arterial (A-a) gradient for oxygen (normally approximately 5 mm Hg) by about 4 mm Hg per decade, leading to a significant decrease in resting PO_2 in the elderly. The respiratory changes with aging are decreased efficiency of gas exchange, decreased expiratory flow rates, and the poor ability to respond to decreased PaO_2 or increased $PaCO_2$. These changes are likely to be exacerbated with analgesics, sedatives, and residual anesthetic agents.

THE GASTROINTESTINAL SYSTEM

Gastrointestinal changes may appear to have little import for outpatient or nonabdominal surgical procedures, but potentially affect patient comfort, metabolism, and the response to medications (Shamburek).

Although there is a decrease in both stimulated and unstimulated salivary flow with aging, most xerostomia is caused by medications or systemic disease. The tongue appears smoother owing to loss of filiform papillae, and only about 30 percent of taste buds remain by the age of 70 years. The teeth are affected more by dental hygiene than aging as such. There are changes in the cement substance that anchors teeth to bone. The resorption of alveolar bone matrix parallels that of the generalized loss of bone mineralization that occurs with age, but accelerates when teeth are removed or lost. Swallowing disorders may be present, which have the potential for leading to malnutrition or aspiration. There is a slowing of the movement of a food bolus through the oropharynx, which is usually asymptomatic. Disease processes such as diabetic neuropathy, polymyositis, Parkinson's disease as well as various neurologic and muscular diseases do affect the swallowing process and can lead to dysphagia. Such disease-associated dysfunction may aggravate any brief swallowing disorder associated with sedation or the onset/offset of general anesthesia and muscle relaxation.

Normal aging is associated with a decrease in the amplitude of esophageal muscular contractions, some increase in the frequency of disordered contractions, and changes in the regularity of primary peristaltic waves after a swallow. Much of this is asymptomatic. In this setting, presumably, disease-related changes such as those seen with diabetes mellitus produce effects much more readily. The problem of gastroesophageal reflux and aging has not been well studied.

In spite of histologic changes of increased fat infiltration and fibrous tissue in the aging pancreas, exocrine dysfunction is not more common, apparently because there is considerable reserve capacity. Digestion, in the absence of systemic illness affecting the gastrointestinal tract or pancreas, is not impaired.

Blood flow to the liver appears to decrease by about 1 percent per year. This may account for the decrease in drug metabolism seen with aging, which is more obvious with microsomal oxidative and hydrolytic functions than with conjugative (e.g., glucuronide) processes. Since serum albumin decreases only by about 0.5 g per L per decade, hypoalbuminemia should not be attributed to aging. The synthetic and enzymatic tests of liver function are not affected by aging. However, amylase and alkaline phosphatase increase to high normal levels past the age of 60 years; the increase in amylase may be partially attributed to a decrease in renal function.

Finally, constipation is a significant complaint of the elderly. For outpatient surgery or for brief hospital stays, it may go unrecognized. It is rather clearly not a problem over which an anesthesiologist has long-term control. Whether related to dietary habits, medications (e.g., narcotics), lifestyle, subtle changes in the physiology of the distal colon and rectum, or various processes affecting neurologic and motor function, it is none the less disconcerting to the patient. Fecal impaction frequently accompanies the problem, and may lead to overflow incontinence. Cognitive impairment from drugs, or dementia and handicaps resulting in poor or infrequent access to toilet facilities may facilitate the problem.

RENAL FUNCTION CHANGES

Renal function deteriorates with aging in a predictable fashion. It is known that both total and cortical mass is lost, with a decrease in the number and surface area of glomeruli, as well as a decrease in the length and volume of the proximal tubules. Vascular changes occur, which may be responsible. The changes seen in glomerular and tubular anatomy mirror the parallel decline in glomerular and tubular function noted with senescence. There are other data to suggest that the reduction in mean blood flow per unit mass with aging is more marked in the renal cortex and that the medullary area is relatively spared. The net result, however, is a progressive decline in total renal blood flow of approximately 10 percent per decade after the fourth decade.

Creatinine clearance decreases steadily from the time the patient is in his or her mid-thirties and accelerates after 65 years of age. This reduction is accompanied by a parallel decrease in daily urinary creatinine excretion, partially reflecting decreased muscle mass. Mean urinary creatinine per kilogram per 24 hours decreases steadily. One needs to remain mindful of the changing relationship between serum creatinine, glomerular filtration rate (GFR), and creatinine clearance. A 20-year-old with a creatinine clearance of 120 ml per minute has a serum creatinine of approximately 1.0 mg per deciliter. However, an 80-year-old with a normal serum creatinine of 1.0 mg per deciliter has a creatinine clearance of only about 60 ml per minute. Since creatinine does not adequately reflect the underlying GFR, it cannot be used as an index for dosing medications. Creatinine clearance is a better guide when known, or one should use age-adjusted renal function tables or formulas (discussed later).

Although age has no significant effect on serum potassium or sodium levels, or on the ability to maintain extracellular volume, acute illness is likely to upset this homeostatic balance and disturb these values. Although incompletely understood, renal sodium handling is abnormal in the elderly. Whether because of changes in renal blood flow or decreased responsiveness of the renin–angiotensin system to acute stimuli, the aging kidney conserves sodium poorly. Alterations of mental status and disorientation are common with acute illness in the elderly. Coupled with a decreased sense of thirst, salt intake may be impaired, while losses proceed without decrement, leading to a decrease in intracellular volume, with attendant changes in cardiac, renal, and mental capacity. Patients on diuretics that alter the handling of electrolytes at the tubular level will be at additional risk. Paradoxically, the aging kidney handles salt loading poorly with the potential for fluid overload from retained water. Medications and fluids with a high sodium content, contrast agents, and dietary excess may lead to an expanded extracellular volume. If cardiac function is impaired, the excess volume may result in dyspnea and pulmonary edema, requiring definitive medical management.

PHARMACOLOGIC CONSIDERATIONS

Alterations of pharmacologic kinetics with aging are of major concern to the anesthesiologist because in the elderly, the incidence of drug reactions is two to three times that in younger patients (Montamat). Little information is available regarding changes in those older than 85 years of age, but presumably there is a progression of those changes seen earlier in the aging process. Greater severity of disease and pathologic conditions as well as polypharmacy certainly contribute to this progression.

Changes in gastrointestinal drug absorption are minimal. Several important cardiovascular preparations are administered through the skin, but the aging effects on percutaneous delivery are uncertain. Drug distribution is a function of body composition, protein binding, and blood flow to organs. As mentioned, there is a relative decrease in total body water and lean mass with aging, and an increase in body fat. The volume of distribution for water-soluble drugs therefore is contracted in the elderly, which leads to higher blood levels (i.e., higher "central compartment levels"). This has been well shown for ethanol, digoxin, and cimetidine, but is not true for the nondepolarizing muscle relaxant pancuronium. Lipid-soluble drugs, on the other hand, have a larger volume of distribution, which in general results in longer elimination half lives.

"Healthy" aging seems to have unimportant effects on the blood levels of the principal drug-binding proteins such as albumin and alpha-1-glycoprotein (chronic disease and/or malnutrition, however, can decrease their levels). In spite of this, the binding of "acidic" drugs is altered in the elderly. For example, free naproxen (Naprosyn, a common nonsteroidal anti-inflammatory agent) levels are twice as high in elderly as in younger patients. Other drugs with similar increases in free, unbound levels include acetazolamide (carbonic anhydrase inhibitor-diuretic, which is used to treat glaucoma), valproic acid (Depakene, an anticonvulsant), and etomidate (common intravenous anesthetic). The volume of distribution decreases for many medications. Doses may need to be smaller and titrated to achieve the desired effect. For lipophilic drugs, moreover, effects may be prolonged because of low blood levels sustained by slow release from the fat compartment. This can be particularly true in the elderly for the benzodiazepines such as diazepam (Valium), lorazepam (Ativan), oxazepam (Serax), midazolam (Versed), and chlordiazepoxide (Librium).

The clearance of drugs, which occurs primarily by metabolism in the liver, depends on both the activity of enzymes responsible for pharmacologic biotransformation and hepatic blood flow. For drugs that are metabolized slowly (low intrinsic clearance), clearance is proportional to the rate of hepatic enzymatic metabolism. Because hepatic mass decreases both in absolute terms and in relation to total body weight with aging, the disappearance of drugs with low intrinsic clearance should also decrease. For drugs with a very high rate of metabolism (high intrinsic clearance), the rate of extraction by the liver is high, and the rate-limiting step is hepatic blood flow (after intravenous administration). Hepatic blood flow decreases by 40 to 45 percent between the ages of 25 and 65 years. This results in a reduction in the metabolism of a number of drugs used by older patients, including propranolol, labetolol, major tranquilizers, tricyclic antidepressants, and antiarrhythmic agents. The phase II reactions of the liver (glucuronidation, acetylation, and sulfation) are essentially unaffected by aging. Phase I reactions (oxidation, reduction, and hydrolysis), however, are reduced or unchanged. There also is evidence that stereoselective metabolism of isomers is altered with aging.

Because of the decline in renal function with aging, there is a reduction in the rate of elimination of drugs and metabolites by the kidney which correlates well with the decline in creatinine clearance with aging. Since creatinine clearance is not always readily measured, a formula such as the following is often used:

$$Cl_{cr} = \frac{(140 - age)\ (kg)}{(6,365)\ (plasma\ creatinine\ in\ mmoles/L)}$$

$\times 0.85$ for women
(may be inaccurate for nursing home patients)

Drugs with predominantly renal elimination frequently used by the elderly include digoxin, lithium, aminoglycosides, cimetidine, procainamide, chlorpropamide (Diabinese), and amantadine.

The target organ effects of drugs, or pharmacodynamics, is less well understood in the elderly than are distribution, metabolism, and excretion. Generalizations are hard to make, and age-related sensitivity may vary with the drug studied and the response measured. Drug levels are extremely important in understanding these effects. Warfarin sensitivity, for example, may increase with aging, and other drugs that inhibit its metabolism (e.g., cimetidine) or displace it from binding proteins (e.g., chlorpropamide) will aggravate this increased sensitivity. Heparin kinetics on the other hand do not seem to change with aging.

The elderly are sedated at lower concentrations of benzodiazepines than younger patients, but tolerance occurs. Dosage reductions are recommended. On the other hand, the dosage of verapamil (a calcium channel blocking agent) required to produce prolongation of the PR interval (short-term intravenous dosing) is increased with aging. However, this is countered by increased sensitivity of the elderly to the vasodilating and negative inotropic effects of verapamil, which produces a greater decrease in blood pressure than in younger patients. Beta-blockade has been well studied in the aging population. In general, the elderly are less sensitive to

both beta-adrenergic stimuli and blockade, and this appears to be a diminished cellular response. Theories offered include a decrease in number of high-affinity receptors or a generalized decrease in affinity of receptors. Impairment of the activity of adenyl cyclase or a reduction in the cyclic AMP-dependent activity of protein kinase may also affect the changes in beta-adrenergic function. Studies of alpha-receptors suggest no change or a decrease in their number and affinity with aging.

Any discussion of drug metabolism in the elderly must emphasize altered effects of psychoactive medications. Major tranquilizers are commonly used, but major side effects are also common and include delirium, arrhythmias, postural hypotension, and extrapyramidal symptoms. The metabolism of antidepressant medications, especially the tertiary amines (e.g., amitriptyline [Elavil], imipramine [Tofranil]) is decreased in elderly patients because hepatic demethylation is altered. Postural hypotension, urinary retention, sedation, and increased incidence of falls are associated with these agents.

Very few anesthesia procedures or surgical interventions can be undertaken without the use of analgesic agents and/or anesthetics. Changes in the elderly population are important here, too. For example, morphine, meperidine, fentanyl, alfentanil, and sufentanil have slower plasma clearance and higher peak levels in the elderly. Although pain relief is potentially improved, side effects such as respiratory depression are more likely. There is a mild decrease in the metabolism of acetaminophen in the elderly. Nonsteroidal anti-inflammatory agents have several side effects of particular importance in the elderly, including increased serum potassium concentration, renal failure, and gastrointestinal hemorrhage. There is a significant increase in the elimination half-life for sodium thiopental, so lower initial as well as maintenance doses are required (Stanski).

Inhalational anesthetics have effects on the CNS, the systemic vasculature, and the myocardium and its conduction system. As mentioned earlier, there are several changes in the nervous system with aging. General anesthesia, unfortunately, results in further depression of brain functions, especially those of the brain stem, reticular formation, thalamus, hypothalamus, and the cerebral cortex. Taken together, these changes are reflected in the decrease in the MAC for inhalational anesthetics seen with aging. In addition, changes in the elimination of other adjunctive analgesics and sedatives result in the potential for exaggerated or prolonged emergence problems such as hypoxia, hypercarbia, sedation, disequilibrium, and delirium. Such problems are especially troublesome in the same-day surgery patient. As mentioned previously, cardiovascular changes with normal aging include a relative slowing of the heart, left ventricular dilation, and increased stroke volume compared with younger individuals. In general, potent inhalational anesthetics flatten the ventricular function curves so that equivalent increases in ventricular filling produce less of an increment in cardiac output than in unanesthetized patients; the rate of rise of left ventricular pressure (dP/dt) decreases significantly. Inhalational anesthetics, as a rule, lower blood pressure, raise systemic vascular resistance, and decrease cardiac output and stroke volume. Any superimposed disease-related myocardial dysfunction obviously further worsens these changes and places the patient at increased risk.

RECENT DEVELOPMENTS IN ANESTHESIA

The 1980s witnessed important improvements in the delivery of anesthesia care. Major strides have been made in the understanding of patients with cardiovascular disease and their tolerance of perioperative stress. Technologic advances have led to the ability to measure reliably patient oxygenation and ventilation in the operating room, in recovery areas, and in intensive care units. At the same time, national standards have been adopted by the American Society of Anesthesiologists for both the preoperative evaluation of anesthesia equipment and for the monitoring of the individual patient receiving general, regional, or monitored anesthesia care. Pulse oximetry is now required during all general anesthetic procedures, regional anesthesia, and sedation. Capnography, to measure end-tidal carbon dioxide, is to be used for all general anesthetic procedures. Free-standing ambulatory surgical centers must use the same intensity of monitoring of oxygenation and ventilation as in a hospital-based setting. Since approximately one-half of critical anesthesia-related incidents involve some difficulty with adequate oxygenation and ventilation, major improvements in morbidity and mortality should be possible with this monitoring. In addition, practical means to measure the concentrations of the inhaled anesthetics are now available using infrared mass spectroscopy or Raman spectroscopy. This information permits quantitative assessment of delivered anesthetic, yielding more rapid emergence (especially useful in outpatients and the elderly) and the potential for monetary savings from the more judicious use of the inhaled anesthetic agents.

Newer drugs for use by the anesthesiologist have also been introduced. Most have been selected because they have rapid onset, shorter durations of action, or both. These agents are uniquely useful for patients receiving anesthesia for outpatient surgery and should become of particular importance for the elderly population. Such agents include narcotics (alfentanil, sufentanil), muscle relaxants (atracurium, vecuronium), and intravenous anesthetics (propofol). One inhalational agent currently in the final stages of clinical trials, Desflurane, should also be of use in the elderly because it is rapidly eliminated when discontinued.

REMARKS

Many of the changes of aging have little to do with the ultimate technical success of a surgical procedure, or for that matter, the administration of anesthetic drugs. They may, however, have a bearing on the patient's overall well being, and his or her perceptions of the "caring" qualities of the medical staff. Stimulated by the burgeoning numbers of older patients, we are challenged to improve both our understanding of the aging process and the care we render. Finally, from a more selfish standpoint, we should remember that we will someday benefit ourselves if we do our job well.

SUGGESTED READING

Brandfonbrener M, Landowne M, Shock NW. Changes in cardiac output with age. Circulation 1955; 12:557–566.

Cole WH. Prediction of operative reserve in the elderly patient. Ann Surg 1968; 168:310–311.

Djokovic JL, Hedley-Whyte J. Prediction of outcome of surgery and anesthesia in patients over 80. JAMA 1979; 242:2301–2306.

Drachman DA. An approach to the neurology of aging. In: Birren JE, Sloane RB, eds. Handbook of mental health and aging. Englewood Cliffs, NJ: Prentice-Hall, 1980:501.

Evans DA, Funkenstein HH, Albert MS, et al. Prevalence of Alzheimers's disease in a community population of older persons: higher than previously reported. JAMA 1989; 262:2552–2556.

Everitt AV. The brain and neuroendocrine system. In: Stephen CR, Assaf RAE, eds. Geriatric anesthesia. Principles and practice. Boston: Butterworths, 1986:87.

Francis J, Martin D, Kapoor WN. A prospective study of delirium in hospitalized elderly. JAMA 1990; 263:1097–1101.

Hosking MP, Warner MA, Lobdell CM, et al. Outcomes of surgery in patients 90 years of age and older. JAMA 1989; 261:1909–1915.

Kenney RA. Physiology of aging. A synopsis. 2nd ed. Chicago: Year Book Medical Publishers, 1989.

Lakatta EG. Health, disease, and cardiovascular aging. In: The aging society: the burden of long-term illness and disability. Washington, D.C.: National Academy of Sciences Institute of Medicine, National Academy Press, 1986.

Larson EB, Kukull WA, Buchner D, et al. Adverse drug reactions associated with global cognitive impairment in elderly persons. Ann Intern Med 1987; 107:169–173.

Lonergan ET. Aging and the kidney: adjusting treatment to physiologic change. Geriatrics 1988; 43:27–33.

Montamat SC, Cusack BJ, Vestal RE. Management of drug therapy in the elderly. N Engl J Med 1989; 321:303–309.

Muravchick S. The aging patient and age-related disease. ASA refresher courses in anesthesiology. 1988; 16:145–153.

Pontoppidan H, Beecher HK. Progressive loss of protective reflexes in the airway with advance of age. JAMA 1960; 174:2209–2213.

Rodeheffer R, Gerstenblith G, Becker LC, et al. Exercise cardiac output is maintained with advancing age in healthy subjects: cardiac dilation and increased stroke volume compensate for a diminished heart rate. Circulation 1984; 69:203–213.

Shamburek RD, Farrar JT. Disorders of the digestive system in the elderly. N Engl J Med 1990; 322:438–443.

Stanski DR, Maitre PO. Population pharmacokinetics and pharmacodynamics of thiopental: the effects of age revisited. Anesthesiology 1990; 72:412–422.

Stephen CR, Assaf RAE. Geriatric anesthesia. Principles and practice. Boston: Butterworths, 1986.

Woodrow KM, Friedman GD, Siegelaub AB, et al. Anesthesia for patients aged over ninety years. NY State J Med 1977; 77:1421–1425.

ANESTHESIA IN CARDIAC SURGERY

FUNDAMENTALS AND COMPLICATIONS OF CARDIAC BYPASS

JOHN R. MOYERS, M.D.

Since its first clinical use in the mid-1950s the basic elements of the cardiopulmonary bypass machine have remained unchanged. However, technologic advances, ongoing research, new anesthetic techniques and agents, and complex surgical procedures have created a different environment for the anesthesiologist. The purpose of this chapter is to discuss the fundamentals, controversial areas, and complications related to cardiopulmonary bypass.

CARDIOPULMONARY BYPASS CIRCUIT

Systemic venous blood is drained by gravity into a venous reservoir and then passes into a blood oxygenator where carbon dioxide is removed and oxygen is added. A heat exchanger is an integral part of the oxygenator. After being cooled or warmed, oxygenated perfusate passes through tubing in a roller pump into a large artery (Fig. 1).

Cannulation

Arterial cannulation of the aorta or femoral artery is usually performed before venous cannulation. This allows for rapid transfusion through the arterial inflow line, if necessary. Also, arterial cannulation is usually less disruptive to the circulation than venous cannula placement. Systemic venous drainage from the body to the venous reservoir is usually accomplished through cannulation of the right atrium or the vena cavae, although the femoral vein can be used, as well.

Venous Reservoir

Systemic venous blood flows into the reservoir by means of a siphon mechanism. Thus "air locks" can be a problem. When they do occur, the problem can often be rectified by having the surgeon or perfusionist simply "milk" the air toward the venous reservoir. Many perfusionists attach a low-level alarm system to the venous reservoir. If the reservoir level becomes too low, the perfusionist can either decrease arterial inflow from the pump while waiting for more venous return or add fluid to the venous reservoir. Most important, the venous reservoir must not become empty; if it does, air may be pumped into the arterial circulation of the patient.

Blood Oxygenator

Disposable bubble and membrane oxygenators are the two types predominantly used today. Oxygen or a

CARDIOPULMONARY BYPASS CIRCUIT

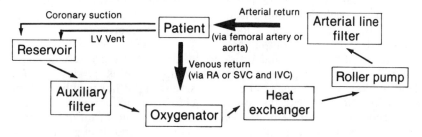

Figure 1 Cardiopulmonary bypass circuit. (Republished with permission from Tinker JH. Cardiopulmonary bypass: technical aspects. In: Thomas SJ, ed. Manual of cardiac anesthesia. New York: Churchill Livingstone, 1984:375.)

mixture of air and oxygen is metered through the devices. Removal of carbon dioxide is usually not a problem. In fact, in some centers, carbon dioxide is added to the gas mixture.

The bubble-type oxygenator is highly efficient and involves direct contact between bubbled oxygen and blood. Before the perfusate passes out of the oxygenator, a defoaming agent or other mechanism removes the bubbles. Generally, more trauma to blood cells is associated with the bubble-type oxygenator.

The membrane oxygenator separates blood and oxygen by means of a thin, gas-permeable, silicone membrane. Because this results in less trauma to blood cells, some recommend the membrane oxygenator for use in all bypass procedures. Others reserve the more expensive membrane oxygenator for when it is anticipated that extracorporeal circulation will exceed 2 hours.

Heat Exchanger

The heat exchanger is integrated with the oxygenator to cool or heat the perfusate. Within the exchanger, heated or cooled water surrounds the perfusate as it passes through the unit. The temperature of the water bath in the heating/cooling unit and the temperature of the perfusate are continuously monitored during bypass.

The heat exchanger allows for hypothermic organ protection during cardiopulmonary bypass. Its function is similar to hybernation, with an approximately 7 percent per degree centigrade reduction in metabolic rate. The metabolic rate is reduced by approximately 50 percent at 30° and by 85 to 100 percent at 20°C. Hypothermia allows for a reduction in bypass flow during extracorporeal circulation and, if necessary, for periods of circulatory arrest (up to 60 minutes at 16 to 18°C). A disadvantage is that hypothermic bypass requires the time at the end of bypass for rewarming. The perfusate can be heated to a temperature approximately 10°C higher than the patient's core temperature during rewarming. There is a limit to the gradient in that the perfusate should not be heated above 41°C because of the danger of enzymatic derangement.

Roller Pump

The roller pump, which drives the perfusate into a large artery, is a double-arm, nonocclusive pump driven by a constant-speed motor. Because the pump is load insensitive, a constant speed and cardiac output are maintained over a wide range of pressures and resistances within the arterial inflow tubing. A totally occlusive pump can lead to blood cell damage and can also damage the pump tubing. Nevertheless, the roller pumps must be occlusive enough to generate pressures of at least 300 mm Hg. Because of the constant-speed mechanism, high pressures generated in the inflow line can cause disconnections or even rupture of the pump "boot" (the plastic tubing carrying the perfusate within the roller head pump).

Additions to the Pump

Many pump set-ups include an arterial inflow filter or a bubble trap. The filter removes debris, clots, and gas bubbles. A bubble trap removes gas bubbles just before the blood enters the arterial inflow line. The arterial inflow filter must have a bypass line around it in case the filter becomes completely occluded. An arterial inflow line pressure gauge is often inserted into the system. Because of the resistance in the inflow line tubing, this arterial line pressure often exceeds systemic pressure. A cardiotomy suction and a ventricular vent or sump return blood from the operative field to the venous reservoir. Suction is generated by roller-head pumps, which often contain filters. These pumps take the place of wall suction and allow for intraoperative blood salvage. Ordinarily, the left ventricular vent is placed in the right superior pulmonary vein, through the left atrium and into the ventricle to decompress it. The cardioplegic solution is often delivered by another roller-head pump on the bypass machine.

Various methods can be used to monitor arterial and venous blood gases. One method is to observe the color of venous and arterial tubing and send intermittent blood samples for arterial and venous blood gas determinations. Saturation monitors may be placed on the arterial and venous pump lines. Monitoring devices allow for on-line continuous measurements of partial pressure of oxygen (Po_2), carbon dioxide partial pressure (Pco_2), and pH on the arterial and venous lines. Finally, a dialysis-type hemoconcentrator to remove water may be incorporated into the bypass system.

Pump Primes

The many recipes for pump primes are more alike than different. The prime is similar in osmolality and electrolyte content to blood. In adults, 1.5 to 2.5 L of "clear," bloodless prime is generally used. This decreases viscosity during hypothermic bypass and reduces the amount of blood and therefore exposure to transfusion-transmitted disease. The benefits of hemodilution (hematocrit 20 to 25 percent) generally outweigh the risk. One is more likely to see the use of blood and osmotically active fluids in the primes for children. The pump primes for children also involve smaller volumes.

At the beginning of bypass, venous blood is allowed to drain into the reservoir and revolution of the roller pumps achieves the desired cardiac output. The perfusionist and other members of the operating room team check for adequacy of venous return, mean arterial pressure, and arterial inflow line pressure. Shortly thereafter and throughout bypass, they monitor arterial and venous blood gases and ensure that signs of adequate patient perfusion exist.

CONTROVERSIAL AREAS OF BYPASS MANAGEMENT

Mean Arterial Blood Pressure and Flow

A range of mean systemic arterial blood pressures (30 to 100 mm Hg) and cardiopulmonary bypass flows (1.2 to 3.0 L per minute per square meter) is used in different institutions. Controversy centers primarily on the mean blood pressure and pump flow that are adequate for perfusion of the central nervous system. Some institutions use low flows (30 ml per kilogram per minute, 1.2 L per minute per square meter) and do not treat blood pressure unless is exceeds approximately 60 mm Hg. Vasodilators would then be used to increase organ perfusion. With these low flows, hypothermia is an important feature of bypass. This "low-flow low-pressure" method reduces noncoronary collateral flow and therefore adds to the preservation of the myocardial protection afforded by cardioplegia and topical hypothermia. The lower flows also reduce trauma to the blood cells. In addition, studies have not shown a definite increase in postoperative neurologic deficits with the use of the low-flow techniques.

Most centers currently use higher flows (60 ml per kilogram per minute, 2.0 to 2.5 L per minute per square meter), with a mean blood pressure of around 60 mm Hg and hypothermia to 28°C. Previously, there was concern that central nervous system damage correlated with the duration of "hypotension" (mean arterial pressure less than 50 mm Hg) during bypass. However, recent evidence shows that, in patients without cerebral vascular disease, a mean blood pressure of 30 mm Hg with moderate or high flows during hypothermia may be adequate. In patients with normal cerebral circulation, cerebral blood flow may be independent of perfusion pressure in the range of 30 to 110 mm Hg during hypothermia and nonpulsatile bypass. In patients with cerebral vascular disease or in older patients (>60 to 70 years of age), however, pressures as low as 30 mm Hg may not be acceptable during normothermic bypass.

Hypertension is also an issue in the higher flow techniques. With pressures greater than 70 to 100 mm Hg, increasing noncoronary collateral flow may lead to premature warming of the heart. As bypass progresses, mean arterial pressure usually increases due to hypothermia and the increased levels of "stress hormones." In many centers, to reduce blood pressure, an anesthetic agent or a specific vasodilator is used to decrease systemic vascular resistance, thus leaving bypass flow constant.

The pressure often drops immediately after initiation of bypass. This may be due to changes in viscosity, anemia, low oncotic pressure of the perfusate, hypothermia, nonpulsatility, or deep anesthesia. A question arises of neurologic damage in a hypotensive, normothermic patient versus the uneven cooling that may accompany administration of vasoconstrictors. Most anesthesiologists wait a few minutes to see if the pressure spontaneously rises in patients without pre-existing central nervous system disease and in those who are not in the geriatric age group. The blood pressure may drop again at the end of bypass during rewarming and after removal of the aortic cross clamp. At this point, concern arises over cerebral perfusion and myocardial perfusion versus the effect of uneven rewarming with treatment by vasopressors. Many anesthesiologists who feel more comfortable with a pressure of 50 to 70 mm Hg at this time either increase pump flow or administer small doses of a vasoconstrictor.

It is difficult to study the proper mean arterial pressure and flow during bypass. Differences among patients, surgical procedures, pump set-ups, temperature, and hematocrit make comparisons elusive. Therefore, the pressure/flow question remains unsettled.

Arterial pH $PaCO_2$

The issue here is the propriety of temperature correction of blood gases during bypass. The "pH-stat" method corrects blood gases to patient temperature. Proponents of this method maintain a temperature-corrected $PaCO_2$ at 35 to 40 mm Hg and a temperature-corrected arterial pH of 7.4. Often, because of oxygenator efficiency, the perfusionist must blend in carbon dioxide with the gases flowing through the oxygenator to achieve this level of $PaCO_2$.

The "alpha-stat" method does not use correction for patient temperature. The "alpha" refers to the alpha-imidazole ring on histidine, which is involved in net protein charges and is part of a major buffer system within the body. Because this method does not use a correction for temperature, during hypothermic bypass at 27°C, the uncorrected arterial pH may be as high as 7.6 and the $PaCO_2$ as low as 20 mm Hg. The pendulum has swung toward the use of the "alpha-stat" method in many institutions. It is simple and makes sense theoretically when comparisons are made with the physiology of poikilothermic animals. There probably is better maintenance of the coupling between cerebral blood flow and metabolism, and this level of acid-based status may better combat myocardial tissue acidosis after removal of the aortic cross-clamp.

Pulsatile Versus Nonpulsatile Perfusion

Pulsatile perfusion during extracorporeal circulation attempts to mimic the normal systemic arterial blood pressure waveform. Some studies show that, when compared with nonpulsatile flow, pulsatile perfusion reduces the level of "stress hormones" and increases renal blood flow. Capillary circulation, oxygen uptake, and lower levels of serum lactate have been found. Furthermore, some investigators have shown that systemic vascular resistance and mean blood pressure are lower during bypass and that lymph flow is better postoperatively. Still, nonpulsatile perfusion is used in most centers. Pulsatile flow occurs only at the expense of a more complicated cardiopulmonary bypass machine. Some studies and experience show that by simply increasing bypass flow, the objections to nonpulsatile flow are countered. Furthermore, there are few, if any, convincing patient outcome studies that favor pulsatile flow. It is very difficult to isolate flow type as a variable in such studies. The procedures and patients for which pulsatile bypass would be a distinct and consistent advantage remain unclear.

COMPLICATIONS OF CARDIOPULMONARY BYPASS

Despite recent advances, cardiopulmonary bypass is still imperfect. Because it is not the ideal replacement for the human heart and lung, it has been said that during bypass the patient is in mild shock and is "gently dying." Approximately 500 reports describe complications of cardiopulmonary bypass. Of these, the more serious and frequent are discussed below. The complications of bypass can be particularly devastating when they affect the lifestyle of a patient whose surgery has been otherwise successful.

Neurologic Complications

The reported incidence of neurologic complications after cardiopulmonary bypass ranges from 0 to 40 percent, with an average of 5 percent. The reported incidence depends on study design and the intensity and timing of the inquiry. Investigations with a small number of neurologic complications are often not prospective in nature and incorporate examinations that were not performed by a neurologist. Fortunately, many postbypass neurologic deficits are temporary, although they may take weeks or even months to resolve entirely.

Fatal cerebral damage is a terrible complication that occurs in less than 1 percent of bypass patients. Patients who remain unresponsive postoperatively after dissipation of anesthetics have a poor prognosis of recovery. Fatal cerebral damage is often the result of periods of severe hypotension or other planned and unplanned episodes of circulatory arrest.

A stroke is a focal neurologic deficit that persists for more than 24 hours. A 0 to 13 percent incidence with an average occurrence of approximately 5 percent has been reported following bypass procedures. Risk factors often associated with stroke after cardiopulmonary bypass are listed in Table 1. Studies of stroke after bypass do not delineate a definite set of risk factors. However, age greater than 70 years, prior central nervous system injury, and open heart procedures appear to predominate in reviews of this issue in the literature. Closely related to the complication of stroke is visual or hearing loss noted postoperatively. This is a rare problem that is believed to be due to emboli causing ischemic optic neuropathy or retinopathy or emboli producing unilateral hearing loss.

Neuropsychological dysfunction occurs in 10 to 50

Table 1 Factors Associated with Neurologic Injury After Cardiopulmonary Bypass

Age
Prior central nervous system injury
Calcified aorta
Intracardiac thrombi
Duration of extracorporeal circulation
Type of oxygenator
Nonuse of filters
Open heart procedures

The factors listed have been associated in some studies, but not all, with neurologic deficit after cardiopulmonary bypass.

percent of patients following bypass. The incidence seems to increase with age. These are not focal cerebral infarctions, but instead are subtle changes detected through interviews with the patient and family and through neuropsychological testings. Deficits range from acute psychosis to mild disorientation, mood change, confusion, and psychomotor dysfunction. Psychological testing reveals intellectual and cognitive changes that include problems with concentration, memory, and learning. Although these defects almost always improve, it may take up to 6 months before complete resolution occurs.

The incidence of peripheral nerve injury varies from 5 to 30 percent. Common within this classification is injury to the brachial plexus at the C8–T1 distribution. A proposed explanation for this problem is that sternal retraction causes a fracture of the first rib, thus damaging the nerves of the brachial plexus. Hypothermia may also contribute to the injury. The ulnar nerve may be damaged at the olecranon from improper arm positioning at the side of the operating room table. Phrenic nerve injuries are occasionally reported. These may occur from stretch or transsection of the nerve, or from hypothermia from the cardioplegic solution or ice placed within the pericardial well. Horner's syndrome and nerve injuries to the lateral femoral cutaneous, median, radial, and common peroneal nerves have also been reported.

Awareness during cardiopulmonary bypass occasionally occurs. Many anesthesiologists believe the risk of awareness is greatest during the rewarming period at the end of bypass, when the anesthetic contribution of hypothermia is gone. Anesthesiologists desire to have as little depressant drug on board as possible so that the myocardium can function well during emergence from cardiopulmonary bypass. Anesthetic depth is difficult to judge because of the effect of muscle relaxants, the artificial physiology imposed by the heart-lung machine, and patient perspiration produced by the hyperthermic perfusate. Any inhalation anesthetics used during bypass have usually been discontinued or reduced in inspired concentration several minutes previously. During bypass using a bubble oxygenator, up to 10 to 25 percent of an inhalation agent may be present 15 minutes after its discontinuation (Fig. 2). Although not well studied, wash-out may be slower with membrane oxygenators.

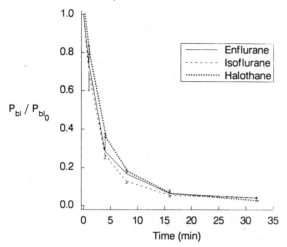

B. Washout of Multiple Anesthetics

Figure 2 Wash-out curves for the three volatile anesthetics, enflurane, isoflurane, and halothane. The partial pressure of each anesthetic in blood (P_{bl}) is expressed as a ratio; the denominator is the peak partial pressure in the sample obtained just before discontinuation of anesthetic administration (P_{bl_0}). (Republished with permission from Nussmeier NA, et al. In vitro anesthetic wash-in and wash-out via bubble oxygenators: influence of anesthetic solubility and ratio of carrier gas inflow and pump blood flow. Anesth Analg 1988; 67:985.)

Despite many studies, a framework for adjusting doses of intravenous drugs during bypass has not been established. Nevertheless, at the end of bypass there is often a need for amnesia but not for myocardial depression. Many anesthesiologists therefore include amnesic drugs such as scopalamine, lorazepam, and diazepam as part of the anesthetic to prevent awareness.

Spinal cord injury and seizures are two other rare neurologic complications that have been reported after cardiopulmonary bypass.

Neurologic Sequelae

As more evidence is accumulated, emboli appear to play a major role in the causation of central nervous system damage after bypass. Filters in the arterial inflow line and venous suction line on the bypass machine have probably helped to reduce emboli, but microemboli and macroemboli remain a major factor in postbypass neurologic problems. Macroemboli occur in both solid and gaseous forms. Solid macroemboli come from intercardiac thrombi, valvular debris, and clamping and cannulation of ascending aorta, which may release atheromatous plaques. Large gaseous emboli are usually in the form of air. Mechanisms of air emboli include depletion of blood in the venous reservoir; resumption of heartbeat before removal of the air from the heart and great vessels; reversal of the pump head and direction of flow; and a pressurized cardiotomy reservoir. Air emboli can also originate from intravenous sites in patients with intracardiac shunts. Microemboli can take the solid or gaseous form. Solid microemboli may come from fibrin and fibrin products; aggregation of platelets and leukocytes; fat and other solids from the cardiotomy suction and cautery; and synthetic material from the oxygenator. Gaseous microemboli include oxygen, air, and nitrous oxide, if used after bypass. As mentioned previously, the presence of microemboli and their association with postoperative neurologic deficit are the impetus for including filters in the bypass system.

Decreased cerebral perfusion has also been considered a cause of postbypass neurologic sequelae, especially in the elderly and in patients with cerebral vascular disease. Patients with a history of a prior neurologic event or with known cerebral vascular disease are three to eight times more likely to suffer central nervous system insult after bypass. Certainly those patients with severe drops in perfusion pressure or no perfusion pressure for extended periods of time are at risk. Another cause of decreased cerebral perfusion pressure is misplacement of the cannula. For example, the tip of the arterial cannula may be misplaced in the innominate artery or in the carotid artery, or the venous cannula can be kinked or misplaced, leading to increased pressure in the superior vena cava and to cerebral congestion.

Attempts have been made to monitor the central nervous system during bypass and to provide therapy once a neurologic deficit has been suspected or known to have occurred. Simply monitoring mean blood pressure or attempting to provide a neurologic examination during bypass are much too unsophisticated. Attempts to monitor the electroencephalogram during bypass have been largely unsatisfactory. The process is complicated, difficult for the untrained to interpret, and confounded by anesthetic agents, hypothermia, false-negatives, and false-positives. Although automated electroencephalographic processing, compressed spectral array, and evoked potentials may be simpler to interpret, they have yet to achieve widespread application in monitoring central nervous system function during bypass. Finally, there is current interest in quantifying cerebral blood flow during bypass to help identify periods of central nervous system risk.

Prevention appears to be the key. Elimination of emboli, and maintenance of cerebral perfusion and hypothermia are the mainstays for many cardiac teams. Other preventative measures include avoidance of hyperglycemia and hypoglycemia and attempts at cerebral protection with barbiturates, calcium entry blockers, or other drugs that may reduce cerebral metabolic oxygen requirements.

Mechanical Complications

A rare but potentially devastating mechanical complication is aortic dissection at the site of arterial cannulation. This problem must be recognized quickly. After arterial cannulation, the team must look for pulsations in the arterial inflow tubing at the blood-prime interface. The perfusionist should check the arterial inflow line pressure gauge for pulsations. When arterial dissection occurs upon initiation of bypass, pressure displayed by the arterial inflow line pressure gauge increases while the patient's systemic arterial pressure decreases. Venous return decreases and the size of the aorta increases.

Failure or dysfunction of the oxygenator, roller head pumps, or bypass tubing may occur. The cardiopulmonary bypass machine, especially the oxygenator, contributes to the destruction of erythrocytes and platelets and inhibition of platelet function. The system may also produce denaturation of proteins and coagulation abnormalities. With the efficiency of a bubble oxygenator, hyperoxygenation and hypocapnia may ensue. Hyperoxygenation can become an issue when aggressive rewarming of the perfusate results in oxygen coming out of solution and appearing as microbubbles in the blood.

Another potential mechanical problem is the failure of wall oxygen or of the oxygenator, which results in hypoxia. As mentioned before, the bypass machine can be a source of gaseous and solid microemboli. Periods of hypoperfusion or no perfusion can occur with the rupture of the plastic bypass tubing, disconnection of arterial or venous tubing, and dislodgement of vessel cannulae. The power source of the cardiopulmonary bypass machine is electricity. An electrical failure at the wall outlet or within the pump prevents circulation to the patient. If this occurs, the roller head pump for the arterial inflow line must be turned by hand with a crank.

A mechanical problem that may occur after emergence from bypass is the discrepancy between the radial arterial line pressure and the central aortic pressure. It is not uncommon for the radial arterial pressure to read lower, not reflecting central aortic pressure (Fig. 3). One study has proposed that a reduction in arterial resistance at the wrist is the reason for this difference. Infusion of vasodilators can compound the problem. If the falsely low blood pressure from the radial arterial line is not recognized, vasopressors may be administered unnecessarily. The blood pressure cuff may be neither accurate nor reliable enough at this critical period. Direct measurement of central aortic pressure with a needle inserted into the aorta can distinguish between real hypotension and a difference between pressure readings in the radial artery and aorta. Usually the discrepancy between the radial arterial pressure and central aortic pressure resolves over 20 to 30 minutes, in time to remove the aortic needle before chest closure. If it does not, a femoral arterial line can be inserted to assure a more accurate measure of central systemic pressure.

Blood Trauma

Damage to the formed and unformed elements of the blood can occur from mechanical trauma, exposure to foreign surfaces, and dilution from the pump prime. The problem can become compounded by long bypass runs and large quantities of blood passing through the cardiotomy suction or vents for extended periods.

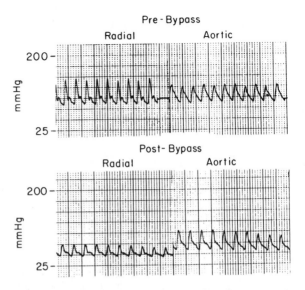

Figure 3 Reversal of the usual relationships between percutaneous radial and aortic pressure after cardiopulmonary bypass. (Republished with permission from Stern DH, et al. Can we trust the direct radial artery pressure immediately following cardiopulmonary bypass? Anesthesiology 1985; 62: 558.)

Damage to the formed elements involves virtually all blood cells. The red cells can be hemolyzed, thrombocytopenia and decreased platelet function may occur, and leukopenia may result from cardiopulmonary bypass. The clotting factors are also affected by bypass. The levels of all clotting factors decrease, but not usually to pathologic levels. Although fibrinolysis and disseminated intervascular coagulopathy occur, these are rare after cardiopulmonary bypass. Also, bleeding complications may result from residual heparin and from preoperative medications such as aspirin, sodium warfarin (Coumadin), or streptokinase, and possibly protamine.

Renal Dysfunction

Depending on the rigidity of the criteria, postoperative renal dysfunction occurs in 2 to 31 percent of bypass patients. Although it is rare, severe, oliguric renal failure has a 67 percent mortality rate. Postoperative renal dysfunction is usually related to low cardiac output after bypass. Prolonged bypass may be a contributory factor. Nonoliguric renal failure has a better prognosis than oliguric renal failure. This has in part prompted the use of mannitol, diuretics, dopamine, and vasodilators during the postbypass period, and even the early use of hemodialysis.

Pulmonary Complications

In adult patients without pre-existing lung disease, pulmonary complications after cardiopulmonary bypass are extremely rare and often of no consequence. This is especially true when patients are ventilated for several hours after bypass. Improvements in pump technology have decreased the occurrence of "pump lung." However, patients with pre-existing lung disease or who experience extended procedures on bypass may develop problems with oxygenation and require some days of mechanical ventilation. In a heparinized patient, pulmonary complications can also be caused by bleeding into the lung or airways as a result of manipulation or trauma. Pulmonary dysfunction may also result from an increase in pulmonary venous pressure, with distention of the left ventricle from inadequate venting or left ventricular failure. Pulmonary dysfunction after bypass is more common in children than it is in adults. Postoperative respiratory dysfunction in children after bypass correlates inversely with age and directly with the duration of bypass.

Gastrointestinal Problems

Gastrointestinal problems occur in less than 1 percent of patients after bypass. Gastrointestinal bleeding has been reported most commonly from duodenal ulcers but occasionally from the gastric mucosa. This is thought to be related to the stress of cardiopulmonary bypass. An increase in serum bilirubin levels and acute cholecystitis are rare occurrences. Pancreatitis and large and small bowel infarction, ileus, obstruction, or perforation have also been reported. Gastrointestinal problems often occur in patients with multisystem disease and dysfunction of other organs. Therefore, it is difficult to attribute these postoperative gastrointestinal problems to cardiopulmonary bypass alone.

Postoperative Hypothermia

Postoperative hypothermia may result from inadequate core rewarming and the redistribution of temperature within the body. In the operating room after bypass, the patient's body temperature may decrease for prolonged periods, while hemostasis or chest closure is achieved and with the transfusion of unwarmed intravenous fluids.

SUGGESTED READING

Hindman BJ, ed. Neurologic and psychologic complications of surgery and anesthesia. Int Anesthesiol Clin 1986; 24:1–265.
Nussmeier NA, Lambert ML, Moskowitz GJ, et al. Wash in and wash out of isoflurane administered via bubble oxygenators during hypothermic cardiopulmonary bypass. Anesthesiology 1989; 71: 519–525.
Ream AK. Cardiopulmonary bypass. In: Ream AK, Fogdall RP, eds. Acute cardiovascular management. Philadelphia: JB Lippincott, 1982:420.
Tinker JH, ed. Cardiopulmonary bypass: current concepts and controversies. Philadelphia: WB Saunders, 1989.
Tinker JH, Roberts SL. Management of cardiopulmonary bypass. In: Kaplan JA, ed. Cardiac anesthesia. Orlando, FL: Grune & Stratton, 1987:895.

CORONARY ARTERY DISEASE

ROBERT G. MERIN, M.D.

A substantial proportion of the patients who present for anesthesia and surgery today in the United States have some degree of coronary artery (or ischemic heart) disease. In particular, it has been estimated that 1.5 million patients being anesthetized for noncardiac surgery have coronary artery disease (1 million overt, 500,000 silent). This is the population discussed in this chapter. I will review (1) preoperative assessment of the patient; (2) the risk of surgery and anesthesia; (3) preoperative therapy that can minimize this risk; and, finally, (4) planning for proper monitoring during the perioperative period.

ASSESSMENT OF THE DEGREE OF CORONARY ARTERY DISEASE

History

As in any patient, one of the most important aspects of the evaluation is the history. Of particular importance in patients with coronary artery disease is the history of symptomatic myocardial infarction and the date of that infarction. In addition, it is important to determine whether the patient has suffered significant sequelae of the infarction, such as persistent angina, left or right ventricular failure, or arrhythmias. Regardless of whether the patient has had an infarction, a thorough evaluation of possible symptomatology is necessary (chest pain or substernal discomfort, radiation of that pain, environmental factors that exacerbate or relieve the pain [including exercise], and any symptoms of congestive heart failure—either respiratory, which indicates left heart failure, or edema, which suggests right heart failure). A most important component of the history in these patients is their prior drug therapy. The physiologic preparation for the patient who is mildly symptomatic or asymptomatic without drug therapy should certainly be totally different from that of a patient taking a beta-blocker, a calcium-channel blocker, and a nitrate in order to produce relief of symptoms. It is important to note whether there has been an acceleration of symptoms and drug therapy and, in particular, which type of drug appears to produce the most symptomatic relief for the individual patient.

Physical Examination

The next logical step in evaluating these patients is the physical examination. On physical examination, evidence of ventricular failure should be particularly noted. For the left ventricle, a finding of basilar rales and/or an S_4 murmur suggests left ventricular failure. In addition, left ventricular enlargement on percussion should cause one to be suspicious. However, a more quantitative method is chest roentgenography. Neck vein distention, hepatomegaly, and peripheral edema suggest right heart decompensation. The other major physical finding of interest would be evidence of an arrhythmia, which must be validated by an electro-cardiogram. In addition, it would be best to assess the adequacy of peripheral pulses, particularly those that are radial, in preparation for monitoring. Again, for monitoring purposes, the ability of the patient to lie flat or, even better, in the head-down position should be ascertained during the preoperative evaluation as well. Of course, blood pressure and heart rate should also be noted. The presence of hypertension—either systolic or diastolic—constitutes an increased risk factor, and for the patient with coronary artery disease, a slow heart rate is to be desired. In particular, if the patient is being treated with a beta-adrenergic–blocking drug, basal heart rate is one index of the adequacy of therapy.

Laboratory Examination

The more complete the laboratory examination, the better able the physician is to assess the risk and the type of monitoring to be used for anesthesia and surgery. Minimum laboratory examination for every patient with a history of coronary artery disease should include measurements of hemoglobin, cardiac enzymes including the MB fraction of the creatinine phosphokinase enzyme, serum creatinine for assessment of renal function (in order to optimize fluid management), and electrolytes if the patient is taking any type of diuretic drug. Of course, an electrocardiogram and a chest roentgenogram are most important. The electrocardiogram is important for assessing the risk (Table 1). In patients with new or changing signs and symptoms of coronary artery disease, a step-protocol of progressively more invasive testing is recommended, beginning with a stress (treadmill or isometric exercise) electrocardiogram. If the results are positive, performing a stress or dipyridamole-thallium perfusion scan is the next step. A positive result dictates coronary angiography and cardiac catheterization. A further positive result with the proper anatomy is an indication for either percutaneous angioplasty or coronary artery bypass grafting before elective surgery. Even if corrective therapy is not possible, the results of these tests can help the anesthesiologist in the perioperative care of patient needing urgent surgery. For example, the classic stress test using treadmill exercise and electrocardiography can also give information about the threshold heart rate and blood pressure at which either electrocardiographic changes or symptoms occur. (Generally speaking, however, the thallium stress test is as useful as the classic stress test and is easier for physician and patient.) In addition to or instead of the thallium scan, echocardiographic or radionuclide estimation of ventricular filling, wall motion, and ejection fraction can also be accomplished non-invasively. Of course, if there is a full-fledged cardiac catheterization, then the degree of coronary stenosis, wall motion abnormalities, left ventricular end-diastolic pressure, cardiac index, and ejection fraction should be noted in this evaluation.

Table 1   Risk of Anesthesia and Surgery in the Patient with Coronary Artery Disease

	Factors	*Risk*
(1)	Angina easily controlled by rest or medication No arrhythmia or signs of heart failure* No myocardial infarction within 1 year prior to surgery	Mild—reassure patient and family
(2)	Symptoms controlled by significant medication No arrhythmia or signs of heart failure* Myocardial infarction 6 months to 1 year prior to surgery	Mild-to-moderate—inform patient and family
(3)	Symptoms *usually* controlled by medication Arrhythmia or signs of heart failure* Myocardial infarction 3–6 months prior to surgery	Moderate-to-severe—if possible, surgery should be delayed until more than 6 months after myocardial infarction, arrhythmia, and congestive heart failure have been treated
(4)	Intractable angina with or without arrhythmias or signs of heart failure* Myocardial infarction less than 3 months prior to surgery	Severe—only emergency surgery should be scheduled and full monitoring is mandatory (see Table 2)

*Ejection fraction <40%, cardiomegaly and/or congestion on chest roentgenogram, moderate-to-severe wall motion abnormality.

ASSESSING THE RISK OF ANESTHESIA AND SURGERY

Several studies on the risk of anesthesia and non-cardiac surgery for the patient with a previous myocardial infarction have been published over the past 20 years. There is amazing agreement among studies disparate in location, patient population, and year as to the important risk factors for these patients. In all studies, a recurrent myocardial infarction carried an inordinate mortality rate (more than 50 percent) when compared with the mortality rate of a primary myocardial infarction not associated with surgery and anesthesia. The risk of recurrent myocardial infarction was related to several factors. The date of the previous myocardial infarction relative to the anesthesia and surgery was the most common risk factor across all studies. Without exception, the retrospective studies from New York Hospital–Cornell Medical Center, the Mayo Clinic, Case Western Reserve University, and St. Vincent's Hospital in New York showed that the risk of recurrent infarction was almost prohibitive in patients who had had their previous infarction within 3 months of surgery and anesthesia. There was still a significant increase in risk at 6 months after the previous infarction, and in most studies, after 6 months the risk was markedly decreased, although even 2 years after an infarction, the risk was considerably (10 to 100 times) greater than in patients without a previous myocardial infarction. However, a publication derived from the coronary artery surgery study (which was not designed for this particular evaluation) denied that previous myocardial infarction, recent or remote, was a factor in perioperative mortality or morbidity in patients with coronary artery disease. Rao's group from Loyola of Chicago claimed that with intensive monitoring and control of myocardial oxygen balance, the incidence of perioperative myocardial infarction and death could be markedly reduced in patients with a previous myocardial infarction. Other risk factors that were not as consistent across studies included intractable angina, evidence of congestive heart failure, and the persistence of arrhythmias following myocardial infarction, especially complete heart block. The famous Goldman study also suggested that the signs and symptoms of congestive heart failure and arrhythmias were important risk predictors for patients with all types of cardiac disease. Studies from the University of California at San Francisco have suggested that patients with severely impaired ventricular function (ejection fractions of less than 40 percent) and/or severe wall motion abnormalities are at considerably greater risk for severe complications during and after aortocoronary bypass surgery. In addition, the same group reported that the presence of cardiomegaly on preoperative chest roentgenograms was also a risk factor. It seems likely that in patients undergoing noncardiac surgery, these same risk factors would apply, although they have not been as well assessed in this group of patients.

Operative Procedure and Choice of Anesthetic

In several studies, the operative site and conditions of operation have also influenced morbidity and mortality. In general, the more extensive the operative procedure, the greater the risk. In both the Cornell-New York Hospital and the Mayo Clinic studies, intrathoracic and upper abdominal surgery carried a substantially higher risk than other more peripheral surgical procedures. In one of the Mayo Clinic studies, the duration of surgery was important. Surgical procedures that lasted for more than 2 hours carried a significantly greater risk of reinfarction and death than those which lasted less than 2 hours. In general, the effect of the anesthetic agent and technique used has not been significant, although the Mayo Clinic and Cornell-New York Hospital studies had very few regional anesthetic procedures. Several studies have documented the high incidence of perioperative ischemia, infarction, and mortality in patients undergoing vascular surgery, both on great and peripheral vessels. Emergency surgery also increased the risk of perioperative myocardial infarction and death. A separate study from the Mayo Clinic in which patients for eye surgery under regional anesthesia were evaluated showed a remarkably low incidence of complications in patients with documented ischemic heart disease; however, it is unclear whether this is also related to the type of surgery, since there were no comparative data for patients having eye surgery under general anesthesia. The interesting study from Loyola of Chicago suggested that the incidence of significant complications in patients with ischemic heart disease was greater when nitrous oxide–narcotic techniques of anesthesia were used, compared with inhalation anesthetic-based techniques. Although there has been some suggestion that regional anesthesia or combined regional and general anesthesia are safer than general anesthesia alone, the evidence is inconclusive.

Several studies have suggested that a patient with symptomatic relief from aortocoronary bypass surgery is in the low-risk (see Table 1) category. Similar data for the patient rated with percutaneous angioplasty and/or thrombolysis are not available as yet.

It is most important to communicate the risk to the patient and his or her family. I do not believe it is possible to actually quantitate this in the individual patient, but certainly a qualitative estimate can be given, depending on the risk factors enumerated above. Many surgeons and internists quote the Goldman index as quantifying the risk. However, it is important to realize that this widely quoted study was from one specific hospital, had several exclusions, and did not deal primarily with patients with ischemic heart disease. Consequently, I do not believe that the Goldman index is particularly useful for this category of patients.

PREOPERATIVE THERAPY

The obvious goal of preoperative preparation and therapy of these patients is to optimize their myocardial oxygen supply/demand ratio. The determinants of oxygen supply—namely coronary blood flow (CBF)—and arterial oxygen content should be greater than the determinants of oxygen demand—namely heart rate, ventricular wall tension (or stress), and contractile performance. In the clinical situation, neither CBF, ventricular wall stress, nor contractile performance can be quantitated. In patients with stenotic coronary arteries, CBF is highly pressure-dependent, so coronary perfusion pressure (diastolic arterial minus ventricular filling) must be maintained. In addition, since most CBF occurs during diastole, a slow heart rate optimizes nutritive CBF. A slow heart rate also decreases oxygen demand, so bradycardia is highly desirable. As long as coronary perfusion pressure (and peripheral perfusion) are adequate, there is no lower safe limit for heart rate in these patients. Ventricular wall tension is a function of ventricular diameter, pressure, and wall thickness. For both hemodynamic and metabolic efficiency, a small heart is desirable. In summary, the goal of therapy for the patient with ischemic heart disease is a small heart that is contracting slowly but generating a high diastolic pressure! As indicated above, the major drug categories that have been useful for achieving this goal include the beta-adrenergic–blocking drugs, the calcium-channel blocking drugs, and the nitrates. In addition, any concurrent pathophysiology (e.g., hypertension, congestive heart failure) must also be treated. Although in the past (and unfortunately sometimes even today) there has been a tendency to discontinue the use of cardioactive drugs before surgery and anesthesia, there is now clear evidence that such a practice in a patient with ischemic heart disease is not warranted. The patient's drug therapy should be optimized. That is, drugs should be titrated to maximum symptomatic and hemodynamic effects. With the use of beta-blocking drugs, the resting heart rate should be no more than 70 beats per minute or, at the outside, 80 beats per minute. The heart rate response to the calcium-channel–blocking drugs is much less consistent, and symptomatic relief of anginal symptoms and control of systolic blood pressure is a more important endpoint for these drugs. When the vasodilating nitrates are used, it is important that the dosage be tailored so that there is not undue systemic hypotension, since these patients are highly pressure-dependent for their coronary perfusion, as mentioned earlier. Consequently, the largest dose of nitrates (long-acting oral preparations or topical nitroglycerin) that is consistent with symptomatic relief and a reasonably diastolic blood pressure should be used. The aim is to have the lowest possible myocardial oxygen demand (heart rate and systolic blood pressure), together with a maintained myocardial oxygen supply (diastolic blood pressure and arterial oxygen content). However, because flow through an orifice (and especially through a stenotic orifice) is also dependent on the viscosity of the fluid, the optimum hemoglobin concentration is probably in the range of 10 to 12 g dl^{-1} rather than in the range of 14 to 16 g dl^{-1} range. The use of the heart rate–systolic blood pressure product to estimate the adequacy of therapy is illogical because the implications of changes in heart rate and blood pressure are not equal. Increases in heart rate uniformly decrease the ratio of myocardial oxygen supply to demand, whereas increases in blood pressure (within limits) actually increase that ratio. Patients are often being treated with a combination of antianginal drugs. Although this can be beneficial, several of these drugs have similar effects. The beta-blockers and the cardioactive-calcium blockers, verapamil and diltiazem, have negative chronotropic, dromotropic, and inotropic effects. The calcium blockers and the nitrates both are potent vasodilators (hypotensive). Consequently, undesirable additive effects can be seen with combinations of these drugs, and one is advised to exercise caution when combining these drug classes.

In addition to treating the primary disease, it is also important to optimize ventricular function. In fact, there is even some evidence to suggest that digitalizing the patient with coronary artery disease who is not in overt congestive failure may be beneficial during the perioperative period. In any event, the patient who is digitalized should certainly continue to receive digitalis throughout the perioperative period unless there is some evidence of toxicity. Of course, systolic hypertension needs to be treated. Except for the most urgent surgery, a patient who presents with uncontrolled systemic hypertension should not undergo surgery until the hypertension is brought under control. An attempt should be made to treat any significant cardiac arrhythmias. In particular, if there is complete heart block, a pacemaker should be inserted before surgery and anesthesia are attempted.

Finally, the inevitable anxiety that the patient experiences from worrying about the disease and contemplated surgery needs to be managed. As was first shown decades ago, the best anxiolytic therapy is a sympathetic and compassionate anesthesiologist. A complete and unhurried preanesthetic visit with adequate explanation for all the patient and family concerns can allay much of the normal preoperative anxiety. However, often additional pharmacotherapy may be helpful. Although the trend in recent years has been not to use preanesthetic medication, in the patient with ischemic heart disease, judicious preoperative psychomedication, usually with a benzodiazepine, can be highly beneficial.

PREOPERATIVE PREPARATION FOR MONITORING

Although monitoring is, strictly speaking, a function of the anesthetic management of these patients, the preoperative evaluation of the patient plays a role in the decision about monitoring (Table 2). The study from the group at Loyola University in Chicago, although not perfect, does indicate that invasive monitoring and, more importantly, the response to that monitoring, can markedly decrease the risk for noncardiac surgery in patients with coronary artery disease. This is the only

Table 2 Planned Monitoring for Anesthesia and Surgery in Patients with Coronary Artery Disease

Risk factors (see Table 1)	Monitoring
1	Multilead electrocardiography; automated blood pressure; central venous pressure for major blood-losing surgery.
2	Multilead electocardiography; automated or direct intra-arterial blood pressure; central venous or pulmonary artery pressure for major blood-losing surgery; intensive care for 2–3 days.
3 and 4	Multilead electrocardiography; direct intra-arterial blood pressure; pulmonary artery catheter; intensive care for 3 days.

study in which the prohibitive risk of reinfarction and death for patients who have suffered a previous myocardial infarction within 3 months of surgery has been effectively managed. Using radial artery and pulmonary artery catheterization, and attempting to maintain heart rate, arterial pressure, and cardiac filling pressures (pulmonary capillary wedge pressure) within 10 percent of the optimal preoperative state, this group was able to anesthetize a significant number of patients for noncardiac surgery with myocardial infarctions within 3 months of that surgery, with a mortality rate of less than 5 percent. Another important finding of that study was that this care should be continued for 3 days postoperatively, since the most common day of postoperative infarction has been Day 3. Consequently, I believe that patients who have a recent myocardial infarction, evidence of congestive heart failure, intractable angina, or perhaps serious arrhythmias should be monitored throughout the perioperative period with direct arterial and pulmonary artery catheterization—primarily because the only logical way to treat hemodynamic abnormalities in these patients is to know what the abnormalities are. If one can monitor only heart rate and blood pressure, then the reasons for changes in blood pressure, especially, cannot be properly assessed. Only by measuring ventricular filling pressures, cardiac output, and calculating vascular resistance can the proper therapy for cardiovascular failure be applied. There is even something to be said for the practice by some teams of instituting this monitoring the night before surgery so that optimal filling pressures and vascular resistances for the individual patient may be estimated without the concurrent complication of surgery and anesthesia.

Monitoring Myocardial Ischemia

A major problem in monitoring these patients is the lack of an exact monitor for detecting myocardial ischemia. The multilead electrocardiogram (ECG) is still our basic monitor, but there is no question that earlier signs of myocardial ischemia can be detected. The

most well-defined of these is abnormal wall motion in the distribution of the stenosed coronary artery. New noninvasive methods, such as cardiokymography and transesophageal echocardiography, are being investigated to try to provide a safe and continuous monitor of wall motion during surgery and anesthesia. The usefulness of the transesophageal echocardiogram seems well established. However, whether the expense and training necessary are cost effective for the average practitioner still remains to be proven. The high incidence of silent myocardial ischemia in patients with coronary artery disease has made angina an imperfect index of ischemia. Although in the patient with coronary artery disease the use of regional anesthesia for surgery of the lower extremities and perineum with the patient conscious may provide an easier method of optimizing myocardial oxygen balance, the absence of angina does not guarantee that such a patient is not suffering myocardial ischemia. Nevertheless, I believe that regional anesthesia is a reasonable choice for extremity, perineal, and perhaps lower abdominal surgery. My rule of thumb is that if the regional anesthetic does not produce profound sympathetic blockade and resultant hypotension, and as long as the patient (and the anesthesiologist) can be made comfortable and free of anxiety, then a regional anesthetic can be the anesthetic of choice for the patient with coronary artery disease.

The preoperative management of the patient with coronary artery disease must focus on optimizing the balance between myocardial oxygen supply and myocardial oxygen demand. This usually involves slowing the heart rate, decreasing systolic arterial pressure while maintaining diastolic arterial pressure, treating any aspect of heart failure (particularly if a dilated ventricle is produced), and allaying the fears and anxieties of the patient, which will otherwise disturb the balance between the myocardial oxygen supply and myocardial oxygen demand. Careful assessment of the patient's history, physical condition, laboratory studies, and the planned surgery allow a certain degree of prediction of risk. This risk prediction also allows planned anesthetic and postanesthetic monitoring for maximizing the changes of a smooth perioperative course.

SUGGESTED READING

Freeman WK, Gibbons RJ, Shub C. Preoperative assessment of cardiac patients undergoing noncardiac surgical procedures. Mayo Clin Proc 1989; 64:1105–1117.

Goldman L, Caldera DL, Nussbaum SR, et al. Multifactorial index of cardiac risk in noncardiac surgical procedures. N Engl J Med 1977; 297:845–850.

Mangano ET. Perioperative cardiac morbidity. Anesthesiology 1990; 72:153–184.

Merin RG. Cardiovascular medications. In: Mangano DT, ed. Preoperative assessment. Philadelphia: JB Lippincott, 1990.

Rao TLK, Jacobs KH, El-Etr AA. Re-infarction following anesthesia in patients with myocardial infarction. Anesthesiology 1983; 59: 499–505.

AORTIC VALVE SURGERY

JAMES M. BAILEY, M.D., Ph.D.
JOHN L. WALLER, M.D.

Aortic valvular dysfunction may arise from congenital, traumatic, infectious, degenerative, and/or collagen-vascular diseases. Regardless of its cause, however, aortic valvular dysfunction reflects either obstruction to outflow, incompetence of the valve, or some combination of the two. This chapter focuses on the pathophysiology of aortic stenosis and insufficiency and how it affects anesthetic and life-support management.

PREOPERATIVE EVALUATION

Preoperative assessment of the patient with aortic valve disease necessitates a detailed evaluation of the cardiovascular system. However, it is important that one not focus on the cardiovascular system to the exclusion of other systems. The usual spectrum of concomitant noncardiac disease will be present. Aortic value surgery is a major physiologic trespass, and it is imperative that concomitant disease be evaluated and treated appropriately. For example, the patient with renal insufficiency should be evaluated by the appropriate consultant before surgery, so that plans for perioperative dialysis may be made, if indicated. The patient with aortic stenosis, who also has symptoms of cerebral vascular insufficiency, should be evaluated for possible carotid endarterectomy before elective aortic valve replacement. Proceeding with elective surgery is seldom justified in a patient whose physical condition has not been optimized.

Data with which to evaluate cardiac status should be available from a variety of sources. A simple assessment of functional disability should be helpful in predicting how the patient will respond to the stresses of the operating room. All patients should be questioned about their exercise tolerance and the extent to which their daily activities are limited. Patients with aortic stenosis should be queried for a history of syncopal episodes and/or chest pain. If there is chest pain, the possibility of concomitant coronary artery disease should be evaluated.

Objective data to be considered include the chest radiograph, electrocardiography (ECG), echocardiographic imaging, and cardiac catheterization report, which will provide information about the extent of disease. It is particularly useful to note the presence of pulmonary edema or pleural effusions, since these affect ventilatory management in the operating room and in the intensive care unit. The ECG allows one to determine the underlying rhythm; to make some judgment about the need for a pacing pulmonary artery catheter; to look for evidence of concomitant coronary artery disease; and, in the case of aortic stenosis, to evaluate the degree of left ventricular hypertrophy.

Specific details about the nature and extent of aortic valve dysfunction are clarified by echocardiographic and catheterization reports. Aortic stenosis is often quantitated by the left ventricle–aorta pressure gradient, but one should bear in mind that this gradient depends on cardiac output and can be misleading. The severity of aortic stenosis can be more directly assessed by calculation — using a formula relating valve area, pressure gradient, and cardiac output — or by Doppler echocardiographic measurement of the valve area. The degree of aortic insufficiency is evaluated qualitatively by visual assessment of the spread of the regurgitant jet and is graded on a 1+ to 4+ scale. This evaluation is subjective, with 1+ insufficiency indicating a regurgitant jet that is barely perceptible, while 4+ insufficiency indicates opacification of the ventricle. For both aortic insufficiency and aortic stenosis, the ejection fraction can provide an index of underlying left ventricular function. However, a decreased ejection fraction in aortic stenosis does not necessarily indicate poor left ventricular function, since ejection fraction is highly afterload dependent. The left ventricular end-diastolic pressure is of interest, since it can provide insight into the extent of left ventricular hypertrophy, and hence, the extent to which acceptable hemodynamic performance depends on adequate preload.

Preoperative assessment should also include notation of the medications that the patient will continue to use through the morning of surgery, except for diuretics and, possibly, digoxin. Digoxin has a low therapeutic index and a long half-life, and may be omitted on the morning of surgery, if not needed for control of arrhythmias.

MONITORING

Before the induction of anesthesia, the placement of invasive monitoring devices is advocated. To accomplish this, the patient must be appropriately premedicated with an efficacious combination such as diazepam, morphine, and scopolamine. It should be emphasized, however, that patients with aortic valve disease can be quite sensitive to the effects of central nervous system depressants, and in general required less premedication than a comparable patient with coronary artery disease. As a rough rule of thumb, it is recommended that one administer a premedication dose of about half that which would be given to a patient of similar age with coronary disease. Standard monitoring includes an ECG with multiple leads (usually leads II and V_5), nasopharyngeal and rectal or bladder temperature probes, an arterial line, and a central venous pressure or pulmonary artery catheter. The question of whether a pulmonary artery catheter should be placed continues to be debated. Several institutions have reported excellent results for cardiac surgery without the routine use of a pulmonary artery catheter. The combination of a central venous pressure catheter and a surgically placed left atrial catheter provides more accurate information about preload than does a pulmonary artery catheter. However, the pulmonary artery catheter offers the capability of thermodilution cardiac output determination, which we believe to be invaluable in the hemodynamic management of patients during the postoperative period. We have found that, if done with great attention to detail, pulmonary artery catheters can be placed successfully with a very low complication rate. Hence they are placed routinely in almost all of our patients presenting for aortic valve surgery.

Other monitoring devices which may be considered include a processed electroencephalographic (EEG) and a transesophageal echocardiographic probe. Aortic valve surgery carries the risk of air or valvular debris emboli. Thiopental sodium may be administered for "brain protection," and the appropriate dose is determined by burst suppression on the EEG. The role of transesophageal echocardiography (TEE) in aortic valve surgery is still unclear. The ability to visualize left ventricular contraction directly can be very helpful in assessing the need for inotropes. Furthermore, many patients with aortic valve disease have reduced ventricular compliance. With TEE, true preload—that is, left ventricular end-diastolic volume—can be directly assessed. TEE is also useful in assessing the efficacy of de-airing maneuvers, and it is invaluable for the detection of subaortic stenosis, facilitating early detection of residual obstruction or iatrogenic ventricular septal defect after the repair.

AORTIC STENOSIS

Pathophysiology

In the healthy adult, the aortic valve area is 2.5 to 3.5 cm^2. Assuming normal cardiac output, flow across this valve generates a pressure gradient from the ventricle to the ascending aorta of 2 to 4 mm Hg. With aortic stenosis, the effective aortic valve area decreases, increasing the resistance to flow and increasing the pressure gradient across the valve. To maintain cardiac output, the left ventricle must generate much higher systolic pressures. Several compensatory responses then follow. Over time, increased afterload stimulates protein synthesis, resulting in concentric hypertrophy of the left ventricle. Increased wall thickness tends to normalize wall stress (equal to wall tension divided by thickness) and enables the ventricle to generate high systolic pressures. Left ventricular ejection time slows as a means of minimizing the pressure gradient. The increasing left ventricular wall thickness results in decreased compliance and increased end-diastolic pressure. Because adequate diastolic filling of the ventricle becomes vital for the maintenance of cardiac output, the patient requires an appropriately timed atrial contraction and a longer-than-normal diastolic filling time. Symptoms and signs of myocardial ischemia often develop, since the

myocardial oxygen demand increases due to the increased pressure work and enlarged muscle mass. At the same time, coronary perfusion decreases as a result of the increased end-diastolic pressure. In addition, there is abnormal distribution of coronary flow, with a deleterious decrease in the subendocardial/subepicardial flow ratio. Myocardial contractility is usually maintained until the onset of ischemia. The end-state of the disease is heralded not only by angina pectoris but also by syncopal episodes caused by the heart's inability to increase its output in the presence of reduced vascular resistance during physical exertion.

It should be noted that patients with both aortic stenosis and insufficiency are sometimes encountered. In this situation, the pathophysiology is usually that of aortic stenosis. Even if the valve is incompetent, the decreased valve area will limit the extent of regurgitation.

Anesthetic Management

For the pathophysiology described above, the goals with regard to anesthetic management are as follows:

1. Tachycardia should be avoided to allow ample time for diastolic filling of a noncompliant ventricle.
2. Sinus rhythm must be preserved or simulated with a pacemaker to maintain the atrial contribution to ventricular filling.
3. Venodilation, with loss of adequate preload, should be avoided.
4. Large decreases in systemic vascular resistance should be avoided, since the patient is often incapable of increasing cardiac output enough to maintain adequate blood pressure (hence coronary perfusion pressure).

To achieve these goals, we usually rely on an opioid for the induction of anesthesia. By carefully titrating the drug to effect, anesthesia can be induced with no depression of myocardial function and with only moderate vasodilation. However, caution must be exercised since there is a decrease in sympathetic activity with the administration of opioids. This can be disastrous in the patient who is dependent on sympathetic tone due to advanced disease or hypovolemia. Hence, one should be very cautious in adding other hypnotics to the opioid induction, since this can result in more precipitous decreases in sympathetic activity. To ensure amnesia during induction, a benzodiazepine and/or scopolamine is included in the premedication.

While opioids are often given to the patient with aortic stenosis, it should be emphasized that the choice of anesthetic agent is less important than the skill with which it is delivered. In many patients, inhalation agents can be tolerated and used either as a supplement to, or as the major component of, maintenance anesthesia. We should also note that the combination of a benzodiazepine and a ketamine has been used successfully for both the induction and maintenance of anesthesia is patients with aortic stenosis.

If hemodynamic instability occurs with induction, it should be treated promptly. In particular, hypotension on induction can be life-threatening for the patient with aortic stenosis. The decrease in coronary perfusion pressure results in myocardial ischemia, left ventricular dysfunction, decreased cardiac output, and further hypotension, with a vicious cycle ensuing. Hypotension on induction should be treated very aggressively, usually with an alpha- agonist to avoid increases in heart rate. Initially, phenylephrine hydrochloride is used. If hypotension does not resolve, norepinephrine is administered. Should this result in an unacceptable increase in filling pressures, low-dose nitroglycerin should be added, with careful titration after blood pressure is stabilized. Such a strategy maintains blood pressure at the expense of cardiac output, but this is usually acceptable for the short time that elapses from induction to institution of cardiopulmonary bypass.

An additional advantage in using an opioid anesthetic is the control of heart rate. Tachycardia should be avoided; this can be achieved via the centrally mediated vagotonic effects of opioids. The choice of muscle relaxants should be dictated by the same concerns. As an initial relaxant, a drug that has little effect on heart rate can be used (usually vecuronium bromide), and then pancuronium bromide can be titrated if there is excessive opioid-induced bradycardia. One important caveat in this discussion of heart rate is that bradycardia that progresses to the point of a nodal rhythm is dangerous. Patients with aortic stenosis are highly dependent on atrial contraction to maintain ventricular filling, and a nodal rhythm should be treated. It may occasionally be helpful to place a pulmonary artery catheter with atrial pacing capabilities in patients who have a very low baseline heart rate, since any further slowing of rate can result in a nodal pacemaker controlling rhythm.

After induction of anesthesia and stabilization, additional hypnotics can be slowly added. Low doses of benzodiazepines or inhalational agents are often tolerated in the presence of surgical stimuli and can ensure lack of awareness. Since patients with aortic stenosis are seldom candidates for early extubation, additional opioids can be given. The report that thiopental given during cardiopulmonary bypass (CPB) reduces the incidence of central nervous system complications has led to an increasing use of thiopental. However, this protection was achieved only when the drug was titrated to burst suppression on the EEG. It is not yet known whether these results will be seen in other institutions where CPB is performed differently (for example, where moderate hypothermia is employed).

Hemodynamic Management

The goals of hemodynamic management during the period before initiation of CPB are the same as those for anesthetic management that are listed above. In general, the main goal during this interval is to maintain coronary perfusion pressure, even at the expense of cardiac output. This is often accomplished by the use of alpha-agonists. During the postbypass period, however, it must be ensured that cardiac output is adequate to maintain normal physiologic function. Thus, management is somewhat different. Patients with aortic stenosis can be expected to show a steady improvement after aortic valve replacement, since the ventricle is effectively unloaded. Filling pressures will be higher than normal. The hypertrophied ventricle of the patient with aortic stenosis will be noncompliant, and a "normal" filling pressure generally implies that preload (i.e., left ventricular end-diastolic volume) is low. However, it is also important to realize that the mean left atrial pressure and pulmonary capillary wedge pressure will be lower than the left ventricular diastolic pressure, which correlates with the peak a wave pressure, a reflection of atrial contraction with ejection into a noncompliant ventricle.

While it is expected that hemodynamic performance will improve after aortic valve replacement, the effects of aortic cross-clamping, even with the best of myocardial protection, can result in transient myocardial dysfunction during weaning from CPB. In this situation, inotropic support is indicated. Institutions vary considerably in the choice of inotropes. Our usual first-line inotrope has been epinephrine, or, for a patient who is significantly vasodilated, norepinephrine. It should be realized that the patient with aortic stenosis will continue to be at risk for coronary hypoperfusion after valve replacement, since left ventricular hypertrophy and high end-diastolic pressures persist during the postoperative period. Thus, perfusion pressure must be maintained. If cardiac output is still inadequate in the face of exogenous inotropic support and if filling pressures are excessively high, a vasodilator may be indicated. However, this should be titrated with extreme care to avoid systemic hypotension. In this situation, nitroglycerin offers some theoretic advantages, since it is purported to improve subendocardial/subepicardial flow ratios. The phosphodiesterase inhibitor amrinone can be very helpful in the treatment of the patient who was in significant heart failure before surgery. These patients frequently exhibit "down-regulation" of beta-receptors because of persistently elevated sympathetic activity. Although their response to exogenous catecholamines is blunted, they may show dramatic improvement in hemodynamic performance when amrinone, acting by a different mechanism, is administered. Again it must be emphasized however, that if amrinone, which is a potent vasodilator, is given, systemic hypotension must be aggressively treated. Also recommended is the insertion of left atrial lines when myocardial performance is significantly compromised. This not only provides a more accurate measure of left ventricular end-diastolic pressure, but enables norepinephrine to be administered, if needed, directly into the left atrium. This route of administration helps ameliorate increases in pulmonary artery pressures that can occur when norepinephrine is being infused into the systemic venous circulation.

Obviously, if there is significant myocardial dysfunction after aortic valve replacement, requiring multiple inotropes, an intraoperative balloon pump should be placed. As we have emphasized, coronary artery hypoperfusion is a significant risk to these patients. The intra-aortic balloon pump will improve coronary perfusion and frequently enables lowering of the rate of exogenous catecholamine administration and thus lowering of myocardial oxygen demands.

After separation from CPB, hemodynamic management will be highly dependent on the maintenance of appropriate preload. This is particularly true during the interval between weaning from bypass and achieving adequate hemostasis. Immediate volume replacement must be initiated as soon as the aortic cannula is removed. In general, if hypovolemia is avoided, hemodynamic performance should be fairly stable during the postoperative period. Impaired function caused by air emboli may occur, and de-airing maneuvers should be carried out before weaning from bypass. Acute malfunction of mechanical valves can also occur during the immediate postoperative period and can result in catastrophic deterioration. Fortunately, this is rare. Closure of the sternum can be associated with some hemodynamic deterioration, although this is usually mild. It is most often caused by increased intrapleural pressure and decreased venous return, and it can be treated by fluid administration. If there is significant compromise, the sternum should be reopened and the possibility of a pneumothorax or accumulation of pleural fluid impairing venous return should be ruled out by exploration.

AORTIC INSUFFICIENCY

Pathophysiology

Aortic insufficiency decreases forward stroke volume due to diastolic regurgitation of some fraction of total stroke volume from the aorta back into the left ventricle. Although assessment of the severity of aortic insufficiency is usually made on a qualitative 1+ to 4+ scale, it is most accurately quantified by calculation of the regurgitant fraction—that is, the fraction of the total stroke volume that regurgitates into the left ventricle. Regurgitant fraction can range from less than 0.1 in trivial aortic insufficiency to greater than 0.6 in severe insufficiency. The magnitude of aortic regurgitation depends on the valve area, the diastolic pressure gradient from the aorta to the left ventricle, and the duration of diastole.

The natural history of aortic insufficiency depends to some extent on whether the condition is chronic or acute. In both conditions, the compensatory mechanism for loss of effective forward stroke volume is volume overload of the left ventricle. However, in chronic aortic insufficiency, the sustained increase in diastolic wall tension (in contrast to the increased systolic wall tension of aortic stenosis) results in eccentric hypertrophy of the left ventricle, and this leads to increased diastolic compliance. Thus, the increase in left ventricular end-

diastolic pressure (LVEDP) is not as great as in left ventricular end-diastolic volume (LVEDV). Stroke volume is generally maintained by the Frank-Starling mechanism. Furthermore, ejection fraction is normal during the early stages of the disease. Since ejection begins at lower left ventricular systolic pressure, afterload is somewhat lower, and this helps maintain ejection fraction. Contractility appears to remain unimpaired initially. However, as the disease progresses, left ventricular contractility eventually decreases. (This can be exacerbated by coronary hypoperfusion, since myocardial oxygen demand increases with dilation and hypertrophy of the left ventricle, while oxygen supply can decrease as a result of lower diastolic aortic pressure.) Stroke volume decreases and both LVEDV and LVEDP increase, resulting in pulmonary congestion. At this point, a vicious cycle often ensues, with compensatory sympathetic stimulation resulting in increased systemic vascular resistance, further impedance to forward flow, and thus increased aortic regurgitation with rapid clinical deterioration.

By contrast, in acute aortic insufficiency, which is usually caused by endocarditis, trauma, or aortic aneurysm, a left ventricle of normal size is suddenly volume overloaded. There is insufficient time for eccentric hypertrophy to occur, with its associated increase in ventricular compliance. Hence, there is not only an increase in LVEDV, but also an increase in LVEDP, which can have several consequences. The increased LVEDP actually decreases the regurgitant volume, since the aortic left ventricular diastolic pressure gradient is decreased. However, the increased ventricular pressure can result in premature closure of the mitral valve, causing stroke volume to decrease. Blood pressure can be maintained only by increasing systemic vascular resistance, which further reduces stroke volume. Furthermore, the increased LVEDP can result in pulmonary edema, and the situation can rapidly deteriorate. Interestingly, in chronic aortic insufficiency, there is usually a greater volume overload of the left ventricle than in acute aortic insufficiency. However, because of better compliance, LVEDP is only mildly elevated, and furthermore, stroke volume is preserved by the Frank-Starling mechanism. In acute aortic insufficiency, LVEDP is elevated and maintenance of stroke volume by the Frank-Starling mechanism is compromised. This often leads to the need for emergent operation.

Anesthetic Management

The goal of anesthetic management is to avoid physiologic changes that will increase the magnitude of aortic regurgitation. Thus we recommend an anesthetic technique that will result in a moderate tachycardia, since this will limit the relative duration of diastole. We also recommend an anesthetic technique that will avoid increases in systemic vascular resistance. Vasodilation can be beneficial by decreasing the impedance to forward flow. One must be careful to avoid excessive vasodilation, however, since further decreases in diastolic blood pressure can result in coronary hypoperfusion.

To achieve these goals, we start with light premedication. Vasodilation caused by heavier sedation could be beneficial, but the response to sedation is highly variable, and it is unwise to allow a patient to become significantly obtunded before he or she arrives in the operating room. Once in the operating room, further sedation can be administered, if necessary, in a controlled fashion.

Monitoring is done as was discussed earlier in this chapter. Two additional points bear emphasis. First, a pulmonary artery catheter with pacing capabilities can be helpful in the management of patients with aortic insufficiency by facilitating heart rate control. Second, in the patient with severe aortic regurgitation, premature closure of the mitral valve may occur, and the pulmonary capillary occlusion pressure may significantly underestimate LVEDP.

We generally use opioids in combination with a hypnotic for the induction of anesthesia. A modest dose of hypnotic, such as a benzodiazepine, can ensure lack of awareness in the presence of a high dose of opioids. Moderate vasodilation caused by the opioid-hypnotic combination can be beneficial, as long as coronary hypoperfusion is avoided. With high-dose opioid anesthesia we also generally use pancuronium as our muscle relaxant to ameliorate opioid-induced bradycardia. As noted earlier, other induction techniques are certainly possible, and the choice depends on the experience and skill of the practitioner. In particular, we would note that the use of a benzodiazepine-ketamine combination has been described, and ketamine-induced tachycardia could be beneficial.

Maintenance of anesthesia can be achieved by several techniques. Further use of opioids, supplemented with low doses of hypnotics, is certainly appropriate. Since many patients who are to undergo surgery have significant disease, it is often not possible to maintain anesthesia primarily with inhalation agents. However, they can be used in conjunction with other agents. In this situation, the best choice is isoflurane because it has less potent negative inotropic effects than halothane or enflurane and because of its effects on systemic vascular resistance and heart rate.

Hemodynamic Management

The need for hemodynamic intervention during the period prior to initiation of CPB is minimized by appropriate anesthetic management. In patients with severe aortic regurgitation, however, hemodynamic instability can occur despite the most carefully administered anesthetic. Bradycardia should be aggressively treated with atropine, beta-agonists, or pacing. Hypotension should be treated with drugs that have beta-agonist activity, in order to increase both heart rate and contractility. The use of a pure alpha-agonist, such as phenylephrine hydrochloride, can increase the severity of regurgitation. If the patient has high pulmonary artery pressures and pulmonary edema, vasodilators are indicated. These should be titrated carefully to avoid diastolic hypotension and coronary hypoperfusion.

The initiation of CPB can be a time of significant risk for patients with aortic insufficiency. Ventricular distention can occur if there is ventricular fibrillation, since there is no ventricular ejection to oppose regurgitation of pump flow from the aortic cannula into the left ventricle. We attempt to delay the onset of fibrillation by administering lidocaine and a beta-blocker shortly after commencing CPB. More importantly, the surgical team must be prepared to vent the left ventricle immediately. After venting, significant hypotension can result, since the systemic circulation is effectively short-circuited, with a significant fraction of the flow passing from the pump, to the aorta to the left ventricle and then back to the pump via the vent. Administration of an alpha-agonist does not increase blood pressure, but simply increases the regurgitant fraction. This situation is resolved only by application of the aortic cross-clamp.

Although not directly responsible for myocardial protection, the anesthesiologist should be aware that simple injection of cardioplegia into the aortic root often does not provide adequate protection because of regurgitation of cardioplegia into the left ventricle. In this situation, direct injection into the main coronary ostia or retrograde cardioplegia via the coronary sinus is necessary. The anesthesiologist should remain alert for electrographic signs of inadequate protection.

Hemodynamic performance following repair depends on the adequacy of myocardial protection and other factors. Before beginning inotropic support, one should ensure an appropriate preload. This is largely a matter of trial and error, with the preload increased during weaning from bypass, and the response observed. One should not fill the heart to the point at which increases in filling pressure do not result in parallel increases in blood pressure and cardiac output. It should be noted that patients with chronic aortic insufficiency often have increased ventricular compliance. Thus, significant increases in pulmonary artery wedge pressure or left atrial pressure are indicative of overdistention. In this situation, inotropic support is necessary. It should be realized that afterload is generally lower in the presence of aortic insufficiency, since systemic blood pressure is lower during the early stages of ejection in this condition. Thus, after repair, the effective afterload on the left ventricle may be increased. Hence, the need for inotropic support should not be surprising. As noted earlier, there is institutional variation in the choice of inotropes. We advocate flexibility in this area, and recommend choosing drugs that are appropriate for the patient's physiologic state at the time. For example, if the patient requires an alpha-agent (e.g., phenylephrine hydrochloride) to maintain blood pressure on bypass before weaning, and then if inotropic support should be required, it would seem logical to choose an agent with both alpha- and beta-activity, such as epinephrine or norepinephrine. On the other hand, if the patient has relatively high blood pressure on bypass, inotropic support, if needed, would be most appropriately provided with drugs that produce vasodilator activity, such as amrinone or dobutamine.

If myocardial contractility is severely depressed, an intra-aortic balloon pump should be placed while the patient is still on bypass. A left atrial line can be very helpful in this situation, both for assessment of left ventricular filling and for administration of inotropes, if pulmonary artery pressures are high.

SUGGESTED READING

Dhadphale PR, Jackson APF, Alseri S. Comparison of anesthesia with diazepam and ketamine versus morphine in patients undergoing heart-valve replacement. Anesthesiology 1979; 51:200–203.

Jackson JM, Thomas SJ. Valvular heart disease. In: Kaplan JA, ed. Cardiac anesthesia. 2nd ed. New York: Grune & Stratton, 1987:589.
Jackson JM, Thomas SJ, Lowenstein E. Anesthetic management of patients with valvular heart disease. Sem Anesthes 1:239–252.
Rackley CE, Edwards JE, Wallace RB, Nevin MK. Aortic valve disease. In: Hurst JW, ed. The heart. 6th ed. New York: McGraw-Hill, 1986:729.
Stoelting RK, Gibbs PS, Creasser CW, Petersen C. Hemodynamic and ventilatory responses to fentanyl, fentanyl-droperidol, and nitrous oxide in patients with acquired valvular heart disease. Anesthesiology 1975; 42:319–324.

MITRAL VALVULAR DISEASE

MICHAEL N. D'AMBRA, M.D.
EDWARD LOWENSTEIN, M.D.

The mitral valve has design characteristics that optimize forward flow at a low driving pressure and minimize regurgitant flow by enabling rapid leaflet closure upon initiation of ventricular systole. The valve contributes significantly to the left ventricular chamber geometry during both systole and diastole. Annulus, anterior and posterior leaflets, chordae tendineae, and papillary muscles constitute a complex device. This complexity can lead to failure modes that go beyond the typical failures of a simple one-way valve: fixed stenosis and/or incompetence. The most common of these is the intermittent incompetence associated with papillary muscle dysfunction. The mitral valve may require surgery in childhood, midlife, or later life.

Mitral regurgitation in children is usually caused by congenital clefting of the anterior leaflet and is most common in association with a primum atrial septal defect. Congenital mitral stenosis is rarely seen as an isolated lesion (usually a supravalvular membrane), but it does appear as a component of complex lesions such as hypoplastic left heart syndrome.

In the United States, rheumatic cardiac valve disease is uncommon during childhood or midlife, but it is the primary cause of mitral disease in less developed nations. During midlife, acute mitral regurgitation may be caused by papillary muscle rupture or dysfunction, failure of a prosthesis in the open position, or rupture of a chorda tendineae in a rheumatic valve. Traumatic rupture of mitral chordae in compression/deceleration injuries may also produce acute mitral regurgitation. Mycotic endocarditis as a result of bacteremia in a

patient with deformed valve or in an intravenous drug user can result in mitral regurgitation, or less commonly, mitral stenosis or mixed mitral stenosis and mitral regurgitation.

In the older age group, rheumatic disease and myxomatous degenerative processes are the most common primary etiologies of mitral valve disease. However, reoperation for failure of a previously placed mitral bioprosthesis is now the most common operation in many tertiary centers. Emergency operation of patients after failed percutaneous mitral valvuloplasty is required increasingly in this age group.

DETERMINING THE PREDOMINANT HEMODYNAMIC LESION

Since cardiac output is optimized by different hemodynamic conditions in stenosis, regurgitation, and mixed lesions of the mitral valve, it is important to determine the predominant lesion before induction of anesthesia. The combination of mitral valve disease with other cardiac lesions (aortic insufficiency and mitral stenosis; coronary artery disease and mitral regurgitation) may make it difficult to determine the optimal management strategy before administration of the anesthetic. For this reason, moment-to-moment monitoring and flexibility in management are needed.

MITRAL STENOSIS

Isolated mitral stenosis is usually caused by rheumatic heart disease. It also occurs with calcification of bioprostheses and with thrombosis of or endothelial ingrowth into mechanical valves. As a rule, the orifice size gradually decreases with this lesion. The decrease is considered severe when the calculated valve area falls below 1 cm^2 from the normal 4 to 6 cm^2.

Mitral stenosis is often accompanied by muscularization of the pulmonary vasculature due to high left atrial pressure. This results in increased pulmonary vascular resistance and compensatory pulmonary hypertension and right ventricular hypertrophy. When left atrial pressure exceeds the level of pulmonary venous pressure at which lung water rises, dyspnea, "congestive symptoms," and/or hemoptysis ensue.

Symptoms often worsen dramatically when atrial fibrillation replaces normal sinus rhythm. Right ventricular loading may lead to elevated venous pressure, tricuspid regurgitation, and the stigmata of right ventricular failure (i.e., hepatomegaly, ascites, and peripheral edema). Hepatomegaly may be associated with coagulopathy following cardiopulmonary bypass, even when preoperative liver function tests have been normal.

The left ventricle is neither hypertrophied nor dilated and is classically stated to be "protected" in pure mitral stenosis. If the left ventricular function is abnormal, other causes should be determined before one proceeds with induction of anesthesia.

Heart rate is especially important in patients with mitral stenosis, as a slow rate will allow for lower pulmonary venous pressure, more effective left ventricular filling, and improved stroke volume. In patients with atrial fibrillation, digitalis should be continued to ensure an appropriate heart rate unless signs of toxicity are present. Adequate premedication is required to prevent tachycardia-associated pulmonary edema. The effects of small doses of sedative medications are exaggerated in patients with cardiac cachexia caused by mitral disease. We prefer to administer 2 to 4 mg of morphine intramuscularly plus 0.2 to 0.4 mg scopolamine intramuscularly. Supplementary oxygen is provided after premedication, and patients are transported in semi-Fowler position.

Transesophageal echocardiography is now used to evaluate patients for suitability for percutaneous mitral valvuloplasty. This diagnostic procedure is rapidly becoming a standard of care to rule out the presence of left atrial thrombus, an absolute contraindication to percutaneous valvuloplasty. Superior laryngeal nerve block plus appropriate monitoring (electrocardiography, pulse oximetry, and automatic noninvasive blood pressure) and sedation constitute an effective management approach in New York Heart Association Class III and IV patients undergoing awake transesophageal echocardiography.

Hemodynamic Management

Control of heart rate is the primary consideration in the hemodynamic management of patients with mitral stenosis as an accelerated rate increases the gradient across the mitral valve, increases left atrial pressure and pulmonary venous pressures, and induces right heart overload. The intraventricular septum is acutely deformed in diastole, and further impinges on left ventricular filling, lowering stroke volume, cardiac output, and

systemic blood pressure. If this course of events continues, right ventricular myocardial oxygen requirements continue to rise because of increasing wall tension. Right ventricular coronary blood supply is dramatically reduced because the normal systolic right ventricular coronary flow is abolished, and diastolic flow is reduced by systemic hypotension.

Other contributory concerns are acidosis, hypercarbia, and decreased oxygen tension, all of which can increase pulmonary vascular resistance and further load the right ventricle. Systemic vascular resistance must be maintained near normal levels since stroke volume is relatively fixed and tachycardia is not tolerated. Declines are treated with alpha-adrenergic agonists and inotropic drugs.

Prebypass Right Ventricular Failure

Treatment of right ventricular failure before bypass differs significantly from the approach used during the postbypass period. The focus of the prebypass approach is primarily ensuring adequate right ventricular coronary perfusion pressure and, secondarily, reducing right ventricular afterload. Alpha-agonists for increasing systemic diastolic pressure are useful in this situation, in combination with low-dose dopamine or dobutamine and the mild pulmonary dilating effects of nitroglycerine (0.2 to 1.0 µg per kilogram of body weight per minute). The use of an intra-aortic balloon pump is effective in refractory situations, even if there is no coronary disease.

Attempts to use potent pulmonary vasodilators, such as prostaglandin E_1 (PGE^1), to reduce pulmonary artery pressures and unload the right ventricle *before* the mitral stenosis has been relieved have been associated with pulmonary edema. This is probably because of sudden exposure of the pulmonary capillary bed to high pulmonary artery pressures when the compensatory pulmonary arteriolar constriction is acutely reversed.

Table 1 Conventional Therapy of Post–cardiopulmonary Bypass Right Ventricular Dysfunction

1. Generously correct any base deficit with bicarbonate *before* termination of cardiopulmonary bypass
2. Administer 5 mg per kilogram calcium chloride bolus into the left atrium
3. Ideal pattern of ventilation: large tidal volume (15 to 20 ml per kilogram) delivered at rapid inspiratory flow rates without positive end-expiratory pressure and with a long expiratory time
4. Administer epinephrine bolus (4 to 10 µg) (right side)
5. Administer dopamine 5 µg per kilogram per minute (right-sided infusion)
6. If systemic blood pressure is acceptable:
   Nitroglycerine, 0.25 to 1.5 µg per kilogram (right-sided catheter)
7. If systemic blood pressure is low:
   Begin selective infusion into right and left circulations
   a. Norepinephrine, 0.01 to 0.3 µg per kilogram via left atrial catheter.
   b. Nitroglycerine, 0.25 to 1.5 µg per kilogram (right-sided infusion)

Postbypass Right Ventricular Failure

A component of right ventricular dysfunction is common after mitral valve replacement, but usually responds to conventional maneuvers (Table 1). The right ventricular impairment may be caused by right ventricular ischemia, increased pulmonary vascular resistance, or a combination of the two. Occasionally right ventricular dysfunction progresses to profound failure and becomes refractory to conventional interventions. Figure 1 presents an algorithm for the treatment of postbypass right ventricular failure, whether it occurs in the operating room or in the intensive care unit. The centerpiece of this therapy is the administration of PGE_1, a potent pulmonary and systemic vasodilator and bronchodilator. Although normally metabolized more than 90 percent during the first pass through the lung blood vessels, pulmonary metabolism is often impaired under these circumstances. It is therefore necessary to administer a potent vasoconstrictor, often at unprecedentedly high doses, into the systemic circulation to prevent systemic hypotension. This may be accomplished via a left atrial catheter (Fig. 2) or the central lumen of an intra-aortic balloon counter pulsator. Once the "selective" infusion therapy has been instituted, it is important to increase the dose of the vasoconstrictor rather than decrease the dose of vasodilator to treat systemic hypotension. Unopposed pulmonary vasoconstriction will occur if the vasodilator is decreased, resulting in further right ventricular distention and acute cardiocirculatory collapse.

This strategy of selective right-sided and left-sided infusions may be lifesaving in refractory right ventricular failure. When a therapeutic effect has been obtained, it is important to continue the drug regimen until hemodynamics are stable. In no event should it be discontinued within less than 24 hours.

Rapid cessation of PGE_1 therapy has been associated with rebound constriction of renal, coronary, and pulmonary vasculature. It is therefore necessary to wean the patient from this drug very slowly. One suggested regimen is to decrease the dose by 3 mg per kilogram per minute every 3 hours.

Anesthetic Management

An anesthetic technique that promotes mild-to-moderate bradycardia without systemic vasodilation, combined with pacing capability, may be an ideal approach; the use of a potent synthetic narcotic (fentanyl or sufentanil) administered either in large induction doses or via continuous infusion with or without diazepam, midazolam, or etomidate is an effective strategy.

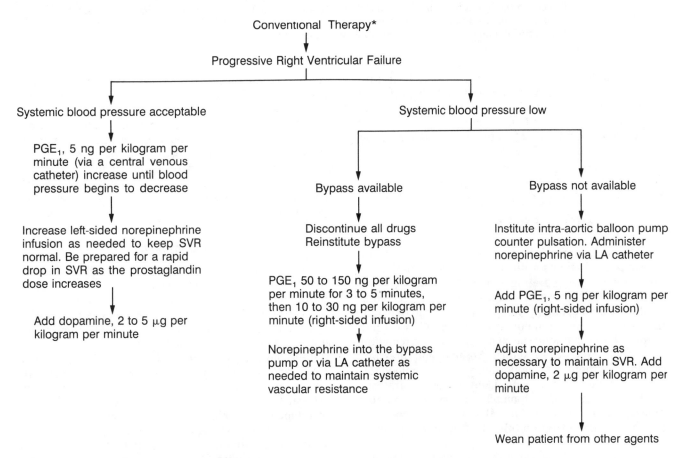

Figure 1 Therapy of refractory post-cardiopulmonary bypass right ventricular failure.
*See Table 1.

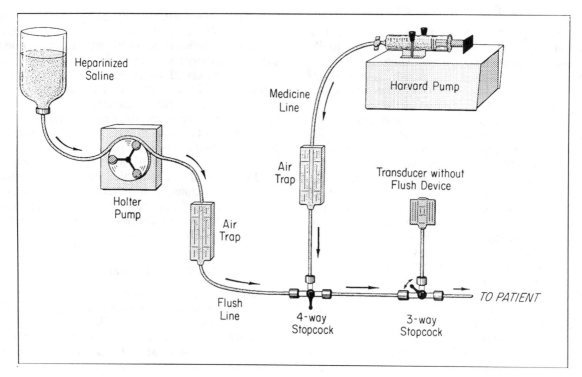

Figure 2 The setup for left-sided infusion of vasoactive/inotropic medications. This technique is applied to maximize effects on the systemic circulation without affecting the pulmonary circulation. It requires measures to prevent systemic embolization. Constant infusion devices that pump against systemic arterial pressures are required if the central lumen of the intra-aortic balloon pump is to be used.

The goal of the narcotic is to slow the intrinsic heart rate so that one can gain absolute control with pacing or relative control with small doses of atropine, gallamine (5 to 20 g), or pancuronium bromide.

Many combinations of intravenous and inhalation anesthetics and muscle relaxants have been used effectively. Knowledge of their pharmacologic effects and rational administration enable safe anesthetic management.

MITRAL REGURGITATION

Mitral regurgitation may be acute, chronic, or intermittent. Patients with acute mitral regurgitation often come to the operating room in pulmonary edema, intubated, and on vasoactive agents. The clinical course is often complicated by compromised renal function, preoperative sepsis, pulmonary edema, and low cardiac output. The right ventricle and pulmonary circulation have been exposed to sudden volume and pressure overload without the opportunity to accommodate. These are the patients most likely to have refractory right ventricular failure upon termination of cardiopulmonary bypass. It is unlikely that these patients will present for any operation other than emergency mitral valve replacement.

Chronic mitral regurgitation develops from enlargement of the mitral annulus, and/or derangements of chordae, leaflets, or papillary muscles. Medical therapy consists of digitalis, diuretics, and afterload reduction with calcium channel blockers and other vasodilators, such as hydralazine.

Intermittent mitral regurgitation is almost always caused by ischemic dysfunction of a papillary muscle. Patients present with a history of "flash" pulmonary edema and often respond to antianginal treatment. These patients can usually be treated effectively by coronary revascularization without mitral valve replacement.

Pathophysiology

During ventricular systole, a portion of the left ventricular ejectate (the regurgitant fraction) flows retrograde through the ineffectively closed mitral leaflets (or around the outside of the annulus of a mitral prosthesis that has a paravalvular leak). The regurgitation jets into the left atrium, creating a characteristic systolic murmur, a regurgitant ("V") wave in the left atrial and pulmonary capillary wedge trace (large regurgitant waves are transmitted to the pulmonary arterial tracing as well), and a distinctive color jet on two-dimensional color-flow Doppler echocardiography. Atrial and pulmonary venous compliance, aortic impedance, and the volume of the regurgitant fraction determine the amplitude of the regurgitant "V" waves. Thus, it is not possible to estimate the regurgitant fraction reliably from the pressure trace alone.

It is especially important to be able to distinguish "V" waves from pulmonary artery (PA) waves in order to avoid fatal PA perforation from balloon inflation in a permanently wedged PA catheter. The left ventricle is dilated in chronic mitral regurgitation. It may or may not also be hypertrophied, but contractility is almost always impaired. Left ventricular ejection fraction is preserved or supernormal, however, because of enhanced end-diastolic volume and the low impedance to ejection. Elimination of the regurgitation by valve replacement or repair increases left ventricular afterload dramatically and may be associated with the requirement for inotropic support.

Hemodynamic Management

Preoperative medical therapy includes vigorous diuresis and afterload reduction, often with combinations of potent intravenous vasodilators such as hydralazine and sodium nitroprusside. Systemic vasodilation affords reduced impedance to aortic ejection and improved "forward flow" into the aorta. For refractory pulmonary edema, the intra-aortic balloon pump provides the best afterload reduction available and should be considered before anesthetic induction in unstable patients and also in patients with severe mitral regurgitation who are undergoing noncardiac surgery.

Because these patients are usually taking digitalis, recognition and treatment of diuretic-induced hypokalemia is important to avoid acute digitalis toxicity. All medications should be continued on the morning of surgery, and a patient scheduled for an afternoon operation should be examined in the morning to determine whether additional diuretics are needed. Digitalis should not be withheld if it is being given for heart rate control in a patient with atrial fibrillation.

Impedance to aortic ejection is considered the single most important determinant for forward flow. Heart rate and ventricular volume are considered secondary factors. Anecdotal observations have been made that the greater the state of systemic vasodilation, the higher the optimal heart rate. However, frequent cardiac output measurement and/or Doppler imaging or regurgitant fraction are essential to confirm the optimization of forward flow. If pulmonary capillary wedge pressure (PCWP) measurement is used to estimate left ventricular filling pressure, the end-diastolic pressure rather than the mean pressure should be used.

Inotropic support is frequently helpful. The first-line agents to be used are those that promote vasodilation (e.g., low-dose dopamine, amrinone, isoproterenol) and those that are relatively neutral with regard to systemic vascular resistance (e.g., epinephrine, dobutamine). In unusual situations and with repeated calculation of systemic vascular resistance and pulmonary vascular resistance, alpha-agonists may have a place in returning systemic vascular resistance to baseline levels.

After repair of the lesion, patients with chronic mitral regurgitation may require inotropic support or afterload reduction in order to tolerate the abrupt increase in afterload. An attempt to establish a paced atrial or A-V sequential rhythm is warranted. Even temporary success will help support the circulation during the crucial early postbypass hours. Patients with acute mitral regurgitation who have suffered preoperative damage to the lungs or right ventricle because of an abrupt increase in volume and pressure load are among the most challenging patients to manage successfully. The right ventricle may have suffered acute distention and have severe contractile impairment. The lung parenchyma may be stiff from water accumulation and the pulmonary vascular bed damaged, causing a high, apparently fixed resistance. Thus, right ventricular failure may become the limiting condition. The regimen outlined previously may then be useful (see Table 1 and Fig. 2).

Anesthetic Management

Premedication should be light in patients with acute or chronic mitral regurgitation. In the patients with acute mitral regurgitation, the anesthesiologist should administer these drugs personally and plan to remain with the patient thereafter. It is important to intervene instantly in the event of sedative-related hypoventilation or hypotension.

Induction of anesthesia requires that attention be paid to the need to reduce the rate of vasodilator infusions as sympathetic tone is abolished with anesthetic drugs. Heart rate must be supported either by pacing, atropine, gallamine, or pancuronium bromide. Pacing may be more predictable. It is best to proceed relatively slowly with anesthetic drugs. Synthetic narcotics, midazolam, etomidate, and ketamine/benzodiazepine have been employed effectively to induce anesthesia. In extremely ill patients, hydromorphone (Dilaudid) in a dose of 0.2 to 0.3 mg per kilogram IV administered over 10 to 15 minutes, along with neuromuscular blockade with vecuronium bromide provides a paralyzed dissociated/euphoric state that avoids sudden alterations in intrinsic sympathetic tone. This regimen must be preceded by the use of drugs that produce amnesia (e.g., scopolomine 0.4 mg IV). Maintenance of anesthesia can be accomplished with high doses of narcotics, constant infusion of narcotic, midazolam or inhalation agents. Isoflurane provides some afterload reduction, while supporting heart rate and contractility. Propofol is an effective vasodilator and may prove useful in the anesthetic management of mitral regurgitation.

Monitoring

Standard monitoring for open heart surgery in most major cardiac surgical centers in the United States, Western Europe, and Japan includes intra-arterial, right atrial, pulmonary artery, and pulmonary capillary wedge pressures; cardiac output; multiple electrocardiographic leads; the capability to obtain frequent, rapid analysis of blood gases, electrolytes, and hematocrit; and a measure of anticoagulation and restitution of coagulation.

Transesophageal two-dimensional echocardiography (TEE) is particularly valuable in monitoring patients with heart valve and congenital heart lesions. Despite its complexity and expense and that it necessitates specific training for its use, it is becoming more commonly accepted. TEE can define the degree of stenosis and regurgitation and the adequacy of repair, and can more accurately reflect ventricular filling volumes than can pressure measurements. Visualization of septal flattening during right ventricular overload is easily appreciated, and response to therapy is immediately apparent. However, considerable controversy still exists with regard to the accuracy of the on-line, intraoperative detection/interpretation of wall motion abnormalities by TEE.

Left atrial catheters are useful both for measuring direct left ventricular filling pressures and for infusion of medications directly into the systemic circuit while minimizing the first-pass effects on the pulmonary vasculature. Pulmonary artery catheters that can continually measure mixed venous oxygen saturation may be useful as an on-line reflection of cardiac output.

Among the most important monitors are the senses. Changes in rhythm and function while the heart is exposed are immediately and dramatically evident to the trained eye. Continuous viewing of hemodynamic trends, either by continuous slow-speed paper-strip chart recording or the electronic equivalent, is important both when the sternum is open and when it is closed. A finger on the pulse or an esophageal stethoscope when the heart is not visible may provide initial clues to changes in heart function. The experienced cardiac anesthesiologist will strive for the elegance of simplicity in managing patients with mitral disease, but will be able to escalate quickly through a series of complex interventions when problems arise.

SUGGESTED READING

D'Ambra MN, LaRaia PJ, Philbin DM, et al. Prostaglandin E (PGE): a new therapy for refractory right heart failure and pulmonary hypertension after mitral valve replacement. J Thorac Cardiovasc Surg 1985; 89:567–572.

Grunkemeier GL, Starr A. Twenty-five year experience with Starr-Edwards heart valves: follow-up methods and results. Can J Cardiol 1988; 4:381–385.

Laver MB, Hallowell P, Goldblatt A. Pulmonary dysfunction secondary to heart disease: aspects relevant to anesthesia and surgery. Anesthesiology 1970; 33:161–192.

Mitchell MM, Sutherland GR, Gussenhoven EJ, et al. Transesophageal echocardiography. J Am Soc Echocardiogr 1988; 1:362–377.

Powderly WG, Stanley SL Jr. Medoff G. Pneumococcal endocarditis: report of a series and review of the literature. Rev Infect Dis 1986; 8:786–791.

Raffa H, Al Khateeb H, Tunisi T. Mitral valve replacement in children. Aust NZ J Surg 1988; 58:647–649.

Risk SC, Fine R, D'Ambra MN, O'Shea JP. A new application for superior laryngeal nerve block: transesophageal echocardiography. Anesthesiology 1990; 72:746.

Sullivan ID, Robinson PJ, de Leval M, Graham TP Jr. Membranous supravalvular mitral stenosis: a treatable form of congenital heart disease. J Am Coll Cardiol 1986; 8: 159–164.

ATRIAL SEPTAL DEFECT PRIMUM AND SECUNDUM

MARK H. GILLIE, M.D.
THEODORE H. STANLEY, M.D.

The presence of an intracardiac, interatrial communication in patients with an atrial septal defect (ASD) creates the potential for blood (and air, if present) to flow through the communication between the left and right sides of the heart. This has several implications that are important in the anesthetic management required for surgical correction of an ASD.

First of all, the anesthesiologist must take special care to minimize the abnormal shunting of blood, particularly right-to-left shunting, and to prevent the occurrence of paradoxical air embolus through the lesion during administration of the anesthetic. Next, the population of patients presenting for surgery represents a spectrum of the pathophysiology and associated clinical manifestations incident to the natural history of an initial left-to-right intra-cardiac shunt. There is great variety in patient presentation due to the variability in the lesion and the slow evolution, usually over many decades, of the pathophysiology associated with an ASD and the consequent subtle development of symptoms. Patients may present at any age, from infancy to old age, and range from those who are asymptomatic to those who manifest congestive heart failure, atrial arrhythmias, and/or pulmonary hypertension. The presence of the ASD therefore creates the challenge of the potential for blood and air shunting through the lesion and for the development of physiologic manifestations that can have an impact on anesthetic management.

The diagnosis of ASD has recently become less invasive and more easily made with the advent of two-dimensional, pulsed Doppler, and color-flow echocardiography. This has resulted in a higher probability of early detection and correction of this defect. Most patients who present for ASD surgery are asymptomatic, and their anesthetic is therefore relatively easily managed and is associated with low morbidity and mortality rates. However, it must be kept in mind that the potential for deleterious intracardiac shunting always exists.

In this chapter we examine the anatomy, pathophysiology, and anesthetic management of two of the more common forms of ASD, ostium primum and ostium secundum.

EMBRYOLOGY

The primitive atrium of the embryo is divided into the right and left atria by the development of two septa, the septum primum and the septum secundum. Initially, the septum primum grows caudally from the roof of the atrium, its free edge forming the superior margin of the ostium primum. Eventually this edge grows downward to fuse with the septum of the atrioventricular canal (which is composed of fused endocardial cushions), effectively obliterating the ostium primum.

Primum ASD results from the incomplete fusion of the septum primum with the endocardial cushions, leaving a patent ostium primum. An abnormal mitral valve usually results from a cleft or commissure in the anterior leaflet of the valve (Fig. 1).

At the time that the septum primum and the atrioventricular septum are fusing, fenestrations appear more cranially within the wall of the septum primum. These coalesce to form the ostium secundum. The septum secundum then begins its development, growing from the roof of the atrium immediately to the right of the septum primum. It grows to cover the opening of the ostium secundum but is essentially an incomplete partition, leaving an opening in its inferior margin called the foramen ovale. The cranial edge of the ostium secundum then begins to regress and eventually disappears, leaving the septum primum to function as the valve of the foramen ovale. Before birth, when pressure in the right atrium exceeds that in the left atrium, blood travels from the inferior vena cava into the right atrium and through the foramen ovale into the left atrium. After birth, when left atrial pressure exceeds right atrial pressure, the septum primum is forced against the foramen ovale, closing it. Eventually tissue from the septum primum and septum secundum fuse, sealing the foramen ovale and leaving a depression in the right atrial septal wall called the fossa ovalis.

Secundum ASD results from inadequate closure of the foramen ovale by the septum primum. This can be secondary to (1) an abnormally small septum primum resulting from excessive resorption, (2) an abnormally large foramen ovale resulting from defective development of the septum secundum, or (3) a combination of both (Fig. 2).

PHYSIOLOGY

Both primum and secundum ASD involve an intracardiac shunt between the left and right atria. In addition, primum ASD may involve a shunt between the left ventricle and right atrium. During the initial stages of the disease, these shunts are almost entirely left-to-

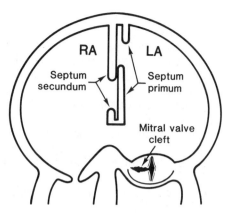

Figure 1 Diagrammatic representation of an ostium primum defect. Note the absence of fusion between the septum primum and the endocardial cushions, leaving an ostium primum defect in the lower atrial septum. Also note the cleft in the mitral valve, which is characteristic of primum ASD. This figure also shows normal development of the septum primum and septum secundum above the superior margin of the ostium primum. Here the septum primum adequately covers the ostium secundum, acting as a valve to seal off the defect when left atrial pressure exceeds right atrial pressure following birth. RA = right atrium; LA = left atrium.

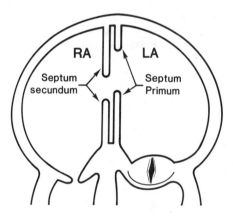

Figure 2 Diagrammatic representation of an ostium secundum defect. Note that the septum primum does not adequately cover the ostium secundum. This figure also shows a normal fusion between the septum primum and the endocardial cushions, thereby obliterating the ostium primum. Note also the normal mitral valve. RA = right atrium; LA = left atrium.

right, as left ventricular and left atrial pressures exceed right atrial pressure during most of the cardiac cycle. A small amount of right-to-left shunt usually occurs, however, during the onset of ventricular systole and early ventricular diastole, particularly in secundum ASD.

Because resistance in the pulmonary circuit remains relatively high during the first several months of life, interatrial shunting is usually minimal. Once pulmonary vascular resistance begins to decrease, right ventricular wall thinning occurs, and right ventricular compliance and interatrial left-to-right shunting increase. During early left-to-right shunting, pulmonary blood flow may be three to four times normal, but it is uncommon for pulmonary hypertension to be present. In fact, it is unusual for pulmonary hypertension to develop before adolescence in patients with primum ASD; in patients with secundum ASD, pulmonary hypertension may not develop until the third or fourth decade, if at all. Fortunately, most patients are diagnosed early in life when pulmonary hypertension is not a concern.

If a patient does not present with pulmonary hypertension (a pulmonary/systemic resistance ratio greater than or equal to 0.7/1), the direction of the shunt and the lability of the pulmonary vasculature are critical in determining if the lesion is amenable to surgical correction. If the shunt is predominantly left-to-right and pulmonary vascular resistance decreases when the patient breathes high concentrations of oxygen, the vasculature is usually sufficiently reactive to justify surgical correction of the ASD. If the patient has developed Eisenmenger syndrome defined as an irreversible right-to-left shunt caused by elevations in the pulmonary vascular resistance to levels that equal or exceed the systemic vascular resistance, accompanied by arterial hypoxemiahe or she is usually considered inoperable.

The concept of dependent versus obligatory intracardiac shunting is useful in the anesthetic considerations of primum and secundum ASD. Dependent shunting occurs between structures in which pressures are nearly equal. The magnitude and direction of the shunt is dependent upon the relative resistances in the circuit, except in cases in which the communication is very small. In the case of interatrial communications, the relative resistances are determined by the relative compliances of the right and left ventricles and resistances of the pulmonary and systemic vasculatures. By contrast, obligatory shunting occurs between structures in which pressure varies widely, such as shunting between the left ventricle and the right atrium that may occur in primum ASD. In this form of shunting, relative resistances are of little importance in determining the magnitude of the shunt. Anesthesiologists have some measure of control over the relative vascular resistances and, therefore, over the amount and often the direction of dependent shunts. This is most critical in a patient who has pre-existing pulmonary hypertension in which a small increase in pulmonary vascular resistance may substantially worsen a right-to-left shunt.

In addition to having an interatrial communication and a possible communication between the left ventricle and right atrium, patients with primum ASD have an abnormal mitral valve, in which there is usually a cleft in the anterior mitral leaflet. Mitral valve insufficiency is almost always present in this condition but varies in degree. If the insufficiency is great, left ventricular volume overload is present as well as right ventricular volume overload secondary to a left-to-right shunt.

Atrial arrhythmias, which are much more common in older patients, may also contribute to right and left ventricular overload (congestive heart failure). Some studies have shown that a few young patients (who are not clinically in congestive failure) nonetheless have depressed left ventricular function. Patients with primum ASD have recently been described as having left ventricular outflow obstruction. This is observed frequently enough to warrant the search for signs of it in the preoperative echocardiogram or during cardiac catheterization.

As suggested earlier, the physiology of the ASD lesion is a major determinant of patients' acceptability for surgery. Surgery should not be performed in patients with small ASDs whose pulmonary/systemic flow ratios (Q_P/Q_S) are less than or equal to 1.5/1, nor should it be performed in patients with severe pulmonary vascular disease (pulmonary/systemic resistance ratio $\geq 0.7/1$) without a significant left-to-right shunt.

Controversy exists as to the ideal age for surgical correction. It is generally agreed that an ASD should be corrected in all patients up to the age of 45 or 50 years who are not excluded by flow ratio or resistance criteria. The operative mortality rates associated with ASD corrections is low (<1 percent), and the benefits in lifestyle and lifespan are impressive. Patients older than 50 years of age who are without symptoms often remain asymptomatic for the remainder of their lives. Patients who are symptomatic (with manifestations of congestive heart failure, pulmonary hypertension, atrial arrhythmias, and/or pulmonary emboli) however, tend to become increasingly disabled. Older patients with symptoms have an increased surgical mortality rate (3 to 6 percent). Several recent reports, however, indicate that most symptomatic older patients (up to 70 years of age) who have their ASD repaired become asymptomatic and enjoy a longer lifespan.

CLINICAL MANIFESTATIONS

As suggested by the discussion on pathophysiology, the clinical manifestations of primum and secundum ASD are caused by congestive heart failure and the development of pulmonary vascular disease.

Secundum ASD tends to be more benign than primum ASD. Left-to-right shunts are usually not as large, and pulmonary volume overload is usually not as prominent. As a result, manifestations of congestive heart failure and pulmonary vascular disease are usually not seen as early in secundum ASD as in primum ASD. It is rare that a diagnosis of secundum ASD is made in infancy. Secundum lesions are usually diagnosed after the age of 2 or 3 years. Quite often the diagnosis is suspected on the basis of a heart murmur rather than on clinical manifestations of the disease. Depending on the extent of the lesion, even older children usually remain asymptomatic even though symptoms tend to be more noticeable to these older children. When symptoms do occur, they are typically those of early fatigue and dyspnea.

The diagnosis of primum ASD is usually (although not reliably) made in younger patients than the diagnosis of secundum ASD because (1) the murmur associated with the shunt is usually louder, and the presence of mitral insufficiency creates a second murmur that can be heard upon auscultation and (2) symptoms are usually present at an earlier age than they are in secundum ASD. Symptoms may occasionally occur in infancy and include growth failure and frequent respiratory infections. As the child grows older, symptoms (early fatigue and dyspnea) become prominent.

It is recommended that for infants and very young children who meet the physiologic criteria for surgical correction and who are asymptomatic or minimally symptomatic, correction be postponed until the patient is 2 to 5 years of age. Patients who reach adulthood without diagnosis and correction of ASD are more likely to develop pulmonary hypertension and subsequent Eisenmenger physiology—although, again, this depends on the extent of the lesion and its concomitant hemodynamic consequences. Severe exercise intolerance with arterial desaturation can result. In most adults whose condition deteriorates acutely, atrial arrhythmias are to blame, particularly atrial fibrillation and flutter. Cyanosis and clubbing may also be present.

DIAGNOSIS

The increased use of echocardiography has enabled even patients with a small ASD to be accurately diagnosed despite the lack of any manifestations other than a murmur. At present, two-dimensional echocardiography is, in fact, the standard technique used to confirm the diagnosis at most major medical centers. With two-dimensional echocardiography, the ASD can be directly visualized. The technique also allows for visualization of the increased right atrial and right ventricular dimensions and the anterior mitral leaflet cleft in primum ASD. Peripheral contrast echocardiography can distinguish the relative degree and direction of shunt. Pulsed Doppler echocardiography is used to confirm the diagnosis of ASD through characteristic flow patterns. Color-flow Doppler techniques have increased the sensitivity of echocardiography (to approximately 99 percent), particularly in the diagnosis of secundum ASD. Color-flow approaches allow the simultaneous display of intracardiac blood flow and ultrasonic anatomy and are comparable to angiographic visualization. They are also useful in demonstrating associated cardiac anomalies.

In most cases, cardiac catheterization is no longer necessary for the diagnosis of primum and secundum ASD because of echocardiographic advances. However, cardiac catheterization is frequently used to document the lesion in an atypical presentation or when multiple cardiac defects of abnormalities confuse the echocardiographic examination.

PREOPERATIVE EVALUATION AND PREPARATION

As previously mentioned, most patients who present for surgical repair of an ASD do so at a time when they are either symptomatic or minimally symptomatic. In other words, most anesthetics will be administered to patients who are relatively healthy despite their cardiac lesion (e.g., robust children between 2 and 5 years of age). Nonetheless, it is important to consider the salient features of the anatomy, physiology, and clinical manifestations of the lesion.

In addition to the routine preanesthetic evaluation, (e.g., attention to medications, allergies), a review of the chart should include attention to specific details regarding the anatomy of the lesion, its location and size, and the presence of associated cardiac anomalies, as well as to details regarding the pathophysiology that are provided by echocardiographic and cardiac catheterization data as interpreted by consultants. Emphasis should be placed on the evidence of pulmonary vascular disease and pulmonary hypertension, relative pulmonary blood flow, the direction and magnitude of the shunt, the presence of congestive heart failure, right and left ventricular function, and the presence of regurgitant lesions. In addition, it is important to note the response of the patient's pulmonary vasculature to 100 percent oxygen as a measure of vascular reactivity. A high degree of pulmonary blood flow relative to pulmonary artery pressure, and the responsiveness of the pulmonary vasculature to 100 percent oxygen are both good indications of the reversibility of pulmonary hypertension.

Reviewing the clinical manifestations of the lesion is important because they document the acute and chronic impact of the pathology. This is of particular significance when a cardiac shunt or valve is involved in the disease. It is also important to know the general health of the patient and how he or she reacts to stress or periods of sedation, sleep, and even anesthesia. This information is valuable because it dictates the type of premedication and/or anesthetic approach that should be avoided or, on the other hand, may be best tolerated.

Patients with ASD rarely present as an emergency because of their cardiac pathology. Therefore, in virtually all cases, medical management should be optimized before surgery. As mentioned, most patients with an ASD are relatively healthy at presentation, but some do present in congestive failure with the primum defect. On occasion, a respiratory infection can add sufficient stress to complicate anesthetic management and should therefore be adequately treated before surgery. Arrhythmias, usually in adults, are another manifestation of ASD that should be controlled preoperatively.

Past anesthetic records should be carefully reviewed and any questions resolved with in-depth discussions with previously responsible anesthesiologists, surgeons, or other physicians. Appropriate laboratory data, including measurements of plasma hemoglobin and/or hematocrit, platelet count, and serum potassium should be carefully evaluated. In addition, radiographs, x-ray reports, and the electrocardiogram need to be reviewed.

Physical examination of the patient should include the usual preanesthetic evaluation of the airway and chest. The airway is of special concern, as inability to ventilate the patient adequately will result in early hypercarbia, hypoxia, and acidosis, which can increase right-to-left shunt fraction and worsen arterial hypoxemia. Auscultation of the precordium typically reveals a systolic ejection murmur at the upper left sternal border, an accentuated first heart sound, and fixed splitting of the second heart sound. In primum ASD, an apical holosystolic murmur may also be heard secondary to mitral insufficiency.

Preoperative psychological preparation of the patient should consist of a discussion with the patient and/or his or her parents (depending on the age of the patient) of what to expect during the perioperative period (e.g., induction of anesthesia, the stay in the intensive care unit). Obviously the idea is to calm the patient (and the patient's family) and relieve as much anxiety as possible.

Premedication, if used, serves to augment psychological preparation. Ideally, the patient should be calm and cooperative without cardiovascular or respiratory compromise. Excitement or, conversely, heavy sedation with consequent hypoxia/hypercarbia in patients who have pulmonary hypertension can result in reversal of left-to-right shunts. The result can be a worsening of arterial oxygenation and the development of cyanosis. Obviously, careful administration of premedication to achieve the desired goals of a calm and cooperative patient is the ideal. Available regimens of preoperative medication for children and adults are numerous. Generally a regimen with which the anesthesiologist is familiar and comfortable and/or one that allows titration is preferred.

MONITORING

In addition to standard monitors (i.e., electrocardiography, blood pressure cuff, pulse oximeter, precordial stethoscope or esophageal stethoscope, and inspired oxygen analyzer), the use of direct continuous arterial blood pressure readings via an arterial catheter, inspired and end-expired gas analysis, multiple-site temperature measurements, and recordings of central venous pressure are all valuable.

ASD lesions that result in intracardiac shunts can be associated with arterial desaturation. Desaturation is easily detected by the use of a pulse oximeter and confirmed by serial arterial blood samples obtained via an arterial catheter. In addition, it is often valuable to determine the impact of changes in ventilation on arterial oxygen and carbon dioxide tensions before and after surgical manipulation.

Continuous arterial blood pressure measurements allow rapid detection and correction of changes in arterial blood pressure. These are valuable after cardiopulmonary bypass, particularly in patients with significant ventricular dysfunction as a result of either manifestations of the primary lesion, coronary artery disease, or cardiomyopathy.

Instantaneous detection of abnormalities in ventilation with end-tidal carbon dioxide monitors can help

prevent postoperative morbidity and mortality and episodes of hypercarbia and hypoxia that can increase right-to-left shunts.

In addition to standard core temperature monitoring, (e.g., esophageal or bladder), most clinicians estimate brain temperature via a nasopharyngeal probe and extremity temperature via rectal or skin probes to ensure completeness of rewarming at the conclusion of cardiopulmonary bypass. A large gradient between temperatures indicates the likelihood of recooling of the central circulation and places the patient at risk for arrythmias and/or circulatory arrest.

Central venous pressure measurements are valuable in assessing right atrial filling pressure in patients with a moderate or large ASD. Pulmonary artery catheters are usually not used before the surgical correction is performed because of the risks of (1) pulmonary artery rupture, particularly in patients with pulmonary hypertension; (2) arrhythmias; and (3) thrombus formation on the catheter. In addition, a pulmonary artery catheter sometimes interferes with surgery. Finally, because of the shunt, determination of a true cardiac output and use of these data for calculation of pulmonary and systemic vascular resistances is difficult. If ventricular failure and/or pulmonary hypertension are problems after surgery, the surgeon can place pulmonary artery and/or left atrial catheters under direct visualization while the heart is open.

ANESTHETIC TECHNIQUE

The impact of anesthetic technique on patient outcome is unknown. However, most clinicians believe that patient age and severity of disease affect morbidity and mortality. The presence of an intracardiac shunt is also important. Prevention of paradoxical air emboli and excessive shunting of blood are key issues in the anesthetic management of ASD corrections.

As previously noted, most patients with either a primum or secundum ASD will be 2 to 5 years old and in relatively good health. In these patients, the best anesthetic approach may be that with which the anesthesiologist is most familiar and comfortable, provided that hemodynamics are stable. In children with congestive heart failure or in adults with pulmonary hypertension, atrial arrhythmias, and/or congestive failure, techniques that do not affect myocardial contractility and/or pulmonary and systemic vascular resistance are best. In addition, high concentrations of oxygen are important for minimizing the impact of right-to-left shunting on arterial oxygen content.

Intracardiac shunts enable air in the venous system to easily pass to the left side of the heart. Although patients with an ASD usually have a predominant left-to-right shunt, it is not uncommon for a small amount of right-to-left shunting to occur during certain parts of the normal cardiac cycle.

The primary causes of air in the venous system are air in the intravenous (IV) infusion and air introduced during cardiopulmonary bypass. It is imperative that all air bubbles from any source be cleared from the IV infusion (including ports) and syringes used for IV injection. Although surgeons are primarily responsible for clearing air from the heart, great vessels, and cardiopulmonary bypass cannulae before reinstating normal cardiac flow, anesthesiologists should be watchful for any air that is missed by surgeons or surgical assistants.

The predominant left-to-right shunt of patients with ASD can be increased, decreased, or changed to a predominant right-to-left shunt by variations in anesthetic management. Shunting of blood away from the pulmonary circulation results in arterial desaturation and cyanosis. Under usual circumstances, good anesthetic management includes maintaining a shunt at the preanesthetic value or minimizing or eliminating it altogether. However, although most patients tolerate increases in left-to-right shunt reasonably well, they do not tolerate increases in right-to-left shunt.

Control of shunting before surgical correction depends primarily on the relative pulmonary and systemic vascular resistances. Table 1 shows manipulations that will result in changes in these relative resistances and therefore in changes in the direction and magnitude of shunting.

Hypoxia, hypercarbia, and acidosis resulting from inadequate oxygenation and ventilation are the most important factors that can change relative shunt. Difficulties in airway control during the induction-intubation sequence constitute the most common cause of decreases in ventilation with subsequent inadequate oxygenation and hypoxia. Adequate preoperative evaluation of the airway and an uneventful anesthetic induction and intubation are therefore of utmost importance.

An uneventful anesthetic induction and intubation begins with proper preoperative assessment, including adequate psychological and pharmacologic preparation of the patient. If anxiety or patient upset are present in the holding area, further reassurance and/or medication may be necessary. Careful titration of appropriate IV medications in those patients with an IV infusion, or the use of light doses of sedatives or hypnotics via other routes in those in whom an IV infusion is not present are valuable. In children, transmucosal routes of drug delivery (e.g., rectal, oral, or nasal) are becoming more common and may provide benefits because of a rapid onset of action. Compounds used with these routes include methohexital, fentanyl, sufentanil, ketamine, and midazolam. Some of the new approaches (oral transmucosal) may enable better titration than others (nasal and rectal). Although intramuscular injection is somewhat less satisfactory and is being employed less frequently, ketamine is still given by this route and is acceptable because of its profound hypnotic and minimal respiratory effects.

Induction of anesthesia in the relatively healthy patient can be accomplished in numerous ways. In patients receiving intravenous infusions, a narcotic induction is fast, blunts the hemodynamic and airway

Table 1 Factors Altering Relative Vascular Resistances

Pulmonary vascular resistance
  Increase
    Hypoxia
    Hypercarbia
    Acidosis
    Elevated airway pressure or positive end-expiratory pressure
    Sympathetic stimulation or vasoconstrictors
    Pulmonary emboli
    Hypervolemia
    Hypothermia
    Surgical manipulation
  Decrease
    High F_{IO_2}
    Hypocarbia
    Alkalosis
    Vasodilators
    Potent inhalation anesthesia
    Low relative airway pressure

Systemic vascular resistance
  Increase
    Sympathetic stimulation
    Vasoconstrictors
    Surgical manipulation
  Decrease
    Potent inhalation agents
    Vasodilators

responses to intubation, and is rarely associated with changes in cardiac output, arterial blood pressure, and the right-to-left shunt fraction. If titrated carefully, sodium thiopental and propofol can be successfully used in patients with congestive heart failure or pulmonary hypertension, but they are more difficult to use. In healthier children who are not receiving an intravenous infusion, a mask induction with a potent inhalation agent with or without nitrous oxide is usually accomplished without problems. Although potent inhalation agents cause varying degrees of myocardial depression and a decrease in systemic blood pressure, they are usually tolerated well in healthier children.

In sick patients (i.e., those who manifest congestive heart failure and/or pulmonary hypertension), it is usually best to induce anesthesia with a narcotic (fentanyl or sufentanil) or ketamine. Virtually all of these patients come to the operating room with an IV infusion, thereby allowing an intravenous induction to proceed without difficulty. In patients who are more ill who are *not* receiving an intravenous infusion, an intramuscular injection of ketamine and an antisialagogue is an appropriate alternative that usually causes little cardiac depression and allows easy airway control. Patients with a primum ASD who have moderate-to-severe mitral regurgitation do not tolerate decreases in heart rate because of increased left ventricular volume and a decreased cardiac output. The decreases in heart rate that are commonly seen with the use of halothane and narcotics can be dangerous. Induction of anesthesia with ketamine and relaxation with pancuronium bromide is effective and has become popular in the treatment of these patients.

In patients with a left-to-right intracardiac shunt, induction with potent inhalation agents results in a more rapid uptake of inhalation anesthetics than in patients without a shunt. Intravenous induction of anesthesia in patients with left-to-right intracardiac shunting results in a slower circulation of the intravenous agents to the brain. This is usually of little practical significance, however, as long as the induction medication is titrated carefully.

Intubation is best accomplished after adequate relaxation has been achieved with the use of a muscle relaxant to optimize airway exposure and minimize coughing and other airway reflexes. Because of hypoxemia, hypercarbia, and acidosis, a prolonged intubation can result in an increase in the right-to-left shunt. Increased intrathoracic pressures developed by coughing or bucking can also result in shunt reversal. It is advisable to blunt airway reflexes with narcotics or with laryngeal or intravenous lidocaine before laryngoscopy.

In healthier patients, maintenance of anesthesia is easily achieved with potent inhalation agents. However, because they lack cardiovascular effects, narcotics are probably easier to use in more ill patients. It is important to remember that maintenance of anesthesia with long-lasting narcotics (e.g., morphine) may result in the need for prolonged postoperative ventilation.

Nitrous oxide can be used for a brief period to facilitate an inhalation induction but is best avoided during anesthetic maintenance because it will enlarge air bubbles that are accidentally introduced into the circulation. Nitrous oxide will worsen the complications resulting from systemic arterial air embolization.

Maintenance of muscle relaxation can usually be safely accomplished with any of the commonly used nondepolarizing agents, such as pancuronium bromide, vecuronium bromide, and atracurium besylate.

The administration of preservative-free morphine, fentanyl, and sufentanil in the caudal epidural space in children and the epidural or intrathecal spaces in adults has become a popular method of providing analgesia during the postoperative period after thoracic surgery. These approaches may even facilitate early endotracheal extubation. These agents can also be useful in reducing analgesic and anesthetic requirements during surgery. Morphine is usually given in a dose of 0.075 mg per kilogram diluted in 5 to 10 ml of preservative-free saline for use in the caudal epidural space in children. In adults, 2 to 5 mg of preservative-free morphine in a total of 5 to 10 ml of preservative-free saline is used in the epidural space, and 0.25 to 0.5 mg of preservative-free morphine is used in the intrathecal space. These doses usually provide 12 to 24 hours of pain relief.

In most patients with an uncomplicated secundum ASD without congestive heart failure or pulmonary vascular disease, cardiopulmonary bypass time is brief and extubation of the trachea can be accomplished in the operating room. However, it may be wise to avoid extubation just before transporting the patient. Once the patient is in the intensive care unit, there is usually little or no reason to leave the patient intubated for an extended period of time if the surgery and anesthesia were uncomplicated. For patients in whom cardiopulmonary bypass is prolonged and/or in whom severe congestive heart failure or pulmonary vascular disease is present, most clinicians recommend that extubation be accomplished later in the intensive care unit.

KEY POINTS OF THE OPERATION

Surgical access is usually accomplished through either a median sternotomy or a right thoracotomy incision. In an uncomplicated secundum ASD, the patient is placed on cardiopulmonary bypass with minimal cooling. Repairs are accomplished quickly through a right atrial incision. Small lesions can often be repaired via suture closure, whereas larger lesions require a patch. Primum ASD repair most often requires that the patient have a more extended period on cardiopulmonary bypass. Deep hypothermia and circulatory arrest are occasionally used in younger patients. The cleft in the mitral valve is repaired via suture and/or plication of the cusp in the valve, while the ASD is usually repaired with a synthetic or pericardial patch.

Air is evacuated from the heart after its closure. This can be facilitated by gently inflating the lungs at the appropriate time to displace air from the pulmonary vasculature.

COMPLICATIONS

The morbidity and mortality rates associated with primum and secundum ASD repair are low, with most complications being of a transient nature. Cerebrovascular accidents resulting from systemic arterial embolization are probably the most devastating of the complications associated with the repair. This problem can usually be prevented by compulsively evacuating air from the intravenous infusions, the cardiopulmonary bypass cannulae, and the heart before resumption of normal cardiac flow. Residual shunting, which usually disappears over the first 5 postoperative days, can be present in patients who have received a thin, porous Teflon patch repair of the ASD.

Perhaps the most common postoperative complications are atrial arrhythmias and residual mitral regurgitation that results from abnormal valve shape after repair of a primum ASD. Arrhythmias are more common in older adults. More than half of the patients undergoing repair after 50 years of age experience new or persistent atrial arrythmias. These usually arise from either established arrhythmias (most commonly in patients with chronic atrial distention and volume overload) or new arrhythmias from surgical damage to conduction tissues. The latter occurs after sutures are accidentally placed through conduction tissue or from the pressure and damage caused by cardiopulmonary bypass cannulae during bypass—for example, cannulation of the superior vena cava through the right atrial appendage.

In patients with severe pulmonary vascular disease, right ventricular failure and prolonged respiratory insufficiency are common postoperatively. Intraoperative and postoperative complications are more common in adults with impaired preoperative hemodynamics. Hemorrhage, atelectasis, and wound infection are also reported after ASD repair.

POSTOPERATIVE CARE

The intensity and duration of postoperative care depends on the preoperative health of the patient, the nature of the anesthetic and surgical management in the operating room, and the incidence and nature of postoperative complications. Tracheal extubation, particularly in uncomplicated secundum ASD repair, is usually accomplished shortly after surgery. In patients with pulmonary vascular disease or with a long or complicated cardiopulmonary bypass, extubation may be delayed.

Patients with postoperative supraventricular arrhythmias, bradycardia, or persistent heart block occasionally require insertion of a pacemaker. Many patients who have symptomatic congestive heart failure preoperatively are asymptomatic or suffer minimal symptoms within 1 year after surgery. Often patients are discharged from the hospital within 1 week of their operation without further need of medical therapy. Although there is usually a dramatic improvement in symptomatology of older patients, right ventricular hypertrophy and problems with cardiac rhythm may continue to persist.

SUGGESTED READING

Behrendt DM. Atrial septal defect. In: Arciniegas E, ed. Pediatric cardiac surgery. Chicago: Year Book Medical Publishers, Inc., 1985:133.

Borow KM, Braunwald E. Congenital heart disease in the adult. In: Braunwald E, ed. Heart disease: a textbook of cardiovascular medicine. Philadelphia: WB Saunders, 1988:976.

Feldt RH, et al. Defects of the atrial septum and the atrioventricular canal. In: Adams FH, Emmanouilides GC, Riemenschneider TA, eds. Heart disease in infants, children, and adolescents. Baltimore: Williams & Wilkins, 1989:170.

Fiore AC, Naunheim KS, Kessler KA, et al. Surgical closure of atrial septal defect in patients older than 50 years of age. Arch Surg 1988; 123:965–967.

Schwartz AJ. Cardiovascular physiology of congenital heart disease. In: Stanley TH, Sperry RJ, eds. Anesthesiology and the heart. Boston: Kluwer Academic Publishers, 1990:25.

VENTRICULAR SEPTAL DEFECT

NANCY SETZER, M.D.

Children, and even young adults, with a ventricular septal defect (VSD) provide a challenge to the anesthesiologist because of the tremendous variety of physiologic effects accompanying the VSD, despite the anatomic similarity of the defects. Patients range from the asymptomatic school-age child who undergoes surgery during school vacation to avoid future health problems such as endocarditis or refractory pulmonary hypertension, to the 1-month-old infant with severe congestive heart failure and cachexia who must undergo surgery urgently as a life-saving measure. The key to choosing a successful anesthetic and planning a smooth perioperative course for these patients is to understand the pathophysiology and planned surgical correction.

EPIDEMIOLOGY AND ANATOMY

Ventricular septal defects are probably the most common congenital heart abnormality, occurring in 1:500 live births and accounting for approximately 20 percent of all congenital heart defects. There are several anatomic types of lesions, including membranous VSD, muscular VSD, and common atrioventricular canal type VSD. Membranous defects are the most common type, comprising approximately 75 percent of the total. Muscular VSD is frequently composed of multiple holes, the so called "Swiss cheese" type of VSD. These muscular defects can close spontaneously during growth of the child, most often before he or she is 6 months of age, because of growth of the muscle borders and fibrous tissue proliferation. Canal-type defects are the least common, and are seen in 50 percent of children with Down's syndrome. These may be associated with mitral and tricuspid valvular clefts.

Supracristal VSD is an uncommon type of VSD, with a 5 percent incidence and unusual physiologic consequences. This VSD is located just beneath the aortic annulus in the ventricular septal wall and is contiguous with the aortic annulus. Progressive aortic insufficiency is found in a large number of the patients because the annulus is unsupported beneath the right aortic leaflet, which prolapses back into the left ventricle during systole. Frank aortic valvular incompetence can ensue as the child grows older, with the valve becoming progressively deformed and fibrotic.

In the majority of instances, ventricular septal defects are isolated cardiac lesions. They can occur with other congenital heart lesions, however, including coarctation of the aorta, atrial septal defect, and the patent ductus arteriosus. They also occur as part of a constellation of abnormalities in some of the complex cyanotic congenital heart diseases, including tetralogy of Fallot, double outlet right ventricle, transposition of the great vessels, truncus arteriosus, and tricuspid atresia.

The majority of children with VSD have no other congenital abnormalities. Less commonly, VSDs can occur as part of a particular syndrome, as for example the Holt-Oram syndrome with digital abnormalities, or as part of the VATER anomaly (*v*ertebral defects, imperforate *a*nus, *t*rache*oe*sophageal fistula, and *r*adial and *r*enal dysplasia) with tracheoesophageal fistula. Anesthesiologists need to be aware that, as with any congenital abnormality, the presence of one defect should alert the clinician to look for other, less obvious problems. Frequently in children with congenital heart disease, these are renal anomalies such as single or horseshoe kidney that are detected as an incidental finding during cardiac catheterization when an abdominal film is obtained after administration of contrast agents.

PATHOPHYSIOLOGY

Prerequisites to predicting a patient's response and tolerance of anesthesia and surgery are understanding the status of the pulmonary vasculature in terms of pulmonary vascular resistance (PVR) and understanding the underlying physiologic abnormalities that accompany the VSD. These vary widely with the size of the defect; the VSD may be restrictive or nonrestrictive. The PVR varies tremendously with the age of the child, the degree of shunting, and coexisting cardiac abnormalities.

When it occurs as an isolated cardiac abnormality, VSD is not detected in the newborn because of the intrinsically high PVR. While in utero, the PVR exceeds the systemic vascular resistance (SVR), leading to the normal intrauterine circulation with bypass of the lungs. Several dramatic changes in the pulmonary circulation occur after the first breath of the newborn and continue during the first few weeks of life. An initial negative inspiratory force, as high as ⁻40 mm Hg, expands the alveoli and thus opens up the pulmonary capillaries for the first time, leading to a sudden decrease in the PVR and the establishment of the adult pattern of circulation. While this recruitment of pulmonary capillaries accounts for the initial decrease in the PVR, a further decrease occurs over the next several weeks. This is related to additional pulmonary arteriolar growth, both in terms of size and number, and to thinning of the pulmonary arteriolar muscular wall.

The child with a VSD, even a relatively large one, is asymptomatic at birth and has no murmur because of the relatively high PVR, which results in little shunt. Only after several weeks, as the PVR decreases, does shunting across the defect occur; it is at that time that frequently a murmur is first noted. Overall, the size of the lesion determines the amount of left-to-right shunting initially, and consequently the rapidity with which the child

becomes symptomatic. With the infant's growth during the first few weeks of life, large defects lead to increases in the pulmonary blood flow compared with the systemic blood flow because the PVR is decreasing while the SVR is maintained. A left-to-right shunt across the VSD as large as 7:1 has been seen in some babies, indicating that seven times as much pulmonary as systemic blood flow is occurring.

The occurrence of this amount of pulmonary blood flow has several consequences. Obviously, these infants will develop congestive heart failure rapidly. However, another more insidious, less clinically apparent change may occur—that is, the development of a secondary increase in PVR in response to this torrential amount of flow. This secondary PVR is characterized by pulmonary arteriolar muscular hypertrophy and is of concern to the anesthesiologist because of the potential for the development of hemodynamic problems at the time of surgery.

If the PVR continues to increase, it can become irreversible, even if the original anatomic defect is corrected. In children with VSD, this increase in the PVR to the point of irreversibility can occur as early as during the 1st year of life, although it is more common in the older child or young adult. Clinically this is manifest by initial improvement in symptoms of congestive heart failure due to decreasing shunt.

If it is left surgically uncorrected, the PVR may become suprasystemic and the child will begin to shunt right-to-left through the ventricular defect. Clinically this is manifest by cyanosis, the so-called Eisenmenger's syndrome (Fig. 1).

Children with lesser degrees of elevated PVR may have episodes of pulmonary hypertension which may transiently reverse shunts and/or lead to right ventricular failure in the operating room and intensive care unit. These episodes may be precipitated by common perioperative events that increase PVR such as hypoxia and hypercarbia, or even by stimuli such as pain, coughing, or

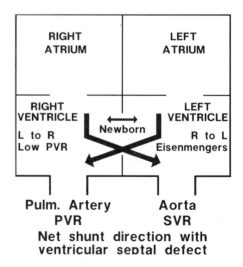

Figure 1 Net shunt direction with VSD.

endotracheal tube suctioning during light levels of anesthesia.

When evaluating cardiac catheterization data, it is important for the anesthesiologist to realize that pulmonary hypertension is not equivalent to elevated PVR. The level of pulmonary hypertension is determined by the amount of blood flow as well as by the PVR. A pulmonary artery pressure of 80 mm Hg in the presence of a 5:1 pulmonary-to-systemic shunt is certainly less foreboding than a pressure of 80 mm Hg with a 1.5:1 shunt. While the absolute pulmonary artery pressures are the same in both instances, the PVR will be much higher in the second patient.

Currently, it is unusual to see a patient with irreversible pulmonary hypertension related to a VSD, except in regions that have limited medical resources. Children with VSDs are ordinarily identified in early infancy, even if asymptomatic, by the presence of a murmur detected during periodic "well baby" evaluations. Since many defects close spontaneously during childhood, they are often followed by a pediatric cardiologist with serial echocardiographic and clinical evaluations. A diminishing murmur may signify closure of the VSD or the development of an elevated PVR with decreased shunting.

PREOPERATIVE EVALUATION

The anesthesiologist most commonly encounters the patient for VSD surgery for the first time on the day before surgery. This is a particularly important preoperative interview because of the magnitude of the operation and the possibility of morbidity or mortality occurring intraoperatively. Although the infant who is to undergo surgery is blissfully unaware of what is about to transpire, information needs to be obtained from and given to the parents. The older, school-age child who is about to undergo surgery needs information also and should be included in a discussion at a level appropriate to his or her level of understanding. It is helpful to review the cardiac catheterization data before speaking to the family so that more accurate information about the expected perioperative course can be given.

The parents should be asked whether the patient has had symptoms of congestive heart failure or cyanosis. Infants express congestive heart failure by feeding intolerance; that is, they become short of breath or diaphoretic during feeding. They may also become dusky or have circumoral pallor that is noted by the mother or primary caretaker. Other clinical signs in the child include growth failure, or the inability to keep up with playmates. Periods of frank cyanosis may have been noted, or even "squatting" episodes, if the child has some element of coexisting dynamic right ventricular outflow obstruction.

Previous hospitalizations for pneumonia or congestive heart failure should alert the anesthesiologist to look for evidence of left lung or left lower lobe atelectasis that is often present preoperatively. The progressive pulmonary circulatory overload that occurs in these infants can lead to enlargement of the left atrium, which in turn compresses the left upper lobe or mainstem bronchus. Left lower lobe or lung collapse can create difficulty for the anesthesiologist in ventilating the infant intraoperatively. Conservative measures aimed at preoperative lung expansion, such as chest physiotherapy, are usually ineffective, although the lung usually expands with positive pressure ventilation and positive end-expiratory pressure. Additionally, copious pulmonary secretions accumulate in the atelectatic segment of the lung. Once the lung is re-expanded intraoperatively, mobilization of these secretions can quickly and unexpectedly plug the small endotracheal tube.

Medical therapy for control of congestive failure should be noted. Generally these children are digitalized and receiving diuretics such as spironolactone and furosemide, or afterload reducers such as captopril. These drugs can create electrolyte imbalances preoperatively that affect dysrhythmias and hemodynamic stability intraoperatively if unrecognized.

Although they occur infrequently, coexisting syndromes can also influence the preoperative course. For example, approximately 10 percent of children with Down's syndrome have atlanto-occipital instability. Quadraparesis following heart surgery, necessitating cervical fusion, has been described in one such child. In a child with a syndrome associated with his VSD, the anesthesiologist should familiarize himself with the features of the syndrome and their anesthetic implications.

Information should be obtained about previous surgeries. Currently, the majority of children with VSD present for primary repair at the time surgical intervention is deemed necessary. Several years ago, however, primary closure of the VSD with cardiopulmonary bypass was deferred in the infant because of size; these infants underwent pulmonary artery banding to control congestive heart failure until large enough to undergo definitive repair. Occasionally, older children still present for VSD repair after having undergone pulmonary artery banding as an infant. The anesthesiologist should recognize that previous thoracic surgery, particularly previous median sternotomy, can create intraoperative problems. These include bleeding from adhesion sites, adherence of the heart to the underside of the sternum during sternotomy, and difficulty in dissection and cannulation with hemodynamic consequences that the anesthesiologist must manage before bypass.

Subtle neurologic deficits have been noted in as many as two-thirds of adults after cardiopulmonary bypass and in a high percentage of children undergoing correction of congenital defects, particularly those with open chamber surgery or those undergoing circulatory arrest as part of their correction. It should be recognized, however, that children with congenital heart disease may also have pre-existing neurologic deficits. It is therefore important to ask about, document, and evaluate neurologic problems, including seizures and developmental delay during the preoperative evaluation.

The preoperative physical examination by the anesthesiologist is generally brief and is concentrated on the airway, cardiac, and pulmonary systems. As with any pediatric patient, it is easiest to listen to the heart and lungs first while the mother is holding the infant. The child perceives auscultation as nonthreatening and usually cooperates, or at least does not cry. While the murmur may be distractingly impressive, it is equally important to assess breath sounds and air exchange, particularly on the left side.

Gentle palpation of the abdomen reveals the degree of hepatosplenomegaly; this is a rough indication of the degree of right-sided cardiac failure. The hands and feet should be examined for evidence of previous cut-downs or femoral cardiac catheterization sites that now may have diminished peripheral blood flow and be unsuitable for arterial cannulation intraoperatively.

Routine preoperative laboratory studies include measurements of electrolytes; a hemoglobin, hematocrit, and platelet count; and coagulation studies (prothrombin time and partial thromboplastin time). These are useful not only in determining the patient's preoperative status, but also in guiding intraoperative decision making.

As mentioned above, cardiac catheterization data should be reviewed before surgery. Important elements to consider include the pulmonary/systemic flow ratio, absolute pulmonary artery pressure, and the PVR. If the PVR is elevated, often supplemental oxygen may be given and a second measurement made during catheterization. The amount of decrease in PVR with oxygen is a rough guide to how much of the pulmonary hypertention is potentially reversible. The presence of extracardiac systemic-to-pulmonary shunts, such as a patent ductus arteriosus, should also be noted. These can lead to excessive pulmonary blood flow and systemic hypotension during bypass if they are not recognized and controlled.

PREOPERATIVE COUNSELING

The final, and in some ways, most important portion of the preoperative interview involves *giving* information, both to the child himself if he is old enough to understand and to the child's parents.

Specific things that the child needs to know are that he is going to undergo an operation, (this is usually, although not invariably, told to the child by the parents ahead of time) and that after the operation he will be in an intensive care unit. The child needs to know that he will be asleep for the operation, but that anesthesia sleep is different from an ordinary nap in that he will not just "awaken" during the middle of the procedure. He also needs to known that he will not be able to speak immediately afterward because of the "breathing tube" but that his caretakers will ensure that he does not have pain or discomfort. The plan for anesthesia induction should be discussed with the child old enough to understand. As with other pediatric surgical patients, rehearsal with an anesthesia mask preoperatively is helpful later on.

Information given to the parents is more detailed, and when the patient is a school-age child who has only partial understanding, should probably be discussed separately. This is often a good time for the patient to be sent to the playroom. Specific anesthetic issues and invasive intraoperative procedures should be reviewed at this time. These include complications related specifically to the anesthetic, such as cardiac compromise, malignant hyperthermia, intubation problems, and those occurring with arterial and central venous cannulation. Serious complications or death may be related to the anesthetic, the procedure itself, cardiopulmonary bypass, or the global perioperative course. According to the study by Hickey et al, when strictly defined, true complications related solely to the anesthetic are rare, with an incidence of less than 1 percent.

A discussion of the anticipated postoperative course is also appropriate at this time. Many parents are more familiar with adult cardiac surgery, particularly bypass surgery, than they are with congenital heart surgery. It is important to emphasize that the drugs used are the same as those used with adults who have "sick hearts," obviously titrated to the age and size of the child, and that they will keep the patient asleep for a period of time postoperatively. The need for postoperative ventilation should be discussed at this time. Many parents have the misconception that all anesthetics are more or less the same, and may be surprised that a child does not emerge from open heart surgery as he does from a tonsillectomy.

Currently, certain high-risk infants with an elevated PVR, (e.g., those with diaphragmatic hernias) may be treated with fentanyl infusions for sedation for several days after surgery to blunt pulmonary vascular responses. Recently, this approach has been adopted in the management of the infant with a high PVR after correction of congenital heart lesions. If a fentanyl infusion is planned, this is also discussed with the parents during the interview.

Preoperative medication is tailored to the needs of the child and anesthesiologist. The infant less than 1 year of age usually does not require sedative premedication, although atropine in a dose of 0.01 mg per kilogram is helpful as an antisialogogue. For the child who is older and fearful of parental separation, a sedative premedication is appropriate. Intramuscular midazolam hydrochloride in a dose of 0.08 mg per kilogram administered approximately 15 minutes before induction frequently works well. This may be combined with atropine in a dose of 0.01 mg per kilogram or scopolamine in a dose of 0.006 mg per kilogram, which has further sedative and amnestic effects. Other agents, such as morphine alone or combined with pentobarbital, have been used.

As with other pediatric patients, the duration of the NPO period should be appropriate to the child's age. To further decrease the risk of aspiration and enhance gastric emptying, many practitioners limit feeding to clear liquids only for the 12 hours before induction in addition to the NPO period.

INTRAOPERATIVE MANAGEMENT

The intraoperative management of the infant or child undergoing VSD repair is actually guided by the patient's underlying pathophysiology and the planned repair. As previously mentioned, the school-age child who is undergoing repair of an asymptomatic defect and the infant with severe congestive heart and pulmonary failure related to a large shunt are vastly different, despite the anatomic similarity of their lesions. Anesthetic management should be tailored to these differences as well as to the age of the child.

INDUCTION OF ANESTHESIA

It has been demonstrated that a wide variety of anesthesia induction methods can be used safely in the child with congenital heart disease who is largely asymptomatic or well compensated. Induction doses of ketamine, thiopental sodium, fentanyl, and halothane have been shown to cause little hemodynamic compromise, and all increase the oxygen saturation in children with both cyanotic and acyanotic disease when carefully administered. This allows the anesthesiologist to induce anesthesia with a mask, intravenously, or intramuscularly, according to the desire of the child and the practitioner's expertise.

Nitrous oxide is also frequently used to facilitate induction when an inhalation induction is selected. Nitrous oxide, however, has been shown to have potentially deleterious, clinically unpredictable effects on the pulmonary vasculature and may worsen an elevated PVR in children. Additionally, it increases the size of any small bubbles of air that may get into the circulation and enhances the possibility of significant air embolus. For these reasons, many practitioners restrict the use of nitrous oxide to the induction period and turn it off once an intravenous line is in place.

Anesthesia induction in children with significant congestive heart failure with or without an elevated PVR is generally carried out with intramuscular ketamine or intravenous agents such as narcotics. Although the cardiac depressant effects of halothane or thiopental may be tolerated for short periods of time, they may exacerbate congestive heart failure significantly when used as the sole agents for induction. Several years ago it was reported that ketamine may elevate pulmonary artery pressure. This has been refuted by Hickey et al, who have demonstrated that the elevation in PVR seen when ketamine is administered is associated with airway obstruction and hypercarbia. In those patients with elevated PVR in whom adequate ventilation is maintained, no elevation of PVR occurs, even with induction doses of ketamine.

ANESTHESIA MAINTENANCE

Although a wide variety of induction techniques can be used, tailored to the child's tolerance and anesthesiologist's expertise, maintenance of anesthesia is generally accomplished with intravenous agents, particularly the narcotics fentanyl and sufentanil. These provide a smooth intraoperative course, but they do not always reliably produce amnesia and may need to be supplemented with a benzodiazepine or a small amount of an inhalation agent such as halothane. Additionally, when used in larger anesthetic doses (e.g., 100 to 200 µg per kilogram of fentanyl), these agents provide sedation into the postoperative period, facilitating mechanical ventilation and initial stabilization in the intensive care unit.

Occasionally, an older, totally asymptomatic child presents for VSD repair. This child may tolerate a total inhalation anesthetic intraoperatively, but will need narcotic supplementation if postoperative ventilation is planned. Additionally, it should be remembered that after bypass and cross-clamping, the myocardium is vastly different than it is preoperatively and may not withstand the myocardial depressant effects of the potent inhalation agents.

INTRAOPERATIVE MONITORING

Monitoring use during cardiac procedures for children, including surgical correction of VSDs, is essentially the same as that used for an adult undergoing cardiac surgery, with the exception of the balloon-tipped, flow-directed pulmonary artery (Swan-Ganz) catheter.

Basic, noninvasive monitors are applied before induction, including electrocardiogram (ECG), blood pressure cuffs, pulse oximeter, precordial stethoscope, and end-tidal CO_2 monitor. At least two leads of ECG, II and V_5, are monitored continuously; in addition to arrhythmias, myocardial ischemia has been well documented in children. Ischemia changes may occur during any portion of the operation, particularly after cross-clamp removal.

After anesthetic induction and intravenous cannulation, invasive monitors, including arterial line and central venous cannulae are placed, using whatever technique the practitioner is familiar with. Percutaneous radial artery cannulations have been performed in infants weighing as little as 400 g, and central access via either the subclavian or internal jugular route is easily accomplished with practice. Pulmonary artery catheters may be placed in the right atrium at this time, but are not advanced because of the intracardiac "holes" and potential for catheter misplacement as well as interference with intracardiac repair. If a pulmonary artery catheter has been placed in the right atrium by the anesthesiologist, this may be manually advanced into the pulmonary artery by the surgeon at the completion of surgery.

After surgical repair, additional transthoracic indwelling catheters in the left atrium and pulmonary artery may be placed by the surgeon for monitoring during weaning from bypass and during the postoperative period. It has long been recognized by anesthesiologists who treat adults and intensive care physicians that isolated left and right ventricular failure can occur, as reflected by widely different filling pressures. Episodic right ventricular failure in children with elevated PVR also occurs; monitors of filling pressures for both sides of the heart are thus important.

Transesophageal echocardiography has recently assumed a position of importance in the monitoring armamentarium for adult cardiac surgery. Currently, application of this technology for examining cardiac function, efficacy of repair, and filling volumes in congenital heart surgery has been limited by the large size of the transducer that is to be inserted into the esophagus. Epicardial echocardiography has been performed in children undergoing congenital heart defect repairs. As a monitoring device, it is limited when used in this way, because views of the heart are obtained only periodically and do not provide continuous on-line information regarding myocardial function or cardiac chamber volumes.

INTRAOPERATIVE MANAGEMENT

In addition to anesthetic maintenance, the anesthesiologist is involved with other facets of intraoperative management, including cardiopulmonary bypass, circulatory arrest (if utilized), and postbypass cardiac and pulmonary support.

Intraoperative management is guided to a large extent by the infant's pre-existing pathology and the surgical repair. It is essential that the anesthesiologist have good communication with the surgeon and perfusionist, and each should be aware of what the other is doing. For example, the period during which aortic and vena caval cannulation are performed is one of potential hemodynamic instability, particularly in the small infant. The aortic cannula can occupy a significant portion of the aortic lumen and act as an impediment to ejection of the left ventricle as well as lead to decreased blood pressure. Similarly, venous return to the heart is limited both during manipulation of the cavae and when the superior and inferior vena caval cannulae are in place. The anesthesiologist should be aware of these trends and be ready to provide a blood transfusion if significant blood loss occurs, and he or she should alert the surgeon if perfusion pressure falls below acceptable levels.

Anticoagulation for cardiopulmonary bypass is accomplished with heparin, given either by the surgeon directly into the heart or by the anesthesiologist through the central venous line. It is important to aspirate blood both before and after heparin injection to ensure intravascular injection. The adequacy of anticoagulation is monitored throughout the bypass procedure and is the responsibility of the perfusionist, anesthesiologist, and surgeon.

Several parameters should be monitored during cardiopulmonary bypass, including perfusion pressure and episodic blood gas analysis. Recently, on-line continuous mixed venous saturation monitoring has become more widespread and may soon be considered a standard of care during bypass surgery. Of critical importance is ensuring adequacy of cerebral blood flow and cerebral autoregulation during cardiac bypass. Blood gases are generally not temperature corrected (alpha stat). It has been demonstrated that temperature correction (pH stat regulation) of blood gases can cause uncoupling of carbon dioxide–regulated cerebral flow, leading to pressure-passive changes in cerebral perfu-

sion rather than normal autoregulation. The clinical significance of this is unknown, although no difference in neurologic morbidity was demonstrated in a prospective study evaluating the two methods of blood gas regulation in coronary bypass patients.

Electroencephalography (EEG) has begun to be studied during bypass surgery as a monitor of adequacy of cerebral perfusion and of "depth of anesthesia." Although it has been speculated that EEG abnormalities can predict postoperative neurologic deficits, this has not been proven. In the experimental setting, EEG monitoring has been undertaken in the adult undergoing a open chamber cardiac procedure as a means of titrating thiopental to burst suppression pattern. Little is known about this type of monitoring in children undergoing open heart procedures, including VSD repair.

Other parameters that should be monitored during the bypass period include the urine output, hematocrit, electrolytes, and acid-base status. These will affect cardiac function after bypass, as well as indicate homeostatic well- being during bypass.

Finally, the approach and ease of surgical correction should be observed during the bypass period. VSD repair can be approached through the atrium, the pulmonary artery, or a ventriculotomy by the surgeon. The approach is important because of the myocardial dysfunction that occurs after ventriculotomy and the need for additional vasopressor support.

CIRCULATORY ARREST

Surgical repair of congenital heart disease is often facilitated by the ability to operate in a quiet, bloodless field. Circulatory arrest is used to create these circumstances. It has been demonstrated that patients, particularly infants, can withstand periods of circulatory arrest of up to 1 hour, without any substantial increased risk of significant neurologic impairment if cooled to a temperature below 20°C. Circulatory arrest is accomplished by surface cooling the infant once anesthesia induction and venous cannulation have been completed. Further cooling is done on bypass and by packing the infant in ice until a uniform temperature below 20°C is achieved. At this time bypass is stopped and the cannulae removed, allowing the surgeon free access to the infant's heart. Once the repair is completed, the cannulae are replaced, the ice bags are removed, and rewarming is accomplished on bypass.

ANESTHETIC MANAGEMENT FOLLOWING CARDIOPULMONARY BYPASS

A great deal of the postbypass management of the patient undergoing VSD repair is determined by preoperative and intraoperative factors. It can be anticipated that in the infant who has had severe congestive heart failure preoperatively, the level of inotropic support necessary will be vastly different than it is in the asymptomatic older child. Chronic congestive heart failure has been shown to decrease beta-receptor density and sensitivity in the myocardium. Similarly, children with elevated PVR preoperatively may be expected to have more problems after bypass, including episodic pulmonary hypertension leading to right heart failure.

Finally, it should be remembered that the composition of the infant myocardium is qualitatively very different from that of the adult or even the older child. Myocardial tissue contains fewer contractile muscle fibers and greater amounts of noncontractile connective tissue. This results in a decreased ability of the myocardium to increase cardiac output by increasing stroke volume and greater dependence on heart rate as a determinant of cardiac output.

Selection of inotropic agents for the postbypass period is based largely on the above-mentioned factors. It can be anticipated that the older child with a normal PVR and an uneventful repair done through an atrial incision will require little if any inotropic support postoperatively, and may be extubated within several hours after surgery has been completed (Table 1).

Infants with chronic congestive heart failure, on the other hand, can be expected to require more inotropic support, specifically designed to lower PVR and lend inotropic support to the myocardium. Beta-agonists (e.g., dobutamine), which lend inotropic support to the myocardium, as well as dilate the pulmonary vasculature, are extremely useful and often constitute the first line of support. Other catecholamines, including epinephrine, are used by some, particularly in the setting of severe myocardial pump failure after bypass.

Isoproterenol may be particularly useful in the child with heart block and bradycardia after VSD repair. Alternatively, ventricular pacing or atrial ventricular sequential pacing may be used. The infant myocardium is limited in its ability to increase cardiac output by increasing stroke volume because of the fewer myofibrils and greater amounts of connective tissue. Bradycardia is particularly detrimental because cardiac output is determined in essence by heart rate.

Amrinone, a type 3 phosphodiesterase inhibitor, has recently been shown to be particularly beneficial in the patient with congestive heart failure and pulmonary hypertension. It is a pulmonary vasodilator, as well as a positive inotropic agent and systemic vasodilator, and it has therefore been described as an ionodilator. Because amrinone works to increase myocardial cellular ionized calcium levels independently of beta-receptors, it can be expected to be effective in the failing heart with decreased beta-receptor density. Additionally, by reducing afterload in both circulations, it can be expected to be especially beneficial in the infant with both congestive heart failure and elevated PVR. In these patients, loading doses of up to 3 mg per kilogram may be needed. Maintenance infusions need to be adjusted to lower levels in infants less than 6 weeks of age.

Other noninotropic pulmonary vasodilators that have been helpful during the postbypass period and in the intensive care unit for these infants include prostaglandin E_1, nitroprusside, and nitroglycerine. Nitroprusside also facilitates even rewarming during and after bypass.

Despite the status of the myocardium, anesthesia will need to continue to be provided during the bypass and chest closure. This can be provided with supplemental narcotics and midazolam as well as with inhalational agents.

POSTOPERATIVE CARE

Anesthetic care of the infant or child with a VSD does not end with the completion of surgery. The period during which the patient is transported from the operating room to the intensive care unit is one in which particular anesthetic vigilance is needed, and full monitoring should be continued. The anesthesiologist should help determine the initial ventilator settings in the intensive care unit since he has been managing the ventilation for a period of hours before the patient's arrival. During the transfer of care, filling pressures as well as blood pressure need to be carefully followed; this is a period of rapid peripheral vasodilatation as the patient continues to rewarm and of ongoing volume losses through the chest tubes and urine output.

During the days after the procedure, the anesthesiologist may participate in postoperative pain management, ventilatory management, and the set-up of fentanyl infusion. Follow-up visits may reveal pulmonary complications such as atelectasis, neurologic complications (often subtle), and cardiac complications such as complete heart block or ventricular failure.

Table 1 Pediatric Vasopressors and Effective Dosages

Vasopressor	Dosage
Dobutamine	2–15 µg/kg/min
Dopamine	2–20 µg/kg/min
Epinephrine	.03–1 µg/kg/min
Isoproterenol	0.1–1.5 µg/kg/min
Norepinephrine	.03–0.5 µg/kg/min
Prostaglandin E_1	.05–0.1 µg/kg/min
Nitroglycerine	0.5–5 µg/kg/min
Nitroprusside	0.5–10 µg/kg/min
Lidocaine	20–50 µg/kg/min
Amrinone	
Loading dose	1–3 mg/kg
Infusion infants <6 wk	3–5 µg/kg/min
Infusion infants >6 wk	10 µg/kg/min

SUGGESTED READING

Hickey PR, Anderson NP. Deep hypothermic circulatory arrest: a review of pathophysiology and clinical experience as a basis for anesthetic management. J Cardiothoracic Anesth 1987; 1:137–155.

Hickey PR, Hansen DD, Wessel DL, et al. Pulmonary and systemic hemodynamic responses to fentanyl in infants. Anesth Analg 1985; 64:483–486.

Lawless S, Burckart G, Diven W, et al. Amrinone in neonates and infants after cardiac surgery. Crit Care Med 1989; 17:751–754.

Liberthson RR. Ventricular septal defect. In: Congenital heart disease: diagnosis and management in children and adults. Boston: Little, Brown and Co., 1989.

Wells WJ, Lindesmith GG. Ventricular septal defect. In: Arciniegas E, ed. Pediatric cardiac surgery. Chicago: Year Book Medical Publishers, Inc., 1985.

TETRALOGY OF FALLOT

ROBERT L. STEVENSON, M.D.

In the United States, approximately 10,000 infants are born each year with cyanotic congenital heart disease. The past 40 years have been a time of rapid advancement in the surgical treatment of this disorder. Since 1945, when a subclavian-to-pulmonary artery shunt for the treatment of tetralogy of Fallot was first described by Blalock and Taussig, several palliative procedures have been introduced. Further progress followed the development of the pump oxygenator by Gibbon in 1953. Extracorporeal support allowed for definitive intercardiac repairs of cyanotic congenital heart defects. Creative surgical approaches were described by Lillehei, Mustard, Rastelli, Senning, and Fontan. The growth of sophisticated surgical repairs has been paralleled by the amelioration of the quality of anesthetic care. Advances in monitoring, a clearer understanding of pathophysiology, and the development of new cardiovascular drugs and anesthetic agents have all played a role in the reduction of anesthetic mortality. This view is supported by a recent report of 500 consecutive pediatric cardiac procedures in which there was not a single anesthesia-related death.

PATHOPHYSIOLOGY

An organized approach to the management of patients with congenital heart disease must begin with an appreciation of the pathophysiology of the defects, which in turn lead to cyanosis. The first category of cyanotic congenital heart disease is caused by reduced pulmonary blood flow. Cyanosis, caused by reduced pulmonary blood flow, results when there is obstruction of blood flow into the pulmonary vascular tree in association with a defect that allows shunting of blood from the right side of the heart to the left. Tetralogy of Fallot is the classic example of this defect. Other examples of lesions that cause reduced pulmonary blood flow are shown in Table 1. They all result in a right-to-left shunting, with a pulmonary-to-systemic blood flow ratio ($Q_p:Q_s$) that is less than 1:1.

The second category of cyanotic congenital heart disease is caused by mixing of pulmonary and systemic blood within the heart. A common example of this

Table 1 Cardiac Defects That Lead to Cyanosis

Classification	Defects
Reduced pulmonary blood flow	Tetralogy of Fallot Pulmonary atresia Tricuspid atresia Double outlet right ventricle with pulmonary stenosis
Mixing of pulmonary and systemic blood within the heart	Atrioventricular canal Common atrium Common ventricle Truncus arteriosus
Subtotal separation of pulmonary and systemic circulations	Transposition of the great arteries
Reversal of left-to-right shunts due to pulmonary hypertension	Eisenmenger's syndrome

problem is truncus arteriosus. In this lesion, the aorta and pulmonary artery fail to separate normally during development, which results in a single arterial trunk from which the pulmonary arteries arise as branches. The aortic and pulmonary valves are combined in one large truncal valve, and there is an associated large ventricular septal defect (VSD), which allows mixing of pulmonary and systemic blood. The ratio of pulmonary blood flow (Q_p) relative to systemic blood flow (Q_s) depends on the degree of stenosis of the pulmonary vascular tree. $Q_p:Q_s$ may be greater than 1:1, but mixing of blood in the ventricles and truncus results in the desaturated blood perfusing within the systemic circulation.

The third category is subtotal separation of the pulmonary and systemic circulations, as occurs in transposition of the great arteries. In this lesion, the aorta arises from the right ventricle and the pulmonary artery from the left ventricle. Total separation of two circulations results in no oxygenated blood reaching the systemic circulation, which is not compatible with life. Survival depends on septal defects at the atrial or ventricular levels that allow some mixing of pulmonary and systemic blood. Balloon septostomy is performed soon after birth in order to enlarge the size of the foramen ovale and to facilitate mixing.

The fourth category is the Eisenmenger complex, which may occur in any situation where there is a large left-to-right shunt—for example, a ventricular septal defect. Such lesions expose the pulmonary circulation to systemic blood pressure and high pulmonary flow, and this results in secondary increases in pulmonary vascular resistance from the hypertrophy of pulmonary vascular smooth muscle. When pulmonary vascular resistance (PVR) exceeds systemic vascular resistance (SVR), the direction of shunting changes to a right-to-left shunt, which causes desaturation of systemic arterial blood and subsequent cyanosis.

This classification system provides an overview of the spectrum of cyanotic congenital heart disease. It is only a limited listing of the many congenital defects that lead to cyanosis. In addition, many lesions display wide variations in anatomy and clinical presentation.

Cyanosis is by definition the presence of 5 g or more of deoxygenated hemoglobin in arterial blood. With cyanosis, the blood that is transported to the periphery has a low oxygen content. This limitation in oxygen delivery may result in delayed growth and development with failure to thrive because of tissue hypoxia. Hypoxia stimulates hematopoiesis, which causes secondary polycythemia. Increases in hemoglobin concentration allow a rise in arterial oxygen content, but as hematocrit rises, the viscosity of the blood increases, which may lead to intravascular thrombosis and infarction.

TETRALOGY OF FALLOT

It is beyond the scope of this chapter to discuss the management of every congenital heart defect. The remainder of this chapter addresses the management of tetralogy of Fallot as an example of cyanotic heart disease. The tetrad consists of a ventricular septal defect, a pulmonic stenosis, an overriding aorta, and a right ventricular hypertrophy. Obstruction of blood flow from the right ventricle into the lung may occur at the right ventricular outflow track, the pulmonic valve, the main pulmonary artery, or the pulmonary artery branches. If pulmonary vascular resistance is greater than systemic vascular resistance, blood is shunted across the VSD and systemic arterial desaturation occurs. The obstruction to right ventricular outflow is caused both by a malposition of the parietal band of the crista supraventricularis as well as by hypertrophy of the ventricle secondary to the exposure of the right heart to systemic arterial pressure.

Pathophysiology

In tetralogy of Fallot, inadequate pulmonary blood flow causes systemic arterial desaturation and tissue hypoxia. The chronic manifestations of inadequate oxygen delivery are delayed growth and development, decreased exercise tolerance, and cyanosis. Hypercyanotic episodes or "tet spells" are a frequent complication of tetralogy of Fallot and are characterized by hyperventilation and worsening cyanosis, which may progress to syncope, seizures, and death. Spells are precipitated by activities that increase oxygen utilization such as feeding, crying, and exercise. The precise mechanism of these attacks remains unclear. Spells may be caused by increased obstruction of the right ventricular infundibulum from increased sympathetic tone. This would cause a further decrease in pulmonary blood flow. Hyperpnea

may maintain the spells by increasing oxygen consumption. Peripheral vasodilation in response to hypoxia may increase right-to-left shunting. Children respond to spells by squatting, which exerts a beneficial effect by increasing venous return and/or by raising systemic vascular resistance. Treatment for spells consists of giving oxygen and morphine and having the patient assume the knee-to-chest position. Phenylephrine hydrochloride (Neo-Synephrine) may be used to reduce right-to-left shunting by raising systemic vascular resistance. Propranolol has been used to block sympathetically medicated right ventricular outflow obstruction. General anesthesia has been recommended as a treatment for refractory episodes.

Anesthetic management is aimed at maintaining adequate pulmonary blood flow. In tetralogy of Fallot, the large VSD allows blood in the combined ventricles to enter either the pulmonary or systemic circulations. The distribution of blood flow is determined by the relative resistances of the two circulations. Right ventricular outflow obstruction in tetralogy of Fallot creates a high, relatively fixed PVR. Factors that can cause further increase in PVR, such as hypercarbia, hypoxia, and acidosis, must be carefully avoided. Increased sympathetic activity may intensify right ventricular outflow obstruction. This may be avoided by ample premedication and adequate levels of anesthesia. A fill in SVR can shunt blood away from the lungs, whereas hypotension from any cause may reduce pulmonary blood flow. Since there is a constant right-to-left shunt in TOF, extreme care must be exercised to exclude and eliminate air bubbles from intravenous lines.

PREOPERATIVE EVALUATION

Successful anesthetic management begins with a thorough preoperative evaluation. As with many cyanotic heart lesions, tetralogy of Fallot presents with a wide spectrum of severity. In reviewing the patient's history, one should assess the degree of cyanosis, exercise tolerance, and frequency of hypercyanotic spells. There may be a history of previous palliative procedures such as a Blalock-Taussig shunt. A careful search should be made for other congenital defects, since the incidence of these defects is high in patients with cyanotic heart disease. In addition to the usual physical examination, a careful inspection of the peripheral vasculature may reveal likely sites for venous access. Pulses may be weak or absent due to previous palliative surgery. Careful review of the history, physical examination, and laboratory findings, including echocardiography and cardiac catheterization, is necessary in order to understand the anatomic lesion completely and to assess the functional severity of the patient. A preoperative conversation with the surgeon may help determine the exact operative plan. Children with cyanotic congenital heart disease may be receiving a variety of medications, which may include diuretics, antiarrhythmics, and sympathetic nervous system agonists and antagonists.

For example, prostaglandins are used as an intravenous infusion in neonates who are dependent on ductal patency for adequate pulmonary blood flow. In patients with tetralogy of Fallot, propranolol may be used to block the hyperdynamic right ventricular outflow tract.

The parents of the patient should be given a clear explanation of the perioperative events, including preoperative fluid restriction, preoperative medications, type of anesthetic induction, intraoperative monitoring (especially invasive monitoring), and the approximate duration of the procedure. They should also be informed of the possible need for postoperative ventilation and of the number of lines and tubes that will be involved in the child's postoperative care. Regardless of the patient's age, one should attempt to establish a rapport with the patient and to explain the perioperative events in a way the child can understand. In older, healthier children, their cooperation can be gained by allowing them to participate in anesthetic decisions, especially with regard to anesthetic induction techniques. The parents should be given a clear understanding of the risks of anesthesia and of the associated procedures.

Within the last 12 hours before the procedure, only clear liquids should be administered orally, and depending on their size, patients should receive nothing by mouth for 4 to 8 hours before the procedure. The choice of premedication depends on the age of the child and on the type of anesthetic induction planned (Table 2). For children younger than 1 year of age, atropine alone may be used. For older children, a combination of narcotic, barbiturate, and atropine given either intramuscularly or orally is a reasonable choice. Meperidine hydrochloride (Demerol) and pentobarbital elixirs are available for oral administration. The oral dose of Demerol is four times higher than the equivalent intramuscular dose because of first-pass metabolism by the liver. In sicker patients, one may choose to omit the barbiturate and administer a somewhat larger dose of narcotic (e.g., morphine, 0.2 mg per kilogram). If an intravenous line is in place, the premedication can be given intravenously over several minutes with the patient under direct observation. In the occasional patient receiving long-term treatment with propranolol, a decision must be made whether to continue the drug on the day of surgery or to withhold it. The benefit of the drug is the possible prevention of hypercyanotic episodes by its blunting of right ventricular contractility. The disadvantages of the drug are the possibility of bradyarrhythmias or asystole (especially during anesthesia induction) and the risk that persistent beta-blockade may interfere with left ventricular performance at the time of termination of cardiopulmonary bypass. Long-term propranolol therapy for tetralogy of Fallot does not appear to have gained wide popularity. Urgent surgery, either palliative or corrective, is the preferred therapy for hypercyanotic episodes.

In the ideal situation, oxygen administration by hood or face mask immediately after premedication is the optimal medical therapy. However, the risks of further agitating an already anxious child outweigh the benefits of oxygen in the majority of patients with tetralogy of Fallot, and it should therefore be reserved for those patients who are unstable or who have been having frequent hypercyanotic spells.

INDUCTION OF ANESTHESIA

For children who weigh less than 10 kg, ketamine is my drug of choice for induction of anesthesia. In order to prevent secretions, atropine should be included in the premedication of all children who are going to receive ketamine. Ketamine, 5 to 10 mg per kilogram, may be administered intramuscularly, followed by oxygen or a nitrous oxide and oxygen mixture by mask. Once the child has become sedated, a peripheral intravenous line is inserted; this is followed by the administration of a muscle relaxant. Additional intravenous anesthetic can be administered at this time (Table 3).

If an intravenous line is already present or can easily be placed, intravenous ketamine, 1 to 2 mg per kilogram, may be used for induction. There are several theoretic disadvantages to the use of ketamine in children with

Table 2 Premedication Alternatives

Indication	Drugs	Dosage	Route
Patients <1 year of age	Atropine	0.02 mg/kg (minimum dose 0.1 mg)	IM
Well-compensated patients 1 year of age and older	Morphine	0.1–0.2 mg/kg	IM
	Pentobarbital and atropine	2–4 mg/kg 0.002 mg/kg	
Oral alternative to IM premedication	Meperidine hydrochloride	4 mg/kg	PO
	Pentobarbital	2–4 mg/kg (maximum dose 100 mg)	PO
	Atropine	0.02 mg/kg	
Sick children under direct observation	Morphine	0.1–0.5 mg/kg	IV over 10 min
	Atropine	0.02 mg/kg	

cyanotic congenital heart disease, particularly those with tetralogy of Fallot. Ketamine has a centrally mediated sympathomimetic effect that has the potential for increasing pulmonary vascular resistance, thereby increasing the amount of right-to-left shunting. There is also a risk that the beta-adrenergic stimulation could cause an increase in right ventricular outflow obstruction. In spite of these concerns, ketamine has been used successfully for the induction of anesthesia in children with cyanotic congenital heart disease without causing a significant increase in pulmonary artery pressure and without precipitating right ventricular outflow tract obstruction. Ketamine may be supplemented with small doses of fentanyl or valium in order to blunt the sympathomimetic effects of the drug. One should bear in mind that ketamine is a direct myocardial depressant so that, in the very sick patient, one may not see the increase in blood pressure and heart rate usually seen with the use of this drug.

In older children who are hemodynamically stable, a mask induction with nitrous oxide, oxygen, and halothane is an alternative to intravenous induction. Because of the decrease in pulmonary blood flow in tetralogy of Fallot, a mask induction is somewhat slower. This can be counterbalanced by having the patient well-premedicated before induction. It is standard practice to begin with nitrous oxide and oxygen inhalation for a short time, and to follow this with incremental concentrations of halothane. Once the child is anesthetized and an intravenous line is established, a muscle relaxant is given, followed by endotracheal intubation. Intravenous or intratracheal lidocaine may be used to blunt the cardiovascular response to endotracheal intubation. Concern exists regarding the use of halothane in patients with tetralogy of Fallot; this is based on fear of increased right-to-left shunting because of hypotension. In a recent study comparing halothane and intramuscular ketamine as induction agents in patients with tetralogy of Fallot, it was found that although halothane causes a decrease in systemic pressure, both drugs maintained arterial oxygen saturation.

Monitoring

A list of monitors used during anesthesia in patients with cyanotic congenital heart disease is given in Table 4. A precordial stethoscope, an electrocardiogram, a pulse oximeter, and a blood pressure–measuring device

should be placed at the time of anesthetic induction. Induction is a vulnerable period because of rapidly changing anesthetic concentrations in the face of minimal monitoring. A reliable, automated blood pressure–measuring device such as the pediatric Dynamapp allows rapid tracking of blood pressure changes. After induction, additional intravascular lines can be placed. In smaller children, the saphenous vein near the medical malleolus is a desirable site for placing a large-bore peripheral intravenous line. For central line placement, the use of the internal jugular vein is recommended. Catheter placement can be facilitated by positioning the child in steep Trendelenburg position with a roll under the shoulders in order to extend the neck. In an anesthetized, paralyzed child, the internal jugular vein can be located by ballottement, Doppler echocardiography, or external landmarks, and cannulation may be performed using the Seldinger technique. Small-diameter, double-lumen catheters are now available, which permit simultaneous drug administration and central venous pressure monitoring. I prefer to cannulate the radial artery percutaneously whenever possible. Alternatively, the femoral artery may be cannulated percutaneously via the Seldinger technique. Recent introduction of pulse oximetry into anesthetic care has been a boon to the management of patients with cyanotic congenital heart disease. It allows an accurate determination of the safe level of inspired oxygen and appropriate concentration of nitrous oxide. End-tidal CO_2 monitoring should be used in all children undergoing surgery for cyanotic congenital heart disease. It is important to appreciate that there can be a wider-than-normal difference between end-tidal and arterial carbon dioxide partial pressures because of mixing of systemic blood from right-to-left shunting.

CARDIOPULMONARY BYPASS

During cardiopulmonary bypass, body temperature is lowered in order to reduce oxygen consumption, thereby allowing a reduction in blood flow through the heart-lung machine. Hypothermia also lowers the requirement for anesthetics. Anesthesia should be continued during the bypass period by the use of either intravenous agents or inhalation agents through the pump oxygenator. Inhalation agents used on the pump should be discontinued well in advance of termination of

Table 3 Induction Techniques

Drugs	Dosage	Route	Indication
Ketamine with	5 to 10 mg/kg	IM	Younger or sicker
O₂ or	100%	Mask	children
N₂O and O₂	50% and 50%		
Ketamine	1 to 2 mg/kg	IV	Sick, older children
Halothane	—	Mask	Older, healthier
N₂O			children
O₂			

Table 4 Monitoring for Cyanotic Congenital Heart Disease

Timing for Placement	Type of Monitor
Monitors placed before induction of anesthesia	Precordial stethoscopy
	Blood pressure
	Electrocardiography
	Pulse oximetry
Monitors placed after induction of anesthesia	Esophageal stethoscopy
	Intra-arterial catheterization
	Central venous catheterization
	Rectal and nasopharyngeal temperature probes
	Urinary catheterization
	End-tidal CO_2 monitor
	Swan-Ganz catheter
	Dye dilution cardiac output
Monitors placed during surgery	Atrial and ventricular pacing wires
	Right and left atrial catheters

cardiopulmonary bypass in order to eliminate the possibility that these anesthetics may inhibit myocardial contractility and thereby interfere with bypass termination. During cardiopulmonary bypass, the aorta is cross-clamped, and the root of the aorta is infused with cardioplegic solution, which perfuses the heart via the coronaries, cools it, and renders it electrically silent. This results in a cold, nonbeating heart with low oxygen consumption and permits a prolonged period for surgical repair, without severely depleting the heart's supply of high-energy phosphates or causing ischemic damage.

POSTBYPASS

At the time of termination of cardiopulmonary bypass, heart action may need to be stimulated by the use of adrenergic agonist infusions. Of the several drugs available, dobutamine and isoproterenol appear to be the most efficacious. Their beta-adrenergic effects increase cardiac contractility and heart rate and dilate the systemic and pulmonary vascular beds. Patients with cyanotic congenital heart disease frequently have reactive pulmonary vasculature after cardiopulmonary bypass. Care should be taken to ensure that hypoxia, hypercarbia, and acidosis do not trigger increases in pulmonary vascular resistance. Once the patient is hemodynamically stable, heparin action is reversed by the use of protamine. The amount of heparin activity is

estimated by means of an activated clotted time or automated protamine titration device. Protamine forms a complex, which heparin renders inactive. Protamine has several side effects; the most common is peripheral vasodilatation, which is related to the rate of administration. Protamine should therefore be administered slowly in incremental boluses or by intravenous infusion, with careful monitoring of blood pressure and, if available, pulmonary artery pressure. Achieving adequate hemostasis is more difficult in patients with cyanotic congenital heart disease. Their high initial hematocrit is associated with a reduction in clotting factors and platelets. After bypass, blood is replaced with packed cells and fresh frozen plasma, and platelet concentrates may be administered as necessary. One should ascertain that the heparin has been adequately reversed with protamine. If bleeding continues, appropriate component therapy can be directed using laboratory information such as platelet count, prothrombin time, partial thromboplastin time, and fibrinogen levels. After surgical hemostasis has been established, the chest is closed, and the patient is transferred to the intensive care unit. The same care and attention to detail should be given during the transport process as are given in the operating room. The electrocardiogram and blood pressure should be monitored by use of a portable monitor, and efforts should be made to maintain body temperature during transport.

Advances in the surgical correction of cyanotic congenital heart defects have been made possible by a growing sophistication in cardiac anesthetic care. Improvement in the quality of care has resulted from better understanding of the anatomy and pathophysiology of congenital heart disease defects, improved techniques of noninvasive and invasive monitoring, and the thoughtful administration of cardiovascular drugs.

SUGGESTED READING

Adams FH, Emmanouilides GC, eds. Moss' heart disease in infants, children, and adolescents. 3rd ed. Baltimore/London: Williams & Wilkins, 1983.
Bland JW, Williams WH. Anesthesia for treatment of congenital heart defects. In: Kaplan JA, ed. Cardiac anesthesia. 2nd ed. Orlando: Grune & Stratton, 1987:281.
Radnay PA, Nagashima H, eds. Anesthetic considerations for pediatric cardiac surgery. Int Anesthesiol Clin 1980; 18.

TRANSPOSITION OF THE GREAT VESSELS

DANIEL P. NYHAN, M.D.

Transposition of the great vessels (TGV) is a common congenital heart defect. It is important to recognize that TGV is not one, or even a few, disease entities but rather represents a wide range of disease complexes. TGV has benefitted greatly from the advances that have been made in the care of patients with congenital heart defects over the last 30 years (Fig. 1). These advances include improvements in the medical management of these patients, new and refined surgical techniques, more sophisticated intraoperative anesthesia care, as well as improvements in the critical area of postoperative care of these patients. However, none of this progress would be possible without an understanding and consideration of the consequences of the progressive adverse postnatal changes that occur as a consequence of transposition anatomy-physiology. Effective participation in the care of these patients at any stage in their illness mandates an understanding of transposition terminology anatomy physiology.

CLASSIFICATION, TERMINOLOGY, AND ANATOMY

A discussion of TGV necessitates that one is conversant with the following pairs of terms: complete transposition versus corrected transposition; the terms SDD versus SLL; concordant versus discordant cavities; and finally, the differential use of the terms simple transposition versus complex transposition by morphologists on the one hand and clinicians on the other.

In the anatomically and physiologically normal heart, deoxygenated blood returns to the right atrium and is subsequently ejected into the pulmonary artery by the right ventricle. Oxygenated blood returns to the left atrium and is ejected by the left ventricle into the aorta. This situation is described in morphometric terms as SDS (solitus atria, D-loop ventricle, solitus normally related great arteries). Solitus indicates usual or normal and "D" indicates dextro- or right to specify the segmental situs of the specific cardiac segments. In the broader sense, solitus denotes the organizational pattern of each of the cardiac segments. In this normal situation, the great vessels are developmentally concordant with their respective ventricles, and the ventricles are concordant with their respective atria. In patients with complete transposition of the great vessels, the aorta arises from the right ventricle and the pulmonary artery from the left ventricle (Fig. 2). This is described as SDD, indicating that the great artery (aorta) has the dextro- or right position. This entity is sometimes described simply as D-transposition. In D-transposition, the atria and ventricles are developmentally concordant, but the great vessels are discordant with their respective ventricles. The term "complete transposition" has, through common usage, come to indicate the transposed great arteries that are physiologically uncorrected.

In physiologically corrected transposition, systemic deoxygenated blood flows to the pulmonary artery and oxygenated pulmonary venous blood flows to the aorta. In alignment terms, this is designated SLL—i.e., transposition of the great arteries with situs solitus atria (S), levo-ventricular segment situs (L), and levo-great artery segment (L). This situation is sometimes described as L-transposition. The atrioventricular alignments are discordant as a result of the abnormal position of the ventricular segment.

Morphologists use the term "simple transposition" to refer to patients with coexisting ventricular septal defects (VSDs), left ventricular outflow tract obstruction (LVOTO), patient ductus arteriosus (PDA), and straddling tricuspid valve, as well as those patients with an intact interventricular septum (IVS). It is important to recognize, however, that most clinical reports now use the term "simple transposition" to designate the largest subgroup of transposition patients—i.e., those with an IVS—and do not use it to refer to patients with hemodynamically significant associated lesions, for example, those with a large VSD, large PDA, and significant LVOTO.

Patients with double outlet right ventricle and a subpulmonary VSD (Taussig-Bing anomaly) may have physiologic and pathologic features and surgical options similar to those of some patients with transposition. These will not be discussed here. Extracardiac anomalies are infrequent in patients with TGV (occurring in 9 percent), compared with their incidence in patients with VSDs (34 percent) and tetralogy of Fallot (31 percent).

PHYSIOLOGY

The physiologic changes that result from transposition are best considered initially in the context of simple transposition of the great vessels (i.e., D-TGV) with an intact IVS without other cardiac anomalies (e.g., VSD, LVOTO). Simple D-TGV represents the single-most common anomaly. The presence of other defects such as VSD, LVOTO, and persistent PDA may profoundly alter the already abnormal pathophysiology and may thus modify therapeutic options and management strategies.

Simple D-TGV is incompatible with life unless there is some minimum adequate mixing between the two circulations. Intracirculatory mixing may occur as a result of shunting at the atrial, ventricular, or ductus arteriosus level, and as a result of bronchopulmonary collateral circulation. In patients with simple D-TGV and intact IVS, intercirculatory mixing can occur only at the ductal level once the foramen ovale has closed. Ductal flow may be promoted by the administration of

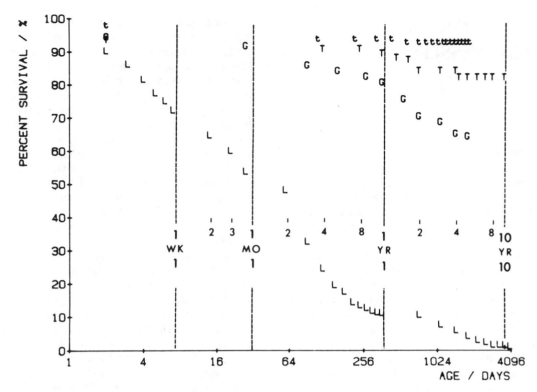

Figure 1 Survival of patients with TGV. L represents survival data antedating the era of the Mustard repair and balloon atrial septostomy. Data are derived from 742 patients with complete TGVs of all subtypes; G represents 4-year survival data derived from 47 infants with TVG and IVS managed with balloon septostomy, subsequent palliative procedure when needed, and finally late Mustard repair; T represents 10-year actuarial survival of 205 children with TGV and intact ventricular septum following Mustard repair; and t represents 5-year actuarial survival of subgroup T, comprising 100 infants operated on with Mustard repair. (Data for L from: Liebman J, Cullum L, Belloc N. Natural history of transposition of the great arteries: anatomy and birth and death characteristics. Circulation 1969; 40:237. Data for G from Gutgesell HP, McNamara DG. Transposition of the great arteries: results of treatment with early palliation and late intracardiac repair. Circulation 1975; 51:32. Data for T and t from Trusler GA, Williams WG, Izukawa T, et al. Current results with the Mustard operation in isolated transposition of the great arteries. J Thorac Cardiovasc Surg 1980; 80:381.)

prostaglandin E_1. However, this may sometimes not provide adequate intercirculatory mixing, and hypoxia with acidosis may ensue. Intercirculatory mixing may be increased at the atrial level by performing an atrial septostomy. However, at best this represents a temporizing therapeutic modality and is used in order to stabilize the patient and plan further treatment. The contrast between systemic arterial and pulmonary venous blood gases in patients with TGV and poor intercirculatory mixing is dramatic. Systemic arterial partial pressure of oxygen (PO_2) levels are rarely greater than 35 mm Hg, while the carbon dioxide partial pressure (PCO_2) is either normal or slightly elevated. By contrast, the pulmonary venous blood has a normal PO_2 but a low PCO_2 (15 to 25 mm Hg), reflecting chemoreceptor-stimulated hyperventilation as a result of systemic hypoxia. The systemic arterial PO_2 response to the administration of a high fractional inspired oxygen (FIO_2) is related partly to the level of intercirculatory mixing. When intercirculatory mixing is poor, adminis-

tration of a high FIO_2 does not significantly change the systemic PO_2.

In TGV, the effective systemic blood flow (i.e., oxygenated pulmonary venous blood perfusing the systemic circulation) is represented by the anatomic left-to-right shunt, while the effective pulmonary blood flow (systemic venous return perfusing the pulmonary circulation) is represented by the anatomic right-to-left shunt. These two flows are equal and constitute the intercirculatory mix that represents the blood flow upon which the patient's survival depends. The extent of intercirculatory mixing in patients with transposition depends on the number, size, and position of the anatomic communications, and also on the total blood flow through the pulmonary circulation. If the anatomic shunt sites are adequate, the level of pulmonary blood flow and thus the arterial oxygen saturation is influenced primarily by the ratio of pulmonary blood flow to systemic blood flow. A high pulmonary blood flow (e.g., that which occurs with a large VSD without LVOTO)

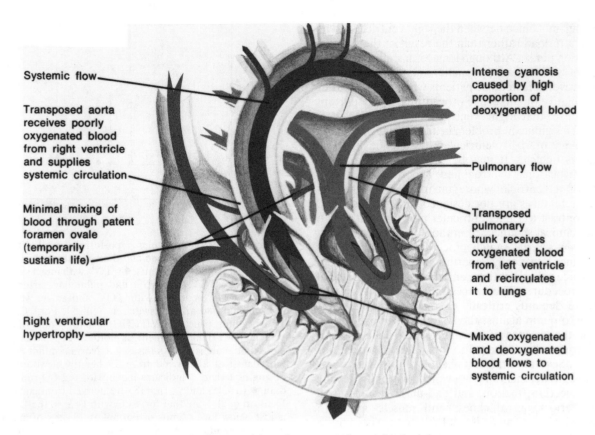

Labels on the figure:

Systemic flow

Transposed aorta receives poorly oxygenated blood from right ventricle and supplies systemic circulation

Minimal mixing of blood through patent foramen ovale (temporarily sustains life)

Right ventricular hypertrophy

Intense cyanosis caused by high proportion of deoxygenated blood

Pulmonary flow

Transposed pulmonary trunk receives oxygenated blood from left ventricle and recirculates it to lungs

Mixed oxygenated and deoxygenated blood flows to systemic circulation

Figure 2   Transposition of great arteries: pathophysiology.

results in a rather higher arterial PO_2 as long as left ventricular failure is avoided. By contrast, if either an anatomic obstructive lesion (e.g., pulmonary stenosis) or secondary increased pulmonary vascular resistance is present, the arterial PO_2 may not be adequate even in the presence of adequately sized anatomic shunts.

Bronchopulmonary Collateral Circulation

Bronchopulmonary collateral circulation, a potentially important variable in patients with TGV, is difficult to quantitate. It is important diagnostically in that it may undermine one's ability to make reliable cardiopulmonary measurements and is important prognostically in that it represents an extracardiac conduit promoting pulmonary capillary blood flow and intercirculatory mixing (which acutely increases systemic arterial PO_2 but chronically may result in significant secondary pulmonary vascular changes). Studies have indicated that bronchopulmonary channels exist in approximately 30 percent of patients younger than 3 years of age with TGV and that these channels fully communicate with the pulmonary circulation proximal to the pulmonary capillary bed.

Assessments of the pulmonary circulation using calculated values of pulmonary vascular resistance have inherent limitations, even in normal individuals. Moreover, in patients with TGV, the calculation of cardiac output using the Fick principle may have major sources of error—for example, oxygen consumption may not be normal in severely hypoxemic patients, and systemic and pulmonary arteriovenous oxygen differences may be quite small. As a result, even small errors in measuring oxygen saturation may secondarily result in large errors in the calculation of flow. Finally, bronchopulmonary collateral circulation represents a significant portion of total pulmonary capillary blood flow but enters the pulmonary circulation distal to the catheter sampling site. Hence, the true pulmonary artery saturation cannot be measured, falsely high pulmonary blood flow calculations will ensue, and falsely low calculated pulmonary vascular resistance values will result.

Ventricular Function

A discussion of the importance of ventricular function (or rather dysfunction) is important in at least two settings in patients with TGV.

Right ventricular dysfunction has been demonstrated repeatedly in infants (although perhaps not in neonates) with TGV. This observation has been made both preoperatively and postoperatively in patients in whom corrective atrial baffle procedures were performed. The presence of right ventricular dysfunction in patients who have undergone atrial corrective procedures (e.g., a Mustard procedure) may represent a continuing imbalance between the right ventricle and its systemic afterload rather than the result of the surgical intervention per se. Although long-term studies indicate that right ventricular dysfunction may eventually be partially reversible in those patients who have had either atrial palliative or corrective procedures, it is important to recognize that right ventricular dysfunction may represent a significant problem in any patient with TGV. The etiology of right ventricular dysfunction in these patients is unclear. It may be a consequence of prolonged myocardial hypoxia and hypertension in the setting of a ventricle whose intrinsic and anatomic-geometric features are not designed for systemic work.

In contrast to right ventricular performance, which assumes clinical significance in those patients who have not had an arterial switch procedure, left ventricular performance is critically important in those patients who are considered potential candidates for an arterial switch procedure. The success of an arterial switch procedure depends critically on the ability of the left ventricle to pump against the systemic afterload, which relies on the absence of the changes that take place in this ventricle when exposed to low pulmonary vascular pressures. Several parameters have been used to assess the left ventricle, including left ventricular end-diastolic volume, ejection fraction, and end-diastolic pressures, and posterior wall thickness and muscle mass. In patients with TGV and an intact IVS, there exists a finite period after birth when left ventricular function would seem adequate to assume its role as a systemic pumping chamber. Coexisting intracardiac abnormalities have the potential of maintaining normal growth in the left ventricle, thus making arterial switch procedures a therapeutic option beyond the neonatal period (Fig. 3).

Pulmonary Vascular Disease

It is now recognized that significant pulmonary hypertension and elevation of pulmonary vascular resistance is a frequent occurrence in patients with TGV. The occurrence and severity of these pulmonary vascular changes is significantly influenced by total pulmonary blood flow. Coexisting anomalies which increase pulmonary blood flow (e.g., VSDs) promote secondary pulmonary vascular changes, whereas lesions which inhibit pulmonary blood flow (e.g., pulmonary stenosis) prevent or slow the progression of pulmonary vascular changes. However, even in patients with an intact IVS, there may be evidence of significant pulmonary vascular changes. A persistent PDA beyond infancy and bronchopulmonary collateral flow may be causally related to this observation. In addition to increased pulmonary blood flow, local and systemic hypoxia, vasoconstrictor influences, and abnormal platelet function may all contribute to the increase in pulmonary vascular resistance observed in these patients.

MANAGEMENT

For patients with TGV, management options are best considered in the context of the underlying ana-

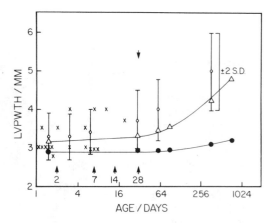

Figure 3 Left ventricular posterior wall thickness (LVPWTH) (echo/M-mode/end-diastolic) from birth to 365 days of age. O = normal infants; ● = TGV with intact ventricular septum; △ = TGV with VSD and pulmonary artery hypertension; x = 19 neonates with TGV and intact ventricular septum who had arterial switch at Willis J. Potts Children's Heart Center, Chicago (WJPCHC) at 2 to 34 days of age and echo LVPWTH measurement, as plotted, at 1 to 30 days of age. Note time scale is in days $\log_2$ scale. Normal infant data from Oberhansli et al derived from 53 healthy newborn infants during first year; O indicates mean with ± 2 SD range; TGV data, ● (n = 25) and △ (n = 18) are derived from equations of Danford et al. Note that for TVG with IVS, ●, the LVPWTH is just below lower limits of normal at 28 days of age and is much below thereafter. Note that most TGV neonate candidates for arterial switch, x, receiving prostaglandin infusions and their LVPWTH, 3.3 ± 0.4 m, was not significantly different from normal values for 1 day of age, 3.3 ± 0.3 mm, or for 30 days of age, 3.7 ± 0.4 mm.

tomic defects and the associated abnormal physiology. The specific intervention in any particular patient at any given point in the disease process is a direct extension of the abnormal physiology of that particular patient. In patients with TGV, the specific intervention is influenced by the presence or absence of any one of several associated anomalies (e.g., VSD, LVOTO, pulmonary stenosis, PDA). Moreover, the development of secondary pulmonary vascular changes also significantly influences management options.

Overall, surgical procedures undertaken in patients with TGV (with or without associated anomalies) can be broadly categorized into two groups: palliative procedures and those aimed at achieving a definitive repair. Palliative procedures include (1) those aimed at improving arterial and venous mixing—for example, an atrial septostomy or surgical atrial septectomy (Blalock-Hanlon procedure) in patients with TGV and intact IVS where ductal blood flow (even with the aid of prostaglandin E₁) is judged inadequate as a temporary method of maintaining a satisfactory arterial oxygen saturation; (2) the placement of a pulmonary artery band in patients with TGV and a large VSD without pulmonary outflow tract obstruction; and (3) conversely, the placement of shunts aimed at promoting pulmonary blood flow in those patients with TGV and pulmonary outflow tract obstruction or pulmonary atresia.

The choice of a definitive surgical procedure is also determined by the combination of anatomic anomalies and associated pathologic changes. Depending on the circumstances, any one of several definitive surgical repairs may be appropriate. In patients with a simple TGV, either an atrial (Senning or Mustard) or arterial switch procedure may be performed. When additional defects are present, the choice of an appropriate corrective procedure is dictated by the specific anomalies in that patient—e.g., a Rastelli procedure is appropriate in patients with TGV and a large VSD with left ventricular outflow tract obstruction. Further discussion in this chapter of the perioperative management of patients with TGV will focus primarily on those patients undergoing either atrial or arterial switch procedures.

Atrial Switch Procedures

Although sometimes used as palliative procedures (e.g., in patients with a large VSD and advanced pulmonary vascular disease), atrial switch procedures were the first to offer long-term survival to patients with TGV. The Senning (described initially in 1959) and Mustard (described initially in 1964) procedures both redirect venous blood via an intra-atrial baffle. Systemic venous blood passes beneath the baffle through the mitral valve and into the left ventricle and thus to the pulmonary artery, while the pulmonary venous blood is directed into the right ventricle and thus to the aorta. In the Senning procedure, the atrial baffle is fashioned from autologous tissue, while in the Mustard procedure the baffle is created from either pericardium or synthetic material.

Atrial switch procedures may be associated with certain specific complications. Right ventricular dysfunction has already been discussed. Dysrhythmias and venous obstruction are seen after both the Mustard and Senning repair procedures. It was initially claimed that these latter complications were seen less frequently with the Senning repair. However, modifications of the original Mustard procedure have resulted in these complications being observed with similar frequency after both operations. As a result, the choice of atrial switch procedure is now one of institutional and surgical preference.

Arterial Switch Procedure for Transposition of the Great Vessels

Arterial switch procedures have become increasingly popular as a means of surgically managing patients with TGV. The arterial switch procedure achieves an anatomic as well as a physiologic correction of the lesions in TGV (in contrast to an atrial switch procedure, which achieves physiologic correction only). Although atrial repair procedures represented a significant advance in the treatment of patients with TGV, long-term follow-up has indicated that there is significant morbidity and mortality (e.g., dysrhythmias with sudden death, right ventricular dysfunction), and an unacceptably high failure rate in those patients with TGV and a large VSD. Hence, efforts were aimed at devising an operation that

would provide total anatomic correction, and for this purpose, an arterial switch procedure was first widely used in those patients with TGV and a large VSD. Such patients do not exhibit the decrease in left ventricular muscle mass and increase in compliance associated with a decrease in pulmonary vascular resistance observed in patients with TGV and an intact IVS (see Fig. 3). Hence, the left ventricle remains a suitable pumping chamber that may successfully tolerate a systemic afterload. This concept was subsequently extended to patients with TGV and an intact IVS by placing a PA band aimed at preparing the left ventricle for a subsequent arterial switch procedure. Finally in 1984, Castaneda began to use the arterial switch procedure before the normal changes occurred in the left ventricle (i.e., in the neonatal period).

The success of an arterial switch procedure depends critically on left ventricular function and its ability to act as a pumping chamber for the systemic circulation. This success in turn depends on the choice of patient and timing of surgical intervention. Other major problems that occur after an arterial switch procedure include the potential for myocardial ischemia secondary to tension, torsion, or kinking of the coronary arteries, or in the longer term, caused by the inability of the coronary arteries to grow. Additional concerns relate to the potential development of aortic insufficiency and obstruction of the reconstructed pulmonary artery. However, short-term and intermediate-term follow-up of all patients, including those who underwent arterial switch procedures during the neonatal period, indicate a high success rate with low morbidity and mortality rates.

Anesthetic Management

The successful perioperative care of patients with TGV mandates a clear understanding of the anatomy, physiology, and procedure contemplated in any particular patient.

The preoperative visit involves a thorough clinical assessment. In addition to the usual concerns associated with all pediatric patients, one should focus the assessment on an evaluation of the degree of systemic arterial oxygenation, the patient's acid-base status, dependence on prostaglandin E_1 infusion as a method of maintaining systemic arterial oxygenation, the proposed surgical procedure, and an evaluation of ventricular function. Right and left ventricular functions are critically important in patients being considered for atrial and arterial switch procedures, respectively. The second objective of the preoperative visit involves a decision as to what preoperative medications, if any, are appropriate for this specific patient. Palliative procedures are considered elsewhere. Arterial switch procedures are now being used increasingly as the definitive mode of surgical therapy. Moreover, these operations are being performed more and more during the neonatal period. Neonates should receive either no premedication or anticholinergic agents only. Infants 6 to 12 months of age may be given morphine (0.1 to 0.15 mg per kilogram IM) plus scopolamine (0.01 mg per kilogram IM). If not in cardiorespiratory distress, infants older than 1 year of age may be given sodium pentobarbital (2 to 4 mg per kilogram) in addition to the above-mentioned doses of morphine and scopolamine.

Induction of anesthesia may be accomplished by any one of several modalities, but is perhaps most safely accomplished by the use of ketamine (intravenously or intramuscularly, 1 mg per kilogram and 8 to 10 mg per kilogram, respectively) or fentanyl. An inhalational agent (halothane) can also be used to induce anesthesia in these patients. Appropriate monitoring is outlined in Table 1.

In addition to the considerations outlined above, where specific complications may be associated with specific surgical procedures (e.g., coronary perfusion following an arterial switch), there are several intraoperative concerns of immediate relevance to the anesthesiologist:

1. Circulatory arrest. Typically, newborns with TGV have normal or high-normal birth weights. However, it is not uncommon for the fine technical details of this procedure to necessitate the use of deep hypothermia and circulatory arrest. It is now common practice to pack the cranium in ice to help maintain cerebral hypothermia. In addition, several authors advocate the practice of steroid administration, with the objective of decreasing cerebral edema in this clinical setting. Steroids are an established treatment modality in patients with raised intracranial pressure as a result of space-occupying lesions (e.g., cerebral tumors). Their role and potential efficacy in other forms of cerebral edema (e.g., trauma) is controversial. Their efficacy as prophylactic agents in patients with potential cerebral edema is not established. Furthermore, the timing of administration is also unclear, and steroid use before circulatory arrest is highly individualized.
2. Use of blood and blood products. The intraoperative use of blood and blood products is a necessity in pediatric cardiac surgery. All reasonable efforts should be made to minimize the total amount of blood and blood products administered, and one should ensure that the infectious risk to the patient is minimized (e.g., irradiated blood, cytomegalovirus-negative). The risk of blood-borne infections (e.g., hepatitus, human immunodeficiency virus) is directly proportional to the amount of blood products administered.
3. Temperature. It is important that patients are kept normothermic during the postbypass and postoperative periods. This is sometimes difficult in a patient who has been subject to deep hypo-

Table 1 Monitoring for TGV

Precordial stethoscope
Blood pressure
Electrocardiogram
Pulse oximeter
Esophageal stethoscope
Intra-arterial catheter
Central venous catheter
Rectal and nasopharyngeal temperature probes
Urinary catheter
End-tidal CO_2 monitor
Atrial and ventricular pacing wires
Right and left atrial catheters

thermic arrest. All reasonable efforts should be made to maintain normothermia (e.g., humidifiers, warming blankets, plastic bags) because hypothermia itself may be life threatening, causing ventricular arrhythmias or severe coagulopathy.

Finally, it is critically important to realize that the pathophysiologic changes observed in these patients following cardiopulmonary bypass continue to evolve during the postoperative period. It is necessary to continue oxygen saturation monitoring as well as electrocardiographic and intravascular pressure monitoring during transfer from the operating room to the postoperative intensive care unit. Complications frequently occur early in the postoperative period. This is a result of the underlying pathophysiology, the surgical procedure per se, and the pathophysiologic changes resulting from anesthesia and cardiopulmonary bypass. To minimize the human error component in these complications, it is important that those individuals responsible for the patient's intraoperative care communicate precisely and effectively the details of the patient's intraoperative course. To do so requires the recognition by both an effective communicator and a responsive listener of the importance of this concept.

SUGGESTED READING

Bland JW, Williams WH. Anesthesia for treatment of congenital heart defects. In: Kaplan JA, ed. Cardiac anesthesia. 2nd ed. Orlando: Grune & Stratton, 1987:281.
Paul MH. Complete transposition of the great arteries. In: Forrest HA, Emmanouilides GC, Riemenschneider Ta, eds. Heart disease in infants, children, and adolescents. Baltimore: Williams & Wilkins, 1989:371.
Van Praagh R, Weinberg PM, Smith SD, et al. Malpositions of the heart. In: Forrest HA, Emmanouilides GC, Riemenschneider TA, eds. Heart disease in infants, children, and adolescents. Baltimore: Williams & Wilkins, 1989:530.

PALLIATIVE SURGERY FOR CONGENITAL HEART DISEASE

EUGENIE S. CASELLA, M.D.

Although the trend in cardiac surgery is toward early complete repair of congenital heart lesions, there remain certain situations in which a patient requires a staged or palliative procedure, with definitive repair performed at a later time. This chapter discusses the indications for palliative surgery, the types of palliative procedures that have been developed, and the anesthetic management of these patients during the perioperative period.

INDICATIONS

Palliative procedures are those that are not intended to be complete repairs. They are used to (1) increase pulmonary blood flow, (2) decrease pulmonary blood flow, (3) improve intracardiac mixing, or (4) alter the hemodynamics in preparation for complete repair.

A palliative operation is performed in infants when a complete repair is not yet feasible. Such patients include cyanotic infants with (1) tetralogy of Fallot who have small pulmonary arteries and/or stenosis of major pulmonary artery branches; (2) transposition of the great arteries with intact ventricular septum and a restrictive atrial septal defect; (3) tricuspid atresia; (4) single ventricle; (5) pulmonary stenosis or atresia with or without other intracardiac defects; and (6) hypoplastic left heart syndrome.

Although cyanosis is the chief reason for a palliative procedure, there may be other reasons as well. In the premature or very small infant, a complete repair requiring cardiopulmonary bypass may impose a significant risk. A palliative procedure would allow time for the child to grow and possibly for the clinical condition to improve so that a definitive repair could be done with a lower risk when the child is older and larger. Children born with poorly developed pulmonary arteries and arterioles are poor candidates for complete repair, so a palliative shunt is used to improve pulmonary blood flow. Some anomalies are so severe that total correction is impossible, and a palliative procedure is the only alternative to improve the hemodynamics. In children of parents of the Jehovah Witness faith, blood transfusions are not acceptable. In these cases, a palliative procedure would delay the need for definitive operation until a time when the operation could be performed with a greater margin of safety without the use of a blood transfusion. For some congenital heart lesions, it is necessary to alter the hemodynamics so that they become more suitable for corrective surgery. An example of this is the use of pulmonary artery banding in infants with transposition of the great arteries with ventricular septal defect. This prepares the ventricle to supply the systemic circulation so that an arterial switch may be performed at a later time. Another example is the Norwood procedure (Stage I) used in children with hypoplastic left heart syndrome.

Finally, there are children who are born with congenital heart disease in conjunction with another illness, frequently due to chromosomal abnormalities, which limits their life expectancy to a few years even with the best cardiac care. These patients include those with trisomy 18, trisomy 13, and recombinant trisomy 8. Because of their shortened life expectancy due to the noncardiac disease, the risk associated with a complete repair outweighs whatever benefit it may have had on prolonging life. In these cases, a palliative shunt to treat cyanosis would be a lower-risk procedure that would improve the child's clinical situation and allow him or her to be discharged home in as good a condition as possible.

TYPES OF PALLIATIVE PROCEDURES

Shunts

Shunts are operations performed to increase pulmonary blood flow (Table 1). Historically, the ability to create a left-to-right shunt was one of the greatest advances in the treatment of congenital heart disease. These systemic-to-pulmonary artery shunts are currently used to treat congenital anomalies associated with inadequate pulmonary blood flow, which at the time of operation are not amenable to complete correction. The chief cyanotic congenital anomalies for which shunt operations are performed are listed in Table 2. In the *classic Blalock-Taussig operation*, the subclavian artery is anastomosed end-to-side to the pulmonary artery (Fig. 1). This operation may be performed through a left or right lateral thoracotomy. The side from which this operation is performed depends on the side of the aortic arch and the need for any additional procedures at the same time. In the *modified Blalock-Taussig operation*, a Gore-Tex (polytetrafluoroethylene) or Dacron graft is used to create the systemic-pulmonary artery shunt. This

Table 1 Operations to Increase Pulmonary Blood Flow

Classic Blalock-Taussig shunt
Modified Blalock-Taussig shunt
Potts aorticopulmonary shunt
Waterston-Cooley shunt
Glenn (cavopulmonary) anastomosis
Central shunts

Table 2 The Most Common Congenital Heart Lesions with Inadequate Pulmonary Flow

Tetralogy of Fallot
Tricuspid atresia
Pulmonary stenosis or atresia (with and without other intracardiac defects)
Transposition of the great arteries

modified technique avoids the need to divide the subclavian artery. In addition, the conduit is generally larger than the infant's distal subclavian artery and provides better pulmonary flow than the native vessel.

The Potts aorticopulmonary shunt is a descending aorta to left pulmonary artery anastomosis made through a left posterolateral thoracotomy incision. The advantage of this shunt is that it does not depend on the size of the subclavian artery. The disadvantages are that the direct aortopulmonary anastomosis makes it difficult to adjust pulmonary blood flow and that it is one of the most difficult shunts to correct during a subsequent definitive repair of the heart defect. It is for these reasons that the Potts shunt is not frequently used today.

Another shunt that is rarely used for similar reasons is the *Waterston-Cooley shunt*. This is an intrapericardial ascending aorta to right main pulmonary artery anastomosis that has a high patency rate. The advantage is that with the anterior approach, there is little dissection of mediastinal structures, although there are still the problems of too much pulmonary blood flow, distortion of the pulmonary arteries, and adhesions which may make subsequent surgery difficult. Despite these disadvantages, there are some surgeons who believe this shunt still has an important role in small infants who require emergency systemic-to-pulmonary artery shunting.

The *Glenn shunt* is an anastomosis between the pulmonary artery and the side of the superior vena cava. This allows approximately 35 percent of the systemic venous return to be directed to the right lung. An advantage of this shunt is that it does not pressure overload the pulmonary circulation. The Glenn shunt and its modifications are currently used for atresia of the tricuspid and pulmonary valves either as a palliative procedure or as part of the Fontan operation. The disadvantages stem from increased pressure in the veins that drain the upper body, which can result in a superior vena caval syndrome and the risk of cerebral edema. Other complications reported are the development of arteriovenous fistulae, dilated lung vessels, and changes in caval blood flow direction.

Central shunts are prosthetic grafts between the descending aorta and the main pulmonary artery. Central shunts are used in infants, usually those younger than 3 months of age with inadequate pulmonary flow who have a patent ductus arteriosus or some other shunt, who have anatomy unsuitable for a modified Blalock-Taussig shunt, or who have had a previous shunt that is failing. The main advantages of central shunts are that they produce less distortion of the pulmonary arteries,

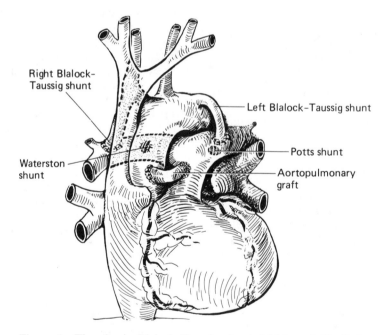

Figure 1 The classic Blalock–Taussig shunt (right or left), Potts shunt, Waterston shunt, and aortopulmonary graft (central shunt). The classic Blalock–Taussig shunt connects the right or left subclavian artery to its respective branch pulmonary artery. The Waterston shunt is an anastomosis of the posterior wall of the ascending aorta to the right pulmonary artery. The Potts shunt is a side-to-side anastomosis of the left pulmonary artery to the descending thoracic aortic. The aortopulmonary graft or central shunt represents the creation of systemic-to-pulmonary shunt using prosthetic graft material. (Republished with permission from Dillard DH, Miller DW. Atlas of cardiac surgery. New York: Macmillan, 1983:191.)

have a lower occlusion rate, and are easier to close at the time of definitive repair. Their disadvantages are that they necessitate opening of the pericardial sac and cardiopulmonary bypass in patients who cannot tolerate occlusion of the pulmonary artery. The use of a short segment of Gore-Tex in creating these shunts has been used with good results.

Other vessels that have been used to create systemic-to-pulmonary artery shunts when other shunt attempts have failed include the internal mammary artery and an anomalous subclavian artery.

All shunts have the disadvantage of distorting peripheral pulmonary arteries. In addition, problems can occur with too much shunt flow causing heart failure or pulmonary vascular disease and with too little shunt flow resulting in unimproved oxygenation and unilateral shunting. These and other postoperative problems are discussed in a later section of this chapter.

Pulmonary Artery Banding

The procedure used to decrease pulmonary blood flow is *pulmonary artery banding*. This operative technique was first described in 1952 for the purpose of alleviating congestive heart failure and preventing pulmonary hypertension. The congenital heart defects for which pulmonary artery banding are indicated are listed in Table 3. Infants with these defects who require pulmonary artery banding have large left-to-right shunts that result in congestive heart failure, pulmonary edema, and recurrent pulmonary infections. These infants show failure to thrive due to decreased systemic blood flow, high resting oxygen consumption, and low energy intake resulting from poor feeding. Pulmonary hypertension can develop at an early age if the pulmonary vasculature is constantly exposed to systemic pressures.

Patients with large solitary ventricular septal defects are now candidates for definitive repair unless their clinical status is such that cardiopulmonary bypass would impose a significant risk. Infants with complex ventricular septal defects, however, often require a palliative procedure early in life. Multiple ventricular septal defects may not be amenable to complete closure. In patients with coarctation of the aorta or interrupted aortic arch and a ventricular septal defect, the aortic

abnormality is initially repaired with pulmonary artery banding and the ventricular septal defect is repaired at a later time, usually when the patient is 1 year of age if it has not closed spontaneously by then. There are cases in which a patient may not tolerate closure of a ventricular septal defect, such as when either the right or left ventricle is too small or if there is an overriding atrioventricular valve that could be obstructed by a patch over the ventricular septal defect.

Pulmonary artery banding may be used to constrict the pulmonary artery in transposition of the great arteries as an attempt to prepare the left ventricle to supply the systemic circulation, so that an arterial switch may be performed at a later time.

It may also be used to treat symptomatic infants during the first year of life who have complex congenital heart lesions that are too difficult to repair. Included in this category are the double outlet right and left ventricles without pulmonary stenosis. In the past, patients with truncus arteriosus would undergo pulmonary artery banding before repair, but with improved surgical techniques, the operative risk for a complete repair is now believed to be no greater than that reported previously for banding.

Pulmonary artery banding is performed through a left lateral thoracotomy in the third or fourth intercostal space. A right thoracotomy may be used if another procedure is to be performed at the same time, such as an atrial septostomy or septectomy. Figure 2 shows a diagram of the placement of a band around the pulmonary artery. In order to reach the pulmonary artery, the lung is retracted and the pericardial sac is opened in front of the phrenic nerve. Damage to the phrenic nerve can produce phrenic nerve palsy, which is discussed in a later section of this chapter. In order to determine how tightly the band should be placed, a pressure monitoring needle is inserted into the pulmonary artery distal to the band. Ideally, the pulmonary artery pressure should be one-third to one-

Table 3 Indications for Pulmonary Artery Banding

Complex ventricular septal defects
  Multiple ventricular septal defects
  Large ventricular septal defect with aortic coarctation or
    interrupted aortic arch
  Ventricular septal defect with small left or right ventricle
  Ventricular septal defect with an overriding atrioventricular valve
Transposition of the great arteries
Double outlet and double inlet ventricles with high pulmonary
  blood flow
Univentricular heart without pulmonary stenosis
Atrioventricular canal
Hypoplastic left heart syndrome (Norwood procedure)

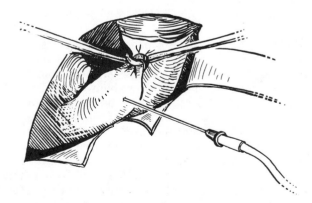

Figure 2 Pulmonary artery banding by placing umbilical tape around the pulmonary artery. The pressure distal to the pulmonary artery band is measured to determine if the band is adequate—i.e., the pulmonary pressure is one-half to one-third the systemic pressure. (Republished with permission from Dillard DH, Miller DW. Atlas of cardiac surgery. New York: Macmillan, 1983:195.)

half the systemic blood pressure. The arterial oxygen pressure (PaO_2) should also be measured to assure that the pulmonary blood flow is adequate.

Operations to Improve Intracardiac Mixing

The procedures to improve intracardiac mixing include balloon atrial septostomy (Rashkind procedure), atrial septectomy (Blalock-Hanlon procedure), and a palliative Mustard procedure. Patients with congenital heart defects that depend on adequate mixing of systemic and pulmonary venous blood for survival include transposition of the great arteries, tricuspid atresia, mitral atresia, complex defects associated with hypoplastic right or left ventricles, and total anomalous pulmonary venous return. In cases where there is restricted flow across the atrial septum, a balloon or blade septostomy may be performed during cardiac catheterization. If a balloon or blade atrial septostomy is not successful in providing adequate interatrial mixing, an atrial septectomy is performed. This operation can be performed under inflow occlusion through a right thoracotomy with the right lung retracted or on cardiopulmonary bypass through median sternotomy. If inflow occlusion is used, it should be realized that pulmonary venous congestion will occur while the pulmonary veins are occluded and can subsequently develop into pulmonary edema.

The palliative Mustard procedure is used to treat patients with transposition of the great arteries and pulmonary hypertension. Because of the pulmonary vascular disease, these patients are not candidates for complete repair, so a Mustard or Senning operation is performed, leaving an intracardiac or extracardiac right-to-left shunt. For example, if a ventricular septal defect is present, it is left open. This clinical situation is not often seen today because of the trend toward early complete repair of transposition of the great arteries during infancy.

ANESTHESIA

The anesthetic care of patients undergoing shunt procedures was first described by Harmel and Lamont in 1946 and later by McQuiston in 1948. Many things have changed since that time, and our ability to care for and monitor these children comfortably is now greatly improved.

There are certain anesthetic considerations that are common to all children with congenital heart disease who are undergoing surgery, as well as factors that are specific for palliative cardiac operations. In this section, the preoperative evaluation, monitoring needs, intraoperative management, and effects of anesthetic agents are discussed. Specific considerations include air bubble precautions and the surgical approach through a thoracotomy incision with partial or total occlusion of major vessels during surgery without cardiopulmonary bypass.

Preoperative Evaluation

The plan for the anesthetic management of a child with congenital heart disease is determined to a large extent by the preoperative evaluation. It is also at this time that the psychological needs of the parents and patient are addressed. Infants undergoing palliative shunts are not cured of their heart disease; the procedure may merely be the first one performed in a sick infant who will need to return for definitive repair at a later time. It may be a repeat procedure in a child with a complex lesion or in whom the first procedure failed. The parents may be undergoing a period of shock and grieving after learning their infant has heart disease. They may be fearful of the outcome and anxious about the procedures the child is to undergo. The parents may withdraw from the child emotionally and/or physically. They may be very angry and antagonistic. Much of the time some degree of denial is exhibited. If the patient is an older child who is aware of the situation, the level of the child's anxiety will be greatly influenced by the parents' feelings. It is during the preoperative visit that these issues need to be discussed and the procedures explained in the hope that the information may dispel some of their fears of the unknown. Parents and patients more often than not appreciate the efforts to reduce their worry, even though it is never completely alleviated.

The preoperative evaluation should focus on assessing the child's cardiorespiratory function. The information obtained from the parents should include (1) how well the child feeds; (2) if the growth and development is appropriate; (3) how frequently the child develops congestion, wheezing, and pulmonary infections; (4) how well the child keeps up with normal children of the same age; and (5) if the patient has cyanosis, how frequently it occurs and if the cyanosis is increasing. If the child is old enough to walk, the parents may give a history that the child squats to relieve the cyanosis. Squatting is thought to increase systemic vascular resistance and thus decrease the amount of right-to-left shunt.

The physical examination should include a cardiac examination of the heart sounds and murmurs; the quality of the peripheral pulses; the quality of the breath sounds and the presence of rales, rhonchi, or wheezes; and an evaluation of the airway. These children may have extracardiac abnormalities that may include airway abnormalities such as cleft lip and palate.

The results of the cardiac catheterization and/or echocardiography should be reviewed. If the patient has had previous cardiac surgery, the records should be carefully reviewed and the anesthetic plan should take into account the possibility of encountering adhesions and unexpected bleeding. More often than not, a review of the patient's preoperative evaluation with the pediatric cardiologist and the cardiac surgeon enhances the anesthesiologist's understanding of the patient's condition and is helpful in further planning the anesthetic management.

Monitoring

During any anesthesia, the patient's oxygenation, ventilation, circulation, and temperature should be continuously monitored. The *basic monitoring* for any cardiac procedure in a child should include: (1) electrocardiography, (2) stethoscope, (3) noninvasive blood pressure measurements, (4) pulse oximetry, (5) capnography, (6) temperature monitor, and (7) an inspired oxygen concentration monitor.

The blood pressure cuff must be of the appropriate diameter. Care should be taken in the case of a Blalock-Taussig shunt not to place the blood pressure cuff on the arm that is on the same side as the shunt. A history of previous shunt may also alter arterial pressures in that arm.

Pulse oximetry may be difficult to obtain if the child has severe cyanosis or poor peripheral perfusion, or if the oximeter probe is exposed to an intense light source. It is, however, an excellent monitor for hypoxemia and can give valuable information about pulmonary blood flow. It can be used to determine the adequacy of pulmonary artery banding. It may also be an early indicator of alterations in cardiac output.

The monitoring of end-tidal CO_2 may be unreliable or misleading in children with cyanotic congenital heart disease. The relationship between end-tidal CO_2 and arterial CO_2 tension is often poor; the arterial CO_2 may be significantly higher than the end-tidal CO_2. This difference usually becomes smaller after complete correction of the congenital heart defect. The end-tidal CO_2 can also be used as an indicator of pulmonary blood flow during shunt procedures as well as during placement of a pulmonary artery band. Decreases in end-tidal CO_2 concentration often occur several minutes before changes in systemic hemodynamics.

Invasive monitoring is usually required during cardiac surgery because the surgical manipulation can often result in hemodynamic instability. Arterial cannulation for continuous blood pressure monitoring and frequent blood sampling is indicated for most palliative surgical procedures. Central venous access is routinely used for the delivery of cardioactive drugs and to monitor right heart filling pressure continuously. It may also be needed for the rapid delivery of blood and blood products when unexpected blood loss is encountered and venous access is inadequate.

Air Bubble Precautions

Air bubble precautions are obviously important in a patient with a right-to-left shunt, since an air bubble introduced into the venous system can pass directly into the arterial circulation at the site of the shunt and result in major organ damage or death. The danger of air bubbles in a left-to-right shunt is not as obvious. One might think that there would be no chance of an air bubble moving from right to left if the blood is shunting left to right. However, the fact is that there are probably no pure left-to-right shunts because of changes in interventricular pressures during the cardiac cycle. In

particular, during the terminal period of ventricular ejection, the right ventricular pressure is greater than the left ventricular pressure. Therefore, if a septal defect exists, left-to-right shunting would cease and shunting would become right to left. During the isovolumic relaxation period that follows, the left ventricular pressure decreases earlier than the right ventricular pressure, accentuating the right-to-left gradient with an even greater chance of an air bubble (or any other embolic material) passing directly from the venous to arterial system.

Air bubbles are best prevented from entering the circulation by the removal of all bubbles from intravenous tubing, stopcocks, and injection ports before connecting to venous or arterial catheters; by the connection of tubing with a free flow of fluid to the catheter with a free flow of blood; and by the removal of air bubbles from syringes. Central venous cannulation should be performed in the Trendelenburg position, if possible, and the catheter should not be left open to air. Many anesthesiologists discontinue the use of N_2O after an inhalation induction in children with congenital heart disease so not to increase the size of an inadvertent air bubble that may enter the circulation during intravenous catheter insertion.

Maintenance of Temperature and Metabolic Status

Because the majority of palliative procedures are performed without cardiopulmonary bypass, it is necessary to keep the child as normothermic as possible throughout the operation. The room should be warm, a warming blanket should be placed under the patient, the gases through the breathing circuit should be warmed, and if necessary, the extremities and head may be covered with plastic to retain warmth.

Operations performed through thoracotomy incisions require that the lung be retracted while the procedure is performed. In addition, major vessels may need to be retracted or clamped. All of these situations can lead to hypoxia, hypercarbia, low cardiac output, and acidosis (metabolic and respiratory). In some cases, intermittently resuming mechanical ventilation of the retracted lung corrects the acidosis. Many patients may have a preoperative metabolic acidosis caused by chronic hypoxemia, poor peripheral perfusion, or congestive heart failure. If a metabolic acidosis persists, an appropriate amount of sodium bicarbonate may be administered ($0.3 \times$ weight in kilograms $\times$ base deficit), with frequent monitoring of blood pH and serum sodium levels.

Hemoglobin Level

Children with cyanotic congenital heart disease often have an elevated hemoglobin level in response to chronic hypoxemia. A child undergoing a palliative shunt procedure may continue to have a lower than normal partial pressure of oxygen (PO_2) and will need to have a higher than normal hemoglobin level to maintain adequate oxygen-carrying capacity and delivery of oxygen to the tissues. A hematocrit of 40 to 50 percent provides maximal oxygen transport in a cyanotic child. Because of the higher hemoglobin level, it is important not to allow the child to become volume contracted or hypothermic, otherwise sludging and thrombosis may occur.

Newborn infants normally have hemoglobin levels of 14 to 20 g per deciliter with varying amounts of fetal hemoglobin. Fetal hemoglobin shifts the oxygen-hemoglobin dissociation curve to the left. Infants with a high level of fetal hemoglobin (>50 percent) do not exhibit cyanosis until the arterial oxygen tension is in the range of 32 to 42 mm Hg, while infants with mostly adult hemoglobin have cyanosis at a PaO_2 of 42 to 53 mm Hg. This is an important point because pulse oximetry is often used as a measure of arterial oxygenation. A baby with a high fetal hemoglobin level may have an oxygen saturation of 85 percent even though the PaO_2 is only 42 mm Hg. (Normally, an oxygen saturation of 85 percent corresponds to a PaO_2 of 53 mm Hg.) Central cyanosis is usually seen when the arterial saturation is 75 to 85 percent and there is more than 3 g of deoxygenated hemoglobin per deciliter of arterial blood.

Prostaglandin E_1

Prostaglandin E_1, a pulmonary artery vasodilator, is used in situations where the child is dependent on flow from the ductus arteriosus. These include (1) right heart outflow obstructions (e.g., pulmonary stenosis, tricuspid atresia) where the ductus arteriosus is supplying the majority of the pulmonary blood flow; (2) left heart outflow obstruction (e.g., hypoplastic left heart syndrome, interrupted aortic arch) where the ductus arteriosus supplies the systemic circulation; and (3) transposition of the great arteries where the ductus arteriosus allows for mixing of arterial and venous blood. The side effects of prostaglandin E_1 include apnea, hypotension, and inhibition of platelet aggregation. It is often used in preparation for surgery and may be continued for 24 to 48 hours postoperatively if there is any question of adequacy of the surgical shunt.

Effects of Anesthetic Agents

It has been well documented in the literature that children with congenital heart disease tolerate both the inhalational and intravenous forms of anesthesia. Studies have been done examining the effects of halothane, isoflurane, N_2O, thiopental, sufentanil, fentanyl, ketamine, and combinations of these agents for both induction and maintenance of anesthesia in infants and children with all forms of congenital heart disease. In general, the results show that the different anesthetics are well tolerated by these patients and can be used safely if the anesthesiologist understands the pharmacology of the anesthetic and the pathophysiology of the lesion.

The choice of anesthetic for a particular case is determined by the condition of the patient, the presence of an intravenous line before induction, and the duration and type of surgery planned. A sick child with cyanosis and/or heart failure may tolerate only light levels of anesthesia. If the patient has intravenous access, fentanyl (30 to 75 µg per kilogram) in divided doses or ketamine (1 to 2 mg per kilogram) can be given for induction. Otherwise, an induction with intramuscular ketamine (5 to 10 mg per kilogram) or an inhalational induction with halothane (0.5 to 1.5 percent) is most often used until intravenous access is established.

The belief that ketamine should not be used in cyanotic congenital heart disease because of increased pulmonary vascular resistance has been disproved by two separate studies. The changes in pulmonary vascular resistance were found to be clinically minor both in patients with previously elevated pulmonary vascular resistance and in those without.

Halothane is widely used in children with congenital heart disease for both cardiac and noncardiac surgery. Isoflurane and enflurane are also used, although not as frequently as halothane. The myocardial depression resulting from halothane may be beneficial to patients with dynamic outflow obstructions, such as in tetralogy of Fallot or hypertrophic subaortic stenosis. Halothane decreases contractility and thereby decreases the amount of outflow obstruction. Of course, if an overdose of the volatile anesthetic is delivered, it can result in hypotension and bradycardia with a severely decreased cardiac output and pulmonary blood flow.

Muscle relaxants used for endotracheal intubation and maintenance muscle relaxation may have a slower onset in children with congenital heart disease. The onset of neuromuscular blockade with pancuronium has been shown to be prolonged in children with right-to-left shunting as well as in those with left-to-right shunting, when compared with normal children. I have found this to be true in my practice as well.

The effect of shunts on an inhalation induction has been examined using a computer model. The results showed that left-to-right shunting had little effect on the speed of induction, a right-to-left shunt slowed induction with a greater effect on the less soluble agents, and that mixing a left-to-right shunt with a right-to-left shunt lessened the effect of the right-to-left shunt on induction.

POSTOPERATIVE PROBLEMS

The postoperative management of infants and children who have undergone palliative surgery is similar to that of infants and children who have undergone complete correction, the main differences being that after palliative surgery, the patients still have a congenital heart defect.

Many of the palliative operations are performed through a thoracotomy incision with necessary retraction of the lung for exposure. This can result in a lung contusion or the obstruction of distal airways by blood and secretions. The inhaled anesthetics are known to decrease respiratory ciliary action and to slow mucous clearance, which may further impair respiratory function during the postoperative period. Pneumothorax on the side of the operation can result from failure of the chest tube to drain due to clotting or obstruction. Pneumothorax on either side can occur from the barotrauma of mechanical ventilation.

Injury to the phrenic nerve is not uncommon after palliative surgery and can result from traction or transection of the nerve. The diaphragmatic paralysis that results from phrenic nerve injury does not usually present until the child is being weaned from mechanical ventilation. The patient will tolerate low-rate ventilation and continuous positive airway pressure, but will exhibit respiratory distress after extubation. The child may have asymmetric chest movement, and the chest radiograph will show elevation of the affected hemidiaphragm. Fluoroscopy confirms the diagnosis with paradoxic upward movement of the involved hemidiaphragm during inspiration. Immediate treatment is reintubation with assisted ventilation until function returns; otherwise a diaphragmatic plication is necessary if function has not returned within a 3- to 6-week period.

Although chylothorax caused by injury of the thoracic duct or its tributaries is unusual, it should be considered, especially with extrapericardial cardiac procedures. The onset of effusion is commonly 2 to 3 days after surgery, but it may not appear until 1 month postoperatively. It usually occurs on the left side, but it can occur on the right or bilaterally. Although chyle is usually milky in appearance, it may be clear in a fasting child. Conservative medical management with pleural drainage and a high-protein, low-fat diet is usually sufficient treatment. If the patient does not respond in 2 weeks, surgical ligation of the thoracic duct may be indicated.

It should be remembered that thoracotomy incisions can be very painful during the postoperative period and that adequate analgesia should be given, especially in a child who needs to cough and deep-breathe to clear secretions and prevent atelectasis.

Several complications are associated with shunt procedures. Shunt failure with too little pulmonary flow and unimproved oxygenation can occur if the shunt vessel is too small or is obstructed by kinking or thrombosis. To ensure the patency of a shunt, maintenance of an adequate blood pressure and cardiac output is imperative during the postoperative period. Thrombosis occurs more frequently with the classic Blalock-Taussig shunt than with the modified technique, and occurs less frequently with aorta-to-pulmonary artery shunts. After a Blalock-Taussig shunt, the arm on the side of the shunt may initially have diminished pulses and perfusion. Arm claudication after Blalock-Taussig shunt has been reported and treated with a reconstructive shunt to the affected subclavian artery.

The Glenn (caval-to-pulmonary artery) shunt also has the disadvantages of occlusion and thrombosis, but in this case, the shunt occlusion can result in a superior vena caval syndrome and subsequent cerebral edema.

The need for a repeat shunt to treat inadequate pulmonary blood flow seems to be related to the age of the child and size at the time of the initial shunt (i.e., if the child is younger than 3 months of age and weighs less than 3.6 kg). If the child develops a very high hematocrit (50 to 60 percent), the viscosity of the blood is increased and blood flow may decrease with eventual thrombosis of the shunt. The overall reported frequency of repeat shunts are 22 percent for central shunts, 23 percent for the classic Blalock-Taussig shunt, and 16 percent for the modified Blalock-Taussig shunt.

Too much pulmonary blood flow can result from a large shunt with subsequent congestive heart failure and the development of pulmonary vascular disease. This occurs more often with aorta-to-pulmonary artery shunts than with the Blalock-Taussig shunt. As stated in the previous section describing the types of shunts, the pulmonary blood flow may be difficult to control in the Waterston, Potts, and central shunts. The shunt may have appropriate flow at surgery, but then may become larger over time.

Distortion of the peripheral pulmonary arteries is a disadvantage of all shunt procedures. This occurs more frequently in the Waterston, Potts, and classic Blalock-Taussig shunts than in central shunts and the modified Blalock-Taussig shunt. Unilateral shunting can occur with the Blalock-Taussig and Waterston shunts, which can lead to uneven growth of the pulmonary arteries.

Some of the shunt procedures may be difficult to correct at the time of definitive repair because of their position. Many of the shunts are created through a thoracotomy incision and may be hard to reach through the median sternotomy incision used for a complete repair. As with any previous surgery, there is the problem of adhesions which add to the difficulty in correcting the shunt. Leakage around the shunt and infection are uncommon with the improved techniques and use of antibiotics. The rates of early mortality after shunt procedures have been reported to be 7.5 percent for central shunts, 4 percent for the classic Blalock-Taussig shunt, and 3 percent for the modified Blalock-Taussig shunt.

Problems with pulmonary artery banding can develop depending on where the band is placed on the artery. If it is too close to the pulmonary valve, the repeated opening of the valve against the band can cause valve thickening and stenosis. If the band migrates to the bifurcation, the distal arteries can become hypoplastic. In addition, subaortic obstruction can develop as early as weeks after banding. During subsequent surgery to remove the band, adhesions may prevent easy removal and a patch may be required to enlarge the area constricted by the band. Pulmonary artery banding will be ineffective if the band is too loose and will result in too little pulmonary blood flow and cyanosis if the band is too tight or if the child grows and the band does not. An attempt to prevent the latter problem that has been reported is the use of a band prosthesis capable of serial dilatation by balloon angioplasty. For these reasons, it is preferable that a ventricular septal defect be corrected early if at all possible, rather than that palliative pulmonary artery banding be performed.

SUGGESTED READING

Adams FH, Emmouilides GC, Riemenschneider TA, eds. Moss' heart disease in infants, children and adolescents. Baltimore: Williams & Wilkins, 1989.

Cooley DA. Palliative surgery for cyanotic congenital heart disease. Surg Clin North Am 1988; 68:477–496.

DeLaval MR. Palliation in congenital heart disease. In: Grillo HC, Austen WG, Wilkins EW, et al, eds. Current therapy in cardiothoracic surgery. Philadelphia: BC Decker, 1989:468.

Lake CL, ed. Pediatric cardiac anesthesia. East Norwalk: Appleton and Lange, 1988.

Radnay PA, Nagashima H, eds. Anesthetic considerations for pediatric cardiac surgery. Boston: Little, Brown, and Company, 1980.

ANESTHESIA IN VASCULAR SURGERY

ABDOMINAL AORTIC ANEURYSM

CHARLES BEATTIE, Ph.D., M.D.

Many clinicians deem aortic aneurysm surgery to be the premier anesthetic challenge. Dramatic physiologic perturbations are superimposed on complex disease states. Aneurysm repair necessitates interruption of aortic blood flow by isolation of the diseased vascular segment with occluding clamps. The resulting tissue ischemia can cause organ damage, while changes in left ventricular afterload, with clamp application and removal, predisposes the patient to cardiac dysfunction and extremes of blood pressure.

This chapter outlines the major considerations surrounding the preoperative evaluation, anesthetic preparation and management, and principles of postoperative care for aortic aneurysm surgery. The basic considerations are applicable to all procedures requiring aortic cross-clamping. The several areas of controversy are discussed, and alternate viewpoints are presented, especially when they might reasonably be expected to improve patient care.

PREOPERATIVE EVALUATION

Because most aneurysmal disease is caused by atherosclerosis, patients usually possess either overt or occult vascular involvement of several organ systems. Prudence dictates a careful consideration of other conditions—most importantly, cerebral, renal, and coronary vascular disease. The specific elements of an appropriate preoperative evaluation have not been studied thoroughly, and current practice varies among institutions. Perioperative morbidity and mortality is significant. The incidence of perioperative death is 1.5 to 8 percent. Myocardial infarction rates range from 4 to 17 percent, depending on the criteria for infraction. Renal failure and pulmonary insufficiency both have an incidence of 4 to 5 percent, while congestive heart failure is observed in 3 percent of patients.

Although the development of improved surgical and anesthetic techniques as well as elevated standards of postoperative management have all served to lower complication rates, serious problems remain. Cardiac morbidity is clearly the greatest concern. The association of coronary artery stenosis with aneurysmal and other peripheral vascular disease has long been appreciated. In a series of 1,000 vascular surgery patients, only 8 percent showed no evidence of coronary involvement on angiography. Currently there is a great deal of interest in identifying preoperative procedures, short of cardiac catheterization, that would identify patients at the highest risk. Delayed filling on dipyridamole thallium reperfusion scans and ST depression on preoperative Holter monitoring have been suggested as high-yield markers. Unfortunately, it is by no means clear what action is appropriate once a patient's risk status has been identified. Preceding aneurysm repair with coronary bypass grafting does not result necessarily in lower *overall* mortality (counting both coronary artery bypass graft and abdominal aortic aneurysm repair). It is possible that instituting medical therapy or using special anesthetic procedures could lower risk to acceptable levels; however, these issues have not been resolved.

A baseline pulmonary evaluation that includes pulmonary function tests and analysis of arterial blood gases is indicated. Some element of lung dysfunction frequently is present because of the high incidence of a history of heaving smoking in this population. This rarely causes intraoperative problems except in the case of bronchospastic disease, but has implications for the postoperative period.

Preoperative consultation with the surgeon is important to establish the anticipated level of aortic cross-clamping (e.g., infrarenal, suprarenal, supraceliac) and the planned sequence of clamp application and removal. Several possibilities exist depending on the extent of the aneurysm and on the surgical technique, and these will influence the choice of monitoring and the timing of intraoperative manipulations. Infrarenal cross-clamping frequently results in minimal hemodynamic and metabolic changes, while supraceliac cross-clamping can cause major cardiac stress and inhibition of organ function. These issues are further elaborated in succeeding sections of this chapter.

Patients who present with leaking or dissecting

aneurysms require special preoperative treatment. Prompt control of hypertension and tachycardia is imperative. The use of nitroprusside, nitroglycerin, beta-blockers, or combined agents should be instituted aggressively to control vital signs. Once the blood pressure has been stabilized, the operation may be planned and then proceed in an orderly fashion.

Aneurysm rupture continues to be associated with an extremely high perioperative mortality (>50 percent). When first encountered by the anesthesiologist, the patient is probably in shock and receiving resuscitative measures (e.g., MAST trousers, intravenous fluids, central line placement) from other medical personnel. Oxygen supplementation, which is often overlooked by surgical and emergency room physicians, should be instituted. Whether or not to intubate the patient before his or her arrival in the operating room is a decision that is frequently difficult (airway protection versus overstimulation). Fluid administration should be as vigorous as required, but it is necessary that caution be exercised. Dilutional anemia, coagulopathy, congestive heart failure, and hypothermia are all real dangers during the poorly monitored preoperative period. If possible, an anesthesiologist should be dispatched to participate in the patient's early care, while others prepare the operating room for his or her arrival.

In elective cases, premedication should be heavy for individuals who are having angina or who are extremely anxious, while it is preferable to administer most of the premedication when the patient is in the operating room, during placement of intra-arterial and venous cannula. Certainly, administration of all significant chronic cardiovascular medications should be continued up to and including the morning of surgery.

MONITORING AND CASE PREPARATION

Routine monitoring for aortic aneurysm surgery includes continuous intravascular measurement of arterial blood pressure and central venous pressure from an intrathoracic cannula. Cannulation of the radial artery or other peripheral arterial sites can occasionally be extremely difficult in these patients with severe peripheral vascular disease. The axillary artery is cannulated easily through the use of a Seldinger technique and is a useful alternative to the standard sites. Use of the axillary artery results in a very low complication rate, although caution is warranted in flushing these lines, since air or particulate matter could be induced to enter the carotid or vertebral system.

Two leads of the electrocardiogram, including inferior and lateral precordial leads, should be monitored continuously, preferably on equipment capable of ST segment analysis. Aortic cross-clamping is capable of inducing a stress to the left ventricle that can result in myocardial ischemia. For patients undergoing cross-clamp procedures above the celiac axis, transesophageal echocardiography may be helpful if this modality is available. The ability of echocardiography to detect regional wall motion abnormalities suggestive of ischemia prior to ST segment changes has been demonstrated in this surgical group.

The use of pulmonary artery catheters in aortic aneurysm surgery varies from institution to institution. Most agree that pulmonary artery catheterization is advisable for patients who are to undergo aortic cross-clamping above the renal arteries. For infrarenal cross-clamping, the majority of clinicians reserve pulmonary artery catheterization for those patients with known heart or renal disease, while others prefer to use catheters in all aneurysm cases. Note that for a patient who is in shock or who is rapidly deteriorating, surgery should not be delayed for the insertion of a pulmonary artery catheter.

Blood loss during aneurysm surgery is highly variable. Routine blood loss for infrarenal aneurysms is usually approximately 2 units but is potentially massive for thoracoabdominal aneurysms. Suitable intravenous access for rapid administration of large blood volumes is necessary. At the least, two well-running large-bore peripheral lines (16- or 14-gauge) should be established. For higher cross-clamps or those cases in which very large blood losses may be anticipated (e.g., reoperation or graft removal), even greater large-bore access should be established; this may include two 7-French catheter sheaths suitable for integration with a rapid transfusion system.

Continuous infusion sets of vasoactive agents, including a vasodilator (usually nitroprusside), are prepared preoperatively. Nitroglycerin is an acceptable alternative. Dopamine is probably the inotrope of choice by virtue of its effect on renal function. Other vasoactive agents that may be useful during the procedure include the alpha-agonist phenylephrine and the standard complement of resuscitation drugs, which includes calcium chloride. Continuous infusions should be administered through a dedicated central line. Rapid response times are necessary in order to control intraoperative events.

ANESTHESIA

Premedication, induction, and maintenance of general anesthesia for abdominal aortic aneurysm repair may be chosen on the same basis as for any major surgery where patients have known or suspected vascular involvement of multiple organ systems. A combined regional anesthesia/general anesthesia technique possesses several theoretical benefits, including a reduced requirement for systemic agents and improved postoperative pain relief. In choosing a technique, one must always consider the anticipated changes in blood volume status and variations in left ventricular afterload caused by the clamping and unclamping process.

Some degree of hypothermia is commonly observed in patients undergoing aneurysm surgery. This is caused by the exposure of abdominal contents, the administration of large amounts of fluid, and the disturbances in thermoregulatory mechanism caused by anesthesia. All intravenous fluids, including those given during induction of anesthesia, should be administered through blood warmers. A heated vaporizer should be connected to the circle absorber system, and the room temperature set as high as possible commensurate with reasonable comfort for the surgical personnel.

General anesthesia should be induced slowly with incremental doses of a sedative hypnotic (e.g., thiopental sodium [Pentothal], etomidate, propofol) or with a continuous infusion of the chosen agent titrated to effect. During induction, narcotics should be administered up to a total of 10 μg per kilogram of fentanyl (or its equivalent) to moderate the stress of intubation and incision. During maintenance of general anesthesia, nitrous oxide supplemented with small amounts of a volatile agent (1 MAC or less) and occasional doses of morphine (2 to 5 mg) or additional fentanyl (50 μg), provide a stable anesthetic. This methodology allows safe and appropriate maintenance of general anesthesia while allowing one to retain the option of early extubation if this should become necessary based on the assessment of factors such as body temperature, fluid status, and renal function. (Extubation is discussed in detail in the last section of this chapter.)

If preoperative epidural administration of a local anesthetic is employed as an adjunct to general anesthesia, it is important to use much lower volumes than would normally be chosen for a pure regional technique. The use of normal volumes (15 to 20 ml) can cause severe problems with intraoperative hypotension. The awkward circumstance can arise of needing to administer a continuous infusion of alpha-pressors to a patient in whom restoration of blood flow to ischemic tissue is the goal of surgery. Also, the preoperative use of epidural opiates limits the amount of intravenous narcotic that may be given to blunt the stimulus of intubation and incision if early extubation is planned. The synergistic effect of even fairly modest doses of intravenous opiates when used in conjunction with neuraxis narcotics can result in profoundly depressed respiratory drive. To counter this difficulty, some authors have proposed the planned titration of a naloxone hydrochloride (Narcan) drip postoperatively. Clearly, the use of combined regional and general anesthesia should be considered very carefully. If careful consideration is given to the use of this technique, however, the superior postoperative analgesic control afforded by epidural administration of narcotics and local anesthetic agents may well contribute to lower morbidity and morality during this highly stressful period.

Vascular patients frequently present in a relatively hypovolemic state caused by recent dye studies, medications, and NPO status. Induction of anesthesia, even when agents are titrated slowly, can result in hypotension unless brisk fluid administration is instituted, frequently resulting in greater than 1 L of crystalloid given during this period. Many individuals benefit from incremental doses of an inotrope or vasopressors during induction, regardless of the agents chosen. In emergency situations, modification of both the techniques and

agents described above is necessary for patients with full-stomach or hypotensive status.

Blood should be available in the operating room early in the procedure as a precaution against the ever-present possibility of major bleeding. Blood scavenging devices have proven useful in abdominal aortic aneurysm repair. This equipment is expensive and requires a certain minimal level of use to be cost effective. Major vascular surgery offers the best opportunity for appropriate employment of blood scavenging units. Three problems must be kept in mind: (1) the surgeon must be alert to the possibility of contamination; (2) the scavenging process is too lengthy to permit rapid blood salvage in the case of major hemorrhage; and (3) the replaced blood is devoid of coagulation factors, and fresh frozen plasma administration should be considered early. For thoracoabdominal aneurysms or other cases in which large blood losses may be anticipated, a rapid transfusion device may be lifesaving. This equipment, which was originally produced for use in liver transplantation, is well designed and requires minimal training for its use. It has the ability of delivering warmed blood at high flow rates from a 2 L reservoir. Myocardial depression may occur when the rapid transfusion device is used secondary to citrate chelation of calcium, a condition specifically treated by calcium chloride administration (300 to 500 mg).

RENAL PROTECTION

Preservation of renal function is a primary concern during aortic aneurysm surgery. Clearly, procedures that require cross-clamping of the aorta above the renal arteries will result in a temporary period of ischemia with the potential for inducing some degree of renal failure. In animal experiments, preischemia administration of mannitol exerts a protective effect on renal function. Because the mechanisms that produce acute tubular necrosis are complex, it is not surprising that controversy exists regarding the exact manner in which mannitol or other agents might inhibit acute tubular necrosis. It is possible that mannitol exerts its protective effect through the scavenging of free radicals produced upon reperfusion of the kidney with cross-clamp release. Even though human studies demonstrating mannitol to have a beneficial effect have not been performed, it is common clinical practice to administer this agent (12.5 g per 70 kg) 10 to 15 minutes before aortic cross-clamping. The use of furosemide is more controversial. Although a protective effect for furosemide per se has not been established, it is generally believed that this agent may result in a conversion of low-output renal failure to high-output renal failure. Because high-output renal failure is much easier to manage during the postoperative period, some clinicians administer furosemide routinely in high cross-clamp cases. For the more common infrarenal aneurysms where cross-clamp application does not impede kidney perfusion, it is interesting that considerable concern regarding the possibility of renal failure remains. The distribution of renal blood flow is altered during infrarenal aortic cross-clamping, and this phenomenon can result in impairment of function. Maintenance of adequate intravascular volume during the surgical procedure has been shown to be the most important factor in avoiding renal dysfunction postoperatively, although most clinicians do administer mannitol but not furosemide in these cases as well. Dopamine in low doses (3 μg per kilogram per minute) increases renal blood flow and has other beneficial diuretic effects that make it attractive for use during aneurysm surgery, especially if some element of renal dysfunction exists preoperatively. Again, clinical practice varies widely.

NEUROLOGIC SEQUELAE

The blood supply to the lower spinal cord is complex, with the critical vessel usually emerging from the aorta above the diaphragm. However, paraplegia has been reported (in approximately 1 percent of patients) in abdominal aneurysm repair, indicating that the anatomy is variable. This incidence increases for abdominal aneurysms that are sufficiently extensive to require supraceliac cross-clamping. Many of the techniques for preserving organ and spinal cord blood flow (shunt, partial cardiopulmonary bypass) for thoracic aneurysm repair may not be useful for abdominal aneurysms. Vessel disease may involve the iliac and femoral arteries, making insertion of cannulae difficult and likely to produce emboli. Abbreviated clamp-times become essential to neurologic preservation. Several modalities to minimize ischemia or the effects of ischemia have been proposed, including the preclamp administration of calcium channel blockers, free radical scavengers, and local vasodilators. Cooling of the spinal cord has been proposed. The administration of intrathecal papaverine hydrochloride has proven protective in animal models. Spinal fluid drainage and maintenance of distal perfusion by shunting or bypass procedures, when technically feasible, is again being practiced. However, at present, none of these interventions has demonstrated sufficient efficacy in clinical studies to be definitively recommended.

PHYSIOLOGY OF AORTIC CROSS-CLAMPING

Acute interruption of aortic blood flow caused by application of a cross-clamp produces an increase in systemic vascular resistance and a rise in the arterial blood pressure. This increase in left ventricle afterload may be followed by a decrease in cardiac output, but the effect is variable. Normal compensatory hemodynamic responses include an increase in preload (preload reserve mechanism) that tends to return the output to preclamp values. Moreover, the vasculature below the clamp can "autotransfuse" its volume into the active circulation since venous return is unimpeded. In many patients, an increase in cardiac output can be observed. If vasodilators that cause venodilation (e.g., nitroglycerin, nitroprusside) are administered, then both cardiac output and stroke-work will consistently fall. Clearly, decreases in these parameters should not necessarily be interpreted as evidence of left ventricular dysfunction. A portion of metabolizing tissue supplied by the arterial system below the clamp has been excluded from the circulation. It has been shown that, under these circumstances, decreases in cardiac output is proportional to the decrease in total body oxygen consumption observed with application of the cross-clamp. It should be remembered however, that the elevations that occur in both preload and afterload may, in fact, result in some degree of left ventricular dysfunction. Regional wall motion abnormalities have been demonstrated during echocardiography during application of an aortic cross-clamp. Careful attention to the electrocardiogram is imperative.

Nitroprusside (50 to 100 μg) administered just before clamping may be useful to prevent cross-clamp hypertension. Actually, the necessity for preclamp vasodilatation is highly variable and depends on the level of cross-clamping. For infrarenal cross-clamps, it may be necessary only to deepen anesthesia. However, for cross-clamp above the celiac axis, repeated doses of nitroprusside or nitroglycerin followed by a continuous of infusion during the clamping period may be required. With regard to blood pressure control, one caveat is worth noting: for cross-clamp procedures in which interruption of the principal anterior spinal cord blood supply is probable, it is desirable to maintain arterial pressures proximal to the clamp as high as possible. It has been suggested, with some corroborating evidence, that blood flow to the spinal cord may be supplied via the anterior spinal artery as fed by the vertebral-basilar system. Proximal arterial pressure becomes the upstream pressure for spinal cord perfusion from this co-lateral supply. A balance of opposing goals is required — hypertension for spinal cord protection and normotension for heart protection.

Metabolic changes during the cross-clamp period range from the trivial to the profound, depending on the extent of the aneurysm and whether or not shunting or partial bypass maneuvers are instituted. During supraceliac cross-clamp, a progressive and substantial increase in blood lactate occurs along with a metabolic acidosis. The extent to which this acidosis is reflected by a decreased pH depends on whether or not ventilation has been altered to account for the changes in total body oxygen consumption. If minute ventilation has been unchanged from preclamp settings, a respiratory alkalosis will be produced that balances very closely the metabolic acid build-up, and thus serum pH may remain unchanged. The respiratory alkalosis results from decreased total body carbon dioxide production, since less tissue is aerobically metabolizing. Presumably, the increase in lactate level is caused by both increased production in marginally profused, anaerobically metabolizing tissues, and by decrease in elimination via the liver and kidney. Bicarbonate administration over the clamp period, while not necessary for stability, results in less acidosis at the time of unclamping.

Release of the aortic cross-clamp can result in a precipitous decline in blood pressure caused by reperfusion of previously closed vascular beds (themselves presumably maximally dilated secondary to ischemia). Computed systemic vascular resistance decreases in proportion to the organ and tissue mass being reperfused. Other mechanisms for declamping hypotension have been postulated, including the release of myocardial depressant factors and a wash-out of acid metabolites. During the immediate postrelease period, an additional acute increase in blood lactate occurs that is superimposed on the progressive increase observed during the clamping period. Carbon dioxide levels in both blood and expired gas increase dramatically at the time of unclamping. This carbon dioxide results from endogenous bicarbonate buffering of organic acid and from a sudden increase in total aerobically functioning tissue. Acidosis can be profound on release of a superceliac cross-clamp. It is probably unwise to administer bicarbonate coincident with cross-clamp release, as this will transiently produce yet an additional source of carbon dioxide.

Both the hemodynamic and metabolic changes are usually minor during the release of infrarenal cross-clamp. The small dip in pressure is well tolerated and usually resolves without vasopressor treatment, and bicarbonate correction of acidosis is seldom necessary. Conversely, hypotension caused by a release of higher aortic clamp can be severe and should be anticipated. Close communication between the surgeon and anesthesiologist is necessary at this time. One or two minutes before the surgeon removes the cross-cramp, administration of vasodilator drugs should be discontinued and fluid infusion increased. As the dilator effect diminishes, vascular tone returns and the blood pressure and filling pressure begin to increase. As the cross-clamp is released, small doses of vasopressors may be administered, commonly phenylephrine (50 to 150 μg). Administration of a vasopressor can be hazardous. It is often necessary for the surgeon to reapply the just-released cross-clamp in order to correct anastomotic bleeding. If this occurs as a vasopressor bolus reaches the vasculature, alarming hypertension may ensue. Some authors counsel against the use of an alpha-constrictor in patients in whom maintenance of distal perfusion is critical. Although this issue has not been investigated systematically, it seems reasonable not to prohibit the use of dilute solutions of vasoconstrictors to maintain systemic pressures and organ perfusion. If cardiovascular support is required on a continuous basis, low-dose dopamine may be beneficial, since return of renal function as demonstrated by urine output is always a primary concern. Intravascular dye administration (5 ml of indigo carmine) can identify true postclamp urine production. Blood gases should be measured shortly after removal of the cross-clamp in order to assess any residual acidosis.

In complicated aneurysm repair that involves su-

praceliac cross-clamping, there are multiple applications and removals of the cross-clamp as the surgeon moves down the vascular tree joining the major vascular runoffs. The sequence of preparation for cross-clamping must be repeated several times. As the clamp is moved more and more distally, there are multiple vessels to graft and anastomoses that are exposed to the systemic arterial pressure. These must be protected from rupture or leakage caused by hypertension.

TERMINATION OF THE PROCEDURE

Decisions regarding the termination of anesthetic care including emergence methodology, extubation versus intubation, and techniques of postoperative pain relief are potentially critical influences to patient morbidity. Several scenarios are possible. Relevant factors include the choice of anesthetic technique, extent of aneurysm repair, and patient stability with regard to the parameters of homeostasis (including body temperature, pulmonary function, urine output, blood loss, and volume status). An additional and important factor in end-of-case management decisions is knowledge of the degree of sophistication and the intensity of surveillance that exists in the postoperative care unit.

Many patients will be ready for extubation at the termination of surgery, having fulfilled all reasonable criteria. Several factors may conspire to complicate what would otherwise appear to be a rational decision to extubate postoperatively the patient with abdominal aortic aneurysm. Many of these patients have a long history of smoking with resulting compromise of respiratory status. The usual and expected postoperative deterioration of pulmonary function superimposed on a marginal baseline state can result in poor oxygenation developing during the hours immediately after surgery. Furthermore, varying degrees of fluid third-spacing commonly occur during aortic aneurysm repair and continue postoperatively. Even if intravascular volume has been carefully maintained, the fluid must be mobilized and eliminated over time. Because it is not always possible to monitor and control this process with a sufficient degree of precision, patients who seem to be doing well may develop problems several hours after procedure and require reintubation.

It is generally conceded that control of the stress response is necessary to reduce the incidence of postoperative cardiac morbidity. Since pain is a major component of stress, its alleviation is an important part of postoperative management considerations. Surgeons and intensivists seem to be progressively gaining an appreciation of this issue. An impressive array of options are available, each of which has its proponents. At one extreme, patients may be given large doses of narcotics with sedative supplementation and planned overnight ventilation, as is commonly done after coronary artery bypass grafting. This approach may be associated with a smoother course for both the intensive care staff and the patient over the first 24 hours postoperatively. Weaving, of course, must eventually occur, and this begins a period of delicate balance in which adequate analgesia for both the surgical incision and presence of the intratracheal tube is given, avoiding the respiratory depression that can be caused by administration of too much of an agent. The effect of extra hours of intratracheal intubation on respiratory complications (including infection) may be serious, resulting in prolonged hospitalization. This has not been resolved.

Several authors have recommended the use of epidural narcotics or local anesthetics as an adjunct to post-operative pain relief in aneurysm patients. One investigation showed that the preoperative administration of morphine (0.1 mg per kilogram) in the epidural space resulted in significantly lower levels of epinephrine and norepinephrine during the postoperative period. Some of these patients were extubated and some were not.

If overnight postoperative intubation is planned, it is not clear that regional techniques offer any advantage, at least during the time of intubation. If an epidural catheter has been left in place, then it is likely that *post*extubation pain relief will be superior using this modality. The role of patient-controlled analgesia versus epidural techniques in postoperative aneurysm patients has not been investigated. If early extubation is planned, then the use of intraoperative opiates or local anesthetics in the epidural space becomes quite rational. Considerably lower doses of inhalational agents may be used during the procedure, and thus the return to mental acuity and reflex-responsiveness is potentially more prompt. As mentioned earlier, supplementation of general anesthesia with epidural local anesthetics may produce serious problems with hypotension that will require administration of vasoconstrictor agents. Provided that this effect is either minimized or accounted for, neuraxis techniques may result in the smallest possible stress response.

The postoperative care of aneurysm patients can be complicated. In addition to the issues discussed above, several other problems may be encountered. Coagulopathies may continue from the operative period or develop anew. Hypothermia may persist and require treatment with heating blankets. Electrolytes and blood gases should be followed carefully, and complete hemodynamic profiles should be determined frequently to ensure optimum control. Patients who have experienced ruptured aneurysm and/or prolonged suprarenal cross-clamping are prime candidates for renal failure. Knowledge of all hemodynamic parameters is necessary in order to provide adequate therapy and to avoid overload.

SUGGESTED READING

Dritz RA. Surgery on the aorta and peripheral arteries. In: Ream AK, Fogdall RP, eds. Acute cardiovascular management: anesthesia and intensive care. Philadelphia: JB Lippincott, 1982:729.

Roizen MF. Anesthesia for vascular surgery. New York: Churchill Livingstone, 1990.

Yeager MP, Glass DD. Anesthesiology and vascular surgery: perioperative management of the vascular surgical patient. East Norwalk, CT: Appleton and Lange, 1990.

THORACIC ANEURYSM

GEORGE J. GRAF, M.D.
PAUL G. BARASH, M.D.

Hypertension and atherosclerosis are the most common etiologic factors in the development of thoracic aneurysms. The peak incidence occurs in persons 50 to 70 years of age, with men outnumbering women by approximately two to one. Atherosclerotic aneurysms are classically described as fusiform and are more common in the lower thoracic aorta, seldom occurring in the arch or ascending aorta. Dissection of the thoracic aorta is a specific clinical and pathologic entity, although the term "dissection" is often used in describing the enlargement and rupture of other types of aneurysms. In addition to being present in cystic medial necrosis, medial degeneration of the aortic wall, which is characteristic of the aging process, is generally considered the primary mechanism leading to aortic dissection. As suggested above, acute dissection of the aorta may *not* be associated with an aneurysm. In addition to hypertension and atherosclerosis, other clinical conditions related to the development of dissection include pregnancy, bacterial infection, Marfan's syndrome, congenital cardiovascular anomalies, such as coarctation and aortic stenosis, and finally trauma. The most common sites of origin for aortic dissection are the ascending aorta, comprising approximately 60 to 70 percent of dissections, the descending aorta, responsible for about 30 to 35 percent, and the aortic arch, comprising the remaining 5 to 10 percent. There are two widely used systems of anatomic classification for aortic dissection. The older DeBakey classification describes three types. Type I dissection starts in the ascending aorta and involves the entire aorta. Type II dissection is limited to the ascending aorta, and type III starts distal to the left subclavian artery and spares the ascending aorta and arch. A recognition of the differences between the clinical presentation, therapeutic intervention, and prognosis of dissection involving the ascending aorta and arch and those of dissection originating distal to the left subclavian artery led to a second classification system.

Dailey et al divide dissections into two groups: Group A includes all patients with dissection involving any part of the ascending aorta, regardless of the site of the intimal tear, and Group B includes those patients with dissection confined to the aorta distal to the left subclavian artery. Type A dissections occur much more frequently than type B dissections and are associated with a higher mortality rate within the first 14 days after the onset of symptoms. Currently all patients presenting with type A dissection are considered to be surgical candidates. At present, most patients with type B aortic dissection are managed medically and surgical intervention occurs on an elective basis. In light of these differences, the anesthesiologist's initial contact with the patient may occur under vastly different clinical circumstances.

DIAGNOSIS AND INITIAL MANAGEMENT

Acute aortic dissection should be considered in the differential diagnosis of any patient who presents with the acute onset of chest pain. This pain is often described as tearing or ripping and occurs in the midchest, neck, jaw, or infrascapular area. The patient often appears pale and diaphoretic, as if in shock, but is commonly hypertensive. Sudden absence of a pulse in an extremity, cardiorespiratory instability, and neurologic or gastrointestinal symptoms are other common clinical features.

The chest roentgenogram is frequently abnormal. It may show mediastinal widening, a pleural effusion, or blurring of the aortic knob. Electrocardiographic findings are similarly nonspecific; ST-segment changes reflecting ischemia or pericarditis are common. The most reliable noninvasive method for diagnosing dissection is computed axial tomography (CT) scan. Magnetic resonance imaging (MRI), like CT scanning, can demonstrate the extent of the disease process and allow one to make the diagnosis without the use of intravascular contrast medium. This is of particular value in patients with known allergies or compromised renal conditions for which intravascular injection of contrast material is relatively contraindicated. Because of inherent difficulties in monitoring critically ill patients during MRI imaging, this technique is reserved for patients who are medically stable. Despite the value of noninvasive radiologic techniques in diagnosing aortic dissection, contrast aortography remains the definitive diagnostic modality for most patients. This technique can identify the extent of the false lumen, the site of the intimal tear, the presence of aortic regurgitation, and vessels arising from the area of the dissection.

The prognosis for patients with acute aortic dissection who are left untreated is poor. Mortality is reported to be 25 to 35 percent within 24 hours, 60 to 70 percent within the 1st week, and 90 percent after 3 months. At present, all patients with type A dissections are considered surgical candidates during the acute stage. The likelihood of surgical mortality is greatly increased with

the emergency resection of type A thoracic aneurysms; when possible, intensive medical therapy is instituted until diagnostic procedures are completed and the patient is stabilized. Most patients with type B aneurysms have been managed medically because surgical intervention resulted in an overall increase in mortality. These patients are considered candidates for surgery if there is evidence of vascular obstruction or compromise of a major branch of the aorta or if continued expansion of the aneurysm occurs despite maximal medical management. The elective repair of type B thoracoabdominal aneurysm is preceded by a thorough medical evaluation. Those patients with symptoms of coronary artery disease undergo coronary angiography and, when indicated, myocardial revascularization before elective repair of the aneurysm. Renal and hematologic function are routinely evaluated, and we obtain a measurement of arterial blood gas and perform formal pulmonary function testing in all patients. Evolving neurologic symptoms suggesting cerebral infarction, poor general health, or extensive systemic disease are all relative contraindications for elective surgery.

The medical management of thoracic aneurysms begins with the admission of the patient to an intensive care unit. Vital signs are monitored continuously using direct arterial pressure monitoring (preferably via the right radial artery), electrocardiography, and a Foley catheter. A pulmonary artery thermodilution catheter is inserted using the internal jugular vein. The initial treatment of choice is vasodilator therapy in an attempt to lower the systemic arterial pressure and ventricular ejection velocity.

Nitroprusside may indirectly increase the heart rate and force of myocardial contraction through afterload reduction and reflex catecholamine release. For this reason, we administer intravenous doses of the beta-blocker propranolol. The drug is given in increments of 0.5 to 1.0 mg and is titrated to the heart rate. Esmolol hydrochloride, a new, ultra-short–acting beta-blocker that is administered as a continuous infusion, may be titrated to assist in the management of heart rate and blood pressure. Trimethaphan camsylate, a competitive ganglionic blocker, is a second-line vasodilator. It has a rapid onset of action, and the hypotensive effect may be accompanied by a reduction in the cardiac index and left ventricular ejection rate. Like nitroprusside, trimethaphan camsylate is administered as a continuous intravenous infusion and continuous blood pressure monitoring is necessary. The usual starting dose is 5 to 10 μg per kilogram per minute adjusted to the desired blood pressure. The parasympathetic inhibition caused by this drug causes an unpleasant loss of visual accommodation, mydriasis (impairing neurologic evaluation), ileus, and difficulty voiding, especially when the drug is administered for more than 24 hours. Other side effects include histamine release, tachyphylaxis, and the remote possibility of respiratory depression. During this period of initial treatment and stabilization, we prefer to sedate the patient using small doses of narcotics or benzodiazepine.

ANESTHETIC MANAGEMENT OF TYPE A ANEURYSM

Patients with aneurysms of the ascending aorta or aortic arch are often hemodynamically unstable when they arrive in the operating room. In most cases, invasive monitoring and medical therapy have already been instituted. We prefer to have two large peripheral intravenous catheters, a radial artery catheter, and a pulmonary artery catheter in place before proceeding with induction of anesthesia. After induction of anesthesia, transesophageal echocardiography is employed to monitor left ventricular wall motion. This modality also has potential as a diagnostic tool for assessing aortic involvement. Additional monitoring includes electrocardiography (leads II, V_5), use of a Foley catheter, end-tidal measurement of all inspired gases and carbon dioxide (mass spectrometry), pulse oximetry (oxygen percent saturation, or SaO_2) and rectal temperature probe.

The anesthetic technique is similar to the technique employed in patients undergoing cardiac surgery with the aid of cardiopulmonary bypass. It is important to consider that patients who present for early and emergent surgical repair may require a rapid sequence induction with cricoid pressure. We use high-dose fentanyl or sufentanil plus a muscle relaxant. We supplement narcotics with a potent inhalation agent or a benzodiazepine. This ensures amnesia, and the additional myocardial depression may be helpful in preventing further dissection. The choice of a muscle relaxant is chiefly based on hemodynamic side effects. Those patients who have received beta-blockers receive pancuronium bromide. When tachycardia is present, we prefer to use vecuronium bromide or atracurium besylate. Ventilation is controlled throughout the operative procedure. After median sternotomy, the temperature is lowered to between 28 and 30°C. The patient is heparinized, and extracorporeal bypass is instituted using the right atrium and descending aorta or femoral artery. If the intimal tear involves the aortic arch, the patient is prepared for possible circulatory arrest by surface cooling and use of cardiopulmonary bypass to achieve a core temperature between 16 and 20°C. The use of high-dose barbiturates (thiopentol) and steroid infusion before circulatory arrest is advocated by some for cerebral protection. Alternatively, the carotid arteries may be selectively infused with cold blood during moderate hypothermia (28°C). The myocardium is preserved by systemic cooling, saline lavage, and cold cardioplegia. When necessary, aortic valve resuspension is carried out. After rewarming (35°C rectal), the patient is weaned from cardiopulmonary bypass and protamine sulfate is administered. The cardiac output and pulmonary capillary wedge pressure (PCWP) are frequently measured and manipulated to optimize cardiac performance. Vasodilators, such as nitroprusside or nitroglycerin, are used during the postbypass period to lower the systemic blood pressure and avoid damage to surgical anastomoses.

Patients are transferred to the intensive care unit where they are sedated and mechanically ventilated for 12 to 24 hours. Muscle relaxants are continued until the patients are fully warmed. Vasodilators and beta-blockade are continued after surgery. Before being discharged from the hospital, patients will have a repeat CT scan to evaluate the aorta for obliteration of the intimal flap. Those patients with complete obliteration of the flap have a good prognosis. Patients with incomplete occlusion of the false lumen are prone to late aneurysmal dilatation and should be carefully followed.

Recent surgical series report a mortality of 10 to 15 percent for repair of type A aneurysms. Preoperative complications increase the operative mortality to approximately 35 percent.

ANESTHETIC MANAGEMENT OF TYPE B DISSECTION

The surgical resection of a thoracoabdominal aneurysm originating distal to the left subclavian artery (type B) is performed with the patient in the right lateral decubitus position. Before induction of anesthesia, invasive monitoring similar to that outlined for type A aneurysms is accomplished (two large-bore peripheral intravenous catheters, right radial artery catheters, and a pulmonary artery thermodilution catheter) using local anesthesia and sedation. Induction is carried out with high-dose narcotic technique and a muscle relaxant. The patient is intubated using a "left-sided" double-lumen endotracheal tube. It is important to remember that placement of a left-sided tube can be difficult because the left mainstem bronchus may be compressed or deviated by the aneurysm. The tube position is confirmed with a pediatric bronchoscope. "One-lung anesthesia" is employed to improve surgical exposure and to avoid damage to the left lung caused by surgical retraction. During one-lung ventilation, a trial of continuous positive airway pressure (CPAP) to the deflated left lung or positive end-expiratory pressure (PEEP) to the dependent lung may be necessary to ensure adequate oxygenation in those patients with hypoxia (an arterial oxygen pressure, or PaO_2, of 60 mm Hg). After the endotracheal tube is secured, the patient is positioned with the left side up (a 60-degree angle to the table) and the hips swiveled to expose the left groin. After positioning the patient, all pressure points are padded and the endotracheal tube position is reconfirmed. All inspired gases are warmed and humidified.

Considerable controversy exists regarding the best operative approach for type B dissections, especially with regard to protection of the spinal cord during aortic cross-clamping. The risk of postoperative paraplegia is reported to be 1 to 11 percent and is directly related to cross-clamp time without shunting. Other possible causes of spinal cord ischemia include: an increase in cerebrospinal fluid pressure associated with proximal aortic hypertension, intraoperative hypotension, and the accidental interruption of critical intercostal arteries.

The hemodynamic consequences of aortic cross-clamping should also be considered. Clamping is associated with a sudden increase in afterload, which causes an elevation in left ventricular wall tension. This leads to increased myocardial oxygen demand. Myocardial oxygen supply is compromised if significant hypotension occurs after unclamping of the aorta. Various shunting and bypass techniques have been employed to preserve the spinal cord and improve hemodynamic stability.

The simplest surgical approach consists of aortic cross-clamping without the use of a shunt. This technique appears best suited for small aneurysms where the anticipated cross-clamp time is less than 30 minutes. A second approach employs a heparin-coated external shunt from the left ventricular apex to the femoral artery. The (Gott) shunt allows for distal perfusion and helps in unloading the left ventricle during the cross-clamp period. Because systemic heparinization is unnecessary, bleeding should be minimized. The use of this shunt is not without complications. Placement of the shunt may be technically difficult, adding significantly to the operative time. In addition, there are reports of paraplegia, congestive heart failure, and an increase in the operative mortality when a shunt is used. Partial cardiopulmonary bypass is another technique that is often used for the repair of extensive thoracoabdominal aneurysms. The patient is heparinized, and either femoral vein to femoral-artery or left atrium to femoral artery bypass is instituted during the cross-clamp period. An arterial catheter is placed in the opposite femoral artery or in the dorsalis pedis artery to measure distal bypass perfusion pressures. Flows are regulated to maintain the mean perfusion pressure at 50 mm Hg. Flows can be adjusted to unload the left ventricle during application of the cross-clamp. This technique provides a margin of safety, but it does not eliminate the possibility of left ventricular dysfunction or paraplegia.

The monitoring of somatosensory-evoked potentials (SEP) to predict anterior spinal cord ischemia during aortic cross-clamping has been recommended, but remains to be verified. Several authors have found a good correlation between SEP changes and neurologic outcome following operations on the aorta; however, anterior spinal cord function (motor) cannot always be assured by the preservation of SEP (dorsal columns) during cross-clamping. When no shunt is used, the production of evoked potentials ceases. We therefore reserve the use of SEP for those procedures when a shunt is employed.

During the pre-cross–clamp period, all patients receive mannitol (0.5 g per kilogram) to aid in preventing renal ischemia. This therapy may also decrease spinal cord edema and improve spinal artery blood flow. The intermittent removal of cerebrospinal fluid through an intrathecal lumbar catheter placed prior to the induction of anesthesia has also been used with the hope of improving anterior spinal artery blood flow. This modality requires further evaluation. Cold renoplegia (Ringer's lactate) may be infused via the left renal artery as an additional method of renal preservation. The patient's temperature is allowed to decrease to 33 to 34°C during the pre-cross–clamp period. Immediately before cross-clamping, a nitroprusside infusion is initiated (2 to 3 µg per kilogram per minute). The cardiac output and PCWP are measured as the surgeon gradually cross-clamps the aorta. The continuous monitoring of mixed venous oxygen saturation (SvO_2) during aortic cross-clamping for type B aneurysms does not correlate well with cardiac output (CO) or oxygen consumption ($\dot{V}O_2$) and cannot substitute for intermittent CO determinations. The use of transesophageal echocardiographic imaging of the left ventricle (short axis) is a particularly effective method for assessing left ventricular function and myocardial ischemia during aortic cross-clamping. This modality is assuming a more prominent role in the anesthetic management of these patients. The nitroprusside infusion is then adjusted to maintain the blood pressure (mean arterial pressure <110 mm Hg) and PCWP (<15 mm Hg) within an acceptable range during the cross-clamp period. The cardiac output is decreased in most patients. Nitroglycerin infusion is an acceptable alternative to nitroprusside when the cross-clamp is applied more distally. Both drugs are often administered simultaneously to patients with clinically apparent coronary artery disease. A constant infusion of sodium bicarbonate (0.05 mEq per kilogram per minute) is delivered during the cross-clamp period. Immediately before unclamping, vasodilators are discontinued and volume loading is increased, using warmed blood or crystalloid. Indigo carmine (50 mg) is administered intravenously to facilitate quantification of urine output after cross-clamp. The blood pressure, PCWP, and CO are closely followed as the clamp is slowly released. Generally, patients with adequate cardiac output and well-controlled intravascular pressure during the cross-clamp period will tolerate unclamping without serious difficulty. We cannot overemphasize the importance of judicious vasodilator and fluid therapy during the pre-cross–clamp and the cross-clamp periods. A cell saver is used to retrieve blood from the operative field. The patient's blood is stored in a reservoir, washed, and concentrated to a hematocrit of at least 50 percent before reinfusion. The cell saver is also employed to "wash" stored packed red blood cells when a large transfusion requirement is anticipated. A rapid infusion pump that warms all fluids is also available. An arterial blood gas is specifically obtained immediately after unclamping, and base deficits are corrected with additional sodium bicarbonate. Furosemide (10 to 20 mg IV) may be administered during the postclamp period if urine output is inadequate.

Recent advances in anesthetic management, surgical techniques, and postoperative care have led to a decrease in surgical mortality for type B aneurysms. In one surgical series, a mortality rate of 11 percent has been reported for uncomplicated cases. With one or more complications before surgery (e.g., stroke, loss of renal or visceral perfusion, paralysis), the operative mortality increases to greater than 70 percent. It is now recognized that many patients receiving medical management will eventually require surgical repair during the chronic phase. The high operative risk following preoperative complications has led many to question the advantage of long-term medical therapy over definitive surgical intervention.

SUGGESTED READING

Crawford ES, Crawford JL, Safi HJ, et al. Thoracoabominal aortic aneurysms: preoperative and intraoperative factors determining immediate and long-term results of operation in 605 patients. J Vasc Surg 1986; 3:389–404.

Crawford ES, Morris GC Jr, Myhre HO, Roehm OF Jr. Celiac axis, superior mesenteric artery, and inferior mesenteric artery occlusion: surgical considerations. Surgery 1977; 82:856–866.

Matsuda H, Nakano S, Shirokura R, et al. Surgery for aortic arch aneurysms with selective cerebral perfusion and hypothermic cardiopulmonary bypass. Circulation 1989; 80:243–248.

Saleh-Shenaq SA, Crawford ES, Bomberger RA. Intraoperative acid-base management for resection of thoracoabdominal aortic aneurysms: a comparison of continuous infusion of sodium bicarbonate versus the bolus. Anesth Analg 1983; 61:213.

Shenaq SA, Chelly JE, Karlberg H, et al. Peripheral vascular disease: use of nitroprusside during surgery for thoracoabdominal aortic aneurysm. Circulation 1984; 70(pt 2):I7–10.

Spargo PM, Cross M. Anesthetic problems in cross-clamping of the thoracic aorta. Ann R Coll Surg Engl 1988; 70:64–68.

CAROTID ENDARTERECTOMY

ROBERT W. McPHERSON, M.D.
ROSS DICKSTEIN, M.D.

Recent studies have questioned whether carotid endarterectomy (CEA) is more efficacious than medical treatment for most patients with carotid atherosclerosis. This controversy has led to a decrease in the frequency with which the operation is performed. Contemporary anesthetic management and monitoring have been developed in studies of patients with widely varying surgical indications and probably mixed pathology of the carotid circulation. Table 1 shows conventional indications for carotid endarterectomy. With a greater selection of patients, modification of anesthetic technique and monitoring may be required.

Under normal circumstances, the carotid arteries supply more than 60 percent of blood to the brain. Disease of the carotid system may disturb brain function by a decrease in cerebral blood flow (CBF) or by emboli producing occlusion of end arteries, particularly in the distribution of the middle cerebral artery. In previous reports of carotid endarterectomy, 60 to 70 percent of patients undergoing surgery had less than 50 percent stenosis of the carotid arteries. Since that degree of stenosis leads to little, if any, decrease in CBF, symptoms were most likely caused by emboli.

Collateral blood flow through the circle of Willis and anastomoses between the external carotid and internal carotid systems may provide adequate blood flow despite high-grade stenosis of one or both internal carotid arteries. In patients with high-grade stenosis, those collateral circuits are probably maximally dilated. Collaterals should be considered non-autoregulating and cerebral perfusion pressure is thus directly related to mean arterial pressure. The patient may be asymptomatic even if CBF is less than normal because cerebral oxygen utilization can be maintained by increasing

Table 1 Indications for Carotid Endarterectomy

Transient ischemic attacks
High-grade carotid stenosis
Embolic phenomenon arising from a carotid lesion
Amaurosis fugax
Large ulcerated plaque
Surgical team with low stroke/death rate

oxygen extraction from normal values (55 percent) to those of 80 to 90 percent.

There is a high incidence of ischemic heart disease and hypertension in patients undergoing CEA. Several studies have suggested that perioperative cardiac complications occur more frequently than neurologic complications. Optimal preoperative preparation requires adequate control of both cardiac disease and hypertension. Because moderate induced hypertension is frequently used intraoperatively to maintain flow through non-autoregulating collaterals, patients should have maximal medical therapy with antianginal medication administered up to the time of surgery. The level of sophistication of cardiac monitoring should reflect the severity of the patient's disease. However, the difficulty of treating these patients aggressively with vasodilators intraoperatively suggests that a lower than normal threshold for use of pulmonary artery catheter insertion is appropriate.

The extent of stenosis, both ipsilateral and contralateral to the proposed operative site, allows an approximation of the hemodynamic consequences of carotid artery clamping. A carotid artery with chronic high-grade stenosis (>95 percent) contributes little to CBF, and cross-clamping will probably alter hemispheric CBF little because blood flow to the clamp hemisphere would be provided by previously established collaterals. The consequences of cross-clamping a carotid artery with a lower degree of obstruction is less clear. In a classic study, Holmes et al studied hemispheric blood flow after unilateral carotid ligation for giant intracranial aneurysms. In that study, carotid cross-clamping resulted in an immediate decrease in flow to about 50 percent of the preclamp value associated with a decrease in the carotid stump pressure. Although stump pressure did not return to control levels, hemispheric CBF returned to control level by 30 minutes. These data support the concept that development of collateral flow is not instantaneous, even if mean arterial blood pressure (MABP) is maintained. It also demonstrates that carotid stump pressure may be an unreliable indicator of blood flow to the clamped hemisphere. Since collateral vessels are probably non-autoregulating, the lower the MABP, the less the flow through those channels. Cerebral vessels are not affected by systemically administered vasopressors, and maintenance of an elevated MABP should promote an increase in blood flow to the clamped hemisphere via collaterals.

ANESTHETIC TECHNIQUE

The choice of an anesthetic technique is the result of physician experience, institutional capabilities (particularly capabilities of neurologic monitoring), and patient preferences. These factors have precluded a well-controlled prospective, randomized study of different anesthetics for CEA. Thus, published comparisons of general anesthesia versus local/regional anesthesia for CEA contain considerable bias. There is little compelling evidence that either type of anesthesia is advantageous in a wide variety of circumstances.

Traditionally, the anesthesiologist has been most concerned with oligemic consequences of carotid cross-clamp, and therefore anesthetic management has evolved to minimize that consequence. The brain has strong homeostatic mechanisms that help protect it when oxygen delivery is limited. Autoregulation is the ability to maintain a constant CBF despite wide changes in cerebral perfusion pressure (mean arterial pressure – intracranial pressure). The cerebral response to oxygen deprivation is vasodilation to increase CBF and maintain cerebral oxygen delivery. This response is sensitive to the arterial oxygen content (hemoglobin × 1.34 × percent saturation) rather than the arterial oxygen tension (PaO_2). Animal studies suggest that autoregulation is obtunded when the vessels are widely dilated because of oxygen limitation. Thus, in the clamped cerebral hemisphere, vessels are probably non-autoregulating, and decreases in cerebral perfusion pressure (CPP), even within the normal range, may decrease flow and oxygen delivery.

Methods of decreasing the risk of ischemic cerebral injury during CEA suitable for intraoperative use are limited in number and are controversial in animal and human studies. Manipulation of cerebral perfusion pressure, arterial carbon dioxide tension, cerebral metabolism, and cerebral arterial oxygen delivery are potential mechanisms. Some or all of these mechanisms may be effected by the anesthetic management. Perfusion pressure is affected by the type of anesthetic, level of anesthetic (particularly in the case of general anesthesia), administration of vasopressors, and insertion of

a temporary intraluminal shunt. The level of cerebral metabolism is depressed by general anesthesia, thus lowering the cerebral metabolic rate of oxygen ($CMRO_2$). Further depression of cerebral metabolism by intravenous administration of short-acting barbiturates has been suggested. However, barbiturate doses sufficiently small to prevent a decrease in arterial pressure have not been shown to be protective in either animal or human studies. Animal studies have suggested that ketamine increases CBF. However, although administration of ketamine immediately before clamping has been suggested, there is no evidence that flow through collateral channels will be increased in such circumstances.

Manipulation of arterial carbon dioxide tension in order to redistribute CBF has been used to decrease the risk of ischemia. Hypercapnia causes cerebral vasodilatation but may cause "steal" from ischemic areas already normally dilated. Hypocapnia is used to decrease flow in normal brain and redistribute flow to the clamped hemisphere. This concept has been reinforced recently by a case report by Artru and Merriman that suggested that the combination of induced hypertension and hypocapnia reversed postclamp ischemia demonstrated by electroencephalographic (EEG) monitoring. There is little proof that either hypocapnia or hypercapnia is universally advantageous, and normocapnia should probably be maintained.

There has never been a randomized, blinded study of different anesthetics on the outcome of CEA. However, historical studies at a single institution have compared halothane, enflurane, and isoflurane in patients undergoing CEA. In a retrospective study, Michenfelder et al found that cerebral ischemia occurs less frequently during isoflurane anesthesia than during halothane or enflurane anesthesia. They also found that the critical CBF for the production of ischemic EEG changes was lower when isoflurane was used than when halothane or enflurane was used (about 10 ml per 100 g per minute versus about 20 ml per 100 g per minute). Young et al have recently compared the CBFs during isoflurane, halothane, and nitrous/fentanyl anesthesia, respectively, in patients undergoing CEA. They found that the $CMRO_2$ was similar with the three anesthetic techniques. Animal studies have shown that autoregulation and cerebral responsivity to changes in carbon dioxide tension are retained during isoflurane anesthesia (1 MAC). Thus, isoflurane anesthesia appears preferable to halothane or enflurane anesthesia.

Local anesthesia has been advocated because neurologic changes can be rapidly appreciated and hemodynamic swings are fewer. Clearly advocates of this technique believe that the major source of neurologic injury is ischemia related to carotid cross-clamping. The advocates of general anesthesia believe that anesthesia decreases cerebral oxygen demand, allows careful control of arterial oxygen and arterial carbon dioxide tension, and provides airway control and a quiet surgical field. In a series of 73 consecutive patients (90 percent symptomatic), regional anesthesia was compared with general anesthesia (with different surgeons for each technique). There was no difference in intravenous pressor or antihypertensive therapy, but the incidence of shunt insertion was much higher in patients receiving general anesthesia (90 percent versus 10 percent for patients receiving local anesthesia). The duration of the postoperative hospital stay was greater with general anesthesia. In a consecutive series in which the first 37 patients received general anesthesia and the subsequent 184 patients received regional anesthesia, the morbidity and mortality were similar for the two groups.

Most anesthesiologists believe that maintenance of a MABP slightly greater than baseline values promotes flow through collaterals to the clamped hemisphere. Methods for accomplishing this include lighter anesthesia, increased intravenous fluids, and the use of vasopressors. Recent studies, however, suggest that the intraoperative use of phenylephrine increases the incidence of postoperative myocardial infarction. Smith et al compared light anesthesia with deep anesthesia in which the MABP was maintained with phenylephrine. They found that in patients who received phenylephrine, the incidence of myocardial ischemia was three times greater: With light anesthesia, myocardial ischemia developed in five of 30 patients, whereas with deep anesthesia plus phenylephrine, 13 of 29 developed ischemia.

NEUROLOGIC MONITORING

Currently available methods for monitoring neurologic function are neurologic examination (local/regional anesthesia), EEG, computer processed EEG, and somatosensory-evoked potentials (SEPs). Because these monitoring modalities have been compared infrequently, the relative efficacy of each is left in doubt. Both EEG and SEP can adequately demonstrate oxygen deprivation to the specific area monitored. With hypoperfusion, changes in the EEG over the parietal area or scalp-recorded SEP will demonstrate changes if oxygen delivery is inadequate. However, injury caused by an embolic phenomenon may be shown only by multichannel EEG, depending on the area where the emboli lodge. Intraoperatively, the most convenient EEG method is computer analysis by Fast Fourier Transformation (FFT) of several channels of EEG. Most monitors available for use in the operating room are limited to two or four channels. Many units are available, and technical advances have made these units functional in the operating room. Alternatively, scalp-recorded SEP responses can be monitored. The scalp-recorded response to median nerve stimulation is generated in the area perfused by the middle cerebral artery, and waveform changes should demonstrate inadequate oxygen delivery to those areas.

The use of neurophysiologic monitoring is controversial and, to a certain extent, tied to the controversy surrounding the use of intraluminal shunts during endarterectomy. Surgical series in which shunts were always used, were never used, and were placed based on

EEG changes with cross-clamp application have been reported with acceptably low morbidity and mortality. The lack of increased frequency of permanent neurologic injury in patients without temporary shunts does not suggest that transient EEG changes do not occur during cross-clamp application. Morawetz et al compared CBF and EEG changes after cross-clamp, with postoperative neurologic deficits present in patients undergoing CEA under general anesthesia. The CBF was measured immediately after the carotid artery was clamped. They found that EEG changes correlated with blood flow changes. EEG changes were frequent but not universal in patients with a CBF of less than 20 ml per 100 g per minute, and the percentage of patients with EEG changes increased as flow decreased. However, the CBF did not correlate with postoperative neurologic deficits; in fact, complications were greater in patients with a flow of greater than 20 ml per 100 g per minute than in patients with a flow of less than 20 ml per 100 g per minute.

Silbert et al compared processed EEG with neurologic assessment in 70 patients undergoing CEA under cervical plexus block. They found that six patients demonstrated neurologic changes associated with carotid cross-clamp application. Only five of the six patients demonstrated simultaneous EEG changes and changes in neurologic function. An additional four patients who did not have changes in neurologic function displayed EEG changes suggestive of cerebral ischemia. They concluded that EEG is less sensitive than the neurologic examination in reliably detecting ischemia. Rampil et al found that computerized EEG predicted postoperative neurologic changes in patients who were neurologically normal (EEG demonstrates ischemia for >10 minutes) but was not predictive in 31 patients who had preoperative neurologic deficits. One patient had no intraoperative EEG changes and developed a new deficit, and one patient with ischemic changes lasting 3 minutes had no neurologic changes.

POSTOPERATIVE PROBLEMS

The immediate postoperative period is a time of extremely high risk for the patient. Immediate risks include myocardial ischemia or myocardial infarction, carotid thrombosis, and cerebral intraparenchymal bleeding (Table 2). In a retrospective study, Cucchiara et al compared the incidence of perioperative myocardial infarction in patients undergoing CEA with halothane anesthesia, isoflurane anesthesia, and enflurane anesthesia. They found a fatal infarction rate of 1 percent with the use of halothane, 0.5 percent with enflurane, and 0.25 percent with isoflurane, with the incidence significantly lower with isoflurane. In a retrospective study of 185 patients, Prough et al showed that no myocardial infarction occurred in patients under regional anesthesia. These two studies suggest that myocardial infarction may be less with local/regional anesthesia. However, this has not been studied directly.

Table 2 Complications of Carotid Endarterectomy

Hematoma with tracheal compression
Supraglottic edema
Cranial nerve injury (cranial nerves VII, IX, X, and XII)
Myocardial infarction
Intraparenchymal hemorrhage
Carotid occlusion

The incidence of postoperative hypertension (an increase in systolic blood pressure >35 mm Hg over the preoperative level) after CEA is about 60 percent. The incidence of hypertension correlates with preoperative hypertensive diabetes, isoflurane anesthesia, prior transient ischemia attacks, and high-grade carotid stenosis. Severe postoperative hypertension (systolic blood pressure >200 mm Hg) occurs in 19 percent of CEAs, with preoperative hypertension the single-most important determinant of postoperative hypertension. The incidence of neurologic deficits is increased in patients with postoperative hypertension (three times greater than in patients who do not have hypertension).

Transient baroreceptor dysfunction may occur after CEA, with hypotension (maximum approximately 5 hours) and hypertension (maximum approximately 2 hours) occurring in different patients. Hypotension has been associated with a decrease in heart rate and may persist for about 12 hours, requiring aggressive fluid therapy. Hypertension usually persists for about 6 hours postoperatively.

In addition to intraoperative embolization or ischemia, transient postoperative neurologic dysfunction may be related to hyperperfusion rather than hypoperfusion. In a report of ten patients who had hyperperfusion, there was typically a history of longstanding symptoms of cerebral ischemia and high-grade carotid stenosis. Hyperfusion occurred after CEA and symptoms of ipsilateral headache and seizures. Typically, the CBF increased to three to four times the baseline CBF. All of the patients in the series recovered, but they were at risk for intracranial hemorrhage.

Fifteen percent of patients undergoing CEA developed cranial nerve paralysis. In half of these patients, the ipsilateral hypoglossal nerve was involved; in one-third, the cervical branch of the facial nerve was involved, and in one-third, the recurrent laryngeal nerve was involved.

Careful cardiovascular control during and after carotid surgery minimizes both cerebral and cardiac complications. Current data suggest that general anesthesia with low-dose isoflurane allows adequate cardiovascular control and minimizes the risk of neurologic injury or myocardial infarction.

SUGGESTED READING

Artru AA, Merriman HG. Hypocapnia added to hypertension to reverse EEG changes during carotid endarterectomy. Anesthesiology 1989; 70:1016–1018.

Cucchiara RF, Sundt TM, Michenfelder JD. Myocardial infarction in carotid endarterectomy patients anesthetized with halothane, enflurane, or isoflurane. Anesthesiology 1989; 69:783–784.

Holmes AE, James IM, Wise CC. Observations on distal intravascular pressure changes and cerebral blood flow after common carotid artery ligation in man. J Neurol Neurosurg Psychiatry 1971; 34:78–81.

McPherson RW, Brian JE Jr, Traystman RJ. Cerebrovascular responsiveness to carbon dioxide in dogs with 1.4 and 2.8 isoflurane. Anesthesiology 1989; 70:843–850.

McPherson RW, Traystman RJ. Effects of isoflurane on cerebral autoregulation in dogs. Anesthesiology 1988; 69:493–499.

Michenfelder JD, Sundt TM, Fode N. Sharbrough FW. Isoflurane when compared to enflurane and halothane decreases the frequency of cerebral ischemia during carotid endarterectomy. Anesthesiology 1987; 67:336–340.

Morawetz RB, Zeiger HE, McDowell HA Jr, et al. Correlation of cerebral blood flow and EEG during carotid occlusion for endarterectomy (without shunting) and neurologic outcome. Surgery 1984; 96:184–189.

Prough DS, Scuderi PE, Stullken E, Davis CH Jr. Myocardial infarction following regional anaesthesia for carotid endarterectomy. Can Anesth Soc 1984; 31:192–196.

Rampil IJ, Holzer JA, Quest DO, et al. Prognostic value of computerized EEG analysis during carotid endarterectomy. Anesth Analg 1983; 62:186–192.

Silbert BS, Koumoundouros EK, Daives MJ, Cronin KD. Comparison of the processed electroencephalogram and awake neurological assessment during carotid endarterectomy. Anaesth Intens Care 1989; 17:298–304.

Smith JS, Roizen MF, Cahalan MK, et al. Does anesthetic technique make a difference? Augmentation of systolic blood pressure during carotid endarterectomy: effects of phenylephrine versus light anesthesia and of isoflurane versus halothane on the incidence of myocardial ischemia. Anesthesiology 1988; 69:846–853.

Young WL, Prohovnik I, Correll JW, et al. Cerebral blood flow and metabolism in patients undergoing anesthesia for carotid endarterectomy: a comparison of isoflurane, halothane, and fentanyl. Anesth Analg 1989; 68:712–717.

ANESTHESIA IN NEUROSURGERY AND NEUROLOGIC DISORDERS

POSTERIOR FOSSA TUMOR

DAVID L. SCHREIBMAN, M.D.
M. JANE MATJASKO, M.D.

Anesthetic management of the patient with a posterior fossa tumor presents the anesthesiologist with an extraordinary challenge. Careful preoperative evaluation and planning and specialized monitoring combined with meticulous surgical and anesthetic technique and attentive postoperative management will maximize neurologic recovery.

ANATOMY

The posterior fossa is enclosed by portions of the sphenoid, occipital, temporal, and parietal bones. The superior boundary is the tentorium cerebelli. It contains one-fourth of the intracranial contents—specifically, the cerebellum, brain stem, cranial nerves III through XII, and the fourth ventricle. The brain stem contains the cranial nerve nuclei, reticular activating formation, ascending sensory and descending motor tracts, and the cardiorespiratory control centers (Fig. 1). The noncompliant and relatively small infratentorial compartment can respond to an increase in volume (tumor, hematoma, edema, obstructive hydrocephalus) by abrupt upward or downward herniation with catastrophic consequences.

PATHOLOGY

Posterior fossa tumor pathology varies according to the age of the patient. Central nervous system neoplasms constitute the second most common cancer of childhood, and 50 percent of pediatric brain tumors occur in the posterior fossa. The most common childhood central nervous system tumor is the benign cerebellar astrocytoma. This slowly growing tumor is usually found in a lateral cerebellar hemisphere and gradually displaces the cerebellum and brain stem. The child may present with nonspecific symptoms or with headache and pro-

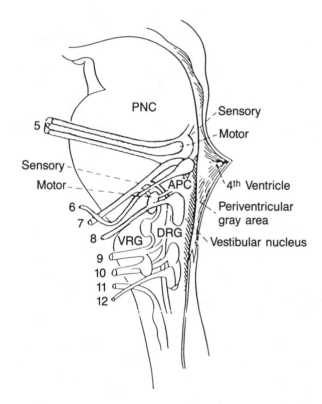

Figure 1 General location of cardiovascular centers (hatched areas), respiratory centers (bold-lettered areas), and cranial nerves in the brain stem. Respiratory centers are designated by the following abbreviations: PNC = pneumotaxic center; APC = apneustic center; DRG = dorsal respiratory group; VRG = ventral respiratory group. (Adapted from Artrou AA, Cucchiara RF, Messick JM. Cardiorespiratory and cranial nerve sequelae of surgical procedures involving the posterior fossa. Anesthesiology 1980; 52:83–86.)

jectile vomiting that may escalate over many months. By contrast, the rapidly growing medulloblastoma arises from midline cerebellar structures and invades the fourth ventricle and surrounding structures, causing symptoms due to obstructive hydrocephalus within 2 months.

The most common adult posterior fossa tumor is metastatic in origin. Metastatic lesions are usually multiple and located in the cerebellar hemispheres.

Cerebellar hemangioblastoma is the most common primary tumor. Cerebellar hematomas are related to long-term systemic hypertension and often constitute an acute neurosurgical emergency.

Brain stem gliomas occur in both adult and pediatric populations. The usual location is the pons, which will appear asymmetric on a computed tomographic (CT) scan. Magnetic resonance imaging (MRI) reveals diffuse tumors to be more frequent than focal tumors. Resection is reserved for discrete tumors, while diffuse tumors are biopsied, usually by a stereotactic technique.

Cerebellopontine angle (CPA) tumors can become as large as 6 cm before producing symptoms for which the patient seeks medical attention, although hearing loss may occur when the tumor is very small. The schwannoma, classically called "acoustic neuroma," tends to arise from the sheath of the vestibular portion of the eighth cranial nerve. CPA tumors may involve multiple adjacent cranial nerves, particularly the trigeminal and facial nerves. It is important to assess the presence of a gag reflex, as its absence will significantly change airway management postoperatively.

SIGNS AND SYMPTOMS

The most common presenting signs and symptoms are related either to the direct effects of the mass itself or to hydrocephalus from obstruction of the fourth ventricle and its outlets. The onset and acuity of presentation depend on the location of the tumor and its speed of growth. Midline tumors present with headache and vomiting, while lateral tumors more often show appendicular cerebellar signs. A slow-growing lateral cerebellar astrocytoma has an insidious onset (years) and its effects may be attributed to migraine, psychological causes, or gastrointestinal disease. Many symptoms occur in the morning as a result of nocturnal hypoventilation and the resultant increased intracranial volume and pressure. Papilledema, headache, vomiting, and ataxia occur in more than 80 percent of the patients.

Headaches are typically frontal at first and become suboccipital as the disease progresses, suggesting tonsillar herniation. They occur more frequently in the morning and may be accompanied by nuchal rigidity. Vomiting, usually projectile and not preceded by nausea, occurs more often during the morning. Persistent vomiting may be indicative of brain stem involvement. Ataxia is often overlooked in children, in whom it is either ignored or described as clumsiness. The ataxia may be accompanied by dysmetria, nystagmus, and a broad-based gait. In lateral cerebellar tumors, the patient veers toward the lesion. Other signs and symptoms of posterior fossa tumor included diplopia from the sixth cranial nerve, palsy, dizziness, morning lethargy, macrocephaly in younger children with unfused sutures that accommodate increased intracranial pressure, cranial nerve palsies, and sudden loss of consciousness.

PREOPERATIVE EVALUATION

The preoperative visit is used to allay anxiety and describe the anesthetic procedures to the patient. The possibility of prolonged intubation as a result of brain stem and cranial nerve dysfunction or postoperative swelling and hydrocephalus is discussed. The use of preoperative sedatives and narcotics is avoided in patients with significant intracranial hypertension because of their exquisite sensitivity to respiratory depressants. In children, a light barbiturate premedication (secobarbital or pentobarbital, 2 mg per kilogram) may be required for particularly anxious patients. Of course, good clinical judgment must be exercised.

Increased intracranial pressure caused by mass effect and hydrocephalus must be closely evaluated. The extent of papilledema may indicate the severity of the reduced intracranial compliance. Herniation (transtentorial or at the foramen magnum) may cause abrupt loss of consciousness. Compression of the superior colliculus causes Parinaud's sign (paralysis of upward gaze). Steroid therapy is used to relieve the symptoms of an infratentorial mass lesion and decrease the need for a preoperative shunting procedure. Hyperglycemia and electrolyte abnormalities are associated with steroid therapy. Cerebrospinal fluid external drainage or shunting procedures were prevalent in the past to ameliorate symptoms of hydrocephalus and allow time for preoperative evaluation and safer anesthetic induction. The risk of upward herniation, tumor seeding, and the small number of patients (20 percent) requiring a postoperative shunt have made preoperative shunting procedures less common.

Tumor location and neurologic deficits must be thoroughly investigated. Dysfunction of cranial nerves IX, X and XII diminish protective airway and respiratory reflexes, which may permit a "silent" aspiration. Involvement of the trigeminal nerve may reduce corneal sensation. The location of the tumor determines whether the operative position will be lateral, prone, or seated. Factors affecting the responses to changes in position, such as cardiovascular disease, hypertension, debility, and obesity should be recognized and treated as necessary to prevent intraoperative hypotension.

The patient with a posterior fossa tumor is often volume-depleted due to vomiting, decreased oral intake, supine diuresis, and the dehydrating effects of intravenous contrast material and mannitol. Preoperative intravenous hydration will optimize cardiovascular stability. Administration of medications such as steroids and histamine$_2$-receptor antagonists should be continued.

MONITORING

Posterior fossa surgery requires the customary monitors used for major neurosurgical procedures: electrocardiogram with appropriate leads for detection of ischemia, intra-arterial blood pressure, pulse oximeter, esophageal stethoscope, temperature probe, urinary catheter, oxygen analyzer, mass spectrometry/capnography (preferably with inspired/end-tidal nitrogen capabilities), and nerve stimulator. Hemodynamic monitoring is begun before induction of anesthesia and continued into the postanesthetic period as necessary. A central venous catheter and precordial Doppler monitor are required during surgery in which the patient is in the sitting position. They may also be required in other positions if significant head-up positioning is planned or if the tumor is vascular or near a major venous sinus. The cardiovascular condition of the patient determines the choice of a central venous versus a pulmonary artery catheter. The presence of sufficient cardiovascular disease is a relative contraindication to the seated position for surgery.

A combination of electrophysiologic monitors—somatosensory evoked potentials (SSEPs) brain stem auditory evoked potentials (BAEPs), and cranial nerve electromyography (EMG)—provides information about multiple vulnerable pathways during posterior fossa surgery (Fig. 2). SSEPs are produced by the stimulation of a peripheral nerve, usually posterior tibial and/or median nerves, and record the evoked response along its course through the ascending posterior columns and brain stem to the cerebral cortex. Compression or ischemia of the brain stem produces attenuation of the amplitude and/or an increase in the latency of the produced potential. BAEPs are performed by applying a click stimulus to each ear, propagating a potential along a diffuse bilateral pathway located exclusively in the pons and midbrain. BAEPs are subcortical in origin since cortical responses to auditory stimuli are not reproducible when the patient is under general anesthesia. If normal or reduced auditory function remains, the BAEP is useful for assessment of eighth nerve function during resection of a CPA tumor. SSEP monitoring is more sensitive and specific for detection of brain stem ischemia than BAEP monitoring. The BAEP is a more global monitor of brain stem integrity by virtue of its bilateral integration. The loss of the bilateral or contralateral BAEP indicates a more ominous neurologic prognosis. An abrupt change in the evoked potentials (i.e., disappearance) has a more disastrous connotation than a gradual change. The presence of cortical air may attenuate the signal acquisition from scalp electrodes. If significant evoked potential changes occur, such as a decrease in amplitude and/or prolongation in latency, the surgeon is advised, a cause for the changes is elicited (e.g., brain stem retraction or ischemia, change in anesthetic depth, hypothermia, hypoxia), and appropriate therapy is instituted.

Electromyography involves the direct stimulation of a cranial nerve in its course through the surgical field and recording the resultant contraction via a needle electrode in the innervated muscle (Fig. 3). The contractions can be visually observed, amplified and viewed on an oscilloscope, recorded on paper, or heard via a loudspeaker. The use of the auditory signal permits the surgeon to have an immediate warning of the proximity of

the monitored nerve to his surgical dissection. Direct stimulation produces a pulse signal while mechanical irritation from surgical dissection results in a burst of electrical activity known as an "injury" potential. Facial and trigeminal nerve EMGs are employed during resection of CPA and laterally located tumors. The use of EMGs has reduced the risk of facial nerve injury during CPA tumor resection, particularly in tumors greater than 4 cm. The accessory nerve EMG is employed for glomus jugulare tumors. Brain stem tumors can involve cranial nerves III, IV, and VI; EMGs of these nerves can be monitored as well.

The effect of individual anesthetic agents on these potentials is beyond the scope of this review. In general, anesthetics increase the latency and decrease the am-

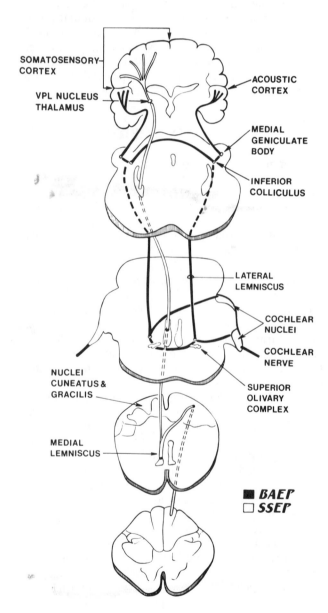

Figure 2 Pathways of the somatosensory- and brain stem auditory-evoked potentials through the brain stem. Note the lateral position and bilateral integration of the BAEP pathway.

plitude of BAEPs and SSEPs. BAEPs are more resistant than SSEPs to these effects because BAEPs are subcortical in origin. We employ a narcotic-based infusion technique to minimize the effects of anesthesia on the evoked potentials. In the past, EMG precluded neuromuscular blockade. However, the use of an atracurium besylate infusion with titration to a 50 percent decrement in the single-twitch amplitude monitored with a nerve stimulator has proven to be satisfactory.

POSITIONING

Tumors in the posterior fossa may be midline or lateral in the cerebellum or lateral to the brain stem (e.g., acoustic neuroma). Some tumors (e.g., meningiomas) may be anterior to the brain stem, surrounding the basilar artery and displacing or stretching many lower cranial nerves. The choice of position is primarily a surgical one. Nonetheless, the anesthesiologist should be prepared to suggest alternative choices of position if warranted by the patient's concomitant disease. For example, severe atherosclerotic or uncontrolled hypertensive disease contraindicates the seated position, while obesity may preclude adequate hemodynamic stability in the prone position. For a tumor located near a major venous sinus, surgery may be more safely performed with the patient in the horizontal rather than seated position (Fig. 4) because of the higher likelihood of significant venous air embolism (VAE).

The seated position offers the advantages of improved venous drainage of the elevated operative site, improved access to the patient compared with the prone position, less blood loss, and better preservation of cranial nerve function. While the incidence of VAE is many times higher with the seated position compared with the horizontal positions, extremely low morbidity and mortality from VAE have been reported in the literature in nearly 9,000 seated patients. Even though the possibility exists for air to reach the arterial circulation via an actual or probe patent foramen ovale or through the pulmonary vessels, appropriate case selection, early detection, and treatment of venous air embolism can render the seated position as safe as horizontal positions. Other complications related to the sitting position include sciatic nerve stretching with extreme hip flexion, and direct compression of the peroneal nerve over the fibular head, both of which result in a foot drop. Failure to support the arms may result in compression of the brachial plexus between the clavicle and the first rib.

Quadriplegia has been reported following extreme neck flexion in the seated position. Presumably, cervical spinal cord ischemia is produced if perfusion pressure is not maintained. The watershed zone in the cervical cord

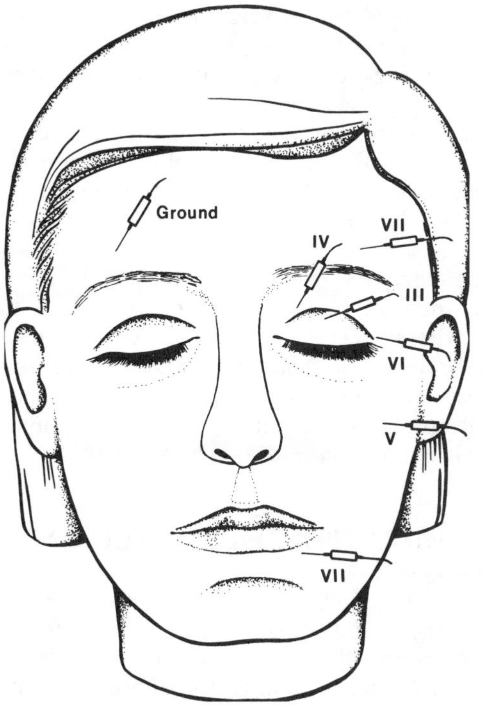

Figure 3 Placement of needle electrodes into the corresponding innervated muscles for recording of cranial nerve EMGs. Cranial nerve III = levator palpebra; cranial nerve IV = superior oblique; cranial nerve V = masseter; cranial nerve VI = lateral rectus; cranial VII = obicularis oris, obicularis oculi, mentalis; cranial nerve XI = sternocleidomastoid, trapezius.

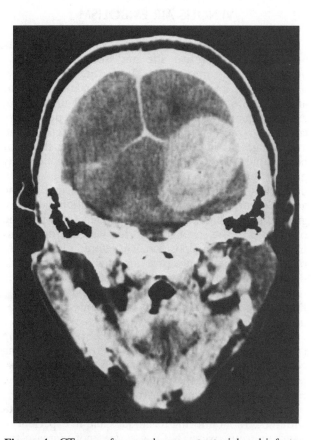

Figure 4 CT scan of a vascular supratentorial and infratentorial meningioma involving the transverse sinus.

circulation is at the C-5 level. Prolonged flexion when the cervical canal is narrowed (<10 mm) due to osteoarthritis is particularly dangerous. If a patient has myelopathic symptoms preoperatively (e.g., spastic gait), evaluation of the cervical spine and spinal cord is performed and the optimal position for intubation and surgery is considered so as to not jeopardize cord perfusion unnecessarily.

Extreme neck flexion may also cause jugular venous obstruction, which can lead to cerebral, tongue, and laryngeal edema and endotracheal tube obstruction. Attention to details of head and neck position as well as protection of the eyes and pressure points are important for sitting, lateral, and prone positions. Careful application of the three-point head clamp is necessary to avoid skull fracture (more likely in children with a thinned cranium caused by long-standing intracranial hypertension), pressure on the eyes, or unexpected head dislodgement because of failure to assure that the pins have penetrated the outer table of the skull. If the seated position is planned, the pin entry points must be wrapped with Vaseline gauze to prevent air entry into emissary or diploic skull veins.

Optimal patient positioning for posterior fossa procedures requires advance planning and a cooperative team approach to avoid patient injury or dislodgement of life support systems.

VENOUS AIR EMBOLISM

VAE is likely when a gradient as small as 5 cm exists between any operative site and the heart. During posterior fossa surgery, most VAEs are of the slow-infusion type, amenable to early detection and treatment and therefore of minimal consequence. If undetected, excessive quantities of air can proceed to the pulmonary circulation where most of the nitrogen is excreted in the alveolar gas. If large quantities of air enter the right heart rapidly, right ventricular outflow obstruction may prevent forward flow. Without left ventricle and coronary artery filling, hypotension, dysrhythmia, and cardiac arrest occur. Once the patient's condition has progressed to this state, resuscitation is unlikely even if the position can be changed to left lateral decubitus head-down (Durant) position. Therefore, it is fortunate that a sensitive noninvasive monitor exists for early detection of VAE. The precordial Doppler placed in the right fourth intercostal space in shorter patients or near the midline lower sternum in taller patients can detect as little as 0.125 ml of air.

In the seated position, the incidence of VAE during craniotomy is between 30 and 40 percent, and during cervical foraminotomy, approximately 10 percent. Most emboli occur within the first hour of surgery when bone removal is performed. Approximately 25 percent of patients with VAE develop hemodynamic changes, but with modern monitoring techniques and in experienced hands, nitrous oxide (N_2O) use does not increase the incidence or severity of VAE.

In addition to the precordial Doppler, monitoring should include end-tidal carbon dioxide ($ETCO_2$). Continuous monitoring of $ETCO_2$ is preferable to intermittent sampling. During VAE, end-tidal nitrogen (ETN_2) increases can occur early and precede decreases in $ETCO_2$ or hemodynamic compromise. Low fresh gas flow in the circle system (e.g., 1 to 1.5 L per minute) allows nitrogen to remain in the circuit and be detected more easily with intermittent sampling. Once changes in precordial Doppler sounds occur, the surgeon should be notified immediately so that hemostatic efforts can proceed. Aspiration through the central line should begin immediately. If the source of air entry cannot be visualized, gentle, short bilateral jugular venous compression frequently allows some back bleeding into the wound so that the vessel can be cauterized or suture-ligated. These maneuvers may eliminate the problem. However, if the source is not apparent and $ETCO_2$ is decreasing and/or vital signs are changing, N_2O, if in use, should be discontinued and the wound packed with gauze saturated with saline. Once vital signs restabilize and $ETCO_2$ and ETN_2 return to normal, systematic inspection of the wound can begin. If recurrent significant emboli occur and the source cannot be identified, the patient should be placed in a horizontal position before surgery is resumed, since there may be an unexpected large and potentially devastating VAE unless the air entry site is eliminated.

Because pulmonary artery pressure increases occur simultaneously with decreases in $ETCO_2$, there is no "early warning" advantage, and the small-bore right atrial orifice does not permit rapid air aspiration compared with a large-bore short central venous line. Transesophageal echocardiography (TEE) is the most sensitive detector of VAE and the only instrument capable of detecting left atrial air. TEE is not widely used because of the expense of the equipment. If arterial air is detected, the hyperbaric chamber, which serves to reduce the size of the nitrogen bubbles, is the only specific therapy. The arterial air may lodge in coronary or cerebral vessels. Small amounts of intracoronary air can result in significant life-threatening arrhythmias, while transient or permanent cerebral ischemia is likely when air enters the carotid-vertebral system.

INTRAOPERATIVE MANAGEMENT

The basic tenets of neuroanesthesia are important during surgery that involves the posterior fossa. Anesthesia must provide brain relaxation, cerebral perfusion in the face of increased intracranial pressure, and stable hemodynamics.

Hydration with a non-glucose–containing balanced salt solution is performed before induction of anesthesia to counteract preoperative dehydration.

Anesthesia is induced with a thiobarbiturate, as this decreases cerebral blood flow, cerebral oxygen consumption, and intracranial pressure in the presence of reduced intracranial compliance. In patients with marked hemodynamic instability, anesthesia is induced with etomidate. After paralysis with a nondepolarizing neuromuscular blocker, a gentle intubation is performed. A balanced N_2O/narcotic technique is employed at our institution, although it is possible to use less than 1 minimum alveolar concentration (MAC) of an isoflurane-based anesthetic. The goal of anesthetic technique is to provide cardiovascular stability that allows intraoperative monitoring of hemodynamic changes that occur during brain stem and cranial nerve manipulation, with a minimal effect on cerebral blood flow, intracranial pressure, and evoked potential monitoring. If preoperative evoked potentials are abnormal, N_2O and volatile anesthetics may attenuate the potential. Before induction of anesthesia, rapid-acting drugs (i.e., esmolol, nitroprusside) should be readily available to treat extremes in blood pressure and pulse that may adversely affect cerebral perfusion.

Controversy exists over the use of N_2O with the patient in the sitting position. However, recent data indicate that its use does not increase morbidity or mortality in seated patients. The presence of N_2O improves the ability to detect embolized venous air. If significant venous air is detected, N_2O is discontinued, and it is avoided in any patient who has undergone a craniotomy within 7 days, since residual intracranial or intraventricular air may expand.

Brain stem integrity can be monitored by hemodynamic changes, respiratory changes, or evoked potentials. Brain stem integrity may be compromised during surgery by direct stimulation (including laser), direct disruption, or indirectly by edema or vascular compromise. There are a myriad of hemodynamic changes noted with brain stem stimulation. Although hypertension and/or tachycardia are the most common of these changes, hypotension, bradycardia, sinus arrhythmia, ventricular ectopy, and asystole have also been seen. Stimulation of the trigeminal nerve produces extreme hypertension, while vagus nerve manipulation causes bradycardia. The surgeon should be advised with regard to this situation; cessation of surgical manipulation usually corrects the problem. Despite adequate muscle relaxation, direct stimulation of cranial nerves VII and XI can result in twitching of the face and shoulder, respectively.

The use of spontaneous ventilation as a monitor of brain stem integrity during posterior fossa craniotomy is also controversial. At our institution, ventilation is controlled to maintain the arterial carbon dioxide pressure ($PaCO_2$) between 25 and 30 mm Hg. The brain stem's cardiac and respiratory centers, although adjacent, are anatomically distinct. The presence of changes in cardiac rhythm, blood pressure, or evoked potentials alerts the anesthesiologist to possible postoperative respiratory difficulties. Because of the risks of hypercarbia or coughing while the head is secured in pins during microscopic surgery, the use of spontaneous ventilation as an intraoperative monitor cannot be justified.

COMPLICATIONS

The postoperative period is fraught with many complications that require intensive management by all concerned in the patient's care. Upon the emergence of the patient from anesthesia, the adequacy of respiration and airway protective reflexes must be carefully assessed. Extubation should only be entertained in an awake, alert patient with spontaneous ventilation and intact cough and gag reflexes. Intravenous lidocaine has been used to prevent hypertensive response during this evaluation. The lack of spontaneous ventilation may be caused by injury to the brain stem respiratory center. Macroglossia or hypoglossal nerve damage can lead to airway obstruction. Macroglossia can be purely mechanical (i.e., venous obstruction), or it may be a brain stem reflex. Injury to the hypoglossal nerve, which provides motor innervation to the tongue, leads to retropositioning of that structure with airway obstruction. Loss of protective airway reflexes is due to glossopharyngeal afferent or vagal efferent innervation injury. During the immediate postoperative period, hypertension may lead to an increased incidence of hemorrhage or edema in the surgical site. Rapid-acting drugs (esmolol, nitroprusside) should be readily available to reduce or prevent extreme hypertension. The major concern is the maintenance of an adequate, but not excessive, cerebral perfusion pressure.

Failure to emerge from anesthesia or a rapidly deteriorating neurologic status may occur during the postoperative period as a result of bleeding, edema, infarction, hydrocephalus, or pneumocephalus. Vascular compromise may occur from direct manipulation or retraction of brain stem blood vessels, leading to brain stem infarction. Patients with a deterioration in neurologic status should be intubated and hyperventilated, and should undergo CT scanning to determine the cause of the problem. Bleeding in the operative site that causes compression of the brain stem is an operative emergency. A subdural hematoma may form in the supratentorial compartment from tearing of bridging veins because of rapid cerebrospinal fluid decompression or brain sag in the seated position. Epidural hematomas caused by skull fracture from pin placement have been seen in pediatric patients.

Cerebellar edema frequently occurs after posterior fossa surgery. This is treated by intubation, hyperventilation, placing the patient in a 30-degree head-up position, and infusing mannitol to decrease the intracranial pressure. Hydrocephalus during the postoperative period may be communicating or noncommunicating. Neurosurgeons frequently place a parietal or occipital burr hole intraoperatively for emergency drainage of cerebrospinal fluid should this be necessary. Approximately 20 percent of the patients will require a postoperative cerebrospinal fluid shunting procedure to treat persistent hydrocephalus.

Pneumocephalus is nearly always found after a craniotomy regardless of the position of the head during surgery, but it is found much more commonly when the ventricular system is open to the atmosphere. As cerebrospinal fluid leaks out of the wound, air enters to replace it. Tension pneumocephalus is a rare but potentially devastating complication and does not appear to be more common when N_2O is used throughout the procedure. Of course, when the cranium is closed readdition of N_2O to the inspired gas can cause the air space to expand. Skull films or a CT scan will diagnose tension pneumocephalus, and aggressive therapy requires decompression of the entrapped air through a burr hole.

Seizures have an incidence of less than 10 percent in these patients, and anticonvulsant prophylaxis is not necessary. Hyperthermia occurs frequently during the first 24 hours after surgery due to blood in the fourth ventricle. Aseptic meningitis is a late complication of posterior fossa exploration due to intraoperative contamination of the fourth ventricle by blood, surgical debris, or cyst fluid.

SUGGESTED READING

Artu AA, Cucchiara RF, Messick JM. Cardiorespiratory and cranial nerve sequelae of surgical procedures involving the posterior fossa. Anesthesiology 1980; 52:83–86.

Black S, Ockert DB, Oliver WC, Cucchiara RF. Outcome following posterior fossa craniectomy in patients in the sitting or horizontal positions. Anesthesiology 1988; 69:49–56.

Drummond JC, Todd MM. Acute sinus arrhythmia during surgery in the fourth ventricle: An indication of brain stem irritation. Anesthesiology 1984; 60:232–235.

Gorski DW, Rao TLK, Scarff TB. Airway obstruction following surgical manipulation of the posterior fossa, an unusual complication. Anesthesiology 1981; 54:80–81.

Hahn JF, Latchaw JP. Evoked potentials in the operating room. Clin Neurosurg 1983; 31:389–403.

Harner SG, Daube JR, Ebersold MJ, Beaty CW. Improved preservation of facial nerve function with use of electrical monitoring during removal of accoustic neuromas. Mayo Clin Proc 1987; 62:92–102.

Lall NG, Jain AP. Ciculatory and respiratory disturbances during posterior fossa surgery. Br J Anaesth 1969; 41:447.

Losasso TJ, Mussi DA, Black S, Cucchiara RF. The "risk" of nitrous oxide in sitting neurosurgical patients: a prospective, randomized study. Anesthesiology 1989; 71:A1137.

Matjasko J, Petrozza P, Cohen M, Steinberg P. Anesthesia and surgery in the seated position: analysis of 554 cases. Neurosurgery 1985; 17:695–702.

Moore JK, Chaudhri S, Moore AP, Easton J. Macroglossia and posterior fossa disease. Anaesthesia 1988; 43:382–385.

Raudzens PA, Shetter AG. Intraoperative monitoring of brain stem auditory evoked potentials. J Neurosurg 1982; 57:341–348.

CENTRAL NERVOUS SYSTEM ANEURYSM

ELIZABETH A. M. FROST, M.D.

Saccular or berry aneurysms develop at arterial bifurcations, probably from medial defects, in patients of all ages who are past puberty. Contrary to previous beliefs, the disease is probably acquired rather than congenital. Evidence for this is based on the failure to find aneurysms on autopsy of infant brains and on the clinical observation that aneurysms are associated with angiographically visible atheromas that form on the internal elastic lamina. There is no racial predilection; however, women are affected slightly more often than men. The genesis has no demonstrable relationship to atherosclerosis, arteritis, or hypertension, although a higher incidence has been associated with smoking. Rarely, mycotic aneurysms may be formed, usually as a complication of heart valve vegetations, associated rheumatic fever, or intravenous drug abuse, or by adhesion of septic emboli to arterial walls that cause necrosis. Traumatic aneurysms develop as a result of direct trauma to an artery. The factors that cause aneurysms to enlarge or rupture are not well defined.

Bleeding may occur at times of extreme physical exercise or, conversely during sleep. An association between rupture and "crack" abuse has been noted.

The most common locations for the occurrence of aneurysms are shown in Table 1. The most frequent sites are on the anterior portions of the cerebral arterial supply. Anterior communicating and internal carotid artery aneurysms are the ones most likely to rupture. Multiple aneurysms occur in 20 percent of patients.

Intracranial aneurysms occur in 5 to 8 percent of the population and are symptomatic in approximately 1 percent. Approximately 25,000 patients annually suffer subarachnoid hemorrhage (SAH). Multiple aneurysms have been identified in 30 percent of these patients. The immediate mortality after rupture of an aneurysm is 43 percent. With conservative management, 35 percent of

Table 1 Incidence of Aneurysms at Various Locations

Site	Incidence (%)
Internal carotid	38
Anterior cerebral system	36
Anterior communicating junction	30
Internal carotid at posterior communicating junction	25
Middle cerebral system	21
Vertebrobasilar system	5

survivors die after another bleed that occurs within 1 year, and 51 percent die within 5 years from complications of the aneurysm. The mortality rate is greatest after recurrent hemorrhage; 64 percent of patients die after the first rebleed and 96 percent die after the second. Neurologic deficits occur in 30 percent of survivors.

Of the approximately 30 percent of patients who undergo surgical intervention, about 10 percent die or are severely impaired. In the nonoperated group, mortality and morbidity figures exceed 60 percent. Outcome is closely related to the initial condition of the patient. A summary of the grading (Botterell, Hess, Hunt and Miller)is as follows:

Grade I: Asymptomatic; minimal headache.
Grade II: Moderate headache; nuchal rigidity; no neurologic deficit except that relating to a cranial nerve.
Grade III: Confusion; facial deficit.
Grade IV: Coma; hemiparesis.
Grade V: Moribund

Perioperative care is aimed at the prevention of further neurologic deficits, which may be caused by vasospasm, rebleeding, intracerebral hematoma, or seizures. Other complications such as hyperglycemia, hyponatremia, or sepsis must be avoided.

REBLEEDING

Following rupture, a clot forms over the dome of the aneurysm. The fibrinolytic activity of cerebrospinal fluid can prevent closure of the leak and cause rebleeding. Several antifibrinolytic agents have been used to inhibit this dissolution. Studies of patients treated with tranexamic acid indicate a lower incidence of rebleeding, which is offset by a higher frequency of cerebral infarction and the development of hydrocephalus that requires shunt replacement. Systemic thrombotic complications of antifibrinolytic therapy, such as subendocardial myocardial infarction and deep venous thrombosis, may occur. Side effects of a similar drug, epsilon-aminocaproic acid, include bradycardia, hypotension, resistance to atropine, and electrocardiographic changes. Thus, for patients to benefit from antifibrinolytic therapy, complications must be minimized without compromising the prevention of rebleeding. Currently, the use of antifibrinolytic therapy has been replaced by other medical therapies including maintenance of normotension, deliberate fluid expansion, adequate oxygenation, and vigilant monitoring in an intensive care unit setting. The incidence of deep vein thrombosis may be reduced by external pneumatic cuff compression. Should deep venous thrombosis develop, an inferior vena cava umbrella should be inserted, as anticoagulation is contraindicated in most neurosurgical patients.

CARDIOVASCULAR ASSESSMENT

Although many patients are hypertensive following SAH, this finding is probably a consequence rather than a cause of the bleeding. Critical to the prevention of rebleeding is control of transmural pressure (TMP) or cerebral perfusion pressure across the aneurysm. (TMP=mean arterial pressure [MAP]−intracranial pressure [ICP]). Maintenance of normotension is achieved by bed rest and administration of sedatives or antihypertensive agents. Such drugs as hydralazine, sodium nitropruside, or nitroglycerine, although rapidly effective in reducing blood pressure, cause cerebral vasodilation, increase ICP, and reduce TMP. Alternative agents include propranolol, labetalol, methyldopa, or hydrochlorothiazide. However, great care should be used in prescribing diuretic therapy, as reduced extracellular volume may predispose the patient to hyponatremia and vasospasm; a possible exception is the patient to whom these drugs have previously been given. In patients in whom hypertension and intracerebral hematoma coexist, acute lowering of the blood pressure, especially if combined with administering mannitol to decrease cerebral edema, may cause further bleeding of the aneurysm into the subarachnoid space. Emergency therapy includes evacuation of the hematoma and clipping of the aneurysm.

Many electrocardiographic (ECG) abnormalities have been associated with blood in the subarachnoid space, the most common being prolonged QT intervals, prominent U waves, and ST wave, T wave, and occasionally, Q wave abnormalities. These patterns are probably related to catecholamine release that is caused by direct stimulation of the hypothalamus or cardiac centers of the brain stem. Occasionally, vasospasm and hemorrhage in small hypothalamic perforating vessels may be related to subendocardial myocardial damage. The patient rarely complains of cardiac symptoms, and enzyme analyses are usually within normal limits. If the patient has a history of cardiac disease, however, further assessment of hemodynamic status by pulmonary artery catheter monitoring, isoenzyme determination, and myocardial nuclear scanning is indicated. Close communication between neurosurgeon, anesthesiologist, cardiologist, and laboratory specialist is essential in order to avoid unnecessary delay in clipping the aneurysm.

Ventricular irregularities may be treated with titrated doses of propranolol to maintain a heart rate of approximately 60 beats per minute.

Respiratory Care

A close association between smoking and SAH has been demonstrated. Preoperative assessment of lung function should include documentation of arterial blood gas values. Pulmonary shunt is increased by both general anesthetics and controlled hypotension. Thus, if baseline values are low, it is prudent to increase the content of inspired oxygen that is administered to modify the degree and duration of the hypotension, to perform frequent blood gas analyses, and to be prepared to adjust ventilatory parameters as necessary.

Although vigorous respiratory therapy exercises should be avoided prior to securing the aneurysm, simple bedside maneuvers can be performed to familiarize the patient with the available equipment. Certainly the patient must be encouraged to stop smoking immediately, as even cessation for 24 hours decreases carboxyhemoglobin levels.

In extreme cases, when the patient is comatose, an impeccable airway must be secured as atraumatically as possible in order to avoid any increase in ICP or change in TMP.

ANESTHETIC MANAGEMENT

Adequate preanesthetic sedation is essential and is achieved by reassurance and pharmacologic means. Ten milligrams of diazepam, given orally approximately 1 hour before the patient arrives in the operative room, is usually adequate. Premedication with atropine is unnecessary since the unpleasant dry-mouth sensation and the tachycardia that are produced outweigh its beneficial effects. Oral administration of propranolol approximately 1 to 1.5 hours preoperatively significantly reduced the hypertensive response to intubation and pinhead insertion.

The primary goals of the anesthetic technique are to maintain a stable transmural pressure and to provide maximal brain relaxation, as visualization of the aneurysm usually requires considerable lobar retraction.

Induction of anesthesia must be achieved with minimal elevation of systemic arterial pressure. During oxygenation, thiopental sodium, 3 to 5 mg per kilogram, and lidocaine, 1 to 5 mg per kilogram, should be given slowly. Also, 1 mg of propranolol may be given intravenously. Adequate muscle relaxation can be achieved with atracurium besylate, 0.5 mg per kilogram, or vecuronium bromide, 0.1 mg per kilogram. Prior to intubation, the cords should be anesthetized by local spraying with 4 ml of 4 percent lidocaine. Anesthesia may be continued with isoflurane 1 percent in air and oxygen. The use of nitrous oxide should be avoided, as this agent increases both cerebral blood flow and metabolism, increases the size of any gas bubbles entrained during surgery, and potentiates the development of tension pneumocephalus. In order to maintain levels of isoflurane that are not deleterious to intracranial dynamics yet allow adequate anesthesia, a continuous infusion of narcotic should be given. Adequate anesthetic depth is achieved by adding fentanyl, 1.5 to 2 µg per kilogram per hour, after a loading dose of 2 µg per kilogram. A reasonable substitute is a sufentanil infusion, 0.2 µg per kilogram per hour, again following an initial bolus injection of 0.2 to 0.3 µg per kilogram. It is important to ensure complete muscle relaxation before administration of even small amounts of these potent narcotics, as thoracic rigidity can increase ICP by 200 to 300 percent.

Routine monitoring includes trend indication by recording the electrocardiogram, arterial blood pressure, temperature, capnograph, pulse oximeter, and fluid balance. Automated data recording ensures accurate records at a time when manual notations may be impractical. Documentation of evoked potentials may also provide important information. Frequently, a needle or catheter is inserted into the lumbar subarachnoid space as a conduit to drain cerebrospinal fluid (CSF) intraoperatively, thereby decreasing intracranial contents. Before the dura is opened, this system may be used to measure spinal subarachnoid pressure. During the course of surgery, more than 100 ml of CSF may be drained. As this volume is quickly replaced postoperatively, and to decrease the risk of infection, the fluid should not be replaced.

The stimulation associated with insertion of the pinhead holder may be mitigated by injection of local anesthesia to the scalp. Also, prior to skin incision, infiltration with 1 percent lidocaine is recommended. Epinephrine should not be added to this solution, since delayed absorption (some 30 minutes later) may cause significant increase in blood pressure—especially in patients maintained on propranolol.

Before the dura is opened, brain volume is reduced by administration of mannitol, 0.5 mg per kilogram, plus furosemide, 0.5 mg per kilogram.

Dissection around the aneurysm may be facilitated by reduction of the blood pressure to increase pliability. Controlled hypotension is best achieved using sodium nitroprusside (SNP) up to 0.4 µg per kilogram per hour. This infusion should not be started until the aneurysm is in view on the monitor. Frequent monitoring of acid-base status is essential to warn of developing cyanide toxicity. Trimethaphan (0.1 percent solution infusion), which has also been used to reduce blood pressure, may cause marked tachycardia, tachyphylaxis, respiratory depression, and pupillary changes. Hypotension that is induced with nitroglycerin may be slightly harder to control. There is also a higher incidence of failed response with nitroglycerin (0.5 to 1.5 µg per kilogram per minute) than is seen with SNP. Adenosine triphosphate (ATP) has a rapid, brief hypotensive action. It does not cause tachycardia or tachyphylaxis. Cerebral blood flow is not altered.

The current trend, however, seems to be away from the use of controlled hypotension. Using temporary clips in aneurysm exposures has minimized and often eliminated the need for systemic hypotension. Temporary clips have a smaller closing force than permanent clips and use a blade design that allows easy placement around vessels and aneurysms. The smaller closing force prevents intimal damage.

Fluid replacement should be done with nonglucose–containing solutions, because the size of a cerebral infarct may be increased in the presence of hyperglycemia. Areas at risk include parts of the brain under the retractors or those supplied by vessels that are necessarily sacrificed during dissection. At all times during manipulation of the aneurysm, blood should be immediately available in case the vessel ruptures. Usually control of bleeding may be achieved by placing a temporary clip. It may be necessary to reduce the systemic arterial pressure briefly to very low levels.

Oxygen administration and monitoring should continue during transfer of the patient to the postanesthetic care unit. If the patient is awake and neurologically intact preoperatively, the same state should be realized immediately after surgery. As the defect is now secured, greater flexibility is possible. The patient should be encouraged to breathe deeply, cough, and move around. In order to decrease the risk of vasospasm, vascular volume should be maintained, and blood pressure should be readjusted to approximately 20 mm Hg above what is the normal value for the individual patient. Optimal rheologic conditions are realized at hematocrit values of approximately 30 percent.

CEREBRAL ISCHEMIA

Rupture of an aneurysm forces blood into the subarachnoid space at the high pressure (70 to 110 mm Hg). As intracranial pressure increases, cerebral perfusion pressure decreases. The presence of blood in the subarachnoid space has been shown experimentally to cause acute vasospasm of short duration (5 to 30 minutes), which is followed by a period of vascular relaxation. A second delayed, long-lasting arterial spasm then develops. In humans, this second stage usually starts on the second or third day after rupture (45 percent of patients), but may be delayed for 10 to 14 days. Spasm usually persists for 7 to 10 days, but may persist for up to 4 weeks. Mentally, patients are drowsy-to-comatose and may exhibit focal neurologic deficits. Although a decreased sensorium is usually associated with vasospasm, considerable arterial constriction has been demonstrated in intact individuals.

Cerebral vasospasm is an exaggerated reaction to vasoconstricting substances such as catecholamines, 5-hydroxytryptamine, angiotensin, bradykinin, histamine, substance P, prostaglandins, calcium, or hemoglobin and its breakdown products. The presence or absence of vasospasm on angiographic studies has frequently determined the timing of aneurysmal surgery. However, current neurosurgical practice suggests that a good outcome is achieved by early operation (within 24 to 48 hours) in patients who are neurologically intact (Grades I to II), regardless of whether vasospasm has been demonstrated (a good outcome is seen in 91 percent of Grade I patients and 73 percent of Grade II patients). Such emergency intervention decreases the likelihood of rebleeding. There is no need for other "traditional" therapies such as administration of antifibrinolytics, sedatives, antihypertensives, bedrest, or fluid restriction, which may cause further complications. However, only 53 percent of Grade III patients achieve a good outcome after early surgery, thereby indicating that the gross neurologic condition preoperatively is the best prognostic indicator of intact survival. Certainly, during the first few days following hemorrhage, the brain is swollen, soft, hyperemic, and prone to contusion and laceration. Impaired autoregulation may decrease cerebral tolerance to retractor pressure. Although removal of subarachnoid clot probably decreases the incidence and severity of delayed arterial narrowing, clearly operative management may be hazardous. In more severely injured patients (Grades III to V), surgery is often delayed in anticipation of resolution of vasospasm and improvement in neurologic status.

Many therapeutic regimens have been developed for decreasing vasospasm. The lack of reproducible beneficial effect may be due to the time-related change of causes of vasospasm. Immediate extravascular blood causes acute cerebral vasoconstriction, which is short-lived and probably a protective mechanism, and is not the phenomenon that peaks 7 to 10 days later. During the acute phase, early vasospasm is readily reversed by vasodilators like SNP. Delayed vasospasm is not. Current data suggest that delayed vasospasm is related more to an anatomic defect, with severe intimal damage, platelet deposits, and endothelial thickening.

Therapeutic prevention of vasospasm is more likely than reversal of the complication once it is established. Work has focused on calcium-entry blockers, specifically nimodipine and nicardipine. These drugs may work either by improving cerebral blood flow or by improving the brain's tolerance to ischemia. A multicenter trial showed that after SAH, patients of Grades III to V had better outcomes after nimodipine therapy (29 percent good outcome at 3 months versus 10 percent in a placebo group). Delayed ischemic deficits occurred in 7 percent of the nimodipine-treated patients compared with 27 percent in those receiving placebo. The beneficial effect does not appear to be preventive of large vessel spasm. When angiography was performed on or about the 8th day after SAH (the study was begun 96 hours posthemorrhage), there was no difference in the incidence of diffuse spasm between the two groups (64 percent for nimodipine-treated patients, 66 percent for those receiving placebo). Although theoretically nimodicarpine preferentially blocks the calcium channels in the heart, this drug has also been shown to have beneficial effects in the treatment of vasospasm.

Other therapeutic regimens include the use of reserpine, 0.2 mg subcutaneously, to reduce the effect of 5-hydroxytryptamine, and kanamycin, 1 g orally three times daily, for its direct vasodilating effect.

Some beneficial results in the effort to reduce late vasospasm have been achieved by means of establishing moderate hypertension and decreasing blood viscosity. Other therapeutic maneuvers have included the use of beta-agonist, alpha- and beta-adrenergic blockers, dopamine hydroxylase inhibitors, serotonin antagonists, nitrites, phosphodiesterase inhibitors, local anesthetics, nonsteroid anti-inflammatory drugs, and stellate ganglion blockade. None of these measures have proven successful on repeated trials.

Giant Aneurysm

Very large aneurysms (>3 cm) may present as space-occupying lesions. Therapy may involve slow ligation of the carotid artery combined with simultaneous or subsequent extracranial-to-intracranial anastomosis. Other techniques use extreme hypothermia or prolonged attempts at cauterization to decrease the size of the defect.

Subarachnoid Hemorrhage Associated with Pregnancy

SAH secondary to a ruptured aneurysm or arteriovenous malformation reportedly causes 12 to 24 percent of maternal deaths. The incidence is estimated to range from one in 2,500 to 1 in 10,000 pregnancies. Aneurysms tend to rupture during the 30th to 40th gestational week and immediately postpartum. Increased blood volume and cardiac output may be contributing causes. The clinical picture resembles severe toxemia with hypertension, proteinuria, headache, and coma.

If surgery to secure the aneurysm is unavoidable during pregnancy, the anesthetic goals include maternal safety, avoidance of teratogenic drugs, fetal well-being, and uterine stability. In terms of anesthetic management, the important physiologic changes in these patients include a 20 percent reduction of functional residual capacity at term and a 20 percent increased oxygen consumption, making the rapid development of hypoxia an ever-present hazard. Cardiac output increased by 30 to 40 percent, and patients develop a relative anemia as the plasma volume increased by 40 percent and red blood cell volume by 20 percent. Aortocaval compression may cause severe hypotension in the supine position, and uterine displacement must be continued during anesthesia.

Inhalational requirements are reduced during pregnancy, as is the effective dose of succinylcholine. Dosage schedules should be adjusted downward. Osmotic diuretics cross the placenta and decrease fetal blood and extracellular volumes, and may cause severe fetal dehydration. Controlled hypotension with SNP has been used successfully. An external Doppler fetal heart rate monitor and an external tocodynamometer should be used in addition to the routine monitors.

NONOPERATIVE CARE

The long-term survival of patients who have recovered from a ruptured aneurysm is signficantly lower than that of the general population. The 10-year survival of patients with posterior circle aneurysms is better than that of patients with anterior circle aneurysms. Although patients with multiple aneurysms have a higher rate of early mortality, the long-term prognosis of these patients does not differ significantly from that of patients with single aneurysms. During the first decade, rebleeding is a significant risk in all patients with aneurysms. The rate of rebleed decreases thereafter to 0.86 percent per year (2.2 percent per year), and thus patients are more likely to succumb to other diseases. Reported rebleeding episodes are fatal in approximately 80 percent of cases. Thus, although surgical management offers a better prognosis, patients who present with other management problems (e.g., a Jehovah's Witness with sickle cell disease or an AIDS patient) may have a greater life expectancy with conservative therapy that includes blood pressure control, cessation of smoking, and avoidance of stressful situations.

SUGGESTED READING

Fox JL. Intracranial aneurysms. New York: Springer Verlag, 1983: 19–26.

Heiskanen O. Risks of surgery from unruptured intracranial aneurysm. J Neurosurg 1986; 65:451–453.

Jacobs GB, Frost EAM. The management of cerebrovascular disease. In: Frost E, ed. Clinical anesthesia in neurosurgery. 2nd ed. Boston: Butterworths, 1990.

Lichtenfeld PJ, Rubin DB, Foldman RS. Subarachnoid hemorrhage precipitated by cocaine snorting. Arch Neurol 1984; 41:223–334.

Petruk KC, West M. Mohr G, et al. Nimodipine treatment in poor-grade aneurysm patients. Results of a multi-center double-blind placebo-controlled trial. J Neurosurg 1988; 68:505–517.

Spetzer RF, Hadley MN, Rigamonti D, et al. Aneurysms of the basilar artery treated with circulatory arrest hypothermia and barbiturate cerebral protection. J Neurosurg 1988; 68:868–879.

Winn HR, Almaani WS, Berga SL, et al. The long-term outcome in patients with multiple aneurysms. J Neurosurg 1983; 59:642–651.

PITUITARY TUMOR

AUDRÉE A. BENDO, M.D.
JAMES E. COTTRELL, M.D.

A pituitary tumor may first become evident because of symptoms related to mass effects, hormonal effects (hyperfunction or hypofunction of the pituitary), or as an incidental finding following skull films. Preoperative preparations, evaluation, and perioperative management of patients with pituitary tumors are challenging to the anesthesiologist because of tumor location and the potential for hormonal derangements. This chapter reviews the anesthetic implications of pituitary tumor surgery.

ANATOMY AND PHYSIOLOGY

The pituitary gland is located at the base of the skull in the sella turcica, a bony cavity within the sphenoid bone. It is divided into anterior (adenohypophysis) and posterior (neurohypophysis) lobes. The anterior bony margin of the sella is the tuberculum sella, and the posterior margin is the dorsum sella. The anterior and posterior clinoids are laterally placed, at the front and back, respectively. The superior surface of the sella is a fold of dura (the diaphragma sella) that is pierced by the infundibular stalk, which connects the posterior lobe to the hypothalamus.

Certain anatomic landmarks of the sella are important. The cavernous sinuses, which occupy the lateral walls of the sella, are traversed by the carotid arteries and cranial nerves III, IV, and VI. The optic chiasm with its associated optic nerves and tracts lies directly above the diaphragma sella in front of the pituitary stalk.

The hypothalamus regulates hormone release from the anterior pituitary through regulatory peptides (hypothalamic releasing and inhibiting factors) that reach the anterior pituitary by a complex portal vascular system. Control of hypothalamic secretion is complex and occurs from neuronal and chemical influences. The neural impulses originate from higher brain centers and are mediated by neurotransmitters such as dopamine, norepinephrine, and serotonin. The chemical influences include the anterior pituitary hormones, target gland hormones, and metabolic fuels (glucose, amino acids, and fatty acids).

The larger glandular anterior pituitary secretes at least seven hormones. The anterior pituitary hormones and hypothalamic regulatory hormones are listed in Table 1. The smaller posterior pituitary secretes two hormones: vasopressin (ADH) and oxytocin. These hormones are synthesized in specialized hypothalamic neurons, transported along axons down the pituitary stalk, and stored in the posterior pituitary gland.

CLINICAL DISORDERS

Based on clinical findings, pituitary tumors can be divided into two categories: nonfunctioning and hypersecreting.

Table 1 Anterior Pituitary Hormones and Hypothalamic Regulatory Hormones

Anterior Pituitary Hormones	Hypothalmic Regulatory Hormones
Growth hormone	Growth hormone release-inhibiting hormone (somatostatin) Growth hormone-releasing factor
Prolactin	Prolactin-releasing factor
Gonadotropins: Follicle-stimulating hormone Luteinizing hormone	Gonadotropin-releasing factor
Adrenocorticotropic hormone Beta-lipotropin	Corticotropin-releasing factor(s)
Thyroid-stimulating hormone	Thyrotropin-releasing hormone Somatostain

Nonfunctioning Tumors

Nonsecreting pituitary tumors are usually diagnosed when they become large enough to produce mass effects by impinging on adjacent structures. Extension can occur into the suprasellar space, sphenoid sinuses, cavernous sinuses, or median temporal lobes resulting in headache, impaired vision, cranial nerve palsies, increased intracranial pressure (ICP), and hypopituitarism. The most common nonfunctioning tumors are chromophobe adenomas, craniopharyngiomas, and meningiomas.

Pituitary tumors can cause selective or global impairment of pituitary function. Although clinically silent in adults, growth hormone (GH) secretion is most vulnerable. In children, GH deficiency results in severe growth failure. Clinical gonadotropin deficiency with amenorrhea in the female or impotence in the male is observed relatively early, because the gonadotropin is also very sensitive to pressure effects. Thyroid-stimulating hormone (TSH) and adrenocorticotropic hormone (ACTH) secretion are usually more resistant to this pressure effect. As the pituitary tumor enlarges, however, hypothyroidism and cortisol deficiency develop. Preoperative diabetes insipidus, although rare, is seen in children with large craniopharyngiomas.

A sudden enlargement of the pituitary caused by spontaneous hemorrhage or infarction into the tumor is referred to as pituitary apoplexy. It is a life-threatening condition characterized by an excruciating headache, cranial nerve deficits, meningeal symptoms, and loss of consciousness. Hypopituitarism and hypotension may also occur. Therapy includes rapid administration of corticosteroids and emergency surgical decompression.

Hypersecreting Tumors

Functioning pituitary adenomas produce an excess of one or more of the hormones of the anterior pituitary. Because of the effects of excessive hormone secretion, patients are usually diagnosed when the tumors are small. The most frequently occurring are prolactin (PRL) and GH- and ACTH-secreting adenomas, with prolactinomas being the most common and ACTH-secreting adenomas the least common. Adenomas secreting TSH or follicle-stimulating hormone (FSH) and luteinizing hormone (LH) are rare. Adenomas secreting both GH and PRL are common, however. Clinical features of hypersecreting pituitary tumors are presented in Table 2. The most significant to the anesthesiologist are the GH- and ACTH-secreting adenomas, which cause acromegaly and Cushing's disease, respectively.

Acromegaly

Excessive production of GH in adults causes acromegaly. Gigantism results from excessive GH production in adolescents, since the epiphyses of the long bones have not closed. Patients with acromegaly exhibit a general overgrowth of skeletal, connective, and soft tissues. Hands and feet become markedly enlarged and

Table 2 Clinical Features of Hypersecreting Pituitary Tumors

Hormonal excess	Syndrome	Clinical features
Prolactin	Amenorrhea-galactorrhea	Amenorrhea or oligomenorrhea; variable galactorrhea; infertility; impotence; decreased libido.
Growth hormone	Acromegaly	Enlarged hands, feet, organs; hypertrophy of facial bones; peripheral neuropathies; gigantism (prepubertal); hypertension; cardiomyopathy; diabetes mellitus; skeletal muscle weakness.
Adrenocorticotropic hormone	Cushing's disease	Truncal obesity; "moon facies"; "buffalo hump"; supraclavicular fat pads; abdominal striae; ecchymoses; hirsuitism; emotional disorders; hypertension; hyperglycemia; osteoporosis.
Thyroid-stimulating hormone	TSH-secreting adenoma (rare)	Features of hyperthyroidism (weight loss, tachycardia, tremor, heat intolerance).
Luteinizing hormone, Follicle-stimulating hormone	LH and/or FSH-secreting adenoma (rare)	No known specific clinical features.

facial features become coarse. All major organs increase in size, including the heart, lungs, liver, and kidneys. Other systemic effects are hypertension, insulin-resistant diabetes mellitus, cardiomegaly associated with an infiltrating lymphocytic cardiomyopathy, and coronary artery disease. If untreated, acromegaly is associated with a markedly increased death rate, with the most frequent cause of death being cardiac complications. Peripheral neuropathies and severe arthritic disease also occur and may predispose the acromegalic patient to postarterial cannulation thrombosis.

The most specific diagnostic test for acromegaly is measurement of GH before and after glucose administration. Normally, glucose suppresses the GH level. In patients with acromegaly, GH is not suppressed and occasionally increases.

Treatment of acromegaly depends on the stage at which the disease is detected. If suprasellar extension of the tumor exists, the conventional transcranial surgical approach is indicated. For small tumors, the transsphenoidal approach is recommended. This approach is associated with lower morbidity (hypopituitarism and diabetes insipidus) and mortality rates than either radiation or transcranial excision. Management of anesthesia in acromegalic patients involves careful attention to the symptoms produced by GH excess, with particular attention to airway management.

Significant anatomic airway changes can occur in acromegalics, making airway management difficult. Facial bone hypertrophy, particularly of the mandible and nose, thick tongue and lips, and hypertrophy of nasal turbinates, soft palate, tonsils, epiglottis, and larynx create difficulties with mask fit and visualization of the larynx. Glottic stenosis caused by soft tissue overgrowth may cause preoperative hoarseness and dyspnea. Besides requiring the use of a smaller endotracheal tube than anticipated based on the size of the patient's facial

features, these patients may be predisposed to post-extubation edema. Vocal cord paralysis may also be present as a result of stretching or compression of the recurrent laryngeal nerves from laryngeal soft tissue enlargement or thyroid gland enlargement.

Because of these anatomic changes, a thorough preoperative airway examination is required. Patients complaining of hoarseness, dyspnea, and/or inspiratory stridor should undergo indirect laryngoscopy and x-ray examination of the neck to analyze airway conformation and lumen diameter. Preparations for difficult airway management and intubation should be anticipated based on this evaluation. Patients without upper airway or vocal cord involvement can be managed in the routine manner. In certain individuals, however, awake or fiberoptic intubation is necessary. For transsphenoidal procedures, only oral intubation is considered, because a nasal tube would obstruct the surgical field. An elective intubation with a fiberoptic laryngoscope is recommended for patients with difficult airways and glottic abnormalities, which obviates the need for tracheostomy in all but the most severe cases.

Cushing's Disease

Cushing's disease develops from an ACTH-secreting pituitary adenoma that causes bilateral adrenal hyperplasia. The term Cushing's syndrome refers to the typical disease complex originally described by Cushing in 1932 and includes Cushing's disease (pituitary adenoma), adrenal adenoma or carcinoma, and ectopic or exogenous ACTH-induced adrenal hyperplasia.

Laboratory confirmation of Cushing's disease is made by measuring elevated serum cortisol, ACTH, and urinary-free cortisol levels. The serum cortisol lacks diurnal variation and is suppressed by large doses of dexamethasone. Serum ACTH is also suppressed after high-dose dexamethasone administration and increases after metyrapone administration.

The clinical features of Cushing's disease are described in Table 2. Increased ACTH and cortisol can produce multiple systemic effects such as diabetes mellitus with insulin-resistant hyperglycemia, hyperaldosteronism with hypokalemia and metabolic alkalosis, hypertension, mild congestive heart failure, and obesity all of which contribute to increased morbidity and mortality. Therefore, surgical excision of ACTH-secreting tumors is recommended. Anesthetic management of these patients requires an awareness of the physiologic effects of excess cortisol secretion. These patients may require control of blood pressure, electrolyte imbalances, and plasma glucose levels preoperatively.

PREOPERATIVE EVALUATION AND PREPARATION

Because of the various medical disorders that may exist in patients with pituitary tumor, a thorough preoperative evaluation is necessary. In addition to the routine physical examination, a visual examination including examination of the visual fields is performed to assess function of the optic nerves and chiasm. The neurologic examination is evaluated for signs of mass effect, local invasion, or compression. When transsphenoidal surgery is planned, an otolaryngologic examination of the nasal passages and nasopharynx is performed, and a nasal culture is obtained to guide antibiotic therapy in the event of postoperative infection.

Preoperatively, anatomic studies of the skull and sella turcica and various endocrine studies, as summarized in Table 3, are performed in these patients. The routine anatomic studies consist of plain skull films and computed tomography (CT) scans. Anteroposterior and lateral skull radiographs are obtained in all patients with suspected sella or parasella lesions to determine whether the sella is normal or abnormal. The CT scan with and without contrast enhancement provides valuable information on the size and extent of the lesion, the degree of suprasellar extension, and the degree of increased ICP. More recently, magnetic resonance imaging (MRI) has been introduced, providing multiple sections of the sella (axial, coronal, and sagittal) with detail on vascular markings. In time, MRI may replace the CT scan in the diagnostic work-up. Cerebral angiograms are also obtained when it is necessary to exclude the presence of an aneurysm or to determine whether major vessels (e.g., internal carotid) are involved by the tumor.

The assessment of endocrine function is an integral part of the diagnostic and therapeutic management of a patient with pituitary disease. Endocrine tests are performed in the basal state and are supplemented by appropriate provocative tests. These tests are used to diagnose hyperfunctioning and hypofunctioning tumors, to delineate the extent of endocrine disturbance, and to assess adequacy of treatment. Kohler's *Clinical Endo-*

Table 3 Minimal Preoperative Testing for Pituitary Tumors

Anatomic studies
  Plain skull radiographs
  CT scan of head with and without contrast material
  MRI
  Cerebral angiography when indicated
Endocrinologic studies
  Basal levels of pituitary hormones: GH, PRL, ACTH, TSH, FSH, LH
  Serum levels: cortisol (AM and PM), thyroxine, testosterone, estradiol
  Urinary levels: 17-ketosteroids, 17-hydroxycorticosteroids, free cortisol, estrogens
  Provocative and suppression tests as indicated:
    GH reserve—glucagon stimulation
    GH suppression—glucose suppression (acromegaly)
    Prolactin reserve—chlorpromazine or thyrotropin-releasing hormone provocative testing
    Low- and high-dose dexamethasone suprression (Cushing's syndrome)
    Metyrapone test (Cushing's syndrome).
  Posterior pituitary function tests:
    ADH reserve—serum and urine osmolality before and after 8–12 hours' water deprivation

crinology provides a more thorough discussion of endocrinologic testing.

During preanesthesia evaluation, the size of the lesion and the patient's endocrine abnormalities are evaluated. The size and location of the tumor determine its effect on intracranial dynamics. Pituitary microadenomas do not produce mass effects. Craniopharyngiomas, other suprasellar tumors, and pituitary tumors with suprasellar extension, however, may exert a mass effect. In these patients, the results of the neurologic examination and CT scan should be evaluated for signs of increased ICP.

The patient's diagnosis and preoperative condition suggest the various systemic disorders that must be medically managed before surgery. Patients who have panhypopituitarism require replacement therapy with appropriate hormones. These patients should be euthyroid before surgery. To avoid stressing an insufficient adrenocortical axis, however, glucocorticoid replacement is required when thyroxine replacement is started. Diabetes insipidus is usually not observed in the patient with anterior pituitary insufficiency, but it may develop after cortisol replacement therapy is instituted. (Glucocorticoids are necessary to facilitate renal excretion of a water load.) Preoperatively, the patient with panhypopituitarism will be receiving oral steroid and thyroxine therapy and, when indicated, intranasal instillation of synthetic vasopressin.

All patients are given supplemental, short-acting glucocorticoid therapy before surgery. Since the surgery involves manipulation or removal of the anterior pituitary, transient or permanent deficiency of ACTH and cortisol secretion may result.

Patients who have Cushing's disease require preoperative evaluation and management of hypertension, diabetes, and electrolyte imbalances, and a cardiovascular evaluation for ischemic heart disease and congestive heart failure. Patients with acromegaly also require an evaluation for systemic hypertension, diabetes, cardiomegaly, ischemic heart disease, and congestive heart failure, with appropriate medical management instituted before surgery.

Premedication that relieves anxiety but does not produce undue sedation is recommended. Diazepam, 5 to 10 mg taken orally the morning of surgery, is often used without problems. Premedication is not administered to patients who exhibit a decreased level of consciousness. When transsphenoidal surgery is planned, the patient is informed during the preoperative visit that he or she will awaken with nasal packing and be required to breathe through the mouth postoperatively.

Since the introduction of the operating microscope, transsphenoidal excision has been recommended for all pituitary tumors that do not have marked suprasellar extension. Advantages of the transsphenoidal approach include lower morbidity and mortality rates; elimination of frontal lobe retraction, damage to olfactory nerves, and external scars; direct magnified visualization of small tumors within the gland; decreased incidence and severity of diabetes insipidus; decreased frequency of blood transfusion; and shorter hospitalization. Relative disadvantages include the possibility of cerebrospinal fluid (CSF) leakage and meningitis (rare with use of antibiotics); inability to visualize neural structures adjacent to a large tumor; inaccessibility of tumors extending into middle and anterior fossae; and the possibility of bleeding from cavernous sinuses or carotid arteries (which can lead to intracranial hemorrhage, brain stem compression, and significant blood loss).

The transcranial approach to the sella permits direct visualization of suprasellar structures (the vascular sinus ring, optic chiasm, hypothalamus, and pituitary stalk). This approach is recommended for pituitary tumors of uncertain diagnosis and those that have significant suprasellar extension and optic nerve or hypothalamic involvement. Overall, the morbidity and mortality rates are higher with this approach. The possibility of permanent diabetes insipidus and anterior pituitary insufficiency is increased. There is also potential for damage to the olfactory nerves, frontal lobe vasculature, and optic nerves and chiasm.

ANESTHETIC MANAGEMENT

The anesthetic management of patients undergoing pituitary surgery is not fundamentally different from those undergoing other craniotomies. Basic neuroanesthetic principles apply whether the transsphenoidal or transcranial approach is used. Intraoperative measures to control ICP are instituted, especially with the transcranial approach, since mass effects, the necessity for brain retraction, and the potential for greater blood loss exist.

In addition to the routine monitors, measurement of intra-arterial blood pressure, arterial blood gases, central venous pressure (CVP), and urinary output is recommended for all major neurosurgical procedures. During transsphenoidal procedures, however, CVP and urinary output are not routinely measured. Air embolism has been reported during this procedure when the patient is positioned with a significant head-up tilt. Therefore, if a significant surgical site–cardiac gradient (15 degrees or more) is unavoidable, precordial Doppler monitoring and right atrial catheterization are recommended for detection and treatment of air embolism.

Fluid intake and urinary output are closely measured intraoperatively and are measured for up to 48 hours postoperatively. If diabetes insipidus is present preoperatively, serum sodium and osmolality and urine specific gravity are also measured.

Evoked potential monitoring of visual evoked potentials (VEPs) has been introduced during pituitary surgery to monitor direct compression or compromise of blood supply to optic nerves and chiasm. Abnormalities in latency, amplitude, and characteristic peaks provide information that guides surgical technique and may prevent permanent neurologic damage. Technical difficulties that cause intraoperative recording problems include changes in pupil size, deviation of eyes, goggle size, and bulkiness, and stimulus delivery (light flashes). Because VEPs are entirely cortical in origin, they are also more vulnerable to the effects of general anesthetics.

The choice of anesthetic technique depends on the patient's general medical condition and pertinent anesthetic history and pathology. The following technique is suggested for either transsphenoidal or transcranial procedures. Although increased ICP is seldom a problem in patients with pituitary microadenomas (excised by transsphenoidal microsurgery), anesthetic management at our institution is similar to that used for patients with increased ICP, with the effects of anesthetic drugs on intracranial dynamics taken into account. The patient is smoothly and deeply anesthetized before laryngoscopy and intubation. Induction of anesthesia is accomplished with intravenous administration of thiopental (4 to 6 mg per kilogram) or midazolam (0.1 to 0.15 mg per kilogram), followed by a narcotic (fentanyl, 3 to 5 μg per kilogram) and muscle relaxant. If no airway difficulties are anticipated, vecuronium bromide or pancuronium, 0.1 mg per kilogram IV, is added while controlled hyperventilation with 100 percent oxygen is instituted. (In patients with potential airway problems, those with acromegaly, for instance — succinylcholine may be preferable. In some cases, intubation with a fiberoptic bronchoscope is advisable.) Oxygen saturation and end-expired carbon dioxide are monitored during both induction and maintenance of anesthesia to assure adequate ventilation. Fentanyl, in 50 μg increments, is administered until a total dose of 10 to 15 μg per kilogram is achieved, depending on the blood pressure response. When the peripheral muscle twitch response disappears, lidocaine (1.5 mg per kilogram IV) and an additional 2 to 3 mg per kilogram bolus of thiopental are given. Ninety seconds later, endotracheal intubation is performed under direct vision as gently and rapidly as possible. After induction of anesthesia, ventilation is controlled mechanically and adjusted to maintain arterial carbon dioxide tension ($PaCO_2$) between 25 to 30 mm Hg if intracranial hypertension is present, or 32 to 37 mm Hg if ICP is normal. (With the transsphenoidal approach, hyperventilation would decrease brain volume and withdraw the suprasellar portion of the tumor out of the surgeon's reach.) After placement of an esophageal stethoscope and thermistor, the oropharynx is packed with saline-soaked gauze to minimize blood pooling in transsphenoidal procedures. The eyes are protected and taped closed.

Anesthetic maintenance must provide hemodynamic stability and rapid emergence for postoperative neurologic evaluation. This can be achieved by using a N_2O-narcotic (fentanyl) anesthetic supplemented with diazepam or doperidol or by using a minimal alveolar anesthetic concentration of 0.5 to 1 percent of isoflurane in oxygen/air supplemented by a narcotic. Current neuroanesthetic practice is moving away from the use of N_2O, especially if the potential for air embolism exists. Muscle relaxation with pancuronium or vecuronium bromide (0.06 mg per kilogram) is recommended with either technique.

Diuretics are not usually necessary during transsphenoidal procedures, but are used during transcranial procedures. The osmotic diuretic mannitol or loop diuretic furosemide may be used separately or in combination to reduce brain volume.

Glucose-free crystalloid solutions are administered so that patients receive their hourly maintenance fluids and replacement of half the urine output and two to three times the blood loss. Blood loss usually does not exceed 200 ml during transsphenoidal procedures, but it can be extensive and acute. Blood should therefore be available. Solutions containing glucose are avoided in all neurosurgical procedures. Hyperglycemia from glucose-containing solutions has been associated with poorer neurologic outcome in the presence of ischemia, aggravation of cerebral edema, and an osmotic diuresis that can be confused with diabetes insipidus.

For transsphenoidal procedures, the nasal mucosa is prepared with 4 percent cocaine pledgets placed in the nares, followed by the injection of 2 percent lidocaine with epinephrine 1 to 200,000 to the submucosa. This combination develops a dissection plane, decreases bleeding, and buffers the hypertensive response to nasal dissection. Initially, however, the cocaine and epinephrine may cause hypertension, tachycardia, and arrhythmias. Drugs to treat these responses should be readily available.

Lumbar cerebrospinal fluid drainage is commonly employed with the transcranial approach, but it is seldom indicated with the transsphenoidal approach unless an intraoperative air study is planned. When the surgical lesion has suprasellar extension, delineation of the superior margin is facilitated by injection of air or N_2O/oxygen mixture into the subarachnoid space during surgery. If air is injected, N_2O must be discontinued from the anesthetic mixture because it rapidly diffuses into the air-filled closed space. Injection of N_2O/oxygen mixture permits continuation of use of N_2O.

Emergence from anesthesia should be smooth, without straining or bucking on the endotracheal tube. Residual muscle relaxant is reversed, and the patient is given 100 percent oxygen to breathe. Intravenous lidocaine (1.0 to 1.5 mg per kilogram) administered approximately 90 seconds before suctioning and extubation helps decrease coughing, straining, and hypertension. After transsphenoidal procedures, the oropharynx is suctioned thoroughly and the pack removed. Before extubation, the patient must follow commands and understand that mouth breathing will be necessary. If the patient is not responsive, the endotracheal tube remains in place until the patient is alert and can follow commands. A brief neurologic examination is performed before and after extubation; pupil size and reaction, visual acuity (finger count), and grasp and movement of extremities are assessed. After this has been successfully completed, the patient is positioned with his or her head elevated 30 degrees and is transferred to the recovery room with oxygen by mask and oxygen saturation monitoring. Close monitoring and care, including neurologic evaluation, are continued in the recovery room.

During the immediate postoperative period, the primary concerns are corticosteroid coverage and fluid balance. Dexamethasone followed by prednisone is given for 5 days after surgery or until postoperative testing shows an intact pituitary-adrenal axis. Fluid balance is assessed by strict attention to hourly fluid intake and output and urine specific gravity. Development of diabetes insipidus is uncommon during surgery but may occur early in the postoperative course.

Diabetes insipidus is commonly seen during the first 12 hours postoperatively and usually lasts for 2 to 4 days. Diagnosis is based on the following: polyuria (2 to 15 L per day); hypernatremia; high serum osmolality (≥ 300 mOsm per kilogram); decreased urine osmolality (≤ 200 mOsm); and decreased urine specific gravity (1.005 or less). Therapy includes replacement of urine losses with intravenous fluids. When urinary volumes are excessive, exogenous vasopressin is given (aqueous vasopressin, 5 to 10 U subcutaneously every 4 hours). In patients who develop permanent diabetes insipidus, vasopressin tannate-in-oil is used every 24 to 48 hours until intranasal desmopressin can be prescribed.

Other complications of pituitary tumor surgery include visual field changes, cerebrospinal fluid rhinorrhea, intracranial hemorrhage, hypothalamic injury or stroke, cerebral ischemia, and meningitis. Patients must be carefully monitored in the recovery room for airway obstruction caused by bleeding and secretions in the pharynx. Frequent neurologic assessments are performed to note any changes in mental status. Patients who have had an uncomplicated hospital course after transsphenoidal surgery are often discharged within 5 to 6 days.

SUGGESTED READING

Kohler J. Clinical endocrinology. New York: John Wiley and Sons, 1986.
Laws ER Jr, Randall RV, Kern EB, et al, eds. Management of pitu-
itary adenomas and related lesions. New York: Appleton-Century-Crofts, 1982.
Matjasko MJ. Anesthetic considerations in patients with neuroendo-crine disease. In: Cottrell JE, Turndorf HE, eds. Anesthesia and neurosurgery. St. Louis: CV Mosby 1986: 224

MAGNETIC RESONANCE IMAGING

MITCHELL TOBIAS, M.D.
DAVID S. SMITH, M.D., Ph.D.

Magnetic resonance imaging (MRI) represents a major advancement in diagnosis through its enhanced resolution of anatomic structures. However, the excellent resolution of MRI can be severely degraded by patient movement. In addition, the intense magnetic fields, which are intrinsic to the technology, create unique problems in the use of physiologic monitors, standard anesthesia machines, and ventilators. As a result, when anesthetizing children and critically ill adults, anesthesiologists are confronted with unique challenges that the restrictive environment of this technology presents. In this chapter we discuss the hazards and limitations imposed on anesthesiologists and their patients by the physical necessities of the MRI instrumentation. We also describe approaches for providing monitored care and anesthesia during MRI.

HISTORY

In 1946, both Purcell and Bloch independently published work, for which they shared the 1952 Nobel Prize in Physics, describing the phenomenon of nuclear induction. Later work by Proctor and others led to nuclear magnetic resonance spectroscopy, an important technique for identifying complex chemical compounds. Use of the nuclear magnetic resonance phenomenon to create images was suggested by Damidian in 1971 and Lauterbur in 1973. A subsequent decade of intense scientific effort produced the currently used high-resolution MRI techniques, which by their nature avoid ionizing radiation or dependency on iodinated contrast media.

PHYSICAL BASIS

Atomic nuclei with an odd number of protons or neutrons have the potential to act as magnetic dipoles. Although this characteristic is true of all paramagnetic elements (^{13}C, ^{31}P, ^{19}F, ^{23}Na, ^{39}K, ^{1}H, and ^{2}H), clinical MRI uses the most abundant element, hydrogen, the nucleus of which consists of a single proton. Normally, the large numbers of hydrogen protons in a given specimen are oriented randomly and there is no net magnetic field. If, however, a biologic specimen is placed within a powerful, homogeneous magnetic field, the hydrogen nuclei align their axes so that there is a slight net magnetization. To produce this alignment, MRI units typically operate with static magnetic fields of 0.5 to 1.5 T. (As a point of reference, the earth's magnetic field measures 0.0006 T.) Pulsed radiofrequency (RF) energy of an appropriate frequency and duration forces these protons out of alignment with the static magnetic field into a higher energy state. When the RF pulse is discontinued, the protons return to the "aligned," lowest energy state. In doing so they emit RF energy that is related to their chemical identity, their chemical relationship to surrounding nuclei, and their quantity. Location within the specimen can be identified by superimposing on the static magnetic field another magnetic field with a specific, changing field strength. The emitted RF signals are received by a large receiver within the bore of the MRI unit or by a surface coil placed directly on the patient's body. These surface coils enhance the signal-to-noise ratio to provide more detailed imaging.

Thus, diagnostic imaging using MRI requires large, powerful, superconducting magnets with a highly homogeneous static magnetic field, controllable electromagnetic coils to create magnetic field gradients, and a source of pulsed energy at specific radio frequencies to change the energy state of the protons. Sophisticated computers are needed to control the timing, strength, and sequencing of the RF pulses and changes in the gradient magnetic field; to collect and process the MRI information; and to construct the resulting images. Because the signals of interest have a relatively low intensity, they may be hard to differentiate from the surrounding "noise."

CONTRAST MATERIAL

Although MRI is not dependent on contrast material, gadopentetate dimeglumine is an injectable paramagnetic agent that develops a large magnetic moment and produces strong signal intensity from intravascular water. Since it does not cross the intact blood-brain barrier, it is useful for revealing areas where the blood-brain barrier is disrupted (abscess, infarct) or where there are vascular lesions (neoplasms, arteriovenous malformation).

Gadopentetate dimeglumine has been shown to alter normal red blood cell membranes in nonhuman species, resulting in increased splenic hemolysis. Patients with pre-existing hemolytic anemia or sickle cell anemia have not yet been evaluated. Irreversibly sickled erythrocytes have been shown to align perpendicular to magnetic fields, and the effect of gadopentetate dimeglumine on this phenomenon is being studied. Hypotension has been reported to accompany rapid intravenous administration of the agent. Headache and nausea are other common side effects. Allergic reactions of varying severity have also been reported.

HAZARDS

The anesthetic considerations for patients having MRI studies reflect both its unique hazards and the problems associated with physiologic monitors used in close proximity to this unique equipment. Hazards may potentially result from the intense static magnetic field, RF energy, the magnetic gradient, released cryogens (used to maintain the low temperatures required for superconductivity), or injected contrast material.

Static Magnetic Field Effects

The potential effects of static magnetic fields on biological tissue may be divided into effects on normal cellular and physiologic function and on implanted prostheses. In addition, the strong magnetic fields attract ferromagnetic material that is on the patient and attending medical personnel, or material introduced into the environment as part of monitoring or anesthesia equipment.

The physiologic effects of exposure to strong, localized magnetic fields in humans have included skeletogenesis, improved bone fracture repair, and changes in erythrocyte rheology. Irreversibly sickled erythrocytes align themselves perpendicularly to a magnetic field in vitro. Nonsickled homozygous erythrocytes have normal flow patterns during MRI. The potential for worsening of an acute sickle cell occlusive crisis by this magnetic effect in vivo is the subject of ongoing investigation. Electromagnetic forces induced from blood flowing in vessels perpendicular to the magnetic field occur, and although these induced voltages produce changes in electrocardiogram (ECG) signals, the changes are not considered to be of physiologic consequence. Induced current is believed to produce visual phosphenes secondary to retinal stimulation. Experiments in lower species have demonstrated magnetically induced alterations in sensitivity of rat pineal gland, *Escherichia coli* enzyme synthesis, and avian navigation sense.

Of greater concern are the potentially dangerous effects of the powerful magnetic field on metallic implants such as (1) pacemakers, (2) automatic implanted cardiac defibrillators (AICD), (3) vascular clips, (4) synthetic cardiac valves, (5) anode endotracheal tubes, or (6) shrapnel. Certain metal alloys have been shown to experience sufficient attraction and movement within magnetic fields to present a risk of dislodgement, hemorrhage, or motile injury to adjacent sensitive structures (e.g., brain). Steel alloys with adequate nickel content (approximately 10 to 14 percent) are not hazardous at the field strengths used for MRI. Suitable alloys are designated Austentitic by the American Iron and Steel Institute, and current vascular and neurosurgical practice is to use clips of this type.

Cardiac pacemakers may have ferromagnetic parts or casings that may be subjected to movement in the magnetic fields. Newly implanted pacemakers may shift position, causing pain or dislodgement. A more likely problem is closure of the reed switch, which changes the pacemaker function from synchronous to asynchronous modes. The magnetic field can induce currents greater than those needed for pacemaker discrimination of native cardiac activity, thus inhibiting discharge of the pacemaker. Magnetic fields may also deactivate AICDs. Direct cardiac stimulation by electrical currents induced by gradient magnetic fields has not been demonstrated. Although measurable current can be induced in pacemaker wires by the changing magnetic fields, the current is well below that needed for depolarization or microshock. However, burns under electrocardiographic (ECG) electrodes have been reported, and high-resistance ECG cables should be used to minimize current generation. Implanted insulin, chemotherapeutic, or intrathecal pumps may malfunction within the magnetic fields. Thus, patients with pacemakers, AICDs, implanted pumps, or vascular clips of an unknown alloy are generally barred from MRI examinations.

Ferromagnetic objects, if brought sufficiently close to the magnet, may launch toward the magnet with considerable force. The force exerted on an object is inversely proportional to the fourth power of its distance from the magnet's center and directly related to the mass of the object. An object too near the magnet may literally fly into the magnet or into an interposed obstruction (e.g., a patient). Numerous anecdotes have been published describing the ballistic actions of ferrous objects ranging from scissors to forklift truck prongs.

Radiofrequency Generation

Absorbed RF energy causes a statistically significant increase in body temperature. Body surfaces absorb markedly more energy than deep tissues. Superficial tissues, which have decreased vascularity and less ability to dissipate heat, may be more subject to heat accumulation. Current MRI machines are unlikely to increase tissue temperature more than 1°C; however, febrile patients or those who are unable to perspire may be at increased risk. The amount of heating of implants is directly related to the size and conductive properties of the implant. Relatively avascular tissue (e.g., the cornea or a hip joint adjacent to a large ferrous implant) may sustain greater RF absorption than highly vascular or deeper tissues. Currents induced by a surface coil near the body are capable of producing local cutaneous burns. This potential problem can be avoided by reorienting the surface coil or permitting air to circulate between the coil and the patient's skin.

Magnetic Gradients

The loud noise generated by switching the magnetic gradient coils on and off frightens some patients. The pulsing sound also creates difficulties in communication between the anesthesiologist and patient. Moreover, it is difficult to see the patient lying in the magnet bore, thus

verbal communication or more detailed monitoring is essential. All patients must be instructed to alert personnel if they experience any problems during MRI.

Cryogen Release

The magnet uses superconductivity to maintain its strong homogenous field. Despite recent advances, superconductors require temperatures approaching 0° kelvin ($-273°C$). These austere cryostatic conditions are maintained by encasing the MRI magnetic coil in liquid helium and nitrogen. In the rare event of a cryogen leak or an emergency shutdown caused by a sudden increase in super-conducting coil resistance with subsequent heating and boiling off of the cryogens (quench), an MRI room could have its available oxygen displaced by the sudden release of this dangerously cold helium and

Table 1 Standards of Anesthetic Care and Magnetic Resonance Imaging*

Standard	Possible Approaches and Problems with Meeting Standard During MRI
Continuous presence of qualified personnel	Can be in room with patient, no known significant hazard to personnel.
Evaluation of oxygenation	
Inspired oxygen	Oxygen analyzers on inspiratory limb have been used. Need to be fixed firmly and sufficiently far from the magnet to minimize attraction. Batteries are ferromagnetic.
Blood oxygenation	
Observation	Observation of lips and fingers is often impossible, especially during head or neck studies. Toes may be outside the magnet and visible.
Pulse oximetry	If not specially designed for MRI, pulse oximetry tends to degrade the image and is unusable.
Evaluation of ventilation	
Observation of clinical signs, chest excursion, reservoir bag, auscultation	Long magnet bore makes observation difficult. Noise generated during imaging makes auscultation difficult or impossible. Observation of reservoir bag, if present, is possible. Placement of a paper cup on the chest may aid in visualization of excursion.
End-tidal carbon dioxide analysis	Has been reported using units that sample the exhaled gas stream by aspiration. All devices have a ferromagnetic risk. Paco$_2$ may be underestimated. Some units may generate EMI.
Volume of expired gas	Respirometers may be used if not ferromagnetic, or if placed and fixed at a safe distance.
Ventilator disconnect alarm	Can be used depending on design and distance from the magnet.
Evaluation of circulation	
Continuous ECG	May be distorted and uninterpretable during image acquisition. Wiring may attract RF; induced currents may burn patient.
Arterial blood pressure and heart rate monitored every 5 minutes	Oscillotonometry and sphygmomanometry, both manual and automated.
Continuous monitoring	
Palpation of pulse	May be difficult or impossible
Auscultation of heart sounds	May be difficult or impossible
Intra-arterial pressure trace	Ferromagnetic risk, many units generate interfering RF radiation
Ultrasonographic peripheral pulse monitoring	No reported experience
Pulse plethysmography	Standard on Siemens Magneton
Measurement of body temperature	Success with thermistor-based units

*Adapted from American Society of Anesthesiologists' "Standards for Basic Intra-operative Monitoring." (Approved by House of Delegates, October 21, 1986.) In these standards, "continuous" means "prolonged without any interruption at any time" and "continual" means "repeated regularly and frequently in steady succession."

nitrogen. Frostbite occurs after only momentary tissue contact with liquid helium or nitrogen. Hair and permeable clothes entrap the liquids, which facilitates skin burning. The eyes are also extremely susceptible to injury. MRI rooms are designed with special venting to help prevent these consequences of cryogen release, although external vents may be blocked by refuse, nests, leaves, and so on.

CLINICAL CONSIDERATIONS

Candidates for MRI are similar to those who come to the operating room. Critically ill adults or infants and children may require general anesthesia and neuromuscular blockade to eliminate movement. Claustrophobic or excitable patients may require sedation. The same careful preoperative evaluation by history and physical examination applies to this procedure as it would to an operative procedure. With varying degrees of difficulty, most of the standards of care adopted by the American Society of Anesthesiologists (Table 1) can be met in the MRI environment.

Specific considerations for the anesthesiologist relate to (1) the impact of the static magnetic field, gradient magnetic fields, RF emission, and electromagnetic interference (EMI) on monitoring equipment; (2) the disruptive effects of physiologic monitors on image quality, and (3) the remote access to the patient. It must be emphasized that the compatibility among monitoring devices and MRI scanners varies not only among manufacturers and types of monitoring devices, but also among the brand of MRI machines employed.

The monitoring equipment commonly used by anesthesiologists in the operating room generates significant amounts of EMI that may degrade the quality of the MR image. Wires from monitors to the patient may act as antennae, attracting ambient or emitted RF energy and contributing to image degradation. A valuable rule learned through clinical experience is that running data or power cables parallel to the Z axis of the static magnetic field aids in limiting artifacts. In addition, locating monitoring equipment, anesthesia apparatus, and so on, beyond the 100 gauss line limits artifacts and the risk of projectiles. Table 2 lists specific equipment that has been used with a General Electric and Siemens magnetic resonance imager.

Ventilatory Support and Inhalational Anesthetic Delivery

Some ventilators and monitoring equipment may not work as a result of EMI or the force of the static magnetic field. Standard anesthesia and intensive care unit ventilators employ electronic and mechanical regulation that may malfunction within the magnetic field. The Siemens 900C Servo ventilator functions within the MRI room, and it has been used to anesthetize patients by introducing the fresh gas flow to its low-pressure inlet. However, it is essential that sufficient distance exist between the ventilator and the magnet because the ventilator has malfunctioned when placed near (within 4 feet of) the magnet. Fluidic ventilators and manual jet ventilators, which do not depend on electronic or ferrous mechanical parts, have been used successfully without compromising either the patient or the image. Metal parts of these monitors must be made of aluminum or another nonferromagnetic material. Spontaneous or controlled ventilation using a reservoir bag obviates the need for any electronic equipment to deliver positive-pressure ventilation. Using oxygen delivered from a central system eliminates the need for pressurized oxygen tanks, which are strongly ferromagnetic. The large amount of oxygen required to drive the bellows of fluidic ventilators makes small tanks impractical for positive-pressure ventilation.

Modifications to pre-existing anesthesia machines to reduce ferric components have been reported. Most magnetic parts are contained within the frame and casters. Most anesthesia vaporizers contain little to no ferromagnetic materials. If kept several feet from the magnet and attached to a fixed support, they function properly and do not become projectile. Ohmeda, Inc., now produces anesthesia machines designed for use with MRI (Ohmeda Excel MRI).

The long circuit involved in providing inhalational anesthesia to the patient deep within the magnet necessitates elevated compression volumes. Tidal volumes need to be adjusted with this in mind, particularly for pediatric patients or patients with low pulmonary compliance. The use of noncorrugated Tygon tubing can reduce compression volumes. The gating of thoracic image acquisition to one point of the respiratory cycle diminishes motion artifacts during positive-pressure ventilation. Consequently, this technique may be preferable to spontaneous ventilation in some patients, although it lengthens MRI scan time appreciably.

Monitoring

Respiratory

The respirometer on the expiratory limb of many ventilators can be used to monitor minute ventilation. The volume data must be interpreted with consideration for the increased compression volumes, as previously discussed. The adequacy of minute ventilation may be accurately monitored by an infrared end-tidal carbon dioxide monitor that aspirates respiratory gas. If the monitor leaks a significant amount of RF energy or is attracted to the magnet, a lengthened sampling tube may be needed to move the monitor away from the magnet. The extra length of tubing distorts the mixture of the capnogram; the carbon dioxide plateau may not be well delineated, and peak measured end-tidal carbon dioxide may be less than the actual value. Placing a paper cup on the patient's chest may facilitate visual verification of thoracic excursion.

Polarographic and fuel cell oxygen analyzers function well in the MRI environment. However, polarographic oxygen analyzers use batteries that may be

Table 2 MRI-Compatible Anesthesia Equipment*

Device	Manufacturer	Model	Experience†	Comments
Anesthesia delivery systems				
Anesthesia machine	Ohmeda, Inc.	Excel MRI	None	
High-impact plastic cart	Eastern Anesthesia, Inc.		S, GE	Can be used as the chassis of a non-ferromagnetic anesthesia machine
Aluminum gas cylinders (size E)	Walter Kidde Division of Kidde, Inc.		S, GE	Standard tanks are strongly ferromagnetic
Anesthetic vaporizer	Ohmeda, Inc.	Fluotec 4	S	
		Isotec 4	S	
Mapelson D type gas delivery system	Vital Signs, Inc.	6098	S	
Mechanical ventilator	Monaghan Medical Corp.	225SIMV	GE	Fluidic, nonelectrical parts, can be next to magnet
	Siemens	900 C	S	Ferromagnetic;‡ may malfunction close to magnet
Physiologic monitors				
Oxygen analyzers	Catalyst Research	Miniox III	S	Batteries are ferromagnetic
Pulse oximeters	Biochem	Microspan 1040 A	S	30 m from center of magnet
	In Vivo Research, Inc.	3100	None	Part of monitoring system designed for MRI use
Capnographs	Ohmeda	5200	GE	Ferromagnetic
Oscillotonometers	Critikon-Dinamap	1846SA	GE, S	Ferromagnetic
	Datascope	Accutorr 2A	GE, S	Ferromagnetic
Temperature detectors	Yellow Springs Instrument Co., Inc.	43TD 43TA	S	Batteries, metallic case
	Protocol Systems, Inc.	Propaq 106	S	Background MRI interference

*These monitoring instruments have been used in either a General Electric Sigma (GE) or Siemens Magneton (S) MRI 1.5 T units. Small changes in room orientation, shielding, design of the monitoring instrument, age of the instrument, and orientation in the room may produce unsatisfactory results. This is not an inclusive list and instruments by other manufacturers may also work well in this environment.

†By the authors or associates.

‡Ferromagnetic materials may be usable if sufficiently far from the magnet and fixed in position.

ferromagnetic. Consequently, the unit should be secured against movement.

RF signals emitted by the pulse oximeter can seriously distort MR images. To improve image quality, the probe can be placed on the toe of selected patients. Shielding the cable or substituting a fiberoptic cable has reportedly minimized the production of artifacts. A specially designed pulse oximeter (Biochem 1042 A) placed 8 feet from the magnet allows continuous and accurate monitoring of oxygen saturation in a Siemens MRI unit. A model is also specifically tailored for use with General Electric MRI units (In Vivo Research, Inc. Model 3109-1).

Cardiovascular

Arterial Pressure. Arterial pressure has been successfully monitored during MRI using both invasive and noninvasive methods. Oscillotonometric monitors may be sufficiently removed from the magnet by using lengthened connecting tubing. Cuff to tubing connectors should be nonferromagnetic.

Pressure transducers connected to intravascular catheters for central venous, arterial, or pulmonary artery pressure monitoring may function near the magnet. However, an increased length of tubing may be required to reach the patient, and this may cause either an overshoot or damping of the pressure wave form. The amplifiers and monitor screens may produce interfering RF signals.

In patients requiring intracranial pressure monitoring, intracranial bolts of plastic are preferable to metallic bolts which, even if not ferromagnetic, have some heating hazard and may produce local artifact during head imaging. Fiberoptic intracranial pressure monitor cables must be disconnected, because the amplifier box contains ferromagnetic parts.

The cathode ray oscilloscope, which uses an electron beam incident on a phosphorous screen, is sensitive to magnetic interference. It must therefore be placed sufficiently far from the magnet to prevent distortion.

Electrocardiography. The ECG is altered by both RF energy and static magnetic fields. The RF creates artifact that may render the ECG unusable. The amount of disturbance depends on electrode and cable material, which act as antennae, and on the frequency of the RF pulsing. Telemetric broadcast of ECG can reduce wiring, improving ECG quality. The quality of the image obtained by MRI is highly sensitive to motion artifact. Synchronization of MRI data acquisition with the ECG permits optimization of image quality, particularly of the thorax and heart, by minimizing motion artifact.

The static magnetic field produces a peaked T wave secondary to the induction of electromotive force by the perpendicular flow of blood. The distortion simply needs to be interpreted in the context of MRI.

Pulse Rate. The patient's pulse may be monitored in many ways. A nonferromagnetic precordial or esophageal stethoscope may be used, but its utility is impaired by the loud gradient coils during image acquisition. The pulse oximeter, oscillotonometer, doppler, or intravascular arterial pressure monitors can also be used to provide information on heart rate.

Temperature. Although body temperature monitoring is a standard of care, its need in most patients during a relatively brief MRI session can be questioned. Liquid crystal devices will be unreadable during scanning because of the remote access of the patient. Remote readout battery-powered monitoring devices are more appropriate, but they must be considered ferromagnetic because batteries are usually encased in such metals. The wires conducting the signal from thermistor or thermocouple may function as antennae for stray RF signals and produce image artifacts.

Neuromuscular Blockade. The use of neuromuscular blocking agents can be valuable since image quality depends to a great extent on patient immobility. Additionally, paralysis can improve pulmonary compliance in some patients, a subject of concern when one is considering the high compression volumes of the long circuits needed to reach the MRI core. The use of nerve simulators is limited in the MRI environment since they are battery powered. Also, the pediatric patient will be so remote from the anesthesiologist that physical contact will be prevented. Visual inspection of the lower extremity undergoing peroneal nerve stimulation remains a monitoring option. Use of strain gauge or pressure bulb transduction also is possible. The wires of the nerve stimulator may act as antennae for exogenous RF signals, degrading image quality.

To ensure patient safety, monitors should be placed close together so that they can be scanned easily and simultaneously. Red light-emitting diode displays make reading easier when monitors are located at a distance from the anesthesiologist and the magnet. The anesthesia machine may be considerably closer to the magnet.

The anesthesiologist should be positioned to enable as good a view of the patient as possible.

Anesthesia Approaches

Intravenous anesthesia, inhalational anesthesia, or sedation may be used depending on the specific needs of the patient.

Sedation

Table 3 lists sedation protocols for patients undergoing MRI. Oral chloral hydrate has been used in younger children when the child is supervised by a nurse and the patient's parent.

General Anesthesia

Our experience with general anesthesia has included adults with head injury, involuntary muscle movement, and claustrophobia. For outpatients we use light sedation as our technique of choice, but we have used general endotracheal tube anesthesia for outpatients as well as inpatients.

We generally induce general anesthesia in an alcove immediately adjacent to the magnet. This area has piped-in oxygen and suction. We supply an anesthesia machine and appropriate portable monitors including ECG oscilloscope, blood pressure oscillotonometer, pulse oximeter, and capnograph. The patient gurney we use can be easily placed in the Trendelenburg position. Thus, our induction area for MRI is equipped similarly to operating room anesthesia locations. After anesthesia induction, intubation, and stabilization, the patient is transferred to the MRI gurney and transported to the MRI room (which is likewise equipped with piped-in oxygen and suction). We have used total intravenous techniques during MRI, thus eliminating the need for an anesthesia machine in the MRI room. We have used combinations of pentobarbital or midazolam, together with fentanyl and vecuronium bromide. Propofol infusions in combination with a narcotic and muscle relaxant

Table 3 Examples of Sedation for MRI in Children* and Adults

Age (Years)	Medication	Dosage (mg/kg)	Comments
<1.5	Chloral hydrate, PO	75–120, not to exceed 2 g	Give 30 min before scan
1.5–6	Pentobarbital, IV or	2–4, not to exceed 150 mg	Give 5 min before scan
	Midazolam, IV or	0.05 to 0.1	
	Pentobarbital + Meperidine, PO	4 3	Give 1 h before scan
>6	Midazolam + fentanyl, IV	0.025 to 0.1 0.75 to 3 μg/kg	Give 5 min before scan

*Many of these approaches are currently used at the Children's Hospital of Philadelphia. The authors would like to thank members of the Anesthesia Department at that institution for sharing this information.

should also work well. We have used the Monaghan MRI ventilator during the MRI study and have monitored the patients with an esophageal stethoscope, automated oscillotonometer, and respirometer, and with capnography. The Monaghan MRI ventilator is not ferromagnetic and can be positioned next to the magnet. By contrast, most monitoring devices are highly ferromagnetic and, if not permanently installed, must be moved into and out of the MRI suite with great care. The equipment should be fixed to a support while it is in the MRI suite. We have found that locating the monitors against the wall near the door of the MRI suite is sufficiently far from the magnet. In our hospital, the magnetic field at this location is about 0.01 T, and the magnetic attraction, although present, tends to be weak. We typically tape the monitors to the floor to decrease the risk of movement. We do not believe that muscle paralysis needs to be monitored, but rather rely on average doses and the fact the vecuronium bromide is relatively short acting. Although we do not monitor body temperature in adults during the MRI study, we do monitor children's temperatures.

After the completion of the study, patients are returned to the anesthesia induction area, allowed to emerge from anesthesia, and are generally extubated before being transported to the recovery room. Because our MRI suite is located at some distance from the recovery room, extubated patients receive supplemental oxygen during transport. Since the MRI examination itself is not painful, the major requirements for the anesthetic are amnesia and elimination of muscle movement; thus, small doses of anesthetic agent are generally used, with emergence from anesthesia being rapid and uncomplicated.

We have anesthetized only patients with head injuries whose cerebral compliance is sufficiently high to allow them to remain in the supine position for the 30 to 60 minutes required for the MRI study. We have used barbiturates (most often pentobarbital) together with narcotics (fentanyl) and muscle relaxants (vecuronium bromide). To minimize hypertension and intracranial pressure increases that may occur during patient movement, we begin administering both the barbiturate and narcotic, and occasionally the muscle relaxant, before the patient is transported to the MRI suite. We typically perform an arterial blood gas analysis shortly after the patient has been transferred into the magnet to assure adequacy of hyperventilation with the Monaghan ventilator.

Resuscitation

For most machines, the time required to decrease the magnetic field to a normal level is 3 to 20 minutes. Thus, the magnetic field will be present if patients require resuscitation. Resuscitation teams are generally not prepared for high magnetic fields in which beepers, hemostats, and laryngoscopes may become unwieldy or ballistic. It is therefore necessary to plan for the rapid removal of the compromised patient from the magnet room. A fully stocked resuscitation cart, defibrillator, and oxygen source should be available just outside the magnet room.

SUGGESTED READING

Budinger TF, Cullander C. Health effects of in vivo nuclear magnetic resonance. In: James TL, Margulis AR, eds. Biomedical magnetic resonance. San Francisco Radiology Research and Education Foundation, 1984:421.

Karlik SJ, Heatherley T, Pavan F, et al. Patient anesthesia and monitoring at a 1.5-T MRI installation. Magn Reson Med 1988; 7:210–221.

Nixon C, Hirsch NP, Ormerod IEC. Johnson G. Nuclear magnetic resonance: its implications for the anaesthetist. Anaesthesia 1986; 41:131–137.

Rao CC, McNiece WL, Emhardt J. Modification of an anesthesia machine for use during magnetic resonance imaging. Anesthesiology 1988; 68:640–641.

Rokey R, Wendt RE, Johnston DL. Monitoring of acutely ill patients during nuclear magnetic resonance imaging: use of a time-varying filter electrocardiographic gating device to reduce gradient artifacts. Magn Reson Med 1988; 6:240–245.

Smith DS, Askey P, Young ML, Kressel HY. Anesthetic management of acutely ill patients during magnetic resonance imaging. Anesthesiology 1986; 65:710–711.

Young SW. Nuclear magnetic resonance imaging: basic principles. New York: Raven Press, 1984:163.

RADIOLOGY AND NEURORADIOLOGY

CECIL O. BOREL, M.D.
TOBY EAGLE, C.R.N.A.

Anesthesia for radiologic studies is fundamentally similar to other anesthetics where basic principles apply, but it is complicated when alterations in technique are required to perform an adequate radiologic study or procedure. The goals of anesthetic management are patient safety and comfort in the radiologic suite, which are, as in any other location, the responsibility of the anesthetist. Because radiologic procedures requiring anesthetics generally cannot be performed in the operating room, the anesthetist is usually in a location away from extra supplies, emergency drugs or equipment, and back-up help. The size or location of radiologic equipment limits access to the patient and his airway during the procedure. Frequent changes in position, movement in and out of scanners, or the movement of contrast agents may be an integral part of the study, and should be anticipated in the planned anesthetic. The radiologist may also require ideal "operating" conditions so that the study can be performed in an optimal fashion. Many radiologic procedures are not particularly painful but require the patient to be absolutely still for a long period of time; deep levels of general anesthesia may not be necessary for successful completion of these procedures. When performed skillfully, anesthetic management during radiologic studies is met with enthusiastic support from radiologists and gratitude from patients.

PREPARATION FOR THE PROCEDURE

Preparing the patient to undergo a radiologic study or procedure involves minimizing or anticipating adverse occurrences particular to the procedure. As in other procedures, the risk of nausea, vomiting, and aspiration is present and may be exacerbated by these studies. There is a particular risk in procedures where the patient is positioned with the stomach higher than the head, or where embolizing material is likely to induce nausea and vomiting. NPO status is required for patients undergoing elective procedures. Where anxiety contributes to nausea, or if nausea is a likely complaint, administration of an antiemetic (promethazine hydrochloride [Phenergan], droperidol, hydroxyzine [Vistaril]), by the oral or intramuscular route is appropriate. Neutralization of gastric acid secretion is an important preventive measure. Histamine-receptor blockers (cimetidine, ranitidine) may be doubly helpful in decreasing gastric acid secretion and providing histamine-receptor blockade in the event of an allergic reaction. When the patient is likely to be positioned so that the stomach is higher than the head, or if the risk of nausea is particularly high (e.g., during embolization procedures), the addition of metoclopramide hydrochloride has been useful in preventing nausea and ensuring an empty stomach. Metoclopramide hydrochloride may be administered orally, intramuscularly, or intravenously, and it should be given at least 2 hours before the procedure to allow adequate emptying to occur.

The risk of allergic reaction to contrast media or therapeutic agents should be considered when one is preparing patients for these studies or procedures. A review of previous reaction to contrast agents or seafood allergy further identifies a patient at risk. In patients at high risk for allergic reaction, pretreatment for prevention of allergic reactions is prudent. Histamine antagonists, such as diphenhydramine hydrochloride (Benadryl), ranitidine, and glucocorticoids are effective for blocking allergic reactions and are indicated in this situation.

Often the assistance of the anesthetist is requested because the patient requests virtual unconsciousness for the procedure. Often this is based on a previously painful procedure or untoward reaction. The compassionate control of anxiety or pain of a procedure is a suitable role for the anesthetist. Most radiologic procedures are not painful but may appear to be very frightening. We prefer intravenous administration of short-acting benzodiazepines supplemented with narcotics for procedures that are mildly to moderately painful. Most patients will have a satisfactory experience when a minor tranquilizer is administered orally 2 hours before the procedure, and supplemental sedation is given intravenously when necessary during the procedure. In patients in whom intracranial pressures may be elevated, neither narcotics nor sedatives may be safely administered because of the risk of raising carbon dioxide partial pressure (Pco_2) and increasing intracranial pressure.

CHOICE OF ANESTHETIC TECHNIQUE

Anesthetics for radiologic procedures are listed in Table 1. Local anesthesia is appropriate for adult patients who are coherent and cooperative, especially when it is anticipated that the procedure will be short, insertion of catheters will be the only stimulation, or neurologic examination will be necessary during the investigation. Local anesthesia is also ideal for the comatose or critically ill patient unlikely to move during investigation. The role of the anesthetist is to monitor airway status and vital signs during the procedure. The anesthetist should be available for emergency airway management or resuscitation in the event of an untoward reaction, and airway equipment, intravenous access, suitable monitoring modalities, and emergency drugs should be available for this eventuality.

Local anesthesia supplemented with intravenous sedation is indicated for adult, cognizant patients when the procedure is likely to be prolonged or uncomfortable but not frankly painful. When mild sedation is used, it is

Table 1 Anesthetic Techniques for Neurodiagnostic Procedures

Procedure	Patient Status	Anesthetic Technique	Monitoring Required	Other Considerations
CT scanning	Child without increased ICP	IV sedation or general anesthesia	ECG, BP, pulse oximeter	All myelograms have position changes; secure ET tube well

CT myelography	Child with increased ICP	General anesthesia, hyperventilation	ECG, BP, pulse oximeter, $ETCO_2$	Light anesthesia primarily to prevent movement
				Procedure time
				  CT scan 1 hr
				  CT myelogram 2–2.25 hr

Stereotactic procedures, diagnostic or therapeutic	Adult with altered mental status (uncooperative, agitated) without increased ICP	General anesthesia	ECG, BP, pulse oximeter, $ETCO_2$	
	Adult with increased ICP, cooperative	Standby (no sedation)	ECG, pulse oximeter, (BP if indicated)	
	Adult with increased ICP, uncooperative	General anesthesia, hyperventilation	ECG, BP, pulse oximeter, $ETCO_2$, ICP monitoring	
	Adult without increased ICP	IV sedation (rarely)	ECG, BP, pulse oximeter	2–3 hr procedure Oversedation can mask neurologic examination Stress good field blocks to neurosurgeon
	Adult with increased ICP	General anesthesia, hyperventilation	ECG, BP (arterial line if needed), pulse oximeter, $ETCO_2$	N_2O/narcotic/pancuronium bromide Poor awakening may be caused by bleed
Angiography Diagnostic	Child	General anesthesia	ECG, BP, pulse oximeter, $ETCO_2$	
	Adult, cooperative	Local with minimal sedation	ECG, BP, pulse oximeter	
	Adult, uncooperative, altered mental status, increased ICP	General anesthesia	ECG, BP, pulse oximeter $ETCO_2$, arterial line, ICP monitoring	
Therapeutic for AVM	Adult, cooperative, without increased ICP	IV sedation	ECG, arterial line, CVP, pulse oximeter, possible PA line, and/or jugular bulb catheter, Foley catheter, eggcrate mattress	3–4 hr procedure Frequent neurologic examinations May need hypotension, hypertension Possibility of rapid change in mental status may indicate bleed
	Altered mental status, increased ICP	General anesthesia, hyperventilation	ECG, arterial line, CVP, pulse oximeter, possible PA line, and/or jugular bulb catheter, Foley catheter, $ETCO_2$, possible evoked potentials	Only done if sedation technqiue is impossible
Giant aneurysm	Adult, cooperative, without increased ICP	IV sedation	ECG, arterial line, CVP, pulse oximeter, Foley catheter, eggcrate mattress	2–3 hr procedure Possible hypertensive therapy after embolization Possible rapid change in mental status caused by rupture
Cavernous carotid fistula, meningioma	Child/Adult	General anesthesia	ECG, BP cuff, pulse oximeter, $ETCO_2$, Foley catheter	2–3 hr procedure Contrast injection, embolization painful External carotid artery branches embolized

BP = blood pressure; CVP = central venous pressure; ECG = electrocardiography; ET = endotracheal; $ETCO_2$ = end-tidal CO_2; ICP = intracranial pressure; PA = pulmonary artery catheter.

possible to maintain enough patient interaction and participation to allow neurologic evaluation. Since the airway will not be controlled during the procedure, access to the airway should be maintained so that it is relatively easy to establish airway control in the event of an emergency. The use of a precordial stethoscope with transmitter, electrocardiographic monitoring, end-tidal carbon dioxide and respiration monitoring, pulse oximetry, and automatic blood pressure cuff enhance the ability to monitor the patient. Measures to ensure comfort during the procedure, such as bladder catheterization, eggcrate mattress padding of the table, and padding of extremities, seem to make long procedures more tolerable.

Although local/sedation techniques are ideal for many radiologic procedures, there are situations in which this anesthetic approach would be quite difficult and for which alternative techniques should be sought. In patients in whom there is increased intracranial pressure, sedation techniques may cause carbon dioxide retention, increasing intracranial pressure and placing the patient at risk for herniation or cerebral ischemia. These patients will need airway control and hyperventilation if sedation is required. Combative, disoriented patients are likely to become more so with light sedation and suffer airway compromise with further control. Since airway compromise may occur at a time when it is difficult to reach the airway, intubation and general anesthesia might be more appropriate for these patients. For very long procedures in which absolute control of patient movement will be important, sedatives are not likely to be adequate. Some procedures are painful at sites remote from the catheter or not controllable by local anesthetics; sedation/narcotic combinations may not be sufficient for control of visceral or vascular pain. In young children who are likely to be frightened, uncomfortable, or uncooperative, general anesthesia may be more beneficial than sedation and local anesthesia.

General anesthesia is indicated in long, difficult procedures; in an uncooperative patient for whom ideal investigational conditions are necessary; in a procedure in which airway compromise or access will be limited or a large part of the procedure; and hyperventilation procedures. A "light" general anesthetic, endotracheal intubation, and moderate relaxation are sufficient for pain management and prevention of movement to optimize imaging. Techniques that do not increase cerebral blood flow are desirable if intracranial pressure is elevated. Nitrous oxide must be avoided if air is injected into a closed space to provide air contrast. The anesthetic should be easily and quickly reversible so that neurologic sequelae can be discovered in the radiologic suite, allowing further diagnostic studies to be performed immediately when necessary.

INDUCTION AND MAINTENANCE OF ANESTHESIA

All of the standard equipment for administering an anesthetic safely should be available before the induction of anesthesia. Because anesthetic administration is not routine in many radiologic suites, extra effort is necessary to ascertain the location and availability of anesthetic equipment before induction: suction, oxygen supply, airway equipment, drugs for anesthesia and resuscitation, and monitoring equipment. Errors in set-up may become greatly magnified by the difficulty of getting emergency or extra equipment from a storeroom located near the operating rooms several floors away.

Special preparation and considerations for anesthetizing patients in radiology suites or scanners where the patient slides in and out of the scanning apparatus include extra-long (at least 6 feet) airway tubing, intravenous tubing with extensions, and monitoring probes sufficiently long to allow this movement. Since the patient's position relative to the radiologic equipment is usually predetermined, it may be necessary to position the anesthesia machine and equipment in unusual positions, such as the left side of the patient. Monitoring equipment with electronic display should remain visible during filming, when the anesthetist will be standing in a protected environment. When there is doubt, reviewing equipment location and changes in patient positioning with the radiologist before induction of anesthesia has avoided the risk and difficulty of correcting problems once the anesthetic is underway.

Induction of anesthesia can usually be carried out with the patient already positioned on the x-ray table. This avoids difficult and potentially risky movement onto the table once the patient is anesthetized. If a problem occurs during the procedure, the patient can be immediately returned to the position assumed before induction so that emergency airway management and resuscitation can take place; if induction of anesthesia took place while the patient was on a stretcher and if he or she was positioned on the table after induction, the stretcher should remain immediately available in the event that emergency management becomes necessary.

Anesthesia should be maintained at a depth sufficient for the rapid completion of investigational and interventional procedures. Judicious use of muscle relaxants can eliminate movement artifact in the anesthetized patient and still allow for a rapid emergence and reversal for neurologic assessment after the procedure. When general anesthesia is required, inhalation, infusion, and nitrous oxide–narcotic have all been used successfully in this situation.

EMERGENCE AND POSTANESTHETIC CARE

The patient should emerge quickly from anesthesia so that any neurologic deficits may be investigated before the patient has been transferred from the radiology suite. There is no better area in which to assess poor emergence due to intracerebral hemorrhage or occlusion of cerebral vasculature than the area in which the studies have been performed. Patients who receive general anesthesia or deep sedation should be observed in the recovery room after emergence to monitor airway and cardiovascular status. Those patients at risk for neurologic or cerebrovascular compromise in the hours following embolization procedures are candidates for overnight monitoring in an intensive care unit where skilled services are immediately available.

ANESTHESIA FOR SPECIAL PROCEDURES

Computed Tomography–Guided Stereotactic Surgery

Using computed tomography (CT) scanning techniques, stereotactic procedures offer an alternative to traditional craniotomy for diagnosis and treatment of tumor, abscess, and other intracranial lesions. Stereotaxis can also be used therapeutically to treat tremors associated with multiple sclerosis. Minimal damage to adjacent structures is possible and is especially important when one is working in the deep structures within the brain.

The lesion is located relative to an external reference frame which is applied with compression pins fitted tightly to the skull. This external frame fits inside the scanner and is included in the scan of the lesion, permitting calculation of the precise trajectory of the biopsy probe. The Leksell frame and the Brown-Robert Wells (BRW) frame are both used for CT-guided stereotactic procedures at our institution. The Leksell is a square frame that allows access to the patient's head and airway. The BRW frame is cylindrical and fits completely around the head, providing little access to the airway once it is in place. Both frames are held in place with four pins in the skull; these pins may be placed with the patient under local anesthesia. The head must remain immobile with reference to the frame because the trajectory of the biopsy probe is calculated by referencing external markers on the frame to the lesion visualized by computed tomography. Airway management becomes difficult once the procedure is underway because of the position of the patient's head and body in the gantry.

Several factors are important to consider when one is selecting anesthetic techniques in this situation. Since the biopsy is usually performed on mass lesions, patients undergoing this procedure are considered to have increased intracranial pressure or the brain is considered to be highly intolerant of changes in intracranial volume. Techniques that increase Pco_2 are not safe in this context. Patients will have the frame placed around the head, and the head will be within the body of the scanner for much of the duration of the procedure, making access to the airway and usual airway management difficult. The procedure itself will involve creation of the burr hole and fixation of pins; painful procedures are often well tolerated with local anesthesia. Once the scanning and passage of the biopsy probe begin, there must be no change in relation of the patient to the frame, a situation facilitated by absolute stillness of the patient as well as head fixation in the frame.

Because of these considerations, we usually choose to anesthetize the patient with a general anesthetic. The airway can be easily controlled with endotracheal intubation, and hyperventilation can be used in the event of increased intracranial pressure. General anesthesia provides excellent analgesia for the burr hole and pin fixation, and will improve absolute patient immobility at crucial periods of the procedure.

Very cooperative and relatively healthy patients can tolerate the procedure under local anesthesia. The benefit of this approach is the continuous assessment of neurologic function as the biopsy probe follows the planned trajectory to the lesion. This approach may be necessary to avoid damage to the speech center when there are biopsying lesions in the left temporal lobe or to assess the response of tremor to thalamotomy. Unfortunately, sedation muddles the neurologic evaluation and may place the airway at risk, so it must be used judiciously, if at all, for these procedures.

Postoperatively, there is a small but significant risk of epidural, subdural, or intracerebral bleeding. The patient should recover in a location where frequent neurologic examination can be carried out.

Computed Tomography Scans/ Computed Tomography Myelograms

In small children, CT procedures frequently require the participation of an anesthetist. For a good quality study, the patient must be completely motionless. In the child older than 12 to 18 months of age, oral sedation is often not sufficient to keep him or her still. Multiple unsuccessful attempts at deepening levels of sedation are not as safe as a light general anesthetic with endotracheal intubation. The general anesthetics place the child at less risk for hypoventilation and hypoxia than do the additive and longer-duration effects of the drugs used for sedation. This is especially true in children evaluated for brain tumors or hydrocephalus where intracranial compliance is poor and the risk of increased intracranial pressure is greater.

Patients undergoing CT scans for extracranial lesions can be managed with intramuscular or intravenous ketamine mixed with a small amount of midazolam and atropine. This causes the child to be quiet, enabling him or her to be scanned easily after the head is positioned and taped in place. Since ketamine does not depress ventilation as greatly as other intravenous anesthetics, less airway support is required during the scan, when the anesthetist must be away from the patient's airway.

Respiratory and cardiovascular monitoring may be performed noninvasively and the patient observed through the leaded glass window while scanning takes place. All patients undergoing CT scans are monitored with electrocardiography with built-in respiratory rate monitor, automated blood pressure cuff, and pulse oximeter. Supplemental oxygen is given by mask to all patients.

Children undergoing myelography usually start in the lateral position for the lumbar puncture and are then turned supine with the body turned from side to side and with the legs elevated to facilitate movement of the dye through the subarachnoid space. During this maneuver, the patient's head is kept flexed to prevent movement of dye through the foramen magnum. Absolute control of the airway must be maintained during this process so that the endotracheal tube does not become dislodged and the child extubated. For the actual scan, the child is supine and the airway is easily secured.

Patients underoing CT scans and CT myelograms recover in the recovery room.

Angiography and Interventional Angiography

Interventional angiography is used to treat disorders such as intracranial arteriovenous malformations (AVMs), spinal cord AVM, facial AVM, carotid-cavernous fistulae (CCF), some intracranial aneurysms, cerebral vasospasm and vascular stenosis, glomus tumors, and meningiomas.

Therapeutic embolization of AVM allows a staged, safe approach to reduction and elimination of arteriovenous flow without the risk of surgery. A variety of embolizing materials are used, including solid particles, detachable balloons, and liquid agents. These materials are not interchangeable, and each has specific indications. Spheres or particles are used for very large AVMs. The principle in using spheres or particles is that they are injected into the internal carotid or the vertebral artery with the expectation that the "emboli" will be directed to the feeders of the AVM because of the higher flow. With this technique, however, particles occasionally go astray and may occlude normal cortical vessels. It appears that cortical tolerance to these particles is high, and neurologic deficit is usually transient. Much recent progress has been made using liquid embolizing agents, such as bucrylate. Potential risks for bucrylate embolization are injection into normal cortical branches; passage of bucrylate into the draining veins with the risk of swelling and bleeding of the AVM; and glueing of the catheter in the vessel being embolized.

There are two types of CCF: spontaneous and traumatic. Spontaneous CCFs result from the rupture of an aneurysm of the cavernous portion of the internal carotid artery or, more frequently, from an AVM of the dura of the cavernous sinus. Treatment is aimed at embolization of the external carotid branches or surgical exposure of the cavernous sinus and induced thrombosis of the sinus. Embolization techniques must be done carefully so that intracranial vessels remain intact. The embolization materials used are either particles or glue. The radiologist releases detachable balloons in the cavernous sinus, allowing preservation of internal carotid artery blood flow in 80 percent of the cases.

Giant aneurysms are also treated by embolization. These aneurysms are often located on the internal carotid artery, are thick walled, and are usually extra-arachnoid. The best treatment is balloon embolization, often with occlusion of the internal carotid artery.

Glomus tumor, nasopharyngeal angiofibromas, and angiomas bleed at the time of surgery. If they are embolized before surgery, the tumor can be devascularized, decreasing the risk for the patient. Because the branches of the external carotid are the vessels being embolized, the radiologist should be as selective as possible when embolizing. These procedures are usually done with particles. Surgery should be carried out within 24 to 48 hours so that recanalization of the vessels does not occur.

Anesthetic management for patients with brain AVMs almost always requires intravenous sedation techniques. The patient may or may not be premedicated, depending on the desires and needs of the anesthetist and the patient. We have found that the addition of metoclopramide (Reglan) to the premedication that the patient receives reduces the incidence of nausea and vomiting associated with the administration of large amounts of contrast media, which almost always occurs during these procedures.

Once the patient is in the angiography suite, we apply routine monitors, including automatic blood pressure cuff, electrocardiography, pulse oximetry, and skin temperature probe. An arterial line and central venous line are inserted for the monitoring and delivery of hypotensive and hypertensive agents that are often used in these procedures. A Foley catheter is useful both for monitoring urine output and because of the duration of the procedure (4 to 6 hours). Because the angiography room is often cold, plastic sheets are wrapped around the patient's legs, torso, and arms to help maintain body temperature. An eggcrate mattress is used to pad the table to keep the patient comfortable during the procedure.

Sedation is usually carried out using a combination of midazolam and fentanyl. Both drugs are titrated slowly, causing the patient to become calm and cooperative and enabling him or her to be easily aroused during the procedure to test neurologic function.

General anesthesia, when indicated, is usually performed using a balanced technique; in our institution, this is accomplished with fentanyl (moderate dose), thiopental, pancuronium, nitrous oxide, oxygen, and the addition of a volatile agent, as needed. Light general anesthesia is sufficient, as the procedure itself is not painful. As in any procedure involving neural tissue, it is important that the patient be awake and capable of being assessed neurologically at the end of the procedure. Somatosensory-evoked potentials are particularly useful in monitoring patients with spinal cord AVMs during embolization, and may be of benefit in patients under general anesthesia who are undergoing embolization of cortical areas in proximity to the sensory motor cortex. The patient should not cough at the end of the procedure before extubation is performed, as a No. 7 French introducer puncture has been made into the femoral artery and coughing can cause hemorrhage at the site.

Magnetic Resonance Imaging

As the magnetic resonance imaging (MRI) scanner becomes increasingly common and useful, more acutely ill and uncooperative patients will become candidates for MRI studies. Because of the high-energy magnetic fields generated, the use of ferromagnetic equipment in the vicinity of the scanner is not possible. Nonmagnetic materials, such as electrocardiographic lead wires, can act as antennae for radiofrequency signals, causing degradation of the electrocardiographic signal and distortions of the image.

Patients requiring mechanical ventilation, intravenous sedation, and general anesthesia can be safely monitored and studied in the scanner as long as there are a limited number of magnetic items in place around the scanner and these items are well secured. Designs for anesthesia machines and equipment have been reported that use few ferromagnetic parts and are securely anchored as far from the magnet as possible. A nonferromagnetic, oxygen-powered ventilator has been developed for use in the scanner, although traditional hand-bagging for ventilation requires few modifications to be effective. Electro-cardiographic electrodes can be connected with short wires to a telemetered signal, but the telemetered signal will show interference from the scanner. Most MRI scanners are now equipped with electrocardiographic monitoring in order to provide gated cardiac images. Automated blood pressure cuff devices have proven satisfactory during scanning when the pump is placed distant from the patient and long tubing is connected to the blood pressure cuff. Transducers and displays for intra-arterial or central pressure monitoring should be located as far from the patient as possible with the use of long extension tubing. Further development of nonferromagnetic devices will allow this modality to be used increasingly in patients requiring general anesthesia and invasive monitoring during MRI procedures.

SUGGESTED READING

Hacke W, Zeumer H. Berg Dammer E. Monitoring of hemispheric or brainstem functions with neurophysiologic methods during interventional radiology. AJNR 1983; 4:382–384.

Kendall B. Results of treatment of arteriovenous fistulae with the Debrun technique. AJNR 1983; 4:405–408.

Karlik SJ, Heatherley T, Pavan F, et al. Patient anesthesia and monitoring at a 1.5-T MRI installation. Magn Reson Med 1988; 7:210–221.

Scialfa G, Valsecchi F, Scotti G. Treatment of vascular lesions with balloon catheters. AJNR 1983; 4:395–398.

Smith DS, Askey P, Young ML, Kressel HY. Anesthetic management of acutely ill patients during magnetic resonance imaging [letter]. Anesthesiology 1986; 65:710–711.

Trankina MF, Houser WO, Cucchiara RF. Neurodiagnostic procedures. In: Cucchiara RF, Michenfelder JD, eds. Clinical neuroanesthesia. New York: Churchill Livingstone, 1990; 421.

ELECTROCONVULSIVE THERAPY

ROBERT W. McPHERSON, M.D.
JOHN R. LIPSEY, M.D.

In the general population, the prevalence of sustained or severe depressive states is approximately 5 percent. The patients who require electroconvulsive therapy (ECT) pose significant anesthetic management problems because of coexisting medical diseases and sequalae of depression such as malnutrition and noncompliance in taking medications. In providing optimal care for these patients, cooperation between the anesthesiologist and the psychiatrist is necessary. Because anesthesia is required for ECT, these patients may not be offered treatment if either the psychiatrist or the anesthesiologist considers anesthesia to pose a greater risk than the complications of untreated severe depression. We have conducted multiple series of ECTs in patients with unstable angina, recent myocardial infarction, pregnancy, intracranial tumor, respiratory failure, and recent stroke. Although these disease entities have been considered relative contraindications to ECT, our opinion has been that the risk to the patient would be greater if ECT were not performed. Although the care of these patients has been demanding, the clinical improvement in each has been gratifying.

Severe depression may be treated either medically (with tricyclic antidepressants or monoamine oxidase inhibitors) or with ECT. Although the choice of therapy (drugs versus ECT) resides with the psychiatrist, ECT may be excluded in the medically complicated patient if the anesthesiologist does not understand the indications for ECT or its therapeutic efficacy. Optimally, in deciding whether to use treatment with drugs or ECT, one should consider the severity of the patient's depression, prior pharmacologic therapy, and potential adverse effects, rather than the coexisting medical conditions.

Although ECT has been used for more than 40 years for the treatment of depression, it continues to have adverse social implications. Thus, antidepressants are frequently the initial therapy even in severe depression and despite a high rate of therapeutic failure (30 to 40 percent), prolonged time for therapeutic effect (weeks), and a significant incidence of complications (orthostatic hypotension, cardiac conduction abnormalities). Therefore, patients who are referred for ECT generally have failed drug therapy, have had significant complications with the use of antidepressants, or require rapid intervention.

In patients who have maintained adequate nutrition and hydration, who are cooperative, and who are neither delusional nor suicidal, antidepressant drugs—tricyclic antidepressants (TCAs) and monoamine oxidase inhibitors (MAOIs) are almost always effective. TCAs are usually more effective than MAOIs and are considered the drugs of choice. Because patients with delusions, hallucinations, and profound psychomotor retardation are less responsive to drugs, ECT is considered early in the treatment of such cases, as it is in the case of acutely suicidal patients. Preanesthetic evaluation of these patients may therefore be hampered because of the patient's inability to give a reliable history.

MECHANISM OF ACTION AND CARDIOVASCULAR RESPONSES

Although the mechanism of action is uncertain, it is the induced generalized seizure rather than the electrical stimulus that is responsible for the therapeutic effect of ECT. Although both unilateral and bilateral electrical stimuli may be administered, unilateral stimulation is preferred because of a lesser incidence of confusion and memory impairment. Generally, a series of six to ten treatments given two to three times per week are required for a good therapeutic effect. As with drug therapy, relapses are common and refractory cases return for ECT at 6- to 12-month intervals.

The ECT stimulus causes a grand mal seizure with an increase in cerebral blood flow and cerebral oxygen utilization. The electrically induced seizure also activates the autonomic nervous system. This is manifested by an initial parasympathetic-sympathetic outflow, beginning immediately after stimulation, that is fairly short-lived (duration of 2 to 5 minutes). This is followed by a second, less dramatic parasympathetic-sympathetic outflow, which persists into the recovery period. The initial parasympathetic outflow occurs immediately after stimulation and generally results in bradycardia (occasionally 3 to 6 seconds of asystole) that is self-limited. Only infrequently is an intravenous anticholinergic agent necessary to treat this bradycardia. The parasympathetic response is followed by a sympathetic outflow that produces hypertension and tachycardia. A secondary parasympathetic-sympathetic outflow frequently follows and lasts 5 to 10 minutes. These hemodynamic changes are usually short-lived and frequently resolve without treatment.

In addition to an increase in heart rate, which averages 35 beats per minute, the autonomic imbalance causes an increase in the PR interval and an increase in the QT interval. Rarely, ECT results in deep T-wave inversion in chest and limb leads, which may last for hours or days, suggesting myocardial infarction. These changes are believed to be caused by the effect of electrical stimulation on the ventral hippocampus and amygdala. The incidence of arrhythmias may vary, with the occurrence of premature atrial contractions, premature ventricular contractions (PVCs), multifocal PVCs, and ST-segment depression having been reported to be 18 percent, 33 percent, 14 percent, and 22 percent, respectively. Again, these changes are usually self-limited and generally do not require specific treatment.

Hypertension is common after ECT, and in many patients, systolic pressures of greater than 200 mm Hg are achieved. Although this blood pressure increase is of fairly short duration (<10 minutes), a short-acting vasodilator may be necessary to prevent myocardial ischemia.

PREOPERATIVE EVALUATION AND LOGISTICAL CONSIDERATIONS

Severe depression occurs as a primary illness or as a component of other major illnesses. For example, cerebrovascular accident, Parkinson's disease, hypothyroidism, Cushing's syndrome, and intracranial tumors may be associated with severe depression. Additionally, the depressed patient may be malnourished, dehydrated, and noncompliant in taking chronic medications. A thorough preanesthetic evaluation must therefore be conducted to rule out anatomic or physiologic/metabolic lesions in patients who may be extremely unreliable historians. Careful evaluation of medical records, history from family, and the aggressive use of diagnostic tests are frequently necessary to overcome the lack of a reliable patient history. Diagnostic tests such as computed tomography (CT) may be necessary to rule out intracranial pathology (stroke, tumor) as the cause of the patient's psychiatric symptoms.

Because many patients must receive repetitive ECT treatment, an efficient evaluation, treatment, and recovery system must be developed in which uncomplicated patients are cared for and in which effective identification, evaluation, and treatment of medically complicated patients are carried out. Ideally, a separate location (meeting all criteria for an anesthetizing location) should be available in which patients undergoing ECT may receive care. This should include a waiting area, a treatment area, and a recovery area. In order to decrease anxiety in this group of patients, the area should be quiet and physically isolated from other activities. The recovery area should have electrocardiographic monitors, piped-in oxygen, and suction.

Because of the repetitive nature of ECT and the frequent need for treatment of relapse, a permanent record of the patient's anesthetic requirements, cardiovascular response to shock, and unusual drug requirements or responses allows rapid and accurate adjustment of drug therapy.

Emergency indications include acutely suicidal patients, patients in whom profound psychomotor retardation increases the risk of atelectasis and deep vein thrombosis, and in patients in whom agitation complicates other medical conditions such as myocardial ischemia. Given these emergency indications for ECT, a close working relationship between the psychiatrist and anesthesiologist is required to facilitate rapid preanesthetic evaluation.

CONTRAINDICATIONS AND MEDICAL CONDITIONS OF INTEREST

The effects of ECT on certain medical conditions are listed in Table 1. As with other medical interventions, all contraindications should be considered relative to the risk of not performing the intervention. In addition to the possibility of suicide and the medical risk of untreated depression, the psychic pain of persisting depression must not be underestimated. Since psychic pain is much more difficult to determine than physical pain and suffering, the psychiatrist must provide the anesthesiologist with an estimate of that pain. The more medically ill patients are, the more important is this estimate of psychic pain. The last days of a depressed terminally ill patient may be salvaged and spent productively in accepting death and completing important business if depression can be successfully treated with ECT.

The cardiovascular changes associated with ECT require careful investigation to determine the presence and extent of cardiovascular diseases such as hypertension and coronary artery disease (CAD). Based on symptoms, CAD may be classified as mild stable angina (e.g., >3 block exercise tolerance), moderately severe angina (<1 block exercise tolerance) and severe angina (e.g., angina at rest). The preoperative management, care during ECT, and postoperative care are different for each degree of angina. The patient with mild stable angina can be safely managed with routine monitoring (blood pressure cuff; electrocardiography), assuming that the patient is receiving adequate antianginal medications. Pretreatment evaluation of patients with more severe angina may include echocardiography and/or coronary angiography. Invasive monitoring should be used during the initial episodes of ECT in these patients.

Arterial catheterization will allow rapid and accurate determination of blood pressure. Continuous measurement of blood pressure will also allow aggressive use of vasodilators to control blood pressure. Pulmonary artery catheterization should be considered in the patients with severe angina to determine the extent of left ventricular dysfunction occurring with ECT-induced hypertension. Patients with CAD are also at risk for ischemia during post-treatment confusion, and this is also associated with hypertension. Recovery following the initial treatment should take place in the postoperative recovery room where invasive monitoring can be continued. The necessity of invasive monitoring usually decreases since the patient's cardiovascular response to ECT and the efficacy of treatment are determined during early treatments. Patients with cardiac pacemakers do not require special treatment except to verify that the pacer is functional.

Depression can be caused by intracranial masses and may occur at any time during the course of the patient's medical treatment. If possible, definitive surgery should be performed before ECT. Although little information is available, postponing ECT for 6 weeks after craniotomy seems reasonable. If ECT must be performed when an intracranial mass is present, blood pressure should be controlled near normal levels and hyperventilation maintained while the patient is anesthetized. Because the sudden increase in blood pressure which usually follows the electrical stimulus will increase intracranial pressure (ICP) and possibly cause brain stem herniation, this response should be blunted. Since both nitroglycerin and nitroprusside increase ICP, they should be used only sparingly in these patients. Beta-blockade with propranolol hydrochloride (Inderal) (1 mg increments, IV) will blunt the hypertensive response without increasing ICP.

Hiatal hernia is common in patients requiring ECT. Since the patients will receive six to ten anesthetics, the decision to intubate the patient should be made carefully. If the patient is asymptomatic, intubation may be avoided. Patients who are mildly symptomatic should receive antacids or drugs to reduce gastric secretions before treatment. Intubation should be reserved for patients who have a history of significant reflux.

Malignant neuroleptic syndrome (MNS) occurs occasionally in patients receiving neuroleptic drugs such as haloperidol (Haldol). This syndrome is characterized by hypertension, tachycardia, hyperthermia, and extrapyramidal signs. Leukocytosis and elevation of serum creatine phosphokinase levels also occur frequently. Treatment is to discontinue the offending drug, and symptoms usually resolve over 1 week. Although the mechanism is unknown, the similarity to malignant hyperpyrexia has raised the issue of whether the patient is at risk for malignant hyperpyrexia. Patients with a history of MNS have been anesthetized for ECT without occurrence of malignant hyperpyrexia. However, we routinely avoid succinylcholine chloride in these patients to decrease the risk of malignant hyperpyrexia and use atracurium besylate instead.

Table 1 Medical Conditions Requiring Special Consideration Prior to the Use of Electroconvulsive Therapy

Condition	Comments
Hiatal hernia	Increased risk of regurgitation
Pregnancy	Supine hypotension syndrome
Angina	Risk of myocardial ischemia caused by hypertension and tachycardia
Myopathy	Increased sensitivity to muscle relaxants
Arterial aneurysm	Postshock hypertension may cause vessel rupture
Carotid stenosis	Inability to increase cerebral blood flow during seizure
Intracranial tumor	ICP increases with seizure; possible brain stem herniation
Perforated viscus	Risk of viscus rupture
Cerebrovascular accident	Hypertension may cause intracerebral bleed

Succinylcholine chloride in the circumstance of upper motor neuron lesion (stroke) or lower motor neuron (spinal cord lesion) may result in hyperkalemia. Short-acting nondepolarizing muscle relaxants should be used in such patients monitored with a nerve stimulator and reversed with an anticholinesterase plus an anticholinergic. Since peripheral nerve stimulation may be unreliable in such patients, adequacy of ventilation must be carefully evaluated. ECT should be postponed for as long as possible following a cerebrovascular accident. The hypertension that follows the electrical stimulus may cause hemorrhage into the area of previous ischemia. In these patients, the increase in blood pressure should be treated aggressively or prevented by administering an intravenous vasodilator immediately before the stimulus is received.

Patients with a history of seizures are particularly difficult to manage for ECT. Antiseizure medication may prevent the induced seizure. Since discontinuation of these medications may lead to spontaneous seizures, a reasonable therapeutic plan is to decrease the medication dose and attempt ECT. If this is unsuccessful, the medication should be further decreased and ECT again attempted. The management goal is to maintain antiseizure medications at the highest level that will allow a therapeutic seizure. There is a theoretical risk of a prolonged seizure after the ECT or recurrence of spontaneous seizures, but these events can be managed with intravenous anticonvulsants (diazepam, thiopental).

Acquired immunodeficiency syndrome (AIDS) is a terminal illness in which severe depression may occur. These patients pose problems for anesthetic management and prevention of spread of the disease if ECT is required. The high incidence of intracranial masses, either neoplasms or abscesses, requires that a CT be performed very soon before ECT. Hospital infectious disease specialists can give suggestions regarding sterilization of equipment, and the use of disposable equipment is strongly advised, as well as treating the patient at the end of the ECT schedule.

Thrombophlebitis may predispose the patient to pulmonary embolus after ECT. If ECT is necessary in a patient with thrombophlebitis, the patient should be stabilized with the use of anticoagulants or heparin before therapy. Management should include complete paralysis prior to the electrical stimulus to minimize the risk of violent muscle contractures dislodging emboli from the pelvic or lower extremity veins.

Skeletal instability requires careful attention to prevent injury during ECT. Patients with recent fractures or postsurgical spinal instability (actual or potential), such as that following extensive laminectomy, are best treated by complete paralysis (verified by nerve stimulation) prior to ECT and by mechanical maintenance in the normal position achieved with the use of neck braces, and casts, for example.

Pregnant patients should be positioned with a wedge under the right hip to prevent the supine hypotension syndrome. Fetal monitoring with Doppler or ultrasonography is useful in assessing the fetal response to treatment.

PSYCHIATRIC DRUGS COMMONLY USED IN THE TREATMENT OF DEPRESSED PATIENTS

Psychiatric drugs and their effects in patients receiving ECT are listed in Table 2. TCAs and MAOIs are commonly used to treat depression. Since many patients have failed drug therapy before being considered for ECT, the anesthesiologist often encounters patients in whom psychotropic drugs have been recently discontinued. Other patients may be taking TCAs or MAOIs concurrently with ECT because of a past history of relapse of depression shortly after a successful ECT course.

According to traditional teaching, MAOIs should be discontinued for 2 weeks before the patient is to undergo anesthesia and surgery. Nonhydrazine derivatives are reversible blockers which, when discontinued, have no pharmacologic effect after 24 to 48 hours. However, the hydrazines (e.g., phenelzine) irreversibly block monoamine oxidase, and the drug effect persists for 14 to 21 days. MAOIs may interact with sympathomimetic drugs to produce hypertensive crises. Although excessive reflex sympathetic activity has been suggested as a possible complication of ECT combined with MAOIs, we have not found excessive increases in blood pressure rises following the stimulus in patients receiving MAOIs, and we continue to administer these drugs if psychiatrically indicated.

Tricyclic antidepressants may interact with anticholinergics (enhanced anticholinergic effects), antihypertensives (enhanced orthostatic hypotension), sedatives (increased sedation), and sympathomimetics (TCA may potentiate blood pressure increases). TCA may also produce cardiac conduction abnormalities.

For medically stable patients, TCAs may be safely continued during ECT if psychiatrically indicated. For patients without a history of rapid post-ECT relapse, however, there is no added antidepressant benefit of combining ECT with TCAs or MAOIs.

ANESTHETIC MANAGEMENT

The anesthetics used during ECT are listed in Table 3. Briefly, the anesthetic requirements for ECT are (1) to make the patient amnestic to the treatment; (2) to prevent hypoxia; (3) to prevent sequelae of the tonic-clonic contracture, such as long bone fractures; (4) to moderate the hemodynamic responses (particularly hypertension); and (5) to allow rapid awakening after treatment. The combination of ventilation with 100 percent oxygen, methohexital, and succinylcholine chloride is widely used to meet these requirements. The doses of both drugs are less than those used for induction of surgical anesthesia. Methohexital (0.5 to 1.0 mg per kilogram) and succinylcholine chloride (0.25 to 0.5 mg

Table 2 Psychiatric Drugs and their Effects in Patients Receiving Electroconvulsive Therapy

Agent	Comments		
Tricyclic Antidepressants	Sedation	Hypotension	Anticholinergic
Desipramine hydrochloride (Norpramin)	+	+ +	+
Nortriptyline hydrochloride (Aventyl hydrochloride)	+	+ +	+ +
Protriptyline hydrochloride (Vivactil)	+	+ +	+ +
Amitriptyline hydrochloride (Elavil)	+ + +	+ + +	+ + +
Doxepin hydrochloride (Sinequan)	+ + +	+ +	+ +
Imipramine hydrochloride (Tofranil)	+ +	+ + +	+ +
Monoamine Oxidase Inhibitors		Risk of hypertension	Orthostatic hypotension
Phenelzine sulfate (Nardil)*		+	+ +
Isocarboxazid (Marplan)*		+	+ + +
Tranylcypromine (Parnate)†		+ +	+ +
Anticonvulsants		Elevates induced seizure threshold	
Phenytoin (Dilantin)		+ + +	
Phenobarbital (Luminal)		+ + +	
Primidone (Mysoline)		+ +	
Carbamazepine (Tegretol)		+ + +	
Ethosuximide (Zarontin)		+	
Valproic acid (Depakene)		+	
Diazepam (Valium)		+ +	

Table 3 Anesthetics for Electroconvulsive Therapy

Anesthetic	Dose	Comments
Hypnotics		
Brevital sodium	1 mg/kg	Lowers seizure threshold
Thiopental	2–3 mg/kg	Longer sleep time than with brevital sodium
Diazepam	0.3–0.5 mg/kg	Raises seizure threshold
Etomidate	0.2–0.4 mg/kg	
Propofol	1.3 mg/kg	Reduces seizure duration by approximately 40 percent compared with brevital sodium
Muscle relaxants		
Succinylcholine chloride	0.5–1.0 mg/kg	Contraindicated in neurologic injury
Atracurium besylate	0.1–0.4 mg/kg	Time to 95% recovery = 23–44 min
Vasodilators		
Diazoxide	200 mg	Administered before treatment
Nitroprusside	50–100 μg	Rapid onset; short-acting
Nitroglycerin	50–100 μg	Rapid onset; short-acting
Esmolol hydrochloride	80-mg bolus plus 24 mg/min for 2 min before and 5 min after ECT	Blunt heart rate increase by 24%, arterial pressure increase by 14%, and rate pressure produce increase by 37%

per kilogram) are widely used. The dosage of each is adjusted to ensure unconsciousness and prevent injury caused by muscle contracture. Medication during the initial ECT should err on the side of the higher doses, and the dosage should be decreased subsequently after evaluation of the response during the initial treatment.

Prestimulus hyperventilation with 20 breaths of 100 percent oxygen decreases arterial carbon dioxide pressure ($PaCO_2$) by approximately 10 mm Hg, and increases seizure duration by approximately 20 percent. Hyperventilation also decreases the incidence of oxygen desaturation. Hyperventilation with 30 percent oxygen leads to a shorter seizure duration than hyperventilation with 100 percent oxygen.

The dose of succinylcholine chloride should prevent sequelae of the convulsion without producing a prolonged period of paralysis. Inflation of a blood pressure cuff above systolic blood pressure on one bicep or calf will prevent succinylcholine chloride from reaching one hand or foot, thus allowing complete motor expression of the seizure. This precaution should be taken in patients who receive a full paralyzing dose of muscle relaxant. A peripheral nerve stimulator can be used to assess the degree of muscle paralysis. In patients without significant risk factors for fracture, 0.5 mg per kilogram of succinylcholine chloride sufficiently blunts the muscular response without preventing identification of the seizure. The incidence of post-treatment muscle pain is not decreased by decreasing the succinlycholine dose.

Although the effects of ECT on the cardiac rhythm are usually self-limited, treatment may occasionally be necessary. Atropine (0.5 mg, IV) is effective in treating bradycardia, and inderal (0.5 to 2.0 mg, IV) may be useful in treating tachycardia. Lidocaine (1 to 2 mg per kilogram, IV) can be used to treat premature ventricular contractions.

Ideally, each patient will respond to a single electrical stimulus with an induced seizure of adequate duration (>25 seconds). Unfortunately, a significant number of patients either fail to have a generalized seizure or have a seizure of insufficient duration. Repetitive stimuli require additional hypnotic and muscle relaxant drugs. Since additional anesthetic agents may significantly prolong recovery, the total number of stimuli to be used should be decided on before therapy. We believe that a maximum of four stimuli should be allowed. If the patient does not respond, attempts should be discontinued and the patient taken to the recovery area. The ECT equipment should be inspected for correct function, and one should seek causes of resistance to seizures (e.g., drugs which elevate the seizure threshold). In patients with severe cardiac disease, even subconvulsive shocks may result in transient asystole.

Prolonged seizure activity is undesirable because of the risk of inadequate cerebral oxygenation and prolonged disorientation that occurs after prolonged seizures. Induced seizures that last at least 25 seconds are effective in treating depression. There is no evidence that prolonged seizures improve recovery of depression, and unusually prolonged seizures should be terminated. Termination of induced seizures at 3 minutes seems reasonable. Although diazepam is the drug of choice for treatment of spontaneous seizures, the prolonged associated somnolence may be undesirable. Thiopental (1 to 2 mg per kilogram) will frequently end the seizure rapidly. Since these patients may have prolonged sedation, they should be carefully observed after treatment.

Each new hypnotic agent and short-acting muscle relaxant has been evaluated for use during ECT. Hypnotics such as thiopental, diazepam, and etomidate have been shown to lower the indicence of seizures and prolonged awakening time. Adequate ventilation returns more rapidly with the use of succinylcholine chloride than with agents such as atracurium besylate.

An increase in oral secretions occurs after ECT. Although drying agents have been recommended, these secretions are of little consequence. Since pretreatment with anticholinergics will enhance the tachycardia and hypertension that follow ECT, these agents are best avoided, especially in patients at risk for myocardia ischemia. Patients with a history of bradycardia, however, may require pre-ECT anticholinergic treatment.

POST-TREATMENT CARE

Immediately after ECT, the patients are generally confused, and, if possible, a psychiatric ward nurse familiar with the patient should be available to help orient him or her. Occasionally, a patient will be severely agitated or combative after treatment. This agitation frequently responds to small doses (1.25 to 2.5 mg) of intravenous intramuscular droperidol. If this emergence phenomenon occurs fairly consistently with each treatment, small doses of droperidol given immediately after treatment may minimize the post-ECT agitation and risk of injury to the patient or staff.

SUGGESTED READING

Bajc M. Medved V, Basic M, et al. Acute effect of electroconvulsive therapy on brain perfusion assessed by ^{99}Tc hexamethylpropyleneamineoxim and single photon emission computed tomography. Acta Psychiatr Scand 1989; 80:421–426.

Barkai AL. Combined electroconvulsive therapy and drug therapy. Compr Ther 1985; 11:48–53.

El-Ganzouri AR, Ivankovich AD, Braverman B, McCarthey R. Monoamine oxidase inhibitors: should they be discontinued preoperatively? Anesth Analg 1985; 65:592–596.

Lew JK, Eastley RJ, Hanning CD. Oxygenation during electroconvulsive therapy: a comparison of two anesthetic techniques. Anesthesiology 1986; 41:1092–1097.

Mielke DH, Winstead DK, Goethe JW, Schwartz BD. Multiple monitored electroconvulsive therapy: safety and efficacy in elderly depressed patients. J Am Geriatr Soc 1984; 32:180–182.

Räsänen J, Martin DJ, Downs JB, Hodges MH. Oxygen supplementation during electroconvulsive therapy. Br J Anaesth 1988; 61: 593–597.

Wells DG, Zelcer J, Treadrae C. ECT-induced asystole from a sub-convulsive shock. Anaesth Inten Care 1988; 16:368–373.

ANESTHESIA IN ORTHOPEDIC SURGERY

KYPHOSCOLIOSIS

ELLIOT J. KRANE, M.D.

The successful repair of kyphoscoliotic curvatures of the spine has been undertaken for the past several decades. The anesthetic management of the patient with kyphoscoliosis includes careful preoperative assessment of coexisting disease and secondary pulmonary impairment, limitation of intraoperative blood loss and therefore transfusion requirement, intraoperative monitoring of spinal cord function, and postoperative respiratory therapy.

ETIOLOGY

Scoliosis frequently is not itself a disease, but rather the result of a disease. A wide variety of processes can result in a pathologic spinal curvature (Table 1). Most patients with scoliosis have the idiopathic variety, an entity that most frequently occurs in healthy teenaged girls. Idiopathic scoliosis first becomes apparent during late childhood and progresses unless intervention is made. Conservative management with bracing or body casts alone may be effective, but if the curve worsens in spite of these measures, surgical intervention is indicated to preserve adequate pulmonary function.

In the remainder of the patients, scoliosis is the result of a defined neuromuscular disease such as myelodysplasia or Duchenne's muscular dystrophy, spinal cord pathology such as neurofibromatosis or syringomyelia, or a discrete anatomic abnormality such as congenital hemivertebrae or spinal fracture(s). In these patients, the indication for surgery may be to improve the level of function in order to allow the patient to sit upright in a wheelchair, or, most important, to arrest the deterioration of pulmonary function, which occurs as the curvature progresses. It has recently been learned that the life expectancy of handicapped patients may be increased and the quality of life improved by postponing or avoiding the inexorable decline of ventilatory capacity that was once so often the slow and excruciating cause of death in this population. To provide optimal anesthetic care, the anesthetist must be familiar with the underlying disease process and all its ramifications.

Table 1 Classification of Scoliosis

Type
I.   Idiopathic (primary) scoliosis
II. Congenital scoliosis (e.g., hemivertebrae)
III. Secondary scoliosis
A. Neuromuscular
1. Neuropathic (e.g., poliomyelitis, spastic cerebral palsy, arthrogryposis, myelodysplasia)
B. Connective tissue disease
1. Congenital (e.g., Marfan's syndrome, mucopolysaccharidoses, osteogenesis imperfecta)
2. Acquired (e.g., juvenile rheumatoid arthritis)
C. Traumatic (e.g., fracture)

SURGICAL PROCEDURES

Kyphosis refers to the round-back deformity seen most frequently in the thoracic spine. Scoliosis refers to the lateral curvature that is associated with a marked rotational curvature of the spine, which may involve either or both of the lumbar and thoracic spines.

Most cases of scoliosis are repaired with a single-stage posterior fusion. If a scoliosis has a significant kyphotic component (kyphoscoliosis), a two-stage procedure is common: the kyphous is usually repaired first through a right-sided thoracotomy, by lysing the anterior ligaments of the vertebral bodies, removing the intervertebral discs, and fusing the released spine. One to two weeks after the anterior fusion, the scoliosis is repaired with a posterior fusion, which often includes the insertion of instrumentation to stabilize the spine. As surgical and anesthetic technique improves, more patients are being subjected to both anterior and posterior fusions during the same period of anesthesia.

The most common methods used currently are the Harrington, Cotrel-Dubousset (CD), and Luque procedures. In these methods, the spinous processes of the involved spine are removed and the lamina of the vertebrae are decorticated, which destroys the facet joints. During the Harrington and CD procedures, a rod is inserted in the concave side of the curve, hooked between facets at the upper and lower ends of the curve, and lengthened, thereby reducing the curve. This procedure is generally reserved for patients with idiopathic scoliosis. The Luque rod technique is performed in patients who have chronic debilitating diseases, in whom osteoporosis and bone fragility limits the use of the Harrington or CD rods. After decortication of the spine, two rods are bent to conform to the curvature of the spine, and a series of wires are passed around each lamina and twisted tightly around the rods. This stabilizes the spine and reduces the curvature, while distributing the force of the rods evenly throughout the spinal column. Because the latter procedure involves more dissection and includes more spinal segments, blood loss is generally greater during Luque fusions. Blood loss is usually not excessive during anterior approaches to repair kyphosis.

REDUCING OPERATIVE BLOOD LOSS

Spinal fusions are extensive operations that result in significant intraoperative bleeding. Several important techniques are at the disposal of the anesthesiologist to minimize blood loss and the consequent need for transfusion.

One of the most important methods is careful patient positioning. The use of the Hall frame or other equivalent four-poster positioning devices permits the weight of the prone patient to be supported on the pelvis and upper thorax, which allows the abdomen to fall freely. Pressure on the abdomen increases intra-abdominal and inferior vena caval pressure and can result in diversion of blood to the vertebral venous plexus. Neuromuscular blockade results in abdominal wall and diaphragmatic relaxation, which further reduces intra-abdominal pressure. Zero or even negative end-expiratory pressure has been advocated by some authorities in order to enhance venous return to the heart, although the latter may theoretically increase the risk of venous air embolism, which is an uncommon but reported complication of spinal fusion.

For the past two decades, controlled hypotension has been successfully used to reduce intraoperative blood loss, and it is now a well-accepted technique. Moderate reduction of mean arterial pressure reduces blood loss by about 40 percent and results in improved operating conditions and shorter operating times. Whereas it is generally accepted that the mean arterial blood pressure may be safely reduced to 60 to 65 mm Hg without producing tissue ischemia in young, fit individuals, the safe lower limit has not been determined in small children. Because young children normally have a mean arterial pressure of only 60 to 70 mm Hg, one may presume that proportional reductions of blood pressure are safe, but confirmatory data are lacking. My practice is to reduce mean blood pressure by 15 to 20 percent below baseline values, but not lower than 50 mm Hg. Because hyperventilation further reduces blood flow to both the brain and spinal cord, every attempt is made to preserve normocapnia during induced hypotension.

Of the several agents in use for this purpose, my preference is for sodium nitroprusside (Nipride). Its immediately onset of action, ease of use, and rapid termination of effect after discontinuation have proved it to be safe and controllable. The rate of administration should be less than 8 μg per kilogram per minute in order to minimize the risk of cyanide toxicity. Occasionally, patients demonstrate resistance to nitroprusside. After inadequate anesthesia has been ruled out, it is useful to administer a beta-adrenergic blocking agent. Propranolol (0.01 to 0.04 mg per kilogram) or esmolol (500 μg per kilogram, followed by 50 to 200 μg per kilogram per minute) blocks the compensatory tachycardia that occasionally meets pharmacologic attempts to lower the blood pressure.

Other hypotensive agents have been used. Nitroglycerin is a less potent hypotensive agent, and several reports suggest that it may interfere with platelet function. Trimethaphan (Arfonad) is a ganglionic-blocking drug with a short duration of action, but its use often results in tachyphylaxis and compensatory tachycardia, which limit the anesthetist's ability to control the circulation with this agent. Experimentally, trimethaphan reduces cerebral and spinal cord blood flow, theoretically making this agent less desirable. Frequently, one need only use deep levels of potent inhalation agents in order to achieve an acceptable depression of arterial blood pressure. This is also an acceptable technique unless spinal cord monitoring is employed, since deep levels of potent inhalation anesthetics can interfere with the veracity of evoked potential recordings and may result in delayed awakening if an intraoperative wake-up test is required.

Other techniques have been used to reduce the requirement for blood transfusion. Autotransfusion of scavenged, washed, and refiltered red blood cells is used at some institutions with success, but requires the use of expensive apparatus and the presence of a trained autotransfusion technician or second physician to operate the apparatus. Although the life span of autotransfused red blood cells after spine surgery and the risk of transfusion of red cell debris and fat globules have not been described, the technique appears to be safe and well tolerated.

Hemodilution for spinal fusion is usually reserved for patients with religious convictions that lead them to oppose blood transfusion. In concert with controlled hypotension and an anesthetic technique that provides a high inspired oxygen fraction, the need for blood transfusion is usually avoided. The method has been described elsewhere.

Controlled hypotensive anesthesia does not imply toleration of hypovolemia, but could more aptly be termed "euvolemic hypotensive anesthesia." Blood and fluid losses are difficult to quantify during spinal fusions. Weighing sponges can contribute to the accuracy of the estimate of blood loss in smaller patients. Evaporative losses from the large open wound are significant. Blood and fluid losses are replaced, accompanied by monitoring of the hematocrit, acid-base status, urinary output, and, in some cases, central venous pressure. In most patients, I begin to replace blood loss with red blood cells when the intraoperative hematocrit falls to below 25 percent.

MONITORING THE PATIENT

Routine monitoring of the patient who is undergoing spinal fusion includes continuous electrocardiography, auscultation of heart tones and breath sounds with an esophageal stethoscope, measurement of temperature and urinary output, peripheral nerve stimulation, and capnography. An intra-arterial cannula for continuous monitoring of blood pressure and intermittent sampling of arterial blood for gas tensions and hematocrit is necessary in the case of anterior fusions or if controlled hypotension or hemodilution is planned. In selected patients, central venous or pulmonary artery catheters are required. Indications include the presence of significant pulmonary disease, cor pulmonale, pulmonary hypertension, or intrinsic cardiac disease. I also routinely monitor pulmonary artery pressure if hemodilution is undertaken, to allow calculation of oxygen delivery and extraction.

A major surgical complication of spinal instrumentation and fusion is spinal cord injury with subsequent paraplegia; this has a reported incidence of 0.1 percent. Over-reduction of the spinal curvature leads to compromised cord blood flow and function. Early detection of cord dysfunction and modification of the surgical correction within 3 hours can prevent permanent sequelae. The anesthesiologist is an important participant in monitoring for this infrequent but devastating problem. Patients without a functioning cord, such as individuals with myelodysplasia or preoperative paraplegia, need not be monitored, but the majority of patients should be. The choice of anesthetic technique profoundly affects the accuracy of cord function monitoring.

Two techniques are presently in use: the intraoperative wake-up test and measurement of somatosensory evoked potentials (SSEPs). The former, a test of long track and anterior horn function, requires the anesthesiologist to awaken the patient on the operating table after the distraction rod is in place and fully lengthened. The patient moves his or her feet on command, and general anesthesia is recommended. If no voluntary movement occurs, the surgeon relaxes the rods. SSEPs are a measure of dorsal column function. Stimulating electrodes are placed on the lower extremities over the posterior tibial nerves, and the evoked potentials are recorded over the cervical spinal cord and the cerebral cortex in order to measure the amplitude and latency of the signal. An increase in the latency predicts neurologic dysfunction, which alerts the surgeon to alter the operative technique and the anesthesiologist to restore the blood pressure to normal levels.

For an intraoperative wake-up test, it is important to inform patients of the planned test during the preoperative visit and to rehearse them in the precise words to be used to command movement of the lower extremities. Patients are informed of the necessity of the test and reassured that recall of intraoperative awakening is very unusual. The surgeon should inform the anesthesiologist 15 to 30 minutes before the anticipated test, in order to allow him or her ample time to partially reverse neuromuscular blockade and discontinue any potent inhalation agents. While monitoring with a peripheral nerve stimulator, half the usual dose of neostigmine and atropine is administered, supplementing the reversal dose as needed in order to achieve four "train-of-four" twitches. At the appointed time, while the anesthesiologist holds both the patient's hands, administration of nitrous oxide is discontinued and an assistant observes the lower extremities under the drapes. After a further 2 or 3 minutes, the patient is instructed to squeeze both hands. When cooperation with this command is certain, the patient is told to move both feet. If absence of movement of one or both feet is observed, the length of the distraction rod is reduced and the test is repeated. On completion of the test, a sleep dose of thiopental is administered concomitantly with an intravenous benzodiazepine (for its putative amnesic effect); neuromuscular blockade is restored by careful titration of relaxant, and any inhalation agents are reintroduced.

Monitoring of evoked potentials provides certain advantages in comparison to the wake-up test. Evoked potential monitoring does not require patient cooperation and therefore can be accomplished in very young or mentally retarded patients. SSEPs measure spinal cord function continuously rather than at one point in time and eliminate the theoretical risks of awakening a patient on the table, with the attendant risk of dislodgment of the endotracheal tube or surgical instruments, air embolism with deep inspiration, or possible adverse psychological effects. However, all commonly used anesthetic agents and drugs may profoundly affect the quality of the SSEP recording, and the anesthetic techniques must be altered if such monitoring is used.

Measurement of SSEPs is affected by the choice of anesthetic agent. It was previously thought that the potent halogenated agents interfered unsatisfactorily with the measurement of SSEPs, but it has subsequently been demonstrated that the latency and amplitude of the signal are not adversely affected by halothane, enflurane, or isoflurane, provided that the end-tidal concentration of the anesthetic is below 1.0 MAC. Indeed, monitoring of evoked potentials is affected less by these agents than by nitrous oxide or thiobarbiturates. Experimental evidence also suggests that equipotent doses of halothane interfere less with the measurement of SSEPs than do enflurane or isoflurane. The effects of etomidate and propofol on SSEPs have not been well defined. Bolus intravenous doses of virtually any opioid or sedative drug transiently depress the SSEPs and confound the information that may be derived from them. For these reasons, anesthetic techniques that provide a continuous and smooth anesthetic effect, without the peaks and valleys of bolus doses of drugs or changes in inhaled concentrations of halogenated agents, are preferred. Short-acting drugs such as fentanyl, alfentanil, sufentanil, thiobarbiturates, and propofol are therefore best administered by continuous infusion during the period of monitoring. If it becomes necessary to administer a bolus dose of an anesthetic drug, it is a wise precaution to inform the technician operating the monitor.

CHOICE OF ANESTHETIC AGENTS AND TECHNIQUES

The following potential requirements should guide the anesthesiologist in selecting the appropriate anesthetic agents during the correction of kyphoscoliosis: (1) reliable and rapid awakening for a wake-up test, (2) a smooth and continuous anesthetic to facilitate evoked potential monitoring, (3) facilitation of intraoperative controlled hypotension, (4) a high inspired fraction of oxygen during anterior fusion, and (5) the need for postoperative analgesia.

Anterior fusions are usually performed without spinal cord monitoring, and the usual considerations for providing anesthesia for thoracic surgery apply. If the patient is of adequate size, the use of a double-lumen endotracheal tube and one-lung anesthesia facilitate the approach to the spine by means of a thoracotomy incision.

A balanced anesthetic with nitrous oxide, thiobarbiturate, fentanyl or fentanyl derivative, and relaxant, or a continuous infusion of propofol, facilitates a rapid intraoperative emergence for a wake-up test. Supplementation with low-dose halothane or another potent inhalation agent facilitates the provision of controlled hypotension without delaying emergence, provided the halogenated agent is discontinued 15 minutes or more before the wake-up test is performed.

At present, I use one of two anesthetic regimens for spinal surgery with SSEP monitoring. A satisfactory result can be obtained by administering an induction dose of 4 to 7 mg per kilogram of thiopental and 10 μg per kilogram of fentanyl, followed by maintenance of general anesthesia with a continuous infusion of thiopental (10 mg per kilogram per hour), nitrous oxide (50 to 70 percent), and D-tubocurarine. Alternatively, I have employed thiopental, 4 to 7 mg per kilogram, and fentanyl, 5 μg per kilogram, for induction, with a continuous infusion of fentanyl (1.5 to 2 μg per kilogram per hour), low-dose halothane or isoflurane (end-expiratory concentration 0.5 to 0.7 percent), and D-tubocurarine. The latter technique allows the delivery of a high-inspired oxygen concentration when clinically indicated. As previously discussed, hypotension with either technique may be induced with nitroprusside and a beta-adrenergic blocker. Evoked potential monitoring is used during hemodilution, provided that administered halothane is kept below 1.0 MAC.

Postoperative analgesia may be accomplished with either a continuous infusion of opioid (most often morphine, 10 to 40 μg per kilogram per hour) or patient-controlled analgesia. Frequently, muscle spasm amplifies postoperative pain, but sequentially increasing opioid therapy to treat this only results in untoward side effects or respiratory depression. When this occurs, small doses of benzodiazepines are usually effective.

Recently, intrathecal injection of morphine (5 μg per kilogram) at the conclusion of surgery before wound closure has been demonstrated to provide prolonged postoperative analgesia without respiratory depression.

Surgery for kyphoscoliosis may be intensely stressful to the patient and may lead to paraplegia in some cases. Anesthetic care should use the most sophisticated and effective means available to minimize intraoperative and postoperative complications and to facilitate monitoring for possible compromise to the spinal cord.

SUGGESTED READING

Friedman WA, Grundy BL. Monitoring of sensory evoked potentials is highly reliable and helpful in the operating room. J Clin Monit 1987; 3:38–44.

Kafer ER. Respiratory and cardiovascular functions in scoliosis and the principles of anesthetic management. Anesthesiology 1980; 52:339–351.

Loughnan BA, King MJ, Grundy EM, et al. Effects of halothane on somatosensory evoked potentials recorded in the extradural space. Br J Anaesth 1989; 62:297–300.

Pathak KS, Ammadio M, Kalamchi A, et al. Effects of halothane, enflurane, and isoflurane on somatosensory evoked potentials during nitrous oxide anesthesia. Anesthesiology 1987; 66:753–757.

Pathak KS, Amaddio MD, Scoles PV, et al. Effects of halothane, enflurane, and isoflurane in nitrous oxide on multilevel somatosensory evoked potentials. Anesthesiology 1989; 70:207–212.

Pathak KS, Brown RH, Cascorbi HF, Nash CL. Effects of fentanyl and morphine on intraoperative somatosensory cortical-evoked potentials. Anesth Analg 1984; 53:833–837.

Peterson DO, Drummond JC, Todd MM. Effects of halothane, enflurane, isoflurane, and nitrous oxide on somatosensory evoked potentials in humans. Anesthesiology 1986; 65:35–40.

Porter SS, Asher M, Fox DK. Comparison of intravenous nitroprusside, nitroprusside-captopril, and nitroglycerin for deliberate hypotension during posterior spine fusion in adults. J Clin Anesth 1988; 1:87–95.

York DH, Chabot RJ, Gaines RW. Response variability of somatosensory evoked potentials during scoliosis surgery. Spine 1987; 12: 864–876.

REGIONAL ANESTHETIC TECHNIQUES FOR SURGERY OF THE UPPER EXTREMITY

DENIS L. BOURKE, M.D.

Virtually all operations confined to the upper extremity can be performed using one of several regional anesthetic techniques. Among these methods, there are regional anesthetic techniques suitable for shoulder surgery as well as for arm and hand surgery. Regional anesthetic techniques offer many advantages over general anesthesia. Operating conditions are ideal with complete anesthesia, muscle relaxation, and sympathetic blockade. Noxious afferent stimuli are blocked before reaching the spinal cord or the central nervous system, thereby preventing initiation of the stress response. Most of the risks of general anesthesia, myocardial depression, respiratory depression, pulmonary complications, renal toxicity, and hepatotoxicity are minimized or avoided completely when regional anesthesia is used.

The benefits of regional anesthesia continue into the postoperative period. With less central nervous system depression, patients ambulate earlier, reducing the risk of pneumonia, thrombophlebitis, and pulmonary embolism. Since regional anesthesia usually provides more postoperative analgesia than general anesthesia, patients require less analgesic medications. As a result, patients receiving regional anesthesia can usually be discharged from the hospital earlier than patients receiving general anesthesia, thereby reducing health care costs.

In certain special instances, highly selective nerve blocks can be performed that spare certain sensory areas or leave specific motor function intact, assisting the surgeon intraoperatively in assessing the results of certain surgical maneuvers.

Overall, for the appropriate operation with a cooperative patient, the risk, discomfort, and cost of surgery can be reduced by the use of a regional anesthetic technique. The use of regional anesthesia, however, does not eliminate the need for thorough preoperative evaluation, careful preparation, appropriate monitoring, and care of the patient. The ability of the anesthesiologist to perform a wide variety of regional anesthetic block techniques for surgery of the upper extremity broaden his or her armamentarium and allows him or her to individualize the anesthetic care more specifically for each patient.

ANATOMY

An understanding of the anatomy of the nerve supply to the upper extremity is essential to the successful performance of regional blocks of the upper extremity. The upper extremity is supplied by the third cervical to the second thoracic spinal nerve roots, with the brachial plexus, composed of C-5 through C-8 and T-1, supplying all of the motor and almost all of the sensory function to the arm. However, the posterior medial aspect of the upper arm is supplied by the intercostal brachial cutaneous nerve, a branch of the second intercostal nerve. The proximal shoulder, both anteriorly and posteriorly, is partially supplied by branches from the cervical plexus, specifically, C-3 and C-4.

The anterior primary rami of the fifth, sixth, seventh, and eighth cervical and the first thoracic nerves, after leaving their respective intervertebral foramina, proceed anteriorly, laterally, and inferiorly to pass between the anterior scalene muscle and the middle scalene muscle. The anterior scalene muscle originates from the anterior lips of the transverse processes (vestigial ribs) of C-3 through C-6 and proceeds laterally and inferiorly to insert on the first rib anterior to the subclavian artery. The middle scalene muscle originates from the posterior lips of the transverse processes of the lower six cervical vertebrae and likewise proceeds laterally and inferiorly, also inserting on the first rib, but posterior to the subclavian artery. As the nerves pass between the scalene muscles, an investing fascia is formed from the posterior fascia of the anterior scalene muscle and the anterior fascia of the middle scalene muscle. This fascia will surround the nerve roots, trunks, divisions, cords, and brachial plexus, forming an investing sheath for the nerves and subclavian artery, and subsequently, the axillary artery all the way into the upper arm. While passing between the scalene muscles, the rami join to form the three trunks of brachial plexus. The fifth and sixth cervical roots unite to form the upper trunk, the seventh cervical root continues itself as the middle trunk, and the eighth cervical and first thoracic roots joined become the lower trunk. The three trunks merge between the scalene muscles and pass caudally and laterally across the base of the posterior triangle, then cross over the first rib where they join with the subclavian artery. Crossing the first rib, each of the three trunks separates into an anterior and posterior division containing innervation for preaxial and postaxial structures, respectively. These six divisions travel together into the axilla, where the anterior division of the upper and middle trunks unite to form the lateral cord; the anterior division of the lower trunk continues on as the medial cord, and the posterior divisions of all three trunks join to form the posterior cord. The cords are named with regard to their relationship to the second part of the axillary artery.

As the three cords pass the lateral border of the pectoralis minor muscle, they divide again, giving rise to the specific peripheral nerves that innervate the upper extremity. The lateral cord gives rise to the lateral head of the median nerve and the musculocutaneous nerve. The medial cord divides into the medial head of the median nerve, the ulnar nerve, and the medial antebrachial and medial brachial cutaneous nerves. The posterior cord divides into the axillary and radial nerves, which provides all of the postaxial innervation for the upper extremity.

Many other nerves arise from the nerves that form the brachial plexus before the formation of the cords. At the root level, the fifth cervical nerve provides a contribution to the phrenic nerve, which can accidentally be blocked during brachial plexus anesthesia. Some other branches from the roots of the brachial plexus include the dorsal scapular nerve, the nerves to the scalene muscles, the suprascapular nerve, the long thoracic nerve, and the lateral pectoral nerve. This simplified overview of the anatomy of the brachial plexus can be a useful clinical framework for nerve blocks of the upper extremity; however, the reader is encouraged to review the more detailed anatomy available in one of the standard texts.

NERVE BLOCK PROCEDURES

Interscalene Block

Although the interscalene block is best suited for surgery of the shoulder, there are several instances where it is the preferred regional anesthetic technique for forearm or hand surgery. Since lymphatic drainage of the arm is to the axillary nodes and not to the cervical nodes, the interscalene block may be preferred to one of the other, lower blocks of the brachial plexus if infection or malignancy exists in the upper extremity. Also, anatomic considerations will occasionally make the interscalene block technically easier to perform. As mentioned earlier, the cervical and brachial plexuses are enveloped in a continuous fascial sheath derived from the interscalene muscles. Therefore, with the injection of a suitable volume of local anesthetic into this sheath at the level of the interscalene groove, this solution can spread to provide both cervical and brachial plexus anesthesia. In this way, the third to the sixth cervical roots can be blocked, permitting surgery to be performed in the shoulder region. An interscalene approach is also useful for upper extremity block in obese patients in whom supraclavicular, axillary, or peripheral landmarks may be obscure; the interscalene groove can usually be easily identified even in very obese patients. The interscalene technique is also useful when the patient is unable to abduct the arm because of injury or pain.

To perform the interscalene block, the patient is placed supine or slightly sitting with the head turned away from the side that is to be blocked. The arm on the side of the block should be extended as though reaching for the knee. It is most convenient for the anesthesiologist to stand on the side that is to be blocked near the head and neck. The interscalene groove can be located by having the patient lift his head slightly, and the posterior belly of the sternocleidomastoid muscle is palpated. The palpating finger can then be rolled just posteriorly off the sternocleidomastoid and into the groove between the anterior and middle scalene muscles. The interscalene groove can also be identified through palpation of the subclavian artery as it passes over the first rib between the insertion of the anterior and middle scalene muscles on the first rib. The groove can then be followed cephalad. The site for the interscalene block is at a point in the interscalene groove lateral to the cricoid cartilage (at the level of the sixth cervical vertebra). At that location, a skin wheal is raised with a 25-gauge needle. A 22-gauge, 3.8 centimeter (1.5 inch) needle is then inserted through the skin wheal perpendicular to the skin. This should provide a direction that is medial, somewhat inferior, and slightly dorsal. The needle is advanced in attempt to elicit a paresthesia into the anterior shoulder, elbow, or thumb. Any of these paresthesias indicate accurate placement of the needle in the fascial sheath. The elicitation of a paresthesia to the back of the shoulder or the shoulder blade may indicate needle placement posterior to the fascial sheath. In this case, the needle should be redirected more anteriorly in an attempt to elicit the appropriate paresthesia. If bone is encountered before a paresthesia, it is usually the transverse process of a cervical vertebra. One should then walk the needle posteriorly or anteriorly across the transverse process until the nerve is found and a paresthesia is elicited. At that location, the local anesthetic can be injected. Once proper needle placement has been confirmed, 20 to 40 ml of local anesthetic solution is injected. The smaller volume anesthetizes the lower cervical plexus and the upper portion of the brachial plexus, but often misses the lower trunk (C-8 through T-1) of the brachial plexus. The larger volume usually anesthetizes C-3 through C-8 and occasionally T-1.

Since the dural nerve root sleeve projects laterally into the foramina above the transverse process, it is possible to inject the local anesthetic into the subdural space using the interscalene technique. Injection into the subdural space produces a total spinal anesthetic. To avoid this complication as well as the possibility of an inadvertent intravascular injection into the vertebral artery or other nearby vessel, aspiration should be performed before injection and intermittently during the injection of local anesthetic. Other possible complications that can occur during interscalene block are stellate ganglion block, phrenic nerve block, laryngeal nerve block, and pneumothorax. The most common of these is laryngeal nerve block. Patients often complain of hoarseness after interscalene block and should be reassured that this is not a serious complication and that it is only temporary.

The specific local anesthetic selected for a regional block should be based on the surgical condition and the duration of the surgery. Table 1 outlines the various blocks suitable for regions of the upper extremity and indicates agents to be used for producing these blocks and for various durations.

Table 2 lists the suggested maximal dose of the local anesthetics that can be used in a healthy middle-aged 70-kg patient. It should be noted that epinephrine retards systemic absorption and therefore lowers blood levels for all of the agents, thereby permitting higher doses to used. Epinephrine should not be used for either digital nerve blocks or intravenous regional anesthesia.

Supraclavicular Approach to the Brachial Plexus

The trunks and divisions of the brachial plexus are grouped closer together as they cross over the first rib, and they can be blocked at this site. There are two basic approaches to nerve blocks in this area: (1) the

Table 1 Guidelines for Upper Extremity Nerve Blocks

Block	Procedure Location	Procedure Duration	Suggested Local Anesthetic
Interscalene	Shoulder and distal	Short (<1 hour)	2–3 percent chloroprocaine (35–45 ml) 1–1.5 percent lidocaine (35–45 ml)
		Medium (1–3 hours)	1–1.5 percent lidocaine with epinephrine 1:200,000 (35–45 ml) 1–1.5 percent mepivacaine with epinephrine 1:200,000 (34–45 ml)
		Long (>3 hours)	0.5–0.75 percent bupivacaine (35–45 ml) 0.5–1 percent ropivacaine (35–45 ml)
Supraclavicular	Arm and distal	Short (< 1 hour)	2–3 percent chloroprocaine (35–45 ml) 1–1.5 percent lidocaine (35–45 ml)
		Medium (1–3 hours)	1–1.5 percent lidocaine with epinephrine 1:200,000 (35–45 ml) 1–1.5 percent mepivacaine with epinephrine 1:200,000 (35–45 ml)
		Long (> 3 hours)	0.5–0.75 percent bupivacaine (35–45 ml) 0.5–1 percent ropivacaine (35–45 ml)
Axillary	Arm and distal	Short (<1 hour)	2–3 percent chloroprocaine (35–45 ml) 1–1.5 percent lidocaine (35–45 ml)
		Medium (1–3 hours)	1–1.5 percent lidocaine with epinephrine 1:200,000 (35–45 ml) 1–1.5 percent mepivacaine with epinephrine 1:200,000 (35–45 ml)
		Long (> 3 hours)	0.5–0.75 percent bupivacaine (35–45 ml) 0.5–1 percent ropivacaine (35–45 ml)
Elbow	Wrist and distal	Short (< 1 hour)	2–3 percent chloroprocaine (5–10 ml per nerve) 1–1.5 percent lidocaine (5–10 ml per nerve)
		Medium (1–3 hours)	1–1.5 percent lidocaine with epinephrine 1:200,000 (5–10 ml per nerve) 1–1.5 percent mepivacaine with epinephrine 1:200,000 (5-10 ml per nerve)
		Long (> 3 hours)	0.5–0.75 percent bupivacaine (5–10 ml per nerve) 0.5–1 percent ropivacaine (5–10 ml per nerve)
Wrist	Digits	Short (< 1 hour)	2–3 percent chloroprocaine (2–5 percent ml per nerve) 1–1.5 percent lidocaine (2–5 ml per nerve)
		Medium (1–3 hours)	1–1.5 percent lidocaine with epinephrine 1:200,000 (2–5 ml per nerve) 1–1.5 percent mepivacaine with epinephrine 1:200,000 (2-5 ml per nerve)
		Long (> 3 hours)	0.5–0.75 percent bupivacaine (2–5 ml per nerve) 0.5–1 percent ropivacaine (2–5 ml per nerve)
Metacarpal	Digits	Short (< 1 hour)	1 percent lidocaine *no epinephrine* (2–3 ml per injection) 1 percent mepivacaine *no epinephrine* (2–3 ml per injection)
		Medium (1–3 hours)	0.5 percent bupivacaine *no epinephrine* (2–3 ml per injection)

Table 2 Maximum Local Anesthetic Dose Guidelines

Anesthetic Agent	Without Epinephrine (mg/kg)	With Epinephrine 1:200,000 (mg/kg)
Lidocaine	4–5	7–8
Mepivacaine	4–5	7–8
Chloroprocaine	7–9	10–12
Etidocaine	4–5	5–6
Prilocaine	5–6	7–9
Bupivacaine	2–3	3–4
Ropivacaine	3–4	4–5

perivascular technique described by Winnie and (2) any of several variations of Kulenkampff's original technique.

With the perivascular approach, the patient lies supine or is placed slightly sitting with his arm by his side. The head is tilted opposite to the side to be blocked and the arm is again extended as though reaching for the knee. The interscalene groove can be identified by either of the previously described methods. After the groove between the scalene muscles has been found, the palpating finger is placed on the pulse of subclavian artery. The point of injection is approximately 1 cm above the finger lying on the subclavian pulse. A skin wheal is made at this point and the block can be performed with a 22-gauge, 3.8-cm needle. The needle is inserted through the wheal in a caudal direction, nearly parallel to the surface of the skin. The needle is advanced and paresthesias are sought. Only paresthesias of the anterior shoulder below the level of the shoulder are acceptable, since a paresthesia to the posterior shoulder indicates contact with the suprascapular nerve, which usually lies outside the investing fascial sheath at this level. If the needle fails to contact any of the three nerve trunks, it will make contact with the first rib and thus prevent the possibility of a pneumothorax. If no paresthesia has been produced at this location, one walks the needle dorsally and ventrally along the surface of the rib until a paresthesia is found. Once the paresthesia is obtained, 20 to 40 ml of local anesthetic is injected (see Table 1). It should be noted that this is the ideal block technique for intermittent or continuous injection of local anesthetic through a catheter, since the catheter direction, nearly parallel to the skin, permits easy and secure taping to the neck in this location.

With the second supraclavicular technique, which relies on boney structures for landmarks, the patients and anesthesiologist are positioned as for the previous, perivascular block. The anesthesiologist locates the midpoint of the clavicle (midway between the acromial and sternal ends). The needle is inserted at the lateral border of the anterior scalene muscle, approximately 2 cm behind the clavicular midpoint. The direction of the needle is dorsal, medial, and caudad. This is virtually at right angles to the plane of the skin at this level of the neck. The needle is advanced until a paresthesia is produced or the first rib is encountered. If no paresthesia is found, one proceeds to walk the needle along the first rib as described for the above-mentioned block.

If the subclavian artery is entered in either technique, it indicates that the needle is located too far anteriorly. The needle should be reinserted or redirected posteriorly, closer to the middle scalene muscle.

Axillary Block

The axillary block, by far the most widely used to anesthetize the brachial plexus, has the advantages of avoiding such complications as pneumothorax, subarachnoid injection, or block of phrenic and laryngeal nerves. The two major disadvantages to this block, as compared with the more proximal approaches, are that the arm must be abducted and that complete shoulder anesthesia is more difficult to achieve. There are two primary techniques for performing an axillary block. Although both methods are essentially perivascular techniques, they differ in the number and specific location of the injections made. The approach popularized by Winnie treats the axillary perivascular space — that space enclosed by the axillary sheath and containing the nerves and vessels — as a single, confluent space. It is assumed that once the axillary sheath is entered, a single large-volume injection of local anesthetic fills the entire space within the sheath and bathes all of the nerves.

Using this technique, the patient is placed supine and the arm is abducted 90 degrees from the body; the forearm may be flexed and the arm externally rotated so that the thumb of the patient's hand lies near his head. The axillary artery, lying just posterior to the coracobrachialis muscle and just anterior to the long head of the triceps muscle, is identified by palpation of its pulse. It is followed proximal as far as possible into axilla. A skin wheal is raised over the axillary artery at this point and a short-beveled, 22-gauge, 3.8-cm needle is inserted through the skin wheal directed proximally at an angle of approximately 45 degrees to the skin surface toward the apex of the axilla. The needle is advanced slowly until a "pop" is felt, indicating that the needle has pierced the superficial fascia and entered the axillary sheath. In experienced hands, this is sufficient confirmation of proper needle placement and 20 to 40 ml of local anesthetic solution is injected, while frequent aspiration is performed to ensure that intravascular injection of local anesthetic does not occur. Alternatively, one may continue to advance the needle in various directions until a paresthesia is elicited and then inject the local anesthetic, again with frequent aspirations. Finally, if the axillary artery is punctured and arterial blood is aspirated during insertion of the needle, the needle is advanced until it just passes through the posterior wall of the axillary artery and no more blood can be aspirated. With the needle in this position, half of the local anesthetic solution is injected. The needle is then withdrawn until the tip lies just superficial to the axillary artery, which is confirmed by the inability to aspirate blood, and the second half of the local anesthetic solution is injected at this location.

More recently, another technique has been advocated based on the assumption that the fascia of the axillary sheath invaginates inward to form septa that may result in compartmentalization of the nerves and vessels that make up the contents of the sheath. The septa are believed to prevent or impede the free spread of local anesthetic throughout the sheath. Therefore a successful axillary block depends on several small-volume injections of local anesthetic into the various individual compartments. With the recommended technique, the patient is positioned as previously described. The axillary artery is located as before and is held against the humerus between the first and second fingers. The palm of the hand is rested flat against the arm and a slight distalward traction is applied to the skin. A skin wheal is made directly over the artery. The needle is inserted immediately adjacent to the artery on the inferior side of the arterial pulse to a depth of 1 to 2 cm, approximately to the depth of the posterior aspect of the artery. After negative aspiration for blood, 3 to 5 ml of solution is injected while the needle is retracted to the subcutaneous tissue. This maneuver is repeated several times while the needle tip is moved away from the artery 1 to 2 cm in a fanlike distribution. The same procedure is performed on the superior side of the artery. If a paresthesia is obtained at any point, 3 to 5 ml is injected at that specific point and the injection pattern is continued. The block is evaluated after injecting approximately 20 ml of local anesthetic solution.

To evaluate the block, a simple four-step test can be used: the so-called push-pull-pinch-pinch sequence. The patient should push to extend the forearm using the triceps muscle, testing the radial nerve block. Next, the patient should be asked to pull with the forearm, using the biceps and brachialis muscles to test the musculocutaneous nerve block. One then pinches the base of the thumb to test the median nerve block, and finally, pinches the tip of the little finger for the ulnar nerve block. One should decide where to reinforce the block, if needed, based on the fact that the ulnar and median nerves are commonly caudal to the artery and the median and musculocutaneous nerves are usually cephalad to the artery.

With either approach to the axillary block, it may be difficult to get a satisfactory block of the musculocutaneous nerve, since it exits the fascial sheath to enter the body of the coracobrachialis muscle earlier than the other nerves. The musculocutaneous nerve can be blocked by injecting 5 to 10 ml of local anesthetic solution into the coracobrachialis muscle high in the axilla. The muscle lies just anterior to the axillary artery.

It should be noted that none of the aforementioned blocks anesthetize the intercostal brachial cutaneous nerve, which provides innervation to the posterior medial aspect of the arm. However, failure to block the intercostal brachial cutaneous nerve is a frequent cause of tourniquet pain. The intercostal brachial cutaneous nerve is easily blocked with a subcutaneous infiltration of local anesthetic high in the axilla from directly over the axillary artery for 2 to 5 cm posteriorly.

Nerve Blocks at the Level of the Elbow

Nerve blocks at the elbow can be used for anesthesia of the hand and wrist when a tourniquet is not used or to reinforce/supplement a brachial plexus block. The ulnar, median, radial, and musculocutaneous nerves can all be easily blocked at the elbow.

The ulnar nerve is blocked where it passes the elbow in the ulnar nerve sulcus on the posterior aspect of the medial epicondyle of the humerus. It can usually be palpated in the sulcus. The elbow is flexed 90 degrees, the nerve palpated, and a 25-gauge needle is inserted 1 to 2 cm proximal to the epicondyle toward the nerve. When a paresthesia is obtained, 3 to 5 ml of solution is injected. The ulnar nerve block is especially useful for supplementing an interscalene block for surgery below the elbow, since fibers from the eighth cervical to the first thoracic nerve root, which are contained in the ulnar nerve, are the most commonly missed during an interscalene block.

The median nerve lies just medial to the brachial artery on the surface of the brachialis muscle in the cubital fossa and can usually be palpated there. An imaginary line is drawn between the medial and lateral epicondyles of the humerus, and a skin wheal is raised at the level of this line (usually corresponding to the cubital crease) just medial to the brachial artery pulse. The needle is advanced at this location perpendicular to the skin. When a paresthesia is elicited, 3 to 5 ml of local anesthetic is injected. If a paresthesia is not obtained with the initial pass of the needle, the needle should be redirected medially and laterally in a fanwise fashion in an attempt to elicit paresthesias, or a nerve stimulator may be used to confirm proper needle placement.

The radial nerve exits the brachial plexus at the lateral border of the pectoralis minor muscle. It then travels down the arm dorsal to the humerus in a medial-to-lateral course. It emerges from behind the humerus in the radial groove at a position approximately 6 to 8 cm above the lateral epicondyle. At this position, the nerve lies in close approximation to and lateral to the humerus. From here it proceeds to a position in front of the lateral condyle, where it divides into four branches. The nerve is most easily blocked approximately 6 to 8 cm (four finger breadths) above the lateral epicondyle, before it divides into these four branches. For blocking the radial nerve, the patient lies with his arm partially abducted and the forearm extended. At the point four finger breadths above the lateral epicondyle, a skin wheal is raised and a 22-gauge needle is inserted through the skin perpendicularly. The needle is advanced until the humerus is contacted or a paresthesia is obtained. If no paresthesia is elicited, the needle may be walked both caudal and cephalad along the long axis of the humerus with multiple injections performed.

The cutaneous branch of the musculocutaneous nerve can be blocked just below the cubital crease at the elbow. At this location, the cutaneous branch of the musculocutaneous nerve, which provides sensation to the radial side of the volar aspect of the forearm, lies in the subcutaneous tissue just lateral to the biceps tendon. The nerve is blocked through a subcutaneous injection beginning at the biceps tendon and proceeding laterally for 2 to 4 cm in the subcutaneous tissue.

Nerve Blocks at the Wrist

Blocks of the ulnar, median, and the radial nerves at the wrist can provide anesthesia for the hand. These nerve blocks can be used for supplementing brachial plexus block or for limited procedures on the hand or digits.

The median nerve lies relatively superficially at the wrist. It can be blocked here as it passes between the tendon of the palmaris longus and a flexor carpi radialis muscle. The patient is asked to flex his hand at the wrist. With this maneuver, the palmaris longus tendon can easily be identified. A skin wheal is raised just lateral to this tendon at the level of the most proximal flexion crease of the wrist (this is approximately at the level of styloid process). The needle is inserted at right angles to the skin and is advanced until a paresthesia is elicited. If a paresthesia is not elicited, the needle is reinserted in a fanwise direction medially or laterally in search of one. When the nerve is identified, approximately 3 to 5 ml of local anesthetic solution is injected.

The ulnar nerve descends in the forearm to a point approximately 2 inches above the wrist, where it divides into a dorsal and a palmar branch. The dorsal branch passes posteriorly under the tendon of the flexor carpi ulnaris, perforates the deep fascia above the wrist, and supplies the ulnar border of the dorsum of the hand. The palmar branch descends along the anterior aspect of the ulnar artery, pierces the deep fascia above the wrist, and crosses the flexor retinaculum to supply the skin over the hypothenar eminence. Ulnar nerve block at the wrist consists of anesthetizing these two branches. To block the palmar branches at the wrist, the patient lies with the arm at his side, palm up. The flexor carpi ulnaris tendon is located by having the patient flex his hand at the wrist. A skin wheal is raised on the radial side of the tendon at the level of the styloid process (approximately at the most proximal crease of the wrist) just medial to the ulnar artery. The needle is inserted at right angles to the skin close to the ulnar artery. The needle is advanced until a paresthesia is obtained. If no paresthesia is elicited, the needle should be advanced in a fanwise fashion medially or laterally until a paresthesia is found. Once the nerve is identified, 3 to 5 ml of local anesthetic solution is injected. The dorsal branch of the ulnar nerve is blocked by a subcutaneous infiltration of local anesthetic in a band from the styloid process around the ulnar aspect of the wrist to the middle of the dorsum of the wrist. The injection is curved around the ulnar aspect of the wrist. From here it is extended to the middle of the dorsal aspect of the wrist.

The radial nerve travels with the radial artery in the forearm to a point approximately 5 to 8 cm above the wrist, where it passes beneath the tendon of the brachioradialis muscle, pierces the deep fascia, and enters the subcutaneous tissue. Just above the wrist, the nerve divides into two branches to innervate the hand. The radial nerve is blocked at the wrist with the arm abducted and the forearm extended. The radial artery is identified at the level of the styloid process. The needle is inserted perpendicular to the skin and paresthesias are sought. If a paresthesia is not found, the needle may be moved in a fanwise fashion laterally, away from the artery, in search of paresthesias. When the nerve is identified, 2 to 3 ml of local anesthetic is injected. To block the branches to the dorsum of the hand, a band of anesthetic is injected subcutaneously in a line at a right angle to the long access of the arm at the level of the styloid process. This injection is performed so that the anesthetic is infiltrated around the dorsal aspect of the radial side of the wrist. It is extended to the middle of the dorsal aspect of the wrist, thus forming approximately a one-half cuff of anesthesia on the radial side of the wrist.

Metacarpal Blocks

For minor procedures on the finger, a digital block can be used. These blocks are simple to perform, safe, and effective. Each digit is supplied by four nerve branches—two dorsal and two palmar—which travel distalward along the respective edge of the digit in close approximation to the bone.

To perform the block, a 25-gauge, 3.8-cm needle is inserted in the dorsal surface of the intermetacarpal space of the hand at the level of the metacarpal head. The needle is advanced into the hand perpendicular to the dorsal surface until the resistance of the palmar aponeurosis is felt. As the needle is withdrawn, 1 to 2 ml of local anesthetic without epinephrine is injected, thereby anesthetizing both the palmar and dorsal nerves.

SUGGESTED READING

Cousins MJ, Bridenbaugh PO. Neural blockade in clinical anesthesia and management of pain. 2nd ed. Philadelphia: JB Lippincott, 1988.

Katz J. Atlas of regional anesthesia. Norwalk, CT: Appleton-Century-Crofts, 1985.

Moore DC. Regional Block. 4th ed. Springfield, IL: Charles C Thomas, 1975.

Winnie AP. Perivascular techniques of brachial plexus block. In: Winnie AP, ed. Plexus anesthesia. Vol 1. Philadelphia: WB Saunders, 1983.

LOWER EXTREMITY NERVE BLOCKS

TERENCE M. MURPHY, M.B., Ch.B., F.F.A.R.C.S.

Nerve blocks of the upper extremity are widely used because the compact nature of the brachial plexus both above and below the clavicle lends itself well to the single-needle insertion technique.

The lower extremity, however, receives its nerve supply from much more widely spaced neural elements. As humans have assumed the upright gate, so large amounts of skin and muscles from the anterior abdominal wall origin have been "incorporated" into the flexor compartment of the lower extremity and carry their nerve supply with them. Therefore, the lower extremity is dually supplied by two separate nerve systems, the "borrowed" femoral and the original sciatic—the true nerve of supply. These arise from spinal levels from L-2 to the distal sacrum S-5 and thus encompass a paravertebral origin some three to four times the spread of the brachial plexus.

Despite the ingenuity of many attempts, at least two and sometimes several needle insertions are necessary to anesthetize the lower extremity via peripheral nerve blocks effectively.

This is in contrast, of course, to the elegant simplicity of a single-needle spinal or epidural anesthetic, which can provide excellent analgesia to the same area. Thus, peripheral lower extremity nerve blocks are usually reserved for those individuals in whom spinal or epidural techniques are contraindicated, as may be the case with the patient receiving anticoagulation therapy or the patient with a contraindication to more central needle trespass (e.g., tumors, prior extensive surgery, unstable spine, patient preference).

GENERAL CONSIDERATIONS

The lumbar plexus contribution to the lower extremity supplies primarily tissue of the anterior thigh. It arises from L-2, L-3, and L-4 nerves, which arrange themselves into the components of the plexus between the psoas major and quadratus lumborum muscles.

The most deeply situated nerve is the obturator, which passes into the pelvis medial to the psoas major and exits through the obturator foramen into the medial-most compartment of the thigh, where it supplies the adductor muscle mass, an area of skin over the medial aspect of the thigh, and provides a terminal twig of innervation to the knee joint.

The femoral nerve forms at the lateral border of the psoas major muscle and enters the thigh under the inguinal ligament immediately lateral to the femoral artery. This supplies the main flexor muscle mass of the thigh and the skin over the anterior aspect of the thigh, and via its terminal sensory saphenous branch, it supplies skin over the medial aspect of the leg from the knee to the medial malleolus and beyond, sometimes even to the great toe.

The lateral femoral cutaneous is the remaining branch of the lumbar plexus that supplies the lateral aspect of the skin of the thigh. It is a purely sensory nerve that pierces the inguinal ligament approximately 1 to

2 cm from its lateral attachment to the anterior superior iliac spine.

The sciatic nerve forms from branches L-4, L-5, S-1, S-2, and S-3 on the anterior surface of the sacrum and exits from the pelvis through the greater sciatic notch, usually passing below the piriformis muscle. Nevertheless, its division into medial and lateral popliteal nerves can occur even within the pelvis, and sometimes the lateral popliteal component pierces the piriformis muscle. It leaves the buttock and enters the thigh approximately halfway between the ischial tuberosity and the greater trochanter, and then pursues a midline course down the posterior thigh to the midpoint of the popliteal fossa, where it is usually divided into its medial and lateral popliteal branches. The medial popliteal branch continues as the posterior tibial nerve situated deeply within the calf. The posterior tibial nerve enters the foot midway between the medial malleolus and the calcaneus. The sural nerve passes laterally below the lateral malleolus to supply sensation to the lateral border of the foot. The posterior tibial nerve supplies sensation to the sole of the foot by the medial and lateral plantar nerves and also supplies motor branches to the short muscles of the toes.

The lateral popliteal nerve (peroneal) leaves the popliteal fossa by crossing below the head of the fibula, where it is often subcutaneously palpable (and therefore easily blocked). This nerve supplies motor power to the dorsal flexors of the distal extremity and sensation to the skin over the dorsum of the foot via its superficial and deep branches.

NERVE BLOCK TECHNIQUES

The above-mentioned nerves can be blocked at many points from their immediate paravertebral origin through to the distal digital branches, depending on the specific need and indication.

Traditionally, the lumbar plexus derivatives are blocked with three separate needling procedures via an anterior approach below the inguinal ligament for the lateral femoral cutaneous nerve, femoral nerve, and obturator nerve, respectively. Individual anesthesiologists have attempted to anesthetize these lumbar plexus derivatives more efficiently by single-needle techniques. These techniques, which have met with varying success, are as follows.

Lumbar Paravertebral Block

The paravertebral placement of anesthetics in the L-2, L-3, and L-4 paravertebral gutter can produce perfectly adequate analgesia of the flexor and adductor compartments of the thigh and of the skin that is covering the same. Because of the communication space in the paravertebral gutter that exists throughout the vertebral column, these three components can often be satisfactorily anesthetized with a single needle stick at L-3 (for instance) and the injection of a large volume that will spread caudad and cephalad in the paravertebral gutter to anesthetize both L-2 and L-4 as well (e.g., 10 to 20 ml of the anesthetic of your choice). This paravertebral block is produced by inserting the needle 2 cm lateral to the craniad end of the lumbar spine of L-3 and inserting a 6-cm needle until it contacts the transverse process. The needle is "walked off" the caudad end of the transverse process, and a paresthesia to the anterior thigh is sought, and/or myotomal contractions of the quadriceps and/or adductor muscle mass are sought with a nerve stimulator.

Attempts have been made to block the lumbar plexus more peripherally from the paravertebral gutter as it forms, "sandwiched" between the psoas major and quadratus lumborum muscles. These approaches have been from below (the "three-in-one" technique by Winnie) and from a posterior approach (psoas compartment block by Chayne).

"Three-in-One" Lumbar Plexus Block

This is a lower limb "equivalent" of an interscalene block, whereby the needle is inserted at the junction of the iliopsoas and iliacus muscles, where the femoral nerve emerges below the inguinal ligament. A large volume (20 to 30 ml) of the anesthetic should be injected somewhat forcefully in a cephalad fashion in the hope that the medication will "dissect" cephalad between iliopsoas, iliacus, and quadratus lumborum, thus bathing the lumbar plexus which is between these muscles.

This technique is usually highly effective at anesthetizing the femoral and lateral femoral cutaneous nerves; however, as in the case of the interscalene block, deficiency is often noted with the more "caudad" elements of the plexus (i.e., the obturator nerve). Fortunately, surgical procedures of the much lower extremity can be accomplished without the necessity of an obturator nerve block, since it supplies only a small area of sensation over the medial thigh (see later). Also, if surgical trespass does not involve that area (or the knee joint), it is often feasible to complete surgery below the knee without an effective obturator nerve block.

Psoas Compartment Block

The psoas compartment block was described by Chayne, who positioned his needle via a posterior approach superior to L-5 transverse process in an attempt to detect a loss of resistance between the quadratus lumborum and psoas major muscles. He distended the space with 20 ml of air, and then injected the blocking dose (30 ml) of local anesthetic. The needle entry for this technique is 5 cm lateral and 3 cm caudal to the L-4 vertebral spine and adjacent to the descending crest of the posterior ilium. The endpoint is less than distinct, although in experienced hands, a very subtle change of resistance can be detected. A nerve stimulator can facilitate contact with the lumbar plexus and an injection at a variable depth, depending on the patient's gneral habitus, can afford highly satisfactory analgesia of all of the roots of the lumbar plexus. This nerve block is particularly suitable for those individuals with significant trauma to the lower extremity because it permits peripheral blockade via just two needle sticks (the sciatic and the lumbar plexus needles), both of which can be accomplished from the same posterior aspect of the patient. Thus the patient does not have to be returned from the prone to supine position to complete the anesthesia, a frequently uncomfortable maneuver in a patient with significant trauma.

Traditional Lumbar Plexus Branch Block

The femoral nerve forms immediately lateral to the femoral artery as they both enter the thigh under the inguinal ligament and is located by identifying the palpations of that vessel at the midpoint of the inguinal ligament (which stretches from the anterior superior iliac spine to the pubic tubercle). The femoral artery is identified and a skin wheal produced immediately lateral. A shallow bevel, short 3- to 4-cm needle is all that is needed in individuals with normal bodily habitus to pierce the skin and deeper structures (fascia lata), and a paresthesia to the anterior and/or medial thigh is sought. If a nerve stimulator is used, then contraction of the anterior or medial muscle mass of the thigh is noted. A dose of 15 ml of the local anesthetic of your choice should be sufficient to anesthetize the femoral nerve.

Lateral Femoral Cutaneous Block

The lateral femoral nerve is entirely sensory and is distributed to the lateral aspect of the thigh. The nerve curves around the iliac fossa within the pelvis and emerges onto the thigh by piercing the inguinal ligament approximately 2 to 3 cm from its lateral attachment. The landmarks for this nerve block are two finger breadths in and down from the anterior superior iliac spine (or two finger breadths down and in). It is of no use to employ a nerve stimulator here, since this muscle does not carry motor components. Therefore paresthesia to the lateral thigh is sought, or if this is not found, a fanlike infiltration of 5 to 8 ml of appropriate local anesthetic at this site will produce analgesia of the lateral thigh (use of this nerve block alone, as opposed to anesthetization of the whole lower extremity, is highly useful for obtaining discrete donor skin graft specimens when such are needed).

If blocked by large volumes which are delivered above the inguinal ligament, it is quite feasible to obtain a "three-in-one" (or "two-of-three") block, whereby the drug spreads to the femoral nerve via the fascial planes over the iliacus muscle. The effect has been used electively to produce thigh analgesia.

Obturator Nerve Block

The obturator nerve is the most deeply situated of all three branches of the lumbar plexus. As it forms in the posterior abdominal wall, it proceeds on a deep intrapelvic course medial to the psoas major muscle and exits from the pelvis through the obturator foramen at its superior and medial border, where it enters the thigh. The traditional insertion point for obturator blocks is two finger breadths out and down (or down and out) from the pubic tubercle. The nerve is deep and usually requires a needle insertion of approximately 3 to 4 cm (sometimes more) before contact with the nerve is obtained. The obturator nerve divides shortly after entering the thigh into a superficial and deep branch. The superficial branch supplies cutaneous distribution to an area about the size of the palmar aspect of your hand and fingers over the medial aspect of the thigh. The deep branch of the obturator carries mostly motor components to the adductor muscle mass but also supplies an articular twig to the knee joint, which, if left unblocked, would compromise patient comfort in surgery on that joint. Once contact with the nerve is obtained, a dose of 10 to 15 ml of local anesthetic is usually an appropriate volume for blockade.

Sciatic Nerve Block

Sacral nerves S-1 through S-3 are joined by a branch from L-4 and L-5 to produce the sacral plexus, which gives rise to the sciatic nerve, as mentioned above. The sciatic nerve is the largest nerve in the body, about the size of the thumb, and emerges into the buttock where it is deeply situated; depending on the degree of steatopygia, it can sometimes be palpated by having the patient relax the gluteal muscles by turning the toes in and the heels out. This palpation is difficult if not impossible to do in all but the slimmest of buttocks. The traditional method for finding the sciatic nerve is to draw a line from the posterior superior iliac spine to the greater trochanter of the femur. This line is now bisected at right angles, and approximately 3 to 4 cm caudad on this second line is the entry point for sciatic nerve block. This level can be checked by drawing a line from the greater trochanter to the sacral hiatus, and where this last line intersects, the bisecting line mentioned above is over the sciatic nerve.

Depending on the dimensions of the buttock, one may need a very long needle, although usually a 6- to 8-cm needle is adequate. As mentioned earlier, the sciatic nerve is the largest nerve in the body and therefore not a difficult target, although it is important not to risk needle trauma. If the nerve is not located with the first needle attempt, it is advisable to attempt to locate the appropriate depth by obtaining contact with the posterior aspect of the ischium and then to "walk" the needle at right angles to the perceived path of the sciatic nerve until either paresthesia or muscle twitches in the hamstrings or calf muscles are identified. Paresthesia caused by needle contact with the sciatic nerve is quite uncomfortable. This is a relative indication for the use of a nerve stimulator whereby appropriate peripheral muscle twitch is identified usually prior to the discomfort of a paresthesia contact.

The sciatic nerve can be blocked once contact is made with the injection of 20 ml of the anesthetic of your choice. Because of the size of the sciatic nerve, a long "soak" time (e.g., 20 to 30 minutes) is often needed for satisfactory block of the peripheral components of the nerve (plantar aspect of the foot).

An alternative site for achieving sciatic nerve block is approximately halfway between the ischial tuberosity and the greater trochanter of the femur.

Alternate Approaches. Just as there have been efforts to find alternative approaches to lumbar plexus block, so attempts have been made to produce sciatic nerve block by anterior and lateral approaches in those cases where it is necessary to minimize patient positioning movement (e.g., because of significant lower extremity trauma).

Anterior Approach. On anterior projection, the sciatic nerve passes posterior to the angle between the neck and the shaft of the femur. At this site, a needle introduced below the medial third of the inguinal ligament can be positioned adjacent to the anterior surface of the sciatic nerve and produce satisfactory sciatic nerve block (although sometimes the posterior cutaneous nerve to the thigh may not be as satisfactorily anesthetized as it would be with the more traditional posterior approach).

The landmarks for this anterior approach are determined by drawing a line from the greater trochanter of the femur parallel to and below the inguinal ligament. A vertical line is dropped from the junction of the middle and medial third of the inguinal ligament, and the point of entry for the needle and anterior approach to the sciatic nerve is where this vertical line intersects the lower line drawn from the greater trochanter parallel to the inguinal ligament. Because of the depth of the sciatic nerve when approached from the anterior aspect, 8 cm or longer is needed.

A lateral approach has also been described in which the needle is introduced posterior to the greater trochanter from the side. This approach is rarely used but, if indicated, should be reviewed prior to use.

Distal Blocks

Distal blocks are infrequently used as a prime anesthetic since most peripheral surgery on the lower extremities involves a proximal tourniquet that will become exceedingly uncomfortable unless analgesia is provided. A peripheral block is sometimes needed, however, either for discrete surgery or to supplement (i.e., "rescue") a more centrally attempted block.

The branches of the sciatic nerve in the popliteal fossa are not difficult to block. The needle is inserted at the apex of the popliteal fossa, and contact with the nerve is usually obtained within 3 to 4 cm. Successful block here would anesthetize all of the lower extremity below the knee, with the exception of that skin over the medial leg and ankle supplied by the terminal saphenous branch of the femoral nerve.

Saphenous Nerve Block

This is the terminal branch of the femoral nerve, which is purely sensory in distribution. It emerges from the subsartorial canal on the medial aspect of the knee joint and it can be anesthetized by a horizontal subcutaneous arc of infiltration across the medial aspect of the tibial condyle. It runs with the long saphenous vein, which when identified can serve as a useful landmark for the block.

Common Peroneal (Lateral Popliteal) Nerve Block

The common peroneal (lateral popliteal) nerve can be blocked as it crosses the head of the fibula for either discrete or supplemental analgesia. The nerve can often be palpated approximately 1 cm distal to the head of the fibula. By infiltration at this site, analgesia of the anterior tibial area and the dorsum of the foot can be achieved.

Nerve blocks of these branches of the sciatic nerve at the level of the knee are associated with significant motor block and inability to walk.

Ankle Block

There has been a resurgence of interest in blocking the foot at the level of the ankle. Techniques for accomplishing this have been available for a long time and have been used often in outpatient offices by physicians and podiatrists for many years. However, with the trend to "day surgery," many anesthesia practitioners in larger hospitals are now called on to use this very valuable block.

The five nerves that are supplied to the foot enter the foot circumferentially. Four of them are terminal branches of the sciatic nerve and the fifth is the terminal branch of the femoral nerve, the saphenous nerve.

Because these nerves are circumferentially distributed around the lower leg and ankle, circumferential anesthetic techniques are needed. The plantar aspects of the foot can be anesthetized by blocking the posterior tibial and sural nerves. The posterior tibial nerve is situated 1 to 2 cm below the medial malleolus and can be identified by localizing the pulsations of the adjacent posterior tibial artery, usually approximately one-third of the distance between the medial malleolus and calcaneum. The infiltration of the posterior tibial nerve at this site will anesthetize the medial and lateral plantar nerves and will produce analgesia of most of the sole of the foot.

The lateral aspects of the foot and part of the lateral sole are supplied by the sural nerve, which enters the foot approximately halfway between the lateral malleolus and the calcaneum. An infiltration of local anesthetic superficially at this site should provide anesthesia.

The dorsum of the foot is supplied by the terminal branches of the superficial peroneal (anterior tibial) nerve, most of which enter the foot superficially to the extensor retinaculum and can be blocked by an infiltration from the medial to the lateral malleolus. This can usually be accomplished by a single needle stick at the junction of the medial and the lateral two-thirds of this line. With the insertion of the needle between the tendons of tibialis anterior and extensor hallucis longus, the branch of the deep peroneal (lateral popliteal) nerve can be identified and anesthetized, producing numbness of the first interdigital cleft. The rest of the dorsum of the foot, however, is supplied by the superficial branches, and these are anesthetized by a subcutaneous infiltration from the lateral to the medial malleolus. Any terminal branches of the saphenous nerve (terminal division of the femoral) are anesthetized over the medial third of this line.

SUGGESTED READING

Beck GP. Anterior approach to sciatic nerve block. Anesthesiology 1963; 24:222.

Ben-David B, Lee E, Croitoru M. Psoas block for surgical repair of hip fracture: case report and description of the catheter technique. Anesth Analg 1990; 71:298–301.

Chayne D, Nathan H, Chayne N. The psoas compartment block. Anesthesiology 1976; 45:95–99.

Dalens W, Tangey A, Vanneville G. Sciatic nerve blocking in children: comparison of the posterior, anterior and lateral approaches in 180 pediatric patients. Anesth Analg 1990; 70:131–137.

Ichiyanigi K. Sciatic nerve block: lateral approach with patients supine. Anesthesiology 1959; 20:601–604.

Parkinson SK, Mueller JB, Little WL, Bailey SL. Extent of blockade with various approaches to the lumbar plexus. Anesth Analg 1989; 68:243–248.

Rorie DK, Byer DE, Nelson DO, et al. Assessment of block of the sciatic nerve in the popliteal fossa. Anesth Analg 1980; 59:371–376.

Schurman DJ. Ankle block anesthesia for foot surgery. Anesthesiology 1976; 44:348–352.

Sharrock NE. Inadvertent three-in-one-block following injection of the lateral cutaneous nerve of the thigh. Anesth Analg 1980; 59:887–888.

DELIBERATE HYPOTENSION

NABIL R. FAHMY, M.D., F.F.A.R.C.S., D.A.

Deliberate (controlled or induced) hypotension is the elective reduction of systemic arterial pressure for the purpose of decreasing blood loss during surgery, which in turn decreases the need for blood replacement and its attendant risks. Utilization of hypotension provides a relatively dry operative field, which may improve operating conditions, thus allowing the surgeon to perform such delicate procedures as middle ear surgery, clipping of a cerebral aneurysm, and plastic surgery. Induced hypotension is also indicated in patients with rare blood groups and those whose religious beliefs preclude the use of blood products (e.g., Jehovah's Witnesses).

ADVANTAGES

Decreased blood loss during surgery diminishes the need for blood replacement. The effect of deliberate hypotension on blood loss is demonstrated readily in major orthopedic procedures (e.g., total hip replacement, excision of bone tumors with allograft bone replacement, Harrington's rod insertion). In these procedures, blood loss may be reduced by 50 percent with the use of induced hypotension. Deliberate hypotension is also useful in head and neck surgery, neurosurgery, radical cancer surgery, plastic surgery, and middle ear procedures. Proper positioning of the patient, with the surgical field uppermost, helps decrease bleeding.

Additionally, the decreased amount of cauterized tissues and number of ligatures may decrease the incidence of wound infection. Requirements for anesthetic drugs are decreased during hypotension. The circulatory effects of bone cement (during total hip replacement) are attenuated or eliminated in patients in whom deliberate hypotension is employed.

A relatively dry operative field is usually obtained when the mean arterial blood pressure is maintained between 50 and 65 mm Hg in healthy individuals. However, a dry surgical field may be obtained at a higher mean blood pressure. In addition to a reduction of arterial pressure, a decreased cardiac output and venous pressure (most surgical bleeding is venous) may help minimize blood loss.

CONTRAINDICATIONS

Vascular insufficiency (determined by clinical and laboratory investigations) to the brain, heart, and kidney represents an important contraindication to the use of deliberate hypotension. The presence of anemia and hypovolemia is also a contraindication. Furthermore, the technique should not be performed by an inexperienced anesthesiologist.

METHODS

Methods include preganglionic blockade, ganglionic blockade, myocardial depression, and peripheral vasodilatation. There is no place in modern-day practice for controlled hemorrhage through arteriotomy.

Preganglionic blockade is produced by a high spinal or epidural anesthesia. Use of high spinal anesthesia requires the concomitant administration of general endotracheal anesthesia to alleviate the manifestations of hypotension. Significant bradycardia occurs (from unopposed vagal activity).

Ganglionic blockade is obtained by either trimethaphan camsylate or pentolinium tartrate. Trimethaphan camsylate may also have a direct vasodilating effect. Histamine release occurs with bolus administration but not during infusion of trimethaphan camsylate. The hypotensive effect of trimethaphan camsylate results from relaxation of capacitance and resistance vessels. Plasma catecholamines and renin activity are not significantly elevated; this is in contrast to nitroprusside. Heart rate may increase, a reflection of parasympathetic ganglionic blockade. Trimethaphan camsylate is probably hydrolyzed by plasma cholinesterase. It is administered through continuous infusion of 10 to 200 μg per kilogram per minute to produce hypotension. Pupillary dilatation accompanies trimethaphan administration.

Controlled myocardial depression can be produced by a high-inspired concentration of halothane. Enflurane and isoflurane produce hypotension through a combination of myocardial depression and vasodilatation.

Vasodilatation may be produced by any of several intravenous drugs. These include sodium nitroprusside, nitroglycerin, hydralazine hydrochloride, adenosine and adenosine triphosphate, prostaglandin E_1, calcium-channel blockers (nicardipine hydrochloride), and labetalol hydrochloride. Recently, a mixture of nitroprusside (25 mg) and trimethaphan camsylate (250 mg) in 5 percent dextrose has been used for deliberate hypotension. A salt, bis-trimethaphan-nitroprusside, has been prepared in Switzerland.

Vasodilatory Agents

Sodium Nitroprusside

Sodium nitroprusside is a rapidly acting vasodilator drug that acts on both resistance and capacitance vessels; it has no direct actions on the autonomic nervous system. It has a short duration of action; blood pressure is rapidly restored when the drug infusion is discontinued. A rapid decrease of arterial pressure by nitroprusside (over 2 minutes) causes a significant decrease in cardiac output and a significant increase in heart rate. However, a slow decrease of blood pressure (over 10 minutes) is associated with minimal changes in cardiac output and heart rate.

Nitroprusside is initially broken down by a nonenzymatic reaction with oxyhemoglobin, releasing its five cyanide radicals; oxyhemoglobin is converted to methemoglobin in this process. The majority of cyanide (60 to 70 percent) is converted to the less toxic thiocyanate in the liver and kidney by rhodanase enzyme, which requires thiosulfate and hydroxycobalamin (vitamin B_{12}) as cofactors. Thiocyanate is excreted by the kidneys (half-life is 4 to 7 days). Cyanide also combines with hydroxycobalamin to form cyanocobalamin, which is more readily excreted in the urine. Excess cyanide, by combining with cytochrome oxidase in the tissues, can interfere with tissue oxygenation. This would increase the mixed venous oxygen tension because of diminished utilization of oxygen by the tissues. Nitroprusside should not be given in doses greater than 10 μg per kilogram per minute or 1.5 mg per kilogram for acute administration, or 0.5 mg per kilogram per hour for chronic administration. Treatment of toxicity consists of the administration of oxygen, sodium nitrite, thiosulfate, and hydroxycobalamin.

Tachyphylaxis or resistance to the vasodilating effect of nitroprusside may develop, particularly in young healthy individuals. The mechanism is not clearly understood. Increased activity of the sympathoadrenal axis may be involved in some patients. This can be attenuated by pretreatment with propranolol (oral or intravenous), captopril, or both. Severe liver disease, Leber's optic atrophy, and tobacco amblyopia may be responsible in other individuals.

Rebound hypertension may follow discontinuation of nitroprusside infusion, reflecting the unopposed actions of vasoconstrictor substances after the vasodilator effect of nitroprusside wears off.

Nitroglycerin

Intravenous nitroglycerin is an effective hypotensive agent, especially in combination with an inhalational anesthetic. It has no known toxic effects. Unlike nitroprusside, nitroglycerin acts on all smooth muscles. It dilates capacitance more than resistance vessels. Venous dilatation causes peripheral pooling of blood, reduction of heart size, and decreased cardiac ventricular wall tension. At comparable systolic pressures, nitroglycerin infusion maintains higher diastolic and mean systemic pressures than nitroprusside. Rebound hypertension is not observed after abrupt discontinuation of nitroglycerin. Intravenous nitroglycerin should be administered via a special delivery tubing to decrease the absorption of the drug by plastic.

Nitroglycerin is metabolized in the liver by nitrate reductase (glutathione dependent) to glycerol and (less pharmacologically active) dinitrate and mononitrate and nitrite, which are excreted in urine.

The continuous infusion of nitroglycerin, 4.7 μg per kilogram per minute (mean dose), in patients anesthetized with halothane produces an adequate decrease in blood pressure that provides a dry operative field for orthopedic procedures.

Hydralazine

Hydralazine acts as a potent direct relaxant of arteriolar smooth muscle, probably by interfering with calcium ion transport in vascular smooth muscle. Hydralazine has been used as a hypotensive drug in neurosurgical patients (5 to 45 mg; mean dose of 17 mg). The associated increase of heart rate requires the administration of propranolol. The drug is metabolized in the liver.

Adenosine and Adenosine Triphosphate

Both are naturally occurring substances that produce a dose-related decrease in heart rate and blood pressure. Hypotension is rapid in onset; rebound hypertension does not occur on discontinuation of these compounds. Severe bradycardia and complete heart block are their serious disadvantages. Alteration of coronary blood flow may occur, leading to ischemic changes.

Prostaglandin E₁

This is a mild hypotensive drug. Renal blood flow increases with this naturally occurring substance.

Labetalol

Labetalol is the only drug currently available with both alpha- (alpha$_1$) and beta- (beta$_1$ and beta$_2$) adrenergic-blocking actions. Intravenous labetalol is a useful drug for the production of deliberate hypotension. The initial dose is 20 mg, and a satisfactory reduction in blood pressure is usually obtained with doses ranging from 60 to 160 mg. It should be used in conjunction with an inhalational anesthetic (e.g., halothane, enflurane, or isoflurane). Tachycardia is not a feature of labetalol-induced hypotension. The duration of action is 3 to 6 hours.

Calcium-Channel Blockers

Verapamil has been used as a hypotensive drug during neuroleptanesthesia (0.7 mg per kilogram). I do not recommend its use for this purpose, however, because it is associated with significant bradycardia and the potential for atrioventricular block. Nifedipine is a potent hypotensive agent, but it is not available for intravenous use. Intravenous nicardipine is a potent hypotensive agent that can be used for induced hypotension and to control hypertensive events during anesthesia and operation.

Nitroprusside-Trimethaphan Mixture

This is a potent hypotensive mixture. The tachycardia and sympathoadrenal stimulation that usually accompany the infusion of nitroprusside alone are attenuated by the ganglionic-blocking activity of trimethaphan. Rebound hypertension is usually not observed after termination of infusion.

MONITORING

Direct monitoring of arterial blood pressure (through a radial artery catheter) is advisable during deliberate hypotension, especially when potent vasodilators are used. Arterial blood samples should be obtained periodically for measurement of blood gases, electrolytes, and hematocrit. Monitoring of the electro-cardiogram (ECG) using a V5 lead (or its equivalent) should be routine. A right atrial catheter is inserted if large blood losses are anticipated. Urine output is measured during lengthy procedures. Blood loss should be assessed by weighing sponges, measuring suction losses, and estimating losses on the drapes. Temperature measurement is important. Other monitors that may be used, such as evoked potentials, electroencephalography (EEG), and tissue surface pH electrodes, depend on the operative procedure.

ORGAN FUNCTION DURING DELIBERATE HYPOTENSION

Most studies of organ function during deliberate hypotension have been performed in animals.

Skin and Muscle. Observations in humans suggest that cutaneous and skeletal muscle blood flows are not deranged.

Central Nervous System. Because of autoregulation, cerebral blood flow is maintained at mean arterial pressures of 50 to 150 mm Hg in healthy normotensive individuals. Volatile anesthetics administered during normocapnia, in concentrations above 0.6 minimum alveolar concentration (MAC), produce dose-dependent increases in cerebral blood flow. The increase is greatest with halothane, is intermediate with enflurane, and is least with isoflurane. Cerebral blood flow is increased with sodium nitroprusside and nitroglycerin but is not changed with trimethaphan camsylate. Normocapnia should be maintained during deliberate hypotension, since a low arterial carbon dioxide pressure ($PaCO_2$) decreases cerebral blood flow.

Intracranial pressure is increased by nitroprusside, nitroglycerin, and trimethaphan camsylate. These drugs should be used after the dura is opened in patients with increased intracranial pressure.

Heart. In dogs with normal coronary arteries, coronary blood flow is well maintained when mean arterial pressure is decreased to 50 to 65 mm Hg with nitroprusside or trimethaphan camsylate. Deliberate hypotension in dogs with coronary stenosis (40 percent reduction in flow) compromises coronary perfusion and depresses the ST segment. Use of this technique should be avoided in patients with compromised coronary blood flow.

Lungs. Physiologic dead space may increase during deliberate hypotension if cardiac output is diminished. Arterial oxygen tension decreases due to increased pulmonary shunting.

Kidneys. The formation of urine is decreased during the hypotensive phase, because of the diminished pressure head necessary for glomerular filtration; urine formation resumes after the blood pressure is restored. Renal blood flow is probably maintained. Renal function is preserved.

Liver. Mild changes in liver functions tests may occur following clinical deliberate hypotension. However, these may be related to the surgical procedure and/or the effect of the anesthetic agents.

Eye. Intraocular pressure decreases with reductions in systemic arterial pressure. Blindness rarely occurs as a complication.

POTENTIATION OF HYPOTENSION

In some patients, especially young, muscular individuals, hypotension may be difficult to induce. Potentiation of the hypotensive technique may be produced by (1) decreasing the heart rate through the use of propranolol or halothane; (2) attenuating the renin-angiotensin system by propranolol, captopril, or both; (3) decreasing venous return by increasing airway resistance; and (4) positioning the operative site uppermost.

COMPLICATIONS

Complications can be avoided if attention is paid to adequate ventilation, monitoring, positioning (head-up tilt), measurement and adequate replacement of blood loss, and limiting the extent and duration of hypotension. Proper selection of patients is also important. The complications that have been reported in the literature include those related to underperfusion of major organs (brain, heart, kidneys, and eyes) and surgical complica-

tions (reactionary hemorrhage, thromboembolism and hematoma formation). In a recent series, my colleagues and I found that the incidence of surgical complications in patients undergoing total hip replacement was not significantly different between hypotension and normotension groups during general anesthesia.

SUGGESTED READING

Bloor BC, Fukunaga Af, Ma C, et al. Myocardial hemodynamics during induced hypotension: a comparison between sodium nitroprusside and adenosine triphosphate. Anesthesiology 1985; 63:517–525.

Fahmy NR. Nitroprusside vs. a nitroprusside-trimethaphan mixture for induced hypotension: hemodynamic effects and cyanide release. Clin Pharmacol Ther 1985; 37:264–270.

Fahmy NR. Nitroglycerin as a hypotensive drug during general anesthesia. Anesthesiology 1978; 49:17–20.

Fahmy NR, Bottros MR, Charchaflieh J, et al. A randomized comparison of labetalol and nitroprusside for induced hypotension. J Clin Anesth 1989; 1:409–413.

Fahmy NR, Soter NA. Effects of trimethaphan on arterial blood histamine and systemic hemodynamics in humans. Anesthesiology 1985; 62:562–566.

Kien ND, White DA, Reitan JA, Eisele JH Jr. Cardiovascular function during controlled hypotension induced by adenosine triphosphate or sodium nitroprusside in the anesthetized dog. Anesth Analg 1987; 66:103–110.

Tinker JH, Michenfelder JD. Sodium nitroprusside: pharmacology, toxicology and therapeutics. Anesthesiology 1976; 45:340–354.

ANESTHESIA IN OPHTHALMOLOGY

OPHTHALMIC ANESTHESIA

MARC FELDMAN, M.D.

Ophthalmic surgery presents challenges to the anesthesiologist not seen in other surgical areas. The anesthesiologist must exercise the best interpersonal skills for the compassionate care of the blind patient or the patient experiencing the anxiety of potential vision loss. The anesthesiologist must also deal with his or her own anxiety in dealing with limited access to the airway in the ill, the elderly, and the dysmorphic child. Most procedures now have the added strain of outpatient anesthetic management. This chapter reviews the anatomy and physiology of the eye, preoperative medical and psychological preparation, regional and general anesthetic techniques, and the anesthetic management of pediatric procedures.

OCULAR ANATOMY

An understanding of ocular anatomy is essential for the anesthesiologist to (1) understand surgical procedures; (2) administer and evaluate regional blocks; (3) diagnose and treat complications of regional blocks properly; and (4) control intraocular pressure.

The eye is a sphere with a diameter of approximately 24 mm (Fig. 1). The eye sits in a pyramidal bony case that is the orbit. The wall of the globe is composed of three layers.

The outermost layer is the sclera, the tough, fibrous "whites of the eyes." The most anterior part of the sclera is the transparent cornea. The radius of the curvature of the cornea is smaller than the rest of the globe. The curvature of the cornea is responsible for most of the focus power of the eye.

The middle layer is the uveal tract. It is composed of three specialized structures: the iris, ciliary body, and choroid. The iris contains muscle fibers that control the central aperture, the pupil. Parasympathetic stimulation causes iris sphincter fibers to contract, causing pupillary constriction or miosis. Sympathetic stimulation causes iris dilator fibers to contract, dilating the pupil. Directly adjacent to and behind the iris is the ciliary body. The ciliary body produces aqueous humor. Ciliary muscles, within the ciliary body, are responsible for fine-tuning focus by releasing tension on the suspensory fibers or zonules of the lens, increasing the refractive power of the lens. The posterior part of the uveal tract is a layer of blood vessels and capillaries called the choroid. Bleeding from the choroid layer is the cause of catastrophic intraoperative expulsive hemorrhage.

The inner layer of the wall of the globe is the retina. The choroid layer provides the retina with oxygen and substrate. Photoreceptors of the retinal layer convert light into neural signals, which are processed and carried to the brain via the optic nerve.

The center of the eye is filled by the vitreous body, a collection of gelatinous fluid, or vitreous humor. The vitreous has attachments to the optic nerve and large blood vessels. Scarring, bleeding, or opacification of the vitreous is treated by its removal, or vitrectomy. Traction of the vitreous on the retina causes retinal detachment.

Extraocular muscles arise from a fibrous ring at the orbital apex and insert on the sclera approximately 6 mm posterior to the corneal-scleral junction. These muscles move the eye within the orbit. The six muscles, four recti and two obliques, form a cone within the orbit, which contains the optic nerve, ophthalmic artery and vein, oculomotor and abducens nerves, and ciliary ganglion. A summary of the function and innervation of the extraocular muscles is provided in Table 1.

The eyelids are composed of an outer layer of skin, a muscle layer, a cartilaginous tarsal plate, and an inner layer of conjunctiva, a mucus membrane that lines the eyelids and covers the globe up to the corneal-scleral junction.

Tears are formed in the lacrimal gland in the superior temporal orbit. Tears pass from the surface of the eye via the puncta, through the canaliculi to the lacrimal sac and duct, to drain in the nasopharynx below the inferior turbinate.

Blood is supplied to the ocular structures primarily through the ophthalmic artery. The ophthalmic artery is a branch off the internal carotid artery just before the circle of Willis. Venous drainage flows through the superior and inferior ophthalmic veins directly to the cavernous sinus.

The innervation to ocular structures is through the cranial nerves. The optic nerve (II) carries the sensory information from the retina. Cranial nerves III, IV, and VI innervate the extraocular muscles.

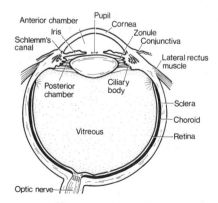

Figure 1 Anatomy of the eye. (Republished with permission from Bruce RA Jr, McGoldrick KE, Oppenheimer P. Anesthesia for ophthalmology. Birmingham, AL: Aesculapius, 1982:57.)

Table 1 Function and Innervation of the Extraocular Muscles

Innervation	Muscle	Function
III	Superior rectus	Elevation
III	Inferior rectus	Depression
III	Medial rectus	Adduction
III	Inferior oblique	Elevation/abduction
VI	Lateral rectus	Abduction
IV	Superior oblique	Depression/adduction

The trigeminal nerve (V) provides sensory innervation to the skin and conjunctiva of the lower lid via the maxillary nerve, and the upper lid and conjunction via the frontal branch of the ophthalmic nerve. The nasociliary branch of the ophthalmic nerve provides sensory innervation to the medial canthus, lacrimal sac, and canaliculi and sends sensory fibers to the ciliary ganglion.

The ciliary ganglion provides sensory innervation to the cornea, iris, and ciliary body. Parasympathetic motor fibers originating from the oculomotor nerve (III) synapse in the ciliary ganglion before supplying the sphincter muscle of the iris and the ciliary muscle. Sympathetic motor fibers originating from the carotid plexus travel through the ciliary ganglion to innervate the dilator muscle of the iris.

The facial nerve arises out of the stylomastoid foramen to innervate the strong orbicularis constrictor of the lids via the zygomatic branch. Local anesthetic blockade of the facial nerve can be important in intraocular surgery.

OCULOCARDIAC REFLEX

The importance of an understanding of ocular anatomy is demonstrated in the pathophysiology of the oculocardiac reflex. First described by Bernard Aschner and Giuseppe Dagnini in 1908, pressure on the globe or traction on the extraocular muscles, especially the medial rectus, results in bradycardia, atrioventricular block, ventricular ectopy, or asystole.

The reflex is trigeminovagal. The afferent limb is from orbital contents to the ciliary ganglion to the ophthalmic division of the trigeminal nerve to the sensory nucleus of the trigeminal nerve near the fourth ventricle. The efferent limb is located in the vagus nerve.

Retrobulbar block is not uniformly effective in preventing the reflex. In fact, retrobulbar block may precipitate the response. Premedication with intramuscular atropine in usual doses is ineffective. The response may be exacerbated by hypercarbia or hypoxia. In the recommended treatment for a single episode, the following steps should be taken:

1. The surgeon is asked to stop manipulation.
2. Ventilatory status is assessed.
3. If bradycardia is severe or persistent, intravenous atropine in increments of 7 μg per kilogram is administered.

Spontaneous return to normal sinus rhythm fre-

quently occurs with cessation of manipulation alone. Bradycardia is less likely to occur with repeated manipulation, possibly because of fatigue of the reflex at the cardioinhibitory center.

Prophylactic intravenous glycopyrrolate can be effective in blocking the oculocardiac reflex and may be indicated in patients with a history of atrioventricular block, vasovagal episodes, or beta-blocker therapy.

REGULATION OF INTRAOCULAR PRESSURE

The retina and optic nerve are dependent on a continuous supply of blood for their survival. Blood flow is driven by the intraocular perfusion pressure. High intraocular pressure (IOP) impairs the capillary blood supply, resulting in the loss of optic nerve function.

The sclera of the eye provides a relatively noncompliant compartment. The volume of the internal constituents is fixed, except for aqueous humor and choroidal blood volume. These two factors account for regulation of IOP and for most acute changes (Fig. 2).

Aqueous humor is formed at a rate of 2μl per minute. Two-thirds is secreted by the ciliary body by an active sodium-pump mechanism, and one-third is produced by passive ultrafiltration through vessels on the anterior iris. From the ciliary body, aqueous flows over the lens and through the pupil, mixing with the aqueous formed by the iris in the anterior chamber. The aqueous bathes the corneal endothelium, then flows through the trabecular meshwork to the canal of Schlemm in the anterior chamber angle. The canal of Schlemm is continuous with venous channels to the episcleral veins. Intraocular pressure is controlled by regulation of the outflow resistance at the trabecular meshwork. Normal IOP is maintained between 10 and 20 mm Hg.

High IOP can result from impairment of aqueous outflow at any point. In open-angle glaucoma, sclerosis of the trabecular meshwork is believed to impede aqueous drainage. Trabeculectomy is a surgical procedure for decreasing IOP by removing the resistance of the trabecular meshwork. Closed-angle glaucoma occurs when the peripheral iris swells or is displaced anteriorly and closes the anterior chamber angle to cause an obstruction to aqueous drainage. The acute rise in IOP may

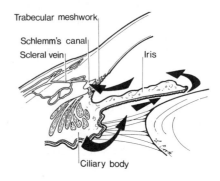

Trabecular meshwork

Schlemm's canal

Scleral vein

Iris

Ciliary body

Figure 2 Anatomy of aqueous flow. (Republished with permission from Bruce RA Jr, McGoldrick KE, Oppenheimer P. Anesthesia for ophthalmology. Birmingham, AL: Aesculapius, 1982:58.)

cause severe pain and is an ophthalmologic emergency.

Acute changes in choroidal blood volume can produce rapid increases in IOP. Hypercarbia can lead to choroidal congestion and increased IOP. The increases in venous pressure associated with coughing, straining, or vomiting can increase IOP to 30 to 40 mm Hg. Similar increases can be seen during intubation. Because these increases are transient, they are relatively innocuous in a closed eye. In an open eye, such as after traumatic injury or during cataract or corneal transplant surgery, such increases can lead to loss of intraocular contents, hemorrhage, and permanent vision loss.

IOP can also be increased by extrinsic compression of the globe. The force of the eyelid in a normal blink may cause an increase of 10 mm Hg. A forceful blink can increase IOP to 40 mm Hg. A poorly placed anesthesia mask could increase IOP to the point of zero bloodflow.

The use of deep inhalational anesthesia or thiopental decreases IOP by 30 to 40 percent in a dose-related manner. Narcotics have little effect on IOP. Atropine in the usual doses is not a problem, even in patients with open-angle glaucoma. Ketamine may cause a modest increase in IOP.

Succinylcholine chloride causes a 6 to 10 mm increase in IOP, which can be sustained for 5 to 15 minutes. Specialized muscle fiber structures in the extraocular muscles appear to respond to succinylcholine chloride with sustained tonic contraction. Self-taming doses and precurarization do not completely abolish the response. The clinical significance of this as regards the deeply anesthetized patient is unclear. The use of succinylcholine chloride for induction of anesthesia in patients with open-globe injury is controversial, although vitreous loss in precurarized patients due to succinylcholine has not been reported.

SYSTEMIC EFFECTS OF OPHTHALMIC DRUGS

Acetazolamide is a carbonic anhydrase inhibitor used to decrease aqueous production and thereby decrease intraocular pressure in glaucoma. It induces an alkaline diuresis that may result in potassium depletion. In patients taking this drug, electrolytes should be checked preoperatively.

Mannitol is an osmotic diuretic that decreases intraocular pressure for 5 to 6 hours. Patients who receive this drug intraoperatively may need a urinary catheter to prevent bladder overdistention. Patients with limited cardiac reserve may develop congestive heart failure due to the increased volume load.

Timolol maleate is a topical beta-blocker used to decrease aqueous production in the long-term treatment of glaucoma. Systemic absorption causes beta-blockade, with possible bradycardia, bronchospasm, or exacerbation of congestive failure.

Phenylephrine is an alpha-adrenergic agonist applied topically to cause pupillary dilitation. Systemic absorption of the 10 percent solution is associated with severe hypertensive reactions. The 2.5 percent concentration is safer, but may still exacerbate hypertension in some patients.

Pilocarpine and acetylcholine are cholinergic drugs used to induce miosis. Toxicity may be manifested in bradycardia or acute bronchospasm.

Anticholinergic eyedrops such as atropine or scopolamine may cause toxic reactions, tachycardia, dry skin, fever, and agitation. Overdosage can be reversed with incremental doses of physostigmine.

Echothiophate iodide (or phospholine iodine) is a topical long-acting anticholinesterase drug used to maintain miosis in the treatment of glaucoma. Systemic absorption leads to inhibition of plasma cholinesterase. Subsequent administration of succinylcholine chloride causes prolonged muscle paralysis. Inhibition of the metabolism of ester-type local anesthetics may lead to toxicity at doses that are lower than usual.

PREOPERATIVE EVALUATION

The first step in planning perioperative management is the preoperative evaluation. Every patient undergoing a surgical procedure under the care of an anesthesiologist must have an appropriate and thorough medical history and physical examination. Further laboratory testing and consultations may be indicated preoperatively depending on the assessed risk of the patient, assessed "stress" of the procedure, and the degree of urgency of the surgery.

Ophthalmic surgery patients tend to comprise a "high-risk" group. These patients are generally elderly, and most have risk factors such as hypertension, diabetes, lung disease, or atherosclerosis. The ophthalmic surgery procedures themselves, however, are "low risk," being associated with no appreciable blood loss or third-spacing and minimal postoperative pain. Despite the fact that the patients comprise a high-risk population, mortality rates for ophthalmic surgery are far lower than for the general surgical population. Even in patients who had previous myocardial infarction, Backer et al found that ophthalmic surgery did not pose the risk of reinfarction seen in general surgery. Nevertheless, high-risk patients do have problems. In a 1-year period at this institution, one patient died and another was admitted emergently to the cardiac care unit after their preoperative evaluations but before the day of surgery.

Where does this leave the anesthesiologist with the high-risk patient undergoing low-risk surgery? We find the following principles helpful for guidance:

1. The patient's personal physician is the consultant of first choice. Every patient seeing a physician for the treatment of chronic medical problems should visit the physician preoperatively.
2. The medical history and physical examination should guide all preoperative testing.
3. The patient should be judged to be at unacceptable risk for elective surgery if (a) the medical condition of the patient indicates the need for acute inpatient medical therapy or (b) the patient presents with a reversible medical condition that is likely to lead to a perioperative complication.

Following these principles, our institution has developed specific guidelines agreed upon by ophthalmologists, medical consultants, and anesthesiologists that have improved rapport, enhanced the consistency of patient care, and increased the efficiency of the operating room.

REGIONAL ANESTHESIA

Unlike some other surgical procedures, ophthalmic surgery requires immobility (or akinesia) and profound anesthesia of the surgical site. Contraction of the lids during a procedure with an open eye may lead to extrusion of vitreous humor and permanent damage. The discomfort associated with incomplete anesthesia of the surgical site is magnified by the patient's anxiety in anticipation of possible vision loss. Safe and reliable regional anesthetic techniques that satisfy the requirements of ophthalmic surgery have been developed. However, because discomfort and anxiety as well as rare but severe complications are associated with these blocks, supplementation of the local anesthetic with intravenous sedation and continuous monitoring of the patient are frequently preferred.

Regional anesthesia offers some advantages over general anesthesia. There is usually less nausea and vomiting, the patient may resume ambulation more quickly, and the local block frequently provides significant postoperative analgesia.

Not all patients are candidates for regional anesthesia. Few children will tolerate being aware of the operation in progress. Regional blocks in patients with a language barrier or with perforated globes, uncontrollable cough or tremor, or bleeding diathesis may be inadvisable. Although procedures lasting 60 minutes or less are easier for patients to tolerate, properly prepared and sedated patients may tolerate procedures as long as 3 to 4 hours.

Communication and rapport between patient, surgeon, and anesthesiologist are crucial to successful regional anesthesia. In preparation, the patient should be told the following:

1. "The planned procedure does not require general anesthesia; it can be performed using local anesthesia without pain.
2. Sedation will be administered in such a manner that the injections will not hurt; in fact, you will probably not remember them at all."
3. You will be awake during the procedure; you will be able to hear people talking, but you will not feel pain. You may doze off during the procedure."
4. It is very important that while the surgeon is operating on your eye, you should not shake your head or try to sit up. Lie still."
5. Someone from the anesthesia department will be with you the entire time. If anything bothers you, let us know. If not, stay quiet because talking causes small movements of the head."

If the patient is prepared before being sedated, the procedure generally goes well. An anxious, talkative patient may be a candiate for general anesthesia.

Before sedation is begun, an intravenous infusion is started and blood pressure, electrocardiographic monitor, and pulse oximeter are applied. Supplemental oxygen is given by nasal prongs. A wedge-shaped pillow is placed under the knees to prevent lower back pain. After sedation, block, and draping, an airblower is turned on and blows 30 L of air per minute under the drapes over the lower face. The purpose of the air blower is to: (1) eliminate carbon dioxide, which can build up under the drapes and cause dyspnea; (2) eliminate excess oxygen, which could be a fire hazard; and (3) decrease feelings of claustrophobia.

For intravenous sedation, a combination of midazolam maleate (0.5 to 2 mg), fentanyl (12.5 to 50 µg), and thiamylal sodium 1.5 to 2 mg per kilogram provides excellent amnesia and unresponsiveness for regional block and leaves the patient only lightly sedated during the surgical procedure.

The local anesthetic solution used most often at our institution is a combination of bupivacaine 0.75 percent and lidocaine 2 percent in 1:1 ratio without epinephrine. Hyaluronidase is added to speed tissue penetration. Akinesis of the eyelids is achieved by blocking the facial nerve through one of the following methods (Fig. 3):

1. *The modified Van Lint block.* The needle is inserted 1 cm lateral to the lateral orbital rim; 2 to 4 ml of anesthetic is injected deeply on the periosteum just lateral to the superolateral and inferolateral orbital rim.
2. *The O'Brien block.* The mandibular condyle is palpated inferior to the posterior zygomatic process and anterior to the tragus as the patient opens and closes the jaw. The needle is inserted perpendicular to the skin up to the periosteum. Three milliliters of anesthetic is injected as the needle is withdrawn.
3. *The Nadbath-Rehman block.* A 12-mm 25-gauge needle is inserted perpendicular to the skin between the mastoid process and the posterior border of the mandible. The needle is advanced its full length, and after careful aspiration, 3 ml of anesthetic is injected as the needle is withdrawn. This blocks the entire trunk of the facial nerve as it exits the skull at the stylomastoid foramen. The patient should be told to expect a lower facial droop for several hours postoperatively.

Akinesis and anesthesia of the eye and the orbit are achieved with a retrobulbar block. A 3-cm 23 gauge blunt Atkinson needle is recommended to protect against ocular perforation. The needle is inserted at the junction of the medial and lateral thirds of the lower lid just above the inferior orbital rim. The needle is advanced along the inferotemporal wall of the orbit until it is about 1.5 cm past the equator of the eye; the needle is then turned superiorly and aimed toward the apex of the orbit. The needle is advanced until it pierces the muscle cone; a rotational eye movement with rebound is seen. After aspiration, 2 to 3 ml of anesthetic solution is injected.

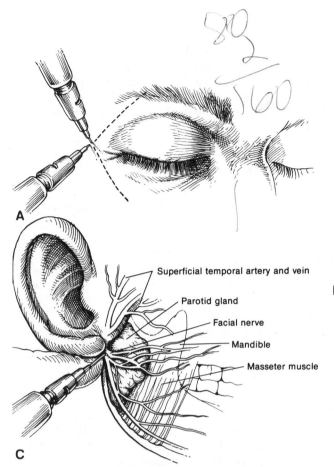

Superficial temporal artery and vein

Parotid gland

Facial nerve

Mandible

Masseter muscle

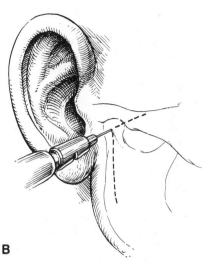

Figure 3 Facial nerve blocks: *A*, Van Lint block; *B*, O'Brien block; *C*, Nadbath-Rehman block. (Republished with permission from Spaeth GL. Ophthalmic surgery: principles and practice. Philadelphia: WB Saunders, 1982:89-90.)

Some intorsion in downgaze is expected, since the superior oblique muscle is outside the muscle cone and may not be blocked.

The most common complication of retrobulbar block is retrobulbar hemorrhage. Proptosis and subconjunctival ecchymosis are seen. Monitoring of intraocular pressure is mandatory. If the pressure becomes markedly elevated, a lateral canthotomy is performed to decompress the orbit. Periocular hemorrhage may be seen as subconjuctival ecchymosis without proptosis. After some monitoring, if no proptosis or increased intraocular pressure develops, the surgical procedure might be safely continued.

The dose of local anesthetic given is not in the toxic range if given intravenously. Accidental intra-arterial injection can cause high levels in the brain via retrograde flow in the internal carotid. This can be seen as central nervous system excitation and seizures. Obtundation and respiratory arrest have been reported and are believed to be caused by injection into the optic nerve sheath, which is continuous with the subarachnoid space. Optic nerve damage and ocular perforations with retinal detachment and vitreous hemorrhage have been reported.

To avoid retrobulbar hemorrhage and other complications, posterior peribulbar anesthesia is becoming more widely used. A blunt 23-gauge Atkinson ⅞-inch needle is inserted at the junction of the middle and lateral thirds of the lower lid just above the interior orbital rim. One milliliter of local anesthetic is deposited just below the orbital septum, 3 ml at the equator, and 2 ml posterior to the equator outside the muscle cone. If no bulging is noted at the superior nasal lid area, a second injection of 2 to 3 ml is given inferior-nasally. Disadvantages of the technique include a longer onset time (9 to 12 minutes) and perhaps a somewhat lower incidence of complete akinesia.

GENERAL ANESTHESIA

The goals of general anesthesia for ophthalmic surgery include a smooth intubation with stable intraocular pressure, avoidance of severe oculocardiac reflexes, maintenance of a motionless field, and an equally smooth extubation. These goals can be accomplished with inhalational anesthesia, balanced narcotic anesthe-

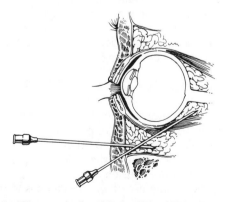

Figure 4 The retrobulbar block. (Republished with permission from Spaeth GL. Ophthalmic surgery: principles and practice. Philadelphia: WB Saunders, 1982:91.)

sia, or intravenous agents, with or without muscle relaxants.

Sulfur hexafluoride (SF_6) is a poorly soluble gas used in vitreoretinal surgery to prolong the resorption of intravitreal air bubbles. In the patient with an SF_6 bubble, nitrous oxide will diffuse in, greatly expanding the bubble and causing huge increases in intraocular pressure. Nitrous oxide should be shut off for 15 minutes before placement of the SF_6 bubble, and nitrous oxide should be avoided for 7 to 10 days thereafter.

ANESTHESIA FOR PEDIATRIC OPHTHALMOLOGY

Pediatric ophthalmic anesthesiology can be considered a subspecialty in and of itself. Certain surgical procedures deserve specific attention. Strabismus surgery is the most common type of ophthalmic surgery in children. Although there is not a great deal of postoperative pain, nausea and vomiting are significant in 50 to 80 percent of these children. Droperidol in a dose of 25

to 75 μg per kilogram seems to decrease the incidence markedly, without prolonging discharge time. Because malignant hyperthermia may be associated with muscle diseases, a careful family history must be obtained, and the anesthesiologist must be psychologically prepared to treat the syndrome aggressively and early. If succinylcholine chloride is used, the surgeon should be told so that he or she may take into account the effect of the depolarizer on forced duction testing.

SUGGESTED READING

Arthur DS, Dewar KMS. Anesthesia for eye surgery in children. Br J Anesth 1980; 52:681–688.
Bruce RA Jr, McGoldrick KE, Oppenheimer P. Anesthesia for ophthalmology. Birmingham, AL: Aesculapius, 1982.
Donlon JV Jr. Local anesthesia for ophthalmic surgery: patient preparation and management. Ann Ophthalmol 1980; 1183–1191.
Jay JL. Functional organization of the human eye. Br J Anesth 1980; 52:649–654.
Murphy DF. Anesthesia and intraocular pressure. Anesth Analg 1985; 520–530.

THE RUPTURED GLOBE

KATHRYN E. McGOLDRICK, M.D.

The challenging situation of the "open eye, full stomach" patient provides a graphic example of conflicting priorities that can complicate the planning and conduct of an anesthetic. Methods employed to protect against aspiration of gastric contents must be balanced against their influence on intraocular pressure (IOP). It must be emphasized that the anesthetic management of the patient with a penetrating eye injury who has recently eaten is controversial, and no one approach is ideal. Although no panacea exists, a comprehensive understanding of the effects of various drugs and manipulations on IOP will assist the anesthesiologist in selecting a course that best offers a satisfactory surgical result without compromising patient safety.

Few would debate what the intraoperative management of the patient with a penetrating eye injury should be. Rather, controversy is focused on induction techniques, specifically the selection of neuromuscular blocking agents for facilitating intubation.

SURGICAL CONSIDERATIONS

Penetrating injuries may be the result of intraocular foreign bodies in the anterior or posterior chambers, the lens, or the vitreous humor, or they may occur after lacerations of the sclera or cornea. Because penetrating injuries can result in extrusion of intraocular contents, a major objective in the use of an anesthetic is to prevent additional increases in IOP that can produce further prolapse and loss of intraocular contents. However, it is important to appreciate that any additional damage to

the eye that occurs after the initial trauma is not necessarily caused by the use of anesthetic drugs and manipulations. In many cases, for example, the patient may have been crying, coughing, vomiting, rubbing the eye, or squeezing the eyelids closed before the induction of anesthesia. All of these maneuvers are guaranteed to increase IOP dramatically.

It is often difficult for the ophthalmologist to assess accurately the prognosis of a penetrating eye injury before surgery. Adequate examination is frequently not feasible until after the patient is anesthetized, prepped, and draped. Moreover, even patients thought to have the poorest prognosis preoperatively may regain useful vision. Factors affecting prognosis include whether the anterior and/or posterior segment is injured, whether there is uveal prolapse, and whether intraocular reaction has resulted. Additionally, recent advances in retinal surgery have improved the visual results following severe posterior segment trauma. Examples of these additions to the surgical armamentarium include techniques to treat vitreoretinopathy, injection of long-acting intraocular gases, silicone oil tamponade, intraoperative endophotocoagulation, and the use of retinal tacks.

Although local or regional anesthesia is often a valuable alternative for the surgical-anesthetic management of trauma patients who have recently ingested food, such an option is not available in the case of penetrating eye injuries. Performance of a retrobulbar block is contraindicated in this setting, since extrusion of intraocular contents is likely to result.

PREOPERATIVE PREPARATION

As in all cases of trauma, attention should be given to the exclusion of other injuries, such as skull and orbital fractures, intracranial trauma associated with subdural hematoma formation, and the possibility of thoracic or abdominal bleeding.

Antacid aspiration prophylaxis is advised. A histamine$_2$ receptor antagonist can be administered to decrease gastric acid production and increase gastric pH. Additionally, metoclopramide is useful to stimulate peristalsis and to facilitate gastric emptying. No attempt should be made to insert a nasogastric tube while the patient is awake, because such a maneuver is guaranteed to trigger a major elevation of IOP.

GERMANE ANESTHETIC CONSIDERATIONS

IOP normally ranges between 10 and 22 mm Hg. In general, the nondepolarizing neuromuscular blocking agents are associated with a decrease or no change in IOP. By contrast, the depolarizing drug succinylcholine elevates IOP. An average peak increase of approximately 8 mm Hg is produced within 1 to 4 minutes after intravenous administration of succinylcholine, with a return to baseline usually within 7 minutes. Several mechanisms have been postulated to explain the ocular hypertensive effect of succinylcholine; these include tonic contraction of extraocular muscles, choroidal vascular dilatation, and relaxation of orbital smooth muscle.

A variety of methods, including prior treatment with acetazolamide, propranolol, nitroglycerin, and nondepolarizers, have been advocated to prevent succinylcholine-induced increases in IOP. Although some attenuation of the increase follows, none of these drugs consistently and completely prevents the ocular hypertensive response. Lively controversy surrounds the purported efficacy of pretreatment with nondepolarizing muscle relaxants. In 1968, using indentation tonometry, Miller et al reported that pretreatment with small amounts of gallamine or curare prevented succinylcholine-associated increases in IOP. However, one decade later, Meyers et al, employing the more sensitive applanation tonometer, failed to obliterate the ocular hypertensive response consistently after similar pretreatment therapy. Furthermore, it is entirely possible that the open eye may react differently from the intact eye in response to drugs.

In addition, stimulation from laryngoscopy and endotracheal intubation also results in an elevation of IOP. In some studies, the ocular hypertensive response to laryngoscopy and intubation has been noted to be blunted through the use of lidocaine (1.5 to 2 mg per kilogram IV) about 4 to 5 minutes before intubation, although another series failed to confirm this. Recently, Badrinath et al claimed that premedication with sufentanil (0.05 μg per kilogram) and pretreatment with a nondepolarizing relaxant plus a high dose of thiopental (7 mg per kilogram) or alfentanil (150 μg per kilogram) for induction effectively block the increase in IOP from succinylcholine and intubation.

Other considerations for the "open globe" patient include (1) avoidance of elevated venous pressure from straining or coughing, which can increase IOP by as much as 60 mm Hg; (2) appropriate preoxygenation (with avoidance of external pressure on the globe from the face mask); (3) application of cricoid pressure to prevent regurgitation; (4) establishing a sufficiently deep level of anesthesia before performing laryngoscopy and intubation not only to prevent coughing but also to avoid a sudden, significant increase in systemic blood pressure; and (5) initiation and maintenance of controlled ventilation after intubation to avoid hypercapnia-associated increases in IOP.

Gentle, short-duration laryngoscopy in the presence of adequate skeletal muscle relaxation and anesthetic depth is crucial in assuring minimal changes in IOP. After the patient is intubated, akinesis is essential for optimal surgical outcome. Hence, nearly complete suppression of the twitch response elicited by a peripheral nerve stimulator should be maintained until the eye is surgically closed. Further, because surgical results may be jeopardized by postoperative vomiting, intraoperative administration of an intravenous antiemetic and passage of an orogastric tube to decompress the stomach prior to extubation are recommended. Patients with a full stomach must be extubated while awake, but intravenous lidocaine and/or an appropriate dose of a narcotic can be given before extubation to attenuate coughing.

INDUCTION OF ANESTHESIA

As previously stated, a rapid-sequence induction with cricoid pressure and a smooth intubation must be accomplished. Ideally, such actions protect the airway and prevent significant increases in IOP. Accordingly, the selection and dosage of a neuromuscular blocking agent are areas of considerable debate.

The use of a barbituate and an intubating dose of a nondepolarizing muscle relaxant is often described as the method of choice for the emergency repair of a ruptured globe because pancuronium bromide, in a dose of 0.15 mg per kilogram, lowers—or at least does not increase—IOP. This technique has serious disadvantages, however, including the risk of aspiration during the relatively long period (varying from 75 seconds to more than 2.5 minutes) during which the airway is unprotected. Moreover, a premature attempt at intubation will trigger coughing, straining, and a dramatic increase in IOP as well as deleterious hemodynamic side effects of concern for those adults with coronary artery disease. The use of a blockade monitor to predict intubating conditions may be unreliable, since muscle groups vary in their response to nondepolarizing relaxants. In addition, the long duration of action of pancuronium bromide may mandate postoperative mechanical ventilation. Furthermore, it is not always possible to predict which patients will be difficult to intubate. The rapid return of spontaneous ventilation is often an invaluable adjunct to assist in the management of a difficult intubation, especially in the setting of recent food ingestion by the patient. Clearly, the use of intubating doses of nondepolarizing agents eliminates this option. Although newer nondepolarizing relaxants such as vecuronium bromide and atracurium besylate have shorter durations of action, in equipotent doses these newer drugs nevertheless have an onset of action as delayed as that of pancuronium bromide. Furthermore, although vecuronium bromide generally has minimal circulatory effects, intubating doses of atracurium besylate may be associated with histamine release and clinically significant hypotension.

Recently, Ginsberg et al reported that the administration of high-dose vecuronium bromide (400 μg per kilogram) reduces the speed of onset from 208 ± 41 seconds, as seen with the usual intubating dose of 100 μg per kilogram, to 106 ± 35 seconds. However, the design of the study did not eliminate the possibility of bias being introduced by factors that could influence the quality of the intubating conditions. For example, the dosages of diazepam, fentanyl, and thiopental given prior to intubation varied greatly among patients.

A few comments on the so-called priming principle are in order. This concept involves using approximately one-tenth of an intubating dose of a nondepolarizing drug, followed 4 minutes later by a full intubating dose. Then, after an additional 90 seconds, intubation can allegedly be performed. However, studies in this area have been characterized by a disconcerting scatter of data. Moreover, it is important to appreciate that priming is not devoid of risk, since aspiration following a priming dose of vecuronium bromide has been reported. Clearly, the priming technique may hasten the onset of neuromuscular blockade, but at the expense of increased morbidity, such as blurring of vision and difficulty with breathing and swallowing, as well as possible mortality.

Another approach involves pretreatment with a nondepolarizing muscle relaxant followed by a barbiturate-succinylcholine sequence. As has already been mentioned, however, the efficacy of pretreatment with small doses of nondepolarizing muscle relaxant to prevent succinylcholine-induced intraocular hypertension remains a moot issue. Nonetheless, in a patient with a full stomach, succinylcholine offers the important advantages of rapid onset, excellent intubating conditions, and short duration of action. Given after pretreatment with a nondepolarizing relaxant (e.g., curare, 0.06 mg per kilogram) and an inducing dose of sodium thiopental (4 to 6 mg per kilogram), succinylcholine (1.5 mg per kilogram) causes only very slight increases in IOP above baseline.

Moreover, the combination of an open eye injury, a full stomach, and limited cardiovascular reserves produces extremely treacherous circumstances for the anesthesiologist. In cases of cardiomyopathy, for example, an intubating dose of thiopental may be ill advised. The use of etomidate (0.3 mg per kilogram IV) may be wise from the viewpoint of cardiovascular parameters, but the very real possibility of myoclonus causes concern. While premedication with diazepam and/or fentanyl may diminish the incidence and severity of myoclonus, these drugs cannot totally eliminate this potentially hazardous complication. A recent report by Berry and Merin suggests that when it is deemed necessary to use the cardiovascular stability provided by etomidate induction in the patient with an open eye, etomidate should be combined with succinylcholine to minimize the time to complete flaccidity. Although these investigators are careful to point out the need for further study in this area, they suggest that the use of etomidate in the patient with an open globe without the rapid muscle relaxation produced by succinylcholine may lead to loss of ocular contents. Others might argue, however, that the problem of myoclonus could be obviated by administering a benzodiazepine or fentanyl in an appropriate dose as the inducing agent in patients with limited cardiovascular reserve.

Libonati et al support the use of succinylcholine in open eye surgery, pointing out that there are no reports in the literature of loss of intraocular contents produced by a nondepolarizing pretreatment-barbituatesuccinylcholine sequence used in this setting. This report, however, has been criticized for being a retrospective analysis without a control group for comparison and for having as its only endpoint the surgeon's report of whether there was extrusion of eye contents. For example, no mention was made of difficulty with uveal prolapse, bleeding, or reformation of the globe. Nonetheless, the study is not without merit, and the aforementioned criticisms are equally applicable to cases where nondepolarizing muscle relaxants were used.

In 1990, succinylcholine is, in my opinion, still the gold standard for rapid, predictable onset of neuromuscular blockade. The anesthesiologist's first and foremost concern must be optimally safe airway management. At this time, succinylcholine with pretreatment probably remains the most tenable compromise in the "open eye, full stomach" challenge.

Acknowledgment. The author thanks her secretary, Miss Jacki Fitzpatrick, for her expert assistance in preparing the manuscript.

SUGGESTED READING

Badrinath SK, Braverman KB, Ivankovitch AD. Alfentanil and sufentanil prevent the increase in IOP from succinylcholine (abstract). Anesth Analg 1988; 67:S5.

Berry JM, Merin RG. Etomidate myoclonus and the open globe. Anesth Analg 1989; 69:256–259.

Ginsberg B, Glass PS, Quill T, et al. Onset and duration of neuromuscular blockade following high dose vecuronium administration. Anesthesiology 1989; 71:201–205.

Libonati MM, Leahy JJ, Ellison N. Use of succinylcholine in open eye injury. Anesthesiology 1985; 62:637–640.

McGoldrick KE. Anesthesia and the eye. In: Barash PG, Cullen BF, Stoelting RK, eds. Clinical anesthesia. Philadelphia: JB Lippincott, 1989; 1049–1065.

Meyers EF, Krupin T, Johnson M, Zink H. Failure of nondepolarizing neuromuscular blockers to inhibit succinylcholine-induced increased intraocular pressure: a controlled study. Anesthesiology 1978; 48:149–151.

Miller RD, Way WL, Hickey RF. Inhibition of succinycholine-induced increased intraocular pressure by nondepolarizing muscle relaxants. Anesthesiology 1968; 29:123–126.

Musich J, Walts LF. Pulmonary aspiration after a priming dose of vecuronium. Anesthesiology 1986; 64:517–519.

ANESTHESIA IN PEDIATRICS

CONGENITAL DIAPHRAGMATIC HERNIA

CHARLES M. HABERKERN, M.D.
ROBERT K. CRONE, M.D.

Since the first description of congenital diaphragmatic hernia (CDH) by Bochdalek in 1848 and the earliest repair of the defect in an infant by Gross in 1946, this surgical entity has been a source of great interest and challenge. Our understanding of the defect and the range of therapeutic modalities available to treat the infant with the defect have increased considerably over the past couple of decades. In the process, the role of the anesthesiologist caring for the infant with CDH has become more important. Yet the chances of survival for the infant with symptoms presenting during the first hours of life have remained generally unchanged—between 40 and 60 percent by most reports. For this reason, distinctly different approaches to the problem are presently being considered, approaches that will involve the anesthesiologist to an even greater extent.

GENERAL CONDITIONS

Embryology, Anatomy, and Pathophysiology

During the first month of fetal development, the pleuroperitoneal cavity exists as a single compartment. Then, between weeks 5 and 10, the gut is normally herniated into the extraembryonic coelom, while the diaphragm develops from the pleuroperitoneal folds and is completely formed by week 9. After this closure of the pleuroperitoneal membrane, its muscularization from the cervical myotomes (2–4) follows. In the developing lung, successive branching of the primitive bronchi and of the vascular segments occurs between weeks 4 and 16, after which time the number of alveoli progressively increases. Thus, if closure of the pleuroperitoneum is delayed or if the gut returns from the coelom early, the gut may herniate into the pleural space and interfere with the growth and development of the lung. Recent ultrasonographic information indicates that this herniation, rather than being fixed, is dynamic: the bowel moves in and out of the chest through the diaphragmatic defect. Although there is some speculation that the primary embryologic event in CDH is failure of growth of the lung bud itself, most experimental evidence is consistent with the diaphragmatic defect being the primary event.

The major result of intrauterine diaphragmatic herniation, then, is hypoplasia of both lungs. Typically, the lungs have diminished volume and weight. They have a decreased number of branches of the bronchial tree and, concomitantly, a decreased number of alveoli; similarly, they have a decreased number of branches of the pulmonary vascular tree (Fig. 1), such that the total cross-sectional area of the pulmonary arterial bed is markedly diminished. A normal alveolus:vessel ratio is retained. In addition, left-sided defects have been shown to be associated with decreased cardiac mass (left atrium, left ventricle, and interventricular septum),

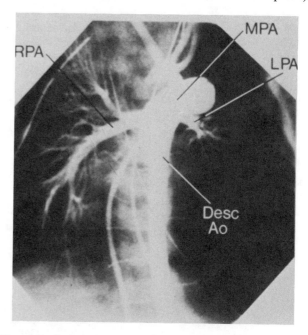

Figure 1 Pulmonary arteriogram showing marked hypoplasia of the left pulmonary vascular tree. Desc Ao = descending aorta; LPA = left pulmonary artery; MPA = main pulmonary artery; RPA = right pulmonary artery.

probably because of intrauterine compression of the developing heart by the herniated bowel.

Lung hypoplasia in CDH is accompanied by alterations in structure that affect the ipsilateral lung more than the contralateral lung. The alveoli are relatively immature, and the amount of surface active material has been shown to be diminished in them. The pulmonary vessels show two impressive changes: the first is an increase in the degree of medial muscle hypertrophy (as much as twofold) of arteries normally muscularized; the second is an extension of muscularization of arteries beyond the normal terminus at the level of the respiratory bronchiole to the level of the alveolar wall itself.

The net result is a pathophysiologic picture in CDH that is the complex interplay between pulmonary hypoplasia and pulmonary hypertension, or between factors that tend to affect gas exchange adversely and factors that tend to affect pulmonary blood flow adversely (Fig. 2). On the one hand, the number of alveoli is diminished in both lungs, and the "good" (or less affected) contralateral lung is compressed by any gas that may be present in the herniated bowel. The decrease in the amount of surface active material may contribute to atelectasis. On the other hand, the pulmonary vascular bed has a high fixed resistance because of its small size, and it has a highly active variable resistance caused by its extensive muscularization. An increase in the pulmonary vascular resistance can be triggered by several factors: hypoxia; respiratory and metabolic acidosis; hypothermia; catecholamines;

thromboxanes (especially TXA_2 and TXB_2); and leukotrienes. Excessive lung volumes achieved with the high airway pressures of assisted ventilation that are often needed in infants with CDH may also increase pulmonary vascular resistance. Finally, pulmonary blood flow is adversely affected by changes seen in the heart: the left ventricle (which may be intrinsically small) tends to fail in the face of the chronic hypoxia and acidosis often seen with CDH, and this failure promotes shunting at the ductal level from the high-pressure pulmonary circulation to the low-pressure systemic circulation; the right ventricle also tends to fail in the face of high pulmonary pressures (in some cases, suprasystemic), and this failure promotes shunting at the atrial level from the right to the left sides. All of these many factors produce a self-perpetuating cycle of hypoxia and acidosis in the infant with CDH.

Clinical Findings

The incidence of CDH is approximately one in 4,000 live births. Most diaphragmatic hernias (80 to 90 percent) occur in the posterolateral aspect of the diaphragm, presumably because the posterolateral part of the pleuroperitoneal membrane is the last part to close during fetal development. These Bochdalek hernias are the focus of this discussion. The remainder of the hernias are anterior (Morgagni hernias) or esophageal. Of the Bochdalek hernias that present during the first day of life, 85 to 90 percent occur on the left side,

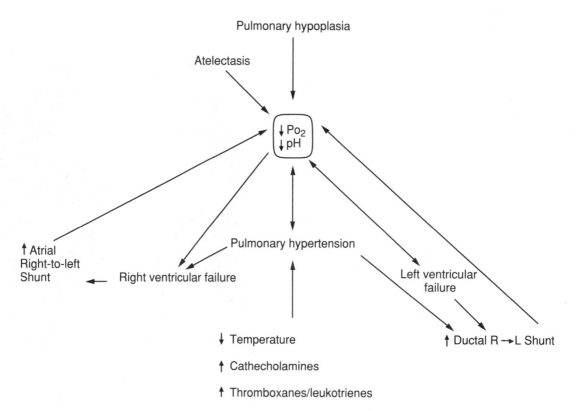

Figure 2 Interplay of factors leading to progressive hypoxia and acidosis in infants with CDH.

presumably because the left side of the pleuroperitoneal membrane closes after the right. The majority of the remaining hernias occur on the right side, and these often have a milder course and present later than left-sided hernias because the presence of the liver on the side of the defect obstructs complete bowel herniation in utero. Less than 2 percent of the defects are bilateral, and these are almost always fatal.

CDH may be apparent during intrauterine life. Maternal polyhydramnios is described as the presenting sign in approximately 30 percent of CDH patients, usually in the third trimester, although Adzick's report of 94 cases of fetally diagnosed CDH indicates a 76 percent incidence of polyhydramnios. Evidence of the defect before 25 weeks' gestation is indicative of a very large defect and a very poor prognosis. Fetal ultrasonography may show the presence of bowel or the stomach in the chest, the latter finding associated with a generally poor prognosis.

The classical clinical presentation in the infant is of cyanosis and severe dyspnea at birth or within the first hours of life. The cyanosis is characteristically worse with crying because the intrapleural bowel becomes more distended. The signs associated with these symptoms are a decrease in breath sounds, especially on the ipsilateral side; the presence of bowel sounds in the chest on the ipsilateral side; displacement of heart sounds toward the contralateral side; and the presence of a scaphoid abdomen. Roentgenographic examination shows a typical pattern of gas and bowel loops in the chest along with a paucity of gas in the abdomen (Fig. 3). If an infant has such a presentation at birth or within the first 6 hours of life, he is considered to be at high risk for significant morbidity and mortality. If an infant presents with the symptoms and signs at a later time, he is considered to be at low risk; in general, the diaphragmatic defect is smaller, the lungs are less hypoplastic, and the outcome is markedly improved.

Anomalies associated with CDH are common: a recent report by Cunniff et al shows that 39 percent of 92 infants with CDH had associated anomalies, including chromosomal, genetic, and nongenetic patterns of malformation. Of particular significance in past reports is frequent occurrence of chromosomal disorders (especially trisomy 13, trisomy 18, trisomy 21, and Turner's syndrome); cardiovascular anomalies (especially atrial and ventricular septal defects, tetralogy of Fallot, and coarctation of the aorta); central nervous system anomalies; and bowel malrotation and atresias. Although CDH usually occurs as a sporadic event, there are reports of recurrence in families, particularly when it is associated with other defects.

PREOPERATIVE PREPARATION

Until recently surgical repair of CDH in infants presenting during the first hours or day of life was considered a surgical emergency, and infants were brought to the operating room as soon as the diagnosis

was made. This approach is presently being reconsidered and preoperatively we generally allow at least sufficient time to complete a thorough evaluation of the infant and to begin appropriate therapies. Many of our basic considerations apply also to the low-risk infant who presents with milder signs and symptoms at a later time.

The most important initial step is the institution of controlled ventilation and oxygenation with endotracheal intubation. Bag and mask ventilation should be specifically avoided, because it usually leads to further distention of the bowel in the chest and, therefore, further compromises lung volume. To minimize bowel distention, institution of controlled ventilation should be accompanied by the placement of a large-bore nasogastric tube and connected to suction (low intermittent). Controlled ventilation should be accompanied by the delivery of 100 percent oxygen to minimize the risk of hypoxia and by the achievement of respiratory alkalosis (pH > 7.45) to minimize pulmonary vascular constriction. Controlled ventilation is optimally provided at mean airway pressures of less than 15 cm H_2O to avoid the risks of barotrauma and to minimize the negative effect of positive airway pressure on pulmonary blood flow. In general, neuromuscular blockade with a long-acting agent like pancuronium bromide facilitates the goals of ventilation.

At the same time that assisted ventilation is begun, basic monitors should be applied in the intensive care setting: electrocardiogram, blood pressure cuff (oscillo-

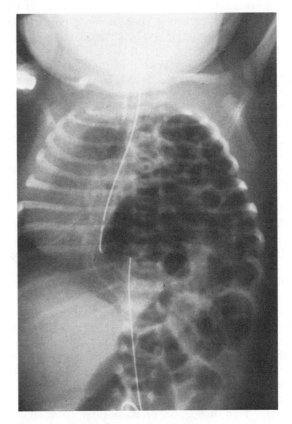

Figure 3 Typical chest roentgenogram of an infant with CDH showing bowel loops in the chest.

metric), temperature probe, and pulse oximeter.Optimally, pulse oximetry should be determined at both preductal (right hand) and postductal sites to help clarify the presence of shunting via the ductus. Invasive arterial monitors should also be placed to follow beat-to-beat blood pressure and to obtain blood gas determinations. An arterial line can usually be placed in an umbilical artery with ease and, although this site will provide postductal blood gas determinations, it is often satisfactory for the early stages of care. An additional arterial line can be placed at some point in the right radial or ulnar artery so that preductal blood gas samples can be obtained. Good peripheral venous access is necessary for infusion of fluids and blood products. Central venous access may be necessary for administration of vasopressor agents. Placement of an indwelling bladder catheter to measure urinary output is also very helpful.

Several other crucial steps should be taken preoperatively. The infant should be placed in a neutral thermal environment (usually on an open warmer) to minimize oxygen consumption and the adverse effects of hypothermia on pulmonary vascular resistance. Sedation should be provided with a narcotic (e.g., morphine sulfate, 10 to 30 μg per kilogram bodyweight per hour, or fentanyl, 1 to 5 μg per kilogram per hour) and perhaps a benzodiazepine (e.g., midazolam, 10 to 20 μg per kilogram per hour) to minimize the effect of handling, noise, suctioning, and other insults on endogenous catecholamine release. Vacanti et al have shown that fentanyl in a dose of 3 μg per kilogram can ablate the pulmonary hypertensive response to tracheal suctioning in infants with CDH who have indwelling pulmonary arterial catheters. Sodium bicarbonate therapy (bolus or infusion) should be used to correct any metabolic acidosis; in fact, along with some degree of hyperventilation, it is used to maintain an alkalotic pH in order the maximize pulmonary arterial vasodilation. In addition, vasopressor support (dopamine, 3 to 10 μg per kilogram per minute) should be used to maintain systemic vascular resistance and minimize the tendency of right-to-left shunting to occur at the atrial and/or ductal levels.

Finally, it is important to complete the preoperative evaluation of the infant with laboratory tests, including blood hemoglobin, serum glucose, and serum calcium. Although blood loss is usually minimal during the repair, it is appropriate to have matched packed red cells available for sudden, unanticipated blood loss. A chest roentgenogram should be obtained preoperatively to confirm the location of the endotracheal tube and the absence of a pneumothorax. An abdominal roentgenogram may be necessary to confirm the location of the tip of the umbilical artery catheter below the level of the renal and inferior mesenteric arteries (L3). Finally, because of the difficulty involved in performing an adequate cardiac examination in an infant with CDH and the high incidence of congenital heart disease associated with the defect, it is optimal to perform an echocardiographic examination prior to surgery.

ANESTHETIC MANAGEMENT

Intraoperative anesthetic management is essentially a continuation of the preoperative management. Complete monitoring should be continued; in addition, end-tidal carbon dioxide monitoring with capnography or mass spectrometry is often used, although it usually does not provide accurate absolute values in this setting.

In the rare situation in which a high-risk infant comes to the operating room on day 1 of life for repair without the airway already secured, induction should proceed expeditiously with preoxygenation and tracheal intubation (awake or rapid sequence with cricoid pressure). Again it is imperative to avoid positive pressure with a bag and mask. Since it is often difficult to assess breath sounds on the ipsilateral side, one must be especially careful to avoid endobronchial intubation. In the operating room, assisted ventilation is best provided by hand with an Ayers T-piece or Mapleson D circuit. This type of circuit allows for rapid, low tidal volume breaths, which are often effective in providing adequate ventilation in infants with CDH. The circuit is relatively sensitive to the changes in lung compliance that often occur during the course of the repair as retractors are placed in the chest or abdomen. Finally, this type of circuit minimizes temperature loss via the airway, although the additional use of active humidification is appropriate. Again, it is best to avoid high airway pressures (i.e., peak pressures > 30 cm H_2O).

Positioning of the infant for the repair depends on whether the surgeon uses an abdominal or thoracic approach. If the latter approach is used, it is important to place an axillary roll and check breath sounds and chest expansion after positioning. It is important also to anticipate that oxygenation may be compromised in this position, since the contralateral, "good" lung will now be down. Use of either operative position demands careful padding of all pressure points.

Maintenance anesthesia is best provided with an oxygen-air-narcotic-muscle relaxant technique. Because fentanyl provides cardiovascular stability and effectively blunts the stress response to surgery, we carefully administer a synthetic narcotic like fentanyl in high doses at induction (20 to 50 μg per kilogram) or in moderate doses at induction (5 to 10 μg per kilogram) followed by intermittent bolus doses. Volatile anesthetics can be used to provide amnestic and pulmonary vasodilatory properties effects; however, throughout the operative period, an infant undergoing CDH repair generally cannot tolerate adequate anesthetic concentrations. The maintenance of anesthesia must be accompanied by meticulous attention to the infant's body temperature, acid-base, glucose, and fluid status. We use airway humidification, fluid warming, head wrapping, and increased ambient warming to help maintain normal body temperature. Since the condition of high pulmonary pressures in a small vascular bed leads to pulmonary edema in infants with CDH, we usually administer a 5 percent glucose-lactated Ringer's solution at a restricted maintenance rate (50 to 60 ml per kilogram per 24 hours), and we administer additional lactated Ringer's solution to replace insensible losses and blood losses.

SURGICAL REPAIR

Surgical repair of CDH basically entails (1) reduction of the hernia and (2) closure of the diaphragmatic defect. In addition, the hernia sac, if present, is removed; the bowel is examined for malrotation or bands; a gastrotomy may be performed; and an ipsilateral chest tube is placed (along with a prophylactic contralateral tube by some surgeons). The ipsilateral chest tube is usually placed only to water seal to minimize the risk of overexpanding the contralateral lung; some surgeons, however, feel strongly that some negative pressure should be applied to help "re-expand" the lungs. Where there is no adequate posterior rim to the diaphragmatic defect, the ribs may be used to anchor the sutures posteriorly; alternatively, a muscle flap (from the anterior abdominal wall or latissimus dorsi) or synthetic patch (Silastic, Teflon, Dacron) may be used. Bax and Collins have argued that patch reconstruction of the diaphragm should always be performed instead of suture closure of the defect because closure alone produces a tight dysfunctional "drum-head" diaphragm. In the uncommon situation in which the abdomen cannot be closed after the reduction of the hernia, the skin only is closed and a ventral hernia is left to be closed at a later date; alternatively, a synthetic pouch may be created.

As noted above, the repair may be performed through either the abdominal or thoracic approach. The abdominal approach is more common and is thought by many to facilitate reduction of the hernia, inspection of the bowel, and creation of an abdominal wall pouch, if necessary. Others believe that the thoracic approach facilitates reduction of the hernia (by pushing rather than pulling) and visualization of the margins of the diaphragmatic defect. The thoracic approach is also associated with less bowel manipulation and edema.

For the anesthesiologist, the operation has several important points. Placing the patient in the lateral position for the thoracic approach may adversely affect oxygenation and ventilation, as noted above. Placement of surgical retractors in the chest and abdomen may also compromise ventilation, as well as venous return and cardiac output. Reduction of the hernia and closure of the defect may adversely affect lung compliance, rather than improve it, since the abdominal cavity will need to accommodate all the abdominal contents when the repair is completed. It is at this point in particular, when one finds that a higher airway pressure may be necessary to ventilate and oxygenate the infant, that a pneumothorax on the contralateral side may occur. This event is often heralded by an acute change in all vital signs and markedly de-

creased lung compliance, and if it is not quickly recognized and addressed, it may be catastrophic. Finally, although an infant's arterial blood gas determinations often improve during the surgical repair, it should be emphasized that the pulmonary vascular bed remains highly reactive and may "clamp down" in the face of any change in oxygenation, acid-base status, or level of anesthesia.

POSTOPERATIVE CARE

The postoperative care continues as a further extension of the preoperative and intraoperative care. After repair of the CDH, an infant may enter a "honeymoon" period of 12 to 24 hours during which oxygenation remains good and the general course remains quite stable. Geggel et al have shown that those infants who do not experience a "honeymoon" generally have smaller lungs and more extensive vascular changes than those who do. Whether or not the infant ultimately survives, this "honeymoon" is characteristically followed by several days of instability that is marked by dramatic changes in oxygenation. During the first 2 to 3 days after the operation, it is important to maintain normal body temperature, maximum oxygenation, normal to alkalotic blood pH, adequate systemic blood pressure, appropriate hydration, and sustained analgesia and neuromuscular blockade.

Postoperative management of the infant may include additional modalities. Although Karl, Bohn, and others have used high-frequency oscillation (HFO) and high-frequency jet ventilation (HFJV) to improve ventilation at lower mean airway pressures, the improvements have been transient only. Pulmonary arterial vasodilation has been attempted by means of various pharmacologic agents, such as chlorpromazine, isoproterenol, acetylcholine, and tolazoline. The latter, an agent that has histaminic, alpha-blocking, and thromboxane-inhibiting qualities, has been used with some reported success (bolus dose of 1 to 4 mg per kilogram followed by an infusion 1 to 4 mg per kilogram per hour). Our experience, however, indicates that not all of these agents have a specific effect on the pulmonary vasculature and may in fact produce unwanted and profound systemic hypotension. Some use pulmonary arterial catheterization and echocardiography to follow changes in pulmonary vascular resistance and to guide therapy postoperatively. Finally, anatomic ligation and balloon occlusion of a patent ductus arteriosus have been attempted to determine if pulmonary arterial blood flow could thereby be increased. As one might expect, in some patients, these manipulations have produced marked adverse changes—i.e., increases in pulmonary pressures, decreases in systemic pressures, and right ventricular failure. The use of extracorporeal membrane oxygenation (ECMO) is discussed later in this chapter.

For the infant who survives CDH, the postoperative course is characterized by gradual improvements in oxygenation, ventilation, and lung compliance, as well as gradual loss of lability despite weaning of imposed alkalosis, vasopressor support, analgesia, and neuromuscular blockade. For the infant who will not survive, the problems of pulmonary hypoplasia and pulmonary hypertension prohibit establishing or sustaining adequate oxygenation and ventilation despite maximum support.

COMPLICATIONS

During the perioperative management of an infant with CDH, the major complications are related to the high airway pressures usually required for adequate ventilation. These include both acute effects (e.g., impaired venous return, pneumothorax, pneumopericardium) and chronic effects (e.g., pulmonary interstitial emphysema and chronic lung disease). Pneumothorax on the contralateral side may be the single event that leads to an irreversible cycle of hypoxia and pulmonary hypertension. Srouji and others have reported a 100 percent increase in mortality in those infants whose course is complicated by pneumothorax. Although the occurrence of pneumothorax may be an expected result of attempting to ventilate hypoplastic lungs, the risk would seem to be lessened by preventing excessive mean and peak airway pressures and preventing overdistention of lung tissue by negative pleural pressure applied through the ipsilateral chest tube.

Other complications related to the perioperative management of CDH include prolonged exposure to high ambient concentrations of oxygen, which may contribute to chronic lung disease; prolonged or episodic hypoxia and acidosis, which may lead to end-organ damage, especially to the central nervous system; and prolonged fluid restriction during the postoperative period, which may contribute to caloric deprivation.

Mortality itself is the major and unfortunately most common complication of CDH. As previously mentioned, the mortality for high-risk infants presenting during the first 6 hours of life has remained between 40 and 60 percent over the last two decades. Various attempts have been made to establish predictors of survival, particularly for high-risk infants. Touloukian correlated the initial radiographs with survival: the side of the defect; the stomach location; the degree of mediastinal shift; the presence of pneumothorax; the

amount of visceral distention; and the volume of aerated lung. Raphaely and Downes showed that infants with a preoperative alveolar-arterial oxygen gradient [(A=a) DO_2] (Table 1) greater than 500 (determined from either preductal or postductal arterial samples) did not survive despite surgery; however, survivors had an improved mean (A=a) DO_2 from 408 preoperatively to 206 postoperatively. Similarly, Harrington showed that postreduction (A=a)DO_2 was predictive: an (A=a) DO_2 less than 400 predicted survival and one greater than 500 predicted death. Bohn et al have correlated survival with both preoperative and postoperative ability to achieve a carbon dioxide partial pressure (PCO_2) of less than 40 mm Hg at a ventilation-index (VI) of less than 1,000 — a result suggesting to the authors that lung hypoplasia is the key to survival. Others have found that an oxygenation index (OI) of greater than 0.40 to 0.45 correlates with a high probability of nonsurvival. Whatever predictor is employed, it is clear that the factors limiting survival are (1) anatomic, the hypoplasia of lung alveoli and vasculature, and (2) functional, the active constriction of the lung vasculature.

NEW APPROACHES TO THERAPY

Given the pathophysiology of CDH and the continuing high mortality associated with its early presentation, a strategy of delaying surgical repair of the defect for hours to days has been adopted by many centers (Fig. 4). Because the primary problem is lung hypoplasia, not atelectasis, it is evident that reduction of the hernia is not curative. In addition, since the early hours of life are the period during which the pulmonary vasculature is normally the most reactive (i.e., the period of the transitional circulation), it makes sense that this is not the best time to subject the infant to the stresses of surgery. Furthermore, although arterial blood gases often seem to improve during and immediately after the surgical repair, Sakai showed in a group of nine infants that gas exchange usually deteriorated immediately after surgery; that only one infant had an increase in respiratory compliance as measured by a passive expiratory flow-volume technique; and that a decrease in respiratory compliance of greater than 50 percent was associated with 100 percent mortality. Distortion of the diaphragm and abdominal distention after repair can account for these changes. Although there is no evidence as yet to confirm that delaying surgery improves survival,

Table 1 Indices of Oxygenation and Ventilation

Alveolar-arterial	
Oxygen gradient	$(Aa)DO_2 = (FIO_2) \times 713 - PaCO_2 - PaO_2$
Oxygenation index:	$OI = \dfrac{FIO_2 \times 100 \times MAP}{PaO_2}$
Ventilation index:	$VI = MAP \times RR$

FIO_2 = fraction of inspired oxygen; MAP = mean airway pressure; $PaCO_2$ = partial pressure of carbon dioxide in arterial blood; PaO_2 = partial pressure of oxygen in arterial blood; RR = respiratory rate.

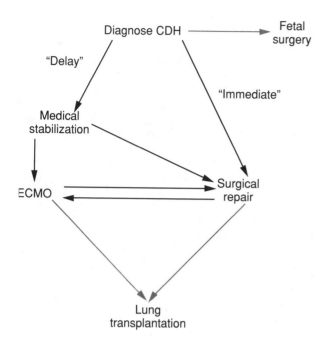

Figure 4 New approaches to therapy for CDH.

there is evidence to show that the delay does not adversely affect outcome and, in fact, may improve the status of unstable patients. During the prolonged period of preoperative stabilization, the principles of care as previously described—monitoring, oxygenation, ventilation, blood pressure support, sedation, and muscle relaxation—are followed.

ECMO has played an increasing role in the management of CDH patients by providing pulmonary "rest": the problems of hypoxia and acidosis are relieved by means of vascular bypass at the same time that the pulmonary vessels can undergo the normal postnatal process of dilating and thinning; the lungs may mature; the work of the right ventricle is alleviated; and the potential for lung injury through barotrauma and oxygen toxicity is reduced. With the current technology of veno-arterial bypass, ECMO is associated with some significant risks (bleeding, embolization, vascular perforation), and certain infants with CDH are not eligible (those less than 35 weeks' gestational age, those with significant intracranial hemorrhage, and those with cardiac, neurologic, or genetic abnormalities associated with a poor prognosis). However, the experience with

ECMO has been encouraging for eligible high-risk infants. As of October 1990, the Extracorporeal Life Support Organization (ELSO) National Registry listed 731 infants with CDH who had been placed on ECMO based on 0 to 20 percent predicted survival with conventional therapy. To date, 61 percent of these infants have survived. ECMO can be used in conjunction with delayed surgery. In this case, an infant is placed on ECMO before repair for a period of days for stabilization and pulmonary "rest," after which the infant may be weaned from ECMO to conventional ventilatory therapy for surgery or even undergo surgery while still on ECMO. For the anesthesiologist familiar with the use of cardiopulmonary bypass, the care of an infant on ECMO before, during, and/or after surgical repair of CDH becomes an appropriate area of involvement.

Whether or not ECMO proves capable of providing significant improvement in the overall prognosis of the high-risk infant with CDH, it is clear that ECMO will do little for the infant whose lungs are severely hypoplastic. For these infants, we may find ourselves turning to two other, potentially more definitive interventions, both of which would entail the crucial involvement of the anesthesiologist: fetal reduction of the hernia, a procedure that has been performed successfully in the experimental animal and in a few instances in humans; and infant lung transplantation.

SUGGESTED READING

Adzick NS, Harrison MR, Glick PL, et al. Diaphragmatic hernia in the fetus: prenatal diagnosis and outcome in 94 cases. J Pediatr Surg 1985; 20: 357–361.

Anderson KD. Congenital diaphragmatic hernia. In: Welch KJ, Randolph JG, Ravitch MM, eds. Pediatric surgery. 4th ed. Chicago Year Book Medical Publishers, Inc., 1986:589.

Bohn D, Tamura M, Perrin D, et al. Ventilatory predictors of pulmonary hypoplasia in congenital diaphragmatic hernia, confirmed by morphologic assessment. J Pediatr 1987; 111:423–431.

Langer JC, Filler RM, Bohn DJ, et al. Timing of surgery for congenital diaphragmatic hernia: is emergency operation necessary? J Pediatr Surg 1988; 23:731–734.

O'Rourke PP, Lillehei CW, Crone RK, Vacanti JP. The effect of extracorporeal membrane oxygenation (ECMO) on the survival of neonates with high-risk congenital diaphragmatic hernia: 45 cases from a single institution. J Pediatr Surg (in press).

Sakai H, Tamura M, Hosokawa Y, et al. J Pediatr 1987; 111:432–438.

Srouji MN, Buck B, Downes JJ. J Pediatr Surg 1981; 16: 45–54.

Vacanti JP, Crone RK, Murphy JD, et al. The pulmonary hemodynamic response to perioperative anesthesia in the treatment of high-risk infants with congenital diaphragmatic hernia. J Pediatr Surg 1984; 19:672–679.

ESOPHAGEAL ATRESIA AND TRACHEOESOPHAGEAL FISTULA

GEORGE A. GREGORY, M.D.

Esophageal atresia (EA) and tracheoesophageal fistula (TEF) are congenital anomalies occurring in approximately one in 3,000 births, with no particular preponderance for a particular sex or race. Neonates with EA and TEF provide major challenges for anesthesiologists because these patients are often premature and have the medical problems associated with prematurity or are small for their gestational age. Furthermore, they often have other congenital anomalies.

ASSOCIATED ANOMALIES

Thirty to fifty percent of infants with EA and TEF have other anomalies. These include hypoplastic lungs, central nervous system abnormalities, and cardiovascular anomalies (ventricular and atrial septal defects, patent ductus arteriosus, tetralogy of Fallot, and coarctation of the aorta). Anomalies of the musculoskeletal system include vertebral malformations, radial aplasia, polydactyly, and wrist and knee anomalies. The associated gastrointestinal anomalies include imperforate anus, midgut malrotation, duodenal atresia, pyloric stenosis, Meckel's diverticulum, and ectopic or annular pancreas. Genitourinary anomalies include renal lobulation or malposition, renal agenesis, hydronephrosis, ureteral abnormalities, and hypospadias. Craniofacial anomalies include cleft lip and cleft palate.

The VATER association is relatively common in these patients and consists of Vertebral and Anal anomalies, Tracheal esophageal fistula with Esophageal atresia, and absent or hypoplastic Radii. The "V" of this acronym can also stand for ventricular septal defect, and the "R" may indicate renal anomalies.

CLINICAL PRESENTATION

Atresia of the esophagus should be suspected prenatally if polyhydramnios is present during pregnancy. Occasionally, EA can be detected prenatally by sonography. However, the diagnosis is usually made at birth when an orogastric tube cannot be inserted into the stomach, or the diagnosis is suggested by the presence of excessive foamy oral secretions. Unfortunately, it is often made when coughing, choking, and cyanosis occur during the first feeding. Aspiration increases the respiratory rate and respirations become labored. When a fistula connects the trachea and distal esophagus, gas is present in the bowels, the abdomen is tympanitic, and bowel gas is seen on the x-ray film. Occasionally the abdomen becomes so distended with gas that breathing is difficult or impossible. The diagnosis of EA is confirmed by inserting a radiopaque catheter into the esophagus and determining whether or not the catheter passes into the stomach. If it does, atresia is absent. If the catheter abruptly stops approximately 10 cm from the gum line, the diagnosis is virtually assured. Posteroanterior and lateral chest radiographs confirm the position of the tip of the oroesophageal tube.

Some authors recommend injecting small quantities of contrast material to outline the proximal esophageal segment and to identify a proximal TEF. Radiopaque material can be aspirated, however, causing respiratory difficulties that vary from barium plugging of a bronchus to chemical pneumonitis. Infants who have esophagograms with contrast material have more respiratory complications and die more often during the neonatal period than those not having these studies.

The entire abdomen should be included on a chest radiograph to determine whether or not there is gas in the stomach or intestines. Air in the stomach is pathognomonic of a fistula between the trachea and lower esophagus in patients with EA. Absence of air in the gastrointestinal tract usually indicates the presence of EA without TEF. Failure of the air column to progress to the anus should lead one to suspect an imperforate anus or rectum.

TEF without EA may not present until much later in life. Choking during feedings, abdominal distention, and recurrent pneumonitis should suggest this diagnosis, which is usually confirmed at bronchoscopy or by contrast cine radiographs of the esophagus. The fistula may sometimes be difficult to demonstrate, and surgical exploration may be necessary to make the diagnosis. The diagnosis can also be made by detecting elevated intragastric concentrations of oxygen during ventilation with 100 percent oxygen. Diagnosis of TEF should also be considered in any patient who develops gastric distention during tracheal intubation and mechanical ventilation with positive pressure.

PREOPERATIVE EVALUATION AND PREPARATION

Since pulmonary complications contribute to infant morbidity and mortality, prevention of these problems is a major goal of preoperative management. Oral feedings are discontinued and the baby is kept in a semi-upright position to reduce the regurgitation of gastric contents through the fistula. Suction is continuously applied to the proximal esophageal segment to reduce aspiration of nasopharyngeal secretions.

Severity of pulmonary disease is evaluated by physical examination, chest radiography, and analysis of arterial blood gases. Because repeated blood gas determinations are required before, during, and after surgery, an arterial catheter should be inserted. Hypoxemia is treated by administering humidified oxygen. Metabolic acidosis is treated by administering sodium bicarbonate (mEq HCO_3^- = body weight [kg] × base deficit × 0.6/4.0; this is the initial dose—further HCO_3^- may be required). Refractory hypoxemia or respiratory failure are treated with oxygen, tracheal intubation, and mechanical ventilation. Infants with TEF and EA are maintained in a neutral thermal environment (30 to 34°C) at all times because hypothermia increases mortality. It also increases pulmonary vascular resistance and causes right-to-left shunting of blood through the ductus arteriosus and foramen ovale.

Prematurity significantly affects the survival of infants with EA and TEF. Abnormalities associated with prematurity (hypoglycemia, hypocalcemia, and hyperbilirubinemia) must be evaluated and treated. In infants with extreme prematurity or severe lung disease, many surgeons will perform a gastrostomy with the patient under local anesthesia and delay the thoracotomy until respiratory function improves.

Associated anomalies also affect survival. Gas in the small bowel rules out duodenal atresia, and gas in the rectum helps rule out coincidental anal atresia. The heart and lungs are evaluated for evidence of congenital heart disease. Echocardiography and/or cardiac catheterization are indicated if a problem is suspected. A ventricular septal defect may be present but may not be clinically evident for several days (when the pulmonary vascular resistance decreases). It may sometimes be difficult to differentiate pulmonary edema from aspiration of gastric contents. Vertebral and other skeletal anomalies may be seen on chest or abdominal radiographs. The abdomen is examined to screen for renal anomalies, and urine is collected for assessment of adequacy and to document urine output. Abdominal ultrasonography or intravenous pylography are used to evaluate suspected lesions. Limb anomalies can be evaluated later, since they are not life threatening.

Reliable venous access should be established before the induction of anesthesia. Central venous cannulation is helpful but not absolutely necessary. Fluid and electrolyte status are evaluated and abnormalities corrected, although depletion of fluid and electrolytes is unusual with EA and TEF if it is detected early and if intravenous fluids are administered. If the patient is several days old and has fed poorly, he or she may be dehydrated. The patient should be typed and crossmatched for whole blood or packed red blood cells preoperatively.

Grouping of patients according to the Waterston classification is helpful (Table 1). Those in Categories A and B usually survive, whereas those in Category C have a mortality of approximately 25 percent. Some surgeons delay surgery in Category C patients or stage the procedures. Patient size alone should not delay surgery. Neonates who are premature but who are otherwise well usually survive.

MONITORING

Monitoring of neonates who have TEF and EA is an important part of their care. Since many of them have

Table 1 Waterston Classification

Category	Description
A	Birth weight > 2.5 kg healthy neonate
B	Birth weight 1.8–2.5 kg May have pneumonia or congenital anomalies
C	Birth weight < 1.8 kg May have severe pneumonia and/or complex anomalies.

respiratory problems, such as hyaline membrane disease or aspiration pneumonia, their oxygenation and acid-base status must be measured and corrected, if abnormal. Measurement of oxygenation can be done by pulse oximetry, skin surface oxygen electrodes, or analysis of blood gases. (Skin surface oxygen electrodes do not work well if halothane is used.) Carbon dioxide concentrations can be determined by skin surface electrodes or analysis of blood gases. pH can be measured only by blood gas electrodes. Therefore, an arterial catheter is required for surgery. Since many of these neonates are premature, there is concern about retrolental fibroplasia (RLF). It is unknown what arterial oxygen pressure (PaO_2) causes RLF, but most experts agree that the PaO_2 should be kept between 50 and 80 mm Hg as much as possible. The oxygen saturation should therefore be kept between 87 percent and 92 percent in neonates at risk for RLF. This may mean ventilating the lungs with room air during some phases of surgery.

An arterial catheter is required for the surgery, not only to measure blood gases and pH but also to measure arterial pressures continually. Compression of the lung or occlusion of the inferior vena cava by retractors can lead to precipitous decreases in arterial blood pressure. These catheters can also be used to measure glucose and electrolyte concentrations during surgery.

Measurements of heart rate, arterial blood pressure, and body temperature are also required before, during, and immediately after surgery. End-tidal gas monitoring is quite useful during surgery if tidal volumes are adequate. A stethoscope (chest piece) is usually placed in the left axilla when the patient is in the left lateral decubitus position to detect changes in the ventilation of the left lung during surgery.

ANESTHETIC MANAGEMENT

The operating room and anesthesia equipment are prepared and the room is warmed to 32 to 37°C before the patient arrives in the operating room. Upon arrival, he or she is placed under a servocontrolled radiant warmer, and monitors (precordial stethoscope, electrocardiogram, blood pressure cuff, and pulse oximeter) are applied. A transcutaneous carbon dioxide electrode is helpful in guiding ventilation. A precordial stethoscope in the left axilla helps detect intraoperative airway obstruction (decreased ventilation of the down lung).

The arterial catheter is connected to a pressure transducer and amplifier, and a rectal temperature probe* and Foley catheter are inserted after anesthesia is induced.

The infant is premedicated with atropine, 0.02 mg per kilogram IV, just before induction of anesthesia. With the patient in a semi-sitting position, the esophageal pouch is suctioned, and awake tracheal intubation is performed. The endotracheal tube is inserted into the right mainstem bronchus. Then, while the lungs are ventilated, the anesthesiologist listens for breath sounds over the stomach as the endotracheal tube is slowly pulled back. When the breath sounds heard over the stomach suddenly increase in intensity, the endotracheal tube is advanced just enough to decrease breath sounds heard over the stomach while still allowing ventilation of both lungs. This positions the tip of the tube just beyond the fistula and avoids gaseous distention of the stomach, a complication that can interfere with ventilation and venous return of blood and can lead to cardiopulmonary arrest or gastric rupture. Because the fistula is usually located just proximal to the carina and because it is usually on the posterior aspect of the trachea, it is helpful to position the bevel of the endotracheal tube so that it faces forward (i.e., the sloping side of the tube should be placed forward to reduce ventilation of the fistula and stomach). Once the position of the endotracheal tube is correct, the tube is taped securely to the face.

Anesthesia is induced with small amounts of halothane, air, and enough oxygen to maintain normal oxygenation. Positive-pressure ventilation is cautiously attempted before a muscle relaxant is administered. If gastric inflation occurs, the patient is allowed to breathe spontaneously while a gastrostomy is performed to decompress the stomach. The position of the endotracheal tube should be adjusted so that the tip of the tube is just beyond the distal edge of the fistula. Higher concentrations of halothane are required when muscle relaxants are not used, so vital signs must be observed carefully. A gastrostomy also can be performed with the patient under local anesthesia before the induction of general anesthesia. Once the gastrostomy is completed, the lungs can be ventilated. If the fistula is large, much of the ventilation will enter the stomach and exit through the gastrostomy. To reduce the amount of ventilation that enters the stomach, place the end of the gastrostomy tube under 5 to 10 cm of water or partially occlude it with a screw clamp. In many patients with TEF and EA, gastrostomy is no longer performed because it is believed that this procedure increases gastroesophageal reflux.

Ligation of the fistula and esophageal anastomosis are performed with the patient turned to assume the left lateral decubitus position. Anesthesia is maintained with a nondepolarizing muscle relaxant and air, oxygen, and halothane in concentrations that do not cause significant cardiovascular depression. Fentanyl and a low-dose inhalational anesthetic can also be used to provide anesthesia. In premature infants, it is important to keep the PaO_2 between 50 and 80 mm Hg during surgery to reduce the risk of RLF. Ventilation is controlled manually. Oxygen saturation is measured continuously by pulse oximetry, and arterial blood gas samples are obtained intermittently to ensure that the PaO_2, arterial carbon dioxide pressure ($PaCO_2$) and pH are normal. Trancutaneous carbon dioxide can also be used to estimate arterial carbon dioxide. However, the value displayed on the monitor is closer to the $PaCO_2$ 90 to 120 seconds earlier, not to the currently displayed $PaCO_2$.

Air entry to the dependent lung is monitored continuously via the stethoscope in the axilla. A suction apparatus, gloves, and catheters should be available for sterile tracheal suctioning because accumulation of secretions or blood may completely occlude the airway. To prevent pulmonary granulomas, talcum powder should be washed from gloves before suctioning of the airway is performed. If the endotracheal tube becomes occluded by secretions or blood, it should be replaced immediately. Although this may be difficult to do because the patient is in the left lateral decubitus position, replacement of the endotracheal tube can be facilitated by advancing a relatively stiff catheter (ureteral stint) through the endotracheal tube, removing the endotracheal tube over the catheter, and inserting a fresh endotracheal tube over the catheter that was left in the trachea. *Care must be taken not to advance the stint into or through the parenchyma of the lung.*

Because hypothermia increases oxygen consumption and can cause metabolic acidosis and pulmonary hypertension, body temperature is maintained with a warming blanket, warmed humidified inspired gases, and an increased room temperature (32 to 37°C). Transfused blood is warmed to 37°C) before it is administered.

Fluid replacement includes Ringer's lactate or saline: 4 ml of fluid per kilogram of body per hour for maintenance plus 6 to 10 ml per kilogram per hour for evaporative and third-space losses. Usually 3 to 5 mg of glucose per kilogram of body weight is required to maintain normoglycemia. Hyperglycemia should be avoided because it increases the likelihood of central nervous system damage if the patient becomes hypoxemic or has a cardiac arrest. Blood loss is quantitated by collecting blood in a calibrated suction bottle and by weighing the sponges. Blood replacement is usually required when the hematocrit decreases to 25 percent. Prior to that time, 3 ml of lactated Ringer's solution or normal saline is administered for each milliliter of blood loss. Urine output, heart rate, blood pressure, serial hematocrits, and sodium and glucose concentrations are followed to evaluate the adequacy of fluid replacement.

At the conclusion of the surgical procedure, the patient should be turned supine, the tip of the endotracheal tube should be placed in the midtrachea, and the tube should be fixed securely in place.

---

*This assumes that the anus is patent.

POSTOPERATIVE CARE

The postoperative management of infants with EA and TEF is influenced by the amount of preoperative pulmonary dysfunction, the severity of associated anomalies, and the degree of prematurity. In vigorous, otherwise healthy term infants, the endotracheal tube can usually be removed shortly after surgery. Enough warmed, humidified oxygen is given to maintain a PaO_2 of 50 to 80 mm Hg. The most frequent complications during the early postoperative period are pneumonia and atelectasis. Nasopharyngeal and oropharyngeal suctioning are performed as needed, but the tip of the catheter should not pass beyond the tip of the endotracheal tube; otherwise, the esophageal anastomosis may be disrupted. If atelectasis occurs after the patient's trachea is extubated, tracheal suction and manual ventilation are performed, when needed, through an endotracheal tube that is inserted for the procedure and then removed. Excessive neck extension should be avoided because it places tension on the esophageal anastomosis.

Infants who have respiratory failure or those who are likely to develop it are returned to the intensive care unit with an endotracheal tube securely fixed in place. Respiration is supported with supplemental oxygen, intermittent mandatory ventilation, and positive end-expiratory pressure (PEEP); or respiration is supported with continuous positive airway pressure. Manual percussion and vibration of the chest are performed every 1 to 2 hours to facilitate removal of tracheal secretions. Ventilator settings and fractional inspired oxygen (FIO_2) are reduced once the infant demonstrates adequate gas exchange and mechanics of breathing. Progress is evaluated through arterial blood gas determinations, chest radiographs, and clinical examination. The endotracheal tube can be removed once intermittent mandatory ventilation has been discontinued, the PaO_2 exceeds 50 mm Hg, and the $PaCO_2$ is less than 50 mm Hg while the patient is breathing 50 percent oxygen.

Tracheomalacia or recurrent laryngeal nerve injury may lead to postoperative respiratory difficulties. When tracheomalacia is present, the soft segment of the trachea collapses either during inspiration (if the defect is above the thoracic inlet) or during expiration (if it is below the thoracic inlet). Tracheostomy may be necessary in neonates who are unable to maintain a patent airway without an endotracheal tube.

Feedings via a gastrostomy or via a small nasogastric tube that was placed at the time of surgery are usually started on the 3rd postoperative day. Unless the esophageal anastomosis is tenuous, oral feedings are begun on the 6th to 7th postoperative day after an esophagogram documents potency of the esophageal lumen.

If an associated anomaly (such as duodenal atresia) or a complication of surgery precludes enteral feedings for more than a few days, intravenous alimentation is begun with glucose, amino acids, trace minerals, and vitamins.

MORTALITY

The survival of patients with EA and TEF is most influenced by the degree of prematurity and the severity of the associated anomalies and pulmonary complications. At present, the overall survival for all patients with EA and TEF exceeds 75 percent. Neonates who fall into the Waterston Category A or B have nearly 100 percent survival. Those in Category C have approximately 75 percent survival. Survival of patients treated with a staged approach—which includes a gastrostomy at the time that the diagnosis is made, division of the TEF 18 to 36 hours later, and definitive repair of the EA when the child has achieved a body weight of 5 to 6 lb and has improved respiratory function—is approximately 85 percent.

OUTCOME OF SURVIVORS

Most survivors of EA and TEF are asymptomatic at 15 to 20 years of age. Nonetheless, the young child who has undergone EA and TEF repair is at risk for dysphagia, esophageal obstruction, and recurrent respiratory infections. During the first year of life, these children are likely to have some degree of esophageal stricture and may require dilatation of the esophagus if the stricture is severe. The esophagus may even become totally obstructed by food, and esophagoscopy may be necessary to remove the obstruction. Strictures seem to be less severe as the child grows. By the second to third decade of life, more than 90 percent of patients are either asymptomatic or have only mild dysphagia. However, almost all patients who survive EA and TEF have demonstrable abnormalities in esophageal motility, which probably accounts for many of the cases of mild-to-moderate dysphagia.

Abnormal esophageal motility also predisposes the child to recurrent aspiration of food and milk, which has been implicated as the cause of recurrent pneumonia, asthma, bronchitis, and upper and lower respiratory infection in survivors (33 to 75 percent). In addition, the findings of squamous epithelium extending from the trachea to the peripheral bronchi in children with EA and TEF who are dying suggests that mucociliary clearance in these patients is impaired. Studies of lung function and bronchial reactivity 7 to 18 years after repair have shown obstructive airways disease in 54 percent of patients, restrictive lung disease in 20 percent, and increased sensitivity to methacholine in 63 percent. It has been postulated that recurrent aspiration and infection damages bronchial walls and leads to airway obstruction and sensitivity. After correction of EA and TEF, a regimen of thickened feeds and upright positioning may reduce the incidence of aspiration during the early postoperative period.

SUGGESTED READING

Pohlson E, Schaller RT, Tapper D. Improved survival with primary anastomosis in the low birthweight neonate with esophageal atresia and tracheoesophageal fistula. J Pediatr Surg 1988; 23:418.

Randolph JG, Newman KD, Anderson KD. Current results in repair of esophageal artesia with tracheoesophageal fistula using physiologic status as a guide to therapy. Ann Surg 1989; 209:526.

Reyes HM, Meller JL, Loeff D. Management of esophageal atresia and tracheoesophageal fistula. Clin Perinatol 1989; 16:79.

Spitz L, Kiely E, Bereton RJ. Esophageal atresia: a five year experience with 148 cases. J Pediatr Surg 1987; 22:103.

Waterston DJ, Bonham-Carter RE, Aberdeen E. Oesophageal artesia. Tracheoesophageal fistula: a study of survival in 218 infants. Lancet 1962; 1:819.

BRONCHOPULMONARY DYSPLASIA

SUSAN A. VASSALLO, M.D.
NISHAN G. GOUDSOUZIAN, M.D.

Bronchopulmonary dysplasia (BPD) is a relatively new clinical entity that was first used to describe the chronic pulmonary changes that occur in some of the premature infants after **respiratory distress syndrome** (hyaline membrane disease). Subsequently, it was recognized that it can occur after other forms of severe lung diseases in newborns. The definition of BPD has therefore been modified to refer specifically to the condition of infants who at 28 days after birth have persistently abnormal chest radiographs while evincing hypercarbia or a continued need for oxygen after a period of mechanical ventilation (if the arterial oxygen pressure $[PaO_2]$ < 60 mm Hg on room air; or if the fractional inspired oxygen $[FIO_2]$ requirement > 0.21; or if the arterial carbon dioxide pressure $[PaCO_2]$ > 45 mm Hg).

Currently, BPD is responsible for the prolonged hospitalization of 10 to 20 percent of neonates who survive with the aid of mechanical ventilatory support. Its incidence is highest in those who require ventilation for respiratory distress syndrome (RDS) and reaches 38 percent in very low–birth weight infants (750 to 1,500 g) with hyaline membrane disease. The majority of neonates with BPD are premature, although rarely a full-term infant develops this condition. The requirement for mechanical ventilation in such patients is necessitated by conditions such as pneumonia, neonatal sepsis, meconium aspiration, tracheoesophageal fistula, and congenital heart disease (e.g., patent ductus arteriosus).

Pathologically, the lungs in these infants show multiple emphysematous areas alternating with atelectasis, bronchiolar mucosal hyperplasia, peribronchial smooth muscle hypertrophy, and interstitial fibroplastic proliferation.

The radiographic abnormalities vary from faint diffuse opacifications to cystic emphysematous changes with air trapping (Table 1). Similarly, the functional impairment can vary from mild carbon dioxide retention to a prolonged need for ventilatory support and oxygen supplementation. With growth, the respiratory function in most infants with this syndrome approaches normal if

Table 1 Characteristics of Bronchopulmonary Dysplasia

Clinical
  Signs
    Tachypnea
    Intercostal and sternal retraction
    Wheezing
    Pulmonary edema
    Cor pulmonale
    Increased airway reactivity
  Arterial blood gas analysis
    Hypoxemia
    Hypercarbia
    Mild respiratory acidosis
  Pulmonary function tests
    Decreased lung compliance
    Increased airway resistance
    Decreased functional residual capacity
Radiographic
  Linear densities
  Atelectasis
  Cystic regions
  Cardiomegaly
  Pneumothorax
Pathologic
  Interstitial fibrosis
  Alveolar septal destruction with coalescence of remaining alveoli
  Bronchiolar smooth muscle hypertrophy
  Medial hypertrophy of small pulmonary arterioles
  Mucosal metaplasia
  Large areas of atelectasis alternating with emphysema

they do not succumb to respiratory infection or cor pulmonale. The unfortunate side of the story is that most of these infants will have varying degrees of growth retardation, reactive airway disease, and retinopathy of prematurity.

MECHANISMS OF INJURY

Multiple factors are believed to be responsible for the development of BPD. The syndrome was originally thought to be caused by pulmonary oxygen toxicity and the barotrauma of mechanical ventilation. However, additional evidence suggests that premature birth, fluid overload, patent ductus arteriosus, damage caused by severe pulmonary disease, and familial predisposition to asthma may all play roles in the pathogenesis of the disease.

Barotrauma is a complication of positive pressure ventilation. Interestingly, peak inspiratory pressures greater than 35 cm H_2O and pneumothorax are in fact both associated with BPD. Further, pulmonary air leak, or movement of air into the interstitium, decreases lung compliance. Exposure to a high PaO_2 induces neutrophil activation and produces damaging free radicals (O_2^-). The premature lung is deficient in antioxidant protective mechanisms, specifically the membrane-bound vitamin E or alpha-tocopherol system and the superoxide dismutase enzyme. The lack of these enzymes may thus be a factor in the development of chronic lung disease.

Infants with a patent ductus arteriosus have an increased incidence of BPD. The subsequent left-to-right shunt results in elevated pulmonary blood flow, which may in itself be injurious to a neonatal lung. More likely, however, the necessity of a high FIO_2 and increased inspiratory pressure are the primary factors leading to BPD in the presence of congenital heart disease. Pulmonary edema may be a cause or result of BPD. It has been shown that infants with RDS in whom BPD develops have a greater fluid intake during the first 5 days of life than those babies in whom BPD does not develop. A family history of asthma has been noted in infants with BPD.

INTERCURRENT MEDICAL PROBLEMS

The infant with BPD may display several other pathologic conditions associated with prematurity. The incidence of *intraventricular hemorrhage* is 54 percent in babies weighing 500 to 1,250 g and reaches 83 percent in infants weighing less than 1,000 g. Hydrocephalus, developmental delay, seizure disorder, and abnormal central respiratory drive are associated with intraventricular hemorrhage. The retina does not reach maturity until 44 weeks postconception. Exposure to high FIO_2 and PaO_2 can result in *retinopathy of prematurity*, which is characterized by retinal neovascularization and recurrent hemorrhage.

Gastroesophageal reflux (GER), which in itself may contribute to chronic respiratory disease, is common in infants with BPD. High metabolic demands may not be met in the presence of GER, with resultant malnutrition and growth delay.

Patent ductus arteriosus is the most common cardiac anomaly seen in infants with BPD. However, acquired disease such as pulmonary hypertension, with or without cor pulmonale, can occur secondary to respiratory-induced hypoxia. Systemic hypertension (defined as a systolic blood pressure > 114 mm Hg) appears in 20 to 40 percent of infants with BPD. Quite frequently, these babies have umbilical arterial catheters, which is considered to be a risk factor for neonatal hypertension.

Metabolic abnormalities are frequently present. The premature infant has lower iron reserves; the hemoglobin determinations remain low in these infants, even with the compensatory efforts for the physiologic anemia seen during the first 3 months after delivery. Furosemide therapy for BPD-associated pulmonary edema can result in increased excretion of sodium, potassium, chloride, calcium, and water. Severe osteopenia, exacerbated by secondary hyperparathyroidism, can result in pathologic fractures.

It seems that there is some type of association between *sudden infant death syndrome* (SIDS) and BPD. In one retrospective study, a sevenfold increase in the incidence of SIDS was noted in infants with BPD. Since the precise mechanism of SIDS is not well understood, the explanation for the association is conjectural. The clinical impression is that infants with BPD suffer respiratory infections more frequently than do healthy infants of similar birthweight. Intermittent unnoticed hypoxic episodes may perhaps occur during the early stages of respiratory infection and act as a contributing factor to SIDS.

FREQUENT SURGICAL PROCEDURES

It is unfortunate that there is no specific form of therapy for BPD. Once the disease develops, all modalities are aimed at preventing further complications. Consequently, surgical intervention is not expected to improve the patient's basic status but only to prevent further deterioration.

It is generally agreed that elective operations should be delayed until any premature infant reaches a post-conceptual age of at least 40 weeks. However, BPD babies often require emergency surgery at younger ages. Insertion of a ventriculoperitoneal shunt for relief of hydrocephalus, inguinal herniorrhaphy, placement of a Broviac catheter, revascularization of peripheral vessels after prolonged catheterization (e.g., femoral artery), and diagnostic bronchoscopy are the usual urgent procedures performed in premature babies.

The appropriate timing for elective surgery depends on analysis of both the infant's pulmonary status and the expected benefits of the proposed operation. A fundoplication is not considered an emergency procedure; however, preventing aspiration may improve the infant's respiratory function and nutritional state. Similarly, re-attachment of the retina via a scleral buckle yields the best chance for vision when performed at the earliest possible age.

PREOPERATIVE ASSESSMENT

The syndrome of BPD can vary widely in magnitude with respect to pulmonary pathology. Many pediatric centers do not routinely perform pulmonary function tests on infants. Therefore, the most common method of preoperative evaluation focuses on the patient's current clinical state. This analysis should include the following questions:

1. Is the infant still dependent on mechanical ventilation? The duration and extent of ventilation should be noted (e.g., continuous support since birth or intermittent periods of ventilation coinciding with recurrent infection). The efficacy of ventilation should be confirmed by the presence of acceptable oxygenation (oxygen saturation or PaO_2) and relative normocarbia with a reasonable pH. Ventilatory settings should be reviewed; a constant need for high inspiratory pressures indicates increased airway resistance. This characteristic may predispose to pneumothorax or air leak.

2. Is the infant still dependent on oxygen? Oxygen delivered at low flow rates (0.25 to 1.0 L per minute) by nasal cannula is frequently needed to maintain oxygen saturation above 90 percent. Oxygenation should be measured during a range of activities such as sleeping, feeding, and crying. A hospital environment is not a requisite for supplemental oxygen therapy. Often, an infant may be discharged home with nasal oxygen into the care of a cooperative family and community.

3. Does the infant have anatomic abnormalities of the airway? Intubation, although necessary, may lead to tracheal stenosis and tracheal granulomata formation. Factors such as duration of intubation, the size of the endotracheal tube, the presence of a leak around the tube, and the number of intubation attempts may all contribute to the development of airway abnormalities. In fact, even a short period of intubation can lead to subglottic stenosis. A tracheostomy may not guarantee absolute airway patency in the presence of heavy secretions (e.g., mucous plug).

The size and fit of the most recent endotracheal tube should be prominently recorded. Chart review by the anesthesiologist should also focus on successful laryngoscopic techniques, including blade style and size, as well as optimal head and neck position.

4. Is the infant gaining weight? Although they have normal head circumference, nearly all infants with BPD exhibit delayed growth in weight and height. Infants with severe BPD are often in the lowest fifth percentile along the weight-growth curve. Poor feeding tolerance and fluid restriction limit the number of calories that can be delivered. Hyperalimentation in the form of intravenous mixtures, or enteral feedings via a nasogastric tube, are often necessary.

Also, it is often difficult to meet the nutritional needs of these patients because of the increased work of breathing that leads to increased oxygen consumption. However, as lung function improves and the respiratory rate declines, oxygen consumption decreases.

5. Does the infant need diuretics? Since infants with BPD tend to accumulate excessive interstitial fluid, daily diuretic administration is often a mainstay of medical therapy. Although blood gases may be slow to improve, diuretic use is associated with a decrease in airway resistance and an increase in lung compliance.

Furosemide's ability to reduce pulmonary capillary pressure by vasodilation is a second mechanism of action, independent of its diuretic effect. Chronic therapy is associated with hypokalemia, hyponatremia, hypercalciuria, and metabolic alkalosis. Electrolytes should be measured preoperatively; correction depends on the magnitude of the deficit. Usually, perioperative infusion of dextrose, one-fourth normal saline with small supplements of potassium, is sufficient.

6. Does the infant need bronchodilator therapy? The traditional anatomist's view maintains that bronchial smooth muscle is poorly developed in neonatal lungs.

Hence, bronchodilator therapy was not universally accepted in the treatment of respiratory distress syndrome. However, infants with BPD have hypertrophy of peribronchiolar smooth muscle, and bronchospasm is a frequent feature of the syndrome. Inhaled beta-agonists such as isoproterenol or isoetharine decrease airway resistance and increase functional residual capacity (FRC). Both theophylline and aminophylline are administered for several reasons: (1) to increase diaphragmatic strength; (2) to stimulate respiration in the infant with periodic breathing; and (3) to bronchodilate constricted airways.

ANESTHETIC MANAGEMENT

Premedication

Sedation is usually unnecessary in the infant younger than 1 year of age. More importantly, the regular medications (diuretics, bronchodilators, steroids) should be continued preoperatively. The infant with gastroesophageal reflux should receive a histamine$_2$ (H$_2$) receptor antagonist (e.g., cimetidine, ranitidine) at least 1 hour before induction of anesthesia. The timing of atropine administration depends on its indication; a preoperative dose can be given to decrease oral secretions, but this agent will also decrease the tracheobronchial secretions and lead to inspissation. (If indicated, intravenous atropine is the most useful route; intramuscular atropine does not reliably prevent bradycardia associated with laryngoscopy.) Of the utmost importance is the continuation of supplemental oxygen during the transport period.

Monitors and Special Equipment

The recent availability of pulse oximetry has made the anesthetic management of infants with BPD much easier than it was a decade ago. Hypoxia must be avoided at all costs; on the other hand, high concentrations of oxygen for prolonged periods may also be deleterious. With the pulse oximeter in place, the oxygen concentration can be adjusted arbitrarily (in the absence of definitive guidelines) to read between 95 and 99 percent. Our preference is to increase the inspired oxygen concentration so as to read a saturation of 100 percent and then decrease the inspired concentration so that the saturation reads approximately 98 percent. The other advantage of the pulse oximeter is that it frequently obviates the need for intra-arterial cannulation; this procedure can be quite difficult to perform at this stage because of its frequent use during the early critical period of the illness.

The presence of a pulse oximeter does not preclude the standard use of other monitors such as precordial or esophageal stethoscope, electrocardiogram, blood pressure cuff, end-tidal carbon dioxide measurements (ETCO$_2$), and the temperature probe. If neuromuscular blockade is to be used, a peripheral nerve stimulator with appropriate low-output settings should be applied. The accuracy of $ETCO_2$ measurements depend on the sampling location. Further, endotracheal tubes with distal aspiration ports minimize the dilution effect seen when regular tubes and small tidal volumes are used; however, the sampling ports are more liable to be obstructed by secretions.

Maintaining *normothermia* is a constant concern with all infants. The smaller the infant, the more critical is this factor. The minimal room temperature should be at least 75°F during induction of anesthesia and surgical preparation, which is the period when most of heat loss occurs; a radiant heat warmer and a warming blanket can also be used. If the infant's body temperature is stable, the room temperature can be lowered when the skin prep is complete and the draping is in place. Intraoperatively, the use of the heated humidifier is extremely important because it decreases the heat loss and helps maintain pulmonary integrity and ciliary activity.

Induction of Anesthesia

There is not and cannot be a "blanket" method for anesthetizing an infant with BPD. The age and size of the infant, the severity of the disease, and the experience of the anesthetist will determine the method of induction. Although it seems superfluous, it is important to stress that more crucial than the anesthetic technique is the avoidance of hypoxia and carbon dioxide retention in the management of these critically ill infants. Both can dramatically increase the pulmonary vascular pressure, inducing right-sided heart failure, one of the most difficult conditions to treat.

Inhalation Induction

If the infant appears vigorous, has mild BPD (i.e., requires low-flow oxygen at night only), is well-saturated on room air, and is gaining weight, then inhalation induction of anesthesia is a reasonable option. Oxygen and halothane by mask is the preferred technique; laryngospasm and coughing are generally less than with inhalation of enflurane or isoflurane. However, myocardial depression and bradycardia are well-known complications of halothane induction. An intravenous catheter should be placed as soon as possible, and fluid deficits should be corrected early. This technique is not appropriate for the infant who is obviously dehydrated or is in congestive heart failure.

Intravenous Induction

An intravenous induction has several advantages in the care of the infant with severe BPD. Atropine can be administered before any manipulation of the airway. Thiopental sodium can be given in fractional doses and oxygen by face mask is readily applied. Once control of the airway is established, a neuromuscular relaxant can be given. The choices include succinylcholine

chloride (2 mg per kilogram), vecuronium bromide (0.1 mg per kilogram), atracurium besylate (0.5 mg per kilogram) and pancuronium bromide (0.1 mg per kilogram). Laryngoscopy is performed after adequate ventilation with high concentrations of oxygen but without the concurrent use of high concentrations of halothane.

This technique is suitable for infants with poor myocardial function (cor pulmonale), infants with increased intracranial pressure or gastroesophageal reflux, and those infants who present for emergency surgery after a recent meal.

Awake Intubation

Awake intubation is usually reserved for those infants with congenital abnormalities of the airway, such as Pierre Robin syndrome or Turner's syndrome. The micrognathia common to these conditions often makes laryngoscopy difficult. This technique is certainly appropriate for the weak infant who has gastroesophageal reflux or for one who has received oral barium for a radiologic study. Awake intubation should be avoided in the premature infant with intracranial hemorrhage because of the fear of inducing a new bleed.

Maintenance of Anesthesia

In a small infant, a good mask airway and assisted ventilation is often difficult to maintain without also inflating the stomach. For this reason, mask anesthesia is indicated only for brief procedures. When adequate oxygenation and ventilation cannot be maintained with a mask, intubation is indicated, even during a simple operation such as myringotomy and tube placement. Mask ventilation is also difficult because very young patients often demonstrate an irritable airway, which predisposes to coughing and hypoxia during the planned surgical procedure. Endotracheal intubation with a muscle relaxant can avoid such problems. In the healthy infant, these complications can be easily treated by positive-pressure ventilation, but in infants with BPD, they are more persistent, and a muscle relaxant is frequently required to overcome laryngospasm.

An understanding of the surgical requirements helps define the plan for anesthetic maintenance. An eye examination, although not extremely painful, mandates relaxation of the extraocular muscles. This can be achieved by deepening the halothane concentration. If the examination dictates immediate surgical intervention, neuromuscular blockade achieves the same results without depressing the cardiovascular system.

The use of nitrous oxide (N_2O) must be considered with respect to both the operation and the respiratory status of the infant. In cases of obstructed bowel, N_2O should be avoided and an air/oxygen mixture used. Severe BPD is characterized by emphysematous alveoli. Positive-pressure ventilation may cause rupture of a bleb. Since N_2O enlarges the size of any gas-filled cavity, an expanding pneumothorax could result.

Regional Anesthesia

The use of regional anesthesia in some BPD-afflicted children can be advantageous. In experienced hands, a spinal anesthetic for a lower abdominal or lower limb procedure of short duration can avert several of the intraoperative and postoperative problems commonly seen in these compromised patients. Further, a caudal or an epidural block can be satisfactorily used to prevent postoperative pain. However, it is of the utmost importance that both the surgeon and the anesthesiologist be experienced in working with regional anesthesia; nothing is worse than finding halfway through a surgical case that the regional anesthetic is unsatisfactory in the absence of a controlled airway. Consequently, if there are any questions, either with regard to one's capability and experience or with the predictability of the surgical course, it is far more advisable to establish control of the airway at the beginning of the procedure than to risk later difficulties.

Postoperative Management

In deciding to extubate the trachea, one should determine the following: (1) that the infant is awake and warm; (2) that the infant is breathing regularly and adequately; (3) that the neuromuscular blockade is fully reversed; and (4) that protective airway reflexes have returned.

If these criteria are met, extubation is indicated even in the tiny (2.0 kg) baby with BPD. However, equipment for reintubation should be immediately available. At our institution, infants of this size return directly to the neonatal intensive care unit (NICU). An alternative approach would be to transport the infant to the NICU while he or she is still intubated. Once vital signs are taken, extubation can be performed. This plan avoids the stress of performing emergency reintubation while in an elevator or deserted corridor. Infants weighing less than 1.5 kg remain intubated and ventilated postoperatively. The NICU staff are familiar with anesthesia recovery and complications and are capable of devising a weaning schedule. Details of laryngoscopic technique are carefully discussed with the covering intensive care physician and nurse.

All infants with BPD should be monitored by both pulse oximetry and electrocardiography in the postanesthetic care unit (PACU). Because the majority of these infants are premature, they are vulnerable to postanesthesia apnea and bradycardia. Infants who are less than 48 weeks' postconceptual age, full-term infants with a history of apnea, and infants with a history of postanesthesia apnea are monitored in the hospital for at least 24 hours after surgery. This approach is followed regardless of the duration of the procedure.

SUGGESTED READING

Bancalari E, Gerhardt T. Bronchopulmonary dysplasia. Pediatr Clin North Am 1986; 33:1–23.

Blanchard PW, Brown, TM, Coates AL. Pharmacotherapy in bronchopulmonary dysplasia. Clin Perinatol 1987; 14:881–910.

Escobedo MB, Gonzalez A. Bronchopulmonary dysplasia in the tiny infant. Clin Perinatol 1986; 13:315–326.

Hoyoux CI, Forget P, Lambrechts L, et al. Chronic bronchopulmonary disease and gastroesophageal reflux in children. Pediatr Pulmonol 1985; 1:149–153.

Motoyama EK, Fort MD, Klesh KW, et al. Early onset of airway reactivity in premature infants with bronchopulmonary dysplasia. Am Rev Respir Dis 1987; 136:50–57.

Nickerson BG. Bronchopulmonary dysplasia: pulmonary disease following neonatal respiratory failure. Chest 1985; 87:528–535.

Northway WH, Rosan RC, Porter DY. Pulmonary disease following respirator therapy of hyaline-membrane disease: bronchopulmonary dysplasia. N Engl J Med 1967; 276:357–368.

NECROTIZING ENTEROCOLITIS IN THE NEONATE

RANDALL C. WETZEL, M.B., B.S., F.C.C.M.

Necrotizing enterocolitis is the most common gastrointestinal emergency to occur in neonatal intensive care units throughout the world. Necrotizing enterocolitis is a disease of small, preterm infants. In contrast to neonatal surgical emergencies, which usually present in full-term infants, these infants are the smallest and sickest infants requiring surgery and anesthesia. The anesthesiologist may be concerned when confronted by a hypotensive, septic, hypovolemic child, weighing usually less than 1,500 g who is in urgent need of resuscitation and surgery. Meticulous anesthetic management and neonatal critical care are the cornerstones of managing the complicated problems of these critically ill neonates.

PATHOPHYSIOLOGY

Necrotizing enterocolitis (NEC) will develop in as many as 10 to 15 percent of all neonates weighing less than 1,500 g who are admitted to the intensive care unit. In some nurseries, the incidence of necrotizing enterocolitis is greater than 5 percent of all admissions. Although frequently NEC can be managed medically with an associated mortality that is quite low, in those infants who require surgery, mortality can be as high as 50 percent.

Although the etiology of necrotizing enterocolitis is not known: it is clearly multifactorial in origin. Four key elements appear to play a role in the pathophysiology of this condition, although not all necessarily occur in each infant with NEC (Table 1): (1) intestinal immaturity (the foremost of the four); (2) intestinal mucosal ischemic injury; (3) enteric feeding; and (4) bacterial and viral pathogens.

Approximately 90 percent of all cases of NEC occur in premature infants. The reason for this susceptibility to NEC in premature neonates is not clear. It seems most likely that the immature immunologic system in the developing gut plays a central role. In addition, NEC usually occurs within the first 10 days of life, even in premature infants, and postnatal maturation therefore also appears to be contributory. This immature host to susceptibility clearly plays a role because NEC does not develop in all infants with the other three factors.

Secondly, gut mucosal injury seems to be a necesary antecedent. As many as 80 percent of all infants in whom NEC develops have an episode indicative of severe hypoxia, asphyxia, mucosal ischemia, and low Apgar scores. These factors have an interesting common link, and that is the diving reflex. At times of stress such as hypoxia and hypotension, the diving reflex is quite active in neonates and leads to shunting of blood flow away from the splanchnic, renal, and peripheral circulations toward the myocardial and central circulations. This diving reflex thus shunts blood away from the gastrointestinal mucosa and, in infants who have been asphyxiated or hypotensive, may result in significant intestinal ischemia. Infants and young children appear to survive significant hypoxic ischemic insults with little myocardial or central nervous system injury, but with profound intestinal mucosal injury. In addition, in the neonatal intensive care unit, respiratory distress, sepsis, and other complicating illnesses of prematurity can clearly aggravate cardiorespiratory instability, leading to further episodes of gut mucosal injury.

Another etiologic factor in gut mucosal injury may well be iatrogenic. The use of umbilical artery catheters, which themselves interfere with the mesenteric blood supply, the role of thromboembolism from these catheters, and the administration of multiple therapeutic agents through the catheters must all be considered. For this reason, umbilical artery catheter monitoring in small premature infants has become less favored in recent years. NEC has also occurred after exchange transfusion and the consequent hemodynamic changes. Additionally, infants with polycythemia with microcirculatory sludging and thromboembolism also appear to be at increased risk for NEC. These multiple insults in the immature gut may set the stage for bacterial invasion.

Although gut mucosal ischemic damage appears to be an important etiologic factor in NEC, it is not the whole story. A large percentage of children in neonatal intensive care units have these antecedent injuries; however, NEC develops in only a small percentage (5 to 10 percent). Other factors have therefore been implicated. The foremost among these is *feeding*. Virtually 100 percent of infants in whom NEC develops have been fed neonatal whole milk derivative formula. Although NEC does occur occasionally in infants who have not had enteric feeding, this is rare. NEC also occurs in infants who have been fed breast milk only, although this is also less common. It is likely that the beneficial properties of breast milk, which contains immunoglobulins, lactoferrin, and macrophages, add some protective effect. Hypertonic and hyperosmolar feedings have also been implicated in NEC. Apart from direct damage caused by milk in the gut, it also provides a substrate for bacterial multiplication. Rapid fermentation with gas production and distention of bowel loops leads to further damage. For these reasons, a cautious approach to the feeding of premature infants is mandatory. Interestingly, it has recently been reported that there has been a shift in the population of infants who develop NEC. This shift is attributed to the fact that feedings in small premature infants are very cautiously undertaken or avoided and that NEC is actually becoming a disease of later infancy, occurring in bigger, healthier infants who are fed earlier.

It must be noted that mucosal enteric injury by and of itself does not lead to NEC. In infants in whom an ischemic intestinal infarction develops in utero, intestinal atresia occurs rather than NEC. NEC does not

Table 1 Causes of Necrotizing Enterocolitis

Prematurity	Mucosal Injury
< 2,500 g	Hyperosmolarity
< 34 weeks (gestational age)	Hypotension
Gut immunodeficiency	Cyanotic heart disease
Prematurity-associated diseases	Hypoxia
Days 1-10	Intravascular catheters
	Respiratory distress syndrome
	Ischemia
	Low Apgars
	Patent ductus arteriosus (PDA)
	Shock
Feeding	Infection
Substrate	Bacterial
Further damage	Viral
Gas production	
Milk allergy	

appear to occur at all in the absence of gut colonization by bacteria. In addition to this observation, several other factors indicate that bacteria have a central role in the development of NEC. NEC can occur epidemically within nurseries; oral treatment with immunoglobins or antibiotics can decrease the incidence of NEC within a given nursery; infection control procedures such as isolation with strict attention to the limitation and spread of infection can control epidemics; and specific viral and bacterial pathogens have been identified in nursery epidemics of NEC. It seems unquestionable that pathogenic infection plays a key role in NEC. Bacterial colonization of the gut is initiated by contact with the vaginal floor during birth and is present within hours after birth. Oral feedings further lead to propagation of gut, and a complete array of anaerobic and aerobic bacteria are noticed in the gut by 10 days of age. Organisms that have been associated with NEC are those that are usually present in normal flora in the neonatal gut. These organisms include *Escherichia coli, Klebsiella, Clostridium perfringens,* and many *Clostridia* species. *C. perfringens* produces a potent exotoxin, associated with fulminant, frequently fatal NEC. *Pseudomonas, Salmonella,* and *Enterobacter* have all been implicated. Among the viral species, corona virus, rotavirus, and enterovirus have been isolated in nursery epidemics of NEC (Table 2).

Table 2 Necrotizing Enterocolitis-Associated Pathogens

Bacterial
  Klebsiella
  Escherichia coli
  Clostridia sp. (*C. difficile; C. perfringens*)
  Salmonella
  Enterobacter
  Pseudomonas sp.

Viral
  Coronavirus
  Rotavirus
  Enterovirus

Pathology

Any part of the intestine from the esophagus to the rectum may be involved in NEC. The ileum and proximal colon are the usual sites of early involvement, and the absence of ileocecal involvement is rare. At laparotomy, the bowel frequently appears dilated and hemorrhagic and is often necrotic and purple (Figs. 1 and 2). The bowel is covered with a purulent discharge and the peritoneum is frequently filled with feculent material. There may be skip lesions, with necrotic involvement of some areas with normal bowel in between. The bowel may feel crepitant due to gas in the intestinal wall (pneumatosis intestinalis) (see Fig. 2). Microscopically, early changes consist of edema and hemorrhage, as well as necrosis and pneumatosis, both submucosally and subserously. Vascular thrombosis and microthrombi in the arteries and veins are common, and inflammation in addition to ischemic injury is frequently seen. In terms of its pathology, NEC is "completed" in the neonate by the multisystem organ failure subsequent to hypoxia, ischemia, and sepsis, which complicates all late cases of NEC.

CLINICAL PRESENTATION

NEC usually occurs within the first 10 days of life. It may occur within the first 24 hours, however, and it has been reported in infants as old as 3 months of age. Although it has a wide spectrum of clinical presentations, the most common is that of feeding intolerance and bloody stools. Other presentations may range from increasing frequency of apnea and mild temperature instability to severe cardiorespiratory compromise with massive hematochezia, disseminated coagulation, and death within hours from fulminant, hemorrhagic, and septic shock. More characteristically, abdominal disten-

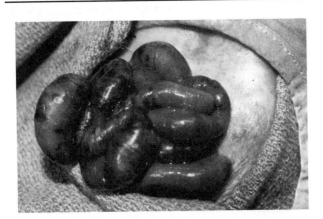

Figure 1 Small bowel exposed at laparotomy in a 1,400-g, 32 weeks' (gestational age) premature infant with NEC. Note the multiple areas of transmucosal necrosis and gangrene. Although intervening areas appear normal, the mucosa in these areas is almost certainly involved.

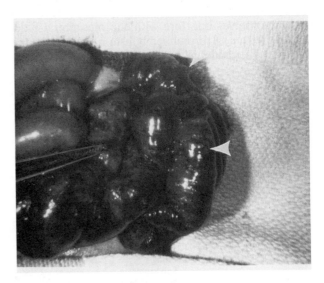

Figure 2 Infarcted bowel from a fatal case of NEC. Extensive bowel gangrene with areas of pneumatoses are seen *(arrows and forceps).*

Table 3 Indications for Surgery for Necrotizing Enterocolitis

Absolute
  Pneumoperitoneum

Relative
  Positive paracentesis
  Abdominal erythema
  Intrahepatic air
  Abdominal mass
  Cardiovascular collapse

tion, feeding tolerance, lethargy, temperature instability, bradycardia and apnea occur. Vomiting and gastrointestinal bleeding follow. At this stage, it may be impossible to distinguish this illness from septicemia. The occurrence of acidosis, oliguria, abdominal wall erythema, and ascites with hemodynamic instability, bilious vomiting, and clinical signs of peritonitis herald cardiovascular collapse and advanced disease.

The diagnosis is assisted by radiologic identification of the pathognomonic pneumatosis intestinalis. Intramural intestinal gas and thickened bowel loops with a bubble pattern (see Fig. 3) is pathognomonic. In addition, portal venous air occurs in 15 to 30 percent of the cases and is usually indicative of severe disease and a higher mortality rate (Fig. 4). The presence of pneumoperitoneum with air under the diaphragm or free air seen on a cross table lateral is an indication for immediate surgery (see Fig. 3). Other radiographic findings include ileus, a fixed loop of distended bowel, ascites, and thickened bowel wall.

The diagnosis of NEC depends on the recognition of the clinical syndrome in the clinically susceptible neonate. Confirmation is made by radiology. The indications for surgery are pneumoperitoneum and the clinical syndrome of septic shock, with a deterioration in vital signs in a child with previously diagnosed NEC. By the time that they require surgery, all patients are hemody-

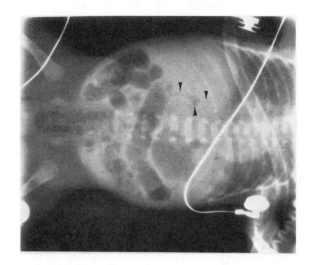

Figure 4 An infant with NEC and intrahepatic air *(arrows)*. Note characteristic linear streaks and large bubble *(white arrow)*.

namically compromised and should be dealt with as if they are in impending septic shock. This is because gangrene and abdominal perforation have occurred in more than 50 percent of surgical patients. Intestinal gangrene is common and, in some centers, may be diagnosed by abdominal paracentesis in the suspected infant. Other centers consider the formation of an abdominal mass indicating a walled-off abscess, portal venous air, and/or erythema of the abdominal wall as indications for urgent surgery (Table 3).

THERAPY

Urgent medical therapy is mandated in all patients suspected of having NEC. The progress of the disease may be fulminant and rapidly progressive; in those infants who respond to medical therapy, however, the survival rate is more than 90 percent. Medical therapy consists of immediate withdrawal of enteric feeding. Gastric suctioning is performed with decompression of the gastrointestinal tract and fluid resuscitation. Efforts to ensure adequate oxygenation and ventilation including intubation, if not previously performed, and monitoring of arterial blood gases are indicated. Massive fluid resuscitation with maintenance fluid given two to three times daily is almost always necessary. Third spacing, peritonitis, and septic shock followed by decreased urine output and hypotension may require volume expansion in blood volume type quantities (70 to 100 ml per kilogram). Because medical therapy also includes efforts to control sepsis, broad-spectrum antibiotics such as ampicillin and gentamicin should be immediately instituted. Antibiotics to cover anaerobic flora such as clindamycin have also been suggested. If a coagulopathy is identified, fresh-frozen plasma, platelets, and blood transfusion may be required. In severely advanced cases,

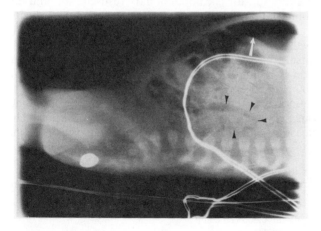

Figure 3 Cross-table lateral of an infant with NEC. *Black arrows* outline a loop of bowel with extensive pneumatosis intestinalis. This picture also demonstrates anterior free air *(white arrow)*.

correction of the acidosis and maintenance of electrolytes as well as treatment for renal failure are indicated. In addition, hemodynamic support with inotropic therapy such as dopamine or epinephrine may also be indicated. It cannot be too strongly emphasized that these small infants may be the most critically ill children managed by the anesthesiologist. A familiarity with neonatal critical care is essential for providing optimal anesthesia in this setting.

Surgical therapy consists of a transverse supraumbilical incision for laparotomy. The surgeon inspects the entire bowel from the stomach to the anus. When the peritoneum is opened, further hemodynamic compromise frequently occurs, and blood loss can be excessive due to inflammation and the coagulopathy. Hypotension may follow manipulation of the bowel with the release of potent enteric vasoactive mediators, the most significant of which are almost certainly eicosanoids, as well as showers of bacteria from the damaged and necrotic bowel. The usual surgical management for isolated lesions consists of resection and primary anastomosis. However, isolated lesions are uncommon, and frequently a dysfunctioning enterostomy of the Mikulicz double-barrel variety is performed. Removal of necrotic and perforated bowel, and a colostomy with peritoneal lavage is the most likely surgery to be performed. In those infants who are severely affected, frequently a "look-and-see operation is performed, with no other surgery other than perhaps a venting jejunostomy. If the infants with this severe disease survive the ensuing 40 to 72 hours, a "second-look" surgery may be performed when the infant is more stable.

ANESTHETIC MANAGEMENT

Frequently these infants are catastrophically ill and must undergo urgent surgery. The principles of optimization of the patient's preoperative condition, preparation for intraoperative management, and meticulous intraoperative monitoring as applied to all neonatal cases are particularly important in this case.

Preoperative Management

It is the anesthesiologist's responsibility to be certain that the patient is as prepared for surgery as time will permit (Table 4). Fluid and inotropic support may be required to ensure a mean arterial pressure of 40 mm Hg or greater and a systolic pressure of between 50 and 60 mm Hg in small premature infants. Heart rates in excess of 160 beats per minute are an indication of severe stress or hypovolemia. Hypovolemia is the leading cause of hemodynamic compromise, poor perfusion, and anuria in NEC. Blood volume expansion consisting of crystalloid, packed red cells and consideration of blood products for treating coagulopathy such as fresh-frozen plasma and platelets before surgery are indicated.

Respiratory status must be evaluated before surgery. It is highly unusual that infants who require surgery for NEC are not already intubated and receiving ventilatory support. The increased incidence of apnea, hypotension, and the pre-existing disease process (e.g., infantile respiratory distress syndrome) have almost certainly necessitated intubation and ventilation before surgery. If the infant requires intubation, however, this should be done with the patient awake to ensure control of the airway and guard against aspiration, as these children all certainly have full stomachs. An examination of arterial blood gas should be carried out before the patient is transported to the operating room. Ventilation should be managed as for all premature infants. To avoid further hypoxemia, specific attention must be paid to arterial oxygenation, but one must also consider the risk of retinopathy of prematurity (ROP) caused by excess oxygen treatment. Infants with NEC are often very premature and a high risk for this complication. In addition, the multifactorial elements that contribute to ROP, such as sepsis, hypotension, and hypocarbia may all be present. Finally, the anesthesiologist should ensure that intravenous access is adequate for transportation to the operating room and that the positions of femoral artery, venous, and umbilical catheters have been identified. Chest x-ray examination should ensure that the endotracheal tube is appropriately placed.

Transportation

Transportation of sick neonates to the operating room is a major part of any surgical procedure. Preparation for cardiopulmonary resuscitation and ongoing fluid and blood product resuscitation during transportation should be ensured. In addition, the availability of the concentration of oxygen appropriate to ensure oxygenation and ventilation during transportation is required. Ideally, means of delivering less than 100 percent oxygen during transport to avoid the risk of retinopathy of prematurity should be employed. Numerous personnel should be assisting in the transport. The anesthesiologist accompanies the infant to the operating

---

Table 4 Preoperative Laboratory Tests for Necrotizing Enterocolitis

Arterial blood gas	
Sodium/potassium	Hemoglobin/hematocrit
Calcium	White blood cell count
Blood glucose	Platelets
Liver function tests/bilirubin	Prothrombin/partial thromboplastin
Preparation of fresh-frozen plasma	time
and platelets	Type and crossmatch

room, ensuring ongoing resuscitation during the transport, and a nurse and a member of the surgical staff should also accompany the infant. Adequate warming during transport to maintain body temperature should be ensured in these infants, who are prone to hemodynamic instability. The anesthesiologist must be thoroughly equipped for all emergencies that could occur (for example, a Miller No. 0 blade, a working laryngoscopy handle, and some means of providing suctioning and oxygenation should be available). He or she should carry not only the usual anesthetic drugs but also resuscitation drugs, including bicarbonate, atropine, epinephrine, calcium gluconate, and lidocaine drawn up in appropriate neonatal doses.

The infant must be monitored during transportation. Insertion of an esophageal stethoscope before transportation and continuous auscultation during transport are recommended. Electrocardiography (ECG) and, if an arterial line is present, a blood pressure monitor are also necessary. In addition, the availability of transport pulse oximetry to ensure adequate oxygenation during transportation is optimal. Continuous monitoring of breath sounds and heart tones is the cornerstone of monitoring during transportation. Frequently, more advanced monitoring is unreliable in transport. These infants are often quite lethargic and immobile during transportation. The provision of anesthesia and paralysis during transport should be considered if the child is highly active.

Preparation for the Operating Room

The operating room should be adequately set up for the management of a critically ill neonate. The room should be warmed to at least 32°C. An overhead radiant warmer is necessary for the infant surgical table. Humidification is also important and the ambient humidity should be more than 80 percent. The preparation of inotropic drips should occur before the infant is transferred to the operating room and the necessary intravenous pumps are provided. All drugs should be drawn up in amounts appropriate for neonates (Table 5).

Adequate volume replacement should be ensured, and large amounts of crystalloid should be warmed to 37°C. In addition, maintenance fluids must contain glucose to avoid the occurrence of hypoglycemia. The glucose content of the maintenance fluid should be the same as that which the infant was receiving in the nursery. If glucose content solutions of 10 percent or more such as those used in hyperalimentation were given preoperatively, they should continue to be given intraoperatively. Fresh-frozen plasma should be thawed and warmed. Packed red cells (30 ml per kilogram) should also be readily available and warmed. The blood bank should be notified of the potentially urgent need for platelets and fresh-frozen plasma, as indicated. A means of warming all fluids should be available. Whether fluids are warmed by preloading fluids in syringes and heating them in a waterbath, or whether all fluids and blood products are drawn through a neonatal blood warmer depends on the anesthesiologist's preference.

Full airway management equipment with replacement endotracheal tubes and laryngoscopes should be available, for any neonatal case. The anesthesia machine should be able to deliver mixtures of oxygen and air so that it is not necessary to give 100 percent oxygen. Nitrous oxide must be avoided in these cases to avoid bowel distention. A means of obtaining rapid hematocrits and determinations of blood glucose and blood gases should be available.

Intraoperative Monitoring

Intraoperative monitoring should include an esophageal stethoscope with constant monitoring of heart sounds, breath sounds, and heart rate (Table 6). An ECG is mandatory. End-tidal carbon dioxide (CO_2) incorporated into an appropriate neonatal circuit is quite valuable, as it can rapidly detect changes in pulmonary perfusion and thus the changes in cardiac output that may occur. Pulse oximetry is clearly useful. Arterial saturation should be maintained at between 90 and 95 percent. A means of measuring blood pressure is essential. In these small premature infants, noninvasive monitoring of blood pressure is frequently difficult, and therefore, intra-arterial pressure monitoring and intra-arterial access for laboratory studies and blood gases are mandatory. The time spent preoperatively to place an arterial line is time well spent. Intraoperative monitoring

Table 5 Drugs for Neonatal Anesthesia for Necrotizing Enterocolitis

Drug	Concentration	Dose
Fentanyl	50 μg/cc*	10–15 μg/kg
Ketamine	10 mg/cc	1–2 mg/kg
Pancuronium bromide	1 mg/cc*	0.1–0.15 mg/kg
Atropine	0.4 mg/cc*	0.15 mg
Succinylcholine chloride	20 mg/cc*	1–2 mg/kg
Lidocaine	20 mg/cc	1–2 mg/kg
Epinephrine	1:10,000	1–10 μg/kg
Calcium chloride	100 mg/ml	10–20 mg/kg
Sodium bicarbonate	1mEq/ml	1–2 mEq/kg
Dopamine		2–10 μg/kg/min

*All drugs drawn up in graduated 1-ml syringes.

Table 6 Intraoperative Monitors

Airway and ventilation
    Esophageal stethoscope
    Pulse oximeter
    FIO_2
    End-tidal carbon dioxide
    Disconnect alarm
    Airway pressure
    Serial blood gases

Metabolic
    Serial blood gases
    Blood glucose
    Electrolyte ($Na^+/K^+/Ca^{+2}$)

Hemodynamic
    Esophageal stethoscope
    Electrocardiogram
    Intra-arterial blood pressure
    Noninvasive blood pressure
    Core temperature
    Urine output
    (Central venous pressure)

in these hemodynamically unstable patients is facilitated. In addition, in the postoperative management of these patients, invasive hemodynamic monitoring and blood gases that will be aided by the placement of an arterial line are frequently required. Favorite sites of placement of an arterial line include radial artery, posterior tibial, or dorsalis pedis. Although recent studies have demonstrated that femoral artery cannulation in children appears to be of low risk, we strongly caution against performing this cannulation, primarily because of the risk of limb ischemia, sepsis, and local infection.

Intravenous access must be obtained to provide large volume resuscitation. At least two well-functioning intravenous cannulae are necessary. If time permits, placing a central line may be beneficial to ensure access for fluid and drug administration. Monitoring of the central venous pressure (CVP) is often not helpful in these small infants. Coagulopathy and the need for surgery may be relative contraindications for placing central lines. Further monitoring is carried out with a Foley catheter, which should be placed to monitor urine output intraoperatively. Temperature monitoring is also mandatory, and a neonatal thermocouple should be applied to the infant's chest or back. Monitors of ventilation, such as end-tidal CO_2 and airway pressure, disconnect alarm, and airway temperature, are also part of routine monitoring in this setting.

Anesthetic Management

As noted above, infants who come to the operating room requiring surgery for NEC are virtually always intubated. If not, they should be intubated while they are awake. The anesthetic choices for a small, premature, hemodynamically unstable infant undergoing a laparotomy for bowel disease are somewhat limited. Because of the risk of bowel distention, nitrous oxide must be

avoided. The anesthetic machine must therefore contain air so that the fractional inspired oxygen (FIO_2) can be titrated to ensure that the arterial oxygen pressure (PaO_2) is greater than 55 mm Hg but not greater than 80 mm Hg and that the arterial saturation is maintained between 90 and 95 percent to avoid ROP.

The use of inhalational anesthesia in this setting is hazardous. All inhalational anesthetics are, to some degree, myocardial depressants and peripheral vasodilators. In infants with the potential for severe hemodynamic compromise, the use of these agents to provide adequate anesthesia is not suggested.

In the past, these critically ill infants may have been anesthetized only with pancuronium bromide (Pavulon). The current evidence is now overwhelming that avoiding adequate analgesia and failing to blunt the stress to surgery worsens the outcome in neonates requiring surgery. Therefore, apart from the obvious humanitarian reasons which by themselves should mandate analgesia, there are sound medical reasons for providing adequate anesthesia. These include greater hemodynamic and cardiorespiratory stability, a better metabolic response to the stress of surgery, and the avoidance of hyperglycemia and postoperative instability. Intravenous anesthesia is indicated. In this setting, barbituates with their hemodynamic depressant effects must be avoided. This also applies to the use of morphine, which may cause catastrophic vasodilation. The narcotic choice for intravenous anesthesia in this setting is fentanyl. One caution is necessary, however: in neonates, fentanyl certainly is associated with blunting of the autonomic response that may be maintaining the infant's perfusion and cardiac output. Even small doses of 2 to 3 µg per kilogram may lead to hypotension. This reveals the underlying need for further fluid resuscitation and hemodynamic support. It should not preclude the administration of adequate analgesia. Adequate analgesia can be provided with doses of 10 to 15 µg per kilogram of fentanyl. Another alternative in a hemodynamically compromised neonate is ketamine. Ketamine in intravenous doses of 1 to 2 mg per kilogram every 20 to 30 minutes provides adequate analgesia intraoperatively. The combination of fentanyl and ketamine is our current preferred choice for hemodynamically compromised neonates. Muscle relaxation is provided with pancuronium bromide (Pavulon). The vagolytic affects of Pavulon and its long-lasting muscle paralysis and nondepolarizing character make it optimal in this setting. Once a safe level of anesthesia has been induced, anesthetic management consists mainly of ongoing cardiopulmonary resuscitation.

The importance of fluid management cannot be too strongly stressed. It is frequently necessary to give 50 to 100 mg per kilogram of volume replacement during surgery for NEC. The overwhelming sepsis and massive multiple organ system failure lead to massive microcirculatory failure and third spacing. Careful monitoring of coagulation factors, hematocrit, peripheral perfusion, urine output, blood pressure, and heart rate will guide fluid therapy. Again, it cannot be too strongly emphasized that, because of this massive volume transfusion, all fluids must be heated to avoid catastrophic hypothermia. The addition of hypothermia to surgical stress in this setting is not acceptable.

At the termination of surgery, the infant again requires meticulous transporation back to the intensive care unit. Although we pride ourselves in being able to resuscitate infants and return them to the neonatal intensive care unit in better condition then they were in preoperatively, these infants are still prone to massive third spacing and all of the complications of sepsis. Therefore the same meticulous monitoring and preparation for ongoing resuscitation are required for transportation back to the neonatal intensive care unit as were required preoperatively. Postoperatively, these patients may continue to be quite unstable in the neonatal intensive care unit, necessitating many days of cardiorespiratory support.

Outcomes

The surgical mortality associated with NEC approaches 50 percent. The overall mortality for NEC is between 20 and 40 percent. Usually the enterostomies that are left during the surgery can be closed between 4 weeks and 4 months of age. If jejunostomies or dysfunctioning ileostomies have been performed, they may necessitate closure earlier due to sodium loss, failure to thrive, and metabolic acidosis. Late complications of NEC include enteric strictures, especially colonic and short gut syndrome from aggressive resection of bowel (Table 7). The long-term outcomes are encouraging. Nearly half of all chidren who require NEC surgery during their prematurity have achieved normal development by the age of 3 years.

Clearly, infants with NEC provide one of the major challenges. The perioperative period is an interlude in which to provide an opportunity to optimally manage

Table 7 Complications of Necrotizing Enterocolitis

Acute
 Hypovolemia
 Shock
 Bacterial sepsis
 Disseminated intravascular coagulation
 Thrombocytopenia
 Acidosis
 Renal failure
 Intraventricular hemorrhage
 Adult respiratory distress syndrome

Chronic
 Strictures
 Adhesions
 Short gut malabsorption
 Recurrent sepsis

these extremely ill children. Successful perioperative management will return them to the necessary state of all preemies—that of growth and development.

SUGGESTED READING

Cashore WJ, Peter G, Lauermann M, et al. Clostridia colonization and clostridial toxin in neonatal necrotizing enterocolitis. J Pediatr 1981; 98:308–311.
Cook DR, Marcy JH, eds. Neonatal anesthesia. Pasadena, CA: Appleton Davies, Inc. 1988.
Covert RF, Neu J, Elliott MJ, et al. Factors associated with age of onset of necrotizing enterocolitis. Am J Perinatol 1989; 6:455–460.
Kosloski AM, Musemeche CA. Necrotizing enterocolitis of the neonate. Clin Perinatol 1989; 16:97–111.
Moss TJ, Adler R. Necrotizing enterocolitis in older infants, children, and adolescents. J Pediatr 1982; 100:764–769.
Tan CEL, Kiely EM, Agrawal M, et al. Neonatal gastrointestinal perforation. J Pediatr Surg 1989; 24:888–892.
Wetzel RC, Nichols DG, Bender KS, et al. Clinical Conference: a premature neonate with necrotizing enterocolitis. Anesthesiol Rep 1988; 1:90–108.

SUPRAGLOTTITIS, LARYNGOTRACHEITIS, AND BACTERIAL TRACHEITIS

I. DAVID TODRES, M.D.

SUPRAGLOTTITIS (EPIGLOTTITIS)

Supraglottitis is a life-threatening infection that requires urgent evaluation and treatment. It is predominantly an infection of children between the ages of 1 and 10 years, but it may occasionally affect older children and adults. The acute inflammation involves the epiglottis and aryepiglottic folds, producing supraglottitis. The organism responsible is usually *Haemophilus influenzae* type B.

The child is acutely ill with a high fever. Inability to swallow (dysphagia) and drooling of secretions are prominent. Inspiratory stridor is not as striking as that seen in laryngotracheitis: it is softer and lower pitched. The voice and cry are muffled. The child sits propped up with the head pushed forward (tripod sign) to achieve a less obstructed airway. Rapid and unpredictable progression of the disease may cause total obstruction acutely.

Differential Diagnosis

Supraglottitis should be differentiated from other significant life-threatening causes of upper airway ob-

Table 1 Differential Diagnosis of Supraglottitis, Laryngotracheitis,
and Bacterial Tracheitis

	Supraglottitis	Laryngotracheitis	Bacterial Tracheitis
Etiology	Haemophilus influenzae B	Viral	Staphylococcus aureus
Age	1 yr–adult	3mo–6 yr	6 mo–10 yr
Preceding symptom	Uncommon	URI	URI
Onset	Sudden	Slow	Slow-to-sudden
Toxicity	Marked	Mild-to-moderate	Moderate-to-severe
Stridor	Mild-to-moderate	Moderate-to-severe	Moderate
Position	Sitting (tripod sign)	Variable	Variable
Drooling	Common	Rare	±
Temperature	High	Moderate	High
Course	Rapid	Slow	Moderate-to-rapid

struction (Table 1). The differentiation from laryngotracheitis (croup) is usually fairly clear, but that from bacterial tracheitis may be more difficult.

Diphtheria, a rare but important bacterial infection occurring in nonimmunized children, may be responsible for acute upper airway obstruction. Foreign body aspiration should always be considered in any such obstruction. The history, clinical examination, and x-ray film findings provide clues to this condition. Retropharyngeal abscess may present with acute upper airway obstruction, which also may occasionally be caused by acute tonsillitis in severely hypertrophied tonsils.

Treatment

A well-organized protocol is necessary to manage the child with supraglottitis. Acute obstruction may be precipitated by crying and agitation. Thus, it is necessary to avoid these reactions; throat examination, arterial puncture for blood gas analysis, and placement of an intravenous line should be deferred until control of the airway has been secured with an endotracheal tube or tracheostomy. An artificial airway should be placed in almost all cases of childhood supraglottitis. The unpredictable progression of the disease and the significant risks of morbidity and mortality make placement of an artificial airway the safest course.

Radiography of the upper airway may be helpful in establishing the diagnosis of supraglottitis or in differentiating it from laryngotracheitis or a foreign body (radiopaque). If the child is in acute distress, however, x-ray procedures may delay lifesaving intervention. If x-ray films of the upper airway are taken (this should be done only in a relatively stable child), skilled personnel should be with the child to intubate the airway should critical obstruction occur.

When the diagnosis of supraglottitis is strongly suspected, arrangements are made to have an artificial airway (usually an endotracheal tube) placed. The child is transferred to the operating room accompanied by the parents (to keep him or her calm) and physicians (prepared to cope with further life-threatening airway obstruction). In the operating room, the child is prepared for general anesthesia. The risk of pulmonary aspiration from a "full stomach" must always be considered. However, this risk is low, and in this life-threatening situation, the benefits of placing an endotracheal tube outweighs this risk.

In the early stages of induction, a parent holds the child upright (the supine position may aggravate the airway obstruction). This helps make the anesthetic procedure emotionally less traumatic and avoids compromising the child's airway by agitation. Induction is generally satisfactory with halothane and oxygen via a face mask. Patient monitoring should include a chest stethoscope, electrocardiography, blood pressure measurement, and oxygen saturation (pulse oximetry). Once a light plane of anesthesia is established, an assistant places the intravenous line (with the aid of locally infiltrated anesthetic) and infuses lactated Ringer's solution (10 to 20 ml per kilogram). The child may be dehydrated from fever and failure to take oral fluids. Atropine (0.02 mg per kilogram) is then administered to block laryngeal reflexes associated with laryngoscopy, dry secretions, and to counteract halothane-induced bradycardia. After a satisfactory depth of anesthesia is reached, the child undergoes laryngoscopy. A laryngoscope (Oxyscope) that can provide supplemental oxygen and anesthesia while laryngoscopy is being performed may prevent serious oxygen desaturation.

With deepening of the anesthesia, careful attention must be paid to maintaining a safe airway. This may be helped by applying 5 to 10 cm H_2O continuous positive airway pressure (CPAP) while allowing the child to breathe spontaneously. With further deepening of anesthesia, the child's respiration will be depressed and should be gently assisted. Induction is carried out with inhalational anesthesia only. I do not generally advocate the use of muscle relaxants because in some patients it may be extremely difficult to intubate the airway, and with loss of spontaneous respiration and possible difficulty in adequately ventilating with a face mask, serious hypoxemia may occur.

Supraglottitis, Laryngotracheitis, and Bacterial Tracheitis / **235**

It may take approximately 10 to 30 minutes to achieve a satisfactory depth of anesthesia because airway obstruction limits the uptake of the anesthetic agent. This process should not be rushed. Detection of the glottic opening may be extremely difficult owing to severe swelling of the epiglottis and aryepiglottic folds. In severely obstructed cases, detection may be aided by chest compression, causing "bubbles" of mucus to escape through the glottic opening. A selection of endotracheal tubes should be available. The use of a stylet within the tube aids intubation. The tube is placed orally. If intubation was carried out without difficulty, conversion to a nasotracheal tube may be considered for preferred stabilization; if it was difficult, however, one should leave well enough alone. The tube is carefully secured in place. The child is kept sedated after the procedure and transferred to the pediatric intensive care unit (PICU). The arms are placed in splints to avoid accidental extubation. Alternatively, in some centers, the endotracheal intubation is performed in the PICU. In skilled hands, the endotracheal tube may be placed nasotracheally with the aid of a flexible fiberoptic bronchoscope.

Cultures of the blood and supraglottic structures are taken. Antibiotics (ampicillin, chloramphenicol, or cephalosporin) are administered, and the appropriate antibiotic is given for 10 days once organism sensitivity has been identified. The tube is left in place for 12 to 36 hours. A leak developing around the tube signals the time for extubation, which is carried out in the PICU. However, if there is no leak, the larynx is visualized (via fiberoptic visualization or direct laryngoscopy with anesthetic agents). Extubation is then performed according to the findings at examination.

Occasionally, pulmonary edema may be seen with supraglottitis, as with other severe forms of acute upper airway obstruction. Metastatic complications of the *H. influenzae* infection are serious and must be suspected when toxicity and fever do not resolve and when new symptoms appear. Metastatic infection may lead to pneumonia, meningitis (rarely), pericarditis, periarticular abscess, and pleural effusions.

Steroid therapy in this disease remains controversial. Rifamycin is administered to intimate contacts and to siblings under 8 years of age.

LARYNGOTRACHEITIS

Laryngotracheitis (croup) is a very common cause of acute upper airway obstruction in children aged 3 months to 6 years. It is most often caused by a viral infection, especially the parainfluenza group. The subglottic area is primarily affected with edema. The swelling leads to an increase in resistance to breathing. Because of the child's relatively small airway and the effect of narrowing on resistance (R):

$$[R \alpha \frac{1}{radius}]_4$$

even modest swelling in this area causes a disproportionate increase in airway resistance compared with the older child and adult.

Differential Diagnosis

The differential diagnosis must consider other causes of a severe acute upper airway obstruction: supraglottitis, bacterial tracheitis, foreign body, and subglottic hemangioma.

Roentgenograms of the upper airway, particularly the anteroposterior view (showing subglottic narrowing), may be helpful in atypical cases.

Treatment

Management usually includes allaying patient and family anxiety, providing oxygen therapy for probable hypoxemia due to associated ventilation-perfusion mismatching, and humidification. Moist air therapy is traditional but is not supported by scientific studies. The use of steroids, although controversial for many years, has recently been shown to be effective in this condition.

Increasing distress in the child (tachycardia, tachypnea, and increasing stridor and cyanosis) warrant more active measures to relieve the airway obstruction. With increasing airway obstruction and fatigue, the child may not generate vigorous respiratory efforts and therefore the stridor may diminish. This may be interpreted erroneously as an improvement in the child's condition.

Inhalation of racemic epinephrine (0.5 ml in 3 ml saline) may provide a short-term benefit. This form of treatment probably does not affect the duration or ultimate severity of the illness. These treatments may need to be repeated every 1 to 3 hours. Close monitoring of the cardiovascular status and airway patency is carried out. Should the obstruction not respond to racemic epinephrine inhalations, tracheal intubation is performed under controlled conditions in the operating room. Helium-oxygen inhalation may benefit the child and provide a "margin of safety" in a deteriorating child before more definitive therapy (namely, tracheal intubation). In some situations, the progressive respiratory distress is compounded by thick inspissated secretions that the child is unable to cough up, and tracheal intubation provides a means for suctioning the airway and maintaining patency. Tracheostomy is an alternative but less commonly performed procedure at this stage. The endotracheal tube should be a size 0.5 to 1.0 mm smaller than would normally be used in order to avoid ischemic necrosis in the subglottitic area and its potential for subsequent stenosis.

Extubation is carried out in the PICU after 3 to 5 days, or earlier if a leak develops around the endotracheal tube.

BACTERIAL TRACHEITIS

Bacterial tracheitis is a primary infection of the trachea, usually caused by *Staphylococcus aureus*. The infection leads to severe subglottic edema and sloughing of the tracheal mucosa. Mucopurulent secretions accumulate and lead to potentially life-threatening airway obstruction.

Children up to about 12 years of age are susceptible. The disease is usually preceded by an upper respiratory infection, which rapidly progresses to stridor and cough with the child becoming acutely toxic. Severe airway obstruction occurs and the child rapidly becomes exhausted and is unable to clear the airway. Urgent placement of an artificial airway, i.e., an endotracheal tube, is necessary. Bronchoscopy may be required to remove obstructing membranes and necrotic tissue. Antibiotics are administered to treat probable staphylococcal infections. Culture and sensitivity tests on the sputum will dictate any necessary changes in antibiotic therapy.

SUGGESTED READING

Banji AS, Asmar BI, Thirumoarta MC. Systemic *Haemophilus influenzae* disease—an overview. J Pediatr 1986; 94:278–279.

Davis HW, Gartner JC, Calvis AG, et al. Acute upper airway obstruction; croup and epiglottitis. Pediatr Clin North Am 1981; 28:859–880.

Friedman EM, Jorgensen K, Healy GB, et al. Bacterial tracheitis: two year experience. Laryngoscope 1985; 95:9.

Henry RL, Mellis CM, Benjamin B. Pseudomembranous croup. Arch Dis Child 1983; 58:180–183.

Kairys SW, Olmstead EN, O'Connor GT. Steroid treatment of laryngotracheitis: a meta-analysis of the evidence from randomized trials. Pediatrics 1989; 83:683–693.

Kilham H, Gillis J, Benjamin B. Severe upper airway obstruction. Pediatr Clin North Am 1987; 34:1–14.

Super DM, Cartelli NA, Brooks LJ, et al. A prospective randomized double-blind study to evaluate the effect of dexamethasone in acute laryngotracheitis. J Pediatr 1989; 115:256–257.

REGIONAL ANESTHESIA

EUGENE K. BETTS, M.D.
MARK S. SCHREINER, M.D.

The attitude of the medical community toward pediatric regional anesthesia changed radically during the 1980s. Earlier concerns over the double risks of two anesthetics, a lack of appreciation for the nonverbalized discomfort of the young infant, and the medicolegal fear that a patient's developmentally delayed walking might be attributed to a caudal or epidural anesthetic received during infancy inhibited the widespread use of regional anesthesia. Parental pressures to relieve their children's postoperative discomfort, combined with Anand's work on the physiologic effects of stress in the neonate, finally broke the resistance to the use of regional anesthesia. With a primary goal of postoperative pain relief, in 1980, Shandling and Steward documented the effectiveness of ilioinguinal/iliohypogastric nerve blocks, performed under general anesthesia, in relieving the postoperative discomfort of inguinal herniorrhaphies.

The use of pediatric regional anesthesia blossomed during the ensuing 10 years. For example, single and continuous caudal and epidural blocks with local anesthetics and/or narcotics gained prominence in providing postoperative pain relief below the nipple line in hospitalized and ambulatory patients. Spinal anesthetics gained popularity as primary anesthetics for premature neonates undergoing herniorrhaphies. Penile nerve blocks were used to relieve the postoperative pain associated with circumcision and hypospadias repair.

In this chapter, we have provided descriptions of the most popular nerve blocks. The practical orientation of the discussion emphasizes what we do in our department and why we do it.

AXILLARY NERVE BLOCK

Axillary nerve block differs little in children and adults. Paresthesias present more of a problem in children than in adults, because an awake child frequently refuses to cooperate after a paresthesia has been elicited. Under general anesthesia, the transarterial and nerve stimulator approaches both produce reliable results.

Transarterial blocks can be done in children 14 to 17 years of age who have been sedated with 1 to 2 μg per kilogram of fentanyl. Moore describes the transarterial approach in his book on regional anesthesia. In children, we modify his technique by using a 5/8-inch 25-gauge needle connected by a "T" piece to the syringe containing the local anesthetic (Winnie's "immobile needle" technique) (Fig. 1). A 23- or 25-gauge Butterfly needle with syringe attached also works well. Although 0.33 ml per kilogram may be sufficient, up to 1 ml per kilogram of 0.25 percent or 0.5 ml per kilogram of 0.5 percent bupivacaine (2.5 mg per kilogram) with 1:200,000 epinephrine may be used. Volume should be limited to 25 ml. For a closed fracture reduction in the emergency room, the quicker onset of 1.5 percent lidocaine, 7 mg per kilogram, with 1:200,000 epinephrine, may be

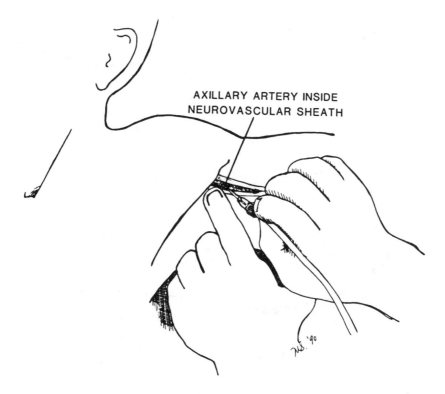

AXILLARY ARTERY INSIDE
NEUROVASCULAR SHEATH

Figure 1 Transarterial axillary nerve block. The axillary artery is palpated high in the axilla. The needle is introduced through the point of maximal pulsation.

preferable. Adding 1 ml of sodium bicarbonate per 10 ml of lidocaine solution reduces the onset time from less than 15 minutes to less than 10 minutes. If the longer duration of action of bupivacaine is desired, the slower onset time of 25 to 30 minutes can be covered by adding 1 to 2 mg per kilogram of lidocaine to the bupivacaine.

The use of a peripheral nerve stimulator is well tolerated by lightly sedated adolescents. With one lead connected to the base of the 22-gauge block needle by an alligator clip, the stimulator can be used to locate the motor nerves within the axillary neurovascular sheath. After the motor nerve has been located with the nerve stimulator set to a low-current setting, a test dose of local anesthetic is injected. If the motor response then becomes absent at a high-current setting, the balance of the local anesthetic dose is injected.

CAUDAL ANESTHESIA

The first report of pediatric caudal anesthesia appeared in the urologic literature in 1933. The anatomy is well delineated in infants and children because of the absence of fat over the sacrum. Thus the block is technically easy to perform. The spinous process of S-5 is not fused, leaving between the two sacral cornu an arched sacral hiatus, which is covered by a firm elastic membrane, the sacrococcygeal ligament. A second difference in anatomy between the infant and the adult is the proximity of the dural membrane to the sacrococ-

cygeal ligament. In the infant, the distance may be as little as 1 cm.

Caudal anesthesia is appropriate for most surgery performed below the umbilicus. Performing the block at the end of the surgery maximizes the duration of analgesia. Alternatively, placing a catheter before starting surgery provides intraoperative and postoperative analgesia for as long as desired.

The block is performed as follows:

1. The patient is placed in the lateral or prone position (Fig. 2).
2. The sacral cornu, the sacral hiatus, and the tip of the coccyx are identified.
3. The sacral area is prepped while gloves are worn, and an aperture drape is placed over the hiatus.
4. A hole is made in the skin with an 18-gauge needle 2 to 3 mm cephalad to a line drawn between the sacral cornu. A 22-gauge block needle is inserted (attached to a short length of small-bore tubing with a Luer Lok connector) at a 60-degree angle to the skin. (Alternatively, a 22-gauge intravenous [IV] catheter is used in children younger than 2 years of age, or a 20-gauge catheter in children 2 years of age or older.) For a continuous caudal catheter, a 24-gauge epidural catheter is inserted through a 20-gauge Medicut catheter. For a 20-gauge epidural catheter, an 18-gauge Medicut intravenous catheter is used. This technique points the

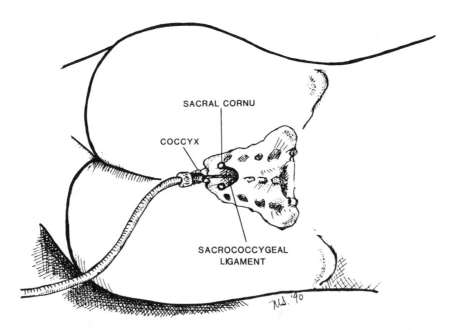

Figure 2 Caudal block. The needle is introduced into the epidural space using an immobile needle and a loss-of-resistance technique. The needle is not advanced after it has entered the epidural space.

epidural catheter up the axis of the epidural space rather than at right angles to it.

5. An obvious and definite "give" will be felt. (If an IV catheter is used, the catheter should be pushed off the stylet.)
6. A syringe is connected to the extension tubing or IV catheter, and a small volume of air is injected to confirm the location of the tip of the needle in the epidural space by loss of resistance to injection.
7. Aspiration is performed for blood and cerebrospinal fluid. Ten percent of the local anesthetic is injected. One should observe for posterior swelling (subcutaneous injection), tachycardia (intravenous injection), or hypotension (subarachnoid injection).
8. One should complete the injection after aspiration for blood has been performed a second time.

Those skilled in the performance of this block may use a no-touch technique, which obviates the need for draping and gloving.

Epinephrine

In children younger than 5 years of age, the addition of 1:200,000 epinephrine prolongs the duration of 0.25 percent bupivacaine from 8.1 hours to an average of 18 hours. The effect is less marked but still present in children 6 to 10 years of age. In addition, the epinephrine is a good marker for intravascular injection.

Volume and Dosage of Local Anesthetic

Bromage and Schulte-Steinberg studied the factors affecting the volume of local anesthetic for epidural and caudal anesthesia. Age, weight, and height were all found to be important in determining dosage. Their formulas simplify to:

$$\text{Dose} = \text{age} \times 0.1 \text{ ml/dermatome} \times \text{number of dermatomes to be anesthetized}$$

A 12-kg, 2-year-old child undergoing a hernia repair would thus require $2 \times 0.1 \times 12 = 2.4$ ml. We have found this formula to be inadequate for most patients. This is not surprising, because both formulas are based on a regression line where 50 percent of the patients receive an inadequate dosage (similar to determinations of minimum alveolar concentration [MAC]). Increasing the dosage, as Hain does in his formula, to:

$$\text{Dose (ml) to block one dermatome} = (\text{age [yr]} + 2)/10$$

produces an adequate block 95 percent of the time.

Takasaki developed a formula based on weight, which simplifies to:

$$\text{Dose} = \text{weight} \times 0.056 \text{ ml/segment}$$

Using Takasaki's formula, the same 2-year-old would receive $12 \times 0.056 \text{ ml} \times 12 = 8$ ml. Eyres studied the pharmacokinetics of caudal bupivacaine and concluded that the maximum safe dosage of bupivacaine is 3 mg per kilogram or 0.6 ml per kilogram of 0.5 percent bupivacaine. This dosage is the same as anesthetizing ten dermatome segments using Takasaki's formula.

McGown studied the sensory level reached after caudal block in children younger than 11 years of age. When a dose of 0.55 ml per kilogram of 1 percent xylocaine with 1:200,000 epinephrine was used, all of the children achieved a level of at least S-3 with no level extending above T-11. With a dose of 1.65 ml per kilogram of the same solution, 1 percent had a level between L-4 and T-12, 5 percent had a cervical level (including 1 percent with total body caudals), and 94 percent had levels between T-11 and T-1. A dose of 1.1 ml per kilogram produced levels between L-2 and T-1 in 100 percent of the patients.

Several studies show there is no advantage to using 0.5 percent instead of lower concentrations of bupivacaine for postoperative analgesia. The lower concentrations of 0.375 percent, 0.25 percent and even 0.125 percent are equally effective. Because concentrations greater than 0.25 percent may delay discharge as a result of the more prolonged motor block, we use 0.25 percent bupivacaine in a dose of 2.5 mg per kilogram. This simplifies to:

$$Dose = 1 \ ml/kg$$

If the patient is to be discharged the day of surgery, 0.125 percent should be used in the same volume as that mentioned above, because the patient is less likely to have a motor block at the time of discharge.

ILIOINGUINAL/ILIOHYPOGASTRIC NERVE BLOCKS FOR HERNIORRHAPHY

Although Hinkle described a combination of ilioinguinal/iliohypogastric and genitofemoral nerve blocks for relief of postoperative herniorrhaphy repair pain, the ilioinguinal/iliohypogastric nerve block provides most of the pain relief. The latter block also provides good postoperative pain relief in orchiopexies. Although the impression is strong, neither we nor others have been able to demonstrate the superiority of these blocks over wound infiltration. Some of our surgeons prefer infiltration because they believe the block distorts the anatomy of the inguinal region.

The ilioinguinal and iliohypogastric nerves run medial to the anterior superior iliac spine and deep to the external and internal oblique muscles. Since it is often difficult to distinguish a "pop" when fascial planes are pierced in young patients, we use the following technique to eliminate the need to identify the fascial layers:

1. The skin is prepped in the region of the anterior iliac spine.

2. A 22-gauge block needle is inserted perpendicular to the skin, one child's fingerbreadth medial from the anterior iliac crest, along a line connecting the crest and the umbilicus (Fig. 3). Going caudad to this line causes the local anesthetic to infiltrate into the incision.

3. The needle is advanced until a "give" is felt, indicating that the fascial planes of the internal and external oblique muscles have been pierced, *or* until the needle hits the inner table of the iliac crest. Two-thirds of the local anesthetic are injected in this region and the balance is injected along the needle tract as the needle is withdrawn, leaving a skin wheal before withdrawal. The skin wheal blocks the perforating branches of T-11 through T-12.

4. 4. Alternatively, half the dose is injected on the first pass. The needle is then redirected approximately 30 degrees from the perpendicular in the plane defined by the umbilicus and anterior superior iliac spine, and the insertion and injection are repeated. Do not attempt to hit the inner table on this second phase.

The block may be performed at the beginning or end of surgery. The usual dose of bupivacaine is 1 mg per kilogram per side with a maximum dose of 2 mg per kilogram. A maximum of 10 ml of local anesthetic should be used per side, with the concentration chosen accordingly (0.25 percent for patients weighing less than 25 kg).

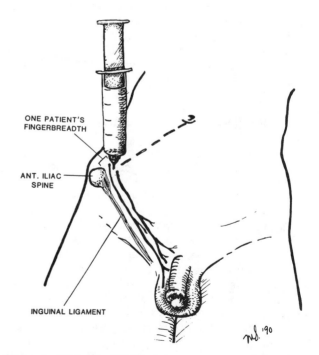

ONE PATIENT'S FINGERBREADTH

ANT. ILIAC SPINE

INGUINAL LIGAMENT

Figure 3 Ilioinguinal/iliohypogastric nerve blocks. The needle is introduced one patient's fingerbreadth away from the anterior iliac spine on a line joining the anterior iliac spine and the umbilicus.

LUMBAR EPIDURAL ANESTHESIA

The recent availability of pediatric epidural anesthesia kits containing a calibrated 20-gauge Tuohy needle and a 24-gauge polyurethane catheter (with stylet) makes lumbar epidural anesthesia a more realistic option in young infants. Although the catheter is difficult to handle, success rates are reasonable. However, it seems prudent in this population to administer the test dose and first anesthetic dose before attempting to place the catheter. If catheter placement is unsuccessful, at least a one-shot epidural is in place.

The spinal cord of the neonate ends at L-3. It assumes the adult position of L-1 around the end of the first year of life. Similarly, the dural sac in the newborn ends at S-3, rising to S-1 by the time the patient is 1 year of age. Thus, lumbar epidurals should be done at L4–5 or L5–S1 during the 1st year of the patient's life.

Although Ecoffey et al recommend an initial dose of 0.75 ml per kilogram of 0.5 percent bupivacaine (3.75 mg per kilogram) with 1:200,000 epinephrine, we prefer to use 0.5 ml per kilogram of 0.25 percent bupivacaine (1.25 mg per kilogram) with epinephrine. If the initial level is too low, an additional dose can be administered. Each injection of the catheter should be preceded by aspiration and the injection of a test dose to ensure that the catheter has not entered a blood vessel.

If you prefer to use the epidural anesthetic as the primary anesthetic, 0.5 percent bupivacaine (2.5 mg per kilogram) with 1:200,000 epinephrine produces a denser block with profound, certain postoperative analgesia and a motor block of the muscles of the hip and upper leg. For knee arthroscopy, use 2 percent lidocaine (7 mg per kilogram maximum—i.e., 0.35 ml per kilogram) with 1:200,000 epinephrine. This also works with a continuous caudal anesthetic where the epidural catheter tip has been threaded up to the lumbar region.

OPIOID CONDUCTION ANESTHESIA

The instillation of opioids epidurally and intrathecally provides long-lasting analgesia. Both the caudal and lumbar regions have been used for epidural anesthesia. Occasionally, the thoracic route has been used. The choice of narcotic influences the spread of the block. For instance, because morphine is hydrophilic, it spreads quite far; caudal epidural morphine relieves the pain that occurs after open heart surgery in children, and intrathecal morphine injected through a lumbar cerebrospinal fluid drain provides relief of postoperative craniofacial pain. On the other hand, fentanyl is lipophilic, and therefore its spread is limited.

Most of the side effects of peridural narcotics, including pruritus, nausea, vomiting, and respiratory depression, can be ameliorated with naloxone, 2 μg per kilogram per hour, mixed in and administered with the maintenance fluids. However, naloxone does not reverse urinary retention. Fortunately, most patients receiving conduction narcotics also have a urinary catheter.

When the catheter tip is kept near its point of entry, preservative-free morphine provides good relief when used in a dose of 0.05 to 0.1 mg per kilogram. Many dilute the morphine in preservative-free saline, 1 ml per kilogram to a maximum of 5 to 15 ml. Preservative-free bupivacaine can be used in place of the saline to confirm the placement of the catheter and to provide a more rapid onset of action. Fentanyl, 1 μg per kilogram in 1 ml per kilogram of 0.25 percent bupivacaine, can also be used and is preferred for patients who will be discharged within 24 hours.

All patients receiving conduction opioids require cardiorespiratory monitoring while the block is in effect. Monitoring may be provided in an intensive care unit, which will limit the use of the block, or in an appropriately equipped and staffed nursing unit. We order hourly nursing observation of these patients and prohibit the use of other narcotics or sedatives while the block is in effect.

Preservative-free narcotics can also be administered intrathecally. For lumbar surgery, 0.002 mg per kilogram (maximum dose 0.2 mg) of preservative-free morphine is diluted with preservative-free saline in a ratio of 1:1 to produce a volume greater than 0.1 ml. The injection is administered by the surgeon via a 27-gauge needle through the dura under direct vision before closure begins. This technique purportedly produces better postoperative analgesia than epidural narcotics. The onset is less than 30 minutes and the analgesia lasts 12 to 24 hours.

PENILE NERVE BLOCK

The dorsal nerves of the penis emerge in the midline from beneath the symphysis pubis and run down the shaft of the penis beneath Buck's fascia at 10 and 2 o'clock. These nerves can be blocked at the base of the penis by piercing Buck's fascia with a small-gauge needle or by performing a subcutaneous ring block, or they can be blocked caudad to the symphysis pubis. We prefer the latter technique because it does not distort the anatomy. In our experience with more than 2,000 penile nerve blocks since 1983, there have been no major complications. The block is appropriate for hypospadias correction as well as circumcision. The technique we use is analogous to an intercostal nerve block. To perform this technique, follow these steps:

1. Use a 22-gauge block needle.
2. Prep the skin at the base of the penis.
3. Standing on the same side of the patient as your dominant side, palpate the symphysis with your nondominant hand.
4. Insert the needle in the midline, perpendicular to the operating room table, until it strikes the symphysis (Fig. 4).
5. Walk the needle *caudad* until it is off the symphysis but not deeper than where the symphysis was last hit. The needle should be midway

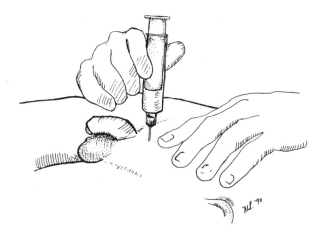

Figure 4 Penile nerve block. The needle is introduced in the midline and "walked off" the pubic symphysis.

between the symphysis and the base of the penis.

6. Aspirate (there are many vessels in this region, but hematoma formation is very rare) and inject a maximum of 1 mg per kilogram of 0.5 percent bupivacaine, *without moving the needle*.

SPINAL ANESTHESIA IN NEONATES

Spinal anesthesia, first used in infants and children during the early 1900s, never achieved widespread popularity. Recently, however, there has been renewed interest in using spinal anesthesia in lieu of general anesthesia for infants, especially the premature infant recovering from neonatal respiratory distress syndrome. We have also found spinal anesthesia useful in hypotonic infants undergoing muscle biopsy. After general anesthesia, infants less than 44 weeks, postconception have an increased risk of postoperative apnea, with an incidence of 18 to 25 percent. In Kurth's study, pneumocardiography, started within 30 minutes of the patient's arrival in the postanesthesia care unit (PACU) and continued for a minimum of 2 hours, revealed prolonged apnea (greater than 15 seconds) in 37 percent of infants younger than 55 postconceptual weeks. An additional 14 percent had apnea for short periods (6 to 15 seconds).

Gregory and Steward have recommended that elective surgery be delayed in preterm infants until they are 44 postconceptual weeks of age. Our policy is to wait until 60 postconceptual weeks of age before performing elective surgery in neonates born before 38 weeks of gestation. Because many surgeons are concerned about the possibility of incarceration, they insist on repairing the hernia before or shortly after discharge. It is in these instances that spinal anesthesia may have a role. Recent publications provide reasonable guidelines for dosage, technique, and treatment of complications. In a review of more than 400 spinal

anesthetics, half of which were performed in former premature infants, Rice and Abajian found no episodes of postoperative apnea.

Because the spinal cord extends down to L-3 in infants, the lumbar puncture should be performed at the L4–5 or L5–S1 interspaces. The block can be accomplished with the patient in the lateral position, but in smaller infants (those younger than 52 weeks postconceptional age), it may be technically easier with the patient in the sitting position. Moreover, Broadman states that the incidence of dry taps is lower. Neonates are premedicated with atropine, 0.04 mg per kilogram, if their weight is less than 4 kg; with 0.16 mg per kilogram if their weight is 4 to 8 kg; or with 0.02 mg per kilogram if their weight is more than 8 kg. The technique we use is as follows:

1. Before the block is performed, the electrocardiographic leads, blood pressure cuff, and pulse oximeter probe are applied. Spinal anesthesia introduces very little hemodynamic change in infants, so the intravenous injection may be started in a lower extremity after the block is established.
2. With the patient sitting or in the lateral position, an assistant should restrain the child and, at the same time, extend the neck to maintain the airway. This may require a second assistant.
3. The skin of the back in the lumbar area is prepped and a lumbar puncture with a 22-gauge, 1.5-inch spinal needle is performed. The average distance to the subarachnoid space is only 1.0 to 1.5 cm. Once through the skin, the stylet may be removed to observe for spinal fluid. If one feels a "pop" but there is no flow of cerebrospinal fluid, then a tuberculin syringe can be attached to the needle and used to gently aspirate.
4. The local anesthetic is injected. One must ensure that sufficient volume is added to account for the dead space in the needle (0.05 to 0.1 ml). The dose of anesthetic is small and the dead space is large relative to this volume. It is important to leave the needle and syringe in place for 5 to 10 seconds after completion of the injection to prevent a cerebrospinal fluid leak.

The dosage recommendations of Rice are greater than those of Abajian, who had several failed blocks in his series. Rice's recommendations are shown in Table 1.

The dosage of epinephrine is described by Broadman as an epinephrine "wash." Epinephrine, 1:1000, is drawn into a syringe and then expressed from the syringe. The amount remaining in the hub of the syringe and in the needle is the appropriate amount.

In infants older than 52 weeks postconceptional age, the anesthetic can be supplemented with ketamine, 1 mg per kilogram IM or 0.25 to 0.5 mg per kilogram IV. In infants younger than 52 weeks postconceptional age, a pacifier with a cotton ball soaked with 25 percent dextrose may be used. At Children's Hospital National

Table 1 Use of Spinal Anesthetics in Neonates Based on Rice's Recommendation*

	5% lidocaine + epinephrine (0.02 ml)	Tetracaine	Tetracaine + epinephrine (0.02 ml)
Dose (mg/kg)	3.0	0.4	0.4
Diluent	7.5% dextrose	0.04 ml/kg of 10% dextrose	0.04 ml/kg of 10% dextrose
Duration of motor block (min)	56 ± 2.5	86 ± 4	125 ± 3
Duration of surgical procedure (min)	≤ 30	≤ 60	60–95

*Adapted from Rice L, DeMars P, Crooms J, et al. Duration of spinal anesthesia in infants under 1 year of age: comparison of three drugs. Anesth Analg 1987; 66:514.

Medical Center (CHNMC), a whiskey nipple is substituted for the sugar water without any reported complication.

DISCHARGE CRITERIA

For these patients, the usual medical criteria for discharge apply—for example, stable vital signs and minimal nausea and vomiting. We no longer require tolerance to clear liquids. If the child has an extremity block, the parents must be aware that he or she will be unable to feel pain. A sling should be provided to protect the upper extremity. The experience at CHNMC demonstrates that children may safely go home after caudal analgesia before regression of their sensory block. They require that children be able to ambulate without assistance and without postural hypotension. They also allow these children to go home before voiding. In more than 1,150 cases, no patient has had to return because of inability to void. Finally, the parents should be given the telephone number of an anesthesiologist on call in case they have any questions about their child's postoperative course. In addition, all parents of patients who have received a regional anesthetic as part of a day surgical procedure should be telephoned and interviewed the following day to ensure that no problems have ensued.

SUGGESTED READING

Amand KJS, Sipple WG, Ansley-Green A. Randomised trial of fentanyl anaesthesia in preterm babies undergoing surgery: effects on the stress response. Lancet 1987; 1:243–248.

Broadman LM. Pediatric regional and postoperative analgesia. In: Barash PG, Deutsch S, Tinker J, eds. ASA refresher courses in anesthesia. Vol. 14:43–60, 1986.

Broadman LM, Rice LJ. Pediatric regional anesthesia and perioperative analgesia. Probl Anesth 1988; 2:386–407.

Dalens BJ. Pediatric regional anesthesia. Boca Raton, FL: CRC Press, 1990.

Ecoffey C, Dubosset A-M Sammi K. Lumbar and thoracic epidural anesthesia for urologic and upper abdominal surgery in infants and children. Anesthesiology 1986; 65:87–90.

Gregory GA, Steward DJ. Life–threatening perioperative apnea in the x-"preemie" (editorial). Anesthesiology 1983; 59:495–498.

Kurth CD, Spitzer AR, Broennle AM, et al. Postoperative apnea in preterm infants. Anesthesiology 1987; 66:483–488.

Shandling B, Steward DJ. Regional anesthesia for postoperative pain for pediatric outpatient surgery. J Pediatr Surg 1980; 15:477–480.

Yaster M, Maxwell LG. Pediatric regional anesthesia. Anesthesiology 1989; 70:324–338.

PAIN MANAGEMENT IN CHILDREN

MYRON YASTER, M.D.
ELIZABETH NICHOLAS, M.D.

The treatment and alleviation of pain is a basic human right that exists regardless of age. Unfortunately, even when their pain is obvious, children frequently receive no treatment, or inadequate treatment, for pain and for painful procedures. The newborn is particularly vulnerable. The common "wisdom" that children neither respond to, nor remember, painful experiences to the same degree that adults do is simply untrue.

Unfortunately, even when physicians decide to treat children in pain, they rarely prescribe potent analgesics, adequate doses, or pharmacologically rational dosing regimens because of their over-riding concern that children may be harmed by the use of these drugs. This is not at all surprising, because physicians are taught throughout their training that opiates cause respiratory depression, cardiovascular collapse, depressed levels of consciousness, vomiting, and, with repeated use, addiction. Rarely, if ever, are the appropriate therapeutic uses of these drugs, or rational dosing regimens, discussed. Indeed, until very recently, it was difficult to find pain and its medical management even mentioned in any of the textbooks of pediatric medicine and surgery.

Nurses are taught to be wary of physicians' orders (and patients' requests) as well. The most common prescription order for potent analgesics, "to give as needed" (*pro re nata*, prn), has come to mean "to give as infrequently as possible." The prn order also means that either the patient must ask for pain medication or the nurse must identify when a patient is in pain. Neither of these requirements may be met by children in pain. Children younger than 7 years of age may be unable to verbalize adequately when or where they hurt. Alternatively they may be afraid to report their pain. Many children will withdraw or deny their pain in an attempt to avoid yet another terrifying and painful experience — the intramuscular injection or "shot." Finally, several studies have documented the inability of nurses and physicians to correctly identify and treat pain even in postoperative pediatric patients.

As anesthesiologists, we have a special, if not unique, role in the treatment of both acute and chronic pain. In our daily clinical practice we use virtually every drug category and method of delivery that is useful in pain and sedation management. We understand, as few others do, that these powerful drugs must be titrated, with appropriate monitoring, to individual patient needs and that dosage is not based solely on weight or on our presumption of how much a procedure "should" hurt. Crossing the boundaries of the operating room and becoming primary care physicians is a "brave new world" for most of us though. However, because of our responsibility of sharing our knowledge and skills and educating our colleagues it is becoming a litmus test of our commitment to better patient care. Fortunately, the past 5 years has seen a virtual explosion in the development of pediatric pain services, primarily under the direction of pediatric anesthesiologists. The pain service teams provide the pain management for patients with acute, postoperative, terminal, neuropathic, and chronic pain.

The purpose of this review is to highlight (1) the component services necessary for a multidisciplinary pediatric pain service and (2) the recent advances in

Table 1 Services Involved in a Multidisciplinary Pediatric Pain Service

Anesthesiology
Hematology–oncology
Neurology
Neurosurgery
Nursing
Oral and maxillofacial surgery
Orthopedics
Pediatrics
Pharmacy
Physical therapy
Psychiatry–psychology
Surgery
Urology

opioid and local anesthetic pharmacology and therapeutic interventions, both in and out of the operating room. Specifically, we (1) review the components of a multidisciplinary pain service; (2) discuss how pain is assessed in children; (3) delineate the role of opioid receptors in the mechanism of opioid analgesia; (4) provide a pharmacokinetic and pharmacodynamic framework regarding the use of opioids and local anesthetics in children; and (5) provide guidelines for pain management using patient-controlled analgesia, methadone, spinally administered opiates, and continuous epidural infusions using bupivacaine alone and in combination with fentanyl.

THE PEDIATRIC PAIN SERVICE

The multidisciplinary approach to pain management has become the most widely accepted model in current clinical practice. Indeed, this is true whether one designs an acute pain service (e.g., for the management of postoperative pain, terminal pain of malignancies, and vaso-occlusive crisis in sickle cell disease) or an acute and chronic pain service (e.g., for the treatment of reflex sympathetic dystrophy, chronic abdominal pain, and headache). The crucial component services involved in a multidisciplinary approach are listed in Table 1. Usually under the medical direction of an anesthesiologist, a pain service can be successful only if the department of nursing is fully integrated into its design and function from the outset. In fact, after deciding to start a pain service, the single most important priority of the director is to select and secure the funding for a dedicated nurse clinician, whose only clinical and administrative responsibilities are the pain service. Anything else will ultimately lead to failure.

The goals of the pain service are to select the appropriate drugs, methods, and techniques of delivery that are appropriate for an individual patient's needs. A 24-hour availability is necessary as well as regular follow up by skilled and knowledgeable physicians. Furthermore, it is the duty of the pain service to provide the medical and nursing services of the hospital with periodic education updates, printed protocols, and standardized orders for the various pain therapy modalities the service uses. Additionally, the pain service must maintain continuing quality assurance reviews of all problems that arise or that may arise.

PAIN ASSESSMENT

The International Association for the Study of Pain (IASP) defines pain as "an unpleasant and emotional experience associated with actual or potential tissue damage, or described in terms of such damage." Pain is a subjective experience; operationally, it can be defined as "what the patient says hurts" and exists "when the patient says it does." Infants, preverbal children, and children between the ages of 2 and 7 years (Piaget's preoperational thought stage) may be unable to describe their pain or their subjective experiences. This has led many to conclude that children do not experience pain in the same way that adults do. Clearly, children do not have to know or be able to express the meaning of an experience in order to have the experience. On the other hand, because pain is essentially a subjective experience, it is becoming increasingly clear that the child's perspective of pain is an indispensable facet of pediatric pain management and an essential element in the specialized study of childhood pain. Indeed, pain assessment and management are interdependent and one is essentially useless without the other. The goal of pain assessment is to provide accurate data about the location and intensity of pain as well as the effectiveness of measures used to alleviate or abolish it.

Validated, reliable instruments currently exist to measure and assess pain in children over the age of 3 years. These instruments, which measure the quality and intensity of pain, are self-report measures and make use of pictures or word descriptors to describe pain. Pain intensity or severity can be measured in children as young as 3 years of age by using either the Oucher scale (developed by Beyer), a two-part scale with a vertical numerical scale (0 to 100) on one side and six photographs of a young child on the other, or a visual analogue scale, or a 10-cm line with a smiling face on one end and a distraught, crying face on the other. Alternatively, color, word-graphic rating scales, and poker chips have been used to assess the intensity of pain in children. In infants and newborns, pain has been assessed by measuring physiologic responses to a nociceptive stimuli, such as blood pressure and heart rate changes or by measuring levels of adrenal stress hormones. Alternatively, behavioral approaches have used facial expression, body movements, and the intensity and quality of crying as indices of response to nociceptive stimuli. Finally, it is important to define accurately the location of pain. This is readily accomplished by using either dolls or action figures or by using drawings of body outlines, both front and back.

OPIOID RECEPTORS

Over the past 20 years multiple opioid receptors and subtypes have been identified and classified (Table 2). An understanding of the complex nature and organization of these multiple opioid receptors is essential for an adequate understanding of the response to, and control of, pain. In the central nervous system there are four primary opioid receptor types, designated mu (μ) (for morphine), kappa (κ), delta (δ), and sigma (σ). The mu receptor is further subdivided into mu_1 (supraspinal analgesia) and mu_2 (respiratory depression, inhibition of gastrointestinal motility, and spinal analgesia) subtypes. Other receptors and subtypes will surely be discovered as research in this area proceeds.

Organizationally, the distribution of the multiple opioid receptors may have significance in the modulation of pain (see Table 2). Nociceptive impulses are transmitted from the periphery to the dorsal horn of the spinal cord where diverse synapses occur with essentially all incoming sensory input. In the substantia gelatinosa of the dorsal horn of the spinal cord, interneurons are activated and release substance P, an 11-amino acid peptide pain transmitter that facilitates nociceptive transmission. Descending fibers also synapse at the interneurons to inhibit or modulate sensory input about an injury as well, via the release of endogenous opioids and other neuropeptides. If unblocked, nociceptive input is transmitted to the brain via the spinothalamic and spinoreticular nerve pathways. Several areas within the brain may further modulate or abolish pain transmission, including the medial and lateral reticular formations of the brain stem, the medullary raphe nuclei, the periaqueductal gray matter, the thalamus, and the cerebral cortex. Binding of either endogenous or pharmacologically administered opiates to receptors in

Table 2 Classification of Opioid Receptors

Receptor	Prototype Agonist	CNS Location	Effects

Mu	Morphine
	Fentanyl
	Meperidine
	Codeine
	Methadone
		Brain
		  laminae III and IV of the cortex,
		  thalamus periaqueductal
		  gray matter
		Spinal cord
		  substantia gelatinosa
			Mu_1 supraspinal analgesia, dependence
			Mu_2 respiratory depression, inhibition of gastrointestinal mobility, bradycardia

Kappa	Ketocyclazocine
	Dynorphin
	? Butorphanol
		Brain
		  hypothalamus periaqueductal
		  gray matter, claustrum
		Spinal cord
		  substantia gelatinosa
			Spinal analgesia, sedation, miosis, inhibition of antidiuretic hormone release

Delta	Enkephalins
	DADL
		Brain
		  pontine nucleus, amygdala,
		  olfactory bulbs, deep cortex
			Analgesia
			Euphoria

Sigma	N-allylnormetazocine Phencyclidine ? Ketamine		Dysphoria, hallucinations

these central locations initiates the modulation of pain transmission. Thus, the organization of opioid systems suggests that there may be a multiplicity of sites at which opioids might modify nociception.

The differentiation of agonists and antagonists is fundamental to pharmacology. A neurotransmitter is defined as having agonist activity, whereas a drug that blocks the action of a neurotransmitter is an antagonist. By definition, receptor recognition of an agonist is "translated" into other cellular alterations (that is, the agonist initiates a pharmacologic effect), whereas an antagonist occupies the receptor without initiating the transduction step (it has no intrinsic activity or efficacy). The intrinsic activity of a drug defines the ability of the drug-receptor complex to initiate a pharmacologic effect. Drugs that produce less than a maximal response have a lowered intrinsic activity and are called partial agonists. Partial agonists also have antagonistic properties, because by binding the receptor site, they block access of full agonists to the receptor site. Morphine and related opiates are mu agonists and drugs that block the effects of opiates at the mu receptor, such as naloxone, are designated antagonists. The opioids most commonly used in anesthetic practice and in the management of

pain are mu agonists (Table 3). These include morphine, meperidine, methadone, and the fentanyls. Mixed agonist-antagonist drugs act as agonists or partial agonists at one receptor and antagonists at another receptor. Mixed (opioid) agonist-antagonist drugs include pentazocine, butorphanol, nalorphine, and nalbuphine. Most of these drugs are agonists or partial agonists at the kappa and sigma receptors and antagonists at the mu receptor (Table 4).

The mu receptor and its subspecies and the delta receptor produce analgesia, respiratory depression, euphoria, and physical dependence. Morphine is 50 to 100 times weaker at the delta than at the mu receptor. By contrast, the endogenous opiate-like neurotransmitter peptides known as the enkephalins tend to be more potent at delta and kappa than mu receptors. The kappa receptor, located primarily in the spinal cord, produces spinal analgesia, miosis, and sedation with minimal associated respiratory depression. Indeed, this may have important clinical significance. As tolerance develops, increasing doses of morphine are required to produce effective analgesia. It is intriguing to speculate that at higher doses, the analgesia produced by morphine occurs by its delta and kappa effects rather than by its mu

Table 3 Commonly Used Mu Agonist Drugs

Agonist	Equipotent IV Dose (mg/kg)	Duration (hour)	Bioavailability (%)	Comments
Morphine	0.1	3–4	20–40	Seizures in newborns; also in all patients at high doses Histamine release, vasodilation→→avoid in asthmatics and in circulatory compromise MS-contin 8–12 h duration
Meperidine	0.1	3–4	40–60	Catastrophic interactions with MAO inhibitors Tachycardia; negative inotrope Metabolite produces seizures; not recommended for chronic use
Methadone	0.1	6–24	70–100	Can be given IV even though the package insert says SQ or IM
Fentanyl	0.001	0.5–1		Bradycardia; minimal hemodynamic alterations Chest wall rigidity (> 5 μg/kg rapid IV bolus). Rx naloxone or a succinylcholine, pancuronium
Codeine	1.2	3–4	40–70	PO only Prescribe with acetaminophen

Table 4 Action of Opioids at Receptor Subtypes

Drug	Receptor Subtype		
	Mu	Kappa	Sigma
Morphine	Agonist	Agonist	
Naloxone	Antagonist	Antagonist	Antagonist
Naltrexone	Antagonist	–	–
Pentazocine	Antagonist	Agonist	Agonist
Butorphanol	–	Agonist	Agonist
Nalbuphine	Antagonist	Partial agonist	Agonist

agonist activity. Finally, the sigma receptor is responsible for the psychotomimetic effects observed with some opiate drugs, particularly the mixed agonist-antagonist drugs. These effects include dysphoria and hallucinations.

A number of studies suggest that the respiratory depression and analgesia produced by mu agonists involve different receptor subtypes. These receptors change in number in an age-related fashion and can be blocked by naloxone. Pasternak and colleagues, working with newborn rats, showed that 14-day-old rats are 40 times more sensitive to morphine analgesia than 2-day-old rats. Nevertheless, morphine depresses the respiratory rate in 2-day-old rats to a greater degree than in 14-day-old rats. Thus, the newborn may be particularly sensitive to the respiratory depressant effects of the commonly administered opioids in what may be an age-related receptor phenomenon. Obviously this has important clinical implications for the use of narcotics in the newborn.

PHARMACOKINETICS

To relieve or prevent pain, the agonist must get to the receptor in the central nervous system. There are essentially two ways that this occurs, either via the bloodstream (following intravenous, intramuscular, oral, nasal, transdermal, or mucosal administration) or by direct application (intrathecal or epidural administration) into the cerebrospinal fluid (CSF). Agonists administered via the bloodstream must cross the blood–brain barrier, a lipid membrane interface between the endothelial cells of the brain vasculature and the extracellular fluid of the brain, to reach the receptor. Normally, highly lipid-soluble agonists, such as fentanyl, rapidly diffuse across the blood–brain barrier, whereas agonists with limited lipid solubility, such as morphine, have limited brain uptake. The blood–brain barrier may be immature at birth and is known to be more permeable to morphine. Indeed, Way and co-workers demonstrated that morphine concentrations were 2 to 4 times greater in the brains of younger rats than older rats despite equal blood concentrations.

Spinal administration, either intrathecally or epidurally, bypasses the blood and directly places an agonist into the CSF, which bathes the receptor sites in the spinal cord (substantia gelatinosa) and brain. This "back door" to the receptor significantly reduces the amount of agonist needed to relieve pain. After spinal administration, opioids are absorbed by the epidural veins and redistributed to the systemic circulation, where they are metabolized and excreted. Hydrophilic agents, such as morphine, cross the dura more slowly than more lipid-soluble agents such as fentanyl or meperidine. This physicochemical property is responsible for the more prolonged duration of action of spinal morphine and its very slow onset of action following epidural administration.

Although it would be desirable to adjust opioid dosage based on the concentration of drug achieved at the receptor site, this is rarely feasible. The alternative is to measure blood or plasma concentrations and model how the body handles a drug. Pharmacokinetic studies thereby help the clinician select suitable routes, timing, and dosing of drugs to maximize a drug's dynamic effects.

Following administration, the disposition of a drug is dependent on distribution ($T_{1/2}\alpha$) and elimination. The terminal half-life of elimination ($T_{1/2}1/2\beta$) is directly proportional to the volume of distribution (Vd) and inversely proportional to the total body clearance (Cl) by the following formula:

$$T_{1/2}\beta = 0.693 \times (Vd/Cl)$$

Thus, a prolongation of the $T_{1/2}\beta$ may be due to either an increase in a drug's volume of distribution or to a decrease in its clearance.

Morphine, meperidine, methadone, and fentanyl are biotransformed in the liver prior to excretion. Many of these reactions are catalyzed in the liver by microsomal mixed-function oxidases that require the cytochrome P_{450} system, NADPH, and oxygen. The cytochrome P_{450} system is very immature at birth and does not reach adult levels until the first month or two of life. This immaturity of this hepatic enzyme system may explain the prolonged clearance or elimination of some opioids in the first few days to weeks of life. On the other hand, the P_{450} system can be induced by various drugs (phenobarbital) and substrates and matures regardless of gestational age. Thus, it is the age from birth, and not the duration of gestation, that determines how premature and full-term infants metabolize drugs. Indeed, Greeley and colleagues have demonstrated that sufentanil is more rapidly metabolized and eliminated in 2- to 3-week-old infants than newborns younger than a week of age.

Morphine and fentanyl are primarily gluronidated into inactive forms that are excreted by the kidney, whereas approximately one-third of meperidine is demethylated into normeperidine, a metabolite that is half as active as meperidine as an analgesic but twice as active as a convulsant. Because of the propensity of normeperidine to produce seizures, we believe that meperidine should not be prescribed for chronic pain management.

Fentanyl is highly lipid-soluble and is rapidly distributed to tissues that are well perfused, such as the brain and the heart. Normally, the effect of a single dose of fentanyl is terminated by rapid redistribution, rather than by elimination, in a manner very much akin to thiopental. However, following multiple or large doses of fentanyl (e.g., when it is used as a primary anesthetic agent), prolongation of effect will occur, because elimination and not distribution will determine the duration of effect (see below). This is particularly important in the newborn, in whom elimination may be further prolonged by abnormal or decreased liver blood flow following acute illness or abdominal surgery. Additionally, certain conditions that may raise intra-abdominal pressure may further decrease liver blood flow by shunting blood away from the liver via the still patent ductus venosus.

The pharmacokinetics of morphine and fentanyl have been extensively studied in adults, older children, and in the premature and full-term newborn. Following an intravenous bolus, 30 percent of morphine is protein-bound in the adult versus only 20 percent in the newborn. This increase in unbound ("free") morphine allows a greater proportion of active drug to penetrate the brain. This may explain, in part, the observation of Way and associates of increased brain levels of morphine in the newborn and its more profound respiratory depressant effects. The elimination half-life of morphine in adults and older children is 3 to 4 hours and is consistent with its duration of analgesic action (Table 5). The $T_{1/2}\beta$ is more than twice as long in newborns less than a week of age than in older children and adults and is even longer in premature infants. Clearance is similarly decreased in the newborn compared to the older child and adult (see Table 5). Thus, infants younger than 1 month of age will attain higher serum levels that will decline more slowly than older children and adults. This may also account for the increased respiratory depression associated with morphine in this age group.

Interestingly, the half-life of elimination and clearance of morphine in children older than 2 months of age is similar to adult values. Thus, the hesitancy in prescribing and administering morphine in children younger than 1 year of age may not be warranted. On the other hand, *the use of any opioid in children younger than 2 months of age must be limited to a monitored, intensive care unit setting.*

Based on its relatively short half-life (3 to 4 hours), one would expect older children and adults to require morphine supplementation every 2 to 3 hours when being treated for pain, particularly if the morphine is administered intravenously. This has led to the recent use of continuous infusion regimens of morphine and patient-controlled analgesia (see below), which maximize pain-free periods. Alternatively, longer-acting agonists such as methadone may be used. Methadone is metabolized extremely slowly in children and has a very prolonged duration of action. The $T_{1/2}\beta$ of methadone averages 19 hours, and clearance averages 5.4 $ml \cdot min^{-1} \cdot kg^{-1}$.

Finally only about 30 percent of an orally administered dose of morphine reaches the systemic circulation. When converting a patient's intravenous morphine requirements to oral maintenance doses, one needs to multiply the intravenous dose by 3 or 4. Oral morphine is available as a liquid, tablet, and sustained release preparations (MS-contin).

Fentanyl and its structurally related relatives sufentanil and alfentanil are highly lipophilic drugs that rapidly penetrate all membranes including the blood–brain barrier. Following an intravenous bolus, fentanyl is rapidly eliminated from plasma as the result of its extensive uptake by body tissues. The fentanyls are highly bound to alpha$_1$ acid glycoproteins in the plasma, which are reduced in the newborn. The fraction of free

Table 5 Morphine Pharmacokinetics

	Premature (<33 wks)	Full-term Infant	Adult
$T_{1/2}\beta$	7.4 ± 1.7	6.7 ± 4.6	3.0
Clearance (ml/kg/min)	9.6 ± 4.0	15.5 ± 10.0	3.2
Vd (L/kg)	5.18 ± 1.6	2.9 ± 2.1	15

unbound sufentanil is significantly increased in neonates and children younger than a year of age (19.5 ± 2.7 and 11.5 ± 3.2 percent, respectively) compared to older children and adults (8.1 ± 1.4 and 7.8 ± 1.5 percent, respectively) and this correlates to levels of alpha$_1$ acid glycoproteins in the blood.

Fentanyl pharmacokinetics differ among newborn infants, children, and adults. The total body clearance of fentanyl is greater in infants 3 to 12 months of age than in children older than 1 year of age or adults (18.1 ± 1.4, 11.5 ± 4.2, and 10.0 ± 1.7 ml · kg^{-1} · min^{-1}, respectively) and the half-life of elimination is longer (233 ± 137, 244 ± 79, and 129 ± 42 minutes, respectively). The prolonged elimination half-life of fentanyl from plasma has important clinical implications. Repeated doses of fentanyl for maintenance of analgesic effects will lead to accumulation of fentanyl and its ventilatory depressant effects. Very large doses (0.05 to 0.10 mg · kg^{-1}, as used in anesthesia) may be expected to induce long-lasting effects, because plasma fentanyl levels will not fall below the threshold level at which spontaneous ventilation occurs during the distribution phases. On the other hand, the greater clearance of fentanyl in infants older than 3 months of age produces lower plasma concentrations of the drug and may allow these children to tolerate more drug without respiratory depression.

PATIENT-CONTROLLED ANALGESIA

Because of the enormous individual variations in pain perception and opioid metabolism, fixed ("Harriet Lane") doses and time intervals make little sense. Based on the pharmacokinetics of the opioids, it should be clear that intravenous boluses of morphine or meperidine may need to be given at intervals of 1 to 2 hours to avoid marked fluctuations in plasma drug levels. Continuous intravenous infusions can provide steady analgesic levels and are preferable to intramuscular injections but are not a panacea because the perception and intensity of pain are not constant. Indeed, the most common method of opioid administration in adults and children is intramuscular injection. It is well known that children will suffer in silence and under-report their level of pain rather than ask for yet another painful stimulus, namely, the "shot." Thus, rational pain management requires some form of titration to effect whenever an opioid is administered. In order to give patients some measure of control over their pain therapy, demand analgesia or patient-controlled analgesia (PCA) devices have been developed. These are microprocessor-driven pumps with a button that the patient presses to administer a small dose of opioid. This treatment modality may be particularly suitable for adolescent patients and patients with sickle cell anemia who present in vaso-occlusive crisis.

Demand analgesia devices allow patients to administer small amounts of an analgesic whenever they feel a need for more pain relief. The opioid, usually morphine, is administered either intravenously or subcutaneously. The dosage of opioid, number of boluses per hour, and the time interval between boluses (the "lock-out period") are programmed into the equipment by the pain service physician to allow maximum patient flexibility and sense of control with minimal risk of overdosage. Generally, because patients know that if they have severe pain they can obtain relief immediately, many prefer dosing regimens that result in mild to moderate pain in exchange for fewer side effects such as nausea or pruritus. Typically, we initially prescribe morphine, 20 µg per kilogram per bolus, at a rate of 6 boluses per hour, with an 8- to 10-minute lock-out interval between each bolus. Variations include larger boluses (30 to 50 µg per kilogram), shorter time intervals (5 minutes), and so forth. The PCA pump computer stores within its memory how many boluses the patient has received as well as how many attempts the patient has made at receiving boluses. This allows the physician to evaluate how well the patient understands the use of the pump and provides information to program the pump more efficiently. Many PCA units allow low "background" continuous infusions (morphine, 20 to 30 µg per kilogram per hour) in addition to self-administered boluses. This is sometimes called "PCA-Plus." A continuous background infusion is particularly useful at night and often provides more restful sleep by preventing the patient from awakening in pain. It also increases the potential for overdosage.

PCA requires that the patient have enough intelligence, manual dexterity, and strength to operate the pump. Thus, it was initially limited to adolescents and teenagers, but the lower age limit in whom this treatment modality can be used continues to fall. In fact, it has been our experience that any child able to play Nintendo can operate a PCA pump. Extensive studies in adult and adolescent patients reveal that patients are extremely satisfied with this mode of therapy. Difficulties with PCA include its increased costs, patient age limitations, and the bureaucratic (physician, nursing, and pharmacy) obstacles (protocols, education, storage arrangements) that must be overcome prior to its implementation. Contraindications include inability to push the bolus button (weakness, arm restraints), inability to understand how to use the machine, and a patient's desire not to assume responsibility for his or her own care.

METHADONE

Primarily thought of as a drug to treat or wean opioid-addicted or -dependent patients, methadone is increasingly being used for postoperative pain relief and for the treatment of intractable pain. It is noted for its slow elimination, very long duration of effective analgesia, and high oral bioavailability (see Table 3).

Methadone has the longest $T_{1/2}\beta$ of any of the commonly available opiates and may provide 12 to 36 hours of analgesia following a single intravenous or oral dose. Pharmacokinetically, children are indistinguishable from young adults. The $T_{1/2}\beta$ of methadone averages 19.2 hours and the clearance averages $5.4 \, \text{ml} \cdot \text{min}^{-1} \cdot \text{kg}^{-1}$ in children 1 to 18 years of age. Because a single dose of methadone can achieve and sustain a high drug plasma level, it is a convenient way to provide prolonged analgesia without requiring an intramuscular injection. Indeed, when administered either orally or intravenously, it may be viewed as an alternative to the use of continuous intravenous opioid infusions (a "poor man's PCA"). Berde and co-workers recommend loading patients with an initial dose of intravenous methadone, 0.1 to 0.2 $\text{mg} \cdot \text{kg}^{-1}$, and then titrating in 0.05-$\text{mg} \cdot \text{kg}^{-1}$ increments every 10 to 15 minutes until analgesia is achieved. Supplemental methadone can be administered in 0.05- to 0.1-$\text{mg} \cdot \text{kg}^{-1}$ increments administered by slow intravenous infusion every 4 to 12 hours as needed. Berde also has reported the use of small incremental doses administered by sliding scale. "Small increments of methadone are administered intravenously over 20 minutes every 4 hours via a 'sliding' scale on a 'reverse prn' (the nurse asks the patient) basis: 0.07-0.08 mg per kg for severe pain; 0.05-0.06 mg per kg for moderate pain; 0.03 mg per kg for little or no pain, if the patient is alert; and no drug if the patient has little pain and is somnolent." The influence of pathophysiology on the pharmacokinetics and pharmacodynamics of methadone are unknown, primarily because its use as an analgesic is a relatively recent phenomenon. Dosing decisions in the very young and in patients with various end-organ diseases must be made conservatively. Finally, because methadone is extremely well absorbed from the gastrointestinal tract and has a bioavailability of 80 to 90 percent, it is extremely easy to convert intravenous dosing regimens to oral ones.

INTRATHECAL AND EPIDURAL OPIOID ANALGESIA

The presence of high concentrations of opioid receptors in the spinal cord makes it possible to achieve analgesia, in both acute and chronic pain, with small doses of opioids administered in either the subarachnoid or epidural spaces. By bypassing the blood and the blood–brain barrier, small doses of agonist are effective because they can reach the receptor by the "back-door." Indeed, CSF opioid levels, particularly for morphine, are several thousand times greater than those achieved by the parenteral route (see below). It is these high levels that produce the profound and prolonged analgesia that accompanies intrathecal and epidural opioid administration.

Yaksh and associates demonstrated, in unanesthetized rats, that intrathecal narcotics produced profound segmental analgesia that is dose dependent and reversible with naloxone. However, after 1 hour, rostral spread was evident, especially at higher doses. The passage of epidurally administered agonists across the dura into the CSF is dependent on the lipid solubility of the drug. Additionally, once in the CSF, opioids must pass from the water phase of the CSF into the lipid phase of the underlying neuraxis to reach the receptor. This too is dependent on lipid solubility. Hydrophilic agents such as morphine will have a greater latency and duration of action than more lipid-soluble agents such as fentanyl. On the other hand, the lipid-soluble agonists produce more segmental analgesia with less rostral spread than the less lipid-soluble agonists.

Even when administered via the caudal route, epidural morphine has been shown to provide effective postoperative analgesia following abdominal, thoracic, and cardiac surgery. Krane and co-workers recently reported that 0.03 mg per kg of caudal-epidural morphine is equally effective as 0.1 mg per kg in providing postoperative analgesia, although the higher dose provides a significantly longer duration of analgesia (13.3 ± 4.7 versus 10.0 ± 3.3 hours, respectively). The incidence of side effects was the same in both groups, although one patient receiving 0.1 mg per kg developed late respiratory depression. Therefore, these investigators suggest starting with the lower dose when using this technique. Whether even lower doses would be effective is unknown.

Spinal opiates produce analgesia without altering autonomic or neuromuscular function. Additionally both light touch and proprioception are preserved. Thus, unlike local anesthetics, spinal opioids allow patients to ambulate without orthostatic hypotension. Common side effects of intrathecal and epidural narcotics include facial or segmental pruritus, urinary retention, nausea and vomiting, and respiratory depression. These side effects occur with greater frequency when opioids are administered intrathecally as opposed to epidurally. Except for urinary retention, reversal of adverse side effects with maintenance of adequate analgesia can be achieved through the use of a low-dose (0.001 to 0.002 mg · kg^{-1}) naloxone infusion. Pruritus and nausea also can be treated with intravenous or oral diphenhydramine (Benadryl), 0.5 to 1.0 mg per kg, or hydroxyzine (Vistaril, Atarax). Urinary retention has not been a reported complication in children because in the majority of pediatric patients studied to date, all patients have had bladder catheters as part of their postoperative management regimen.

Although rare, respiratory depression is a major risk when intrathecal and epidural opioids are used. Attia and colleagues demonstrated that the ventilatory response to carbon dioxide is depressed for as long as 22 hours following the administration of 0.05 mg · kg^{-1} of morphine epidurally. Following intrathecal morphine administration (0.02 mg per kg), in children between 3 month and 15 years, Nichols and co-workers demonstrated significant depression of the ventilatory response

to carbon dioxide for up to 18 hours. The greatest respiratory depression correlated with the highest CSF morphine levels (2,863 ± 542 ng per ml), which occurred 6 hours after administration. This depression persisted despite a fall in CSF morphine levels 12 (641 ± 219 ng per ml) to 18 (223 ± 152 ng per ml) hours later. This confirms the clinical impression that respiratory depression usually occurs within the first 6 hours after the administration of epidural or intrathecal morphine but may occur as long as 18 hours afterward.

In clinical practice, respiratory depression most commonly occurs when intravenous or intramuscular narcotics have been administered to supplement the intrathecal opioid. The risk of respiratory depression can be minimized if smaller doses of supplemental narcotics are used, or through the epidural use of shorter-acting, more lipid-soluble agents (fentanyl, sufentanil), which produce more segmental analgesia, with little rostral spread. On the other hand, because of their shorter duration of action, fentanyl and sufentanil are increasingly being administered by continuous epidural infusion, either alone or in combination with very dilute (1/16 percent, [0.0625 mg per ml] or 0.1 percent [1.0 mg per ml]) bupivacaine concentrations. Typically, the epidural solution contains 1 to 2 µg per ml of fentanyl, with or without bupivacaine, and is administered at rates ranging between 0.2 and 1.0 ml per kg per hour. This provides effective analgesia for both postoperative and chronic cancer pain. Sufentanil (0.1 to 0.2 µg per kg), the only drug approved for epidural use by the FDA, has been shown to provide effective analgesia in children ranging between 4 and 12 years for about 2 hours.

Regardless of the opioid and route of administration a regular system of monitoring for respiratory depression is required. Clinical signs that predict impending respiratory depression include somnolence, small pupils, and small tidal volumes. We also insist on the use of oxyhemoglobin saturation monitoring (pulse oximetry), particularly in the first 24 hours after institution of this therapy.

LOCAL ANESTHETICS

The use of local anesthetics in pediatric practice has recently undergone a revolutionary metamorphosis. For decades children were considered poor candidates for regional anesthetic techniques because of their overwhelming fear of needles. However, once it was recognized that regional anesthesia could be used as an adjunct, and not a replacement for general anesthesia, its use has increased exponentially. Furthermore, because catheters placed in the epidural, pleural, and other spaces can be used for days or months, local anesthetics are increasingly being used for postoperative, neuropathic, and terminal pain relief. To be used safely, a working knowledge of the differences in how local anesthetics are metabolized in infants and children is necessary.

The ester local anesthetics are metabolized by

plasma cholinesterase. Neonates and infants up to 6 months of age have less than half of the adult levels of this plasma enzyme. Clearance may thereby be reduced and the effects of ester local anesthetics prolonged. Amides, on the other hand, are metabolized in the liver and bound by plasma proteins. Neonates and young infants (less than 3 months of age) have reduced liver blood flow and immature metabolic degradation pathways. Thus, larger fractions of local anesthetics are unmetabolized and remain active in the plasma than in the adult. More local anesthetic is excreted in the urine unchanged. Furthermore, neonates and infants may be at increased risk for the toxic effects of amide local anesthetics because of lower levels of albumin and alpha-1 acid glycoproteins, which are proteins essential for drug binding. This leads to increased concentrations of free drug and potential toxicity, particularly with bupivacaine. On the other hand, the larger volume of distribution at steady state seen in the neonate for these (and other) drugs may confer some clinical protection by lowering plasma drug levels.

The metabolism of the amide local anesthetic prilocaine is unique in that it results in the production of oxidants that can lead to the development of methemoglobinemia. This occurs in adults with doses of prilocaine greater than 600 mg. Because premature and full-term infants have decreased levels of methemoglobin reductase, they are more susceptible to developing methemoglobinemia. An additional factor rendering newborns more susceptible to methemoglobinemia is the relative ease by which fetal hemoglobin is oxidized compared to adult hemoglobin. Because of this, prilocaine can not be recommended for use in neonates. Unfortunately, this may limit the use of an exciting new topical local anesthetic, EMLA (eutectic mixture of local anesthetics), in the newborn.

Finholt and co-workers found that the volume of distribution, clearance, and elimination half-life of an intravenous bolus of lidocaine, 1 to 2 mg per kg, used to facilitate tracheal intubation or to treat arrhythmias, are similar in children older than 6 months of age and in adults. They recommend that lidocaine doses need not be altered based on age alone when lidocaine is administered intravenously. The elimination half-life of intravenously administered lidocaine in infants less than 6 months of age is prolonged, however. Since neonates have reduced protein binding, repeated administration of lidocaine may predispose these patients to toxic concentrations of drug. The routine administration of intravenous lidocaine in children with right-to-left intracardiac shunts may produce systemic toxicity. Normally,

approximately 60 to 80 percent of an intravenous lidocaine bolus is absorbed on the first pass through the lungs, then subsequently released over time. In patients with right-to-left intracardiac shunts, venous blood enters directly into the systemic circulation through the intracardiac defect, bypassing the lungs. Peak arterial concentrations of lidocaine would be expected to be higher and occur more rapidly. In fact, in lambs with right-to-left intracardiac shunts, lidocaine levels were double those of normal controls.

Fortunately, cardiovascular and central nervous system toxicity have rarely been observed in children following local anesthetic administration. The hemodynamic response to regional anesthesia, even after fairly extensive epidural blockade (cutaneous analgesia below T4 to T5), is minimal in children compared with adults. Convulsions have rarely been noted to date, probably because they may be masked or the seizure threshold may be increased by the concomitant use of sedatives, particularly the benzodiazepines. Alternatively, children may be less sensitive to the toxic effects of local anesthetics than adults. This is unlikely though. Several animal studies have demonstrated that there are no significant differences in the sensitivity to the toxic effects of local anesthetics between newborn and adult animals. Indeed, we have recently seen bupivacaine toxicity (seizures, arrhythmias) following prolonged epidural infusions of concentrated (0.25 percent) bupivacaine.

SUGGESTED READING

Anand KJ, Hickey PR. Pain and its effects in the human neonate and fetus. N Engl J Med 1987; 317:1321–1329.
Berde CB. Pediatric postoperative pain management. Pediatr Clin North Am 1989; 36:921–964.
Beyer JB, Wells N. The assessment of pain in children. Pediatr Clin North Am 1989; 36:837–854.
Cousins MJ, Mather LE. Intrathecal and epidural administration of opioids. Anesthesiology 1984; 61:276–310.
Shannon M, Berde CB. Pharmacologic management of pain in children and adolescents. Pediatr Clin North Am 1989; 36:855–872.
Shapiro BS. The management of pain in sickle cell disease. Pediatr Clin North Am 1989; 36:1029–1045.
Yaster M, Deshpande JK. Management of pediatric pain with opioid analgesics. J Pediatr 1988; 113:421–429.
Yaster M, Maxwell LG. Pain management. In Hoekelman RA, Friedman SB, Nelson NM, Seidel HM, eds. Primary pediatric care, 2nd ed. (in press).
Yaster M, Maxwell LG. Pediatric regional anesthesia. Anesthesiology 1989; 70:324–338.
Yaster M, Nicholas E, Maxwell LG. The use of opioids in pediatric anesthesia and in the management of childhood pain. Anesthesiol Clin North Am (in press).

ANESTHESIA FOR OTOLARYNGOLOGIC PROCEDURES

ENDOSCOPY

ROGER GRAYSON, M.D.

Broadly defined, anesthesia for endoscopy includes a discussion of bronchoscopy, esophagoscopy, thoracoscopy, and mediastinoscopy. The last two are discussed in other chapters. For most surgical procedures performed in the operating room, the airway remains the exclusive responsibility of the anesthesiologist; yet when anesthesia is required for endoscopy of the pharynx, larynx, bronchi, or esophagus, the anesthesiologist is required to share the airway but remain its protector at the same time. No matter what procedure the surgeon or endoscopist plans, and no matter which technique the anesthesiologist chooses, avoidable and possibly catastrophic problems can arise unless the endoscopist and anesthesiologist have collectively discussed each other's needs and plans on a case-by-case basis. Preoperative communication between the two clinicians will help clarify (1) whether the endoscopist needs to have the patient asleep; (2) what the position of the bed will be in relation to the anesthesia machine; (3) where the anesthesiologist will be positioned; (4) what kind of bronchoscope will be used; (5) whether muscle relaxants can be used; (6) what kind of endotracheal tube (ETT), if any, will be required, and whether it should be inserted via the nose or the mouth; (7) where the ETT will be secured (taped or sutured); (8) whether a tracheostomy will be required, and if so, at what point during the procedure; (9) what were the findings of indirect laryngoscopy, and (10) what is the known extent of airway pathology: is it friable or obstructing air flow, and is there vocal cord paralysis or significant tracheal distortion? Knowing these details will help the anesthesiologist and endoscopist estimate the duration of the anticipated procedure, determine whether intubation is required and whether it should be done awake or after induction, decide which induction agents and relaxants are best, choose a method of ventilation (e.g., Venturi jet vs. intermittent apneic vs. uninterrupted positive pressure mechanical vs. high frequency vs. assisted spontaneous), and decide how to manipulate the agents to best enable a smooth emergence that maintains airway patency after airway ma-

nipulation. Ready access to and maintenance of the airway is a cardinal principle for the safe practice of our specialty, but during these procedures this tenet is compromised. Preoperatively, therefore, the operating room team should establish a coordinated plan for unequivocally securing the airway in the event of intraoperative airway compromise.

PREOPERATIVE EVALUATION

As with all patients, a thorough review of the history and preoperative work-up, a physical examination, and a review of laboratory data are required. Particular attention must be paid, of course, to data relating to airway patency and pulmonary function. The patient should be questioned about stridor, wheezing, snoring, mouth breathing, and sleep apnea and examined for neck mobility, mouth opening, Mallampati signs (visualizable uvula), receding mandible, and tracheal deviation. The results of indirect laryngoscopy, previous awake fiberoptic examinations, magnetic resonance imaging (MRI) or computed tomography (CT) scans, arteriography, fluoroscopy, or pulmonary function tests can all help determine the size and location (intrathoracic vs. extrathoracic) of masses, tumors, and foreign bodies. Previous medical records document the use of radiation or operations, including whether intubation was difficult and the size of ETT used. If nasal intubation is anticipated, it is appropriate to check the clotting status.

Special attention should be directed toward detecting stridor or wheezing, especially if the patient complains of such symptoms. Inspiratory stridor is associated with extrathoracic lesions, while expiratory stridor suggests intrathoracic obstruction. Stridor may also be absent with quiet respiration but become apparent with varying levels of exertion. In any case, the symptom connotes airway narrowing. Wheezing, on the other hand, often reflects smaller airway narrowing and may be unilateral, as with foreign body aspiration. Clearly, a patient with additional known reactive airway disease who is about to undergo a stimulating airway procedure is at significant risk of experiencing generalized wheezing. Rhonchi (retained airway secretions) may reflect generalized pulmonary insufficiency with impaired mucociliary transport, or may be secondary to an inability to clear secretions distal to an obstruction. The assessment of these factors may actually help direct the choice of anesthetic technique. A severely obstructed upper airway may require securing the airway first (e.g., fiberoptic intubation, tracheostomy) with the patient awake. Jet ventilation may not be indicated in patients who have a foreign body that might be blown more distally down the airway, or in patients with significantly decreased overall pulmonary or chest wall compliance where it may not be possible to deliver an adequate tidal volume. Patients with sleep apnea (including children with, for example, chronic tonsillitis) may have pulmonary hypertension and marginal right heart function due to chronic hypercarbia. Further elevation of $PaCO_2$ or depression of contractility, as might occur during induction with spontaneous assisted ventilation and a volatile agent, may be enough to precipitate heart failure.

PREMEDICATION

Premedication is usually thought of as pharmacologic only (in the form of antisialagogues, anxiolytics, narcotics); an additional psychological concept should be stressed. If flexible bronchoscopy or esophagoscopy in the awake patient is being considered, a calm and unhurried preoperative discussion with the patient of what is likely to happen in the operating room can be most helpful in ensuring maximal patient cooperation. Most adults respond very positively to a quiet, nonthreatening explanation of the need to use topical and local anesthetics (oropharyngeal spray, IX and X nerve blocks, transtracheal injections) to maximize their comfort intraoperatively. The use of intravenous benzodiazepines and narcotics, which may critically impair a patient with marginal respiratory drive, can often be kept to a minimum or occasionally eliminated entirely. The elderly are especially sensitive to the respiratory depressant effects of these agents.

Antimuscarinic agents (atropine, glycopyrrolate, scopolamine) to diminish oropharyngeal secretions and maintain a clear dry endoscopic view of the airway are indispensable. When local anesthetics are used in a dry airway, they are more effective by directly reaching the airway mucosa itself and not being washed away or diluted with secretions and removed during suctioning. By decreasing the need for suctioning, functional residual capacity and oxygenation may also be better maintained. The unpredictable dysphoria seen with scopolamine makes this agent less ideal.

If spontaneous ventilation is deemed adequate, carefully titrated doses of benzodiazepines (midazolam, diazepam) can provide effective angiolysis and even some amnesia. For use in children, 0.5 to 1.0 mg per kilogram of midazolam (diluted to 5 to 10 ml in sodium chloride) per rectum has resulted in remarkably acceptable sedation for fiberoptic bronchoscopy without respiratory depression. While narcotics do have the abovementioned deleterious effects, they inhibit the cough reflex and provide some analgesia. Although analgesia in the awake patient should be primarily achieved with local anesthetics, small doses of narcotics in closely monitored patients may be helpful.

The use of histamine$_2$ blockers the morning of surgery and perhaps the evening before should be considered, especially in patients with a known risk of reflux. For the patient whose airway has been anesthetized with topic sprays or nerve blocks, protective reflexes are compromised as well, and histamine$_2$ blockers afford some protection.

SPECIAL MONITORING CONSIDERATIONS

A careful preoperative assessment, as is done for any patient, will help determine which hemodynamic monitors are necessary. A few special comments are in order for endoscopy.

During the course of either fiberoptic or rigid bronchoscopy, periods often arise when the resistance to ventilation increases. This may be due to the bronchoscope obstructing the existing airway or the ETT, because the rigid ventilating scope is electively placed down a mainstem bronchus, or because of tumor disruption, bleeding, or secretions. From the beginning of the procedure, the airway pressure gauge should be closely followed for sudden increases (obstruction, pneumothorax) or decreases (extubation, airway leak, or disconnect).

Breath sounds heard with the usual precordial stethoscope may largely reflect an air leak around the cords during rigid bronchoscopy. True alveolar ventilation may not be indicated by transmitted tracheal noise. Movement of the chest, both up and down, is at least another indicator of inspiration and expiration. Chest movement should be carefully noted at the beginning of the procedure so that any subsequent changes (pneumothorax, air trapping) can be more easily recognized.

When each lung is to be examined separately, placing a different precordial stethoscope on each side of the chest and connecting them using a three-way stopcock can allow either selective or simultaneous auscultation of the lungs.

Jet ventilation may quickly lower the temperature of infants if cool dry gases are used.

LOCAL ANESTHESIA FOR THE AIRWAY

The effective use of local anesthetics for the airway is an indispensable part of the anesthetic management of patients undergoing fiberoptic bronchoscopy in the awake/sedated state. They may also be used to help block the sympathetic responses provoked during rigid bronchoscopy in fully anesthetized patients. Once airway reflexes are blocked, patients are at increased risk for aspiration, whether in the awake state or emerging from general anesthesia.

Preparing the nasopharynx for passing a fiberoptic bronchoscope and endotracheal tube involves gradually passing a series of Q tips soaked in 2 to 5 percent cocaine, or a lidocaine and phenylephrine mixture, progressively deeper into the nose. This serves to anesthetize and vasoconstrict the nasal mucosa, thereby diminishing bleeding during intubation or endoscopic manipulations. This is especially crucial if nasal intubation is required in a patient with a clotting disorder. After one Q tip has been passed to the back of the nose, two and then three soaked Q tips together should be gradually advanced to further dilate the passageway. Then progressively larger nasal airways (from No. 26 to No. 34 French in adults) may be coated with anesthesia and gently inserted to further dilate the nasopharynx if nasal endotracheal intubation is planned. It is vital to note that blood in the airway greatly impairs the visual field during fiberoptic-guided endotracheal intubation, whether via the nose or mouth. Therefore the above process should not be rushed, and force should be avoided if an obstruction is felt during these steps. Cocaine is an effective topical anesthetic and vasoconstrictor. Were it not for the occasionally severe cardiac (hypertension, tachycardia, even angina) and central nervous system stimulatory side effects, cocaine would be an ideal topical agent. Lidocaine (4 percent) mixed with phenylephrine (0.5 percent) can achieve the same combination of anesthesia and vasoconstriction. Alternatively, 30 to 60 ml of lidocaine jelly may be mixed with 10 to 20 mg of phenylephrine and five to ten sprays of 10 percent lidocaine spray to form a slurry that is an effective topical anesthetic, vasoconstrictor, and lubricant with negligible systemic side effects. This slurry is used to coat the Q tips, nasal airways, and then ETT before their insertion and is probably our preferred technique.

Topical anesthesia to the oropharynx may be achieved with anesthetic sprays, lozenges, ultrasonic nebulizers, soaked cotton balls, or an oral airway coated with lidocaine jelly or ointment. The last-named is sometimes useful in children, while adults and many children readily accept anesthetic sprays or nebulized anesthetics via a face mask or mouthpiece. This route is also effective in delivering anesthetic to the trachea and larger bronchi. It is questionable, however, how much of the nebulized drug is actually delivered to the distal respiratory bronchi, since commonly used nebulizers generally produce droplets larger than the size of these bronchi (1 to 2 μm). Depending on patient size, nebulizing 2 to 4 ml of 4 or 5 percent lidocaine usually gives satisfactory results. A portion of the drug is lost during its administration in the expiratory phase of respiration, although some nebulizers deliver drug only during inspiration.

Topical (mucosal) anesthesia to the oropharynx, however, does not block submucosal pressure receptors at the base of the tongue that provoke the gag reflex. Blocking this requires glossopharyngeal (cranial nerve IX) and superior laryngeal nerve (SLN) blocks. The lingual branch of nerve IX may be readily blocked with 1 to 2 ml of 1 percent lidocaine injected at the lateral base of each side of the tongue in the palatoglossal arch.

A 25-gauge or smaller needle should be inserted only 1 cm while aspirating to guard against an intravascular (e.g., carotid artery) injection. The posterior third of the tongue and the pharyngeal surface of the epiglottis will be anesthetized, facilitating use of a MacIntosh blade for gentle laryngoscopy. This block is best done after using anesthetic spray to the oropharynx. The superior laryngeal nerve (internal branch) of the vagus (X) may be blocked topically by placing an anesthetic-soaked sponge gently along the curve of the tongue into each pyriform sinus. This is effective because the SLN is submucosal at this location. Again, this is best done after use of an oropharyngeal anesthetic spray. This peroral (topical) approach may be best when a carcinoma or infection prevents the safe installation of an SLN block percutaneously through the thyrohyoid membrane. This approach may be difficult to perform, however, if the patient has restricted mouth opening. Alternatively, the SLN can be blocked with 1 to 2 ml of 1 percent lidocaine injected percutaneously into the thyrohyoid membrane on each side just anterior to the superior thyroid cornu. Since this site is just anterior to the carotid artery, the artery should be gently retracted posteriorly and, of course, one should aspirate before injecting. This blocks the base of the tongue, the laryngeal (posterior) surface of the epiglottis, and the laryngeal aperture, thereby permitting use of a Miller blade usually without provoking a cough. The trachea may be anesthetized with nebulized anesthetics as described above, or by a transtracheal injection through the cricothyroid membrane. A safe technique includes first making a skin wheal, then puncturing the membrane with a 22- or 20-gauge catheter over needle connected to a syringe being aspirated. Once air is aspirated, the needle is removed, the catheter is aspirated to reconfirm the intratracheal location of the catheter, and 3 to 4 ml of 2 to 4 percent lidocaine is rapidly injected. The injection usually provokes a cough and deep inspiration, which serves to further distribute the anesthetic to the underside of the vocal cords and down the airway. Gently restraining the patient's head by having an assistant place a hand on the forehead will help minimize patient movement during the cough. If a fiberoptic bronchoscope is being used, lidocaine may be instilled via the suction port into the airway at any level. To minimize patient coughing and bucking when the scope of the ETT enters the trachea, it is useful to first inject 2 to 4 ml of 2 to 4 percent lidocaine at the cords and down the trachea when the cords come into view. (However, a transtracheal injection often obviates the need for this.)

GENERAL ANESTHESIA

When general anesthesia is necessary for either rigid or flexible fiberoptic bronchoscopy, the first requirement is to assess airway patency and determine whether supraglottic access will be adequate to permit intubation with either the rigid bronchoscope or a standard ETT. The use of local anesthesia to the supraglottic structures as described above will permit gentle laryngoscopy in most awake and sedated patients, especially if they have been informed beforehand of this plan. A sufficient view of the supraglottic structures can usually be obtained by direct vision with a MacIntosh blade to decide whether intubation can be achieved. If doubts exist, general anesthesia is more wisely induced after first securing the airway by awake intubation (usually with fiberoptics) or tracheostomy. A MacIntosh may be the blade of first choice since it is generally considered slightly less likely to cause trauma to airway tissues, but other blades may be used. The Miller blade may be more capable of compressing glottic tissue into the space behind the mandible and ultimately providing a better view. The key words for such a laryngoscopy are "gentle" and "atraumatic," because obstructing tissues may be very friable and bleeding may be provoked with surprisingly little instrumentation. Once the airway becomes bloody, both direct and fiberoptic intubation quickly become very difficult, and loss of the airway due to edema and blood is a risk. Before the introduction of fiberoptics, induction was often produced by spontaneous assisted ventilation and a volatile agent with 100 percent oxygen or an oxygen-helium mixture. Muscle relaxants were avoided until adequate mask ventilation could be demonstrated. Although this is still an option, total loss of the airway can sometimes occur only after induction, as the tone of airway structures is decreased and the narrowed airway is further compromised. In neonates with suspected severe congenital airway pathology (web, vocal cord paralysis, laryngomalacia, coanal atresia), protecting the airway may require that endoscopy be performed with the patient awake and restrained. The endoscopist will also thereby be able to observe abnormal airway movement.

Once the airway is secured, anesthesia may be maintained with volatile agents or a combination of narcotics and neuroleptics. Muscle relaxants are usually advisable, because the consequences of a patient bucking violently during airway instrumentation, especially with a rigid bronchoscope, are severe: e.g., unnecessary bleeding, airway rupture. The choice of maintenance agents should also take into account the need for good spontaneous ventilation and the end of the procedure. Excessive use of narcotics with benzodiazepines may cause unwanted depression of respiratory drive. Excessive residual volatile agent may require a prolonged period to eliminate after extubation if a partially obstructed airway is compromising alveolar ventilation. Indeed, the airway may be worse postoperatively than preoperatively owing to airway edema. Nitrous oxide would usually be considered in an attempt to decrease the required dose of narcotics, neuroleptics, or volatile agents. However, the use of nitrous oxide obviously decreases the FiO_2 delivered and may exacerbate a pneumothorax should it occur. If less than 100 percent oxygen is preferred, air or helium may be substituted for nitrous oxide. Therefore, knowledge of the patient's airway pathology and general medical condition, the surgeon's plan, and the expected duration of the procedure are all important in choosing maintenance agents. Communication is crucial.

Ventilation may be maintained by a variety of techniques, depending on whether the endoscopist plans to use a flexible fiberoptic or rigid bronchoscope. Ventilation for flexible bronchoscopy may be accomplished either by placing an ETT large enough to permit the bronchoscope to be passed through the ETT (via a special diaphragm connector), with ventilation continuing around the scope through the narrowed ETT lumen, or by placing a small enough ETT through the cords to permit the bronchoscope to be passed adjacent to the ETT through the cords (often causing some gas leak around the cuff). In either case, ventilation during the endoscopy is achieved through a lumen smaller than would otherwise be used for a given patient. This may require larger than usual ventilatory pressures from the anesthesia machine during inspiration, although actual airway pressures may be lower. Ventilating by hand during this period is often more effective than machine-delivered breaths, and chest excursion should be closely followed, especially in children. It is important to allow sufficient time between breaths to permit adequate expiration, because decreased flow rates through the narrowed ETT lumen can lead to an overexpanded chest with decreased venous return or pneumothorax. The pulse oximeter usually accurately reflects oxygenation. However, the end-tidal carbon dioxide, if measured at the ETT connector, may read falsely low if dead space to tidal volume ventilation has proportionally increased owing to incomplete expiration of alveolar gas through the narrowed ETT.

Continuous ventilation for rigid bronchoscopy may be achieved via a side-arm attachment that allows either jet ventilation, high-frequency ventilation, or use of the usual circle system for controlled or assisted ventilation. High-frequency ventilation has the advantage of providing a nonmoving surgical field and is potentially less risky when bullous emphysema or airway rupture is suspected. However, it makes the detection of airway obstruction more difficult. Ventilating via a side-arm using a circle system allows for humidification and warming of gases, which is especially important in children. Furthermore, scavenging exhaled vapor is possible. The anesthesiologist can also sense changes in compliance in the reservoir bag that may reflect either less than ideal positioning of the scope in the bronchus or true lung compliance changes.

Intermittent apneic ventilation may be used to ventilate for either flexible or rigid bronchoscopy. The patient is hyperventilated with 100 percent oxygen for a few minutes to drive the $PaCO_2$ down (preferably to 30 mm Hg or below) and raise the PaO_2 to a very high level. Ventilation is then stopped while bronchoscopy proceeds for a few minutes. In the case of rigid bronchoscopy, ventilation usually takes place through the bronchoscope side-arm or down the center lumen, using a jet apparatus. When ventilation is interrupted, this scope remains in place for endoscopy. For flexible bronchoscopy, ventilation must take place via an ETT, which is then removed during endoscopy, and reinserted when further ventilation is required. Periods of apnea will be accompanied by rising $PaCO_2$ (5 to 10 or even 15 mm Hg in the first minute and 3 to 4 mm Hg per minute thereafter) and falling PaO_2. Because a pulse oximeter reading 100 percent can reflect such wide variations in PaO_2, following oxygen saturation alone may not be sufficient to predict when ventilation should resume. Elevated $PaCO_2$ with acidosis, elevated pulmonary artery pressure, and the risk of arrhythmia may be of greater concern. The duration of apnea should be carefully followed with an eye toward estimating the $PaCO_2$. To minimize the drop in PaO_2 during periods of apnea, low-flow oxygen may be insufflated through the flexible scope suction part or through the bronchoscope side-arm. Such flow should be discontinued if the bronchoscope is wedged tightly in a smaller bronchus, to avoid a pneumothorax. Alternatively, a separate catheter insufflating oxygen may be placed at the carina.

Unique problems during anesthetic emergence can occur after bronchoscopy. Edema, bleeding, or bronchospasm may result in worse pulmonary function than before surgery. If a preoperative check of arterial blood gases on room air was marginal, it may be worse postoperatively. Intraoperative pneumothorax is also more likely with these procedures than with others. Therefore, supplemental humidified oxygen, a chest x-ray examination, and oxygen saturation monitoring with a pulse oximeter should be standard postanesthesia practice. Steroids, nebulized racemic epinephrine, and other bronchodilators should be immediately available and may need to be used in the operating room. Ultimately, a few patients may require reintubation. One might initially decide not to extubate in the first place.

Anesthesia for laser surgery is discussed elsewhere, but two recent developments merit comment. In an effort to minimize the risk of ETT ignition, ETTs are often wrapped. Until recently, no ETT wrap had been sanctioned for use by the FDA; in fact, none of the former wraps (e.g., foil tapes) was ever considered a medical device. Recently one wrap (Laser Guard, Merocel Corporation) has received FDA acceptance and has received generally positive testing reports by the nonprofit Emergency Care Research Institute (ECRI). To be effective, however, the ETT must be carefully wrapped to avoid any gaps between the seams of the Laser Guard, and the ETT should not be sterilized once the wrap has been applied because sterilization (e.g., with ethylene oxide) will cause the wrap to peel away from the ETT. Also, the wrap (essentially a foam sponge with a sticky metal backing) must be kept moist throughout the procedure.

A new laser technique, the holmium laser, may prove a useful addition to ENT surgery. This laser is especially useful in resecting bone and therefore may be well suited to endoscopic nasal surgery, which could be performed under local anesthesia with sedation. For such procedures, it is common to provide patients with insufflated supplemental oxygen by mouth when lasers are not employed. If the laser is used, such added oxygen should be discontinued.

ESOPHAGOSCOPY

Esophagoscopy may be performed for problems referable to the esophagus (e.g., achalasia, foreign body obstruction, hiatal hernia) or problems arising from the airway that may involve the esophagus (e.g., an infiltrating neoplasm). Esophagoscopy may be performed with a flexible esophagoscope and local topical anesthesia in a sedated patient, or may be done on an anesthetized patient with either a flexible or rigid esophagoscope. In either case, these patients have frequently had a period of poor dietary intake before the procedure, and yet the nature of the lesion requires the anesthetist to consider the patient at risk for aspiration of gastric or retained esophageal contents. The patients may be hypovolemic and hypoalbuminemic, predisposing them to hemodynamic instability and local anesthetic toxicity. Irrespective of which scope or anesthetic technique is used, preoperative administration of H_2 receptor blockers and clear antacid, such as 30 ml of sodium citrate, helps reduce the sequelae of unintended aspiration. A large retained esophageal volume including undigested food may be waiting to greet the endoscopist. It is therefore reasonable to attempt to remove this volume, especially before general anesthetic induction. Only a soft-suction catheter should be used for this, however, since the thin-walled, serosal free esophagus is indeed at risk of perforation if the more standard, stiffer nasogastric tubes or plastic suction catheters are used. After such suctioning, the sodium citrate is administered.

The performance of esophagoscopy with local anesthesia usually requires the use of a topical spray to the oropharynx and swallowed anesthetic reaching the esophagus. However, a large retained esophageal volume may limit the effectiveness of any anesthetic that reaches this area. If coughing ensues during esophagoscopy, the patient is at risk of perforation, especially if the objective is to remove a sharp foreign body. Therefore, general anesthesia using a rapid-sequence induction and muscle relaxation is often preferred, although this incurs new hazards. The risks include aspiration and esophageal perforation during the application of cricoid pressure or during placement of the ETT owing to anterior compression of the esophagus. Removal of an upper esophageal foreign body appears to involve a special risk of such esophageal perforation during rapid sequence induction. If the maintenance of airway integrity during a rapid-sequence induction is considered uncertain, an awake fiberoptic-guided intubation is necessary.

SUGGESTED READING

Gaskill JR, Gillies DR. Local anesthesia for peroral endoscopy. Arch Otolaryngol 1966; 84:654–657.

Laser-resistant endotracheal tubes and wraps. In: Bond PM, ed. Emergency care research institute (ECRI) health devices. 1990; 19:109–139.

Mallampati SR. Clinical sign to predict difficult tracheal intubation. Clin J Anesthesiol 1985; 32:429–434.

Norton ML, Brown ACD. Evaluating the patient with a difficult airway for anesthesia. Otolaryngol Clin North Am 1990; 23:771–785.

Ovassapian A. Fiberoptic airway endoscopy in anesthesia and critical care. New York: Raven Press, 1990.

Woods A. Pediatric bronchoscopy, bronchography, and laryngoscopy. In: Berry FA, ed. Anesthetic management of difficult and routine pediatric patients. New York: Churchill Livingstone, 1986.

HEAD AND NECK CANCER

DEVANAND MANGAR, M.D.
ENRICO CAMPORESI, M.D.

Providing anesthesia for head and neck surgery in which the surgical field may surround or directly involve the airway greatly challenges the ingenuity and expertise of the anesthesiologist. The anesthesiologist must provide general anesthesia for the patient, an uninterrupted airway during surgery and recovery, and an unobstructed field for the surgeon. Patients with head and neck cancer are often fragile, high-risk noncardiac surgery patients. Medical consultation for patients with chronic concomitant disease should be elicited in all cases.

Endotracheal general anesthesia is the preferred technique for these patients. Rapid induction and intubation using short-acting barbiturates and intravenous muscle relaxants are not employed unless a patent airway is ensured. In the event of abnormal tissue obscuring the airway, restriction of jaw motion, or distortion of the face that precludes a satisfactory mask fit for oxygenation, endotracheal intubation must be accomplished before induction of general anesthesia.

Surgical procedures may last 8 to 12 hours in patients who often have a history of tobacco and alcohol abuse. These patients are usually older and may have associated cardiopulmonary diseases. Such factors intensify the potential problems related to increased blood loss, fluid and electrolyte changes, dysrhythmias, and airway difficulty. Moreover, both the surgeon and anesthesiologist are working in the same anatomic area and the anesthesiologist is usually physically separated from the airway. Hence, the endotracheal tube must be carefully secured.

The choice of techniques and drugs for general anesthesia depend on condition of the patient. The mode of intubation to be used is determined by the presence of extremely friable or exophytic lesions in the airway and the possibility of dislodging cancerous tissue into the tracheobronchial tree. Previous radiotherapy may cause complications of osteoradionecrosis of the mandible and trismus caused by soft tissue scar contraction.

Prophylactic antibiotic therapy for endocarditis and postoperative wound infection may be necessary.

PREOPERATIVE EVALUATION

The patient's history is taken, and a physical examination and careful review of organ system function affected by coexisting disease are carried out. The anesthesiologist should review current drug therapy and elicit details relating to previous anesthetic experience of the patient or the patient's blood relatives. It is also important to inform the patient and family about what to expect on the day of surgery. The anesthetic technique should be discussed, including a description of potential complications. A good preoperative visit reduces patient anxiety and thereby also reduces the need for heavy premedication. This is especially important in patients with obstructive airway disease.

The physical examination should primarily involve evaluation of the upper airway, lungs, and cardiovascular system. Special attention should be directed to detection of cardiac murmurs, carotid bruits, and abnormal breath sounds. Appropriate preoperative studies to evaluate the airway fully enables the anesthesiologist and surgeon to devise an optimal plan of management.

Cardiac Evaluation

In patients who have experienced an infarction less than 3 months before surgery and anesthesia, the incidence of perioperative infarction is 27 to 37 percent, while patients with a history of previous myocardial infarction more than 6 months before surgery have a 6 to 7 percent overall risk of reinfarction during the perioperative period. In this population at risk, evaluation of the ejection fraction by nuclear V-gram is of paramount importance to assess ventricular function. Preoperative optimization of the patient's status coupled with aggressive invasive hemodynamic monitoring may decrease perioperative morbidity.

Cardiac evaluation should concentrate on detection of hypertension, rhythm disturbances, jugular venous distention, third heart sounds, significant murmurs, edema, critical aortic stenosis, and diminished peripheral pulses.

Pulmonary Evaluation

Since many patients presenting for head and neck surgery are heavy smokers, the preoperative pulmonary evaluation should include screening for chronic obstructive pulmonary disease (COPD), dyspnea, cough, wheezing, rhonchi, abnormal sputum production, and prolonged expiratory phase.

Indications for preoperative pulmonary function tests (PFT) include a history of smoking, chronic cough, age greater than 70 years, obesity, history of thoracic or upper abdominal surgery, and pulmonary disease. The test provides a baseline and aids in identifying patients at risk for postoperative pulmonary complications.

Arterial blood gases should be obtained in elderly patients, those with obvious pulmonary disease, or with moderate-to-severely affected PFTs. Postoperative oxygen therapy needs can be better anticipated if the chronic arterial oxygen pressure (PaO_2) and arterial carbon dioxide pressure ($PaCO_2$) are known. The importance of incentive spirometry should be discussed preoperatively, especially since postoperative pulmonary complications after general anesthesia may be decreased with this technique when combined with chest physiotherapy and other treatment modalities.

Patients with asthma should have bronchodilators continued during the perioperative period. If necessary, aminophylline and steroids may be administered to patients with severe disease.

The anesthesiologist will also encounter patients who have received bleomycin in their chemotherapy regimen. Occasionally these patients develop interstitial lung disease, and the risk of perioperative adult respiratory distress syndrome (ARDS) must be considered. Minimizing inspired oxygen concentration and avoidance of fluid overload may reduce this risk.

Airway Evaluation

A careful preoperative evaluation of the patient's airway is necessary to minimize the risk of loss of airway patency during induction of anesthesia. It is imperative to consult with the surgeon and to review radiologic examinations such as computed axial tomography (CAT) scans and the reports of prior endoscopy in order to predict potential airway problems during induction of anesthesia.

Examination of the neck and face will help identify patients in whom difficult laryngoscopy and intubation can be expected. The presence of micrognathia (receding chin), large tongue and small mouth, short and stout neck, or limited cervical spine motion indicate that visualization of the larynx may be difficult or impossible. Prior irradiation, surgery, scarring, and contractures may make tracheal intubation difficult.

Patients may have deeply invasive tumors of the tongue that are not markedly large to the eye. Palpating the tongue can give a better estimate of the size of the lesion. Tumors of the tongue cannot be compressed by an upward lift of the laryngoscope. Lesions of the epiglottis, vocal cords, or piriform sinus may be large, edematous, and friable, and may make intubation of the trachea challenging if not impossible. Radiologic evaluation or CAT scan of the upper airway and appropriate consultation with the surgeon is of utmost importance to minimize risk of airway disaster. During the preoperative evaluation, one seeks to identify patients who may be more safely anesthetized by first securing a patent airway either by (1) topical local anesthesia, retrograde intubation, and awake, fiberoptic, or rigid laryngoscopy, or by (2) tracheostomy with the patient under local anesthesia.

Laboratory Evaluation

Laboratory tests should be obtained based on positive findings elicited during the history and physical examination as well as indicated by the complexity of the procedure and the age of the patient.

The minimum preoperative evaluation is a matter of controversy. For head and neck surgery patients receiving anticoagulants and as indicated by physical examination, the minimal preoperative laboratory tests should include a measurement of hemoglobin, a white blood cell count, and coagulation profiles. The need for baseline arterial blood gas and pulmonary function tests is based on the patient's pulmonary status. Patients with cardiopulmonary disease should undergo chest radiography and electrocardiography. Patients taking digoxin, aminophylline, and procainamide should have their plasma drug levels confirmed. Liver function tests can be helpful in patients at risk for hepatic disease secondary to alcohol abuse.

Nutritional Evaluation

Patients with head and neck cancer usually have a history of decreased appetite and oral intake, often resulting in a poor nutritional status. Inadequate intake may be manifested by tachycardia and orthostatic hypotension. It is important to initiate appropriate treatment for malnourished patients to improve immunocompetency and allow healing of surgical wounds. Patients who cannot take food by mouth can be nourished through a feeding tube or, in extreme cases, by hyperalimentation. If hypovolemia is present, anesthetics may not be well tolerated and the anesthesiologist will need to make appropriate alterations. Metabolic derangements (i.e., electrolyte disturbances and acid-base abnormalities) should be corrected preoperatively.

ADJUNCTIVE HYPERBARIC OXYGEN THERAPY

Hyperbaric oxygenation is presently used as a major adjunctive therapeutic tool in the management of postradiation syndrome of the head and neck. This modality requires repetitive exposure of the patient to increased oxygen tension inside an hyperbaric chamber, usually to a level of 2 atmospheres absolute. Most frequently, the patient is exposed to hyperbaric oxygen for 2 hours daily, for 20 to 40 treatments. The resulting microvascular growth in areas of postradiation tissue ischemia prepares the tissue for major flaps healing during the postoperative period. A special subset of patients who benefit from hyperbaric therapy suffer from mandibular osteoradionecrosis. In these patients, hyperbaric oxygenation often induces a dramatic relief of pain accompanying this complication after only a few treatments.

MONITORING

Intraoperative monitoring requirements include monitoring of blood pressure, heart and breath sounds, body temperature, electrocardiography, pulse oximetry, and capnography. Depending on the patient's cardiopulmonary status and the extent of planned neck dissection, an arterial cannula may be indicated for blood pressure monitoring. Arterial line placement is appropriate for the multiple arterial blood gas sampling required for patients with significant COPD. Also, depending on the patient's cardiac function and expected blood loss and the duration of the procedure, central venous lines or a pulmonary artery catheter may be indicated. In placing a central venous catheter, internal jugular vein access is inappropriate, since the line would be in the operative field. Therefore, subclavian access or antecubital access, which is frequently more difficult, may be required. It is recommended that subclavian access be obtained the night before surgery and that an x-ray film then be obtained in order to avoid unnecessary delay in the operating room.

A Foley catheter should be placed to monitor urine output and avoid bladder overdistention. Blood loss should be carefully monitored, and the use of weighing sponges should be included for this purpose. The placement of one or two large-bore peripheral intravenous lines will enable the anesthesiologist to replace blood and fluids rapidly.

Special attention should be paid to body positioning to prevent pressure sores and nerve injury. The head should be cradled in a soft headrest and maintained in the neutral position. Cerebral ischemia may result from venous or arterial occlusion secondary to extreme extension or lateral rotation of the neck. The eyes are particularly susceptible to damage and should be protected by lubrication and sealed with hypoallergenic tape or tarsorrhaphy. The upper extremities should be adequately padded to prevent brachial plexus injury, and the buttocks and heels should be padded to avoid pressure sores.

The greatest loss of body heat occurs by convection and radiation when the patient is anesthetized and uncovered. This can result in hypothermia and adverse physiologic effects including cardiac arrhythmias, decreased perfusion and oxygen delivery, prolongation of anesthetic drug action, and central nervous system depression. Techniques to avoid hypothermia include limiting skin exposure, warming intravenous fluids, increasing the environmental temperature, using heated mattress pads, and humidifying and warming anesthetic gases.

TECHNIQUES OF GENERAL ANESTHESIA

General anesthesia is administered endotracheally after the airway has been carefully surveyed by direct visualization and x-ray studies and following consultation with the surgeon. In the event that tracheostomy is performed with the patient under local anesthesia, the incision is usually located low in the neck and the distance from the tracheal stoma to the carina is relatively short. If warranted, the patient may be endotracheally intubated and a tracheostomy then performed. A polyvinylchloride (PVC) endotracheal tube is used, and once the tracheostomy has been performed, an anode tube is placed and secured by sutures to prevent accidental extubation. The anode tube is reinforced with a spiral wrapped wire embedded in the wall which resists kinking when bent. If a tracheostomy is required, the use of muscle relaxants is usually avoided until the tracheostomy is in place to allow spontaneous respiration. Administration of 100 percent oxygen before tracheostomy is advisable to build up oxygen reserve in case the airway is lost. Continued coughing and bucking after intubation may suggest that the tube has advanced too far and is irritating the carina or is lodged in one of the major bronchi.

It may be convenient to fix the connecting tube and adapters to the patient rather than to the operating table to prevent accidental extubation of the trachea when the surgeon moves the patient's head. Longer breathing circuits and tight-fitting connections will allow the anesthesiologist to move a distance from the patient's head, permitting unobstructed surgical access.

For cases in which the carbon laser will be used to vaporize a lesion, care must be taken to prevent combustion either of the tube or in the airway. PVC tubes support combustion, and metallic or muslin-wrapped tubes are preferable. Because both nitrous oxide and oxygen support combustion, helium with 30 percent to 40 percent oxygen can be administered.

Once the airway is safely secured, anesthesia can be induced with either intravenous or inhalation anesthesia. The three most commonly used inhalation agents—enflurane, isoflurane, and halothane—cause dose-related cardiovascular and respiratory depression. Depending on the patient's condition, the choice of an anesthetic agent may be that which least decreases cardiac output. Thus low-dose isoflurane and intravenous narcotics may provide the greatest hemodynamic stability. For patients with poor cardiac function, hemodynamic stability may be supported with the use of short-acting narcotics such as alfentanil and muscle relaxants such as vecuronium bromide. However, the use of muscle relaxants may be limited by the surgeon's need to evaluate nerve integrity during neck dissection. Nitrous oxide may also be used since it decreases the requirements for narcotics and potent inhalation agents. Intraoperatively, every effort should be made to maintain normovolemia.

Potential complications faced during head and neck surgery include pneumothorax, cardiac dysrhythmias, prolongation of the QT interval, cardiac arrest, and venous air embolism. Pneumothorax can result from the dissection and also from the tracheostomy with accompanying subcutaneous emphysema. Manipulation of the carotid sinus can result in cardiac dysrhythmias, wide fluctuations in blood pressure, and frequently, vagal slowing of the heart rate. The latter can be counteracted by supplemental intravenous doses of atropine. As much as 2 mg may be required in the adult. The surgeon must be informed about these complications and asked to stop surgical manipulation, thus eliminating the inciting stimulus. Occasionally a patient may exhibit hypotension that is unresponsive to atropine and cessation of surgical stimulus. In this situation, 5 to 10 mg of intravenous ephedrine may restore the patient's normal blood pressure and heart rate. Repeated difficulties may be circumvented by perivascular infiltration with a local anesthetic such as lidocaine to block the reflex.

Prolongation of the QT interval and cardiac arrest have been reported following right radical neck dissection. This increase in the QT interval has been shown to persist in patients for more than 2 months postoperatively. Patients may exhibit intraoperative episodes of atypical ventricular tachycardia known as "torsades de pointes." Prophylaxis of this phenomenon can be achieved by administration of beta-adrenergic blockers to prevent generation of ventricular extrasystole. If prolonged QT interval persists in cardiac pacing, left stellate ganglion pharmacologic blockade or left cervical thoracic sympathetic ganglionectomy may be beneficial.

Venous air embolism may occur during radical neck dissection since major vessels are exposed, allowing atmospheric air to enter the circulation. If the amount of air is sufficient to interfere with the ability of the right heart to pump blood to the lungs, the amount of expired carbon dioxide will decrease, the central venous pressure will increase, and the cardiac output will decrease. The presence of air will be immediately audible by precordial Doppler monitoring. The air can be removed by an in situ right atrial catheter or the patient may be rapidly placed in the Trendelenburg position to force the bubbles out from the heart through the superior vena cava and retrograde through the neck veins to exit at the surgical site. Other treatment modalities include raising the central venous pressure by forced inspiration, the use of inflatable G-suit, or positive end-expiratory pressure (PEEP).

Tumors may involve major vessels of the neck and require sacrifice of one or both internal jugular veins. Cerebral edema may occur secondary to decreased cerebral perfusion pressure and increased cerebral venous pressure. In cases in which tumor involvement requires sacrifice of the carotid artery, preoperative temporary occlusion of the artery by balloon during angiography in the conscious patient may determine the patient's tolerance of loss of blood flow from the involved vessel. Intraoperative electroencephalographic (EEG) monitoring should be instituted if the surgeon may sacrifice the carotid artery. Care should be taken to maintain adequate cerebral blood flow and normocarbia in these patients.

EXTUBATION AND RECOVERY

In patients who are shivering postoperatively, 25 to 50 mg of meperidine hydrochloride (Demerol) is effective in abolishing the shivering and also helps control pain.

Depending on the cardiopulmonary status of the patient and other organ systemic dysfunction, the anesthesiologist may decide to continue heavy narcotic sedation and mechanically support ventilation in the intensive care unit overnight. Patients should be fully awake when extubated, preferably by an anesthesiologist who has managed the case. In the patient who has undergone extensive surgery (in the oronasal cavity, pharynx, or lateral neck region), the surgical site may be swathed in bandages deliberately applied firmly to serve as pressure dressing and occasionally to limit neck motion. The tongue may be grossly edematous and the swallowing mechanism impaired by the presence of long sutures, packs, or prosthesis, thereby severely compromising the airway. The possibility of postoperative airway obstruction should be anticipated. An emergency tracheostomy set and a variety of intubation equipment should be readily available in the recovery area. In cases in which total laryngectomy was performed, the surgeon may decide to extubate the patient immediately after surgery, depending on the preoperative pulmonary function tests. In this case, extubation is carried out in the presence of the surgeon and the patient is allowed to breathe through the stoma.

The recovery room nurse should be thoroughly familiar with providing good tracheobronchial hygiene and pulmonary toilet, since these patients are prone to aspiration of secretions. Patients with excessive coughing secondary to tracheal tube irritation can be treated with 1.5 mg per kilogram of lidocaine intravenously or 2 ml of 2 to 4 percent lidocaine injected into the trachea. The antitussive, sedative, and analgesic properties of intravenous morphine can also be beneficial.

Good communication with the patient is essential to assess the patient's medical condition throughout the recovery period. Communication can be facilitated with a writing pad or an alphabetic board for patients who are unable to speak.

A postoperative chest x-ray examination may be ordered to rule out atelectasis, pneumothorax, and effusion and to verify feeding and tracheal tube position.

These patients are usually most comfortable sitting up, and as soon as their anesthetic status permits, they can be gradually raised to this position. Cyanosis of the lips and face is common because of the tight dressings and ligation of the external jugular veins. Edema of the face occurs early but may be minimized by a 30-degree head elevation. Patients who have undergone intraoral surgery, particularly that involving the tongue, breathe more easily and comfortably in the lateral position.

Patients with head and neck cancer usually do not require intensive care postoperatively, and it is preferable that they be taken from the recovery room to the surgical floor to a room where they can be watched closely for airway compromise. The drains and dressings are observed carefully for excessive bleeding, and the neck is observed for hematoma formation. Patients with major organ dysfunction requiring invasive monitoring should be observed in the intensive care unit.

ACUTE PAIN MANAGEMENT

Acute pain following head and neck surgery is not as great as might be anticipated and patients are fairly comfortable with moderate doses of narcotics. In our experience, these patients do not usually require patient-controlled analgesia (PCA) since their narcotic requirements are minimal.

CHRONIC PAIN

It is extremely important to establish a good rapport with the patient to provide effective pain relief. The fear of death is always present, but many times the fear of pain is more profound in these patients. A trusting relationship can help control the patient's pain by decreasing anxiety and insecurity. The patient who participates in working toward pain relief is much more likely to achieve that goal.

The treatment of head and neck cancer may sometimes require radical surgery that significantly alters the patient's appearance. The accompanying loss of pride and dignity may increase depression and intensify the pain. This, along with the physical and financial drain faced by the patient, may result in emotional upheaval leading to uncontrolled pain.

Pain originating from head and neck tumors is often difficult to treat effectively since these tumors may infiltrate deeply into areas of overlapping cranial or cervical innervation. Areas involved may be supplied by the fifth, seventh, ninth, and tenth cranial nerves or by the first, second, and third cervical nerves. In addition, the trigeminal nerve has extensive sensory supply to the skin and mucous membrane of the head with three primary sensory divisions: ophthalmic, maxillary, and mandibular. The tenth cranial nerve is especially important in the airway, since the superior laryngeal nerve conveys sensation to the epiglottis and structures above the cords. The recurrent laryngeal nerve supplies the larynx below the vocal cords.

The cause of pain should be carefully analyzed since it may involve factors other than the tumor itself. It must be remembered that patients with incurable cancer may have other sources of pain. Many of these patients are treated with excessive medication when, in fact, the pain of sinusitis may be relieved by appropriate treatment. Tension headache is not an unusual finding in patients who have been treated for cancer of the head and neck. Biofeedback and autorelaxation techniques have been found to be useful in treating some of these headaches. Herpes zoster (shingles) can occur in and around nerve

ganglia, including the trigeminal nerve. Rheumatic neuritis, dental problems, trismus, and cervical spine lesions are not infrequent causes of pain in the neck or head after tumor removal. Pain that can be described in a simple and crisp manner is organic in origin, whereas pain described more elaborately and vaguely may be a result of psychological factors.

Obviously the tumor may be the cause of the pain, especially when inflammation develops. Tumors of the intraoral and pharyngeal regions are prone to ulceration and infection and may therefore cause excruciating pain. Bulky tumors compressing nerves also produce pain.

Shoulder pain, often experienced after radical neck dissection with resection of the spinal accessory nerve, is believed to be a result of limited postoperative shoulder motion resulting in the development of an adhesive capsulitis. A shoulder sling for support and elevation of the affected arm is usually helpful in relieving the pain.

Patients with severe pain from bony metastases (especially to the vertebrae) who have a life expectancy of at least 2 months may benefit from irradiation to that site. Pain relief is usually obtained within 2 to 3 weeks after onset of treatment. However, poor results are obtained when metastases to the vertebrae cause significant nerve compression.

Chemotherapy may be helpful to treat some types of squamous cell carcinoma. As many as 35 percent of patients respond to treatment with methotrexate or cisplatin, and pain relief may be seen within 1 to 2 weeks. However, the use of this drug must be weighed against potential side effects.

In patients with a life expectancy of greater than 3 months, a major surgical denervation procedure may be contemplated. Local nerve blocks and peripheral neurectomy can be performed. Local anesthetics can be injected to evaluate the effectiveness of the proposed nerve resection.

Overall, it is very important for the patient to understand what is wrong, why the pain is present, and how long the pain may last. The addition of pain may be devastating to the patient who has to deal with cancer. Some of these patients may feel guilty, demoralized, and rejected because of the intensity of the pain. They should be kept constantly informed of the treatment modalities that are being employed and of future treatment plans.

SUGGESTED READING

Hermens JM, Bennett MJ, Hirschman CA. Anesthesia for laser surgery. Anesth Analg 1983; 62:218.

Mangano DT. Perioperative cardiac mortality. Anesthesiology 1990; 72:153–184.

Marx RE. Osteoradionecrosis of the mandible: a new concept in its pathophysiology. J Oral Maxillofac Surg 1983; 41:283–288, 351–357.

Myers EN, Suen JY, eds. Cancer of the head and neck. 2nd ed. New York: Churchill Livingstone, 1989.

Otteni JC, Pottecher T, Bonner G, et al. Prolongation of the Q-T interval and sudden cardiac arrest following right radical neck dissection. Anesthesiology 1983; 59:358–361.

CRANIOFACIAL RECONSTRUCTION

JACOB SAMUEL, F.F.A.R.C.S.
PHILIP D. LUMB, M.B.B.S.

Craniofacial surgery (CFS), a relatively young speciality, has been practiced as a distinct medical specialty for only the past 25 years. By definition, it is surgery in and around the orbit(s), at the junction of the face and cranium. Patients present for craniofacial reconstruction with congenital defects or with acquired disfigurement caused by trauma, radical cancer surgery, or radiotherapy for a malignancy, or with cancrum oris, a form of gross facial pathology prevalent in West Africa.

The pioneering work of Tessier showed that gross congenital abnormalities (e.g., hypertelorism, hypotelorism, craniofacial dysostosis) could be corrected by mobilizing and rearranging cranial and facial bones. Fundamental to this surgical approach was the observation that the optic foramina are always normally situated and therefore the orbital bones could be moved without compromising vision. CFS procedures may be intracranial or extracranial, relatively limited and therefore of short duration, or quite extensive, sometimes lasting as long as 24 hours and involving several surgical subspecialties. The craniofacial team draws its surgical expertise from ophthalmology, otolaryngology, neurosurgery, maxillofacial, plastic, and dental surgery. Because a relay of teams may be involved, communication and coordination between personnel is particularly important in the delivery of care to the patient.

Maxillofacial trauma is caused largely by motor vehicle accidents. The increased use of seat belts has resulted in fewer injuries to the torso but more facial fractures. With blunt injuries to the face, the maxilla serves as a shock absorber. The fracture patterns are consistent and fall into three categories: Le Fort fractures I, II, and III (Fig. 1). Le Fort I is the simplest, with the fracture line passing along the floor of the maxillary sinus at the junction of the thin sinus cortex with the dense palatal bone and extending into the pterygoid plates. Le Fort II has a triangular appearance, with the base at the palate and the apex at the root of the nose and involves the floor of the orbit. Le Fort fracture III is also called craniofacial dysfunction, because the fracture involves all the buttresses that anchor the maxilla to the rest of the skull, the maxilla lies free. The cribriform plate, ethmoidal arteries, optic nerve, and maxillary artery are all at risk of injury. Le Fort fractures II and III are compound fractures complicated by gross facial edema and cerebrospinal rhinorrhea. Any of these injuries may be associated with cerebral edema, cervical instability, or injuries to more distant parts of the body (e.g., pneumothorax, pelvic fracture, or splenic rupture).

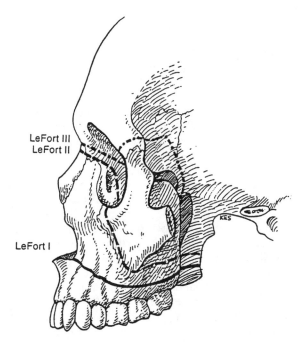

Figure 1 Le Fort Fractures. (Reprinted with permission from Holt GR. Maxillofacial trauma. In Cummings CW, Fredrickson JM, Harker LA, et al, eds. Otolaryngology—Head and Neck Surgery. St. Louis: CV Mosby, 1986:329.)

Irrespective of the underlying etiology, paramount anesthetic considerations during surgery involve the airway, blood loss, and hypothermia. The anesthesia plan begins with the preoperative assessment and should address the following issues: (1) choosing a safe method to secure and maintain the airway; (2) the need for invasive monitoring; (3) the need for controlled hypotension; (4) the position of the patient and location of staff and equipment in the operating room; (5) the duration and extent of surgery; and (6) the possibility of soft tissue edema, maxillomandibular wiring, or prolonged surgery, which warrant continued tracheal intubation and intensive care nursing into the postoperative period. Because of the unique nature of each repair, a discussion with the surgical team is essential to draft a comprehensive anesthesia plan.

PREOPERATIVE ASSESSMENT

The anesthesiologist must be aware of the psychological trauma that patients suffer with facial disfigurement. Also, the parents of children with congenital abnormalities of the face may be especially sensitive to comments and may be similarly afflicted themselves.

Surgery should be postponed for patients with otitis media or respiratory tract infections or for patients in the prodromal phase of one of the childhood illnesses. Wound infection is a disastrous complication in craniofacial surgery. With bronchorrheal respiratory tract infections, secretions may occlude the endotracheal tube, especially in children, and the need for frequent suctioning is a nuisance when working space is at a premium.

Adenoidal hypertrophy predisposes to a chronic obstructive state and may rarely cause cor pulmonale. The upper airway obstruction may not be relieved immediately by adenotonsillectomy and can take 1 to 2 weeks to improve. When the postoperative airway is the focus of concern (e.g., because of maxillomandibular wiring) elective preoperative adenotonsillectomy at least 2 weeks before surgery is indicated.

Craniofacial synostosis, or premature fusion of skull sutures, may involve the sagittal suture (scaphocephaly); the metopic suture (trigonocephaly); the coronal suture, one (plagiocephaly) or both (brachycephaly) or all the -sutures (cloverleaf deformity). The cloverleaf deformity is usually associated with abnormal facial bones (e.g., retrusion of the maxilla). The condition is then categorized as a craniofacial dysostosis that usually forms part of a syndrome complex (e.g., Apert's, Crouzon's, or Pfeiffer's). Especially with regard to cloverleaf deformity, failure to treat leads to raised intracranial pressure (ICP) from the rapidly expanding cerebrum. Surgery between the ages of 3 and 6 months favors brain growth, and even when no signs of raised ICP are noted, children show accelerated growth postoperatively. With some syndrome complexes, abnormalities may be found in other organ systems. For example, Goldenhar's syndrome (hemifacial microsomia) is associated with a 50 percent incidence of tetralogy of Fallot. Therefore, a cardiology referral to define or exclude possible congenital heart lesions is important. A patient with a Blalock-Taussig shunt may present for CFS. An accidental intraoperative endobronchial intubation may favor the poorly perfused lung, thus inducing hypoxia.

It is important to recognize the potentially difficult airway. Mask fit can be compromised by an abnormal contour to the face seen, for example, in the cleft-like extension of the mouth with the Goldenhar variant. Congenital cervical vertebral defects (e.g., Kippel-Fiel syndrome) restrict full movement of the neck. Difficulty with feeding may suggest an inadequate nasal airway. False or bony ankylosis of the temperomandibular joint may make mouth opening impossible, in which case the distance between the upper and lower incisions must be measured and documented. In adults, a thyromental distance (thyroid notch to chin) of less than 6 cm is believed to make laryngoscopy impossible. No such dimension has been described in children. Restricted cervical motion with prominent upper incisors may make an otherwise easy laryngoscopy impossible in the adult with a thyromental distance of 6.5 cm. Protruberant upper incisors, micrognathia, macroglossia, or a cleft palate may contribute to difficult laryngoscopy. Missing upper incisors or a cleft palate create similar problems. The laryngoscope blade tends to slip into the gap so that teeth or gums intrude into the line of vision or the path of the endotracheal tube.

Although fortunately children with severe craniofacial anomalies, airway obstruction, and sleep apnea are rare, their management in general is extremely difficult. They are notoriously difficult to intubate, show poor weight gain, and are prone to the sudden death syndrome. Cine fluoroscopy and radiographic profile studies show that the airway is compromised by the retruded maxilla, leaving little room for the tongue. Le Fort fracture III midface advancement by about 15 mm has been recommended as a means of improving the airway. Autologous rib grafts and a halo frame applying traction on a palatal splint have been used to maintain the advanced position of the maxilla. However, maintaining this position is extremely difficult in small edentulous children, because maxillomandibular (interdental) wiring is not possible. Partial or complete relapse commonly occurs. Therefore, some authorities believe that a tracheostomy with the intent of prolonged tracheal cannulation should be performed early in the management of these infants, who may need to undergo several surgical procedures (including ventriculoperitoneal shunts and their revision), sedation for computed tomographic scans, and fundoscopies. Some of these infants show weight gain after a tracheostomy has relieved their chronic airway obstruction. This suggests that chronic airway obstruction causes a catabolic state that is promptly converted to an anabolic state with tracheostomy. A waiting period to allow for weight gain before more definitive surgery contributes to surgical success.

The main purpose of defining a preoperative plan and alternative means of securing the patient's airway is to avoid life-threatening situations in which ventilation by mask or tracheal intubation is impossible. If an alternative plan is not available, then death is inevitable, even if the physician is aware of the danger. The three modes of securing the airway are (in diminishing order with regard to safety): (1) with the patient awake; (2) with the patient anesthetized but breathing spontaneously; and (3) with the patient anesthetized and *paralyzed* with breaths delivered via face mask by manual intermittent positive pressure ventilation (IPPV). The choice of mode depends on the anticipated difficulty with the airway; and on the patient's ability to cooperate, which is largely determined by age. Having made the choice, the anesthesiologist should explain the details of the method to the patient. This generally elicits better patient cooperation at the time of induction of anesthesia.

Laboratory tests should include complete blood count and measures of serum electrolytes, prothrombin time, partial thromboplastin time, blood urea nitrogen (BUN), and creatinine levels to provide baseline reference values. Because aspirin compromises platelet function for the duration of the platelets' lifespan and bleeding is a cause for concern with CFS, a recent history of aspirin ingestion warrants that a planned case be rescheduled to 7 days postingestion.

Typed and crossmatched blood must be made available for use in the operating room. As a rule, an adequate volume of available blood equals half the patient's estimated blood volume. As a working rule, an adequate volume of available blood would equal half the patient's estimated blood volume (EBV). In surgery for craniosynostosis a preoperative estimate of blood loss (EBL) and arrangements for replacement can be made depending on the suture or sutures involved. For the sagittal suture the EBL is 24 percent of EBV; the unicoronal, 24 percent of EBV; the metopic, 40 percent of EBV; and the bicoronal, 65 percent of EBV. If the patient has access to an autologous blood donation program, the use of predeposited blood will minimize the frequency of homologous transfusion, thus reducing the risk of transfusion-related infections. The use of autologous blood is to the patient's advantage in cancer surgery, when homologous transfusion may encourage the growth and spread of neoplastic tissue by suppressing the patient's immune system. Intraoperative red blood cell salvage using a cell saver, acute preoperative normovolemic hemodilution, controlled hypotension, and autologous predeposits minimize red blood cell loss. However, a combination of techniques is probably most effective.

Invasive monitoring is indicated in prolonged surgery, massive blood loss, and controlled hypotension. In syndromes associated with syndactyly, difficulty with radial arterial cannulation may be foreseen, especially when wrist extension is impossible. Venous access can be limited when limbs are encased in plaster.

Older children and adults must be told if their eyes will be bandaged shut, if maxillomandibular wiring will prevent mouth opening, or if a period of postoperative endotracheal intubation and intensive care nursing is to be expected.

Preoperative medication should include (1) sedation if the neurologic and airway status allows it (sedation can be omitted in patients younger than 1 year of age); (2) an antisialogogue to eliminate saliva during difficult intubation; (3) dexamethasone to minimize postoperative facial edema; (4) prophylactic anticonvulsant therapy; and (5) antibiotics to sterilize the nasopharynx.

ANESTHETIC MANAGEMENT

Anesthetic management starts with the layout of equipment in the operating room (OR). Because induction of anesthesia and intubation are conducted with the patient in the supine position, equipment may have to be rearranged when the patient is subsequently repositioned for surgery. A sheepskin mattress and heating blanket should be placed on the OR table before the patient arrives. Basic equipment should also be prepared beforehand: a working suction apparatus, an anesthesia machine that has been checked and will deliver 100 percent oxygen, a leak-free breathing system that can generate and sustain positive pressure, and a working laryngoscope, mask, and endotracheal tube. A simple breathing system with a minimum of possible disconnection points is all that is required for induction of anesthesia. A humidification system and extension tubing for remote delivery of fresh gas may be added to

the breathing system while the patient is being positioned for surgery. Whether an oral or nasal endotracheal tube is used depends on the surgical site. An oral Rae tube is convenient for surgery of the upper face; for the lower face, a nasal Rae tube is convenient. The oral Rae tube is preformed to angle over the lower teeth and lip in the caudad direction, and the nasal Rae tube goes over the forehead in a rostral direction. Both are attached to the breathing circuit by the standard 15-mm connector. When surgical access to the whole face is essential but a tracheostomy will not be performed, a standard endotracheal tube with a swivel angle piece is included in the surgical skin preparation and covered by a transparent adhesive drape. All endotracheal tubes used for prolonged procedures should be anchored with a suture to the teeth, lip, or nasal septum.

Management of the Difficult Airway

The difficult airway is rare. Preparation in the management of the difficult airway is focused on avoiding a situation in which the patient cannot be ventilated or intubated. Preparation means that all equipment is available and ready for use before such a situation develops. A selection of endotracheal tubes, laryngoscope blades, stylets, Magill forceps, suction catheters, and masks are made available and neatly arranged in an area dedicated to airway management. To avoid confusion during a crisis, neatly arranged equipment is as important as a well-thought-out plan and alternative plans. Although a flexible approach is essential, the plan must include provisions for (1) emergency percutaneous tracheal cannulation, and transtracheal jet ventilation (TTJV); and (2) emergency cricothyroidotomy or tracheostomy, which requires that an otolaryngologist be ready to perform the procedure at a moment's notice.

Securing the Airway with the Patient Awake. This method is indicated when the airway cannot be safely maintained while the patient is anesthetized. However, it requires a cooperative patient and thus may not be applicable in children. Patient anxiety can be counterproductive to attempts at awake intubation, but whatever mechanisms maintain the airway in the awake state will be preserved nevertheless. Sedation should be used judiciously and be titrated to effect. A clinically useful rule is to ensure that one is able to maintain verbal contact with the patient at all times. Methods used for intubation are listed in Table 1.

Topical anesthesia may be supplemented with superior and recurrent (transtracheal) laryngeal nerve blocks. When combined with sedation, these blocks permit assessment of the airway by awake laryngoscopy.

The fiberoptic laryngoscope may be passed nasally or orally. When nasal instrumentation is expected, a local anesthetic agent containing 1:200,000 epinephrine may minimize bleeding. Bleeding and secretions make fiberoptic laryngoscopy difficult. Attempts at blind nasal intubation should not precede fiberoptic laryngoscopy. Efficient suction and a dry field are the key to success with the fiberoptic laryngoscope, especially since the

Table 1 Methods Used for Intubation

1. Topical anesthesia → laryngoscopy → intubation.
2. Topical anesthesia → fiberoptic laryngoscopy → intubation.
3. Percutaneous transtracheal cannulation → TTJV → induction of anesthesia → fiberoptic laryngoscopy → intubation.
4. Topical anesthesia → retrograde catheter technique → intubation.
5. Topical anesthesia → blind nasal intubation.
6. Tracheostomy under local anesthesia.

instrument restricts the field of vision. Only endotracheal tubes with an internal diameter greater than 4.5 mm can be mounted on a fiberoptic laryngoscope that also has a suction channel.

Retrograde and blind nasal methods are accepted techniques for managing a difficult intubation, although they carry a recognized failure rate. With the retrograde technique, a guide wire is passed retrograde via a transtracheal cannula and through the Murphy's eye of a lubricated endotracheal tube, which is then threaded into the trachea. However, obstruction may be encountered while the tube is negotiating an acute bend near the epiglottis. A combined technique allows the tube to be placed by guiding a fiberoptic laryngoscope along the wire via the suction channel of the instrument.

Fiberoptic laryngoscopy, retrograde or blind nasal techniques are entirely compatible with TTJV in an anesthesized patient after securing the airway by awake percutaneous cannulation of the trachea, and demonstration of satisfactory lung expansion. A weal with a local anesthetic agent is raised in the midline over the cricothyroid membrane or first and second tracheal rings. The anatomic landmarks are accentuated by hyperextending the neck on a sandbag. A 14- or 16-gauge intravenous cannula mounted on a syringe containing saline is passed caudally and posteriorly. The cannula is threaded over the needle when bubbles are aspirated into the barrel of the syringe. The cannula must be anchored with a stitch to avoid dislodgement. A preassembled jet ventilation system provides a leur lock connection to the cannula. The optimal jet ventilation system consists of a dedicated source of high-pressure oxygen, a pressure regulator that can vary the working pressure of the system between 10 and 50 psi, a flow interrupter, and noncompliant tubing with a leur lock attachment for the cannula. Small jets at 15 psi are followed by increasingly larger ones while the working pressure is gradually increased until satisfactory lung expansion is observed. Breath sounds may not be audible, as the turbulance of jet ventilation is considerable. Expired gas escapes via the natural passages. There is a very rare possibility that total obstruction to expiration occurs with induction, in which case the chest remains in the position of inspiration and subsequent breaths risk barotrauma and pneumothorax. In such cases, the narrow-bore transtracheal cannula does not provide a satisfactory route for expired gases, and an emergent tracheostomy must be performed while apneic oxygenation is provided via the transtracheal cannula.

Other methods of providing transtracheal ventila-

tion are considered suboptimal. The least efficient method, often described as a life-saving maneuver, delivers 100 percent oxygen by manual intermittent positive-pressure ventilation (IPPV). This method amounts to apneic oxygenation and arterial carbon dioxide pressure ($PaCO_2$) increases at a rate of 4 mm Hg per minute. The barrel of a 3-ml syringe (without the plunger) is attached to the hub of a transtracheal cannula. The barrel accepts a connector for a 7-mm endotracheal tube and thereby provides a standard 15-mm diameter port for a breathing circuit or self-inflating bag. However, jets of 100 percent oxygen delivered by the flush valve of the anesthesia machine approximates to TTJV—an assembly that requires a noncompliant delivery system.

Transtracheal cannulation can be repeated with a minimum of patient discomfort. Although the incidence of serious complications is low, it is higher with emergent cannulation than with planned cannulations. Subcutaneous and mediastinal emphysema are the most common complications. The anesthesiologist must be alert to the possibility of a pneumothorax, which may present with tension (hypotension, bradycardia). Craniofacial procedures of short duration may be safely completed with TTJV and total intravenous anesthesia.

Securing the Airway with the Patient Anesthetized While Spontaneous Respiration is Preserved. This method is especially useful in children when a difficult intubation is anticipated. Establishing venous access before gaseous induction of anesthesia is performed is ideal but may not always be possible. When an abnormal facial contour (e.g., hemifacial microsomia) compromises mask fit, an oversized mask may provide a better seal. A soft air-filled cushion improves mask fit in patients with distorted facial anatomy. With increasing depth of anesthesia, the introduction of a small positive pressure into the circuit (3 cm H_2O) splints the airway. This, however, may cause gastric distention if the airway is not entirely clear.

Young children tend to have a large head that lolls on the occiput. It can be stabilized and brought into the classic sniffing position for laryngoscopy by placing the occiput in a doughnut-shaped padded ring. Close attention must be paid to the depth of anesthesia by watching the pattern, depth, and rate of respiration. A modest decrease in blood pressure usually indicates that safe laryngoscopy is possible without provoking the gag or laryngeal reflex. Ideally, venous access must be established before laryngoscopy. If peripheral venous access is poor, the femoral vein may be cannulated percutaneously or under direct vision by means of a cut-down. The femoral artery may then also be cannulated for intraarterial pressure monitoring. The demonstration of lung inflation by manual IPPV indicates that muscle relaxants may be safely administered. This converts to securing the airway in the anesthetized-paralyzed method. If the glottic chink is not visible but the epiglottis is, a stylet that acutely angles the tip of the endotracheal tube may aid successful intubation. If not, fiberoptic laryngoscopy may be employed via the port of an endoscopic mask or while inspired gases maintaining anesthesia are delivered by nasal prongs. A blind nasal technique with an endotracheal tube too small to be mounted on a 3-mm fiberoptic laryngoscope may be modified and the tube passed with fiberoptic aid if the instrument is passed via the other patent nostril. Small fiberoptic catheters (1.3 to 3.6 mm) lack suction ports and cannot be deflected. Retrograde techniques have also been described in children older than 6 years of age but have not been uniformly successful. Although experience with percutaneous TTJV in small children is limited, principles similar to jet ventilation during bronchoscopy apply. For example, a child-size Negus bronchoscope delivers jets of 100 percent oxygen via a 19-gauge cannula. Therefore, for percutaneous transtracheal cannulation in a small child, a 19- or 20-gauge IV cannula is appropriate.

Securing the Airway with the Patient Anesthetized and Paralyzed. The anesthetized-paralyzed method is employed when no difficulty with the airway is anticipated. Most patients are managed with this technique.

Fewer tracheostomies are currently performed during CFS than in the past. However, tracheostomy is indicated when a basal skull fracture precludes nasal intubation and when the need for maxillomandibular wiring requires the removal of the oral endotracheal tube at the end of the procedure (during some cases of Le Fort fracture II and most cases of Le Fort III fracture).

During craniofacial surgery, a well-secured endotracheal tube does not guarantee a safe airway. It may be violated by an osteotome or included in a suture, thus making subsequent extubation difficult. When a Le Fort III fracture osteotomy and advancement of the maxilla are required, as in Treacher Collins syndrome, a nasal endotracheal tube moves 1.5 to 4 cm (depending on the age and size of the patient). To minimize the danger of extubation, the tip of the tube should be positioned immediately proximal to the carina, either fiberoptically or by intentional endobronchial intubation, and subsequently withdrawn until breath sounds are heard over the left hemithorax. Contrary to intuition and what has been previously described in the literature, there is radiological evidence to suggest that flexion (not extension) of the neck will favor endobronchial migration of a nasal endotracheal tube. A stethoscope placed in the infra-axillary region of the left chest will warn the anesthesiologist of an accidental endobronchial intubation. A moist throat pack should surround the endotracheal tube in the pharynx and should be packed tightly with the aid of a Magill forceps. The throat pack serves two purposes. First, it reduces or prevents ingestion of blood which, as an irritant, promotes postoperative nausea. Secondly, it protects the airway in case of cuff rupture or if an uncuffed endotracheal tube is in use, as is the practice with children.

An orogastric or nasogastric tube ensures gastric decompression, which is especially important during prolonged procedures. Gastric dilatation encourages a high end-expiratory position for the diaphragm. Children with gastric dilatation are especially prone to respiratory embarrassment and arterial desaturation.

Monitoring

The primary objective of monitoring is to make sure that no avoidable harm befalls the anesthetized patient. Ensuring the adequacy of gas exchange, circulation, organ perfusion, and acid-based balance depends on several considerations in CFS. These include the duration of surgery, anticipated blood loss, the position of the patient (which determines the risk of air embolism), the need for controlled hypotension, and the presence of any coexisting disease.

During CFS the airway is often part of or close to the surgical field. Although danger to the airway is ever present, the anesthesiologist has no direct access to it. Therefore, the anesthesiologist must warn the surgeon as soon as he or she suspects a compromised airway. This is possible only with obsessive vigilance and adequate monitoring of airway pressure, end-tidal carbon dioxide concentration, ($ETCO_2$), and breath sounds over the left hemithorax. Monitoring will warn of a disconnection, a severed, kinked, or blocked endotracheal tube, bronchospasm, accidental endobronchial intubation, or extubation. Also, because the anesthetized patient is excluded from the atmosphere, he or she is at risk for hypoxia. Continuous monitoring of inspired or expired oxygen concentration and pulse oximetry are therefore essential.

In controlled hypotension, intra-arterial pressure monitoring and infusion of the hypotensive agent via a central venous catheter minimizes blood pressure oscillations. With the use of sodium nitroprusside, serial blood gas estimations showing increasing metabolic acidosis suggest early cyanide toxicity. Arterial cannulation is indicated in prolonged CFS surgery, which is usually associated with massive blood loss. It allows intermittent sampling of arterial blood for blood gas analysis, serum electrolytes, and hematocrit, and it allows beat-to-beat pressure monitoring with minimal morbidity. In CFS, blood loss is often difficult to estimate. Monitoring central venous pressure and hematocrit allows more accurate fluid and red blood cell replacement. Measures of hourly urine output (0.5 ml per hour) may provide indirect evidence of adequate organ perfusion. However, in simple suture surgery, which constitutes most cases of craniosynostosis, empiric transfusion practices without invasive monitoring are considered adequate.

Venous air embolism was once believed to be a rare event with a high mortality. However, the routine use of precordial Doppler ultrasound and $ETCO_2$ monitoring has confirmed that it is a common event with a low mortality. It can occur whenever a pressure gradient exists between the open veins of the operative site and the right atrium. A pressure gradient of 5 cm H_2O, which is sufficient to predispose to embolism, is easily achieved by the head-up position routinely used during CFS to minimize bleeding. The routes of entry may be via severed diploic veins, scalp veins, or the venous lakes of the skull. $ETCO_2$ is an early and sensitive indicator. A more specific indicator may be end-tidal nitrogen if air is not already present in the inspired mixture. More recently, transesophageal Doppler ultrasonography and echocardiographic techniques have proved to be especially useful in detecting paradoxic embolization — that is right atrium to left atrium via a patent foramen orale. The foramen ovale, although functionally closed, is probe-patent in 35 percent of the population. Flow from the right to the left atrium can occur when right atrial pressure exceeds left atrial pressure (e.g., as in air embolus). A volume of air greater than 300 ml for a 70-kg individual is potentially fatal. Large pockets of air form "air locks" in the right ventricular outflow tract. Air, being compressible, does not allow the right ventricle to generate sufficient pressure to open the pulmonary valve. Smaller bubbles that generate froth may have an air-blood interface area large enough to trigger the complement cascade, resulting in lung injury, pulmonary hypertension, edema, and hypoxia. Hypotension and cardiovascular collapse are late signs. Once air embolism is suspected, the surgeons should be told to flood the field with saline, the head should be lowered to the level of the heart, and nitrous oxide (N_2O) should be discontinued in favor of 100 percent oxygen. Aspiration of a central venous catheter does not usually yield air but may be attempted. Large-bore central venous catheters with multiple ports especially designed for aspiration of air have become available. However, preventing further embolization may be more important than retrieving already embolized air. Most air emboli resolve by dissipation into the periphery of the pulmonary arterial tree. The application of positive end-expiratory pressure, although recommended as a means of acutely elevating central venous pressure, may encourage paradoxic systemic embolism. Closed chest cardiac massage is indicated if hemodynamics are not restored promptly. This may force air out of the right ventricle. If all measures fail and the outlook is grim, the chest should be opened for direct cardiac massage and aspiration of intracardiac air.

An anesthetized patient is at risk for hypothermia and pressure sores. Although malignant hyperthermia may be associated with some syndromes, hypothermia is the usual consideration. Core temperature should be monitored with a rectal or esophageal probe. The effort to minimize heat loss should start early during anesthesia, by using a heating lamp for infants and by warming the OR. Heat loss can be minimized by using warm intravenous fluids, warm humidified inspired gases, warm fluids for surgical skin preparation and irrigation, and a heating mattress. The skin over the sacrum heel and occiput are in danger of pressure necrosis. Padding pressure points offers some protection. Traction on the endotracheal tube may cause ulceration of the mucous membrane over the lower lip or nostrils.

Electrocardiographic monitoring, which is mandatory for all cases, will warn of the bradyarrhythmic effects of the oculocardiac reflex arc. This is especially active in children and likely to be triggered by manipulations in the orbit. Intravenous atropine affords protection against this cholinergic reflex.

Anesthetic Technique

For most patients, anesthesia can be maintained with a combination of N_2O, a muscle relaxant, a narcotic, and a minimal concentration of an inhalation agent. Controlled ventilation is adjusted to achieve normocarbia or moderate hypocapnia. With intracranial procedures or in cases with raised intracranial pressure, osmotic diuretic therapy (mannitol 0.5 to 1.0 g per kilogram) and hyperventilation to a $PaCO_2$ of 25 to 30 mm Hg reduces brain bulk. Isoflurane may be considered the agent of choice because it reduces the cerebral metabolic rate of oxygen while it does not completely ablate sensitivity of the cerebral vessels to $PaCO_2$. The anesthetic technique must be modified when branches of the facial nerve need to be identified by electrical stimulation in the surgical field. This precludes the use of muscle relaxants. Anesthesia is maintained with a potent inhalation agent or supplemented with a short-acting μ receptor opioid agonist such as sufentanil or alfentanil hydrochloride. Controlled ventilation can be instituted without neuromuscular blockade either by depressing the respiratory drive with narcotics or by rendering the patient hypocapnic.

Controlled Hypotension

Controlled hypotension is not universally practiced in CFS for small children, although it has been safely employed. Because controlled hypotension has only a small effect on blood loss during craniectomy for craniosynostosis, some pediatric anesthesiologists consider the risk unjustified in small children. Teenagers or young adults however, are unlikely to have the relative contraindications (e.g., coronary artery and cerebrovascular disease) to controlled hypotension. This makes the risk/benefit ratio more favorable. Deliberate hypotension for Le Fort I fracture maxillary osteotomy in young adults reduces blood loss by 40 percent and provides an improved surgical field. However, it has not been found to affect operating time or postoperative edema.

Several drugs and combinations of drugs are used in the induction of controlled hypotension. Simple physical principles make useful adjuncts to its pharmacology. The anti-Trendelenburg position reduces the hydrostatic pressure of blood in the capillaries of the operative site. It also promotes venous drainage. Free venous drainage can occur only when the veins are not kinked, as can happen when the head is flexed on the neck. Sodium nitroprusside (SNP) is a potent vasodilator with a quick onset and offset of action. However, it triggers a reflex sympathetic response and high angiotensin II blood levels, which tend to restore blood pressure, especially in young patients. This response increases the dose requirements of SNP, risking toxicity. Esmolol, a B_1 cardioselective antagonist, potentiates SNP-induced hypotension in a dose-related manner. Because of their short half-lives, the pharmacokinetic profiles of esmolol and SNP are well matched. Beta-blockade is also known to reduce intrapulmonary shunting. It improves arterial oxygen pressure (PaO_2 during SNP infusion and prevents rebound hypertension with its cessation. Other competing vasodilators are nitroglycerine and labetalol. Alternative techniques employ controlled cardiovascular depression with potent inhalation agents that may also be combined with intravenous vasodilators. Organ perfusion, particularly cerebral, is of particular concern during controlled hypotension. The transducer of the intra-arterial pressure monitoring system, when placed at the level of the head, reads the pressure in the carotid siphon. The goal should be to maintain this at 50 mm Hg. The arterial pressure should be allowed to return to normal values before skin closure to avoid reactionary hemorrhage.

Management of Blood Loss

Estimation of blood loss is extremely difficult. A significant proportion of shed blood is lost on the surgical gowns and drapes. The goal of the anesthesiologist should be to have a normovolemic patient with a hematocrit of 0.3 who has had minimal exposure to homologous blood product donors by the end of surgery. Several factors, such as controlled ventilation, controlled hypotension, scalp infiltration with epinephrine (1: 200,000 solution), and hemostatic scalp sutures, may reduce blood loss. Much of the hemorrhage arises with periosteal stripping. It is therefore questionable whether the use of interstitial scalp epinephrine is truly hemostatic. Initially, blood loss can be allowed to reach 20 percent of blood volume or a hematocrit of 0.3. Normovolemia is maintained with 3 ml of Ringer's lactate for every 1 ml of blood lost. Subsequent losses are managed with packed red blood cells for red blood cell deficits, and crystalloids and/or colloids for volume deficits, which are guided by frequent hematocrit determinations and central venous pressure measurements. Red blood cell loss as well as the need for homologous transfusion can be reduced by autologous predeposits; acute preoperative hemodilution; and intraoperative red blood cell salvage using a cell saver. It is important to plan adequately for the use of these methods. The cell saver is not indicated for cancer surgery or when sepsis is present, as retransfusion may spread malignant cells and infection. An estimate of red blood cell loss can be made in the normovolemic patient at the end of the procedure by using this formula:

$$ERCM_{deficit} = ERCM_a + ERCM_b - ERCM_c$$

Where ERCM = estimated red cell mass = hematocrit × estimated blood volume; and where a = before surgery; b = transfused blood; hematocrit of packed cells = 0.6; hematocrit of reconstituted or whole bank blood = 0.3; and c = after or during surgery.

With massive bleeding, the dilutional effects of transfusion reduces clotting factor activity and the platelet count. The onset of a coagulopathy is an indication for substitution therapy with fresh frozen plasma, cryoprecipitate, or platelets.

Particulary in infants and small children, the transfusion of citrated blood binds serum calcium. The resulting decrease in ionized calcium levels (Ca^{++}) may be manifested as hypotension with a slow upstroke on the arterial pressure trace. Empirical administration of calcium chloride, which may also be titrated to periodic ionized calcium determination, will maintain Ca^{++} in the normal range. The chloride salt, not the gluconate, consistently increases plasma ionized Ca^{++}. The usual recommended dose for a low-output state is 10 to 20 mg per kilogram.

POSTOPERATIVE CARE

The timing of extubation is a major postoperative consideration. With a decision to extubate, the anesthesiologist has no doubts about the adequacy of the airway or the patient's ability to sustain the required level of respiratory work. After short procedures in which the operative site was some distance from the nasopharynx or oropharynx (e.g., craniostenosis), the decision is simple. The patient may be extubated in the OR after removal of the pharyngeal pack, bronchial and pharyngeal toilet, and adequate reversal of neuromuscular blockade. With small infants who are obligatory nose breathers, the nares must be clear of secretions.

When patients have had maxillomandibular wiring, a wire cutter must be taped to the bed, where it is readily available to release the lower jaw if airway compromise caused by emesis or edema occurs. Potent antiemetics (e.g., droperidol) may be used to reduce nausea. Ingestion of blood that accumulates in the pharynx postoperatively promotes nausea. A nasopharyngeal airway provides a route for pharyngeal suction without mucosal trauma.

If autologous rib grafts were taken, a postoperative chest film should be obtained to rule out a pneumothorax. Patchy atelectasis or lobar collapse is common after long procedures.

After prolonged procedures, hypothermia, or when soft-tissue edema is expected (e.g., following a bilateral sagittal mandibular osteotomy or Le Fort fracture III maxillary osteotomy), the patient should be transferred to the intensive care unit with the endotracheal tube in place. Steroids may be helpful in hastening the resorption of edematous fluid, but it may take 3 to 4 days before the edema subsides enough to consider extubation. The patient should be alert and cooperative at the time of extubation and, as always, equipment for airway management must be checked and ready for use at the bedside.

SUGGESTED READING

Biebuyck JF. The importance of transtracheal jet ventilation in the management of the difficult airway. Anesthesiology 1989; 71: 769–778.

Christianson L. Anesthesia for major craniofacial operations. Int Anesthesiol Clin 1985; 23:117–148.

Kearney RA, Rosales JK, Howes WJ. Craniosynostosis: an assessment of blood loss and transfusion practices. Can J Anaesth 1989; 36:473–477.

Lauritzen C, Lilja J, Jarlstedt J, et al. Airway obstruction and sleep apnea in children with craniofacial anomalies. Plast Reconstr Surg 1986; 77:1–5.

Lessard MR, Trepanier CA, Baribault JP, et al. Isoflurane induced hypotension in orthognathic surgery. Anesth Analg 1989; 69: 379–383.

Sitigeyuki S, Shuji D, Hiroshi N. Alteration of double lumen endobronchial tube position by flexion and extension of the neck. Anesthesiology 1985; 62:696–697.

Sumner E, Hatch DJ. Craniofacial surgery in textbook of paediatric anaesthetic practice. Philadelphia: Bailliere Tindall/WB Saunders, 1989:392.

TRACHEAL RECONSTRUCTION

ROGER S. WILSON, M.D.
STEVEN M. FRANK, M.D.

Surgical resection and reconstruction of the trachea are performed to correct several types of abnormalities. The plan for anesthetic management must consider the existence of preoperative pulmonary and systemic disease and the tracheal pathology. It is incumbent on the anesthesiologist to understand the nature and extent of the lesion and to have a clear idea of the proposed surgical approach to be used for correction. Under most circumstances, anesthesia can be safely accomplished using standard anesthetic techniques as long as forethought is given regarding special needs. This involves selection of endotracheal tubes, tube position, and limitations to ventilation and secretion removal in the immediate postoperative period. This chapter reviews the important causes of major airway disease, considers the preoperative evaluation, and formulates a systematic approach for anesthetic management.

ETIOLOGY OF TRACHEAL PATHOLOGY

Although the most common cause of tracheal injury is benign stricture following laryngeal intubation or tracheostomy, several other less common causes must be considered. Congenital lesions vary in severity from those that are incompatible with life, such as tracheal atresia or agenesis, to less severe involvement with regional stenosis. Congenital stenosis can be associated with a number of other abnormalities, including aberrant left pulmonary artery or pulmonary artery sling, which can compress the posterior tracheal wall. Vascular ring malformations that compress the trachea, such as those occurring with double aortic arch, a right aortic arch, or ligamentum arteriosum, are generally amenable to surgical correction.

Primary surgical repair of tracheal abnormalities in the pediatric patient must be considered with great caution. The limited cross-sectional area of the airway in the infant increases the potential for obstruction from secretions and edema in the immediate postoperative period. Under certain circumstances it may be preferable to provide an adequate airway with temporizing methods such as tracheostomy and to delay definitive surgical repair until later stages of childhood.

Primary and secondary tracheal tumors are an infrequent cause of airway obstruction. Although squamous cell carcinoma is the most common primary lesion, a wide variety of cell types are possible, especially adenoid cystic carcinoma. Although there is limited experience concerning the natural history of airway tumors, it would appear evident that both squamous and adenoid cystic tumors are best treated with early and aggressive surgical therapy for potential cure. Squamous cell tumors may present as well-defined exophytic or ulcerating lesions. Distant spread occurs first into regional lymph nodes and then by direct extension into mediastinal structures. Adenoid cystic carcinoma generally infiltrates the airway within the submucosa, frequently for longer distances than are evident on initial gross examination. Early spread of the more malignant cell types occurs with direct involvement of pleura and lung by the time the diagnosis is established.

Primary tracheal tumors present in a variety of ways, often at a late stage of tumor development. Nonspecific symptoms such as shortness of breath, especially with exertion, may be the first presenting evidence of disease. Wheezing, which is often misdiagnosed and treated as bronchial asthma, may precede audible stridor. Occasionally, patients may present with a history of position-dependent airway obstruction; this is especially true when lesions are exophytic in nature. History of obstruction, which may be better or worse in various positions, is important to ascertain during the preanesthetic visit. The induction of anesthesia in such patients must take into account optimization of airway caliber by use of the best position. Other nonspecific findings such as unilateral or bilateral pneumonias, frequently recurrent in nature, may be one of the late-stage presenting signs. Hemoptysis, an infrequent finding, is governed by the extent, cell type, and character of the neoplasm.

A variety of metastatic neoplasms may occur throughout the airway. Common primary sites producing secondary lesions include bronchogenic, laryngeal, and esophageal carcinomas. These tumors can involve the trachea and mainstem bronchi by direct invasion. Thyroid malignancies also may involve the larynx and trachea by direct invasion. The surgical approach to metastatic tumors is dictated in part by the type and extent of the primary lesion and the degree of involvement of the tracheobronchial tree. With the exception of thyroid lesions, which may be directly invasive and slow growing, many secondary tracheal neoplasms are associated with very advanced disease. This may obviate surgery except under circumstances in which palliation is the primary intent. A variety of other tumors can involve the trachea, including carcinoma of the head, neck, and breast.

Trauma to the larynx and trachea can result from penetrating and blunt injuries. Damage occurs throughout the airway from the larynx to the major bronchi. Blunt injuries to the larynx and cervical trachea frequently result from high-speed injuries such as sudden deceleration during automobile accidents with direct contact with fixed objects such as the steering wheel. In addition, motorcycle and skimobile injuries, resulting from contact with wires and cables, may produce a localized but severe, life-threatening dissection of the cervical airway. Penetrating wounds from high-velocity objects such as gunshot, shrapnel, and knives may produce injury throughout the major airway.

Tracheal and bronchial disruption can occur during direct closed-chest trauma. The posterior membranous wall of the trachea, especially immediately proximal and distal to the carina, is an area particularly susceptible to injury. Lacerations to the membranous wall at this location are usually in a vertical direction with extension into the right or left posterior mainstem bronchus.

Both blunt and penetrating injuries are frequently difficult to diagnose because of the variety of presentations. Direct trauma to the laryngeal or cervical area may be sufficient to disrupt the airway completely. Under such circumstances, it is possible for the supporting tissues to hold the transected airway close enough together to provide an adequate path for gas flow to enable the patient to reach the hospital. If not properly diagnosed and appropriately managed, total disruption and loss of airway may occur at the time of attempted intubation or emergency tracheostomy. Under such circumstances of upper airway trauma, especially when the airway is adequate to provide gas exchange, all invasive maneuvers should be delayed until clinical and diagnostic evaluations are performed to define the precise location and extent of injury.

Intrathoracic injuries due to closed-chest trauma or penetrating injuries frequently present in combination with a pneumothorax. Major tracheal or airway disruption should be suspected when a pneumothorax fails to resolve with closed-tube thoracostomy with suction or with inability to re-expand a collapsed lung in the presence of persistent and excessive air leak. Incomplete and undetected separation of the bronchi may occur at the time of injury. It can be missed on clinical examination and chest radiography, only to present at a later stage as stenosis of the airway when healing and scarring occur.

Pathology resulting from endotracheal intubation and tracheostomy has been described in a number of recent reviews and monographs. Lesions may be produced throughout the airway as a result of pressure, tissue necrosis, and formation of scar tissue.

Endotracheal intubation potentially can produce injuries extending from the nares into the pharynx, larynx, and trachea. Necrosis of the nares secondary to direct pressure from the tube may be cosmetically disfiguring and painful but not life threatening. Laryngeal injury ranges from mild edema and local irritation of any or all laryngeal structures to more serious and extensive ulceration, erosion, and scarring. Such injuries commonly involve vocal cords and the area of the posterior commissure. Injury to the larynx should be suspected whenever hoarseness, extensive soreness, and stridor are present following extubation. A more distal lesion, subglottic stenosis, results from erosion of the mucosa, frequently at the level of the cricoid cartilage. Laryngeal and subglottic lesions are troublesome because they are potentially life threatening, may produce long-standing alteration in vocal function, and in their severe form, may not be amenable to surgical repair.

Lesions occurring with the use of inflatable cuffs on both endotracheal and tracheostomy tubes have been the subject of extensive animal and human investigation. A cuffed airway is presumed to produce injury as pressure is applied directly to the tracheal wall, resulting in an area of ischemic necrosis. The extent of injury may vary from mild superficial mucosal ulceration with no long-term sequelae to more extensive destruction of soft-tissue and supportive cartilagenous structures. The degree of injury produced by the cuff appears to be dependent on a number of factors. The cuff material and design and the pressure produced between the cuff and the tracheal wall have been cited as major elements in producing injury. Other factors such as the length of time the device is used, the patient's nutritional status, and the ability of the tissues to withstand local trauma and infection must be considered. In general, the natural evolution of this injury is a loss of tissue with resulting scarring that reduces the cross-sectional diameter of the airway. Endotracheal tubes characteristically produce a circumferential lesion of dense scar that is concentric and fixed in nature. Stenosis, occurring as a result of tracheostomy, is frequently located at the site of surgical entry into the anterior tracheal wall. The stomal lesion produces minimal impairment, since the damage is frequently located in the anterior tracheal wall with a normal and movable posterior membranous portion.

Tracheal malacia occurs when there is an unstable segment of trachea without fixed cartilagenous support. It results from direct destruction of these structures secondary to the cuff or possibly from prolonged local inflammation. Tracheal malacia may be found to lie adjacent to the area where the cuff contacts the tracheal wall. When a tracheostomy has been done, malacia occurs in a position between the cuff and the tracheostomy stoma. The likely origin is the pooling of secretions between cuff and stoma, producing local infection, thinning of the cartilagenous structures, and loss of support. This can occur without extensive injury to the tracheal mucosa itself.

Granulation tissue may be produced by local trauma throughout the full extent of the airway. This tissue results from local irritation and is often most extensive at the area of the tracheostomy stoma. Less frequently, it may be produced by excessive motion and contact of the tip of the tracheostomy or endotracheal tube with the anterior tracheal wall. Such lesions produce progressive airway obstruction as they enlarge. They may result in intermittent hemoptysis with additional trauma produced by the tube or as a result of endotracheal suctioning. Tissue may be dislodged to produce obstruction in the distal airway.

More extensive lesions such as tracheoesophageal fistulas, fistulas between the airway and major vessels in the juxtatracheal location, are additional sources of problems and are usually life threatening.

DIAGNOSTIC EVALUATION

The preoperative evaluation of a patient with an obstructive airway lesion includes history and physical examination, pulmonary function studies, radiography, and bronchoscopic evaluation. The specific indication for each study must be based on the potential benefit gained from the information, balanced against the urgency to proceed with the operative procedure. This is especially true in cases of acute life-threatening airway obstruction, when it often is necessary to abbreviate any preoperative evaluation. It is most important to use the objective data obtained from the studies above to determine the precise location, nature, and extent of the tracheal pathology.

History

The symptoms produced by airway obstruction are affected by several factors, including anatomic location, the degree of airway impairment, and the possible presence of pre-existing cardiopulmonary disease. Dyspnea, especially on exertion and often preceded by difficulty in clearing secretions, is an early finding in patients with tracheal pathology. Wheezing and stridor are usually signs of more advanced and serious airways disease. Although these are simple nonspecific findings, they are frequently misdiagnosed. As previously mentioned, this is especially true when dealing with slow-growing tracheal tumors that are often misdiagnosed as asthma. Only after the condition has failed to respond to conventional therapy is the suspicion of tracheal pathology raised. It is important to consider the presence of tracheal stenosis in any patient who gives a history of intubation and/or tracheostomy within recent months or even years. Any of the symptoms mentioned above

should be considered a result of an organic lesion until proved otherwise.

Physical Examination

Physical examination is often of marginal value. Audible stridor that may occur with exercise, forced inspiratory and expiratory flow, or at rest is a common finding in the advanced stages of airway pathology. Auscultation of the chest often reveals diffuse inspiratory and expiratory wheezing, which may clearly mimic that heard with bronchospasm. Auscultation of the upper airway (trachea) produces characteristic sounds of obstruction to airflow, based on the extent and nature of the lesion.

Pulmonary Function Tests

The use of the flow-volume loop has been shown to be a valuable diagnostic tool in patients presenting with obstructive lesions of the airway. Maximal expiratory and/or inspiratory flow is significantly reduced with a resulting characteristic plateau pattern. Depending on the nature of the airway obstruction, this pattern occurs on inspiratory, expiratory, or both segments of the loop. With fixed lesions that are either intrathoracic or extrathoracic, the inspiratory and expiratory flows are reduced. In cases in which there is a variable obstruction (i.e., with tracheal malacia), the maximal plateau occurs either on inspiratory or expiratory flow alone, depending on the location of the lesion within or outside of the thorax. Extrathoracic or cervical lesions characteristically produce a plateau during inspiration as airway pressure falls below atmospheric pressure, producing narrowing of the lumen. In the case of intrathoracic lesions, the opposite effect occurs on inspiratory and expiratory loops as governed by the negative or positive changes in pleural pressure during inspiration and expiration relative to the pressure within the airway.

Components of standard spirometry are of limited value in the specific diagnosis of large airway obstruction. In the absence of the ability to carry out a flow-volume loop, one indicator of such obstruction is the relationship between the 1-second forced expiratory volume (FEV_1) and the peak expiratory flow rate. Since the FEV_1 is generally affected to a far less degree than is the peak expiratory flow, the ratio of peak expiratory flow to FEV_1 has been used as an index of obstruction. When this ratio is 10 to 1 or greater, it is suggestive, but not diagnostic, of airway obstruction.

Radiography

Both routine and special radiologic studies are important in demonstrating the extent and location of tracheal pathology. The standard anteroposterior and lateral chest roentgenograms, combined with oblique views, are often of value in delineating tracheal pathology. An anteroposterior copper-filtered view of the trachea accentuates the detail of the air column. Lateral cervical views are often useful to demonstrate the pathology. Fluoroscopy is frequently helpful to determine the functional nature and the extent of dynamic change in the airway column during inspiratory and expiratory maneuvers. Tomograms and computed tomography (CT) of the chest are of value in demonstrating clearly the precise location and extent of pathology.

Bronchoscopic Evaluation

Bronchoscopy is the ultimate diagnostic procedure in cases of airway pathology. The decision to use a flexible or rigid bronchoscopic technique is determined by factors including the experience of the endoscopist, available equipment, and the location of the airway pathology. In general, we rely primarily on use of rigid bronchoscopy, which, when combined with straight and angled telescopes, provides a better definition of the extent and nature of the lesion. Bronchoscopy is usually deferred until the time of the proposed operative procedure, because it is possible for the procedure to precipitate an increase in airway obstruction secondary to edema or hemorrhage.

Special precautions must be taken in the evaluation of patients with pre-existing endotracheal or tracheostomy tubes. When the tube lies within the area of pathology, flow-volume studies and radiologic evaluation may be of limited value. Under such circumstances, it is generally necessary to decannulate patients to obtain adequate information from the studies. When these procedures are carried out either in the x-ray or pulmonary function laboratory, they should be performed under the close supervision of an individual trained in the use of equipment and techniques necessary to reinstitute tracheal intubation.

ANESTHETIC MANAGEMENT

At the time of the preoperative evaluation, it is assumed that the important aspects of the tracheal pathology such as location and extent have been clearly delineated. Several surgical approaches for abnormalities in different portions of the airway are considered in this section.

As previously indicated, bronchoscopy is usually performed at the time of proposed surgical correction. This is done to reduce the incidence of airway compromise as a result of the bronchoscopy and to require only one anesthetic for both diagnosis and surgical correction.

Since these patients already present with potentially life-threatening obstructing airway lesions, it is incumbent to note additional anatomic abnormalities in the face, pharynx, and jaw. This is especially true when these pose problems with mask fit and visualization with direct laryngoscopy. In such patients one can anticipate a prolonged and difficult induction with a combination of inhalation and intravenous agents; one must rely heavily on the ability to maintain an adequate natural airway with a mask. Tracheal tumors, especially those of a pedunculated nature, must be evaluated with a careful preoperative history. The position used during the induction may be modified (semi-Fowler's, sitting, lateral, etc.) to minimize airway obstruction by the tumor mass.

Preoperative Medication

Choice of preoperative medication is dictated by a variety of factors. The potential complications of heavy sedation with tranquilizers, barbiturates, and narcotics must be considered. Any central nervous system depression, when superimposed on airway obstruction, could further compromise respiratory gas exchange. When little or no airway obstruction exists, the need for sedation and/or drying agents is usually dictated by conventional criteria. Anxiety can generally be averted with small doses of tranquilizers and/or barbiturates following arrival in the operating room. Drying agents are generally avoided, based on the experience that airway obstruction worsened as mucus became less viscous and produced occlusion at the site of tracheal pathology.

When tracheal obstruction is bypassed with use of endotracheal, tracheostomy, or T-tube, the use of premedication is determined by the needs exhibited by the patient and the anticipated induction technique.

Monitoring

In most uncomplicated approaches to tracheal resection and reconstruction, standard monitoring techniques are employed. These include the use of the electrocardiograph (ECG), radial arterial (or alternative site) cannulation, blood pressure cuff, and when feasible, esophageal stethoscope. Intravenous access is generally achieved with an appropriate-sized catheter placed in the distal aspect of the upper extremity used for arterial cannulation. The selection of the site of cannulation is governed not only by the availability of vessels but also by the potential need to sacrifice one of the major vessels leading to the extremity. This is especially true for the right upper extremity, because the arterial supply is through the innominate artery, which lies in a position anterior to the cervical trachea. Retraction and digital dissection of the trachea through a cervical incision can cause temporary compression of the innominate artery and temporary loss of the arterial pressure trace. Occasionally it is necessary to sacrifice the innominate artery; thus, when given the choice, the left radial artery is the preferred site for cannulation. Alternative sites, such as femoral, dorsalis pedis, and axillary arteries, can be used under special circumstances.

In general, central venous and pulmonary artery catheters are selected when pre-existing cardiovascular pathology dictates the use of such monitoring or when there is need for central drug administration. When such catheters are placed in neck vessels, one must drape the site in a manner that does not interfere with the surgical approach.

Use of an esophageal stethoscope not only provides information pertinent to the character of heart sounds and airflow but also serves as a foreign body to guide the surgeon in identifying the esophagus in the surgical field.

Other noninvasive techniques such as end-tidal carbon dioxide monitoring, and pulse oximetry provide obvious additional information that can be of value during periods of airway compromise. These monitoring techniques may be helpful during induction or during the operative procedure itself.

Airway Equipment

Special consideration must be given to the selection of unusual equipment prior to administration of anesthesia. It is beneficial to have an anesthesia machine with the capability of delivering oxygen at a high flow rate (in excess of 20 L per minute). This is useful if air leaks pose problems during rigid bronchoscopy.

The choice of laryngoscope and blade is governed by the experience of the anesthesiologist and the anatomy of the upper airway. An appropriate atomizer with a long (6- to 8-inch) limb is useful for topicalization of the pharynx and upper airway. A 4-percent lidocaine solution is preferred.

The selection of endotracheal tube size and type is the most important issue to be considered. In our experience, the most suitable tube for the uncomplicated procedure is the red rubber nondisposable type. These are left uncut—that is, they are kept the length supplied by the manufacturer. The optimal tube size is one that provides an adequate airway and ability to suction secretions and that allows surgical manipulation of the trachea. It is advisable to have a variety of sizes available (20, 22, 24, 26, and 28 French); the last two sizes are used most frequently. Since the small diameter endotracheal tubes have a proportionately shorter length, it may be necessary to use an MLT R tube (Mallinckrodt). These tubes are long and narrow and are designed for adults with airway lesions, allowing sufficient length to advance the tube beyond the lesion. The extra length is also useful when intubation is done via the nasal approach. The tube size is selected following visualization of the airway with bronchoscopy. As will be discussed later in this chapter, a decision must be made as to whether to intubate through the stenosis or to rely on a tube placed proximal to it.

Induction of Anesthesia

The patient is placed in the supine position with the limb used for intravenous catheter and arterial monitoring extended at about a 45-degree angle from the trunk. The other upper extremity may be tucked in at the side. In patients with minimal airway obstruction and a good natural airway, anesthesia may be induced with thiopental or a similar agent. When airway conditions are lim-

ited by a high degree of obstruction, it is desirable to use a more controlled inhalation induction with a volatile agent. In either case, patients are denitrogenated prior to induction. With an inhalation induction, choice of agent is somewhat arbitrary. Halothane, because it is somewhat better tolerated, is probably slightly superior to either isoflurane or enflurane. Muscle relaxants are usually not necessary. Use of spontaneous respiration is advisable, because the ability to intubate the trachea and to provide an airway is not always guaranteed with tracheal pathology. In cases of severe airway obstruction, it is often possible to maintain minimal yet marginal satisfactory gas exchange with a combination of spontaneous and assisted positive-pressure breaths. If ventilation is difficult after induction of anesthesia, a rigid bronchoscope may be used to dilate strictures or bypass the tumor mass. These bronchoscopes have a side-arm that may be connected to the anesthesia breathing circuit.

Anesthesia is induced until the patient is able to tolerate laryngoscopy. At this time, laryngoscopy serves to visualize the upper airway, to ascertain otherwise unforeseen difficulties in laryngeal intubation, and to apply topical anesthesia to the upper airway for anticipated bronchoscopy. During bronchoscopy, it is important for the anesthesiologist personally to inspect the airway to evaluate the nature and extent of the lesion. Thus, one can better anticipate difficulty with endotracheal tube placement.

A decision is made at the time of rigid bronchoscopy whether to pass the endotracheal tube distal to the lesion. Lesions involving the upper third of the trachea, especially those in the subglottic area, pose special problems in allowing placement of the tube distal enough into the airway to position the cuff below the level of the cords. Use of extremely small tubes (20 or 22 French) carries the potential risk of obstruction due to foreign material such as secretions and blood. Surgical dilatation of the airway must be undertaken with caution because trauma is possible, including bleeding, dissection of mucosa, and potential for perforation. The standard approach has been to dilate strictures if the diameter of the airway measures less than 5 mm. Such dilatation is done under direct vision with small rigid pediatric ventilating bronchoscopes; dilators passed through a larger bronchoscope may easily perforate the tracheal wall and create life-threatening situations. If the airway is more than 5 mm in diameter, the endotracheal tube is passed through the lesion into normal distal trachea.

When the pathology is located in the lower or middle third of the trachea, and when it is possible to place a cuff below the level of the cords, the lumen is evaluated. Again, if the airway is 5 cm in diameter or less, and if it can be done with minimal trauma, the airway is dilated. Strictures of the anterior tracheal wall generally occur following tracheostomy, because the previous stoma produces airway narrowing due to scarring. This problem is usually dealt with easily because the posterior membranous wall is not involved and hence provides enough mobility for the endotracheal tube to pass beyond the lesion into the normal distal trachea.

Once bronchoscopy is completed, intubation is carried out with the appropriate-size tube. Standard laryngoscopic techniques are employed, with the only difference being that one tries to sense the point at which the distal end of the tube passes through the narrowed area of the trachea. The tube is secured, the eyes are protected, and an esophageal stethoscope is passed. Anesthesia is then maintained with an inhalation agent and oxygen, and when normal pulmonary function exists and an adequate airway is present, with use of nitrous oxide.

ALTERNATIVE AIRWAY MANAGEMENT TECHNIQUES

There are several other approaches to the airway in patients with obstructive tracheal lesions. In the presence of an abnormal upper airway or a severely stenotic trachea, an awake intubation may be the safest method of establishing a secure airway. This can be accomplished with a fiberoptic endoscope used as a stylet inside of an endotracheal tube. With adequate sedation, topical anesthesia of the upper airway, and a transtracheal injection of lidocaine, this technique is well tolerated by the patient.

When appropriate, some lesions may be amenable to laser excision. This can be performed through a fiberoptic bronchoscope using a Nd:YAG (neodymium-yttrium-aluminum-garnet) or KTP (krypton) laser in an awake or sedated patient. Laser surgery can also be performed through a rigid bronchoscope or suspension laryngoscope with a carbon dioxide laser with the patient under general anesthesia. The use of Venturi jet ventilation can help provide adequate oxygenation and ventilation without an endotracheal tube impinging on the surgical field during the procedure. This technique uses a high-pressure oxygen source (50 psi) with a manually triggered valve and a small-bore cannula to provide high velocity flow into the airway. The cannula can be attached to the suspension laryngoscope and directed at the glottic opening. The cannula also can be passed down an endotracheal tube to bypass large tracheal tumors and provide gas exchange distal to the lesion.

There are several reports of successful tracheal surgery using partial and full cardiopulmonary bypass, especially in small children in whom intraoperative selective endobronchial intubation may be physically difficult. Some would claim, however, that these patients should be treated with a Silastic stent with surgical repair delayed until the child has grown, thus facilitating surgical repair.

Surgical Reconstruction of the Upper Trachea

For uncomplicated lesions involving the upper third of the trachea, the surgical approach uses a short collar incision with the potential for a vertical extension with partial sternal division. Airway patency must be continually assessed, especially if intubation was not carried through the diseased portion of the trachea, because surgical dissection and release of the external support can produce a more complete airway obstruction. At this point in the procedure, the diseased portion of the trachea is identified and the site of surgical entry into the trachea is determined. Nitrous oxide, if previously used, is eliminated from the inspired gas mixture.

Lateral traction sutures are placed through the full thickness of the tracheal wall at the midline on either side, above and below the diseased portion of the trachea. It is important to deflate the cuff on the endotracheal tube to avoid having the needle puncture the tracheal wall. Sterile "connecting equipment," consisting of two corrugated anesthesia tubes, a Y-piece, and an appropriate-size flexible armored (Tovell) endotracheal tube, should be available on the surgical field. The trachea is now transected, generally at a site below the lesion. The distal trachea is intubated across the operative field with the flexible armored tube. The two limbs of the corrugated tubing, passed back under the head drapes, are then connected to the anesthesia machine. The oral endotracheal tube is advanced into the surgical field and a soft sterile rubber catheter is sutured to the tip so that the tube can be drawn back up into the proximal trachea with the catheter lying in the surgical field. This catheter prevents malpositioning of the tube out of the larynx and facilitates repositioning of the endotracheal tube back down into the trachea at the time of the reanastomosis of the tracheal ends.

Once surgical dissection has been carried out and the diseased portion of the trachea has been removed, the feasibility of reanastomosis without undue pressure is decided with use of traction sutures and head flexion by the anesthesiologist. When it is not possible to bring the ends together owing to a high degree of tension, surgical laryngeal release is performed.

Intermittent sutures are placed through the proximal and distal tracheal ends with gas exchange provided by the armored tube placed into the distal trachea. Once all sutures are in place, the armored tube is removed and the oral endotracheal tube is advanced through the anastomosis into the distal trachea. Care must be taken at this point not to pass the tube too far distally into the surgically foreshortened trachea. Subsequent flexion of the neck would increase the likelihood of mainstem bronchial intubation. The appropriate, previously used, corrugated tubings are reconnected to the anesthesia machine and connected to the proximal end of the original endotracheal tube. Once all sutures are tied securely, the anastomosis is tested by applying positive airway pressure (cuff deflated) using sterile saline in the surgical field.

In most cases, an attempt is made to extubate the patient in the operating room. This may be accomplished with the patient under deep anesthesia or in the awake state. The selection of a technique must be balanced against the potential complications of each approach.

The advantages of extubation at deep levels of anesthesia is the reduced potential for bucking, struggling, and extensive neck motion during the excitement stage, with injury to the suture line. In patients in whom intubation was difficult because of upper airway pathology, it is prudent to allow the patient to awaken with the tube in place and to support the head and neck during the excitement phase. In general, it is easier to reintubate when necessary with a level of anesthesia than it is when the patient is partially or completely awake. Once the airway and ventilation are judged to be adequate, the patient is transported, using supplemental oxygen, to the intensive care unit.

Reconstruction of the Lower Trachea

The general principles followed for intubation and maintenance of anesthesia for surgery in the upper trachea are applied to most lesions involving the distal area, including the carina. The major differences are tube placement and ventilation of individual lungs independently. Thoracotomy is generally necessary for lesions in the distal airway. In most cases the initial anesthetic management involves placement of the endotracheal tube proximal to the lesion, which potentially can produce increased airway obstruction as surgical exposure with dissection and compression is carried out. Once the trachea is divided, it is fairly common to find that the distal tracheal stump is too short to accommodate both endotracheal tube and cuff. Thus, endobronchial intubation, either unilaterally or bilaterally, is necessary. In the lateral position, the dependent lung is generally preferred if one lung is to be used, because the distribution of blood flow should be to that area. When one lung (the dependent one) is not sufficient to maintain oxygenation or carbon dioxide elimination, the nondependent lung is ventilated with a separate endotracheal tube and a second anesthesia machine. If oxygenation is a limiting factor, then continuous positive airway pressure to the nondependent lung without ventilation is often adequate. High-frequency ventilation and insufflation to the nondependent lung can also be useful.

During resection of the carina, reanastomosis of the distal trachea to both bronchi can be carried out in a variety of ways. In general, the first bronchus is anastomosed in an end-to-end fashion to the distal trachea. This anastomosis is carried out in a manner similar to that used for the upper trachea. Once the sutures are in place, the endotracheal tube is advanced from its proximal position through the anastomosis into the distal bronchus and the sutures are tied to secure the airway. During this time, the unattached lung may be left collapsed, inflated, or ventilated, depending on need with respect to gas exchange. The second lung is then reanastomosed in an end-to-side fashion either into the distal trachea or into the bronchus of the other lung. Once this anastomosis has been completed, the endotracheal tube is pulled back into a more proximal position and both lungs are ventilated simultaneously using this route.

The surgical approach using a thoracotomy may limit the adequacy of spontaneous ventilation or pulmonary toilet in the postoperative period. The need for continued intubation and positive pressure ventilation poses several potential problems including disruption at the suture line, direct trauma from the tube itself, and a source of infection. In most cases in which there is no pre-existing lung disease, it is generally possible to extubate patients in the operating room following major carinal reconstruction. Choice of extubation in the awake state or at a deeper level of anesthesia carries the same considerations as were previously discussed.

POSTOPERATIVE CARE

All patients are admitted to the intensive care unit following tracheal resection and reconstruction. A chest radiograph is obtained immediately following admission to ensure that pneumothorax was not inadvertently produced even though the approach was through a collar incision. The patient is maintained in a semi-Fowler's position with the head in a flexed attitude and a number of firm pillows placed directly under the occiput; support is aided by the suture placed from chin to anterior chest. The patient should receive supplemental oxygen with a high-flow humidified face mask system. Analgesia in most cases is easily accomplished with parenteral narcotics. Following thoracotomy, supplementation with intercostal nerve block is often advantageous.

Routine nursing procedures are dictated by the nature and extent of underlying disease and the ability to maintain gas exchange and pulmonary toilet. Chest physical therapy is routinely administered to such patients. This includes encouragement to cough, chest percussion and vibration, and blind nasotracheal suctioning to remove secretions from the airway when necessary. In selected cases in which pulmonary toilet is inadequate, flexible fiberoptic bronchoscopy on a daily or more frequent basis is used to obviate a need for intubation. In individuals for whom secretions cannot be removed or ventilation is necessary, intubation of the trachea is required. This procedure obviously must be done with a great deal of caution to avoid direct trauma to the fresh anastomosis. In most cases, this is accomplished by maintaining the head in a flexed position with use of intravenous sedation, topical anesthesia, and local nerve block. A careful, controlled, blind nasotracheal approach is usually tried first. The advantage of the nasotracheal route is that the tube, once in position, is easily secured in relation to the anastomosis. When blind intubation fails, direct visualization with either fiberoptic technique or standard laryngoscope is carried out.

Upper airway obstruction secondary to laryngeal edema is a possible complication in the immediate postoperative period. This is especially true when a high surgical anastomosis has been carried out. Specific therapy when this occurs includes use of racemic epinephrine (0.5 ml of a 1-to-200 dilution) administered every 2 to 4 hours, with or without use of inhaled or intravenous steroids every 4 to 6 hours. This therapy is generally carried out for a minimum of 24 hours, or longer if there is persistent evidence of laryngeal edema with stridor.

Discharge of patients from the intensive care unit to the floor is determined by the ability to discontinue monitoring, the lack of a need for serial blood gas measurements, the ability to clear secretions, and the presence of an adequate airway with respect to gas flow.

SUGGESTED READING

Geffin B, Bland J, Grillo HC. Anesthetic management of tracheal resection and reconstruction. Anesthes Analg 1969; 48:884–894.

Grillo HC. Reconstruction of the trachea. Experience in 100 consecutive cases. Thorax 1973; 28:667–679.
Grillo HC. Tracheal tumors: surgical management. Ann Thorac Surg 1978; 26:112–125.
Grillo HC. Congenital lesions, neoplasms, and injuries of the trachea. In: Sabiston DC Jr, Spencer FC, eds. Gibbon's surgery of the chest. Philadelphia: WB Saunders, 1982.
Grillo HC, Mathisen OJ. Surgical management of tracheal strictures. Surg Clin North Am 1988; 68:511–524.
Grillo HC, Mathisen DJ. Primary tracheal tumors: treatment and results. Ann Thorac Surg 1990; 49:69–77.
Heitmiller RF. Tracheal stenosis. In: Cameron J, ed. Current Surgical Therapy-3. Philadelphia: B.C. Decker, 1989:516–519.
Wilson RS. Tracheostomy and tracheal reconstruction. In: Kaplan J. ed. Thoracic anesthesia. New York: Churchill Livingstone, 1983: 421–445.

TONSILLECTOMY, ADENOIDECTOMY, AND PRESSURE-EQUALIZING TUBES

SUSAN G. STRAUSS, M.D.

In the world of pediatric surgery, ears, nose, and throat (ENT) procedures represent the largest category of the operative case load. At the Children's Hospital and Medical Center (CHMC) in Seattle, Washington, in the fiscal year 1989, they accounted for more than 33 percent of the total number of operating room cases and 58 percent of the day surgery cases. Insertion of pressure-equalizing (PE) tubes, alone or in combination with tonsil and adenoid surgery, accounted for 62 percent of those ENT procedures. Adenotonsillectomy remains the most common major pediatric surgical procedure, and insertion of PE tubes is the most commonly performed minor surgical procedure.

TONSILLECTOMY AND ADENOIDECTOMY

Athough it has long been the most common operation performed in children, there has been a significant reduction in the number of tonsillectomies and adenoidectomies performed over the past two decades. In the United States, the frequency of tonsillectomies and adenoidectomies declined 80.7 percent during the 16-year period from 1971 to 1987. Despite the overall reduction in recent years, these surgical procedures continue to comprise more than 50 percent of cases scheduled in most active pediatric day surgery centers. Any anesthesiologist whose practice includes the pediatric population will inevitably provide anesthesia for tonsil and adenoid surgery. The anesthesiologist will therefore require a full understanding of the child's pathophysiology and the anesthetic implications in order to tailor an anesthetic that is both safe and appropriate.

The marked variation in the attitude and practice of tonsil and adenoid surgery that existed in the past has lessened in recent years. This can be explained in part by the more stringent criteria now employed by the authorities in the medical community recommending surgery. Until recently there had been little convincing evidence supporting the efficacy of surgery over conservative management. With an improvement of study design and focusing on more severely affected children, a current study from the Children's Hospital of Pittsburgh has shown tonsil and adenoid surgery to have several benefits. In this study, three main issues were addressed:

1. The efficacy of tonsillectomy in reducing the frequency and severity of episodes of pharyngitis.
2. The efficacy of adenoidectomy in reducing the frequency and severity of otitis media.
3. The effect of adenoidectomy on the course of nasal obstruction due to large adenoids.

Most of the benefits from surgery were statistically significant for the first 2 years postoperatively when compared with conservative medical management.

In contrast to popular belief of the past, when tonsillectomy and adenoidectomy were carried out as a single, combined operation, it is currently believed that the two procedures are separate entities that may be performed individually. Each component of the operation has its own specific indications and requires individual attention. Nevertheless, for the sake of discussion throughout the remainder of this chapter, I will refer to tonsil and adenoid surgery as a single procedure.

The indications for performing adenotonsillectomy fall into two major categories: *infection* that is recurrent or chronic and *obstruction*. In addition to infection of the tonsils and adenoids, there may be infection of the middle ears, mastoid air cells, paranasal sinuses, peritonsillar tissues, and cervical lymph nodes. Obstruction involves the nasopharyngeal and oropharyngeal airways. Tonsillectomy has generally been considered the component of tonsil and adenoid surgery that is beneficial with regard to recurrent pharyngitis, and adenoidectomy the component that is efficacious with regard to chronic otitis media with effusion. The indications for performing adenoidectomy are found more often than for performing tonsillectomy, and the rate of adenoidectomy alone has significantly increased in recent years.

Adenotonsillar surgery is clearly indicated for obstructive symptoms in those *rare* patients in whom massive tonsillar and adenoidal hypertrophy causes ventilatory obstruction resulting in alveolar hypoventilation and cor pulmonale consistent with obstructive sleep apnea (OSA). (These severe cases are discussed in greater detail elsewhere in this text.) [There is a large patient population in whom although obstructive symptoms are present to varying degrees, the secondary pathophysiology has not yet occurred or its symptoms are not clinically appreciated.] It has been argued that the incidence of patients presenting for surgery with upper airway obstruction has increased as the criteria for tonsillectomy and adenoidectomy have become more stringent. This patient population can be quite challenging to the anesthesiologist.

Risks

The anesthetic concerns for tonsil and adenoid surgery fall into one major category: appropriate airway management. Partial airway obstruction caused by adenotonsillar hypertrophy may worsen during induction of anesthesia. Postoperatively, uvular and palatal swelling may occur, causing yet another source of airway obstruction. In the young toddler, particularly, uvular and palatal swelling may be severe enough to require reintubation and hospitalization until the swelling subsides.

Patients with chronic partial airway obstruction may be more sensitive to the ventilatory depressant effects of narcotics. Patients with obstructive sleep apnea may have an abnormal ventilatory response to carbon dioxide (i.e., the carbon dioxide response curve is shifted to the right) in addition to chronic carbon dioxide retention. Narcotics must be administered *gingerly*, if at all, in this particular patient population.

Bleeding from adenotonsillar surgery is actually a surgical risk, although its anesthetic implications are ever present. Fluid resuscitation may be required. Blood in the airway is a noxious stimulus that can promote laryngospasm if caution is not taken. Swallowing blood can cause profound postoperative nausea and vomiting.

Preoperative Evaluation and Preparation

Preoperative evaluation of the patient about to undergo tonsil and adenoid surgery should attempt to identify those patients with obstructive airway symptoms and bleeding disorders. In most cases, a careful history identifies these patients; the physical examination and appropriate laboratory evaluation will most often be confirmatory. Important questions to ask in order to assess the degree of airway obstruction include the following:

1. Does the patient snore while sleeping?
2. If the patient snores, does he or she have periodic apneic episodes? Does the apneic period last for 10 seconds or more?
3. Is the patient's snoring exacerbated or relieved by any particular sleeping position?
4. If pauses in breathing occur, has the patient ever been noted to appear cyanotic during these episodes?
5. Is the patient's sleep pattern restless?
6. Is the patient not well rested in the morning?

These questions attempt to identify those patients with increasing severity of obstruction. The latter three questions identify the rare patient with obstructive sleep apnea. Patients with severe obstructive symptoms will require further medical investigation. The severity of snoring does not imply severity of the disorder. Loud snorers may have little or no apnea, whereas quiet snorers, especially infants and young toddlers, may have extended apneic periods. Physical examination may reveal a mouth-breathing patient with a "hot potato" voice, adenoidal facies, and marked tonsillar hypertrophy.

Questions to elicit a bleeding disorder may include the following:

1. Is there a family history of bleeding tendency (e.g., childbirth, trauma, surgery)?
2. Does the patient bruise easily or have frequent epistaxis or gingival bleeding?
3. Have there been problems with excessive bleeding from previous surgery (e.g., dental extractions or circumcision)?
4. Has the patient been using aspirin or a nonsteroidal anti-inflammatory drug during the past 2 weeks?
5. Does the menstruating female have prolonged or excessive bleeding?

A positive answer to any of the above questions suggests the possibility of a coagulation disorder. Appropriate laboratory testing should begin with a platelet count, bleeding time, prothrombin time, and partial thromboplastin time. Recognizing these possible problems in advance allows the anesthesiologist to tailor the patient's anesthetic and be prepared to treat the problems as they arise during the perioperative period.

The anesthetic plan should encompass the aforementioned concerns as well as address any other ongoing medical problems. In addition, the anesthesiologist needs to consider not only the patient's problems, but the presence or absence of support staff at the particular surgical center. Physicians and nurses at a hospital caring exclusively for children may be more comfortable caring for, anticipating, and handling the various pediatric problems that may arise perioperatively than the staff at a primarily adult hospital. For example, the availability of nurses and technicians with an expertise in pediatric intravenous cannulation may allow an anesthesiologist to feel more secure in performing an inhalation induction, which, when followed by intravenous cannulation, avoids the usual emotional trauma of awake intravenous insertion in the child. Similarly, if the recovery room nurses are trained and comfortable in providing temporary airway support, an anesthesiologist may opt for a plan that includes deep extubation at the end of the case. The ideal anesthetic plan should maximize patient safety, minimize emotional trauma and be expeditious and efficient.

Induction of Anesthesia

The anesthetic induction should ensure airway safety as a priority; patient acceptance and comfort, although important, are secondary. The safest anesthetic induction will maintain spontaneous ventilation until airway control is established. Sufficient monitoring includes a precordial stethoscope, pulse oximetry, capnography, electrocardiography, and measurement of blood pressure and body temperature. Capnography, although currently not mandatory, is quite helpful as an indication of adequacy of ventilation and unintentional circuit disconnection.

Most children will readily accept an inhalation induction with halothane, with or without nitrous oxide, especially if a parent or guardian is present. At the beginning of an inhalation induction, during spontaneous ventilation, the patient maintains his or her own patent airway. As the level of anesthesia deepens, the anesthesiologist may then assist or manipulate the airway as needed, should partial obstruction occur. *Gradual* control is the key to successful airway management. It avoids confronting the dangerous situation of airway obstruction in an apneic and/or paralyzed patient. Should an intravenous line be placed before induction, the anesthesiologist may combine small increments of short-acting intravenous barbiturate with an inhalation induction. This, too, provides a smooth induction while still maintaining spontaneous ventilation and may offer the advantage of passing through the excitement phase, during which obstruction most often occurs.

Occasionally a child accepts neither an intravenous line nor a mask for an inhalation induction, and alternative methods of induction must be sought to avoid both a physical struggle and emotional trauma. If airway obstruction is not an anticipated problem, other reliable modes of induction may include rectal barbiturates and more recently, nasally or orally administered midazolam.

Of all the rectally administered sedative-hypnotic drugs, methohexital has received the most attention because of its short half-life. When a 10 percent solution is used, a dose of 20 to 25 mg per kilogram provides adequate sedation in 90 percent of children within 6 to 8 minutes. Among the side effects, respiratory depression (2 to 3 percent) and laryngospasm (< 1 percent) warrant extreme caution in its use in any patient with a compromised airway. Resuscitation equipment and individuals with airway skills should be available. Rectal sedation as a mode of induction in patients 6 months to 6 years of age is an excellent alternative to an intravenous or inhalation induction: it is effective, relatively safe, and generally well accepted by parents and patients alike. Its use is limited by the patient's weight, and hence the volume of drug administered. Disadvantages of rectal barbiturates may include a prolonged awakening and recovery room stay for a relatively short operation.

Recently, nasally administered drugs have received a lot of attention, particularly for the pediatric population. Midazolam, in particular, with a half-life of 45 minutes, is quite effective in changing a previously apprehensive, uncooperative child into an accepting, cooperative child. A dose of 0.2 to 0.3 mg per kilogram of a 5 mg per milliliter midazolam solution administered intranasally is effective within 8 to 10 minutes. The patient is often awake but very relaxed and will readily accept a mask for inhalation induction or intravenous cannulation. Less than 10 percent of children actually sleep as a result of this dose. As with any central nervous system depressant, caution must be taken when administering this agent to a patient with a compromised airway. Small volumes of the midazolam are well tolerated, although a transient postnasal "stinging" usually occurs due to its low pH. Occasionally, even intranasal administration of midazolam is fraught with terror, in which case it may be administered orally in a dose of 0.5 to 0.75 mg per kilogram. It is more palatable if diluted with 10 ml of a clear, sweet juice. Effects are less reliable after oral administration due to the first-pass effect through the liver giving more variable blood levels. The relatively large dose and volume required for oral administration also limits its use in patients weighing less than 20 to 25 kg.

Children who are chronic mouth-breathers with obstructed nasal passages may become obstructed during the early phase of induction when the mouth closes under the mask. Mask ventilation with the patient's mouth open can be accomplished by placing the lower end of the mask under the lower lip, which partially opens the mouth. This technique is useful when obstruction occurs, yet the level of anesthesia is still too light to tolerate airway instrumentation. Other maneuvers that may be employed to overcome airway obstruction, should it occur, include (1) jaw lift; (2) 5 to 10 cm H_2O mask continuous positive airway pressure; (3) changing the head position (e.g., side-to-side, extension, flexion); and (4) creation of an artificial airway (oropharyngeal or nasopharyngeal). Insertion of an artificial airway almost always relieves the obstruction. To avoid laryngospasm, care must be taken not to introduce the artificial airway before the laryngeal reflexes are obtunded.

Airway manipulation is better tolerated at a lighter level of anesthesia if topical anesthesia has been applied to the base of the tongue and oropharynx before induction. Topicalization is most easily performed on the cooperative patient; therefore, it has its limitation in the young child. It is quite beneficial for the older patient should the need for early airway manipulation be anticipated.

Intubation may take place with the patient under deep anesthesia or with the aid of a muscle relaxant. The preformed oral-reverse-angle-endotracheal tube (ORAE) allows the anesthesia circuit to be connected and positioned below the chin, away from the operative field. The midline groove of the tongue blade of a self-retaining mouth gag holds the ORAE tube in place (Fig. 1). Maximal opening of the mouth gag may cause compression or caudal displacement of the endotracheal tube and endobronchial positioning. Compression or malposition can be adjusted easily by releasing the tension and repositioning the endotracheal tube.

Intraoperative Management

The goal of intraoperative anesthetic management for adenotonsillectomy is to deliver a safe anesthetic that enables prompt awakening at the end of the case yet provides an adequate level of anesthesia for a particularly noxious surgical procedure. The addition of narcotics offers the advantage of decreasing the concentration of the volatile agent needed for anesthetic maintenance, which facilitates more rapid awakening. Such a balanced technique may be used in combination with a short-acting muscle relaxant. The addition of a muscle relaxant may allow further reduction of the volatile agent required for an adequate anesthetic. Without the use of muscle relaxation, despite what appears to be an appropriate level of anesthesia, the patient may sometimes swallow, disrupting the surgical field.

The most commonly used narcotics are morphine, meperidine hydrochloride (Demerol), and fentanyl. A morphine dose of 0.05 to 0.10 mg per kilogram or a Demerol dose of 0.5 to 1.0 mg per kilogram will allow a progressive reduction in the concentration of volatile agent required. Likewise, a fentanyl dose range of 2 to 5 μg per kilogram will provide the same benefit. It is most effective to administer the entire dose of a short-acting potent narcotic, such as fentanyl, at the beginning of the anesthesia. Given as a bolus up front, the marked respiratory depressant effects are minimized, and the patient readily resumes spontaneous ventilation at the end of the case and within a couple minutes is awake and ready for extubation.

By and large, most patients presenting for adeno-tonsillar surgery benefit from the addition of a narcotic to their anesthetic. However, the anesthesiologist should *always* consider the possibility of unappreciated, undiagnosed obstructive sleep apnea in *all* children presenting to the anesthesia department for adenotonsillectomy. As a rule, the use of narcotics should be avoided in any patient with symptoms suggestive of moderate-to-severe chronic partial airway obstruction. These particular patients, although uncommon, often display an exquisite sensitivity to the respiratory depressant effects of narcotics. Once a patient is extubated and maintaining a patient airway in the recovery room, then—and only if necessary—one may carefully administer very small incremental doses of a narcotic of approximately 0.025 mg morphine or 0.25–0.5 μg of fentanyl.

The most commonly employed muscle relaxants are the short-acting nondepolarizing agents, vecuronium bromide and atracurium besylate. Usually only the initial intubating dose is necessary for adequate relaxation for the entire surgical procedure. In fact, for some surgical techniques only two-thirds to three-fourths of an intubating dose of a muscle relaxant is needed, because the procedure is so brief. Familiarity with particular surgeons and their preferred techniques gives the anesthe-

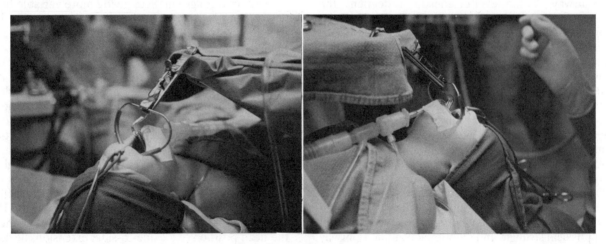

Figure 1 *A,* The oral RAE tube is secured over the center of the lower lip. The midline groove of a self-retaining mouth-gag firmly holds the tube in place. *B,* The surgeon may insert a soft red rubber catheter through the nasopharynx to retract the soft palate and provide better visualization for performing an adenoidectomy.

siologist foresight to formulate the optimal anesthetic plan.

Extubation

Before extubation, the anesthesiologist should inspect the hypopharynx to evaluate hemostasis and remove any blood clots or loose fragments of lymphoid tissue. Inspection and suctioning by direct visualization with a laryngoscope avoids traumatizing the surgical field, which may exacerbate bleeding. If adenoidal tissue has been excised, it is helpful to assess bleeding in the nasopharynx by elevating the head, thus promoting drainage toward the hypopharynx. If there is doubt as to the rate of oozing, the anesthesiologist should not hesitate to call it to the surgeon's attention. Once the patient is wide awake, the endotracheal tube may be removed. The patient should be transported to the recovery room with the head down in the lateral position. This position promotes drainage away from the hypopharynx and larynx, which aids in decreasing the stimulus for laryngospasm and the possibility of aspiration. Placing a pillow under the hips of a small child while in the lateral position will accomplish the head-down position and facilitate drainage away from the hypopharynx.

Some anesthesiologists prefer a technique that allows assisted spontaneous ventilation and removal of the endotracheal tube with the patient under deep anesthesia. Spontaneous ventilation is maintained throughout induction, and intubation takes place with the patient under deep anesthesia. Supplemental narcotics given 15 to 20 minutes before the end of surgery helps provide a smooth, nonstressful anesthetic effect and may facilitate deep extubation.

Recovery Room and Postoperative Care

Because of the recent demand for reducing health care costs, most tonsil and adenoid surgery is performed on an outpatient basis. In this particular setting, the recovery period has two phases.

During phase one of recovery, the patient receives immediate postanesthetic care and is closely monitored. Particular attention is paid to blood loss and the adequacy of the airway, hydration, and analgesia. The patient is ready for phase two of recovery once he or she meets the following criteria:

1. Hemodynamically stable.
2. Maintains a good airway.
3. Easily aroused.
4. Comfortable.
5. Can communicate to some degree at a level appropriate for his or her age or baseline ability.

In phase two, the patient may be joined by a parent/guardian. He or she continues to awaken and is observed by nursing personnel. Additional analgesics and antiemetics may be administered if necessary. It is usually during this phase that primary postoperative

hemorrhage (bleeding within the first 24 hours) is observed. Intravenous infusion is continued until oral fluids are fairly well tolerated and the patient is assessed to be adequately hydrated. Some patients, especially toddlers, may refuse any oral intake because of discomfort while swallowing. Before discharge from the Day Surgery facility, the youngster should be encouraged to swallow so that both he and his parent know that it can in fact be done, and the behavior can be continued at home. It is only with incessant encouragement that patients in this age group will attempt the oral intake that is important in maintaining adequate postoperative hydration. Good analgesia often aids the ability to swallow.

Recurrent emesis may be a cause for a prolonged recovery period. These patients are best treated by ensuring good hydration through intravenous infusion and fluid bolus. In this case, it is best not to encourage the use of oral fluids until the patient so desires, at which time he or she will most likely tolerate the oral intake. The average duration of both phase one and phase two is approximately 3 hours, although the recovery period is highly individualized. Ultimately, the decision to discharge a patient to home depends on physician judgment as well as on factors such as parent reliability, and distance and transportation from the home to the hospital.

Postoperative Hemorrhage

Postoperative bleeding is a surgical risk of adenotonsillectomy. Hemorrhage may be primary or secondary, depending on when the bleeding occurs. Primary hemorrhage occurs within the first 24 hours; usually it is noted within the first 2 to 3 hours of the recovery period. In recent reports, the rate of primary hemorrhage has ranged from 0.5 to 2.2 percent. Secondary hemorrhage occurs from 5 to 10 days postoperatively and represents dislodgement of the eschar. The extent of bleeding can range from very mild to quite brisk. Secondary bleeding may be more worrisome, because the situation initially takes place in an uncontrolled out-of-hospital environment without the availability of immediate intravenous access. The rate of secondary hemorrhage ranges from 0.1 to 3 percent.

Bleeding following adenotonsillectomy usually presents as a persistent ooze rather than acute brisk hemorrhage. The extent of blood loss is often unappreciated and underestimated, because the slow trickle is quietly swallowed during the recovery period. Often, it is not until the patient suddenly vomits a large, bloody emesis that the bleeding is appreciated as significant. Vomiting may be infrequent, however, and therefore is not a reliable sign of postoperative bleeding.

Anesthesia for reoperation involves careful evaluation and preparation. The patient may be pale, tachycardic, hypotensive, orthostatic, and possibly restless and hypoxemic from partial upper airway obstruction. Patients who have postoperative hemorrhage require an indwelling intravenous catheter before anesthesia is induced, which is why the intravenous line should be left in place for several hours after the initial surgery. Preinduction intravenous volume resuscitation with a balanced salt solution is paramount until vital signs indicate the patient is normovolemic. One may consider obtaining a hematocrit and type and crossmatch if bleeding is thought to be extensive for that particular patient. When the patient is sufficiently rehydrated, he or she may be taken to the operating room. Premedication should be avoided. If the patient is cooperative, the pharynx is examined and gently suctioned to remove large clots. Attempts to suction the stomach are likely to be unsuccessful in the child and cause more harm than good. The patient is considered to have a full stomach, even if vomiting has occurred.

A rapid-sequence induction following the use of intravenous atropine, 0.02 mg per kilogram, and preoxygenation is the induction method of choice. A large tonsillar suction must be immediately available to suction the hypopharynx in order to provide better visualization upon laryngoscopy. Induction agents of choice include thiopental, 4 mg per kilogram, or ketamine 1 to 2 mg per kilogram, if the volume status is more tenuous, followed by succinylcholine chloride for intubation. Cricoid pressure is maintained until the trachea is intubated. The stomach should be suctioned before extubation. Extubation should take place when the patient is fully awake and protective airway reflexes are intact.

A thrashing, uncooperative child with postoperative hemorrhage may somehow dislodge his or her intravenous line and make it close to impossible to start another. In this challenging, less than ideal situation, further combativeness may worsen bleeding and delay reoperation, which must take place sooner rather than later. A few options are available. One may consider a "stun dose" of ketamine (2 to 5 mg per kilogram IM) followed by intravenous placement. Because even this low dose of ketamine may obtund airway reflexes, equipment for airway management must be readily available. Another option is to proceed with a controlled inhalation induction. As the patient is anesthetized with the head down in the lateral position, with suction immediately available, gentle cricoid pressure is applied. Very close attention is paid to blood pressure and heart rate as the patient's volume status may be tenuous and unable to tolerate much inhaled anesthetic. Preinduction atropine, 0.02 mg per kilogram IM, may aid hemodynamic stability during induction. Intravenous cannulation is then performed as soon as possible, followed by a rapid infusion of crystalloid and intubation either with the patient under deep anesthesia or with succinylcholine chloride.

CHRONIC AIRWAY OBSTRUCTION

Obstructive Sleep Apnea

Obstructive sleep apnea (OSA) is part of a clinical spectrum that includes snoring and other sleep-related obstructive disorders. In OSA, there is a narrowed airway due to anatomic, congenital, neuromuscular, or other miscellaneous factors. In order to maintain adequate airflow through a decreased lumen, the patient increases his respiratory effort, causing an increase in intraluminal negative pressure. Collapse of the airway with cessation of airflow occurs when the collapsing force of negative inspiratory pressure exceeds the dilating force of pharyngeal airway-maintaining muscular contraction. Subsequent physiologic changes ensue, including hypoxemia, hypercarbia, and acidosis. Sufficient changes in arterial oxygen pressure, carbon dioxide partial pressure, and pH then stimulate central and peripheral chemoreceptors and baroreceptors, resulting in arousal from sleep. Once awakened, the patient will usually gasp, resume airflow, and then return to sleep. This cycle of repeated awakenings and restless sleep may occur many times in a night. Disturbed sleep associated with chronic hypoxemia, hypercapnia, and acidosis may induce secondary physiologic changes, including pulmonary hypertension and cor pulmonale. The quality of sleep (i.e., psychologically restful sleep) is markedly disturbed, and this may lead to behavioral disturbances such as hyperactivity, aggression, depression, and hypersomnolence. Longstanding obstructive sleep apnea may impair growth and development.

Adenotonsillar hypertrophy is the most common cause of upper airway obstruction during sleep in children. It has been suggested that in recent years, as the approach to tonsil and adenoid surgery has become progressively more conservative, there may be an increasing tendency for children to develop the sequelae of adenotonsillar hypertrophy. The diagnosis of OSA can be suspected from a thorough history. A detailed history usually requires very specific and direct questioning. The history usually reveals a chronic, gradually worsening condition. Snoring is a cardinal finding; loudness does not imply severity. Any history of snoring should prompt immediate questioning that may elicit a history of apnea. Parents, when specifically questioned, may describe restless sleep with frank apneic episodes (> 10 seconds) followed by gasping for air. They may also report unusual sleeping positions. Both nocturnal and daytime symptoms occur in OSA (Table 1).

Table 1 Features Commonly Found in Obstructive Sleep Apnea

Daytime	Nocturnal
Mouth-breathing	Snoring
Behavioral changes	Apneic episodes
aggression	Restless sleep with frequent
hyperactivity	awakenings
Depression	Nightmares
Excessive daytime sleepiness	Nocturnal enuresis
(hypersomnolence)	Nocturnal diaphoresis
Failure to thrive; obesity	
Frequent upper respiratory	
tract infections	
Chronic rhinorrhea	

Upon physical examination, one may observe the prognathic mandibular position of a chronic mouth-breather and a hyponasal speech quality. OSA is more common in males and blacks. Vital signs may reveal systemic hypertension. Marked tonsillar hypertrophy is frequently apparent when the oropharynx is examined. The severity of OSA is evident when the secondary changes have occurred (Table 2). If severe OSA is suspected, an electrocardiogram (ECG) may reveal right ventricular hypertrophy and possible arrythmia; a chest radiograph may show cardiomegaly; an arterial blood gas may show a chronic partially compensated respiratory acidosis (e.g., pH of 7.36, PCO_2 of 69, PO_2 of 68 base excess (BE) + 13). Polycythemia often occurs from chronic hypoxemia.

At present, the most sophisticated method of assessing respiration in a sleeping patient is polysomnography. By measuring various parameters such as eye movement, chest movement, airflow at the nose and mouth, electroencephalogram, ECG, and oxygen percent saturation, a complete sleep picture may be obtained. Central neurogenic apnea can be differentiated from peripheral or obstructive sleep apnea. The severity of obstruction can be categorized on the basis of associated oxygen desaturation and the frequency of cardiac arrythmias. Although polysomnography provides a complete sleep picture, it may not be a cost-effective or practical method for deciding who has significant airway compromise from adenotonsillar hypertrophy and who does not.

In most cases, adenotonsillectomy is highly effective in alleviating the symptoms associated with upper airway compromise. Relief can be quite dramatic. There may be episodes of sleep apnea after surgery, but these are likely to be of a "central" variety and likely to be far fewer in number. Snoring and mouth-breathing resolve, and patient disposition, growth, and development may improve dramatically.

The anesthetic management of patients with OSA follow the same basic principles for any patient with airway compromise (see earlier). Emergency airway equipment should be immediately available, including that for a temporizing cricothyroidotomy or tracheostomy. An intravenous infusion is mandatory before induction. Sedative hypnotics should be administered with *extreme* caution and in very small doses *only if*

necessary. Narcotics should *not* be given until the patient is fully awake after surgery, and at that time only in very small incremental doses. Very recently, Ketorolac tromethamine, a new injectable nonsteroidal anti-inflammatory drug has received some attention as an appropriate alternative to narcotics for pain relief. It may be beneficial for patients in whom analgesia is necessary, but the sedative and respiratory depressant effects of narcotics are of concern. It may be administered intramuscularly only and has yet to stand the test of time; however, its efficacy in patients of OSA is quite hopeful. Death during anesthesia has been reported in children with OSA and may be precipitated by hypoventilation during induction in those patients with right heart strain. Before a child with severe OSA undergoes surgery, it is advisable to identify such cardiac abnormalities. Irregular respiration and apnea may occur during the early postoperative period but quickly diminish within the next 24 to 48 hours. Patients should be observed overnight in a hospital setting with a cardiorespiratory monitor and oximetry. Frequently the child requires little to no analgesia, and may sleep almost continuously for the next 18 to 24 hours. The prolonged sleep is the result of the chronic preoperative sleep deprivation. Once sleep disturbance from intermittent airway obstruction is no longer an issue postoperatively, good quality sleep may finally ensue.

PRESSURE-EQUALIZING TUBES

Otitis media is the most frequently diagnosed illness during childhood. In the usual course, after several days of an upper respiratory tract infection, a child suddenly develops otalgia and fever consistent with acute otitis media. Some children develop recurrent acute episodes of otitis media with almost every upper respiratory infection that completely resolve after an appropriate course of antimicrobial therapy. Other children may develop persistent middle ear effusion and suffer recurrent episodes of acute otitis media superimposed on the chronic disorder. These patients may require myringotomy and ventilatory tympanostomy tubes (also known as pressure-equalizing tubes or PE tubes) to promote middle ear drainage and prevent subsequent accumulation of effusion.

Myringotomy and insertion of tympanostomy tubes (M & T) is a very short procedure (5 to 10 minutes) in the hands of a skilled otolaryngologist. More time may be required when performed by inexperienced trainees. With the aid of an operating microscope and an ear speculum, the surgeon visualizes the tympanic membrane, evacuates the middle ear effusion, and inserts the tympanostomy tube (Fig. 2).

M & T is almost exclusively performed on an outpatient basis. Premedication may be administered at the discretion of the anesthesiologist but is not routinely administered. An inhalation induction with oxygen, nitrous oxide, and halothane is generally well accepted and is the induction method of choice. Mask adminis-

Table 2 Clinical Features and Physiologic Changes Seen in Obstructive Sleep Apnea

Physiologic Response to Apnea with $\downarrow O_2$, $\uparrow PCO_2$, $\downarrow pH$	Clinical Manifestations of Physiologic Changes
Arrhythmia	Pulmonary hypertension
Vagal bradycardia	and cor pulmonale
Ectopic beats	Systemic hypertension
Pulmonary vasoconstriction	Polycythemia
Systemic vasoconstriction	Behavioral changes
Erythropoeisis	Restless sleep
Sleep fragmentation	

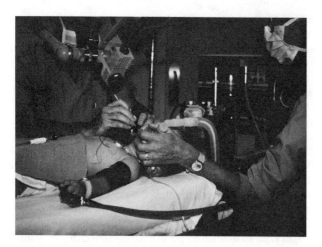

Figure 2 PE tubes are easily inserted under mask anesthesia. The anesthesiologist turns the patient's head from side to side to provide surgical exposure.

tration of halothane with or without nitrous oxide for anesthetic maintenance proves to be a smooth and efficient anesthetic. It provides an adequate surgical anesthetic without undue delay and allows prompt postoperative awakening and recovery.

Most patients presenting for M & T are otherwise healthy infants and children. However, not infrequently the anesthesiologist is confronted with two particular problems. The first problem is the patient with ongoing, chronic symptoms of an upper respiratory tract infection (to be distinguished from the acute phase with a fever). Frequently the symptoms will not subside until the effusion is drained. Although an upper respiratory tract infection is associated with an increased incidence of early postoperative hypoxemia, waiting for a window in the patient's symptoms may be inappropriate and offers no additional benefit. In these particular children, surgical intervention is often needed to improve the symptoms. The second problem is nasal obstruction during induction of anesthesia. These children commonly have adenoidal hypertrophy with eustachian tube and nasal airway obstruction causing the frequent episodes of otitis media with effusion. In these patients, it may be necessary to keep the mouth open during

induction in order to maintain a patent airway. Once the child is adequately anesthetized, an oropharyngeal airway may be inserted.

M & T is one of the very few procedures in the current practice of pediatric anesthesia in which an intravenous infusion is not routinely started intraoperatively. The decision to place an intravenous line depends not only on the patient's health, but on the comfort of the anesthesiologist with doing so and the skill and reliability of the support staff at the operating center. Routine monitoring, including precordial stethoscope, ECG, blood pressure measurements, and oximetry, is sufficient for providing a safe anesthetic.

Usually a short, uneventful anesthetic, anesthesia for M & T should never be taken for granted. This "simple and straightforward" anesthetic allows little room for error, especially if it is performed without an intravenous infusion in place for the rapid administration of emergency drugs. Potentially, severe laryngospasm may develop if the procedure commences before adequate surgical anesthesia is established. Observing the patient's response to insertion of the ear speculum is helpful in assessing the depth of anesthesia and proves to be a worthwhile maneuver before one proceeds with the surgical procedure. If an intravenous line is not in place and a laryngospasm occurs that is not responsive to positive airway pressure, atropine in a dose of 0.02 mg per kilogram IM, followed by succinylcholine chloride in a dose of 3 mg per kilogram IM or administered intralingually may help regain ventilatory control.

SUGGESTED READING

Grundfast KM, Wittich DJ Jr. Adenotonsillar hypertrophy and upper airway obstruction in evolutionary perspective. Laryngoscope 1982; 92:650–656.

Maddern BR. Snoring and obstructive sleep apnea syndrome. In: Bluestone CD, Stool SE, eds. Pediatric otolaryngology. Philadelphia: WB Saunders, 1990:927.

Paradise JL. Tonsillectomy and adenoidectomy. In: Bluestone CD, Stool SE, eds. Pediatric otolaryngology. Philadelphia: WB Saunders, 1990:915.

Richardson MA, Seid AB, Cotton RT, et al. Evaluation of tonsils and adenoids in sleep apnea syndrome. Laryngoscope 1980; 90: 1106–1110.

Swift AC. Upper airway obstruction, sleep disturbance, and adenotonsillectomy in children. J Laryngol Otol 1988; 102:419–422.

ANESTHESIA IN THORACIC SURGERY

ENDOBRONCHIAL INTUBATION

R.J.N. WATSON, M.A., M.B., B.Chir., F.F.A.R.C.S.
COLIN F. MACKENZIE, M.B., B.Chir., F.F.A.R.C.S.

Endobronchial intubation is useful during thoracic surgery and sometimes during intensive care. The objectives of endobronchial intubation are (1) to ventilate (or collapse) one lung independently of the other, and (2) to protect one lung from contamination by the other. These objectives can be achieved by using a bronchial blocker, single-lumen endobronchial intubation, a double-lumen tracheal tube, or a combination of single-lumen tube with bronchial blocker. This chapter summarizes the techniques and apparatus for performing endobronchial intubation and the physiologic and pharmacologic consequences of anesthesia during one-lung ventilation.

ENDOBRONCHIAL INTUBATION

Indications

Endobronchial intubation during thoracotomy is used to isolate the dependent lung, allowing one-lung ventilation and preventing contamination from blood, abscess, tumor and bronchiectatic sputum, or empyema. Collapse of the operative lung also improves surgical conditions by providing access to the mediastinum and hilum. The indications for endobronchial intubation are listed in Table 1.

Techniques

The most frequently used equipment for endobronchial intubation is a double-lumen tracheal tube, one lumen of which has a cuffed endobronchial extension. The range of double-lumen tubes includes the nondisposable left-sided Carlens (the White tube is the right-sided equivalent), the Robertshaw (Leyland), and several brands of disposable polyvinylchloride (PVC) tubes. The Carlens and White tubes differ from other double-lumen tubes in having a small rubber carinal

hook that gives a very positive "feel" to correct placement but makes the passage through the larynx more difficult and mucosal damage more likely. The nondisposable tubes employ low-volume, high-pressure cuffs and require greater care in establishing correct inflation than the higher-volume, lower-pressure cuffs used on the PVC tubes. Nevertheless, the high-pressure cuffs may provide superior protection against aspiration. The red rubber used in constructing the Robertshaw tube has been associated with mucosal irritation when used in long-term application. During short-term use, however, this tube has not been shown to cause greater airway damage than disposable tubes.

Double-lumen tube sizes are traditionally reported in the French scale (divide by pi for the outer diameter) and are commonly available in 28- to 41-Fr sizes. Generally the 35- or 37-Fr tube is suitable for most women and adolescents, while the 37- or 39-Fr are appropriate for men. The largest tube that will easily pass the larynx is preferred for optimal endobronchial placement. A common mistake is to use a small tube that is not long enough to seat in the correct endobronchial position.

Whether right-sided double-lumen endobronchial intubation should be used is controversial. Some practitioners advocate left-sided tubes for both left and right

Table 1 Indications for Lung Isolation or One-Lung Ventilation

Absolute	Relative
Control of ventilation	Surgical exposure in order of
Large bronchopleural	priority
fistula	Thoracic aortic aneurysm
Giant unilateral lung	Pneumonectomy
cyst or bulla	Upper lobectomy and sleeve
Disruption of the	resection
tracheobronchial tree	Middle and lower lobectomies
	Esophageal surgery
Control of contamination	Differential ventilation and
or spillage	PEEP requirements of
Massive unilateral pulmonary	each lung
hemorrhage	
Infection (or tumor)	
Unilateral bronchopulmonary	
lavage	

thoracotomies. Left-sided double-lumen tubes are easier to place than right-sided double-lumen tubes because the left upper lobe bronchus to carinal distance is 44 mm in women and 49 mm in men. The corresponding distances to the right upper lobe bronchus are 15 mm and 19 mm. The left-sided endobronchial tube is therefore less likely to be dislodged during surgery than the right-sided tubes. Left endobronchial intubation can be used satisfactorily in all right and most left thoracic procedures. The exceptions include a left pneumonectomy or left upper lobectomy with sleeve resection. Even during these procedures, the left-sided tube can simply be pulled back into the trachea. However, some anesthesiologists believe that contamination of the right lung in the right lateral position is more reliably prevented by using a right-sided tube. There are, therefore, some indications for right-sided as opposed to left-sided double-lumen tubes.

The difficulty with right endobronchial tubes concerns obstruction of the right upper lobe bronchus, which results in hypoxemia and collapse of the right upper lobe. The margin of safety is the range of position, relative to the carina, over which a double-lumen tube will perform without obstructing a major airway. Measurements of all types of left-sided tubes indicate a fairly consistent and adequate margin of safety between 16 and 19 mm. By contrast, right-sided tubes have a much smaller margin of tolerance, and also, there is a much greater variation with this type of tube. Although the Robertshaw (Leyland) tube has an 11-mm margin, margins of the disposable PVC tubes vary from 1 to 7 mm. The implication is that satisfactory ventilation through a right-sided PVC tube is difficult to achieve without obstructing the right upper lobe. Thus, the indications for checking placement by bronchoscope are much stronger than if a Leyland tube is used.

Bronchial blockers are an alternative to double-lumen tubes and consist of a balloon-tipped catheter (often water-filled) that is positioned under bronchoscopic control in the bronchus. The catheter has a central lumen and an inflation port for the balloon that is filled when one-lung ventilation is required. Bronchial blockers may be valuable in controlling hemorrhage from a lung (e.g., after major lung contusion) or in reducing air leaks (caused by bronchopleural fistula or traumatic bronchial tears, for example). However, bronchial blockers are easily dislodged and, as traditionally used, require further intubation with a single-lumen cuffed tracheal tube to hold the blocker in position and allow ventilation. A new single-lumen tube, the Univent, has a balloon-tipped, moveable endobronchial blocker with a diameter of 2 mm within the wall of the tube. The blocker can be extended 8 cm beyond the tip of the main tube and is rotated into the mainstem bronchus under fiberoptic control. The balloon tip is inflated to isolate the lung. The blocker lumen (or the upper lumen of a double-lumen tube) may be used for insufflation of oxygen, application of continuous airway pressure (CPAP), high-frequency ventilation (HFV), or for suctioning, draining secretions from the diseased lung, or

pulmonary lavage. The Univent tube has advantages of simplicity and safety. When compared with a double-lumen tube, it is less traumatic to place, offers lower airway resistance, and allows prethoracotomy fiberoptic bronchoscopy without the use of a pediatric-size bronchoscope. Any endobronchial trauma that does occur is limited to the operative side.

Endobronchial intubation and one-lung ventilation can be achieved in emergencies and in pediatric patients with airways too small for endobronchial tubes by advancing a conventional tracheal tube into the mainstem bronchus. A right-sided intubation is easier to perform, but obstruction of the right upper lobe bronchus and refractory hypoxemia are likely to occur. Left-sided placement, technically more difficult because of the more acute carinal angel of the left bronchus, may require fiberoptic bronchoscopy. Ventilation on the left lung is usually satisfactory after left endobronchial intubation. The disadvantages of using endotracheal tubes in this manner include difficulty with correct positioning, even with bronchoscopy, and loss of access to the opposite lung for suctioning and ventilation.

PHYSIOLOGY AND PHARMACOLOGY OF ONE-LUNG VENTILATION

Physiology

A large intrapulmonary shunt occurs when the chest is opened and the operative lung partially collapses, because pulmonary blood flow continues to both lungs. The shunt is further increased when only the dependent lung is ventilated. In addition, during general anesthesia with the patient in the lateral position, the upper lung is preferentially ventilated with spontaneous and positive-pressure ventilation because of the higher compliance of the upper lung and hemithorax. However, pulmonary blood flow increases to the dependent lung because of the effects of gravity on the pulmonary vasculature. There is greater shunt with a right thoracotomy than with a left thoracotomy, because the right lung contains 55 percent of the combined lung tissue, whereas the left contains only 45 percent.

The occurrence of hypoxemia during one-lung ventilation is also influenced by regional differences in ventilation and perfusion ($\dot{V}/\dot{Q}$) in both lungs. There may be nonuniformity of the disease process and $\dot{V}/\dot{Q}$ mismatch in the lung to be resected; $\dot{V}/\dot{Q}$ mismatch and disease may also occur in the dependent lung. During surgery, pulmonary blood flow is influenced by surgical manipulation of the lung and the use of vascular ligatures, both of which may alter shunt from time to time. The function of the dependent lung may deteriorate during surgery because of compression, anesthesia, secretions, or inadequate ventilation. Changes in cardiac output and pulmonary artery pressure alter blood flow through the nondependent lung. A decrease in cardiac output can be particularly hazardous during one-lung ventilation because mixed venous denaturation occurs and hypoxemia is exaggerated. Oxygenation during one-lung ventilation correlates significantly with preoperative perfusion of the operative lung. Greater than 45 percent perfusion of the operative lung predicts an arterial oxygen pressure (PaO_2) of less than 175 mm Hg on 100 percent oxygen. Malposition of endobronchial tubes, accumulation of secretions, excessive manipulation of the lung, and a decrease in cardiac output must be avoided, because these intraoperative risk factors cause hypoxemia during one-lung ventilation, and they cannot be predicted by preoperative screening.

Hypoxemia may be particularly troublesome if ventilation to the dependent lung is reduced because of malpositioning and partial obstruction by an endobronchial blocker or a double-lumen tube. Oxygenation can be improved by positioning the tube or blocker correctly and by other methods, including increased fractional inspired oxygen (FIO_2); positive end-expiratory pressure (PEEP) to the dependent, mechanically ventilated lung; CPAP of 5 to 10 cm H_2O or high-frequency ventilation at 15 lb per square inch driving pressure to the upper lung, or discontinuation of one-lung ventilation. Reduced output can contribute to hypoxemia and may be improved by transfusion, management of dysrhythmias, and reduction of excessive anesthesia (Table 2).

Hypoxic pulmonary vasoconstriction (HPV) reduces blood flow to the collapsed nondependent lung by constructing the precapillary pulmonary arteries. The magnitude of the HPV response is inversely proportional to the volume of lung made hypoxic. Because the operated nondependent lung is collapsed during one-lung ventilation, alveolar hypoxia causes increased pulmonary vascular resistance. Blood flow to this lung is reduced by approximately 50 percent. There is therefore a total shunt of at least 20 percent so that 100 percent oxygen will normally produce a PaO_2 of approximately 250 to 300 mm Hg. Many patients who present for thoracic surgery have chronic obstructive pulmonary disease (COPD) with significant $\dot{V}/\dot{Q}$ mismatching. Elevated pulmonary artery and left arterial pressures and respiratory alkalosis impair the HPV response. Patients with cirrhosis or pneumonia also have impaired HPV for reasons that are poorly understood. Application of PEEP to the lower lung during one-lung ventilation increases blood flow to the upper lung. If lower lung PEEP and increasing FIO_2 fail to reverse hypoxemia, it is advisable to insufflate oxygen and to maintain CPAP in the upper lung until the pulmonary vessels can be tied off and shunt can be reduced.

HFV of the upper lung may be achieved with low mean airway pressure and little lung distention. Oxygenation and carbon dioxide removal are improved during one-lung ventilation. Oxygenation may be better than can be achieved with CPAP to the upper lung because HFV may actively recruit collapsed alveoli. HFV may also be used during thoracotomy to ventilate the dependent lung.

Pharmacology

All of the major volatile agents impair HPV in a dose-dependent fashion in laboratory studies. Vasodilators also impair precapillary pulmonary artery constriction and increase blood flow to the collapsed lung. Intravenous anesthetics, narcotics, and benzodiazepines preserve HPV. Theoretically, ketamine is beneficial as a continuous infusion anesthetic for one-lung ventilation because it does not depress HPV and may potentiate it.

Table 2 Causes and Management of Hypoxemia During One-Lung Ventilation

	Causes	Management
Ventilatory		
	Tube malposition	Adjust tube position, if necessary with bronchoscopy
	Lung manipulation	Communicate difficulty to surgeon
	Secretions	Suction secretions; lavage if necessary
	Bronchospasm	Determine cause and provide appropriate treatment
Pulmonary		
	Greater than 45 percent perfusion of operative lung	Control blood flow to operation lung by collapse or vascular compression
	Intrapulmonary shunting	
	Nonuniform pulmonary disease; $\dot{V}/\dot{Q}$ mismatch	Try PEEP to ventilated lung
	Drug effect on HPV	Reduce concentration of inhaled anesthetics and vasodilators
	Pleural effusion or pneumothorax around ventilated lung	Drain chest tube of ventilated lung
Circulatory		
	Reduction in cardiac output	Avoid cardiodepressants; Treat cardiac dysrhythmias
	Pulmonary hypertension	Maintain blood volume; Transfuse to maintain oxygen-carrying capacity
	Mixed venous desaturation	Reduce body oxygen consumption

Histamine release from neuromuscular blocking agents such as *d*-tubocurare and atracurium besylate can be detrimental to patients with known obstructive disease. Supplementation of an intravenous technique by up to 1 MAC of either halothane or isoflurane does not usually cause a decrease in PaO_2. Provided that endobronchial ventilation is technically adequate and that lung traction, changes in $\dot{V}/\dot{Q}$, pulmonary artery pressure, and cardiac output are minimal, the inhalation agents do not produce clinically relevant reversal of HPV. This information is important because inhalational agents decrease bronchomotor tone in patients with reactive airway disease. Unlike intravenous agents, they can be rapidly eliminated, and they can be used easily with 100 percent oxygen. The inhalational agents are the most frequently used anesthetics for thoracotomy; however, reduction of the inhalation component of an anesthetic may be beneficial in hypoxemic patients resistant to other means of improving oxygenation.

Endogenously produced prostanoids such as prostacyclin, thromboxane A_2 and prostaglandin F_{2a} may contribute to HPV. Surgical manipulation of the nonventilated lung and positive-pressure ventilation of the dependent lung increases release of vasodilating prostaglandin E_2 (PGE_2). With PGE_2, HPV is decreased and deterioration in oxygenation occurs. During HPV, arachidonic acid cascade metabolism shifts from cyclooxygenase to lipoxygenase and vasoconstrictor leukotrienes are produced. Drugs blocking these vasoconstrictor pathways may also adversely affect oxygenation during one-lung ventilation. Table 2 summarizes reasons for the development of hypoxemia during one-lung ventilation.

PREOPERATIVE PREPARATION AND MONITORING

A history and physical examination of the patient should be performed to identify symptoms and signs of the disease process requiring thoracic surgery. (The complete medical evaluation and preoperative preparation of the patient is covered elsewhere in the text.) The patient's cardiorespiratory function is assessed and, where possible and necessary, it is optimized before endobronchial intubation and anesthesia are begun. Some of the preoperative assessments and preparation for elective thoracic procedures are summarized in Table 3. Routine pulmonary function tests that examine both lungs are not as helpful as measurements of independent lung function such as $\dot{V}/\dot{Q}$ scans. Unimpaired perfusion of the operative lung on $\dot{V}/\dot{Q}$ scan, with the patient in the lateral position, correlates well with low intraoperative PaO_2 during one-lung ventilation.

Monitors

Because of the potential for considerable hermorrhage during thoracotomy involving lung or tumor resection and during repair of intrathoracic structures, at least two large intravenous lines (16-gauge or larger)

Table 3 Preoperative Assessment and Preparation for Elective Thoracic Procedures

Assessment	Preparation
History and physical examination	Chest physiotherapy
Current medications	Cessation of smoking
Past medical history	When indicated:
Past aneshtetic history	Antibiotics
Laboratory studies	Bronchodilators
Chest roentgenography	Digitalization
Electrocardiography	Antihypertensives
Pulmonary function testing	Antianginal drugs
$\dot{V}/\dot{Q}$ scans	Premedication
	Blood transfusion

should be placed. Routine monitors include electrocardiography, pulse oximetry, esophageal stethoscope, and end-tidal carbon dioxide analyzer ($ETCO_2$). There is a significant incidence of dysrhythmias if the mediastinum is manipulated (e.g., during hilar carcinoma resection). Pulse oximeters and end-tidal carbon dioxide analyzers are continuous monitors helpful in detecting hypoxemia and inadequate ventilation. Invasive arterial blood pressure monitoring is advisable in patients during one-lung ventilation and in patients with impaired cardiorespiratory function who undergo thoracotomy. Right-sided radial artery cannulation is used during major vascular procedures, such as repair of traumatic rupture of the aorta, to allow blood pressure monitoring during aortic cross clamp. A central line, either in the superior vena cava (CVP) or pulmonary artery (PA), allows estimation of reserve cardiac function, monitoring of venous blood pressures and gases, and central drug administration. The choice of a CVP or PA line is determined by the patient's preoperative cardiopulmonary status and the type of surgery. The anesthesiologist should be aware that artifacts occur in pressure, cardiac output, and blood sample measurements from a PA catheter positioned in the collapsed lung. Since the tip of a percutaneously placed PA catheter most frequently goes to the right pulmonary artery, the problem occurs more often with the right than left thoracotomy. Because neuromuscular blockade is used during thoracotomy to prevent coughing or straining during airway manipulation, monitoring by peripheral nerve stimulator is advisable. Both CVP and intra-arterial blood pressure monitoring may be unnecessary for patients who are otherwise healthy and require only a brief period of one-lung ventilation for node biopsy or a similar intrathoracic procedure that is unlikely to cause blood loss. The monitors used during endobronchial intubation and one-lung ventilation are listed in Table 4.

ANESTHETIC INDUCTION AND MAINTENANCE

Although endobronchial intubation is usually associated with general anesthesia, there are indications for awake intubation with topical airway anesthesia only. Topical anesthesia is sprayed in the mouth, pharynx, and

Table 4 Monitors and Equipment Used During Anesthesia for Thoracotomy

Electrocardiography
Noninvasive blood pressure or arterial line
Central venous pressure
Esophageal stethoscope
Thermometer
Blood warmer
Humidifier
Inspired oxygen analyzer
Pulse oximeter
Arterial and venous blood gas monitor
End-tidal carbon dioxide capnography or mass spectrometry
Urine flow
Airway pressure monitor
Peripheral nerve stimulator

larynx together with transtracheal lidocaine with or without a superior laryngeal nerve block. Awake double-lumen tube intubation is used in patients with florid empyema and bronchopleural fistula. It is also used when lung protection is required but the airway is difficult to manage or the patient has a full stomach. The awake technique has been described both with and without fiberoptic bronchoscopy. The Carlens tube was originally designed for differential spirometry after blind placement in the awake patient.

Several induction techniques are advocated for general anesthesia. Thiopental (3 to 5 mg per kilogram), ketamine (2 mg per kilogram), or thiamylal sodium (3 to 5 mg per kilogram) is frequently used as the induction agent. Succinylcholine chloride (1 mg per kilogram), pancuronium bromide (0.1 mg per kilogram), vecuronium bromide (0.1 mg per kilogram), or atracurium besylate (0.5 mg per kilogram) is used for tracheal intubation. The longer-acting nondepolarizing neuromuscular blockers have the advantage of allowing plenty of time for endobronchial placement of a double-lumen tube or blocker. Mechanical ventilation is used after intubation, and minute ventilation is adjusted to obtain a $PaCO_2$ of 35 to 40 mm Hg. Inhalation agents such as halothane, enflurane, and isoflurane may be used to supplement nitrous oxide-oxygen anesthesia or they may be used in combination with narcotics. The patient should be in the lateral position and deeply anesthetized and fully paralyzed during endobronchial intubation to prevent coughing and straining that may dislodge the endobronchial tube. Premedication with an antisialagogue such as atropine, hyoscine, or glycopyrrolate is advisable.

Laryngoscopy occurs after optimum positioning of the head and neck. A double-lumen tube is placed in the larynx with the endobronchial extension rotated 90 degrees anteriorly from its final position in the bronchus. This facilitates passage under the epiglottis. If a stylet is used, it is removed after the tip of the tube has passed through the cords to prevent tracheal damage. Once through the cords, the entire double-lumen is rotated back 90 degrees so that the oropharyngeal curve points directly up. The endobronchial portion is then posi-

tioned against the left or right side of the trachea, depending on whether it is a left or right endobronchial tube. Advancing the tube in this position results in endobronchial intubation, which is indicated by increased resistance that suggests the tube is seated against the carina. Correct placement of the tube may be assisted by turning the patient's head and neck away from the bronchial side to be intubated and rotating the tube slightly toward the bronchus.

The first priority is to inflate the tracheal cuff and ventilate the lungs with 100 percent oxygen while listening bilaterally for breath sounds. If breath sounds are only heard unilaterally or if the patient is very difficult to ventilate, the tube should be withdrawn 2 to 3 cm and breath sounds rechecked. Both lumens may have passed down the same bronchus, causing unilateral ventilation. Alternatively, the endobronchial extension may have folded back on itself during forceful insertion and obstructed the other lumen, thus resulting in high airway resistance. Partial withdrawal and reinsertion may correct the problem. Otherwise, the tube should be completely removed and the patient should be ventilated with a mask.

If bilateral and equal breath sounds are heard, the bronchial cuff should be inflated carefully with no more than 5 ml of air. The bronchial cuff is often marked with *B* or is colored blue on PVC tubes. Overinflating the bronchial cuff may result in bronchial rupture and associated patient morbidity. If bilateral and equal breath sounds remain after the bronchial cuff is inflated, correct placement may be confirmed by unilateral clamping and auscultation over the midaxillary line. If the tracheal lumen is clamped, ventilation will go only to the endobronchially intubated lung. Release of the clamp placed across the tracheal lumen while one is listening is helpful in identifying breaths sounds transmitted from the contralateral lung. The cross-clamp is taken off the tracheal lumen and then placed across the endobronchial lumen and the process is repeated. Clinical examination should also distinguish ventilation of the upper lobes from the lower lobes. The acid test of whether the bronchial cuff is providing an airtight seal and that it is not underinflated is to cross-clamp the tracheal lumen and deflate the tracheal cuff. If gurgling sounds or air leaks are heard when ventilating down the endobronchial lumen, the bronchial seal is inadequate. In this case, bronchial cuff should be deflated and the tube repositioned. The tube usually requires advancement. The bronchial cuff should then be slowly inflated until all leaks and gurgles disappear. The procedure for confirming correct placement of the double-lumen tube or endobronchial blocker before and after turning the patient is summarized in Figure 1.

Controversy exists over the need for bronchoscopic confirmation of position. Some anesthesiologists believe that this should be performed in all cases, because clinical evaluation alone does not detect about half of the left-sided and most right-sided malpositioned tubes. Nevertheless, many thoracic anesthesiology groups believe that bronchoscopy is less frequently indicated. In

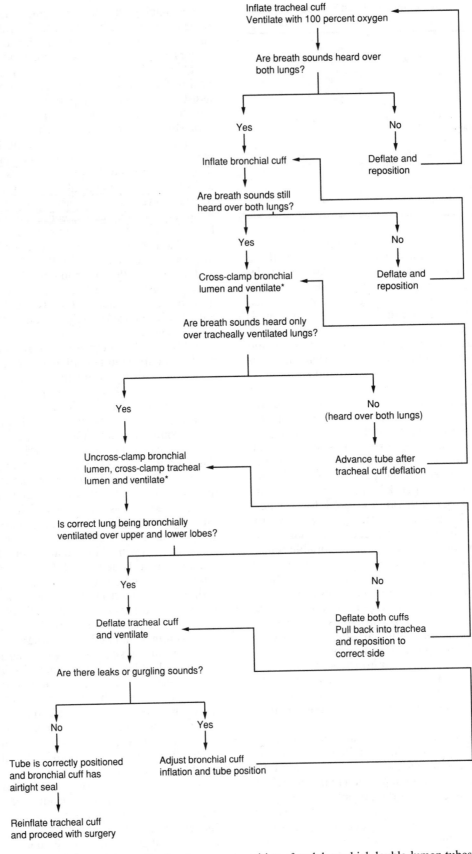

Figure 1 Protocol for confirming the correct position of endobronchial double-lumen tubes. *Repeat this step after turning the patient.

the case of left-sided double-lumen tubes, there is some consensus that the incidence of clinically evident malpositioning is not likely to be affected by routine use of bronchoscopy. With right endobronchial intubation, the type of tube used is of considerable importance. If disposable tubes are routinely employed, malpositioning reaches clinical importance without bronchoscopic confirmation. Whether placement is checked clinically or bronchoscopically, it is imperative that it be checked when the patient is turned, after major mediastinal manipulation, or when a change in ventilating airway pressure occurs. The anesthesiologist should also guard the patient's head, neck, and tube position, because tube movement of 28 mm with head extension or flexion has been recorded.

POSTINDUCTION MANAGEMENT

In addition to checking the placement of the double-lumen tube after lateral positioning, the right- and left-sided pulmonary static compliances may be checked and recorded for later comparisons. One-lung ventilation should be postponed until required. When one-lung ventilation is initiated, 100 percent oxygen is delivered and the desired lumen of the ventilator tubing is clamped. The suction port of the double-lumen tube connector is opened to the atmosphere to allow complete decompression of the lung. A tidal volume of 8 to 10 ml per kilogram is delivered to the dependent lung unless airway pressures of more than 30 cm H_2O mandate a reduction. If airway pressures exceed 30 cm H_2O, the ventilatory pattern is changed to a higher respiratory frequency with lower tidal volumes. The airway pressures must be continuously monitored throughout this phase. An arterial carbon dioxide pressure ($PaCO_2$) of approximately 40 mm Hg is desirable and, because of the increased physiologic dead space, an increase in minute ventilation of approximately 20 percent may be required. The impact of one-lung ventilation on patient gas exchange is unpredictable; the degree of vascular collapse and HPV in the operative lung will depend to some extent on the disease process and on patient variability. Finally, any tube that is malpositioned can severely affect gas exchange. Therefore, both the arterial partial pressure of oxygen (PO_2) and carbon dioxide partial pressure (PCO_2) should be closely followed. PaO_2 decreases initially as oxygen is absorbed from the atelectatic lung. PaO_2 may fall further as atelectasis and $\dot{V}/\dot{Q}$ mismatch develop in the contralateral lung. Pulse oximetry is valuable in monitoring oxygenation. The end-tidal carbon dioxide, however, does not accurately reflect the $PaCO_2$ because of significant changes in dead space. In clinical practice, $PaCO_2$–end-tidal carbon dioxide differences of 15 mm Hg are sometimes recorded.

Progressive hypoxemia may develop during one-lung ventilation despite measures to optimize ventilatory parameters. The steps described in Table 2 may reverse this situation. The ventilated lung may require suction clearance or treatment for bronchospasm. Application

Table 5 Differential Diagnosis of Bronchospasm During One-lung Ventilation

Double-lumen tube displacement
Partial airway obstruction by secretions
Light anesthesia
Lung contamination
Intrinsic bronchopulmonary disease
Cardiogenic pulmonary edema
Pneumothorax in ventilated lung

of PEEP to the ventilated lung may then be initiated and may help if the functional residual capacity can be raised above the closing volume, thus preventing premature airway and alveolar closure. Intra-alveolar pressure is frequently increased significantly by PEEP, a condition that may worsen shunt by directing blood away from ventilated alveoli, thus causing a further deterioration in PaO_2. The effect of PEEP on the ventilated dependent lung is therefore somewhat variable. The most commonly used successful maneuver to reduce hypoxemia is to apply CPAP to the upper operative lung using 100 percent oxygen. Although oxygen insufflation at atmospheric pressure does not help at all, low levels of CPAP (5 to 10 cm H_2O) cause appreciable increases in PaO_2 without changing blood flow to the lung and therefore without affecting the surgical field. Maximum efficacy is gained, as in apneic oxygenation, when the lung is fully denitrogenated. Therefore, brief reinflation of the operative lung should be considered when surgically appropriate, both as a reliable way of reversing the trend toward hypoxemia and as an adjunct to CPAP. A variety of CPAP devices have been used; the most convenient is probably a Mapleson pediatric circuit with an airway pressure gauge and an independent oxygen supply.

Wheezing is a potentially serious development during one-lung ventilation. If possible, the cause should be ascertained (Table 5) and appropriate treatment started. If bronchodilators are indicated, volatile anesthetic or nebulized sympathomimetic agents can be administered via the airway until intravenous aminophylline can be started. Inspissation of secretions and postoperative atelectasis can be reduced by active humidification of inspired gases. For short procedures, however, passive airway humidifiers ("artificial noses") may be adequate.

When suctioning is performed, left and right endobronchial suction catheters should be clearly identified and separated to minimize cross contamination.

POSTOPERATIVE CARE

Postoperative management after thoracotomy generally involves prompt reversal of neuromuscular paralysis and anesthesia, with extubation following re-establishment of spontaneous ventilation. Objective measurements helpful in determining whether extubation will be successful include maximum inspiratory force greater than -20 cm H_2O, vital capacity greater than 1,000 ml or 15 ml per kilogram, and PaO_2/FIO_2 greater than 250. The chest radiograph should be checked for unexpected abnormalities such as pleural effusions, pneumothoraces, lung infiltrates, and mediastinal position. In very debilitated patients in whom intraoperative oxygenation is impaired despite clamping and ligature of the pulmonary vessels, the extubation criteria are often not met, and positive pressure or high-frequency ventilation is required after thoracotomy. Double-lumen tubes are poorly tolerated by patients postoperatively and should be replaced by single-lumen tubes if postoperative ventilation is necessary.

PAIN RELIEF

Adequate pain relief may permit early extubation and can help the patient cough well enough to clear tracheobronchial secretions. Intrathecal or epidural narcotics or bupivacaine should be considered for pain relief because they are usually more effective than intercostal or paravertebral blocks. There is little additional benefit to using thoracic rather than lumbar

MEDIASTINOSCOPY AND THORACOSCOPY

PETER ROCK, M.D.

Mediastinoscopy and thoracoscopy are surgical procedures used to diagnose chest and mediastinal masses. Mediastinoscopy was originally described by Carlens in 1959 and has been used extensively since its introduction. Thoracoscopy was originally described by Jacobeus in 1910. Although thoracoscopy has been used less frequently than mediastinoscopy, there has been renewed interest in this procedure with the resurgence of endoscopic surgery. These procedures have in common direct visualization of either the mediastinum or pleural cavity to obtain a tissue diagnosis of an abnormality detected through radiographic techniques, which in turn determines whether the patient is a candidate for surgical resection. While mediastinoscopy is primarily a diagnostic tool, thoracoscopy may be used for certain therapeutic maneuvers such as pleurodesis and ablation of lung blebs causing pneumothorax.

MEDIASTINOSCOPY

Cervical mediastinoscopy involves a small transverse incision one fingerbreadth above the sternal notch and

narcotics. Self-administered infusions of analgesics, which are controlled by the patient, or intravenous or intramuscular narcotics may also be helpful. Most forms of pain relief can cause respiratory depression, so a spontaneously breathing patient should be monitored. Pulse oximetry is a noninvasive way to monitor oxygen saturation during the immediate postoperative period. Naloxone should be available to reverse narcotic-induced depression if intrathecal or epidural narcotics are used. Early mobilization, encouraging the patient to breathe deeply, and chest physiotherapy can help reduce the incidence of postoperative pulmonary complications.

SUGGESTED READING

Benumof JL. Anesthesia for thoracic surgery. Philadelphia: WB Saunders, 1987.
Gothard WW, Branthwaite MA. Anaesthesia for thoracic surgery. Oxford, Boston: Blackwell Scientific Publications, 1982.
Kaplan JA. Thoracic anesthesia. New York: Churchill Livingstone, 1983.
Voelkel NF. Mechanisms of hypoxic pulmonary vasoconstriction. Am Rev Respir Dis 1986; 1186–1195.

subsequent blunt dissection of the pretracheal space down to the carina. A short rigid lighted mediastinoscope is then introduced. By this method, the superior and middle mediastinum and contained structures may be visualized and biopsies obtained. It is important to note that only this portion of the mediastinum may be visualized. A related procedure that sometimes uses the same rigid mediastinoscope is anterior mediastinoscopy. This procedure, described by Chamberlain (often called the Chamberlain procedure) uses a 5- to 7-cm anterior thoracotomy through the second or third intercostal space, which allows access to the anterior mediastinum, aortopulmonary window, anterior aspect of the hilum, and both the superior vena cava and azygous vein. Usually, insertion of the mediastinoscope is not done, and digital inspection is performed. The remainder of this section discusses cervical mediastinoscopy. Originally, an operating laryngoscope was used to allow inspection of the mediastinal structures revealed by this procedure. However, special instrumentation for this expressed purpose is now available.

Most frequently, mediastinoscopy is used to stage patients with lung cancer by sampling tissue from enlarged paratracheal or subcarinal nodes. Because plain chest roentgenography or computed tomography (CT) cannot provide a tissue diagnosis, mediastinoscopy is one way of determining if the enlarged lymph nodes are reactive or contain malignant cells without subjecting the patient to a formal thoracotomy. Moreover, the demonstration that the nodes are not involved at the time of mediastinoscopy may allow the patient to undergo a potentially curative pulmonary resection.

Numerous studies have attested to the value of mediastinoscopy in both sparing patients from thoracotomy and permitting resectional surgery to proceed.

Other indications for the use of mediastinoscopy exist. Superior mediastinal masses that have not been diagnosed by other means may be biopsied if they are not vascular and if biopsy, as opposed to excision per se, is a reasonable alternative. Granulomatous disease involving mediastinal adenopathy such as infection or sarcoid may be diagnosed. There are case reports of mediastinoscopy used to retrieve left atrial catheters (implanted at the time of cardiac surgery) that could not be removed in the normal fashion and to implant left atrial pacing catheters.

No absolute contraindications to mediastinoscopy exist. Formerly, an absolute contraindication to mediastinoscopy was prior mediastinoscopy. It was thought that the fibrosis and inflammation that accompanied the healing obliterated the necessary tissue planes. However, recent experience in a limited number of patients indicates that repeat mediastinoscopy may be performed safely in experienced hands. Clearly, repeat mediastinoscopy requires that the anesthesiologist be prepared for massive bleeding or emergency thoracotomy should the surgeon encounter difficulty.

Relative contraindications to the performance of mediastinoscopy include the superior vena cava syndrome, in which engorgement of veins and tissues may result in bleeding. In this situation, some surgeons prefer to perform mediastinoscopy *before* x-ray therapy, as the resulting inflammation may make mediastinoscopy even more difficult. A thoracic aortic aneurysm is also a relative contraindication, as are other vascular anomalies in the area of the arch of the aorta. Other anatomic conditions, such as involvement of the recurrent laryngeal nerve or deviation of the trachea, may render the procedure difficult or impossible. Tracheotomy or laryngectomy are also relative contraindications to mediastinoscopy. Prior x-ray therapy may produce fibrosis and distortion of the mediastinum; performance of mediastinoscopy under such circumstances will be related to the experience of the surgeon and the necessity to obtain a tissue diagnosis by that route. Finally, coagulopathy may necessitate delay or inability to perform this procedure.

The surgical field includes not only the neck but the chest so that a thoracotomy or sternotomy can be performed in the event of a complication. A 3- to 5-cm cervical incision is made one fingerbreadth above the suprasternal notch. Depending on the preference of the surgeon, mediastinoscopy may be performed at the head of the patient on either side. The incision is carried down to the trachea, and using blunt dissection, a finger is advanced along the anterior trachea into the superior mediastinum. The rigid mediastinoscope is then inserted through the incision under direct vision, with care taken to keep the mediastinoscope in the midline and identify appropriate anatomic landmarks. Inspection and biopsy of lymph nodes in the paratracheal areas, tracheobronchial angles, and the anterior subcarinal region for lymph nodes is performed. Bleeding of a minor nature frequently occurs and is controlled by packing and/or cautery.

The surgical experience of the last 30 years with this procedure attests to its safety. Several recent surgical series comprising thousands of cases have had no surgical mortality, although in Carlens' large series of more than 11,000 mediastinoscopies reported in 1971 there were 16 deaths. The most common reported complications are bleeding, vocal cord paralysis, and pneumothorax. Arterial bleeding is usually from the innominate artery and may require a median sternotomy or upper sternal split in order to repair the laceration to the artery. The superior vena cava, azygous vein, or pulmonary artery can also bleed and require thoracotomy if local control is not obtained. Vocal cord paralysis occurs with an incidence of approximately 0.3 percent. It results from damage to the left recurrent laryngeal nerve. This may occur if the nerve is unintentionally damaged when a lymph node close to it is biopsied, if edema develops from the electrocautery, or from hematoma formation around the nerve. Bilateral recurrent laryngeal nerve damage is very rare. Other reported complications include wound infection, mediastinal infection, esophageal perforation, and tumor seeding along the path of the mediastinoscope. While obviously very important, these latter complications are usually delayed in their presentation and have no immediate anesthetic implications.

This procedure has two other important potential complications. The mediastinoscope may impinge on the innominate artery and compromise blood supply to the vessels supplying the brain. If undetected, this may result in a left hemiparesis. For this reason, it is essential to monitor perfusion to the right arm. This may be done by placing an arterial line in the right radial artery; a decrease or loss of waveform can be taken as evidence of impingement of the innominate artery. This should be ruled out before a diagnosis of cardiac arrest is made. Alternatively, a pulse oximeter, placed on a digit of the right hand, can be used to indicate adequacy of perfusion of the right arm. The negative pleural pressure in a spontaneously ventilating patient may result in venous air embolism, although this appears to be a very rare complication of this procedure. However, the recommended method of anesthetizing patients for this procedure requires positive-pressure ventilation, and air embolism should not occur under these conditions.

Local anesthesia and sedation have been used in the performance of mediastinoscopy. However, in such cases the airway is not controlled, the patient may not be fully cooperative, patient movement may result in displacement of the mediastinoscope into a vascular structure, and the patient is not immediately ready if an emergency thoracotomy is required. It might be argued that mediastinoscopy performed with the patient under local anesthesia spares the patient with little pulmonary reserve general anesthesia and its consequent negative effects. The effects of general anesthesia on lung function, however, are limited compared with the effects of a thoracotomy on lung function. Also, general anesthesia ensures control of the airway, patient cooperation, and positive-pressure ventilation and the decreased chance of air embolism, and enables a potentially lifesaving thoracotomy to be performed immediately should a complication arise. Because there are many disadvantages to local anesthesia for this procedure and few advantages, we do not employ it for mediastinoscopy and do not recommend it.

Preoperative evaluation focuses on several aspects of the patient's condition. Mediastinoscopy is frequently employed for the evaluation of mediastinal tumors or adenopathy. Recently it has been recognized that anesthetic catastrophe may follow induction of anesthesia in patients with large mediastinal tumors or nodes that compress the major bronchi or impinge upon the pericardium. It is therefore essential to review the diagnostic studies in which such findings were sought, and if there is any question, to discuss the anatomy with the surgeon. If present, the finding of airway or pericardial impingement may warrant a different diagnostic approach.

Similarly, evaluation should be performed to exclude tracheal deviation that might render either intubation or the performance of mediastinoscopy difficult. The presence of superior vena cava syndrome, suggested by facial suffusion or edema, arm swelling, or engorgement of upper extremity veins, should be known. Since innominate artery impingement may occur during the course of mediastinoscopy, a history and findings of a physical examination suggestive of cerebrovascular disease should be sought. There are case reports of prolonged neuromuscular paralysis following mediastinoscopy in patients with bronchogenic carcinoma and unsuspected Eaton-Lambert syndrome; similarly, patients with previously undiagnosed myasthenia gravis undergoing mediastinoscopy for a mediastinal mass may have prolonged action of nondepolarizing muscle relaxants.

Monitoring requirements for mediastinoscopy include routine electrocardiography, noninvasive blood pressure monitoring, pulse oximetry, end-tidal capnography, and precordial or esophageal stethoscope. We frequently employ intra-arterial monitoring for the reason described above because of the potential for massive bleeding and progression to a thoracotomy. Adequate intravenous access is essential, and we commonly insert a second intravenous catheter after the induction of general anesthesia. Central venous or pulmonary artery monitoring is not required unless dictated by the patient's medical condition. Obviously, the blood bank must have available cross-matched blood for the patient.

There is no one specific anesthetic technique for this operation. In general, the technique and agents used should be relatively short acting, as this procedure may be completed within 1 to 2 hours. Once the surgeon has completed the biopsies, the time for closure of the wound is short, and agents with a short half-life may therefore be desirable. As usual, preoxygenation is employed, followed by administration of a short-acting barbiturate for induction of anesthesia. A short-acting muscle nondepolarizing relaxant, such as atracurium besylate or vecuronium bromide may then be used. In the past, a succinylcholine chloride bolus followed by an infusion were used; the above-mentioned nondepolarizing agents may obviate the use of succinylcholine chloride. Muscle relaxation, although obviously not required for surgical exposure, is desirable since it prevents the patient from moving and thus causing displacement of the mediastinoscope, and since it prevents coughing and straining, which distend venous structures. We routinely use small doses of a short-acting narcotic (e.g., fentanyl, 5 to 7 µg per kilogram, IV) to blunt the hemodynamic response to intubation, provide analgesia, and further suppress the cough reflex. Some authors advocate the additional use of intravenous lidocaine (1 to 2 mg per kilogram) to decrease the hemodynamic response to laryngoscopy and prevent further coughing.

We routinely use a regular endotracheal tube, although an armored (Anode) tube may better resist kinking caused by the mediastinoscope. In our experience, this is not an issue. A volatile agent is inhaled; isoflurane may be desirable owing to its rapid elimination. However, as mentioned earlier, a variety of agents and techniques may be used successfully, and enflurane is well suited to this procedure. Nitrous oxide may be used as tolerated by the patient. At the termination of the case, neuromuscular blockade is reversed, and when the patient is awake and strong, extubation is performed. Unless there has been a complication, patients do not require intensive care unit observation. In fact, currently some patients undergo mediastinoscopy as outpatients.

In summary, mediastinoscopy remains an essential diagnostic tool for the evaluation of resectability in patients with bronchogenic lung cancer as well as in the evaluation of patients with unexplained mediastinal masses. Usually the procedure is well tolerated. Serious complications can occur but fortunately are infrequent. Careful anesthetic care can minimize some of these complications and help ensure the safety of the patient during the procedure.

THORACOSCOPY

Thoracoscopy, sometimes referred to as pleuroscopy, is the direct visual examination of the pleural surfaces of a hemithorax. It is undertaken most frequently to evaluate undiagnosed pleural space disease, especially in cases in which cancer seems likely. The goal of this examination is to ensure that no metastases are present that would preclude surgery. Patients with spontaneous pneumothoraces may also undergo this procedure in an attempt to locate and ablate, by electrocautery, laser coagulation, or fibrin glue, the emphysematous blebs that result in this condition. Other conditions that may be diagnosed by pleuroscopy include tuberculosis and connective tissue disorders. Intrapleural foreign bodies (e.g., segments of catheters) may be removed. Finally, thoracoscopy may be used as part of pleurodesis, in which either talc or tetracycline are introduced into the pleural cavity of a patient with debilitating pleural effusions, usually malignant, so as to obliterate the pleural space and reduce or eliminate the effusion.

Compared with mediastinoscopy, the literature available from which to judge thoracoscopy's role in patient management is limited. It would appear that it is of value in selected patients meeting the above-mentioned criteria. However, because there are no studies comparing this procedure with other forms of diagnosis and therapy, no firm conclusions can be drawn. There are few contraindications to the performance of pleuroscopy. Patients with dense pleural adhesions that would prevent collapse of the lung and hinder or prevent inspection of the pleural membranes are not candidates for this procedure. The presence of coagulopathy may make this procedure hazardous.

Thoracoscopy is performed in a fashion similar to that of closed chest tube thoracotomy. A small incision is made in an appropriate interspace, blunt dissection is carried out down to the pleura, and a small rent is then created in the pleura. In order for the thoracoscope to visualize the pleural cavity adequately, a pneumothorax must be created and the lung allowed to collapse. Two approaches to this have been described. A Veres needle is used to fill the pleural space with a gas such as carbon dioxide to create and maintain a pneumothorax. Alternatively, a double-lumen endotracheal tube may be employed and used to collapse the lung in the pleural cavity of interest. A variety of instruments are available for this purpose, including a specially designed thoracoscope and mediastinoscopes, bronchoscopes, and laparoscopes. Obviously, at the end of the procedure, a chest tube is inserted and attached to suction.

Thoracoscopy is a safe procedure and there has been only one death reported that was directly related to its performance. Reported complications include hemorrhage in the pleural space, infectious complications such as empyema and pneumonia, subcutaneous or mediastinal emphysema, persistent air leak, and tumor seeding along the thoracoscopy site.

This procedure may be performed with the patient under either local or general anesthesia. However, the procedure requires a pneumothorax in order to be successful. This may be poorly tolerated by many patients undergoing this study, who may have pulmonary parenchymal disease or be otherwise debilitated by cancer. In such a setting, general anesthesia, which allows better control of ventilation and oxygenation, may be preferable. A young, otherwise healthy patient undergoing thoracoscopy for treatment of recurrent pneumothoraces may be better suited for local anesthesia with sedation. The choice of anesthetic technique must be dictated by individual patient considerations.

The patient is generally placed in the lateral decubitus position. Regardless of the type of anesthesia, routine monitoring with electrocardiography, noninvasive blood pressure measurements, precordial stethoscope, and pulse oximetry are essential. Oxygen supplementation is desirable as well. More invasive monitoring, such as intra-arterial catheterization or central venous pressure monitoring, is not required unless dictated by the individual patient. If local anesthesia and sedation are chosen, a variety of agents are suitable as long as care is taken to monitor the adequacy of ventilation and oxygenation. Thus ketamine, droperidol, benzodiazepines, and narcotics may be used alone or in combination.

Similarly, if general anesthesia is chosen, a variety of agents may be used. Like mediastinoscopy, thoracoscopy may be a short procedure. Short-acting agents are therefore preferable. It is not essential to paralyze the patient for this procedure, but paralysis may be employed as part of the anesthetic technique, if desired. Nitrous oxide may be used but should be discontinued if pneumomediastinum, a recognized complication of this procedure, occurs. The concentration of nitrous oxide that is used may be limited by hypoxemia, especially if one-lung ventilation is used to assist the surgeon. If a double-lumen endotracheal tube is used, an intra-arterial catheter may be desirable in order to ensure proper oxygenation of the patient. Unfortunately, pulse oximetry does not allow detection of high degrees of shunt, as normal saturations are seen with arterial partial pressure of oxygen greater than 80 to 90 mm Hg. Such an arterial partial pressure of oxygen in a setting of a high fractional inspired oxygen implies a high degree of shunt. No one specific anesthetic technique is preferable, and induction and maintenance of anesthesia with suitable agents is acceptable. When general anesthesia is chosen for this procedure, the above-mentioned monitors and end-tidal capnography are essential. It is important to note that, regardless of the type of anesthesia chosen, intercostal nerve block should be performed, as this should provide a certain measure of analgesia.

In conclusion, thoracoscopy is a safe, well-tolerated procedure for diagnosing pleural diseases. It may also be used for therapy of recurrent pleural effusions and pneumothoraces and spares the patient a more extensive thoracotomy.

SUGGESTED READING

Goldstraw P. Mediastinal exploration by mediastinoscopy and mediastinotomy. Br J Dis Chest 1988; 82:111–120.

Jay SJ. Diagnostic procedures for pleural disease. Clin Chest Med 1985; 6:33–48.

Kaiser LR. Diagnostic and therapeutic uses of pleuroscopy (thoracoscopy) in lung cancer. Surg Clin North Am 1987; 67:1081–1086.

Oakes DD, Sherck JP, Brodsky JB, Mark JBD. Therapeutic thoracoscopy. J Thorac Cardiovasc Surg 1984; 87:269–273.

Page RD, Jeffrey RR, Donnelly RJ. Thoracoscopy: a review of 121 consecutive surgical procedures. Ann Thorac Surg 1989; 48:66–68.

Prakash UB, Abel MD, Hubmayr RD. Mediastinal mass and tracheal obstruction during general anesthesia. Mayo Clin Proc 1988; 63:1004–1011.

Puhakka HJ. Complications of mediastinoscopy. J Laryngol Otol 1989; 103:312–315.

Puhakka HJ, Liippo K, Tala E. Mediastinoscopy in relation to clinical evaluation. Scand J Thor Cardiovasc Surg 1990; 24:43–45.

Rusch VW. Thoracoscopy under regional anesthesia for the diagnosis and management of pleural disease. Am J Surg 1987; 154:274–278.

Swain JA. Surgical techniques in the diagnosis of pulmonary disease. Clin Chest Med 1987; 8:43–51.

Thermann M, Loddenkemper R, Schroder D. Thoracoscopy: a forgotten endoscopic procedure? Endoscopy 1985; 17:203–204.

Trastek VF, Piehler JM, Pairolero PC. Mediastinoscopy. Br Med Bull 1986; 42:240–243.

UNILATERAL BRONCHOPULMONARY LAVAGE

JONATHAN L. BENUMOF, M.D.

Unilateral bronchopulmonary lavage, or massive irrigation of the tracheobronchial tree of one lung, has been employed with good success in patients with pulmonary alveolar proteinosis as a means of removing the enormous accumulation of a lipoproteinaceous material that these patients characteristically have in their alveolar space. The lipoproteinaceous material is thought to be surfactant, and the abnormal accumulation is due to failure of clearance mechanisms rather than to enhanced formation. The abnormal accumulation of alveolar lipoproteinaceous material is bilateral and symmetrical and causes the classic chest roentgenographic picture of air space consolidation with patchy, poorly defined shadows throughout the lung; the roentgenographic picture parallels the course of the disease. The air space consolidation causes progressive hypoxemia, shortness of breath (first on exertion and then finally at rest), and poor compliance. The diagnosis of alveolar proteinosis is made by correlating the above clinical, roentgenologic, and laboratory data with the results of a lung biopsy. The indications for lavage consist of PaO_2 less than 60 mm Hg at rest or hypoxemic limitation of normal activity. Infrequently, lung lavage may be performed in patients with asthma, cystic fibrosis, and radioactive dust inhalation.

Unilateral lung lavage is performed with the patient under general anesthesia and with a double-lumen endotracheal tube in place, allowing lavage of one lung and ventilation of the other. In patients with alveolar proteinosis, lavage is performed on one lung and then, after a few days of rest, on the other lung. Following lung lavage, these patients usually have marked subjective improvement that correlates with increases in PaO_2 during rest and exercise, vital vapacity and diffusion capacity, and clearing of the chest roentgenogram. Some patients require lavage every few months; others remain in remission for several years and the disease may even eventually remit completely.

The unilateral lung lavage technique for patients with pulmonary alveolar proteinosis is discussed below. On admission to the hospital, ventilation-perfusion scans of the lung are obtained. Ventilation can be maximized during lung lavage by performing the first lavage on the most severely affected lung, allowing the healthier lung to provide gas exchange. If the scan indicates relatively equal involvement (the usual case), the left lung is lavaged first, leaving the larger right lung to support gas exchange.

Unilateral lung lavage is performed in the operating room, where the appropriate amount and type of equipment and ancillary personnel are present to enhance safety. Patient safety is also increased if a relatively constant team, composed of members of the departments of anesthesia and pulmonary medicine, becomes familiar with the nuances and technique of unilateral lung lavage. Patients are usually cooperative and require only light premedication. Because many of these patients are hypoxemic at rest, they are given oxygen by face mask following premedication and during transport to the warmed operating room.

Since the procedure takes several hours to complete and lavage fluid temperature cannot always be precisely controlled, some patients require external warming (e.g., heating blanket) to maintain normal body temperature. The monitoring system consists of a blood pressure cuff, electrocardiogram, precordial stethoscope, temperature probe, pulse oximeter, and peripheral arterial and central venous pressure catheters. Patients with compromised cardiovascular function are monitored with a pulmonary artery catheter in place of the central venous catheter.

After several minutes of preoxygenation (see below), general anesthesia is induced with 3 to 4 mg per kilogram of thiopental in divided doses and inhalation of either isoflurane or halothane in 100 percent oxygen. Isoflurane is more often indicated in patients in whom therapeutic levels of theophylline (and the risk of dysrhythmias) are present. Neuromuscular blockade is monitored with a peripheral nerve stimulator and is induced with intravenous pancuronium, 0.1 mg per kilogram. When a suitable level of anesthesia has been reached, the trachea is topically anesthetized with lidocaine and intubated with the largest left-sided, double-lumen endotracheal tube that can be passed atraumatically through the glottis. A clear plastic disposable left-sided, double-lumen tube is used because of the ease and certainty with which it is positioned correctly, because of the reliability of obtaining the left cuff seal (the right endobronchial cuff is small and inflates asymmetrically), and because of the ability to observe continuously the tidal movements of respiratory gas moisture (ventilated lung) and the lavage drainage fluid for leaking air bubbles (lavaged lung). The largest tube is used because the left endobronchial cuff makes contact over a greater bronchial mucosal area with less air in the left cuff (compared to a small double-lumen tube), and a large tube facilitates suctioning, which is an important consideration at the end of the case when the lungs need to be made as clear as possible. Precise placement of the tube and detection of leaks are essential because of the serious hazard of spillage during the lavage procedure. The position of the double-lumen tube must be confirmed with a fiberoptic bronchoscope, and the cuff seal must be demonstrated to hold against 50 cm H_2O pressure using a catheter underwater technique. The patient's eyes should be protected with a lubricant and eye pads.

The question of patient position during unilateral lung lavage is important, for there are major advantages and disadvantages related to each position (Table 1). The lateral decubitus position with the lavaged lung dependent minimizes the possibility of accidental spillage of lavage fluid from the dependent lavaged lung to the nondependent ventilated lung. However, during periods of lavage fluid drainage, pulmonary blood flow, which is gravity dependent, would preferentially perfuse the nonventilated dependent lung and the right-to-left transpulmonary shunt would be maximal. The lateral decubitus position with the lavaged lung nondependent minimizes blood flow to the nonventilated lung, but, on the other hand, increases the possibility of accidental spillage of lavage fluid from the lavaged lung to the dependent ventilated lung. As a compromise, the supine position is used in order to balance the risk of aspiration against the risk of hypoxemia.

Following insertion and checking of the double-lumen endotracheal tube and positioning, baseline total and individual lung compliance should be measured. Airway pressure can be electronically transduced and continuously recorded on a paper write-out, and a Wright spirometer should be placed in the expiratory limb of the anesthesia circle system in order to measure tidal volume accurately. A volume ventilator that can deliver relatively high inflation pressures is required, because these patients have diseased and noncompliant lungs. Prelavage total dynamic compliance (chest wall and lung) of both lungs together (using 15 ml per kilogram per breath) and then of each lung separately (using 10 ml per kilogram per breath) are measured. Following measurement of total and individual lung compliance, and with the patient breathing 100 percent oxygen, baseline arterial blood gases are measured.

The patients are completely preoxygenated prior to the induction of anesthesia and lavage for two reasons. First, as with induction of any general anesthetic in any patient, an oxygen-filled functional residual capacity greatly minimizes the risk of hypoxemia during the apneic period required for laryngoscopy and endotracheal intubation. This consideration has increased importance for patients with alveolar proteinosis, because

Table 1 Unilateral Lung Lavage: Position of Lavaged Lung

Position	Advantage	Disadvantage
Lavaged lung nondependent	Minimized blood flow to the nonventilated lung	Maximizes possibility of spillage
Lavaged lung dependent	Minimizes possibility of spillage	Maximizes blood flow to the nonventilated lung
Supine	Balances spillage and blood flow distribution problems	

they are already severely hypoxemic. Second, preoxygenation denitrogenates the lung that is to be lavaged. Alveolar gas is then composed only of oxygen and carbon dioxide. During fluid filling, these gases are absorbed, which usually allows the lavage fluid maximal access to the alveolar space. Failure to denitrogenate the lung prior to filling with lavage fluid may leave peripheral nitrogen bubbles in the alveoli and thus may limit the effectiveness of the lavage.

Warmed isotonic saline is used as the lavage fluid and is infused by gravity from a height of 30 cm above the midaxillary line. After the lavage fluid ceases to flow (i.e., lung filling is complete), drainage is accomplished by clamping the inflow line and unclamping the drainage line, which runs to a collection bottle placed 20 cm below the midaxillary line. The inflow and outflow fluid lines are connected to the appropriate endotracheal tube lumen by a Y-shaped adapter. Each tidal lavage filling is accompanied by mechanical chest percussion and vibration to the lavaged hemithorax prior to drainage. The lavage fluid that is drained is typically light brown, and the sediment layers out at the bottom of the collection bottle after a short period of time. Filling and drainage of approximately 500- to 1,000-ml aliquots are repeated until the lavage effluent clears. Volumes delivered and recovered from each tidal lavage are recorded. Total lavage fluid volumes of 10 to 20 L are usually employed.

Most patients studied have been hemodynamically stable throughout the entire lavage procedure. In particular, lavage itself has caused no significant changes in systemic and pulmonary artery pressures and cardiac output. In these patients, the arterial saturation as measured by oximetry has increased and decreased, respectively, with each lung filling and lung drainage. Arterial saturation increases during lung filling because blood flow to the nonventilated lung is decreased by the lavage fluid infusion pressure. The opposite set of events (increased nonventilated-lung blood flow, decreased arterial oxygen saturation) occurs during drainage. Adequate neuromuscular blockade must be maintained, because unexpected vigorous coughing during the procedure could alter double-lumen endotracheal tube position.

If a small leak should occur during lavage, the following sequence may be observed: (1) the appearance of bubbles in the lavage fluid draining from the lavaged lung, (2) rales and rhonchi in the ventilated lung, (3) a difference between the administered and the drained lavage volumes (the former exceeds the latter), and (4) a fall in arterial oxygen saturation. If a small leak is suspected or detected by any of the above signs and the lavaged lung has been only minimally treated, the lavaged lung should be drained of all fluid, and the endotracheal tube position and the adequacy of cuff seal and lung separation should be rechecked. Before beginning the lavage procedure again, and no matter what solution to the possible leak problem has been used, the functional separation of the two lungs should be tested and found adequate by using an underwater air bubble leak detection method.

Massive spillage of fluid from the lavaged lung to the ventilated lung is not a subtle event and results in a dramatic decrease in ventilated lung compliance and a rapid and large decrease in arterial oxygen saturation. Under these circumstances, the lavage procedure must be terminated no matter how much treatment has been accomplished. The patient should be moved quickly to the lateral decubitus position with the lavaged side dependent and the operating room table placed in a head-down position in order to facilitate removal of lavage fluid. Vigorous suctioning and inflation of both lungs should be carried out. The double-lumen tube should be changed to a standard single-lumen tube, and the patient should be mechanically ventilated with positive end-expiratory pressure (PEEP). Timing of further unilateral lung lavage attempts is dictated by the patient's subsequent clinical course and gas exchange status.

After the effluent lavage fluid becomes clear, the procedure is terminated. The lavaged lung is thoroughly suctioned and ventilation to it is re-established. Since the compliance of the lavaged side is much less than that of the ventilated side at this time, large tidal ventilations (15 to 20 ml per kilogram) to that side alone (with the nonlavaged side temporarily nonventilated) are necessary to re-expand alveoli. Arterial blood oxygenation may decrease precipitously during this time, but this can be minimized by clamping the nonlavaged side after a large inspiration of 100 percent oxygen.

After lavage, the recovery procedure consists of repetitive periods of large tidal ventilations with PEEP, postural drainage, chest wall percussion, and functioning while intermittently measuring combined (total) and individual lung dynamic compliance. As the compliance of the lavaged lung returns toward prelavage values, ventilation with an air-oxygen mixture may help lavaged lung alveoli with low ventilation-perfusion ratios to remain open. When the compliance of the hemithorax of the lavaged side returns to its prelavage value, the neuromuscular blockade is reversed. Mechanical ventilation and extubation guidelines are the same as for any patient with pulmonary disease; I find most patients are able to be extubated while still in the operating room. If the patient is not considered a candidate for extubation, the double-lumen tube is changed to a single-lumen tube and the patient is mechanically ventilated with PEEP in a conventional manner.

During the immediate postextubation period, deep breathing (incentive spirometry), coughing exercises, chest percussion, and postural drainage are used to remove remaining fluid and secretions and to re-expand the lavaged lung. After 3 to 5 days of recovery, the patient is returned to the operating room to have the opposite side lavaged. The anesthetic considerations for the second lavage are the same as for the first lavage, although oxygenation is usually not nearly as severe a problem as during the first lavage.

ALTERNATIVE METHODS

There are two special problems associated with pulmonary lavage that may be encountered. First, a few very critically ill adult patients may be unable to tolerate the conventional procedure. Second, unilateral lavage through a double-lumen tube is not possible in children and very small adults.

There are three alternative (and more complicated) ways of accomplishing lung lavage in adult patients who simply cannot tolerate one-lung ventilation under any circumstances. First, extracorporeal membrane oxygenation (ECMO) has been used to provide support of gas exchange during standard unilateral lung lavage. Partial venoarterial cardiopulmonary bypass has been used for a few hours during unilateral or bilateral lung lavage, but the distribution of oxygenated blood from the venoarterial bypass can be markedly inhomogeneous and dependent on the site of blood return, and it requires major arterial cannulation. Venovenous bypass provides uniform arterial distribution and the safety of not requiring major arterial cannulation. During either kind of bypass, the nonlavaged lung may also be mechanically ventilated with PEEP (through a double-lumen tube).

The second method of accomplishing lung lavage in patients who cannot tolerate conventional unilateral lung lavage is the use of lobar lavage through a fiberoptic bronchoscope inserted with topical anesthesia. With this technique, a cuffed fiberoptic bronchoscope is inserted into a lobar bronchus and saline irrigation is carried out. The patient remains awake and breathes high-flow oxygen delivered through a face mask. One or two lobes may be done at a time, and lobar lavages can be repeated as many times as necessary. Ventilation-perfusion scan of the lung can be used to dictate which lobes are most severely affected and should thus be lavaged first. This technique has been used successfully, and some feel that the relative ease with which it can be done makes it a preferable alternative to the use of an ECMO support system.

Third, there are patients who cannot tolerate the periods of lavage drainage when nonventilated lung blood flow markedly increases (because there is no alveolar pressure) and PaO_2 decreases, but who can tolerate the periods of lavage installation, when the high lavage fluid pressure decreases the blood flow to the nonventilated lavaged lung and increases PaO_2. In an effort to reduce this particular risk, pulmonary blood flow has been diverted away from the lavaged lung during drainage by inflation of a pulmonary artery catheter balloon in the main pulmonary artery of the side being lavaged. The pulmonary artery catheter should be inflated only during periods of lung drainage and only until the phasic pulmonary artery trace just begins to dampen (is not wedged). The deflection of blood flow away from the drained nonventilated lung to the ventilated lung by the partially inflated balloon decreases shunt through the drained lung and increases PaO_2. Because of the potential hazard of pulmonary artery rupture, and because patients who cannot selectively tolerate periods of lung drainage cannot be ordinarily predicted, this technique should be reserved for patients who had unacceptable oxygenation during lung drainage on a first lavage attempt.

Lavage performed in the conventional manner is not possible in children (or very small adults) in whom double-lumen endotracheal tubes are too large to be inserted. This problem routinely occurs in persons weighing less than 25 to 30 kg, because the smallest double-lumen endotracheal tube made is 28 French, with each lumen being slightly less than 4.5 mm. In this situation, partial cardiopulmonary bypass has been used successfully to provide oxygenation during unilateral or bilateral lavage. In one of these reports, the technique was used in two brothers aged 4 and 2.5 years. Both these patients underwent whole-lung lavage, during which time blood was removed from both femoral veins, oxygenated, and returned to the left femoral artery. Both patients were eventually discharged from the hospital, although they continued to require supplemental oxygen by face mask. In another report the technique was used to support gas exchange during whole-lung lavage in a ventilator-dependent 3.7-kilogram, 8-month-old child. The extracorporeal oxygenation system was again venoarterial (right internal jugular-right atrium catheter to right axillary artery catheter). Marked improvement in pulmonary function was noted after lavage (total 420 ml per kilogram); bypass was able to be discontinued 3 hours after lavage, and the patient was extubated 48 hours after lavage. In the last report, partial venoarterial bypass with a bubble oxygenator permitted bilateral simultaneous lung lavage in two siblings aged 3 and 4 years. Bypass in these patients was carried out with femoral vein and femoral artery cannulation. During bypass, radial artery PaO_2 ranged between 25 and 30 mm Hg; this may, in part, have been related to continued cardiac output of desaturated blood into the proximal aorta. No neurologic sequelae were noted. Oxygenation and functional levels were improved after lavage. These various efforts to treat pulmonary alveolar proteinosis in children with bilateral lung lavage support by extracorporeal oxygenation must be regarded as successful, in view of the fact that in children without this kind of treatment the average survival from the time of severe symptoms is less than 1 year.

SUGGESTED READING

Alfery DD, Benumof JL, Spragg RG. Anesthesia for bronchopulmonary lavage. In: Kaplan J, ed. Thoracic anesthesia. New York: Churchill Livingstone, 1982:403.

Alfery DD, Zamost BG, Benumof JL. Unilateral lung lavage: blood flow manipulation by ipsilateral pulmonary artery balloon inflation. Anesthesiology 1981; 55:376–381.

Blenkarn GD, Lanning CF, Kylstra JA. Anesthetic management of volume controlled unilateral lung lavage. Can Anaesthesiol Soc J 1975; 22:154–163.

Freedman AP, Pelias A, Johnston RF, et al. Alveolar proteinosis lung lavage using partial cardiopulmonary bypass. Thorax 1981; 36: 543–545.

Rogers RM, Levin DC, Gray BA, et al. Physiological effects of bronchopulmonary lavage in alveolar proteinosis. Am Rev Respir Dis 1978; 118:255–264.

Smith LJ, Ankin MG, Katzenstein A, et al. Management of pulmonary alveolar proteinosis. Chest 1980; 78:765–770.

Warr RG, Hawgood S, Buckley DI, et al. Low molecular weight human pulmonary surfactant protein (SP5): isolation, characterization, and cDNA and amino acid sequences. Proc Natl Acad Sci USA 1987; 84:7915–7919.

PNEUMONECTOMY

W. DAVID WATKINS, M.D., Ph.D.

Anesthesia for noncardiac thoracic surgery is uniquely challenging. The patient undergoing pulmonary resection usually has several coexisting medical problems with specific anesthetic implications, and the surgical procedure itself demands special considerations. Postoperatively, these patients must compensate for a relatively fixed reduction in cardiopulmonary capacity. Pneumonectomy is usually prescribed for malignant diseases of the lung, although occasionally it is performed for hemorrhage, drug-resistant infections, and bronchiectasis. Although this chapter focuses on pneumonectomy, it is equally applicable to partial pulmonary resections. Patients undergoing less extensive resections are dependent on one-lung ventilation intraoperatively and may have significant embarrassment of the operated lung postoperatively. Hence, these patients may be considered to have undergone functional pneumonectomies during the perioperative period. This chapter reviews the current practice of anesthesiology as it applies to pneumonectomy, with emphasis on preoperative assessment, intraoperative management, and postoperative complications.

PREOPERATIVE ASSESSMENT

In no field of anesthesia are appropriate preoperative evaluation and optimization as important as in noncardiac thoracic surgery. By its very nature pulmonary resection permanently reduces cardiopulmonary reserves in addition to producing the transient reduction seen with any surgical procedure requiring general anesthesia. It is the goal of any preoperative evaluation to identify problems that may be avoided, or at least optimized, and thus limit intraoperative complications and postoperative morbidity. As such, this assessment should view the patient in totality.

The preoperative history and physical examination should include evaluation of the patient's general status, such as the state of nutrition, presence of obesity or wasting, and history of recent weight loss. The patient's mental status should be such that he or she can understand and cooperate with preoperative testing and therapeutic interventions. Neurologic disorders that involve the upper airway or thorax should be noted. A history of dysphagia or esophageal reflux has obvious implications for airway management. Advanced age (> 60 years) and male gender have also been associated with increased postoperative complications. Additionally, an estimate of the exercise tolerance and level of daily activity gives subjective information regarding the patient's ability to tolerate the surgical procedure and postoperative recovery.

A history of tobacco abuse is almost invariably present in patients who present for pneumonectomy. Numerous studies document a link between smoking and postoperative pulmonary complications and have shown that the patient must abstain from smoking for approximately 8 weeks to reduce that risk. Patients with a history of smoking are also at increased risk for coronary artery disease, the presence of which dramatically increases the likelihood that the patient will require pulmonary surgery. Any symptoms attributable to coronary insufficiency, such as angina or cardiac asthma, require evaluation. In addition, left ventricular failure suggested by symptoms such as dyspnea on exertion places the patient at high risk for perioperative complications.

Bronchopulmonary symptoms with significant anesthetic implications include wheezing, chronic cough, and excessive sputum production. A change in sputum quality or quantity may indicate a concurrent pulmonary infection, which should be treated. Symptoms of hyperreactive airways should be treated as serious and assessed with the goal of finding and treating any reversible component. Unilateral wheezing or dyspnea may indicate compression of a major bronchus, and hoarseness may result from recurrent laryngeal nerve paralysis, indicating proximal tumor involvement and airway management difficulties. Recurrent laryngeal nerve palsy may prevent the patient from generating an effective cough or predispose the patient to aspiration, adding potential postoperative complications.

Symptoms attributable to compromised cardiovascular reserve include those of right ventricular failure and cor pulmonale, such as edema, ascites, and right upper quadrant abdominal pain. Superior vena cava obstruction presents as upper body edema, and superior sulcus tumors may present with Horner's syndrome or arm pain secondary to brachial plexus involvement. Anesthetic implications of these findings include altered pharmacokinetics of hepatically metabolized drugs, variable volumes of distribution and protein binding, and difficulties with vascular access. Chronic renal disease, vascular disease, and diabetes also require careful perioperative management and monitoring. The use of preoperative medications such as bronchodilators, antihypertensives, diuretics, and hypoglycemics should be noted as well as any drug allergies.

The physical examination of the patient who presents for pneumonectomy should concentrate on identifying signs of compromised cardiopulmonary reserves and areas of potential optimization. Findings of airway obstruction or cardiac failure warrant further evaluation. Preoperative laboratory testing should include chest radiography, arterial blood gas determination, electrocardiography, serum electrolytes with creatinine and glucose, and complete blood counts. Pulmonary function testing by timed spirometry is also indicated.

PULMONARY EVALUATION

Functional assessment of the pulmonary system before thoracic surgery should be that of a staged approach with advanced studies done as indicated by routine tests or physical symptoms or findings. The pulmonary system may be divided into three functions: gas exchange, control of breathing, and pulmonary mechanics. Gross performance of gas exchange and control of breathing may be assessed by arterial blood gas determination while the patient is breathing room air. Arterial hypoxemia or hypercarbia indicates severe dysfunction. When reversible airway obstruction is adequately treated and in the absence of neuromuscular dysfunction or drug-induced hypoventilation, persistently elevated arterial carbon dioxide pressure ($PaCO_2$) (> 45 mm Hg) reliably predicts high perioperative pulmonary complication and death rates. Although studies evaluating this limit in pulmonary surgery are few, it is nonetheless frequently used as a cutoff for operability in routine practice. While arterial oxygenation may improve, worsen, or remain unchanged after pulmonary resection, resting hypoxemia (particulary arterial oxygen pressure [PaO_2] <50 mm Hg) indicates a high likelihood of significant pulmonary artery hypertension that should be evaluated with more invasive studies.

The ventilatory mechanics of the pulmonary system

are elevated initially by timed spirometry (commonly called pulmonary function tests or PFTs). This simple test provides the forced vital capacity (FVC) and forced expiratory volume in 1 second (FEV_1). The normal FEV_1/FVC ratio (expressed as 1 percent = FEV_1 percent) should be greater than 70 percent; a result of less than 50 percent indicates severe obstructive lung disease. Any deviation from normal should warrant repeating the test with the addition of an inhaled bronchodilator to evaluate a reversible component of airway obstruction. Significant (> 10 percent) improvement in any parameter after bronchodilation indicates incomplete optimization that should be corrected prior to surgery. Table 1 lists accepted minimal PFT parameters for specific surgical procedures as recommended by Benumof. Inspiratory capacity (IC) as well as expiratory reserve volume (ERV) can be easily calculated from the spirograph. Maximum voluntary ventilation (MVV) or maximum breathing capacity (MBC) can be obtained by integrating expired volume over a set time period at maximum ventilation. Although this test is highly effort dependent, it has a significant predictive value owing to its assessment of qualitative variables such as motivation, endurance, and cooperation. Functional residual capacity (FRC) can be determined by nitrogen wash-out, helium dilution, or body plethysmography and used to calculate total lung capacity (TLC) and residual volume (RV).

In an effort to predict postoperative pulmonary function, regional lung function tests have been developed using nuclear medicine techniques. In these tests, a radioactive tracer is used to quantitate percent regional function of perfusion, ventilation, or volume by means of an external detector. For perfusion determination, the radioisotope (either a poorly soluble gas or microaggregate) is injected intravenously, and its appearance in the lung fields is detected by a gamma camera. The percent perfusion can be determined as the fraction of counts in the particular lung region divided by the total counts. A similar technique is used for ventilation measurements except that the bolus of tracer is inhaled instead of being introduced into the bloodstream. If the inhaled radioisotope is rebreathed and allowed to equilibrate, the lung units with long time constants will be included and regional volume may be determined. The results thus obtained only provide fractional distribution, but by multiplying by quantities such as PFT determined flows or volumes, an absolute contribution to total lung function can be made for

individual regions. For example, postoperative FEV_1 or a pneumonectomy can be calculated by multiplying the fractional blood flow of the residual lung and the preoperative FEV_1. It should be remembered, however, that these predictions frequently overestimate pulmonary function during the immediate postoperative period due to residual lung dysfunction and underestimate compensatory function after recovery. These techniques are most accurate for whole lung (right versus left) function, but by using sequential views (anterior, right and left lateral), lobar function can also be determined. Postoperative pulmonary function tests have a high correlation with the predictive results of these regional function tests. The usefulness of these tests is in evaluating patients with borderline pulmonary function and in determining operability for the proposed resection.

A staged approach to preoperative pulmonary function testing is intended to limit invasive (and expensive) tests to that population shown by routine testing to be at high risk for complications. The patient should be medically optimized before the testing so that any transient (e.g., infection) or treatable (e.g., reversible airway obstruction) factor is excluded. If routine tests such as arterial blood gas determinations and spirometry are acceptable, further testing is not necessarily required. Factors shown to be predictive of postoperative complications include baseline hypercarbia ($PaCO_2$ > 45 mm Hg), FVC, or MVV less than 50 percent of the predicted value, FEV_1 less than 50 percent of the FVC or less than 50 percent of the predicted value and RV/TLC greater than 50 percent. If significant disease is indicated by routine whole lung tests, determination of regional lung function should be employed. Common practice is that patients with a resting $PaCO_2$ greater than 45 mm Hg or a predicted postoperative FEV_1 less than 40 percent of the predicted value are at such high risk that surgery should be performed only under extreme circumstances, although justification for these cutoffs is limited. Prediction of postoperative lung function for the proposed resection should be used as guide in determining the operability for a particular patient.

Several invasive tests have been developed to simulate postoperative physiology after pulmonary resection. These include selective pulmonary artery occlusion and bronchoscopically placed endobronchial blockers. With pulmonary artery occlusion, proximal pulmonary artery pressures are recorded at rest and during

Table 1 Minimal Pulmonary Function Test Parameters

Test	Unit	Normal	Pneumonectomy	Lobectomy	Biopsy or Segmental
MBC	liters/minute	>100	>70	40–70	40
MBC	% Predicted	100	>55	>40	>35
FEV	Liters	>2	>2	>1	>0.6
FEV_1	% Predicted	>100	>55	40–50	>40
FEV_{25-75}	Liters	2	>1.6	>0.6–1.6	>0.6

From Benumof JL. Anesthesia for thoracic surgery. Philadelphia: WB Saunders, 1987.

exercise in an effort to determine the compensatory ability of the remaining vascular bed. Elevated pulmonary artery pressure indicates a high probability of residual pulmonary hypertension and risk of cor pulmonale. With bronchial blockers, pulmonary function testing is repeated to simulate postoperative ventilatory capacity. Both of these tests are highly invasive and are not commonly performed, even though right heart catheterization provides information that cannot be obtained with routine noninvasive testing.

Recently, variations on exercise testing have been employed to further define patients at high risk for pulmonary resection. These techniques evaluate systemic functions of the lung with respect to blood flow and gas exchange. The stress imposed by exercise is used to simulate more closely the increased blood flow and ventilatory requirements of residual lung tissue following resection. Patients with elevated pulmonary vascular resistance or reduced maximum oxygen consumption during exercise have been shown to be at very high risk for death or developing complications regardless of whole lung or regional function test results. While such testing is currently not routine practice, with further study, the promise of a specific preoperative predictor of complications may be realized.

INTRAOPERATIVE MANAGEMENT

Anesthesia for pulmonary resection has made significant advances through the years because of better understanding of pulmonary physiology, monitoring equipment, and management of double-lumen endotracheal tubes. Universal acceptance of pulse oximetry has made the utilization of double-lumen tubes safer and the practice widespread.

Silvay surveyed 126 major medical centers in 1983 and reported that only 39 centers use double-lumen tubes in more than 50 percent of their cases. Thirty-three centers handled pulmonary resections with single-lumen endotracheal tubes. The reluctance to use double-lumen tubes prior to monitoring with pulse oximetry was largely due to the risk of hypoxia during one-lung ventilation. The development of polyvinyl chloride double-lumen

tubes has reduced the incidence of tracheal bronchial damage. Double-lumen tube design lacks the carinal hooks and uses high-volume and low-pressure bronchial and tracheal cuffs that inflate symmetrically, avoiding the deviation of the tips against the walls of the airway. Use of the double-lumen tubes provides improved surgical exposure and is now considered a high priority for pulmonary resection.

Intraoperative anesthesia management entails several major maneuvers, including induction of anesthesia, placement of the double-lumen tube, lateral positioning of the patient, and maintaining adequate gas exchange during one-lung ventilation.

Choices of induction agents vary and all have been used successfully. Agents that minimize bronchomotor tone are useful in the management of the patient with limited pulmonary reserve and concurrent airway irritability. Intravenous lidocaine can be a useful adjunctive induction agent. Lidocaine does not attenuate hemodynamic responses to intubation but has been demonstrated to reduce reflex bronchoconstriction. Intratracheal lidocaine may be of particular benefit when a double-lumen tube is used because the carina has been demonstrated to have the highest concentration of sensory receptors in the tracheal bronchial tree. Case reports of intratracheal instillation of lidocaine causing airway constriction are uncommon, provided that adequate general anesthesia is administered concurrently. If no contraindications exist to ventilation during induction (full stomach, delayed gastric emptying, reflux), potent inhalation agents are also useful for blunting airway reflexes and hemodynamic changes.

Placement of the double-lumen tube has been extensively studied, described, and reviewed by Benumof. A brief overview of methods for confirming placement of double-lumen tubes is shown in Table 2.

When one is positioning the patient laterally, it is important to ensure that the brachial plexus is protected from compression and stretching by placing an axillary roll under the upper chest wall. Pillows are placed between the knees to protect both the saphenous nerve and lateral peroneal nerve (sensory medial distribution to the lower leg and foot and dorsiflexion to the foot, respectively).

Table 2 Methods Used for Checking Position of Double-Lumen Tubes

Method	Advantages	Disadvantages
Auscultation	Quick and easy Confirms bronchial intubation	May not detect upper lobe obstruction Does not ensure adequate seal or complete isolation of lung
Holloway test: After placement, both cuffs are inflated and tracheal port is tested.	Quick and easy Confirms bronchial intubation, adequacy of seal, and isolation	Cannot determine which bronchus is intubated Will not detect upper lobe obstruction
Fiberoptic bronchoscopy	Confirms appropriate placement and upper lobe patency; repositioning may be done under direct vision	Requires skill with bronchoscopy equipment Secretions or blood may obscure vision

Two-lung ventilation should be maintained when possible. One-lung anesthesia is begun by increasing the fractional inspired oxygen (FIO_2) to 1.0 and ventilating with tidal volumes of 10 ml per kilogram. Normocapnia is maintained by adjusting the respiratory rate. Inspiratory pressures are noted, and compliance of the lung is estimated.

Decreases in PaO_2 generally occur immediately and continue to decline with time. A decrease in oxygenation may occur for many reasons during one-lung ventilation. Shunt fraction through the nonventilated lung is a major contributor to changes in oxygenation and varies from 20 to 50 percent. This major factor to the decrease in PaO_2 cannot be predicted by preoperative evaluating tests. Pulmonary hypoxic vasoconstriction (HPV) will decrease the shunt fraction but may be blunted by clinical conditions or anesthetic drugs. (Tables 3 and 4).

The weight of the mediastinum, pressure on the diaphragm by abdominal contents, axillary rolls, and opening of the nondependent pleura all decrease the functional residual capacity (FRC) of the dependent lung. The decline in FRC to closing volume leads to ventilation and perfusion (V/Q) mismatching and also contributes to a reduction in PaO_2.

Larson studied patients undergoing thoracic surgery and observed that the FRC decreased by 10 percent with lateral positioning and fell an additional 10 percent with opening of the nondependent pleura. During one-lung ventilation, the FRC returned to baseline and the FRC of the remaining lung after pneumonectomy increased by 30 percent.

Decreases in cardiac output that lead to a reduction in mixed venous oxygen (MVO_2) content may further compound the reduction in FRC, causing PaO_2 to fall further. Cardiac output can be maintained satisfactorily during one-lung ventilation, provided that plateau inspiratory pressures are limited to less than 30 cm H_2O and extremes of positive end-expiratory pressure (PEEP) are avoided. Pulmonary vessels are capable of recruitment and readily accept the increase in blood flow to the dependent lung.

Hypoxia during these procedures can be problematic. Maneuvers to remedy intraoperative hypoxia during one-lung anesthesia are outlined in Table 5.

PEEP to the dependent lung can increase or decrease PaO_2. Improvement in V/Q mismatch will increase PaO_2. However, the diversion of blood flow to the nonventilated lung may increase the shunt fraction and cause a further decline in PaO_2. Therefore, this is not recommended as the first choice to improve oxygenation. High-frequency positive-pressure ventilation has not gained widespread usage, but reports indicate success in maintaining oxygenation and a motionless operative surgical field.

Intraoperative hypotension occurs more frequently during pneumonectomy than during other thoracic procedures because of the proximity of the hilar region to the heart. Surgical retractors against the heart can effectively reduce venous return and left ventricular end-diastolic (LVEDV) volume, leading to a decrease in cardiac output. Dysrythmias, such as atrial fibrillation, can be triggered during hilar resection, decreasing LVEDV and causing hypotension in patients with limited cardiac reserve. Perioperative digitalization remains controversial but may prevent rhythm disturbances in certain patients with marginal cardiac reserve.

Hemorrhagic complications were reviewed by Peterffy, who concluded that pneumonectomy and nonspecialist operators were associated with a higher incidence of intraoperative bleeding. Significant hemorrhage occurred in 40 of 428 cases. Bleeding from the pulmonary artery or vein accounted for 37 of the 40 episodes. Hemorrhagic complications must always be excluded when perioperative hypotension occurs.

Inadvertent spinal anesthesia has been reported following intraoperative intercostal nerve blocks for postoperative analgesia. Hypotension with bradycardia, Horner's syndrome, and total paralysis confirm the diagnosis. Injections in the dural cuff, which can extend 8 cm beyond the vertebral foramen, or intraneural injections via the perineural space have been proposed for distributing local anesthetics to the spinal roots. Recommendations of limiting the volume of local anesthetic to 3 ml per intercostal nerve and injecting at the angle of the rib (outside the dural cuffs) will reduce the occurrence of this complication.

Thoracic epidural regional anesthesia has been used in combination with general anesthesia for thoracic surgical procedures. Advocates of this technique claim that its advantages include reduction of stress response

Table 3 Clinical Conditions That Blunt Hypoxic Vasoconstriction

Mitral valve stenosis
High pulmonary art pressure
Hypocapnia
Hypothermia
Volume overload
Positive end-expiratory pressure
Leukotrienes

Table 4 Drugs That Attenuate Hypoxic Vasoconstriction

Calcium channel blockers
Nitroglycerin
Nitroprusside
Isuprel
Beta$_2$ agonists
Aminophylline
Potent inhalational agents
Hydralazine hydrochloride

Table 5 Mechanisms for Improving Intraoperative Oxygenation

1. Oxygen sufflation with 5 to 10 cm/H_2O continuous positive airway pressure to nonventilated lung
2. Positive end-expiratory pressure to dependent lung
3. Intermittently two-lung ventilation
4. Early clamping of pulmonary artery and vein
5. High-frequency positive-pressure ventilation

and excellent intraoperative and postoperative analgesia. The lower concentrations of potent inhalation agents required with epidural regional anesthesia may preserve hypoxic pulmonary vasoconstriction. Postoperative maintenance of transdiaphragmatic pressures with the use of epidural narcotics will reduce the degree of atelectasis in the remaining lung. Also, in a recent study by Blomberg, myocardial perfusion improved with the use of thoracic epidurals because the endocardial to epicardial blood flow ratio improved.

Those opposed to the use of thoracic epidural anesthesia argue that combined regional and general anesthetic techniques expose the patient to increased anesthetic complications such as dural puncture and spinal cord injury. The decrease in tissue metabolism by epidural anesthesia is short lived and is equivalent to general anesthesia 12 hours after the neuroblockade has dissipated. Thrombotic complications are reduced with prostatic and limb surgery. Mellbring recorded no statistical difference in postoperative thrombotic complications for major abdominal surgery with or without the addition of epidural anesthesia, and this probably applies to the thoracic procedures as well.

The thoracic epidural catheter should be placed before induction of general anesthesia so that any symptoms of parasthesia can be noted, and the epidural needle or catheter repositioned. After induction of general anesthesia, the epidural anesthetic can be titrated to effect. The thoracic epidural space is smaller than in the lumbar region and generally requires only 1 ml of 2 percent lidocaine per segment (five to six segments are required pending level of placement of catheter). Epidural narcotics are used concurrently to control postoperative pain while minimizing sedation.

No conclusions can be drawn at this time as to whether or not a combined regional and general anesthesia technique offers any distinct advantage over a well-controlled general anesthetic. Further outcome studies are required.

Extubation at the end of the surgical procedure is desirable in order to minimize airway pressures on the bronchial stump. Thorough preoperative and intraoperative evaluation aid in making the decision as to when to extubate. The patient should be alert, cooperative, and should be able to maintain adequate respiratory gas exchange and clear secretions. If tidal volumes, vital capacity, and inspiratory effort are inadequate and if shunt fraction is excessive, the patient is maintained under anesthesia and the double-lumen endotracheal tube is replaced by a single-lumen tube. A relatively large-bore single lumen tube (9 mm for most adult male patients) will minimize airway resistance and ease the clearance of secretions until weaning parameters are achieved.

POSTOPERATIVE MANAGEMENT AND COMPLICATIONS

Postoperative complications following pneumonectomy are probably unrelated statistically to the site of operation, the presence of an abnormal preoperative electrocardiogram, a preoperative functional vital capacity less than 2.8 L, FEV_1 less than 1.7 L, a preoperative PaO_2 less than 60 mm Hg, and the seniority of the surgeon (resident versus attending). Hence, routine preoperative spirometry is not a significant predictor of postoperative complications, an opinion shared by Smith and co-workers, who suggested additionally that on a cycle ergometer, maximal oxygen uptake of greater than 15 ml per kilogram per minute is predictive of a decreased complication rate for thoracotomy itself. The major complications associated with pneumonectomy include pneumonia, respiratory failure, and cardiac dysrhythmia. In addition, postoperative morbidity and mortality seem to be increased in male patients (47 percent versus 29 percent for female patients), in patients who underwent operation for carcinoma (45 percent), and in patients older than 60 years of age (50 percent versus 36 percent for patients younger than 60 years of age). The risk of pulmonary complications increases with hypercapnia, severe dyspnea on exertion, and prolonged anesthesia time. Prevention of postoperative complications in these patients should begin during the preoperative period, with cessation of smoking for at least 8 weeks before surgery, vigorous pulmonary toilet, and prophylactic lung expansion maneuvers.

After pneumonectomy, the remaining lung undergoes compensatory growth, which, in animal studies, is greater in younger patients. Stretch is thought to be the initial stimulus for lung growth, although postoperative distention of the pulmonary vasculature seems to play a role. Therefore, favorable respiratory mechanics appear to be important. Compensatory lung growth is promoted by evacuation of the empty hemithorax, whereas the presence of air (e.g., pneumothorax) inhibits it. The rate of nature of lung growth appears to be influenced by adrenocorticosteroids and growth hormone. Hypoxemia appears to play a minimal role in determining increased lung mass. When compensatory growth is complete, the volumes and thickness of alveoli and capillaries, and the surface area of the blood-gas barrier are maintained. Whether new alveoli are formed remains controversial. No new major airways develop. However, the contralateral (remaining) lung increases dimension to compensate for the loss of lung tissue (i.e., to re-establish functional capacity). In fact, the FRC has been reported to increase by 30 percent in the dependent (remaining) lung after pneumonectomy.

During the immediate postoperative period, the major emphasis is placed on resumption of spontaneous ventilation, reversal of residual neuromuscular blockade, and removal of the endotracheal or endobronchial tube. Excessive postpressure ventilation and vigorous suctioning through the endotracheal tube before its removal should be avoided in order to minimize the possibility of disruption of the bronchial stump, as well as to diminish air leakage into the thoracic cavity. Postoperative mechanical ventilation presents unique problems. The use of high FIO_2 may promote absorption atelectasis. Mechanical ventilation may also contribute to deconditioning of respiratory muscles, leading to prolonged weaning. Endotracheal tubes are associated with decreased clearance of secretions and may promote tracheal erosion if cuff pressures are excessive.

Postoperative respiratory insufficiency may be caused by loss of lung tissue, sputum retention, or infection of the remaining lung. The maximum strength of the diaphragm decrease in patients undergoing pulmonary resection, and the impact of this on respiratory mechanics may set the stage for further pulmonary complications. Respiratory failure during the postoperative period, defined as the inability to wean the patient from mechanical ventilation, is a particularly ominous sign. Possible causes include pneumonia or atelectasis, fluid overload or congestive failure, aspiration, drug or blood component reactions, opportunistic infections, and sepsis. Nearly all of these conditions can be treated successfully if intervention is early and aggressive and is aimed at the cause rather than merely the symptoms. Atelectasis is the most frequent respiratory problem in post-thoracotomy patients and occurs when the FRC falls below the pulmonary closing volume. Conditions promoting postoperative atelectasis include the use of high FIO_2, a history of smoking, and obesity. Atelectasis promotes acute shunting, hypoxemia, hypoventilation, and infection. Postoperative atelectasis may be prevented by the use of blow bottles or incentive spirometry. Patients are particularly prone to postoperative hypoxemia and hypercapnia after pneumonectomy. Since most of these patients have some form of significant chronic pulmonary disease, increasing the FIO_2 may correct the hypoxemia, but may lead to a worsening of the hypercapnia. A respiratory stimulant might be useful in this circumstance, and in one study, both doxapram hydrochloride (acting centrally and peripherally) and Almitrine (acting only on aortic and carotid chemoreceptors) produced a decrease in $PaCO_2$ of 15 to 20 percent, with an increase in PaO_2 of 20 percent; this was statistically significant relative to placebo-treated patients after 60 minutes.

A rare but ominous insidious pulmonary insufficiency has been reported in the postpneumonectomy patient who develops pulmonary hypertension. The cause is unclear. The clinical signs include a loud, fixed pulmonic valve component (P_2), third heart sound (S_3), and arterial denaturation. The treatment is aggressive therapy for airway disease, such as the use of bronchodilators, oxygen, and possibly steroids and pulmonary vasodilators, and antibiotic treatment of proven infections. Platypnea, the dyspnea induced by the assumpton of an upright position and which is reduced by recumbancy, is another rare complication, and is believed to be caused by increased anatomic right-to-left shunt. This may lead to a postural hypoxemia. There may be an actual mechanical distortion of the intra-atrial septum, with the blood from the inferior vena cava entering the left atrium directly, presumably through the foramen ovale, and leading to venous admixture of the arterial blood.

Pulmonary blood loss and hemorrhage during the postoperative period are not usually problems, unless a major pulmonary artery or vein is involved. Most often, the blood loss is due to bleeding from systemic vessels in the chest wall or mediastinum or to diffuse bleeding. However, when one observes massive, acute hemorrhage occurring after pneumonectomy, the pulmonary artery, and to a lesser extent the pulmonary vein, is most likely to be involved, with the cause of bleeding being slipping or cutting through of ligatures applied to the divided major vessels. To control the hemorrhage, emergency thoracotomy may be required in some cases—a procedure associated with a high operative mortality rate (up to 22.5 percent).

Tension pneumothorax caused by the breakdown of the bronchial suture line may lead to bronchopleural fistula, which is associated with a high mortality rate. In these cases, the technique of bronchial suturing itself probably makes little difference, although a lower bronchopleural fistula rate has been observed with stapling as opposed to hand-suturing techniques. The incidence of bronchopleural fistula formation is higher after right pneumonectomy than it is after left pneumonectomy, because the right bronchial stump is less protected. The complication usually occurs during the first 2 weeks postoperatively. High-frequency ventilation techniques have been used successfully during fibrin-sealant repair of bronchial stump fistulae, because the technique avoids stress on the sealed site, which generally requires approximately 60 seconds to stabilize. Bronchial rupture is exceedingly rare, but has been reported to be more likely to occur with the older, red rubber Robertshaw double-lumen endobronchial tubes or with the Carlens tube with a carinal hook.

Dysrhythmias may be caused by surgical manipulation of the mediastinum, or by the presence of chest tubes, pulmonary artery catheters, hypoxemia, or pericarditis. Atrial fibrillation or flutter, the most common dysrhythmia, is serious and difficult to manage because it is often associated with respiratory insufficiency and decreasing cardiac output. It is also related to increasing age and an increase in the amount of lung resected. However, pretreatment with digoxin may reduce the frequency and severity of the problem. Myocardial infarction and pulmonary embolus may occur and are often fatal in the pneumonectomy patient. Intraoperative myocardial function and irreversible ventricular arrhythmias can be caused by large swings in intravascular volume and blood pressure. Intraoperative blood loss is poorly tolerated. Therefore, fluid replacement and management must be managed aggressively both intraoperatively and postoperatively.

Cardiac herniation can be life threatening; the mortality rate associated with this condition is approximately 50 percent, and it usually manifests itself within the first 24 hours. Herniation occurs through a pericardial defect. Contributing factors include suction applied to the evacuated hemithorax; positioning of the patient postoperatively with the operative side dependent; positive-pressure ventilation; coughing; and vomiting.

Signs of cardiac herniation may demonstrate sudden hypotension, atrial or ventricular dysrhythmias, superior vena cava syndrome, cardiovascular collapse, and rarely, airway obstruction. Treatment includes repositioning of the patient so that the nonoperative side is dependent; decreasing tidal volumes to avoid hyperinflation of the remaining lung, which will otherwise worsen the herniation; therapeutic pneumothorax; and perhaps surgery.

Because of the rich vascularity of the chest wall, infections are rare, except in mediastinal incisions and wounds. Empyema is a late surgical complication that may be caused by bronchopulmonary fistulae in 50 percent of patients. For this reason, early extubation and meticulous disposal of secretions have been recommended. It is usually seen in patients who have intracurrent pulmonary infections or those patients with prolonged air leaks or incomplete expansion of the remaining lung. Empyema is particularly troublesome in postpneumonectomy patients in whom the remaining lung, although expanded, fails to fill the entire chest. Nonspecific prophylactic antibiotic therapy does little to prevent either intraoperative or nosocomial infection. By contrast, specific antibiotic therapy against proven infective agents is appropriate.

Other rare complications in postpneumonectomy patients include renal failure, most often caused by pre-existing disease; inadequate volume replacement; or decreased cardiac output and glomerular filtration rate during the perioperative period, the paraplegia caused by interruption of the vascular supply to the spinal cord.

Postoperative pain is a most important consideration in these patients and is associated with splinting, reduced tidal volume, tachypnea and increased work of breathing, and decreased FRC that is compounded with the administration of respiratory depressant analgesics. Pain relief can be problematic. Tranquilizers, rather than parenteral narcotics, and the use of nonsteroidal anti- inflammatory agents, such as indomethacin, have been suggested for relief of post-thoracotomy pain. The paraspinous or intercostal use of long-acting local anesthetics such as bupivacaine may preserve FEV_1, although intrathecal or epidural narcotics may be more effective than either intercostal or paravertebral blocks. Thoracic epidural narcotics seem to have no advantage over lumbar epidural narcotics, and there may be more risk associated with thoracic epidural placement. Epidural narcotics will provide analgesia without motor neuron block, although respiratory depression is rare (occurring in < 1 percent of patients). Such respiratory depression is biphasic, due to an initial systemic absorption of the narcotic, and later to central distribution. The more lipid-soluble narcotics (e.g., fentanyl) have been recommended for epidural use because they may produce less respiratory depression than do other local agents, and their effects may last 6 to 8 hours. Finally, patient-controlled analgesic regimens may be helpful in controlling postoperative pain.

SUGGESTED READING

Benumof JL. Anesthesia for thoracic surgery. Philadelphia: WB Saunders, 1987.

Benumof JL, Alfery DD. Anesthesia for thoracic surgery. In: Miller RD, ed. Anesthesia. 3rd ed. New York: Churchill Livingstone, 1990.

Brodsky JB, ed. Problems in anesthesia: thoracic anesthesia. Vol 4, No. 2. Philadelphia: JB Lippincott, 1990.

Eisenkraft JB, Cohen E, Kaplan JA. Anesthesia for thoracic surgery. In: Barash PG, Cullen BF, Stoelting RK, ed. Clinical anesthesia. Philadelphia: JB Lippincott, 1989.

Kaplan JA, ed. Thoracic anesthesia. New York: Churchill Livingstone, 1983.

ANESTHESIA IN ABDOMINAL SURGERY

SURGICAL TREATMENT OF PORTAL HYPERTENSION AND ASCITES

WILLIAM T. MERRITT, M.D.
SIMON GELMAN, M.D., Ph.D.

Obstruction to venous flow through the liver develops secondary to the fibrotic changes that occur with progressive destruction of liver tissue by chronic liver diseases. Portal hypertension then results in an array of collateral channels around the liver, which often leads to repeated episodes of esophageal variceal bleeding and the production of ascites. Variceal hemorrhage is often life threatening. In addition to transfusion and optimal replacement of coagulation factors and platelets, several types of surgical therapy have evolved (Table 1). Because patients undergoing operations for treatment of variceal hemorrhage are often extremely ill, morbidity and mortality rates can be high, and for a given patient,

Table 1 Surgical Treatment of Portal Hypertension and Ascites

Nonshunting procedures
  Esophageal sclerotherapy
  Percutaneous variceal embolization
  Surgical variceal ligation
  Portal-azygos disconnection

Portosystemic shunting procedures
  Nonselective
    Portacaval
      End-to-side
      Side-to-side
    Mesocaval
    Proximal splenorenal
  Selective
    Distal splenorenal
  Mesoatrial

Ascitic fluid shunting procedures
  Peritoneovenous shunts

controversy may arise as to the correct procedure or whether any procedure is indicated.

NONSHUNTING PROCEDURES

The nonshunting procedures include transesophageal sclerotherapy, percutaneous embolization of variceal vessels, some forms of surgical ligation of varices, and portal–azygos disconnection procedures.

Transesophageal sclerotherapy is currently considered the treatment of choice for acutely bleeding varices. It can be performed with either a flexible fiberoptic scope or with a rigid esophagoscope. Because the procedure often requires only mild sedation (especially in adults) and can take less than 1 hour to perform, the fiberoptic approach is more often used. Drugs commonly used for sclerotherapy are sodium morrhuate, ethanolamine, and polidocanol. These drugs are "inflammatory, vasoconstrictive, thrombogenic, protein-precipitating lipid liquids that induce tissue necrosis" (Conn). Sclerotherapy involves injection of one of these agents either directly into the varix or into the perivariceal area. Visibility is often impaired by active bleeding in spite of the local or systemic vasopressin that is administered to those patients who are actively bleeding. With systemic injection, these chemicals have been associated with (1) decreased mean arterial pressure, (2) decreased cardiac output, (3) decreased hepatic blood flow (probably secondary to decreases in mean arterial pressure and cardiac output), and (4) acute respiratory failure. Acute and chronic complications of sclerotherapy can be severe. They include bleeding, esophageal rupture, pneumothorax, chest pain, mediastinitis, esophageal stricture, small pleural effusions, and adult respiratory distress syndrome (ARDS). Overall, the mortality rate associated with injection sclerotherapy is approximately 10 percent. This rate is relatively low when the seriousness of underlying disease is considered. The mortality rate for esophageal rupture, which occurs in approximately 9 percent of cases, is high. Some centers regard sclerotherapy as inferior to emergency portacaval shunting, even though the latter procedure is considerably more invasive. In addition, patients who have undergone previous sclerotherapy should be considered as having an abnormal gastroesophageal junction. Occasionally, embolization of varices, collateral vessels, and feeding veins is undertaken by way of a transhepatic catheterization of the portal vein and its branches as a temporary measure to control hemorrhage.

Open transesophageal variceal ligation and various esophagogastric transection/reanastomosis procedures for the same purpose are considerably more invasive nonshunting procedures for decompression of the portal system. Only an open approach to the stomach, however, addresses gastric varices. Operative mortality for the transesophageal variceal ligation procedure is high, and some form of elective shunt is usually performed at a later date. Various esophagogastric devascularization procedures have been described (under general heading of "sugiura procedure"), which can include splenectomy; extensive ligation of veins around the distal esophagus and upper stomach; and ligation of the hepatic, left gastric and splenic arteries. The value of these procedures is difficult to evaluate, and they are performed primarily in Japan. Long-term survival rates have been low. In the United States, esophagogastric devascularization procedures have been associated with considerable mortality and a high rate of recurrence of variceal bleeding.

PORTOSYSTEMIC SHUNTS

Various portosystemic shunting procedures have been performed in an effort to decompress the splanchnic–portal venous system. Considerations that may lead to the use of one shunt rather than another include emergency versus elective surgery, size and age of the patient, and individual anatomic configurations. Blood flow to the liver is also affected by the nature of the shunt.

Nonselective, or total, shunts, such as the end-to-side portocaval shunt (Fig. 1), essentially deprive the liver of splanchnic flow and may produce encephalopathy even in normal patients. In patients with long-standing portal hypertension, side-to-side portocaval, proximal splenorenal (with splenectomy), mesocaval, and portal–renal shunts have the potential to be functionally total (i.e., because of reversed flow). Whether they are "total" or not depends on the relative inflow pressures, intrahepatic and intravascular resistances, shunts between the hepatic arterial system and the portal system (e.g., at the sinusoidal level), and any collateral vessels present. A selective shunt (Fig. 2), on the other hand, does not deprive the liver of splanchnic–portal flow because only the coronary (gastric) and splenic veins are diverted. Even these shunts may become nonselective with time. Because intraoperatively measured pre- and post-shunt portal pressures may not reliably characterize measured flows, operative assessment of flow is the better standard. In general, the hemodynamic effects of opening a portosystemic shunt are modest at best and include a mild and very temporary increase in central venous pressure and cardiac output and imperceptible changes in systemic pressure. The anesthesiologist can assist the surgical team in measuring the necessary pressures during shunt surgery; a recording system that permits well-calibrated paper recording is preferred.

Patients with the Budd-Chiari syndrome have partial or total thrombosis of the hepatic veins that may extend into the upper inferior vena cava. They may present with subacute disease (several weeks to several months) or less commonly after a more chronic course. The obstruction to venous flow can lead to necrosis of hepatocytes secondary to the marked increase in sinusoidal pressure and decreased hepatic arterial and portal blood flow. In these patients, a variety of shunts have been attempted, but the most successful appear to be side-to-side portocaval shunts and both mesocaval H grafts and C shunts. Obviously, the success of any shunt depends on the presence of a patent inferior vena cava that permits flow to reach the right atrium as well as the portal to systemic pressure gradient that drives the flow. If the liver is so congested that the caudate lobe enlarges and compresses the inferior vena cava, or if the thrombotic process extends into the inferior vena cava and blocks venous return, these procedures do not help because collateral vessels around the obstructed vena cava are inadequate to decompress the system. Patients with obstruction of the vena cava have been treated with a mesoatrial shunt. For these, a long synthetic graft is extended from the superior mesenteric vein into the chest for anastomosis with the right atrium. Appropriate pressure gradients and myocardial contraction facilitate flow. Results of this operation appear promising.

Of interest to the anesthesiologist are the hemodynamic changes associated with the acute opening of the shunt. Patients with Budd-Chiari syndrome usually have a normal cardiac index and systemic vascular resistance prior to surgery and do not manifest the hyperdynamic, low-resistance state of chronic cirrhosis. Upon opening of the mesoatrial shunt, there is roughly a 50 percent increase in the cardiac index and a 40 percent decrease in systemic vascular resistance. Both right atrial and pulmonary capillary wedge pressures increase sharply by approximately 5 mm Hg. Shunting, then, appears to alter hemodynamics in the direction of those seen in patients with chronic liver disease and cirrhosis. This is postulated to result both from the volume effects of the shunt and from the release into the general circulation of a vasodilator substance.

PALLIATIVE SHUNTS FOR TREATING ASCITES

Peritoneovenous shunting can be used to treat intractable ascites. Two basic types of shunt, the LeVeen and Denver, both have a pressure-sensitive valve with an opening pressure of 3 to 5 cm of water that permits one-way flow of ascitic fluid. The Denver shunt, in addition, has a small pumping chamber designed to allow the patient to pump and flush the tubing and pressure chamber. There is no particulate or bacterial filter in either shunt. Insertion may be performed in

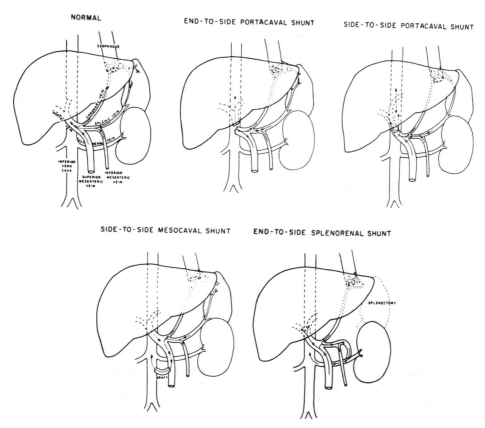

Figure 1 Four types of nonselective shunts. Arrows indicate the direction of blood flow. (Reproduced with permission from Conn HO. In Schaffner F, et al, eds. The liver and its diseases. New York: Intercontinental Medical Books, 1974:289.)

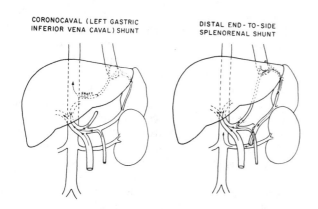

Figure 2 Selective portosystemic vascular shunts. Arrows indicate portal and systemic flows after selective shunting. (Reproduced with permission from Conn HO. In Schaffner F, et al, eds. The liver and its diseases. New York: Intercontinental Medical Books, 1974:289.)

extremely ill patients and is often done under local anesthesia or light sedation. An incision is made for tunneling the catheter into the peritoneal cavity at the distal end and into a neck vein at the proximal end. The proximal tip of the catheter rests at the right atrium. The hemodynamic effects seen acutely with the opening of these shunts range from minor increases in the central venous and mean arterial pressures to intravascular fluid overload. Other complications of peritoneovenous shunting include thrombosis and failure of the shunt, peritonitis with generalized septicemia, endotoxemia, central venous thrombosis and embolism, and a post-shunt coagulopathy similar to disseminated intravascular coagulation.

Anesthetic management during these procedures can be complicated by this coagulopathy. When blood is instilled into the peritoneal cavity, it clots secondary to the presence of soluble collagen procoagulants in peritoneal fluid, a process which consumes platelets and fibrinogen. Subsequently, the clots are lysed by tissue plasminogen activator (TPA). Similar events presumably happen when ascitic fluid reaches the general circulation. This may result in a DIC-like state with a prolonged PT and PTT, increased concentration of fibrin degradation products, and a decrease in platelet count and fibrinogen levels. Treatment is facilitated by replacement of factors (FFP), platelets, ϵ-aminocaproic acid (Amicar) and fibrinogen.

SUGGESTED READING

Beattie C, Sitzmann JV, Cameron JL. Mesoatrial shunt hemodynamics. Surgery 1988; 104:1–9.

Camara DS, Caruana JA, Chung RS, et al. The hemodynamic effects of the sclerosant sodium morrhuate in dogs. Surg Gynecol Obstet 1985; 161:327.

Conn HO. Complications of portal hypertension. In Gitnick G, ed. Current hepatology. Chicago: Year Book, 1985.

Fleig WE, Stange EF, Ruettenauer K, et al. Emergency endoscopic sclerotherapy for bleeding esophageal varices: a prospective study in patients not responding to balloon tamponade. Gastrointest Endosc 1983; 29:8.

LeVeen HH, Christoudias G, Moon IP, et al. Peritoneo-venous shunting for ascites. Ann Surg 1974; 180:580–591.

LeVeen HH, Moon IP, Ahmed N, et al. Coagulopathy postperitoneovenous shunt. Ann Surg 1987; 205:305–311.

Malt RA. Elective portosystemic shunts. In McDermott WV, ed. Surgery of the liver. Boston: Blackwell Scientific, 1989: 353.

Mitchell MC, Boitnott JK, Kaufman S, et al. Budd-Chiari syndrome: etiology, diagnosis and management. Medicine 1982; 61:199–218.

Monroe P, Morrow CR, Miller E, et al. Acute respiratory failure after sodium morrhuate esophageal sclerotherapy. Gastroenterology 1983; 85:693.

Orloff MJ, Krims P, UCSD Gastroenterology Division. Effect of endoscopic sclerotherapy on rebleeding and survival of cirrhotic patients with bleeding esophageal varices [abstr]. Gastroenterology 1986; 90:1574.

Roussel JGJ, Kroon BBR, Hart GAM. The Denver type for peritoneovenous shunting of malignant ascites. Surg Gynecol Obstet 1986; 162:235–240.

Sanfey H, Boitnott JK, Cameron JL. Surgical management of patients with the Budd-Chiari syndrome. World J Surg 1984; 8:706–715.

Steegmuller KW, Marklin H-M, Hollis HW. Intraoperative hemodynamic investigations during portacaval shunt. Arch Surg 1984; 119:269–273.

Sugiura M, Futagawa S. Further evaluation of the sugiura procedure in the treatment of esophageal varices. Arch Surg 1977; 112: 1317–1321.

Terblanche J, Yaleoob E, Bornman P: Acute bleeding varices: a five-year prospective evaluation of tamponade and sclerotherapy. Ann Surg 1981; 194:521.

HEPATIC RESECTION

WILLIAM T. MERRITT, M.D.

The majority of patients who undergo some degree of hepatic resection have essentially normal liver function. Most will have a primary liver tumor or a metastasis from a gastrointestinal cancer (Table 1). Some patients will have more than one lesion that is deemed resectable, either from the preoperative evaluation or after discovery at laparotomy. Another large group of patients who may require some degree of hepatic surgery are patients with traumatic abdominal injury; often the liver insult is part of multisystem trauma. Patients with extensive malignant disease who are not candidates for resection often have a chemotherapy infusion pump inserted prior to the conclusion of surgery.

Preoperative assessment involves attempts to obtain a tissue diagnosis and to look for metastases or a primary tumor as appropriate. Some lesions such as suspected hemangiomas, hydatid cysts, and highly vascularized tumors are dangerous to biopsy percutaneously. Ultrasonography should be used to distinguish cystic from solid lesions. The results of computed tomography (CT) and magnetic resonance imaging (MRI) scans can better serve to determine the size and number of masses better, as well as the potential for involvement of major vascular structures such as the inferior vena cava, portal venous system, and major arteries. Often, however, the results of these tests are not completely definitive, and final decisions about the extent of disease and appropriate procedures are not possible until a thorough evaluation has been conducted at laparotomy. The necessity for preoperative arteriography is debated, but knowledge of an aberrant vascular supply is usually helpful, especially if drug infusion devices are placed.

The initial incision for hepatic resection procedures is usually a right subcostal one. Following this, a major portion of the surgery involves extensive evaluation of the nonhepatic abdominal contents for evidence of additional lesions, as well as a thorough examination of the liver for disease not recognized preoperatively. This can entail the use of intraoperative ultrasonography. For large or inaccessible right-sided lesions, the incision may need to be extended into the right side of the chest. Occasionally, the sternum may be partially divided for similar considerations. During the process of assessing the liver many ligamentous attachments are severed. After a decision to proceed with a resection is made, additional mobilization may be required. At some point, the hilar vessels are usually completely dissected free for eventual hemorrhage control or ligation if necessary.

The goal of curative resection is to remove the tumor completely. This generally means that a 1- to 2-cm margin is desired. Wedge resections are usually possible for smaller lesions located peripherally along the free edges of the liver. Sometimes concern for viability of remaining tissue demands a more formalized lobectomy than a wedge resection. There are no avascular planes for dissection in liver resection. Although the portal triad vessels branch together and become the basis for dividing the liver into segments and lobes, the hepatic veins cross these planes at right angles. As dissection proceeds with blunt instruments or with the ultrasonic dissector (e.g., Cavitron), numerous vessels are encountered. If they tear or bleed prior to ligation with suture or clips, they may retract into the liver parenchyma and continue to bleed. Manual pressure on the liver tissue usually will control this bleeding.

Several clues should alert the anesthesiologist to more extensive surgery and the potential for more

Table 1 Potentially Resectable Hepatic Lesions

Benign
    Hemangioma
    Focal nodular hyperplasia
    Liver cell adenoma

Malignant
    Metastatic
        From possibly widespread metastasis
            Lung
            Breast
            Esophagus
            Stomach
            Pancreas
            Upper GI tract
            Melanoma
        From possibly hepatic only metastasis
            Colon
            Rectum
            Pancreatic islet cell
            Carcinoid
            Gastrointestinal sarcoma

    Primary hepatic
        Hepatocellular
        Cholangiocarcinoma
        Hepatoblastoma
        Angiosarcoma
        Lymphoma

    Local extension into liver, gallbladder and extrahepatic bile ducts
        Colon
        Stomach
        Duodenum
        Adrenal gland

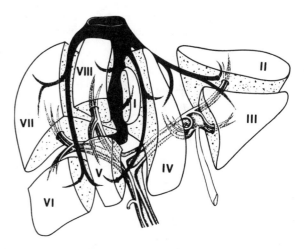

Figure 1 A stylized interpretation of hepatic segments 1 through 8, with their respective blood supplies. (Republished with permission from Bismuth H. Surgical anatomy of the liver. World J Surg 1982; 6:3.)

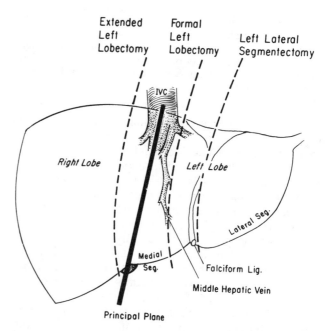

Figure 2 The definition of formal right hepatic resections. (Reprinted with permission from Steele G Jr, "Technique of hepatic lobectomy, trisegmentectomy, and a variety of hepatic wedge resections." In McDermott WV, ed. Surgery of the liver. Boston: Blackwell Scientific, 1989; 452.)

extensive bleeding. A lobectomy is usually associated with more bleeding than a wedge resection, although large wedge resections violate the planes referred to previously and can lead to blood loss as well. Although eight segments in the liver are described (Fig. 1), major liver resection is usually divided into wedge, lobe, right or left extended lobectomy, and left lateral segmentectomy (Figs. 2 and 3). The extended right lobectomy (a trisegmentectomy if dissection proceeds as far as the sulcus of the falciform ligament) is a major resection with potential for significant bleeding. A left trisegmentectomy, which includes resection of the left hepatic lobe and an anterior segment of the right lobe near the right hepatic vein, has been termed by Steele an anatomic fantasy, and generally leads to significant intraoperative blood loss. Tumor near major vessels always presents the potential for sudden catastrophic blood loss. Some surgeons routinely, and others in emergencies, will clamp the inflow vessels in the hilar area (Pringle maneuver) to control bleeding. Occasionally, the hepatic veins or the suprahepatic inferior vena cava is clamped to gain control of hemorrhage. Either of these tactics leads to warm ischemia. Clamping of the suprahepatic inferior vena cava has profound hemodynamic effects in patients without major shunting from portal hypertension. If tumor extends into the diaphragmatic tissue, it may be removed with portions of the diaphragm. This

defect is then closed primarily or with prosthetic material.

ANESTHESIA CONSIDERATIONS

In planning the anesthetic management for this category of surgery, it is important to know what procedure is thought to be necessary. It is useful to question the surgeon as to the likelihood of any resection

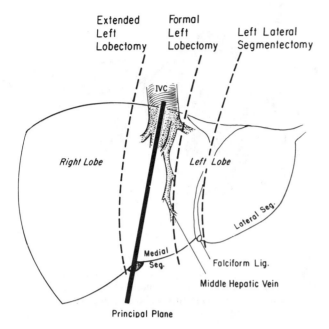

Figure 3 Definition of formal left hepatic resections. One should note that the plan of dissection for the extended left is anterior to the right hepatic vein. (Reprinted with permission from Steele G Jr, "Technique of hepatic lobectomy, trisegmentectomy, and a variety of hepatic wedge resections." In McDermott WV, ed. Surgery of the liver. Boston: Blackwell Scientific, 1989; 452.)

at all. When evidence suggests that a resection will not be possible, it may be reasonable to postpone invasive monitoring until that decision has been made. Obviously, time must then be allocated intraoperatively to place an arterial line, a central line, and large-bore transfusion lines. Significant bleeding can occasionally occur during the evaluation phase if a major vessel is torn; therefore many anesthesiologists prefer to establish at least a portion of the potentially necessary lines prior to, or shortly after, the induction of anesthesia. Even if preoperative liver function is entirely normal, it should be anticipated that liver function will be impaired postoperatively, either from loss of hepatocellular mass or from the direct trauma of manipulation during surgery. Intraoperatively, medication doses of both narcotics and muscle relaxants should be titrated to desired effect. Extremes of carbon dioxide tension should be avoided. Hypocarbia appears to lower hepatic arterial blood flow during abdominal surgery, whereas hypercarbia is associated with increased portal and total hepatic blood flow and appears to depress both hepatic function and hepatic oxygen uptake. Isoflurane often is recommended for liver surgery because it is associated

with better maintenance of liver blood flow. Patients usually experience traction on their upper abdomens and diaphragms for extended periods. Most, except those patients undergoing very limited procedures (e.g., a small wedge resection), should be cared for in an intensive care setting postoperatively. Even with this management, more than 90 percent of patients develop some pulmonary complication (i.e., pleural effusion, atelectasis, or pneumonia). For patients with prior upper abdominal surgery or portal hypertension, the bleeding should be anticipated to be more than routine. For those patients with some element of cardiac disease or for the elderly in whom the perioperative stress of this type of surgery may uncover coronary artery disease, additional monitoring, such as with a pulmonary artery catheter, may be warranted. Additionally, if the surgery is extensive, the blood sugar concentration should be monitored to detect the infrequent patient who will develop intraoperative hypoglycemia. If the right side of the chest is entered, the surgeon may ask for a brief increase in inflation pressures during evacuation of air from the pleural space prior to closing the chest wound. Such maneuvers can decrease venous return profoundly and should be done cautiously. As in other abdominal procedures, it is quite important to keep the patient warm; the use of good fluid, blood warmers, and warming blankets and raising the temperature of the operating room are all useful.

SUGGESTED READING

Biondi JW, Schulman DS, Soufer R, et al. The effect of incremental positive end-expiratory pressure on right ventricular hemodynamics and ejection fraction. Anesth Analg 1988; 67:144–151.

Bismuth H, Houssin D, Castaing D. Major and minor segmentectomies "reglees" in liver surgery. World J Surg 1982; 6:10–24.

Foster JH. Liver resection techniques. Surg Clin North Am 1989; 69:235–249.

Fujita Y, Sakai T, Ohsumi A, et al. Effects of hypocapnia and hypercapnia on splanchnic circulation and hepatic function in the beagle. Anesth Analg 1989; 69:152–157.

Gelman S. Carbon dioxide and hepatic circulation. Anesth Analg 1989; 69:149–151.

Gelman S, Dillard E, Bradley E. Hepatic circulation during surgical stress and anesthesia with halothane, isoflurane or fentanyl. Anesth Analg 1987; 66:396.

Goldfarb G, Debaene B, Ang E, et al. Hepatic blood flow in humans during isoflurane-N$_2$O and halothane-N$_2$O anesthesia. Anesth Analg 1990; 71:349–353.

Schulman DS, Biondi JW, Matthay RA, et al. Effect of positive end-expiratory pressure on right ventricular performance. Importance of baseline right ventricular function. Am J Med 1988; 84:57.

Starzl TE, Bell RH, Beart RW, et al. Hepatic trisegmentectomy and other liver resections. Surg Gynecol Obstet 1975; 141:429–437.

Steele G. Technique of hepatic lobectomy, trisegmentectomy, and a variety of hepatic wedge resections. In McDermott WV ed. Surgery of the liver. Boston: Blackwell Scientific, 1989; P451.

LIVER TRANSPLANTATION

LAWRENCE M. BORLAND, M.D., F.A.A.P.
D. RYAN COOK, M.D.

Homologous orthotopic liver transplantation is the only successful nonpalliative therapy available to patients in hepatic failure and for selected patients with hepatomas and biliary tract tumors. In patients with certain inherited metabolic disorders, metabolic pathways and reactions may be returned to normal after hepatic transplantation.

Since 1980, advances in anesthetic and surgical techniques have dramatically improved intraoperative survival. Cyclosporin A, which selectively inhibits the clonal proliferation of helper T cells by preventing synthesis of interleukin-2 and interferes with suppressor T cells, has profoundly decreased postoperative mortality by muting the body's immune response.

SURGICAL TECHNIQUE

During the first stage of an orthotopic liver transplantation, the recipient's liver is dissected to its vascular pedicle. The anhepatic phase (stage 2) commences with the clamping of the suprahepatic inferior vena cava, the infrahepatic inferior vena cava, the portal vein, and the hepatic artery. After the diseased liver is removed, the donor liver is revascularized with complete anastomosis of the suprahepatic inferior vena cava and partial anastomosis of the infrahepatic inferior vena cava. The donor liver is flushed via the portal vein with 300 to 500 ml of Ringer's lactate solution, which is allowed to drain from the incompletely anastomosed infrahepatic inferior vena cava. Flushing of the donor liver removes the transport infusate (Collin's solution), the intrinsically high potassium concentration of which has been augmented by the intracellular to extracellular movement of potassium from the ischemic donor liver. It also serves to clear the liver vasculature of entrapped air. The infrahepatic inferior vena cava and portal vein anastomosis are then completed.

Clamps on the portal vein, the infrahepatic inferior vena cava, and the suprahepatic inferior vena cava are released in rapid sequence, incorporating the donor liver into the recipient's circulatory system. During stage 3, the hepatic artery anastomosis is performed. In 15 to 20 percent of pediatric cases, cross-clamping of the abdominal aorta is required to complete this anastomosis. After adequate hemostasis has been achieved, the bile duct is reconstructed. If the patient has a normal extrahepatic ductal system, a duct-duct anastomosis with a T tube or indwelling stent may be performed. If the extrahepatic bile ducts are abnormal, a Roux-en-Y choledochojejunostomy is done. An intraoperative cholangiogram is usually obtained to assess the patency of the biliary drainage system.

PREOPERATIVE ASSESSMENT

The emergency nature of this surgery rarely allows time for correction of preoperative abnormalities in the patient's laboratory values. Hemoglobin levels less than 10 g per deciliter are frequently the result of nutritional deficiencies, coagulation abnormalities, or upper gastrointestinal bleeding due to portal hypertension. Coagulation profiles are usually abnormal: 30 percent have an elevated prothrombin time (more than 15 seconds); 33 percent have an abnormal partial thromboplastin time (more than 30 seconds); and 21 percent have a platelet count of less than 100,000 per mm. Moderate-to-massive ascites are treated with loop diuretics and oral replacement of potassium. Although serum electrolyte concentrations are reported to be with-in the normal range, total body potassium stores are low.

Previous renal tubular injury, inadequate renal preload, and hepatorenal syndrome may contribute to pretransplantation renal dysfunction and failure.

Patients in liver failure usually have a restrictive lung defect as the result of simple lung compression from chronic ascites. More significantly, an increased alveolar arterial oxygen difference may exist as a result of diffuse pulmonary arteriovenous shunting; indeed, the presenting clinical signs of liver failure may be cyanosis and clubbing.

ANESTHETIC AND INTRAOPERATIVE CARE

In children, intramuscular premedication is frequently contraindicated because of abnormally elevated coagulation times. Under these circumstances, atropine (10 to 30 μg per kilogram) is given intravenously immediately before induction of anesthesia. When intramuscular injections are not contraindicated, atropine (10 to 30 μg per kilogram) or scopolamine (10 μg per kilogram), morphine sulfate (0.1 mg per kilogram), and pentobarbital (3 to 5 mg per kilogram) are given by this route. Before the induction of anesthesia, a precordial stethoscope, electrocardiographic leads, and blood pressure cuff are put in place.

In adults, preoperative counseling and occasionally hepatic encephalopathy make intramuscular premedications unnecessary in most instances, which is fortunate, since pre-existing coagulopathies are relative contraindications to such injections. The small number of patients who are anxious can easily be calmed with intravenous sedatives given in the operating room under the supervision of the anesthesia team.

If aspiration precautions are required because of intake of food, drink, or cyclosporin A (in orange juice), or because of delayed gastric emptying as a result of severe abdominal distention, the patient should be preoxygenated before intubation, and the Sellick maneuver used after administration of thiopental sodium (3 to 5 mg per kilogram) or ketamine hydrochloride (1 to 2 mg per kilogram) and succinylcholine chloride. When aspiration precautions are not required, anesthesia may be induced with thiopental (3 to 5 mg per kilogram), ketamine (1 to 2 mg per kilogram), or fentanyl (as part of the maintenance anesthetic), or by inhalation with isoflurane.

After induction of anesthesia, rectal and esophageal temperature probes, an esophageal stethoscope, an indwelling urinary catheter, and systemic arterial and central venous pressure cannulae are placed. In children, arterial sites below the diaphragm are avoided, because the abdominal aorta may be cross-clamped during the hepatic artery anastomosis. Central venous pressure catheters are placed via the external or internal jugular route. A sheath-type catheter is frequently chosen to allow for the rapid infusion of large volumes of blood components or for introduction of a flow-directed, balloon-tipped pulmonary artery catheter. Ample padding of extremities, the occiput, and the pelvis is used to avoid pressure-induced injuries during the long operative course.

Although the duration of surgery and the cardiovascular status of these patients vary greatly, an isoflurane relaxant is currently the most frequently used anesthetic for this surgery at our institution. The use of halothane is usually avoided. A fentanyl relaxant anesthetic may also be utilized; however, massive bleeding and transfusions required during liver transplantation lead to hemodilution, which in turn increases the dose of intravenous narcotic agents required to maintain anesthesia. Nitrous oxide should not be used because bowel distention interferes with surgical dissection and vascular anastomosis. The risk of air embolization during stage 2 would also preclude its use. During narcotic relaxant anesthesia without nitrous oxide, patient awareness may occur as a result of the wash-out of intravenous anesthetic agents, and it may be desirable to administer intravenous amnesic agents such as diazepam or lorazepam.

Although production of pseudocholinesterase is disturbed, prolongation of the action of succinylcholine chloride is not a clinical problem because of the duration of surgery. The duration of neuromuscular blockade after administration of pancuronium may be significantly prolonged (by more than 100 percent), since its hepatic and renal routes of elimination are frequently impaired. The kinetics of atracurium besylate are not appreciably altered, but the short half-life of this agent makes it clinically cumbersome unless it is administered by constant infusion. The action of neuromuscular blocking agents must be carefully monitored by train-of-four determination.

Measurements of arterial blood gas tension and pH, hemoglobin, hematocrit, colloid osmotic pressure, and serum concentrations of sodium, potassium, and ionized calcium should be available from the laboratory within 5 to 10 minutes. Serum concentration of glucose, platelet count, and prothrombin and partial thromboplastin times should be obtainable from the central laboratories within half an hour. Coagulation may also be monitored with a thromboelastograph, a device that rapidly assesses the onset of clot formation, the quality of the clot, and the presence of accelerated fibrinolysis. When the clinical situation requires immediate estimation of serum glucose, Dextrostix analysis of whole blood may be used in the operating suite.

INTRAOPERATIVE PROBLEMS

Preservation of intravascular volume and of myocardial stability is the anesthesiologist's most immediate challenge during homologous orthotopic liver transplantation. Correction of abnormal coagulation may require the administration of at least 1 ml of fresh frozen plasma for each 1 ml of packed red blood cells. Pre-existing or dilutional thrombocytopenia or both occur uniformly, and platelet infusion is almost invariable. The infusions of crystalloid and colloid (fresh frozen plasma) solutions should be carefully titrated using colloid osmotic, central venous, and pulmonary artery wedge pressures in order to minimize the incidence of intraoperative pulmonary edema. In patients weighing less than 35 kg, conventional methods of fluid administration are usually successful. In patients weighing 35 kg or more, a rapid infusion device capable of transfusing up to 2,000 ml per minute is used to replace blood loss. The reservoir of the rapid infusion device is filled with 2 U of packed red blood cells, 2 U of fresh frozen plasma, and 500 ml of Plasma-Lyte, resulting in a total volume of 1,500 ml with a hematocrit of approximately 28 percent. The citrate added to the blood products for preservation precludes the need for additional anticoagulants in this system. Plasma-Lyte is used because it resembles intracellular fluid and contains neither calcium, which might cause clotting, nor glucose, which might cause rouleaux formation.

Intraoperative hypotension occurs as a result of inadequate replacement of massive amounts of fluid and blood lost during the procedure; cardiac dysfunction secondary to decreased serum concentration of ionized calcium (presumably as a result of increased citrate concentration after massive transfusion with packed red cells and fresh frozen plasma); surgical manipulations that disturb preload, including occlusion of the inferior vena cava during the anhepatic stage; life-threatening arrhythmias; and, rarely, pre-existing myocardial disease. The mean blood loss for all pediatric patients is 4.3 blood volumes; the range is 0.22 to 45 blood volumes. Patients with biliary atresia lose the most blood (mean blood loss of 5.77 blood volumes; range of 0.26 to 33.2 blood volumes). Lysing adhesions that have developed as a result of the Kasai procedure (as well as during stage I) increase the total blood loss and increase the duration of surgery. The mean blood use for adult patients is 17 Units or about 3.5 blood volumes; the range is 1 to 200 U.

Although the preoperative diagnosis, severity of preoperative coagulation dysfunction, and surgical technique would appear to influence total blood loss, none of these factors correlates well with the blood loss in our pediatric group. In our adult population, disease processes with widespread destruction of parenchymal liver cells adversely influence the total intraoperative blood loss. It may be possible to limit the quantities of blood products administered by using a cell-saver device; however, these devices cannot be used when scavenged blood is contaminated with bowel contents. If clinically appropriate, scavenging of blood should continue while blood is being processed.

In adults and selected pediatric patients, venoveno bypass with heparin-bonded tubing is a means of maintaining the systolic pressure during the anhepatic period. Heparin-bonded polyvinylchloride tubing delivers blood from the portal and femoral veins into a centrifugal flow pump (Bioconsole, Biomedicine), which returns the blood to the axillary vein. Decompression of the portal system with venoveno bypass may also decrease blood loss during this period. Since blood loss during stage 2 is far more significant in the adult than in the pediatric patient, this technique has wider applicability in the former group.

Citrate intoxication and the ensuing myocardial dysfunction may occur as a result of massive blood transfusion of citrate phosphate dextrose blood. Because of hepatic dysfunction (or the absence of the liver in stage 2), the serum citrate concentration is significantly higher than after a comparable transfusion in a normal patient. Decreased body temperature serves to prolong the cardiovascular depression. Hypothermia ($<35°$ C) has occurred more than half of the time. A warming blanket, administration of heated humidified gases, and application of a head wrap are techniques used to maintain the patient's temperature. Blood products may be prewarmed in a water bath and then transfused through an in-line warmer. Decreased concentrations of serum ionized calcium consistently cause systemic arterial hypotension during or immediately after the rapid administration of blood products (500 ml of whole blood contains 1.656 g hydrated trisodium citrate). Calcium chloride is administered by bolus or constant infusion to normalize the ionized calcium concentration. Calcium gluconate is not recommended because it is reported to require hepatic metabolism.

Pre-existing myocardial disease occurs infrequently in the pediatric population, although 50 percent of those with Alagille-Watson syndrome presented with a cardiomyopathy. Several children requiring retransplantation have had myocardial infarctions after the first liver transplantation. Hypotension, hypoxemia, or systemic air embolism had not occurred, although such patients had experienced significant acute systemic hypertension (as a result of cyclosporin A treatment). In adult patients, significant cardiovascular disease is uncommon.

Significant cardiovascular changes may occur at the time of vascular clamping and anastomosis. When the inferior vena cava is clamped at the onset of the anhepatic phase, preload to the heart may decrease. In adult patients, despite infusion of almost a whole blood volume, cardiovascular stability returned only with the infusion of significant quantities of vasoactive compounds. The routine use of venoveno bypass in our adult patients has significantly lessened this problem. Inter-

estingly, in most pediatric patients, collateral circulation secondary to portal hypertension modulates this decrease. At the time of vascular unclamping (at the end of stage 2), there is a transient (5 to 10 minute) decrease (20 to 30 mm Hg) in the systolic and diastolic arterial pressures or in the diastolic pressure only. When the vessels are unclamped after completion of the vascular anastomosis, myocardial contractility decreases as a result of perfusion of the heart with acidotic, cold blood and serum potassium increases transiently. However, even when the pH and serum potassium remain stable, a decrease in systemic vascular resistance is observed as a result of the release of unknown vasodilating agents from the revascularized liver. This occurs with or without the use of venoveno bypass. If the filling pressures are low, hypotension should be treated by administration of crystalloid or colloid. A bolus of calcium chloride is usually necessary, and occasionally an infusion of dopamine (10 to 15 μg per kilogram) for up to 30 minutes is required.

Profound metabolic derangements (especially decreased ionized serum calcium) and the requirement for infusion of massive quantities of fluids almost invariably result in cardiac dysfunction during liver transplantation. However, intraoperative measurement of central venous and pulmonary artery wedge pressures has rarely demonstrated right-to-left heart dissociation. Cardiac output determination and calculation of systemic vascular resistance may be useful in managing the cardiovascular alterations at the time of vessel unclamping. In our pediatric population, surgical manipulation of the right diaphragm and heart usually displaces the pulmonary artery catheter.

During late stage 3 and the postoperative period, profoundly elevated systemic arterial blood pressure resulting from cyclosporin A therapy may be observed and must be treated in order to accomplish the transition of the patient to the intensive care unit safely. Neither volume overload nor inadequate anesthesia is causative. Various therapeutic agents have been used, including morphine sulfate (up to 2 mg per kilogram), hydralazine, nitroglycerin, nitroprusside, diazoxide, beta-blocking agents, and calcium channel–blocking agents. Currently the exact pathophysiologic mechanism is unknown.

Life-threatening arrhythmias may also occur when vessels are unclamped. At this time, wash-out of the cold Collin's solution may produce hyperkalemia and cardiac arrest. Diligent flushing of the donor liver before revascularization is most important. After cardiac arrest, normal sinus rhythm and systolic arterial blood pressure can usually be restored by external cardiac compressions, hyperventilation, and administration of sodium bicarbonate, calcium chloride, and regular insulin. During stage 3, potassium is taken up by the donor liver and all other cells because of the extracellular to intracellular shift of potassium secondary to metabolic alkalosis and temperature rewarming. Supplemental potassium is usually required at this time.

Hyperglycemia uniformly occurs as a result of impaired or absent (during anhepatic stage) hepatic gluconeogenesis. Peripheral uptake is markedly decreased from the lowered basal body temperature. At the same time, the patient receives an enormous glucose load in the transfused blood products (each unit of whole blood contains 0.5 g glucose before processing). After revascularization of the donor liver is complete, serum glucose concentration decreases gradually and spontaneously.

Maintenance of adequate urine output is difficult, especially in those patients who have previously had acute tubular necrosis or hepatorenal syndrome. Cross-clamping of the inferior vena cava (without the use of venoveno bypass) and the abdominal aorta compromises the best attempts to maintain urine output. Despite the osmotic diuretic action of the elevated serum glucose, more vigorous therapy (furosemide and dopamine at 5 μg per kilogram per minute) is often required.

Although the preoperative metabolic status may vary widely, in most patients a significant metabolic acidosis develops that increases through the end of stage 2. This stagnation metabolic acidosis during stage 2 is not as severe if venoveno bypass is utilized; it should be treated conservatively (based on arterial blood gas tension and pH and the degree of cardiovascular instability), since a moderate-to-severe metabolic alkalosis will appear during stage 3 as a result of the metabolism of the exogenously administered citrate and the vigorous use of furosemide throughout the postoperative period.

Large arterial-to-alveolar oxygen gradients may be present from pre-existing arteriovenous shunting, and lung compression may be seen from massive ascites. In children, surgical traction severely displaces the right diaphragm cephalad. Suitable oxygenation can usually be maintained with conventional ventilation and an inspired oxygen concentration of 50 percent with 5 cm or less of positive end-expiratory pressure. Pneumothorax may occur during internal jugular cannulation, or more commonly, from the surgical dissection. Bowel disten-

tion and an oversized liver may prevent immediate closure of the abdomen. In these instances, temporary abdominal closure with a Silastic silo similar to that used to repair large omphaloceles in the newborn infant is recommended.

Despite the massive blood loss and the duration of the surgical procedure, most patients are ready to attempt spontaneous respiratory effort on arrival at the intensive care unit. Many are extubated within 24 hours postoperatively. Respiratory failure is rare except in those patients with multiorgan failure, sepsis, and/or intracranial hemorrhage. On postoperative days 2 to 3, major fluid shifts may occur, and a pulmonary artery catheter may be required for clinical management. A moderate-to-severe metabolic alkalosis persists for weeks postoperatively. The degree of alkalosis seems to be more severe in the pediatric patient. Systemic arterial hypertension is common in all patients who receive cyclosporin A. Hydralazine, captopril, beta-blocking agents, calcium channel–blocking agents, and sodium nitroprusside are employed to control the hypertension. Intracranial hemorrhage from severe arterial hypertension has occurred in several patients.

SUGGESTED READING

Borland LM, Roule M, Cook DR. Anesthesia for pediatric orthotopic liver transplantation. Anesth Analg 1985; 64:117–124.
Ellis D, Avner ED, Starzl TE. Renal failure in children with hepatic failure undergoing liver transplantation. J Pediatr 1986; 108:393.
Gelman S, Fowler KC, Smith LR. Liver circulation and function during isoflurane and halothane anesthesia. Anesthesiology 1984; 61:726.
Lawless S, Ellis D, Thompson A, et al. Mechanisms of hypertension during and after orthotopic liver transplantation in children. J Pediatr 1989; 115:372–379.
Mallett SV, Kang Y, Freeman JA, et al. Prognostic significance of reperfusion hyperglycemia during liver transplantation. Anesth Analg 1989; 68:182–185.
Shaw BW Jr, Martin DJ, Marquez JM, et al. Venous bypass in clinical liver transplantation. Ann Surg 1984; 200:524.
Starzl TE, Demetris AJ, Van Thiel D. Liver transplantation. N Engl J Med 1989; 321:1014–1022; 1092–1099.

PHEOCHROMOCYTOMA

PETER ROCK, M.D.
ROSE CHRISTOPHERSON, M.D., Ph.D.

Anesthesia for resection of a pheochromocytoma remains one of the most daunting challenges anesthesiologists face. Patients with pheochromocytoma require appropriate preoperative evaluation and therapy in order to minimize perioperative complications. Unrecognized, this condition can pose serious risk of cardio-

vascular or neurologic complications during or after a surgical procedure. The anesthesiologist plays a major role in the perioperative management of patients with this disorder.

PATHOPHYSIOLOGY AND DIAGNOSIS

Pheochromocytoma is a catecholamine-secreting tumor of the adrenal medulla that occurs in one to two individuals per 100,000. Although pheochromocytoma must be considered in patients with hypertension, this entity accounts for only 0.1 percent of such patients. The majority of such tumors secrete both epinephrine and norepinephrine, although the norepinephrine/ epinephrine ratio is higher than normal. Usually a solitary tumor arising in the right adrenal, 10 percent such tumors may be bilateral in adults and 25 percent may be bilateral in children. Familial cases of pheochromocytoma are often bilateral in presentation. The germ cell origin of this tumor parallels that of the adrenal gland, which is chromaffin tissue. Thus, extra-adrenal sites of pheochromocytoma are found in as many as 10 percent of patients; these are usually in the abdomen but may occur in the neck, chest, or bladder. In patients with this disease it is imperative to ensure that both adrenals have been studied to ascertain that the condition is not bilateral. It is also important to exclude extra-adrenal sites of involvement before surgery.

Pheochromocytoma also occurs in association with other endocrine diseases. Multiple endocrine neoplasia includes pheochromocytoma in association with medullary thyroid carcinoma, parathyroid hyperplasia, and oral mucosa neuromas. Pheochromocytoma may also be associated with von Recklinghausen's neurofibromatosis and von Hippel-Lindau disease. The importance of the familial association of pheochromocytoma with other disorders is that these should be looked for in any patient suspected of having pheochromocytoma.

The secretion of catecholamines is responsible for the characteristic signs and symptoms of this disease. Most pheochromocytomas are recognized in either early to mid-adulthood. Hypertension is a hallmark of pheochromocytoma which may either be sustained or paroxysmal in nature. A small number of patients (10 percent) with pheochromocytoma are normotensive. Paroxysmal elevations in blood pressure may occur spontaneously or in association with physical stress on the tumor (e.g., palpation of the abdomen). The diagnosis of pheochromocytoma should be sought in the following patients: (1) those with sustained or difficult-to-treat hypertension; (2) hypertensive children; (3) those in whom there is an association between glucose intolerance and hypertension; and (4) those with a familial history of pheochromocytoma or the multiple endocrine neoplasm syndrome. An unexplained episode of severe hypertension during anesthesia and surgery should also prompt investigation for pheochromocytoma.

Other manifestations of pheochromocytoma also relate to excess catecholamine secretion. Patients may complain of diaphoresis, palpitations, and headache. Chronic hypertension leads to intravascular volume contraction, and these patients will frequently have orthostatic hypotension.

The diagnosis of pheochromocytoma requires measurement of elevated catecholamines, either in plasma or by urinary metabolites. Progress in plasma assays of catecholamines has now achieved sufficient accuracy to allow the diagnosis to be made in this fashion. The finding of normal blood catecholamine levels does not exclude pheochromocytoma, however, since there may be intermittent catecholamine secretion. Thus, urinary metanephrine and vanillylmandelic acid (VMA) are used as indicators of daily catecholamine secretion.

There are other tests that involve provocation of catecholamine release by histamine, but this entails an element of risk and is not usually required. Clonidine will suppress catecholamine release of central nervous system (CNS) origin but not that which originates from a tumor.

The tumor may be localized by computed tomography (CT) of the abdomen or magnetic resonance imaging (MRI). Selective venous catheterization may be necessary for catecholamine determination. Usually, arteriography is avoided because an intravenous contrast agent may precipitate release of catecholamines.

PATIENT PREPARATION

The goal during the preoperative period is to ameliorate the adverse effects that excess catecholamine secretion has on various organ systems. One major goal is to render the patient normotensive and allow restoration of intravascular volume. There are a variety of agents available for this purpose. An underlying rationale behind antihypertensive therapy in this setting is that alpha-blockade must be performed before beta-blockade can be instituted. Failure to use alpha-blockade in the patient adequately may result in unopposed alpha activity (severe hypertension, malignant arrhythmias) if beta-blockade is begun.

Commonly, the patient is started on a regimen of oral phenoxybenzamine as an outpatient, beginning with a dose of 10 to 20 mg twice daily. The dose is increased until the blood pressure is controlled or symptoms such as orthostatic hypotension or tachycardia develop. Guidelines for acceptable control in patients with pheochromocytoma include (1) control of blood pressure to less than 150/90 mm Hg; (2) decrease or elimination of symptoms such as headache or palpitations; and (3) mild orthostatic hypotension. The use of this agent usually results in acceptable control of blood pressure. Tachycardia, a sign of decreased systemic vascular resistance due to this agent, may be deleterious in the patient with coronary artery disease. If blood pressure is not adequately controlled with this agent or if tachycardia must be treated, additional agents may be used. If the patient is adequately alpha-blocked, a beta-receptor blocker such as propranolol may be used. Labetalol, because of its combined alpha- and beta-blocking properties, may also be used. Prazosin, which is a pure alpha$_1$-receptor blocker, may also be used, although with caution because severe hypotension may result. This phenomenon is related to the fact that feedback inhibition of norepinephrine release occurs with alpha$_1$ blockers in contrast to combined alpha$_1$ and alpha$_2$ blockers such as phenoxybenzamine. This also helps explain the tachycardia that is observed with phenoxybenzamine, which does not cause feedback inhibition of norepinephrine release.

Several weeks may be required for the adequate treatment of hypertension and to allow time for restoration of intravascular volume. It is unclear whether alpha- and (if used) beta-blockers should be continued right up until the time of surgery. The use of long-acting agents may complicate postoperative management because hypotension may result once the excess secretion of catecholamines stops. Our practice is either not to give the morning dose of the blocking agent or to give a lesser amount. Because of the variety of potent, short-acting agents available for use in the operating room, it is not necessary for patients with pheochromocytoma to continue to take oral medications right up until the time of surgery.

The effects of excess catecholamine secretion may be observed in other organ systems. Both catecholamine cardiomyopathy and myocardial ischemia can occur in patients with pheochromocytoma. The latter may be caused by underlying atherosclerotic disease as well as hypertension and catecholamine-induced increases in myocardial oxygen demand. Patients with pheochromocytoma may have ventricular arrhythmias, which should be looked for and treated, if present. Hypertensive renal disease may also be present and may complicate perioperative management. Glucose intolerance may also occur related to catecholamine excess and may be managed with diet or appropriate hypoglycemic agents. Alpha-methyl-tyrosine inhibits tyrosine hydroxylase and thus decreases catecholamine synthesis. Unfortunately, significant toxicity prevents its routine use.

MONITORING

These patients may be formidable management problems, both in the operating room and later in the intensive care unit. Routine monitoring should include noninvasive blood pressure, pulse oximetry, end-tidal capnography, and use of either a precordial or esophageal stethoscope. Two leads of the electrocardiogram should be monitored for arrhythmias and for electrocardiographic evidence of myocardial ischemia. Because tumor manipulation or other stress may cause release of catecholamines, with consequent rapid and marked increase in both blood pressure and heart rate, intra-arterial catheterization is essential. It also permits periodic determination of oxygen tension, electrolytes, and glucose.

Central venous pressure monitoring is also desirable since it allows administration of vasoactive substances and measurement of right atrial pressure. In a child or extremely healthy adult, this may be sufficient. It is our experience, however, that a pulmonary artery catheter (PAC) is desirable in most cases of pheochromocytoma. It aids with fluid management in a patient who may not have been adequately intravascularly repleted before surgery. Pheochromocytoma surgery involves a laparotomy and attendant third-space fluid loss. The PAC permits more precise fluid administration in this situation. Most importantly, the marked and often dramatic increases in blood pressure and heart rate, frequently requiring the administration of large amounts of potent vasodilators and/or beta-blockers, make determination of hemodynamic parameters essential to appropriate

anesthetic management. Finally, the postoperative period can be complicated by hypotension that may be caused by hypovolemia, inadequate catecholamine secretion in the event of a bilateral adrenalectomy, or the residual effects of vasoactive substances administered during surgery. The PAC can help determine the etiology of the hypotension.

Finally, the PAC is essential in those cases where preoperative control of blood pressure has not been achieved. In this situation, measurements from the PAC will guide vasodilators, beta-blockade, and fluid therapy.

CARDIOVASCULAR DRUGS

A variety of vasoactive drugs have been used in surgery for pheochromocytoma, and nearly every vasodilator has its proponents. Our experience is that patients with pheochromocytoma may be managed intraoperatively with a relatively few drugs. Originally, phentolamine was used, since it is a specific alpha-blocker. However, sodium nitroprusside (SNP) has many advantages over phentolamine. It is easy to titrate the doses of SNP, as it has a rapid onset and short half-life, and it is extremely potent. Also, most anesthesiologists are familiar with its use in contrast to phentolamine, which may be used only during pheochromocytoma surgery. Another reasonable approach is to use the two drugs in combination. After placement of the PAC and determination of hemodynamic parameters, phentolamine is infused, if appropriate, to produce a slight degree of peripheral vasodilation. Then, without producing marked alpha-blockade, SNP may be used for further fine control, working against a background of mild alpha-blockade. There may be the occasional patient in whom other agents may be required, such as the ganglionic blocker trimethaphan camsylate.

Beta-blockade is frequently required, particularly when tumor manipulation produces profound increases in heart rate. This can be accomplished safely with the help of the PAC, which can allow the anesthesiologist to determine if alpha-blockade or SNP-related vasodilation is present. Once satisfied that the patient will not develop hypertension with beta-blockade, this can be performed with any of the available beta-blockers. Our preference is to use propranolol, titrated to the desired effect. In a fashion analogous to that of vasodilators, beta-blockade may be accomplished in two phases. During the first phase, propranolol is titrated until some reduction in heart rate occurs. During the second phase, esmolol, with its rapid onset and short half-life, can be used to produce further changes in heart rate. The advantage of using this method is that although the tachycardia seen in association with tumor manipulation may be life threatening in its magnitude, it is brief in duration. The use of sufficient amounts of propranolol to blunt such tachycardia may have effects lasting for hours. Labetalol has also been used with good effect in the intraoperative management of these patients, since it has both alpha- and beta-blocking effects.

Other agents that may be useful include phenylephrine and norepinephrine. Once the tumor is removed, there may be hypotension related to low levels of catecholamines. Hypovolemia must be excluded, but once this has been done, hypotension may be treated with either phenylephrine, an alpha-agonist, or norepinephrine. Usually, these agents will be needed for a brief period, if at all.

ANESTHETIC MANAGEMENT

Many techniques can be safely used to anesthetize a patient with a pheochromocytoma provided that certain principles are adhered to. These include the following: (1) the patient should be relatively deeply anesthetized so that nonsurgical stimulation, such as that provided by laryngoscopy and an endotracheal tube, does not lead to marked catecholamine secretion by the tumor; and (2) the use of agents known to release catecholamines or stimulate sympathetic ganglia should be avoided. Thus, regional anesthesia using epidural agents in combination with general anesthesia have been described. General anesthesia using enflurane or isoflurane alone or with narcotic supplementation has also been successfully employed. Because halothane may sensitize the myocardium to the effects of catecholamines, this agent is generally avoided.

Premedication may be used depending on the patient's overall medical and psychological condition. Since morphine may cause histamine release, which is a potent stimulant to catecholamine release, its use should be avoided, especially since other appropriate agents are available. Vagolytic or sympathomimetic drugs should be used with caution as they may exacerbate tachycardia caused by catecholamine release or cause catecholamine release directly. However, as with morphine, once the anesthesiologist is in the position to evaluate the hemodynamic parameters, and in the presence of SNP and beta-blockade, these agents may be used albeit with caution. Other agents that may potentially result in catecholamine release include droperidol, metoclopramide, ephedrine, and the tricyclic antidepressants. Although some authors recommend that intravascular catheters be placed after anesthesia is induced and the patient is deeply anesthetized, in our experience, these catheters may be placed successfully in conscious patients with the judicious and appropriate use of sedation and local anesthesia. The hemodynamic parameters obtained before the patient is anesthetized may be of help in later management.

Our induction technique includes a moderate dose of fentanyl (approximately 15 to 20 μg per kilogram IV) and small doses of thiamylal (approximately 2 mg per kilogram IV) to produce amnesia. Etomidate is thought to be safe for use in this condition. Once the airway is secured, muscle relaxation may be achieved through the administration of pancuronium bromide or vecuronium bromide. An inhalational agent may be used to deepen the anesthetic state. Prior to intubation, intravenous lidocaine (1 to 2 mg per kilogram IV) should be used to attenuate further the hemodynamic response to laryngoscopy and intubation. Because manipulation of the tumor may result in significant turbulence in blood pressure and heart rate, agents with rapid onset and offset are desirable. It is for this reason that we favor the use of moderate doses of narcotics as described above, low concentrations of volatile agents to provide amnesia, and SNP and esmolol to control perturbations in heart rate and blood pressure.

At the end of surgery, the patient may be extubated, assuming that the usual criteria for extubation have been met. However, it is not uncommon for large amounts of crystalloid to have been administered, and occasionally there may be significant blood loss. The decision to extubate must therefore be based on the condition of the patient, including body temperature and fluid requirements during surgery. It may be necessary to supplement glucocorticoids intravenously if both adrenals are to be removed, using hydrocortisone in a dose of 50 mg IV every 8 hours for the first 24 hours.

As mentioned earlier, the removal of circulating levels of catecholamines combined with the effects of alpha-blockers, SNP, and beta-blockers can result in hypotension after tumor removal. Chronically elevated levels of catecholamines preoperatively may result in insensitivity of the alpha-receptor to normal levels of catecholamines. The use of the PAC allows determination of appropriate therapy, including the use of vasopressors and/or fluid administration. The tendency in this situation is to attribute hypotension to the removal of catecholamines. It cannot be overemphasized that hemorrhage must be excluded. Because pheochromocytoma surgery involves manipulation and dissection of the inferior vena cava, unrecognized bleeding may occur.

SUGGESTED READING

Braude BM, Leiman BC, Moyes DG. Etomidate infusion for resection of pheochromocytoma. S Afr Med J 1986; 69:60–62.

Bravo EL, Gifford RW. Pheochromocytoma: diagnosis, localization, and management. N Engl J Med 1984; 311:1298–1303.

Goldfien A. Disorders of the adrenal medulla. In: Stein J, ed. Internal medicine. Boston: Little, Brown and Co., 1990:2208.

Hull CJ. Pheochromocytoma. Br J Anaesth 1986; 58:1453–1468.

Nicholas E, Deutschman CS, Allo M, Rock P. Use of esmolol in the intraoperative management of pheochromocytoma. Anesth Analg 1988; 67:1114–1117.

Van Heerden JA, Sheps SG, Hamberger B, et al. Pheochromocytoma: current status and changing trends. Surgery 1982; 91:367–373.

Roisen MF, Hunt TK, Beaupre PN, et al. The effect of alpha-adrenergic blockade on cardiac performance and tissue oxygen delivery during excision of pheochromocytoma. Surgery 1983; 94:941–945.

ANESTHESIA IN GENITOURINARY SURGERY

TRANSURETHRAL PROSTATECTOMY

ALAN W. GROGONO, M.D. (Lond), F.F.A.R.C.S.

Urologic surgery, both perineal and transurethral, antedated the introduction of anesthesia. Approximately 2,000 years ago, a midline incision in the perineum was employed for vesical calculi, and during the first century A.D., a semielliptical perineal incision was used to perform partial prostatectomy. Apart from the use of catheterization to relieve urinary retention, however, transurethral surgery was not developed until the 16th century, when Ambrose Pare developed the curette and hollow sound to relieve urethral stricture.

The fundamental discoveries and inventions that were to permit modern transurethral surgery were all made before 1900. Thanks to Morton and others, general anesthesia was introduced clinically in 1846; Bottini described his galvanocautery incision in 1877; Edison invented the incandescent lamp in 1879; Bousseau du Rocher made the first attempt to introduce an optical system into the cystoscope in 1885; and Hertz produced the very high–frequency oscillating current in 1888. The modern cystoscope was refined during the 1920s, and despite vicious controversy, the use of transurethral prostatectomy spread rapidly during the 1930s. General surgeons, comfortable with the open approach to the prostate, were quite understandably reluctant to concede the superiority of a procedure that was difficult to learn, that was performed seated, solo, out of the view of others and, to add to the indignity, that incurred the risk of partial flooding. The diminished stress for the patient and the reduced short-term mortality were sufficient to persuade the doubtful, however, and transurethral resection became the routine approach for most prostatic surgery. A recent review by Mebust et al reports a mortality rate of 0.23 percent, with the majority of the deaths being attributed to sepsis and occurring with multisystem disease more than 30 days postoperatively. Most of the deaths occurred in carcinoma patients.

PATIENT CHARACTERISTICS

Although transurethral surgery is performed on patients of all ages, surgery on the prostate is confined almost entirely to older men.

Enlargement of or tumor of the prostate commonly causes urinary obstruction that may lead to urinary tract infection and potentially, renal damage. Instrumentation of an infected prostate gland should be expected to cause bacteremia. Before the routine use of antibiotics, gram-negative sepsis was a significant risk and this possibility should be kept in mind today as one of the possible causes of pyrexia, rigors, and shock.

Because of the patient's advanced age, various other diseases are commonly encountered. Cardiovascular disease, including myocardial infarction and heart failure, require careful evaluation as well as optimization of the patient's therapy. Although postponement of the surgery might be warranted from a cardiac standpoint, a protracted delay is rarely practical for these patients. The benefits of waiting because of a recent myocardial infarction may have to be weighed against the advantages of prompt surgical intervention. The patient with valvular disease of the heart is at risk for endocarditis and warrants treatment with prophylactic antibiotic therapy because of the incidence of bacteria as discussed earlier.

Respiratory disease is also frequently encountered in these patients and may warrant specific preoperative therapy. For example, the patient with chronic bronchitis or bronchiectasis may benefit from 2 to 3 days of preoperative therapy with bronchodilators, pulmonary physiotherapy, and, if indicated, antibiotics.

Other diseases of the older age group, such as diabetes mellitus, arthritis, and vascular insufficiency, also require appropriate evaluation and optimization before, during, and after surgical intervention.

SURGICAL PROCEDURE

The nature of the surgery itself imposes constraints, stresses, and requirements, some of which are nonspecific, and some of which are peculiar to this type of surgery.

Lithotomy Position. The lithotomy position is required for a period of about 1 hour. This position autoinfuses approximately 500 ml of blood from the legs. In the obese patient, this position diminishes the functional residual capacity, the inspiratory capacity, and the vital capacity. Airway closure may occur, particularly in the elderly. The position may also exacerbate symptoms of backache or arthritis, and it tends to increase the risk of damage from pressure or electrical burn caused by contact with metal parts of the table or stirrup assembly. Also, it may increase the risk of pulmonary aspiration because the position delays placing the patient in a lateral decubitus position if he regurgitates during the procedure.

Continuous Irrigation of the Urethra. Continuous irrigation of the urethra required to maintain visibility causes several problems. Blood loss caused by transurethral resection is usually not measured because the blood is carried away with the effluent irrigating fluid. The fluid is commonly cooler than the body, and the cooling effect of the irrigation may therefore lower the patient's body temperature. Finally, and perhaps most critically, the irrigating fluid may enter the veins of the area being resected and, depending on the type of fluid, may cause hemodilution, hemolysis, dilutional hyponatremia, elevated central venous pressure, dyspnea, changes in the electrocardiogram, water intoxication, visual disturbances, coma, and cardiac arrest. Various irrigating fluids have been employed. These include distilled water (which causes hemolysis), saline solutions (which are too conductive electrically), and various organic solutions, including urea, sorbitol, mannitol, and glycine, a nonessential amino acid that is metabolized to ammonia. Although glycine is probably the most commonly employed irrigating solution, it is not without risk and has been blamed for causing symptoms such as blurred vision, transient blindness, and pupillary dilation. In a diabetic, sorbitol is probably best avoided as an irrigant solution. This is because sorbitol is converted to fructose, which introduces an error into the estimation of blood sugar levels. However, the blood glucose oxidate test is specific for glucose and could therefore be used to assess a diabetic in such circumstances.

Obturator Nerve Stimulation. This occasionally occurs during transurethral resection. However, this is uncommon when the surgery is confined to the prostate and the cautery pad is grounded adequately. When it occurs, the violent spasms of the adductor muscles may prevent further surgery in the area until they are prevented (see later).

Cystoscopy Tables. Some cystoscopy tables limit access to the patient and may make it difficult to position him for certain procedures. In addition, in some cystoscopy suites, the space and anesthetic facilities are limited.

Preoperative Anesthetic Assessment

In addition to the routine requirements, the preoperative anesthetic evaluation of the patient requires that one pay attention to the above mentioned factors. Commonly recommended preoperative studies include complete blood count, chest radiography, electrocardiography, and the measurement of fasting blood glucose and serum creatinine levels. Other testing is predicated on the patient's condition. If there is any question as to the patient's ability to tolerate the lithotomy position, it should be tried at the time of the preanesthetic assessment.

Premedication

The routine preoperative use of sedative or parasympatholytic drugs are not indicated in these patients. Older patients are often familiar with hospital routines or have acquired a stoicism that will not be improved by impairing their mental faculties; moreover, requirements for analgesia and anesthesia appear to be reduced with increased age. Pain caused by transurethral surgery is more moderate than that following some other procedures. Risks such as respiratory depression accompany the use of opioid analgesics in the elderly, and the discomfort of a dry mouth caused by the administration of atropine preoperatively is not balanced by any commensurate benefit. As in other patients, the choice of preoperative sedation should be based principally on the anesthesiologist's preoperative information and counseling with the patient.

Any medications that the patient is receiving, such as cardiac drugs, antihypertensives, antiasthmatics, and steroids, should generally be continued uninterrupted. The period of surgery and anesthesia is not the time to withhold necessary therapy. The exceptions to this general rule are the anticoagulants, monoamine oxidase inhibitors, and aspirin and other nonsteroidal anti-inflammatory drugs; significant adverse drug interactions between this latter group of drugs and drugs employed during anesthesia have been described. Ideally, nonsteroidal anti-inflammatory drugs should be withheld for approximately 2 weeks before the intended surgery.

Positioning the Patient

Appropriate positioning is important for the patient undergoing cystoscopy. The lithotomy position tends to eliminate the normal lumbar lordosis. For this reason, some authorities recommend that the patient have a small pillow or roll of sheeting placed under the back to maintain the normal curvature. Because of the lack of sensation and muscle tone while the patient is under the influence of anesthesia, the extremities may be forced into an inappropriate position or may be subjected to pressure against the stirrups or other objects. The legs should be positioned without force and be adequately protected against injury caused by pressure.

Because electrocautery is employed, the usual precautions are required to ensure that the patient is appropriately grounded and not touching any metal parts of the table, arm boards, or infusion poles.

ANESTHETIC MANAGEMENT

Regardless of the anesthetic technique employed, the patient should have at least one intravenous cannula. Its bore should be large enough for use during resuscitation (e.g., at least 18 gauge or larger). Because significant fluid uptake is anticipated, fluid administration should be minimized.

Although general anesthesia can be satisfactorily employed, there are various advantages to spinal and epidural anesthesia. In particular, it is possible to discuss with the patient his sensations and feelings while he or she is under this form of anesthesia. This facilitates the assessment and prompt management of potential disasters such as water intoxication, fluid overload, heart failure, and bladder perforation during the critical period of maximum risk. In addition, problems with the airway intraoperatively are usually avoided; the bladder is relaxed and easily filled with minimal hydrostatic pressure; blood loss is reduced; and the patient is comfortable during the initial postoperative period.

Despite the advantages of having the patient conscious during the procedure, there are many contraindications to spinal and epidural anesthesia. These include a coagulopathy (which would, of course, also be a contraindication to the surgery), the wishes of the patient, localized infection in the area of the intended injection, and previous injury or disease affecting the back or lower limbs.

During spinal or epidural anesthesia, abductor spasms caused by simulation of the obturator nerve may be controlled by relocating the grounding pad or by the infiltration of a local anesthetic around the obturator nerve in the obturator canal. If the patient is under general anesthesia, neuromuscular blockade may be required.

Spinal Anesthesia

Spinal anesthesia is the quickest and most reliable way of providing conduction anesthesia for transurethral resection of the prostate. It is predictable and requires a relatively low dose of local anesthetic solution. Postspinal headache is less common in the age group of these patients, and the use of a small, 25- or 26-gauge needle further decreases its incidence.

The level of anesthesia should reach T-10 to permit distention of the bladder without discomfort. This is not particularly high, and it is therefore appropriate to perform the block with the patient seated. This position is usually more comfortable for the elderly patient on a hard cystoscopy table. It also facilitates the identification of the midline and enhances the patient's efforts to flex his or her spine.

Various drugs may be satisfactorily employed to produce spinal anesthesia (Table 1). Unless dextrose is included in the ampule, a solution of 10 percent dextrose is added to make them hyperbaric.

The use of spinal anesthesia has several potential disadvantages. Stress from the surgery itself may be reduced, but the patient may be subject to other stresses

Table 1 Examples of Drugs Used to Produce Spinal Anesthesia for Transurethral Resection of the Prostate

Local Anesthetic Drugs without Epinephrine	Dose (mg)	Concentration (%)	Duration (minutes)
Bupivacaine	15–20	0.75	75–150
Lidocaine	80–100	5.00	45–60
Tetracaine	8–10	1.00	120–180

instead. Rapid onset of sympathetic blockade may cause hypotension, which can cause nausea, vomiting, and other complications. Although the hypotension may respond adequately to the intravenous infusion of electrolyte solution, it will occasionally require therapy with a vasopressor such as ephedrine (5 to 10 mg as required). Some patients dislike undergoing surgery while conscious and may benefit from sedation; therefore a benzodiazepine such as diazepam (2 to 10 mg intravenously), midazolam (0.5 to 3 mg intravenously), or, particularly in the aged, diphenhydramine (20 to 50 mg intravenously) may be employed. Two disadvantages are peculiar to and inherent in spinal anesthesia. One is that when the single-injection technique customarily employed is used, it is not possible to alter the duration of the anesthesia once the agent and dose have been selected. Fortunately, urologists commonly limit the duration of the procedure to 1 hour because of the risk of fluid overload or intoxication with water or glycine. The other disadvantage is that there is, as mentioned earlier, an incidence of spinal headache. Nevertheless, transurethral resection remains one of the procedures in which spinal anesthesia is most widely and appropriately employed.

Epidural Anesthesia

Although epidural anesthesia shares many of the features, advantages, and disadvantages of spinal anesthesia, it has some distinctive characteristics. The remarks made earlier about placing the patient in the sitting position for the procedure are even more applicable here; placing the epidural tray on the table against the seated patient creates a large sterile work area, which minimizes the risk of contaminating the catheter. It is advisable to allow the patient to remain seated for few minutes after the initial injection. This facilitates the spread of solution down toward the sacral roots. A selection of suitable agents for epidural anesthesia, with suggested dosage ranges and durations of action, is shown in Table 2.

The principle advantages of epidural anesthesia are that headache following lumbar puncture is almost entirely eliminated and that, by inserting a catheter, supplementary doses may be administered to prolong the duration of the anesthetic. The principle disadvantages are that significantly higher doses are being injected into a vascular area, with the attendant risks of toxicity. The dose required for elderly patients is variable since less volume escapes through the intervertebral

Table 2 Examples of Drugs Used to Produce Epidural Anesthesia for Transurethral Resection of the Prostate

Local Anesthetic Drugs without Epinephrine	Dose (mg)	Concentration (mg)	Duration (minutes)
Bupivacaine	40–225	0.5–0.75	180–360
Chloroprocaine	400–900	2.0–3.0	30–90
Lidocaine	150–500	1.0–2.0	60–180

foramina. In addition, a slower onset and a higher incidence of failure are associated with the technique. It is employed less often than spinal anesthesia for transurethral resection, probably because the procedure is reasonably predictable in duration and because it is usually feasible and appropriate to induce general anesthesia if a spinal anesthetic wears off.

General Anesthesia

Despite the reasons for considering conduction anesthesia, general anesthesia is still widely employed for transurethral resection of the prostate. Convenience, familiarity, rapidity, medical or legal contraindications to conduction anesthesia, and patient preference are undoubtedly the explanation. In addition, with some of the more severe complications such as water intoxication or heart failure, the presence of an endotracheal tube makes it possible to provide intermittent positive pressure ventilation and positive end-expiratory pressure promptly.

The type of general anesthesia selected varies widely. It is influenced by many factors, including past anesthetic history, concomitant disease, bodily habitus, age, physical strength, and the access available for the anesthesiologist to intubate the patient in an emergency. The healthier, stronger, younger patient who is not overweight can be managed using spontaneous ventilation and a face mask. If regurgitation occurs, however, it is not practical to turn the patient, because the legs are constrained by the stirrups. The risk of pulmonary aspiration is therefore somewhat higher. This, together with the ill health commonly encountered in these patients and the fact that they are usually older, explains the prevalence of endotracheal intubation when general anesthesia is employed. The actual anesthetics, neuromuscular blocking agents, and other adjuvant drugs selected are rarely significant and commonly reflect the preference of the anesthesiologist.

Monitoring During Anesthesia

The patient should be appropriately monitored whether under general or conduction anesthesia. Pulse oximetry is now standard practice and, with it, the electrocardiographic findings, blood pressure, pulse rate, and body temperature should be monitored. When general anesthesia is employed, the precordial or esophageal stethoscope should be used as well. Because of the risk of water intoxication, there should be facilities for the rapid determination of serum sodium level, osmolarity, hemoglobin level, and free hemoglobin level. Although attempts have been made to limit the hemorrhage associated with the prostatectomy by administering epsilon-aminocaproic acid; recent controlled studies (e.g., by Smith et al) have not substantiated that this provides any valid advantage.

Treatment of Water Intoxication

Severe hyponatremia is treated by infusing hypertonic saline. In a study by Ayus et al, a reduction in mortality was associated with rapid correction (2 mmol per liter per hour) when compared with slow correction (0.6 mmol per liter per hour). However, the definition of "rapid" may need to be modified in the light of a more recent report by Worthley and Thomas in which excellent results were obtained using 29.2 percent saline and mannitol to obtain a correction averaging 7.4 mmol per L in 10 minutes.

Therefore, in addition to the usual drugs, supplies, and equipment found in any safe anesthetizing location, there should be specific provision for treating the untoward effects of hemodilution, hyponatremia, and water intoxication. Mannitol 1 to 1.5 g per kilogram may be used to treat cerebral edema. Hypertonic sodium chloride 5 percent should be available to treat hyponatremia; when required, 100 to 300 ml should be administered cautiously, as needed. Although sodium bicarbonate 8.4 percent may also be employed to provide sodium, it causes an unneeded metabolic alkalosis. The effects of fluid overload may necessitate the use of furosemide or a raised pressure in the airway. Because hemodilution lowers the level of ionized calcium, hypotension may respond to the intravenous administration of calcium chloride.

SUGGESTED READING

Ayus JC, Krothapalli RK, Arieff AI. Changing concepts in treatment of severe symptomatic hyponatremia. Am J Med 1985; 78:897–902.

Butt AD, Wright IG, Elk RJ. Hypo-osmolar intravascular volume overload during anesthesia for transurethral prostatectomy. S Afr Med J 1985; 67:1059–1061.

Mebust WK, Holtgrew HL, Cockett ATK, Peters PC, and committee. Transurethral prostatectomy: immediate and postoperative complications. A cooperative study of 13 participating institutions evaluating 3885 patients. J Urol 1989; 141:243–247.

Mei-li J, Wong KC, Creel DR, et al. Effects of glycine on hemodynamic responses and visual-evoked potentials in the dog. Anesth Analg 1985; 64:1071–1077.

Restall CJ, Faust RJ. Anesthesia for transurethral surgery. In: Greene LF, Segura JW, eds. Transurethral surgery. Philadelphia: WB Saunders, 1979.

Smith RB, Riach P, Kaufmann JJ. Epsilon-aminocaproic acid and the control of post-prostatectomy bleeding: a prospective double-blind study. J Urol 1984; 131:1093–1095.

Steinmetz PR, Balko C. The sorbitol pathway and the complications of diabetes: Seminars in Medicine of the Beth Israel Hospital, Boston. Engl J Med 1973; 288:831–836.

Stjernstrom H, Henneberg S, Eklund A, et al. Thermal balance during transurethral resection of the prostate. Acta Anaesthesiol Scand 1985; 29:743–749.

Worthley LIG, Thomas PD. Treatment of hyponatremic seizures with intravenous 29.2 saline. Br Med J 1986; 292:168–170.

RENAL TRANSPLANTATION

DONNA LYNN DARK-MEZICK, M.D.
JOHN N. MILLER, M.B., B.S.

Renal transplantation is an accepted and viable treatment for end-stage renal disease. The kidney was the earliest internal organ transplanted, with the first human allografts performed during the 1930s and 1940s. Almost four decades have passed since the first transplantation was performed between identical twins. Only recently, however, has immunosuppression dramatically improved the results of nonrelated cadaveric donor transplants. The introduction of cyclosporine has improved long-term survival such that cadaveric donor transplants are almost as successful as those from living-related donors.

In the early days of renal transplantation, anesthetic administration was challenging because the patients were not dialyzed and because their chronic renal failure was severe and was associated with other diseases and sequelae. Effective dialysis techniques, first peritoneal dialysis, and later, hemodialysis, allowed patients to survive long enough to be considered for transplantation. These patients still present challenges due to the effects of uremia on multiple organ systems, but because of better preoperative preparation, we can focus more closely on anesthetic techniques more favorable for the transplanted kidney.

PREOPERATIVE EVALUATION

Because renal failure impacts on every organ system in the body, special attention must be paid to anemia, cardiovascular disorders, metabolic disturbance, and concurrent drug therapy.

Anemia is universal and develops as serum creatinine exceeds 3 mg per deciliter. Decreased erythropoietin production occurs with the loss of renal parenchyma. Bone marrow suppression, hemolysis, lessened iron absorption, deficiencies in folic acid, vitamin B_6 and B_{12}, and secondary hyperparathyroidism all contribute to anemia. Moreover, excessive fluid retention commonly reduces the hematocrit to 20 to 25 percent. Many centers prefer a hematocrit of 24 to 25 percent before transplantation to provide some reserve oxygen-carrying capacity. During the early years of transplant procedures, preoperative blood transfusion was contraindicated because of concern about sensitizing the recipient to donor antigens. Recent data, however, seem to indicate that pretransplant transfusion has a beneficial effect. Nevertheless, transfusion does carry the risk of circulatory overload. Anemia causes an increase in the serum level of 2,3-diphosphoglycerate in end-stage renal disease, but not to the same extent as in nonrenal anemia. These patients have increased cardiac output and a change in oxygen-hemoglobin affinity to boost tissue oxygenation.

Platelet dysfunction is a problem in end-stage renal disease that can be treated with dialysis.

Most patients with end-stage renal disease are hypertensive, with many taking potent antihypertensive drugs. Approximately 10 to 15 percent have refractory hypertension. Left ventricular hypertrophy and congestive heart failure are associated problems. These result from hypertension, anemia, hypervolemia, atherosclerosis, pericarditis, and negative inotropy from acidosis and hyperkalemia. Dialysis fistulae may also have high flow rates which contribute to high output cardiac failure. Uremic pericarditis may occur but can be treated with dialysis; but pericarditis continuing in the face of dialysis is unresponsive and leads to the development of cardiac tamponade.

The circulating blood volume of the pretransplant patient is variable, depending on the time of last dialysis. Indeed, the patient may be hypovolemic if recently dialyzed, or hypervolemic before dialysis, or normovolemic. Most patients who are to undergo elective renal transplantation are dialyzed the day before surgery.

The patient's serum potassium level is critical and should be measured just before the operation. Although the postdialysis serum potassium level is low (approximately 3.5 mEq per liter), this rapidly increases. If the serum potassium level is 5.5 mEq per liter or greater, succinylcholine chloride should be avoided. Succinylcholine chloride administered during rapid-sequence induction may increase the serum potassium level by 0.5 to 1 mEq per liter. The serum potassium level frequently increases during surgery, especially when the surgery is prolonged and associated with significant tissue trauma. Vascular clamp release allows reperfusion of ischemic and acidotic tissues high in potassium. Also, with initial arterial perfusion of the transplanted kidney, potassium from the storage solution may be washed into the systemic circulation.

Gastrointestinal symptoms are often the earliest manifestations of uremia. They include anorexia, nausea, vomiting, diarrhea or constipation, and hiccups. Gastric emptying is delayed, and duodenitis, gastritis, and gastrointestinal bleeding are common. Many of these symptoms can be alleviated by dialysis or by decreasing protein intake.

These patients are at high risk for hepatitis B infection. Many patients receiving dialysis are chronic carriers of hepatitis B surface antigen, and preoperative testing should be done.

Uremia is associated with various psychiatric and neurologic abnormalities. Patients may be irritable, depressed, or anxious. Overt psychoses may occur. Dialysis may improve these initially, but frequent episodes of depression often follow. Uremic encephalopathy with subtle changes in neurologic function may occur despite adequate dialysis. Uremic peripheral neuropathy occurs, as do abnormalities in autonomic nervous system function. As in diabetes, autonomic neuropathy in uremia may prevent the normal sympathetic response to hypotension.

Secondary hyperparathyroidism occurs in end-stage renal disease. Serum phosphate increases as a a function of renal failure. As phosphate increases, serum calcium decreases and parathyroid hormone (PTH) secretion increases. PTH liberates calcium from bone, thereby contributing to osteoporosis. Metastatic calcification occurs in various parts of the body, including the skin, eyes, and arteries. Vitamin D deficiency results in osteomalacia. Because of the various bone diseases associated with end-stage renal disease, transplant recipients should be positioned on the operating table carefully and have pressure points well padded.

End-stage renal disease is associated with alterations in pharmacokinetic and pharmacodynamic variables. The renal excretion of drugs and their metabolites are decreased, changes in protein binding occur, and the bioavailability of the active agent is altered. Generally, the loading dose of a drug remains the same, but subsequent doses must be decreased or have an increased dosing interval. If a drug is greater than 90 percent protein bound, changes in protein binding are important. There is decreased protein binding in end-stage renal disease due to a relative hypoalbuminemia so that free fraction of drug increases. Patients with end-stage renal disease often take numerous medications. Insulin regimens may require alteration. Digitalis therapy must be carefully regulated and signs of toxicity sought. Antihypertensive medication is normally continued until the time of surgery.

Preoperatively, the recipient's immune system is suppressed with either azathioprine or cyclosporine. Azathioprine is given orally if the transplant is from a living related donor and orally or intravenously just before cadaver transplantation. Cyclosporine, given orally diluted in milk or juice, is the agent preferred by many for cadaver transplants. Gastric retention of either of these agents presents a serious risk of aspiration during general anesthetic induction; however, the intravenous preparation of cyclosporine takes several hours to administer and could prolong the storage of the cadaver kidney beyond its viable limit. Corticosteroids are usually administered intraoperatively before vascular clamp release.

Although preoperative medication must be tailored to the individual patient, the anesthesiologist should be aware that patients often have unexpected sensitivity to central nervous system depressants. Delayed gastric emptying and increased gastric volumes should also be considered, particularly with respect to the induction of general anesthesia. Metoclopramide and ranitidine or cimetidine may be given as part of the preoperative regimen.

MONITORING

Recommended monitoring includes measurements of oxygen saturation end-tidal carbon dioxide, intermit-

tent arterial blood pressure, and body temperature, and the use of precordial stethoscope, electrocardiography, inspired oxygen analysis, and neuromuscular blockade. Continuous electrocardiographic monitoring aids in the diagnosis of hyperkalemia. Noninvasive blood pressure monitoring is generally preferred, as the cannulation of a peripheral artery may prohibit its subsequent use for dialysis access. Central venous pressure monitoring is routine. Pulmonary artery catheterization in these immunosuppressed patients is not routine because it is associated with higher infection rates and tissue friability.

The patients usually have an arteriovenous fistula for dialysis access, which should be monitored and protected throughout surgery. The blood pressure cuff should not go on the arm with the fistula, and no intravenous lines should be placed in that arm. Sterile technique should be used for placement of all lines, since susceptibility to infection is increased by uremia, immunosuppression, and steroids. The presence or absence of a bruit can be recorded on the anesthesia record. If hypotension occurs, the arteriovenous fistula may be threatened by thrombosis.

ANESTHETIC TECHNIQUE

Patients awaiting renal transplantation may be called to surgery on short notice. Therefore, rapid sequence induction is recommended. Pretreatment with metoclopramide and ranitidine or cimetidine is recommended. Drugs that blunt the cardiovascular response to intubation, such as narcotics and beta-blockers, may be given, but the hemodynamic response will likely be exaggerated. Thiopental has been recommended as the induction agent of choice in most renal transplant patients, with no change in induction dose required. Although the unbound fraction of thiopental is increased in end-stage renal disease, volume of distribution and clearance are increased, and the half-life is therefore unchanged. However, etomidate may be the preferred induction agent in patients with cardiac disease.

Narcotics should be used as necessary in renal transplant patients. When doses are increased, morphine and meperidine tend to accumulate, as does fentanyl. Sufentanil appears to be an acceptable opioid in renal failure. Sear found renal failure to have no effect on sufentanil binding and no difference between groups in either free drug clearance or free drug apparent volume of distribution. In patients undergoing renal transplantation, Fyman et al also reported pharmacokinetics similar to those found in healthy patients.

Inhalational agents are most commonly used for maintenance of general anesthesia. All inhalational anesthetics decrease glomerular filtration rate and water and electrolyte excretion in a dose-related fashion. Halothane was used extensively in the past, as were enflurane and fluroxene. However, when metabolized, enflurane produces free fluoride that is associated with nephrotoxicity. Isoflurane now predominates, since only 0.1 percent is metabolized and cardiac depression is less than with halothane and enflurane.

Nitrous oxide is not specifically contraindicated, but its use is declining, as it is associated with nausea and vomiting, always a problem with these patients. Besides, in therapeutic concentrations of nitrous oxide, oxygen delivery is restricted and pneumothorax from a misplaced central venous catheter is dramatically exacerbated.

Neuromuscular blockers are likely to undergo altered responses in patients with end-stage renal disease. Although succinylcholine chloride provides rapid intubating conditions, in renal failure, pseudocholinesterase levels are reduced and serum potassium may increase by 0.5 to 1.0 mEq per liter. Often, this may be of little clinical importance; however, in the recently dialyzed patient, serum potassium may not reflect intracellular levels and the use of succinylcholine may produce ventricular fibrillation. Moreover, succinylcholine chloride has also been associated with a variety of other cardiac dysrhythmias.

Although pancuronium and d-tubocurarine have frequently been used successfully in renal transplantation, reports of prolonged neuromuscular blockade have lessened their use. Vecuronium bromide has a short half-life (1 hour) and a rapid rate of clearance. Only 10 to 25 percent of this agent is excreted in urine. Cumulative effects are seen with repeated small doses, but with neuromuscular blockade monitoring, these effects should be reversible. Furthermore, vecuronium bromide offers a stable hemodynamic profile as well. Atracurium besylate is also a competitive nondepolarizing neuromuscular blocker. It undergoes Hoffman elimination and ether hydrolysis and is therefore unaffected by hepatorenal function. No apparent cumulative effect occurs after administration of multiple doses of atracurium besylate. High doses of atracurium are known to cause histamine release that may be detrimental to patients with coronary artery disease. We would recommend the use of either vecuronium bromide or atracurium besylate in renal transplantation, with atracurium besylate perhaps having the advantage because it does not accumulate. Neuromuscular blockade may be successfully reversed with the usual doses of neostigmine, edrophonium, and pyridostigmine bromide.

Spinal and epidural anesthesia have both been used successfully for renal transplantation. They represent attractive alternatives because intubation and the attendant risk of aspiration may be avoided, and anesthetic agents that induce hyperkalemia need not be chosen. Moreover, immediately after the operation, the patient is awake and comfortable, and spinal narcotics can be administered effectively. However, the duration of action of local anesthetic agents in end-stage renal disease is decreased because of the hyperdynamic circulatory state, and more frequent dosing is required. Epinephrine should also be avoided in a hyperdynamic circulatory state. Nevertheless, in a patient who is emotionally labile, these advantages must be balanced against a possible prolonged surgical procedure.

Reasonable intraoperative fluid management is of paramount importance, since transplanted kidneys function better when optimally hydrated. A central venous pressure (CVP) of 10 cm H_2O, and a systolic blood pressure of 120 mm Hg usually assures adequate hydration. Before release of the vascular clamps, the CVP should be increased to 15 to 17 cm H_2O, and systolic pressure should be raised to 130 mm Hg or the pulmonary artery pressure to 20 mm Hg or greater. The object here is to provide an increased perfusion pressure initially for the ischemic, cold, transplanted kidney. Dopamine may be used, especially in low doses, but other vasopressors should be avoided because of the risk of splanchnic vasoconstriction. Normal or half-normal saline is preferred, since Ringer's lactate solution contains additional potassium. Diabetic patients are given a glucose-containing solution, as indicated. Blood should be replaced, generally as packed red cells, with the goal being a hematocrit of 24 to 25 percent. Seldom are more than 2 U of packed cells needed.

Hemodynamic and pharmacologic status should be optimized before release of the vascular clamps. Furosemide and mannitol are given before the renal vascular clamps are released, and they are said to decrease the oxygen demand of the kidney. Furosemide decreases glomerular filtration rate and protects areas of the kidneys vulnerable to mild ischemic insults. Mannitol increases plasma volume, filling pressures, and cardiac output; it also decreases systemic vascular resistance and, specifically, is a renal vasodilator.

Hyperkalemia may occur at the time of vascular clamp release of the newly transplanted kidney with reperfusion of ischemic, acidotic tissue and washout of potassium from the cold storage solution. Spiking of the T wave on the electrocardiogram may be noted. If hyperkalemia is severe, cardiac conduction slows, accompanied by a flattened P wave leading to atrial asystole, a widening QRS complex with intraventricular block, and finally, cardiac standstill.

The hyperkalemic patient under general anesthesia should be hyperventilated with 100 percent oxygen and given sodium bicarbonate (50 to 100 mEq). Increasing the pH redistributes potassium from the serum into the cells. On the other hand, in the event of hypernatremia, bicarbonate dosage should be decreased.

Intravenous regular insulin (10 to 20 U) administered with 25 ml dextrose 50 percent shifts potassium intracellularly as well. Calcium is a physiologic antagonist of the cardiotoxic effects of potassium, and 1 g should be given intravenously. This therapy does not remove potassium from the body but is useful until cation-exchange resins and dialysis can be employed postoperatively.

After unclamping, hypertension may occur secondary to renin release from the reperfused kidney. The CVP may then decrease, and fluid replacement is usually required. Urine output volumes should be replaced, one to one, to help ensure continued renal perfusion.

Postoperatively, close monitoring of gas exchange and cardiovascular status is essential. The newly transplanted kidney may fail to function, leading to anuria and pulmonary edema. Respiratory depression caused by the residual effects of narcotics and neuromuscular blockers may also occur. Technical problems such as ureteral obstruction or renal arterial stenosis, although not common, may require early repeat surgical intervention. Protecting the patient from infection is quite important.

SURGICAL TECHNIQUE

In an adult, the kidney is transplanted into the iliac fossa. The entire procedure is extraperitoneal, allowing less complex vascular anastomoses and ureteral implantation. The right iliac fossa is preferred since the right iliac vein is more superficial. The renal vein is anastomosed to the side of the external iliac vein, and the renal artery is anastomosed to the end of the hypogastric artery or to the side of the external iliac artery. The ureter is implanted directly into the bladder via a neoureterocystotomy after the vascular clamps are released.

POSTOPERATIVE COMPLICATIONS

Postoperatively, these patients should be monitored in an intensive care setting usually for at least 24 hours. Although the list of possible complications is long, sudden death, myocardial infarction, and serious dysrhythmias remain the most serious. Acute tubular necrosis occurs to some degree in nearly all cadaveric transplants, and dialysis may be required. The incidence is much less in living-related donor transplants. Hypertension should be vigorously controlled and hypotension avoided.

Sodium nitroprusside is given for hypertensive crises during the immediate postoperative period. Since cyanide is liberated during the degradation process, biotransformed to thiocyanate, and excreted in the urine, there is concern if the kidney fails to function. However, data seem to indicate that no change or reduction in sodium nitroprusside dose is required, although signs of cyanide toxicity should be sought. These are metabolic acidosis, tachyphylaxis, and increasing oxygen tension in mixed venous blood. If these occur, nitroprusside is easily dialyzed.

Patients who undergo renal transplant require immunosuppressant agents that present a host of possible problems. Cyclosporine interacts with drugs that increase liver microsomal metabolism (e.g., phenytoin and phenobarbital), and levels may decrease. Antibiotics such as erythromycin, ketoconazole, and possibly rifampin inhibit liver microsomal enzymes and increase the half-life and toxicity of cyclosporine. Dose- and time-related nephrotoxicity occurs with cyclosporine and is difficult to distinguish from acute tubular necrosis or rejection. Other problems include transient hepatotoxicity and nausea and vomiting. Steroids delay wound healing and increase the risk of infection, but they may also increase insulin requirements in diabetics and cause gastrointestinal ulceration.

Despite immunosuppression, rejection of the transplanted kidney may begin within hours, and it may be irreversible and require transplant nephrectomy.

Surgical complications may necessitate another surgical procedure during the early postoperative period. Ureteral obstruction certainly occurs, but at this time only rarely. Vascular complications occur in as many as 12 percent of transplants, the most common being renal artery stenosis. Worsening diastolic hypertension without other signs of rejection is characteristic, and bruit may be present.

POSTOPERATIVE CARE

Good data comparing various postoperative pain control modalities in patients undergoing renal transplant do not exist, but postoperative pain does not seem to be great, and most patients ambulate readily.

The use of narcotics may be desirable, but narcotics may accumulate if the grafted kidney does not function. Spinal narcotics offer an alternative to the large doses of narcotics that may be required intravenously or intramuscularly. Although epidural catheters allow continued dosing, they should be removed postoperatively because of risk of infection.

Patients with end-stage renal disease remain an anesthetic challenge. However, with careful preoperative preparation, vigilant intraoperative monitoring, reasonable drug selection, and strict postoperative care, these patients can do well. Expected survival now may be 10 or more years, with patients leading active, productive lives.

SUGGESTED READING

Fyman PN, Reynolds JR, Moser F, et al. Pharmacokinetics of sufentanil in patients undergoing renal transplantation. Can J Anaesth 1988; 35:312–315.
Graybar GB, Tarpey M. Kidney transplantation. In: Gelman S, ed. Anesthesia and organ transplantation. Philadelphia: WB Saunders, 1987.
Linke CL. Anesthesia considerations for renal transplantation. In: Brown BR, ed. Anesthesia and transplantation surgery. Philadelphia: FA Davis, 1987.
Moore PJ, ed. Kidney transplantation: principles and practice. 3rd ed. Philadelphia: WB Saunders, 1988.
Sear JW. Sufentanil disposition in patients undergoing renal transplantation: influence of choice of kinetic model. Br J Anaesth 1989; 63:60–67.
Strunin L, Davies JM, Filshie JJ. Anesthesia for renal transplantation. Int Anesthesiol 1984; 22:189–202.

MAJOR GENITOURINARY PROCEDURES

JUDITH L. STIFF, M.D.

Unlike many other major procedures, a major genitourinary procedure in and of itself does not have major anesthetic-related consequences. However, many of these procedures entail the use of physiologically significant patient positioning; are lengthy, with large fluid requirements; and may cause patients to become hypothermic. All of these situations should be managed as in any other major operative procedure. With any of these procedures, there is the potential for sudden and/or persistent blood loss. The anesthesiologist has to decide beforehand how much blood loss can be tolerated by the patient, because transfusion of homologous blood is not without risk. Additionally, there is some evidence that the survival time of patients with solid tumors, including those of the genitourinary tract, may be decreased if the patient received homologous blood during the perioperative period. Many patients who are to undergo major genitourinary operations are candidates for donating autologous blood and should be encouraged to do so.

Often these procedures are performed in older patients, who have the pre-existing conditions prevalent in that population. The anesthesiologist should therefore consider patient factors—how a particular patient will be affected by compromise induced by the operative position, the duration of the procedure, and the fluid shifts and replacement involved.

KIDNEY PROCEDURES

Before a patient undergoes a procedure that may result in the loss of a kidney, pre-existing renal function should be defined. If significant renal compromise will result, care must be taken with the use of drugs, both those dependent on renal excretion and those that could cause further renal damage. Many procedures, such as renal vascular operations and procedures for stone removal, may require a period of renal ischemia. The anesthesiologist needs to be prepared for this by optimizing renal blood flow, and many favor the administration of mannitol before the clamping of the renal artery. Because of the proximity of the large blood vessels to the kidney, sudden major blood loss is always a risk. Occasionally a radical nephrectomy includes extraction of tumor thrombus from the inferior vena cava. The patient needs to be adequately volume expanded to avoid hypotension with caval clamping. Kidney operations are almost always done with the patient under general anesthesia because an awake patient is very uncomfortable in the usual lateral "kidney position." However, a combined epidural-general anesthetic can be used; this has the advantage of the availability of the catheter for postoperative narcotics, provided that there will be adequate monitoring of the patient for late respiratory depression.

Placing the patient into "kidney position" is potentially very physiologically compromising. Not only is the patient moved from the supine to lateral decubitus position, soon after that shift, the table is flexed and the kidney rest is raised. In addition to causing the shifts in blood volume, these maneuvers may cause impedance to venous return to the heart, either by kinking of the vena cava when the patient is on the right side or by stretching and thinning of the vena cava if the left side is down. Placing the kidney rest at the iliac crest, rather than more cephalad, minimizes the problems. Any position change can lead to hemodynamic instability due to shifts in intravascular volumes in the face of vasodilatation with either regional or general anesthesia and the blunting of normal homeostatic mechanisms. Position change in the anesthetized patient should be undertaken slowly, with blood pressure checked frequently so that the positioning may be stopped or reversed if significant hypotension develops. Patients with cardiac disease, particularly where there is a relatively fixed cardiac output, and patients who are hypovolemic are most susceptible to the hypotension caused by position change. Usually, slow position change and some extra fluids prevent decreases in blood pressure, but occasionally pressors are needed, and rarely, an "extreme" position (e.g., having the kidney rest fully elevated) cannot be safely achieved.

Nerve damage caused by pressure on the brachial plexus in the lateral position should be prevented by the placement of an axillary roll slightly caudad to the axilla to allow the vessels and nerves to be free from pressure. It is inadvisable to secure the "up" arm to the ether screen, as this may easily involve pressure to vulnerable points or stretching of the brachial plexus. Pillows or pads between the arms will allow adequate positioning. In this position, the most vulnerable point of the lower extremities is on the "down" leg, where the common peroneal nerve comes laterally around the head of the fibula. This should be checked for the necessity of extra padding, for pressure here can result in foot drop and sensory deficit along the lateral aspect of the leg.

Once this position has been achieved safely, there are additional considerations. The "down" lung, because of the impaired descent of the diaphragm, can become atelectatic at the base, and although this is not a problem during the procedure because the patient's ventilation will be controlled, it may lead to respiratory problems postoperatively. Also, the pleura may be entered on the side of the operation, and, if the air is not sufficiently evacuated at the end or a chest tube is not placed, the patient is left with another potential for respiratory difficulty after a seemingly straightforward operation.

OPEN OR RADICAL PROSTATECTOMY, RADICAL CYSTECTOMY WITH URINARY DIVERSION

Some patients undergoing prostatectomy may have presented with urinary obstruction. Although this will have been resolved by a urinary catheter before the operation, some degree of renal failure and electrolyte imbalance may remain. The vascularity of the prostatic bed and the bladder makes significant blood loss a possibility. In these operations, the anesthesiologist is unable to monitor fluid status by urinary output. Therefore, hemodynamic monitoring of volume status by a central venous pessure catheter or pulmonary artery catheter is needed. These operations can be performed with the patient under continuous spinal or epidural anesthesia. Regional anesthesia may help reduce blood loss because of the relative hypotension included. Some patients receiving regional anesthesia may require the addition of light general anesthesia because of the duration of the procedure and the position.

Although the patient is supine for transabdominal approaches to the bladder or prostate, usually ante-flexion and Trendelenburg positioning is also used to aid in surgical exposure. Placing the patient in the Trendelenburg position in addition to any other position can cause aberrations in physiology that are proportional to the degree of the head-down tilt. It can mask uncompensated blood loss and lead to hypotension when the patient resumes a level position. If adequate ventilation is not maintained in this position, the weight of the abdominal contents will lead to hypoventilation and atelectasis. The head-down tilt can cause venous distention of the upper body, which can lead to facial edema if this position is maintained for long periods of time. If there is significant edema of the tongue, extubation may need to be postponed until the swelling resolves. More importantly, with the head-down tilt, the increased venous pressure leads to decreased intracranial perfusion pressure. This is not a problem as long as other factors that can decrease pressure are not present, such as previously increased intracranial pressure or an inadequately maintained arterial blood pressure. In theory, having the pelvis higher than the heart could lead to air entrainment through open veins and resulting air embolus; however, this does not seem to occur.

Perineal prostatectomy requires that the patient be put in extreme lithotomy position, with the legs flexed on the abdomen. This can cause respiratory embarrassment. In all of these unusual positions, the adequacy of ventilation should be monitored. An end-tidal carbon dioxide monitor for general anesthesia and a pulse oximeter for either regional or general anesthesia are helpful. Blood gases should be checked in patients receiving general or regional anesthesia if there is any question of problems with ventilation and oxygenation. In a patient with pre-existing pulmonary disease in which blood gases need to be checked frequently intraoperatively and postoperatively, an arterial line can be placed.

Radical cystectomy also entails a urinary diversion, most commonly an ileal loop. Thus the procedure is additionally lengthened and fluid requirements are increased as in any major bowel procedure. Some patients undergo cystectomy following chemotherapy. The specific drug regimen should be determined, in order to look for possible complications of chemotherapy. In particular, doxorubicin (Adriamycin), which is often part of the protocol, can cause toxic effects on the heart. If a patient shows any signs of myocardial compromise or early congestive heart failure, he or she will need further cardiac evaluation.

URINARY DIVERSION REOPERATION

While an initial urinary diversion operation is quite straightforwrad, the long-term consequences of such a procedure are of concern when the patient comes for reoperation. A revision may be proposed because of a mechanical problem. However, rediversion may be necessary because of metabolic problems, the most common being hyperchloremic acidosis. Electrolyte imbalances are worse in patients with overlying renal compromise and worse in patients who have a jejunal conduit.

RETROPERITONEAL LYMPH NODE DISSECTION

Patients who undergo retroperitoneal lymph node dissection, too, may have undergone chemotherapy for the testicular tumor before the operation. Knowing the drug regimen is important because it may have included bleomycin, which can cause pulmonary fibrosis. Any dyspnea needs further evaluation. This is especially important because of the large incision, often thoracoabdominal, which adds to respiratory compromise during the postoperative period. Because the operation is close to the large blood vessels, sudden bleeding must be considered a risk. Fortunately, almost all of these patients are young and recover well from this operation.

POSTOPERATIVE CONSIDERATIONS

The proper postoperative management of patients who have undergone major genitourinary procedures is important. Hematocrit and possibly electrolytes should be checked postoperatively. Any patient undergoing such a major procedure should remain in the recovery room for a sufficient length of time to ensure that vital signs are stable and that there are no signs of bleeding. The sympathetic block from regional anesthesia should be resolved, so that one can be sure the patient has tolerated the intraoperative fluids without overload.

All of the patients will have a reduction in their vital capacity and one second forced expiratory volume. Those having undergone transabdominal operation may have a reduction of up to two-thirds of their vital capacity. Thus, any patient with pre-existing pulmonary disease is at risk for respiratory complications in proportion to the degree of preoperative pulmonary impairment. A postoperative overnight stay in a monitored unit should be considered for patients with pulmonary disease, and when the pre-existing compromise is significant, elective ventilatory support may be necessary. As in many long procedures, these patients get cold. Rewarming is demanding on the heart, and leaving a patient with cardiac disease anesthetized and with ventilatory support to wake up slowly after rewarming has occurred may be wise.

Fortunately, with meticulous attention to intraoperative and postoperative care, the mortality rate associated with these major genitourinary procedures is low.

SUGGESTED READING

Lieber MM, Utz DC. Open bladder surgery. In: Walsh PC, Gittes RE, Perlmutter AD, Stamey TA, eds. Campbell's urology. 5th ed. Philadelpha: WB Saunders, 1986:2639.

Smith RB. Complications of renal surgery. In: Smith RB, Ehrlich RM, eds. Complications of urologic surgery: prevention and management. Philadelphia: WB Saunders, 1990:128.

Stiff JL. Respiratory complication and complications of anesthesia. In: Marshall FF, ed. Urologic complications: medical and surgical, adult and pediatric. St. Louis: Mosby–Year Book, 1990:116.

Walsh PC. Radical retropubic prostatectomy. In: Walsh PC, Gittes RE, Perlmutter AD, Stamey TA, eds. Campbell's urology. 5th ed. Philadelphia: WB Saunders, 1986:2754.

Welborn SG. Anesthesiology consideration: urology. In: Martin JT, ed. Positioning in anesthesia and surgery. Philadelphia: WB Saunders, 1978:170.

ANESTHESIA IN OBSTETRICS

SURGERY IN THE PREGNANT PATIENT

RHONDA L. ZUCKERMAN, M.D.

In the United States, each year there are approximately 50,000 anesthetics administered to pregnant women having surgery other than delivery. The most common procedures include cervical suture placement, appendectomy, ovarian cystectomy, breast biopsy, and trauma-related procedures. The goal during anesthetic care of these patients is to ensure both maternal and fetal safety and well-being. To provide optimal anesthetic care for the pregnant patient, one must consider the implications of the physiologic changes of pregnancy during the preoperative, intraoperative, and postoperative management of the patient. Since the physiology changes dynamically during pregnancy, the patient's period of gestation should be kept in mind when one is estimating the extent of expected physiologic changes. The principles of fetal physiology must also be understood, including the teratogenic potential of anesthetic agents. Taking all of these factors into account, the anesthesiologist must tailor the anesthetic to meet the different needs of the pregnant patient.

ESTABLISHING THE DIAGNOSIS OF PREGNANCY

Since pregnancy, even very early pregnancy, has implications with regard to both the anesthetic and often the surgical care of a patient, it is important that this diagnosis be made preoperatively. Certainly all women who undergo menses should be questioned about the possibility of being pregnant preoperatively. Specifically, they should be asked when their last menstrual period occurred and whether or not they have been sexually active since that time. Physical examination can also be helpful in diagnosing pregnancy in some cases. After the first trimester, the pregnant uterus can usually be palpated above the pelvis. In addition, fetal heart tones can be detected using Doppler techniques after approx-

imately 12 weeks' gestation. Laboratory testing to diagnose pregnancy involves either urine or blood analysis for the presence of beta-human chorionic gonadotropin (beta-hCG). The serum beta-hCG radio-immunoassay is used to detect suspected early pregnancy since in some laboratories it may be accurate as early as 4 days after conception.

Although no universal policy exists, in many surgical centers, all female patients of childbearing age must have a documented negative beta-hCG prior to an elective procedure. A prudent policy would include obtaining a careful history and measuring serum beta-hCG if the date of the suspected pregnancy would be within detectable range for the hospital laboratory.

If the diagnosis of pregnancy has been established or if pregnancy is suspected but might be too early to detect, a decision must be made regarding the timing of surgery. For reasons discussed later in this chapter, elective surgery that must be done prior to delivery is usually postponed until the second trimester or, if possible, until the period of fetal viability (with the exception of elective cervical suture placementa procedure done during early pregnancy to treat cervical incompetence). Once the decision has been made to proceed with surgery during pregnancy, optimal care of the patient involves consideration of the maternal physiologic changes of pregnancy and fetal physiology.

PHYSIOLOGIC CHANGES OF PREGNANCY

Respiratory Changes

Changes in the respiratory system begin early in pregnancy and clearly affect anesthetic management. The capillaries of the airway become engorged and swollen secondary to hormonal influence. As a result, the airway is more fragile and manipulation, especially of the nasal airway, can easily result in trauma and bleeding. Therefore, during pregnancy, neither nasal airway placement nor suctioning are recommended. Oral intubations are comparatively less traumatic, but even for this procedure, smaller-than-average endotracheal tubes should be used to minimize the risk of bleeding. In addition to upper airway capillary engorgement, the pulmonary vasculature becomes engorged during pregnancy. In fact, chest x-ray images during pregnancy may resemble pulmonary edema.

Other important respiratory changes include lung volumes and capacities. Although often assumed to decrease markedly concomitant with the increasing size of the uterus, the total lung capacity of the parturient is at most only 5 percent lower than that of nonpregnant individuals. There are, however, significant changes in other lung volumes and capacities, as illustrated in Figure 1. The tidal volume is increased by 40 percent. The increase in tidal volume occurs partially at the expense of the functional residual capacity (FRC), which decreases by 20 percent by term.

Since the FRC can be thought of as the patient's "oxygen tank" if an emergency occurs, this physiologic change has profound implications in anesthesia, especially if the anesthetic technique used involves transient cessation of maternal respirations. A combination of decreased oxygen supply in the FRC and the increased oxygen demands of pregnancy result in the presence of little reserve, with oxygen desaturation occurring readily during apnea. Therefore, supplying supplemental oxygen and protecting and maintaining the airway and ventilation are especially important principles in these patients. Another implication of the decreased FRC in pregnancy is that the FRC can approach the closing volume, especially when these patients are supine. The

potential resultant airway closure can further decrease maternal oxygenation reserve. The time course of ventilatory changes is shown in Figure 2. The 20 percent increase in oxygen consumption that occurs by term is accompanied by an increase in alveolar ventilation of 70 percent. The respiratory rate increases by 15 percent.

During pregnancy, arterial blood gases change due to the increase in maternal alveolar ventilation. These changes occur after the first trimester and reflect hyperventilation and the resulting hypocapnia. By term, arterial carbon dioxide pressure ($PaCO_2$) decreases to 28 to 32 mm Hg. Since the respiratory quotient does not change during pregnancy, but alveolar carbon dioxide pressure ($PACO_2$) decreases, arterial oxygen pressure (PaO_2) increases to 100 to 105 mm Hg. Because of metabolic compensation (a decrease in serum bicarbonate), the normal arterial pH remains 7.4 during pregnancy. These arterial blood gas values should be kept in mind during interpretation of blood gases of parturients, and when mechanical ventilation parameters are being set for a pregnant patient (e.g., a $PaCO_2$ of 40 mm Hg should not be considered normal).

Cardiovascular Changes

The changes in cardiac output that occur as pregnancy progresses are illustrated in Figure 3. Specific

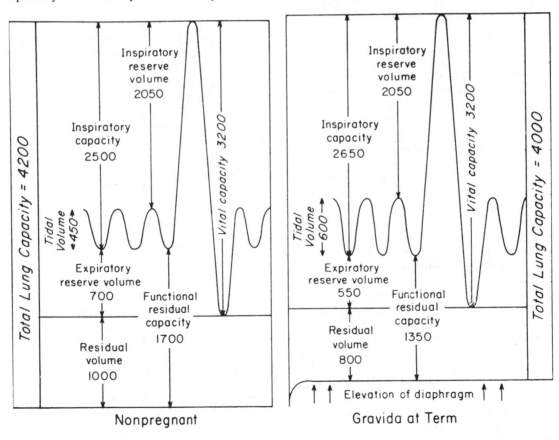

Figure 1 Lung volumes and capacities in the nonpregnant subject and the gravida at term. (Republished with permission from Bonica JJ. Principles and practice of obstetric analgesia and anesthesia. FA Davis, Philadelphia, 1967.)

hemodynamic changes during pregnancy include an increase in cardiac output and blood volume, both of which begin to increase early in pregnancy and continue to rise until delivery. By term, cardiac output is increased by 50 percent. Although the increased cardiac output is due predominantly to an increase in stroke volume, there is also a slight increase in heart rate. The systemic vascular resistance is decreased by approximately 15 percent and the central venous pressure is unchanged during pregnancy. The blood volume is increased by 40 percent overall, with a 50 percent increase in plasma volume and a 30 percent increase in red blood cell volume by the end of pregnancy. The peak blood volume occurs at about 8 months of pregnancy but is already significantly elevated from normal levels by the midpoint of gestation. Patients who have cardiovascular compromise often begin to have difficulties when the blood volume begins to peak during the late second trimester. This may be manifest as worsening exercise tolerance, orthopnea, or frank dyspnea.

The discrepancy between the percent increase in plasma volume and the percent increase in red blood cell volume leads to a normal decrease in hematocrit over the course of pregnancy, often referred to as the "physiologic anemia of pregnancy." Pre-existing anemia exacerbated by pregnancy will result in a greater burden on the cardiopulmonary system to meet the increased energy requirements of pregnancy.

Perhaps the most important cardiovascular physiologic change of pregnancy is aortocaval compression. By approximately 20 weeks' gestation, the uterus has grown to a sufficient size to begin to compress the great vessels when the patient is supine. This compression occurs between the uterus and the spine. The vena cava is more easily compressed than the aorta since it is a thin-walled vessel. An uncompensated decrease in venous return resulting from vena caval compression can profoundly decrease maternal cardiac output and blood pressure.

Usually vena caval compression has no harmful effect on the mother, since baroreceptor reflexes result in adequate vasoconstriction and tachycardia to offset the hypotensive effects of the decrease in venous return. Patients who are able to compensate often have a normal blood pressure and slight tachycardia when they are supine. However, approximately 2 to 10 percent of parturients are unable to reflexly compensate for the decreased venous return that occurs, and develop symptoms when supine that are consistent with the supine hypotensive syndrome. Those symptoms include lightheadedness, nausea and vomiting, sweating, and palpitations. Patients with supine hypotensive syndrome are noted to be hypotensive and bradycardic when supine.

It is important to realize that even if the supine hypotensive syndrome is not present (i.e., the mother is able to maintain her blood pressure while supine), this may be at the expense of intense vasoconstriction of many vascular systems, including those to the uterus. Decreased uterine blood flow and decreased fetal oxygenation may occur.

Another cardiovascular change that occurs during pregnancy is the presence of a systolic heart murmur on physical examination. This is thought to be secondary to the increased flow that occurs during pregnancy. In addition, pregnant patients can have characteristic electrocardiographic changes. The heart is displaced upward and leftward during pregnancy and slight left axis deviation as well as T-wave flattening in lead III are commonly seen.

Central Nervous System Changes

Although it is frequently stated that the minimum alveolar concentration (MAC) to produce anesthesia is decreased during pregnancy, this may vary from species to species. For instance, although a 25 to 40 percent decrease in MAC has been measured in pregnant ewes,

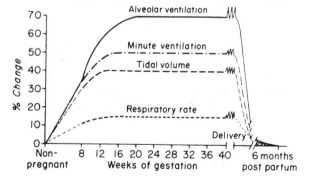

Figure 2 Time course of ventilatory changes during pregnancy. Note that near-maximum hyperventilation occurs as early as the 2nd or 3rd month of gestation. (Republished with permission from Bonica JJ. Obstetric analgesia and anesthesia. 2nd ed, revised. World Federation of Societies of Anesthesiologists, Amsterdam, 1980.)

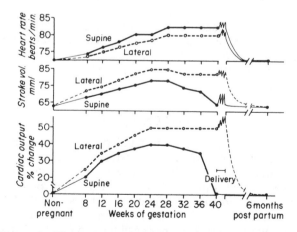

Figure 3 Time course of changes in cardiac output during pregnancy. Changes in heart rate and stroke volume through gestation are shown. Note the difference in values when the pregnant patient is supine compared with when the patient is lateral. (Republished with permission from Bonica JJ. Obstetric analgesia and anesthesia. 2nd ed, revised. World Federation of Societies of Anesthesiologists, Amsterdam, 1980.)

this could not be demonstrated in mice. The reason for this decrease in MAC is unclear. Progesterone and other hormonal influences as well as pregnancy-induced changes in endogenous opioids may be involved.

There is a decrease in spinal and epidural local anesthetic dose requirements during pregnancy. Three possible explanations for this observation exist. Both increased engorgement of epidural veins and increased epidural pressure caused by pregnancy could play a role. These effects would decrease the volume of the non-blood vessel epidural space and the subarachnoid space, respectively. Therefore, a given volume of local anesthetic would theoretically distribute over more levels. A final explanation for the decreased local anesthetic requirement during pregnancy is that a decrease in the minimum blocking concentration (C_m) occurs; that is, there is an increased sensitivity to local anesthetics during pregnancy. This effect has been demonstrated to be present in the median nerves of parturients who underwent nerve conduction studies.

Gastrointestinal Changes

Several changes occur in the gastrointestinal system during pregnancy. Delayed gastric emptying occurs secondary to both hormonal and mechanical effects. Both increases in progesterone and decreases in motilin levels occur, which lead to delayed gastric emptying as well as decreased lower esophageal sphincter tone. The change in the position of the stomach during pregnancy results in displacement of the pylorus and relative incompetence of the gastroesophageal junction (allowing gastric reflux). This can result in delayed gastric emptying. Increased intragastric pressure occurs secondary to obstruction of the gastric outlet by the growing uterus. These effects combined with the increased incidence of hiatal hernia during pregnancy all lead to an increased risk of acid aspiration during loss of airway reflexes. Steps must therefore be taken to avoid acid aspiration in parturients. Gastric chemoprophylaxis should be used preoperatively. Heavy sedation should be avoided since protection of the airway may be compromised, and difficult airways in particular must be well protected.

Renal Changes

There is an increase in renal plasma flow during pregnancy. During the first trimester, the increase is 68 percent, and during the third trimester, 46 percent. The glomerular filtration rate is increased by 50 percent throughout pregnancy. Creatinine clearance is also increased. During pregnancy, the normal BUN and creatinine are 9 ± 1 mg per deciliter and 0.5 ± 0.1 mg per deciliter, respectively (versus 13 ± 3 and 0.7 ± 0.2 mg per deciliter in nonpregnant patients). Therefore, a serum creatinine of 1.0 mg per deciliter during pregnancy is abnormal. Proteinuria up to 250 mg per day and glucosuria up to 150 mg per day is considered normal during pregnancy.

Table 1 Hepatic Changes During Pregnancy

Liver Function Test	Effect	Trimester of Maximum Change
Albumin	Decreased 20%	Second
Cholinesterase	Decreased 28%	Third
	Decreased 33%	3 Days Postpartum
Bilirubin	Normal to slightly increased	Third
Alkaline Phosphatase	2–4 × increased	Third
LDH	Slightly increased	Third
Cholesterol	2 × increased	Third
AST	Normal to slightly increased	Third
ALT	Normal	—

ALT = alanine aminotransferase; AST = aspartate aminotransferase; LDH = lactate dehydrogenase.

Hepatic Changes

Liver blood flow is unchanged during pregnancy. A list of the changes in liver function tests are given in Table 1. The elevations in lactic dehydrogenase (LDH), alkaline phosphatase, and cholesterol are considered normal. The marked increase in alkaline phosphatase is thought to be caused by its placental production.

Serum pseudocholinesterase levels and activity are decreased during pregnancy. However, the clinical effect of this has not been consistently demonstrated. Therefore, alterations in the dosage of succinylcholine chloride during pregnancy are not recommended.

Hematologic Changes

The changes in plasma volume and red blood cell mass with the resultant decrease in hematocrit have been described above. The white blood cell count can normally be elevated by the end of pregnancy.

Major changes in the coagulation system occur during pregnancy. In fact, pregnancy has been described as a hypercoagulable state, since an increase in activity of many of the coagulation factors, including factor I (fibrinogen), occurs. During pregnancy, the normal range for fibrinogen is 400 to 650 mg per deciliter, compared with 200 to 450 mg per deciliter in nonpregnant patients. The hypercoagulable state is also potentiated by a decrease in antithrombin III during pregnancy. The platelet count can decrease during pregnancy, although no change in platelet function should occur.

FETAL PHYSIOLOGY

Fetal Oxygenation

Maintenance of adequate fetal oxygenation depends on two factors: maternal oxygenation and uteroplacental function. Adequate maternal oxygenation, in turn, depends on maternal respiratory function. Since pregnant patients have decreased respiratory reserve due to decreased FRC in the setting of increased oxygen demand, any respiratory dysfunction may have profound effects on both maternal and ultimately fetal oxygenation. Intrinsic pulmonary disease and airway closure due to changes in lung capacities and volumes may contribute to maternal respiratory dysfunction.

Adequate uteroplacental function facilitates sufficient oxygen delivery from oxygen-rich maternal blood to the fetal circulation. Since autoregulation of blood flow has not been observed in the uterine circulation, blood flow on the maternal side is believed to be proportional to uterine perfusion pressure and inversely proportional to uterine vascular resistance. Maintenance of adequate maternal mean arterial pressure is therefore of great importance to fetal oxygenation. Factors that may decrease maternal mean arterial pressure, such as hypovolemia, aortocaval compression, and profound sympathectomy during major regional anesthesia must be anticipated and properly managed to avoid detrimental fetal consequences.

Likewise, increased venous pressure, as can occur with supine positioning, decreases uterine blood flow by decreasing perfusion pressure independent of its effect on arterial pressure or vascular resistance.

Uterine vascular resistance is thought to rely mainly on alpha-adrenergic tone. Exogenous administration of alpha-adrenergic agents can lead to uterine arterial vasoconstriction and decreased uterine blood flow. For similar reasons, increased endogenous alpha-adrenergic output secondary to stress, untreated hypovolemia, or the reflex vasoconstrictive response to aortocaval compression can be detrimental to the fetus.

The fetal side of the placental unit remains vasodilated at all times. In fact, during periods of fetal distress from decreased oxygenation, vasoconstriction occurs in all fetal systems except the brain, heart, adrenals, and placenta.

The adequacy of fetal oxygenation is usually indirectly assessed by continuously monitoring the fetal heart rate using the methods described later in this chapter.

Teratogenesis

Teratogenesis is a major concern only during the first trimester of pregnancy. During the early first trimester, the response to any insult is usually pregnancy loss rather than fetal malformation at birth. Later in the first trimester, during the classic teratogenic period, major organogenesis occurs. This period spans days 31 through 71, with cardiac and CNS development occurring early in the period and ear and palate formation occurring relatively late in the period (Fig. 4). After the first trimester, the teratogenic potential of drugs is absent or greatly diminished, with the exception of their

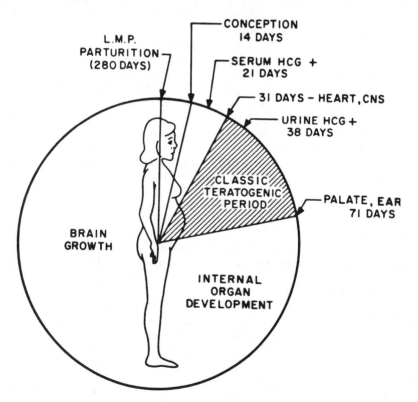

Figure 4 Gestational "clock" illustrating the classic teratogenic period. (Republished with permission from Gabbe SG, Niebyl JR, Simpson JL, eds. Obstetrics: normal and problem pregnancies. New York: Churchill Livingstone, 1986.)

potential on the gametes and perhaps on cerebral myelinization.

ANESTHETIC MANAGEMENT

Preoperative Evaluation

History

Preoperative evaluation of the pregnant patient should be performed with consideration of the above physiologic changes and their influence on perioperative risk.

The pregnant patient should be questioned carefully about acute or chronic respiratory problems. If a patient has a history of respiratory disease, it is important to evaluate the adequacy of their treatment. For example, a patient with a history of asthma should be asked when they were last evaluated for this condition; what medications were prescribed, and whether the medications (if any) are being appropriately taken.

During evaluation of the pregnant patient with a history of cardiovascular disease, the specifics of her problem should be noted and the degree of compensation evaluated. Specifically, a history of dyspnea, orthopnea, or impaired exercise tolerance should be elicited. If gestation is more than 20 weeks, the patient should be questioned about symptoms of supine hypotensive syndrome. When supine, some affected patients may only experience lightheadedness, while others may also have associated nausea and vomiting, sweating, and palpitations.

Since the pregnant patient is at increased risk for acid aspiration during anesthetic induction, NPO status should be verified carefully preoperatively. Although pregnant patients are still at some risk for aspiration if they are kept NPO, it is recommended that they not be anesthetized within 8 hours of ingesting solid food or within 6 hours of ingesting liquids. Symptoms of gastrointestinal reflux such as heartburn and a history of hiatal hernia should be elicited.

Physical Examination

Physical examination should focus first on the airway (regardless of the type of procedure or anesthesia planned). During pregnancy, obesity and enlargement of the breasts may contribute to difficulty with intubation and ventilation. The condition of the teeth, extent of mouth-opening, and mandibular size should be noted; one should also keep in mind that oral rather than nasal intubation is preferable during pregnancy. Any abnormality on pulmonary examination should be noted.

During cardiovascular examination of the pregnant patient, a systolic flow murmur, which is usually of no consequence, is frequently noted. If pregnancy has progressed past 20 weeks, the patient's blood pressure and heart rate should be checked while the patient is in the lateral position, and again while they are supine

to diagnose supine hypotensive syndrome. If the patient is considered at risk for hypovolemia (e.g., if they have undergone trauma and blood loss), orthostatic blood pressure and heart rate determination should be made.

Laboratory Evaluation

Before surgery, laboratory evaluation of the pregnant patient should include a hematocrit. Although the physiologic anemia of pregnancy itself may not be detrimental, coexisting problems such as iron deficiency may result in severe anemia. Since both maternal and fetal oxygenation depend on maternal blood oxygen content, severe anemia can contribute to perioperative oxygenation problems. Other laboratory tests should be done if indicated based on maternal disease and medication use. Results of blood count and liver and renal function tests must be interpreted, with consideration given to normal values during pregnancy. Adequate levels of prescribed medications such as aminophylline and anticonvulsants should be documented preoperatively.

Preoperative Medication

Preoperative medication can be used for the pregnant patient when sedation or analgesia are considered necessary or desirable. During the first trimester, the use of barbiturates and narcotics rather than benzodiazepines and phenothiazines is recommended. The latter have been associated in some studies with teratogenic effects when administered during the first trimester and therefore are best avoided.

Preoperative medication should always include gastric chemoprophylaxis. Antacids, histamine$_2$-blockers, and gastric motility enhancers are recommended for use during pregnancy. If surgery is emergent, antacids alone are usually used since histamine$_2$-blockers and gastric motility inhibitors require a relatively long onset interval to be effective. Nonparticulate antacids, such as sodium citrate, are preferred since particulate antacids may cause pneumonitis if aspirated. The dose of sodium citrate is 15 to 30 ml of 0.3 M solution. The optimal time to administer sodium citrate is immediately before the induction of anesthesia, since in some patients its protective effect may persist only for minutes. If ranitidine is used, the recommended dose is 50 mg IV administered at least 30 minutes before induction or 150 mg orally administered at least 60 minutes before induction. Metoclopramide, 10 mg orally or IV, can be given with ranitidine, with the caveat that this agent has been associated with a prolongation of action of succinylcholine chloride.

Monitoring

Regardless of the anesthetic technique planned, all routine monitors appropriate for use during general or major regional anesthesia should be present. These include electrocardiography, blood pressure measurements, pulse oximetry, oxygen analysis, measurements of end-tidal carbon dioxide, and temperature monitoring. Further monitoring may be needed, depending on the mother's state of health. If maternal illness or features of the operative procedure dictate the use of a pulmonary artery catheter, hemodynamic measurements must be interpreted relative to normal values during pregnancy and must be obtained with left uterine displacement.

Use of additional monitors may be indicated. These include a fetal heart rate monitor and a tocodynamometer, with the latter used to measure uterine contractions. The fetal heart rate monitor is important because it allows indirect assessment of the adequacy of fetal oxygenation. Doppler technology is often used to measure the heart rate. A probe can be placed on the skin, on the uterus itself (if it is exposed during surgery), or intravaginally. It may be necessary to move the probe to follow the heart rate signal as the fetus moves intraoperatively. Intermittent intraoperative fetal heart rate monitoring can also be done using ultrasonographic techniques.

A tocodynamometer can be used alone or in conjunction with a continuous fetal heart rate monitor. Use of the tocodynamometer involves placing a relatively tight belt around the abdomen with a pressure sensor over the uterus that would detect contractions if and when they occur. This is often not practical for use during surgery on the abdomen because the belt may disrupt the surgical field.

The tocodynamometer can be helpful for two reasons. First, periodic changes in fetal heart rate that may be indicative of fetal distress can best be interpreted when the association of heart rate changes to uterine contractions is known. Second, this monitor can detect the onset of preterm labor, which can occur independently of fetal heart rate changes.

When deciding whether to use fetal heart rate monitoring and tocodynamometry, the likelihood of reliable interpretation and intervention should be considered. There are no definite guidelines or requirements for fetal heart rate or uterine activity monitoring during nonobstetric surgery. However, the following practice is often recommended: if the surgery is to be performed before the period of fetal viability, fetal monitoring should include documentation of a fetal heart rate just prior to surgery and again postoperatively in the recovery room. More frequent or continuous monitoring is usually used only when the fetus is viable and acute intervention might be considered in the setting of fetal distress.

During use of continuous fetal heart rate monitoring, consideration should be given to the fact that normal values for fetal heart rate and normal patterns of variability are well described for term or near-term infants only. Interpretation of fetal heart tracings during the early stages of gestation is therefore difficult. Consultation with an obstetrician can help determine whether this monitoring is indicated and how it can best be interpreted perioperatively.

INTRAOPERATIVE MANAGEMENT: ANESTHETIC TECHNIQUE

Fetal Considerations

When one is choosing an anesthetic technique, a major concern is maximizing fetal safety, since the fetal loss rate is known to be greater for pregnant patients who undergo anesthesia and surgery than for parturients who do not. The potential causes of fetal compromise during surgery and anesthesia include decreased oxygen delivery to the placenta (secondary to decreased uterine blood flow and/or decreased maternal blood oxygen content), preterm labor, and teratogenicity.

Placental Oxygen Delivery

Regardless of the specific anesthetic technique chosen, fetal oxygenation can be optimized by providing adequate oxygen to the mother (as assessed by maternal pulse oximetry) and also by achieving left uterine displacement by placing a "wedge" under the parturient's right hip so that uterine blood flow will not be compromised. This latter maneuver is indicated after approximately the 20th week of gestation. The "wedge" can be a specific reusable one or simply a taped roll made of bed sheets.

Intraoperatively, adequate fetal oxygenation depends on some factors specific to particular anesthetic techniques. Patients who receive general anesthesia often require mechanical ventilation that can affect maternal cardiac output and central venous pressure. The decrease in maternal cardiac output and increase in central venous pressure can result in decreased uterine blood flow and poor fetal oxygenation.

During epidural or spinal anesthesia, often accompanied by sympathectomy, the fetus may be at increased risk for decreased oxygenation if severe maternal hypotension with decreased uterine blood flow occurs. Adequate fluid management and optimal positioning to potentiate venous return (i.e., legs elevated) can help prevent severe hypotension. Left uterine displacement is especially important in these patients.

Preterm Labor

The risk of perioperative preterm labor is estimated to be approximately 8 to 11 percent and is believed to be higher when pelvic surgery is involved. The risk may be highest in individuals who undergo cervical suture placement, since by definition these patients have an underlying risk of cervical incompetence. A concern of the anesthesiologist might be whether or not certain anesthetic techniques are associated more often with preterm labor than others. In fact, there is no evidence that either regional or general anesthesia is associated with a higher incidence of perioperative preterm labor.

The effects of specific anesthetic agents on uterine activity have been studied. It is well known that potent inhalational anesthetics are tocolytics. However, this effect is beneficial only when the agent is being administered in the operating room and therefore is not protective during the equally high-risk postoperative period. High-dose ketamine is the only general anesthesia induction agent that increases uterine activity. The local anesthetics commonly used for regional anesthesia have no significant effect on uterine activity. Epinephrine, which is often added to local anesthetics, is a known tocolytic agent.

Perhaps the most basic way in which the anesthesiologist can help prevent preterm labor (regardless of the anesthetic technique used) is to ensure adequate perioperative hydration status for the parturient. Dehydration can lead to decreased uterine perfusion. Prostaglandin release and uterine contractions may occur. Therefore, adequate perioperative fluid management can protect against preterm labor.

If a surgical procedure is planned during the period of fetal viability, intraoperative delivery of the fetus may be necessary in the event of preterm labor or fetal distress. Therefore, it is essential not only that an obstetrician be available, but also that a pediatrician or perhaps a second anesthesiologist be present to resuscitate the neonate. Pediatric resuscitation equipment must be available, including a warmer, airway and oxygenation/ventilation equipment, and appropriate resuscitation drugs and fluids.

Teratogenesis

Several points need to be made regarding the studies on the teratogenic potential of anesthetic drugs. First, there is evidence that chronic exposure to anesthetic agents may lead to increased risk of pregnancy loss in humans. This is of more significance to personnel who work in the operating room on a steady basis than it is to a patient having one acute exposure to anesthetic agents. Second, extrapolation of results of animal studies to humans may be misleading. For example, it is well known that although thalidomide was not found to be teratogenic in rodents, it is teratogenic in humans. And finally, the studies on acute human exposure to anesthetic agents indicate that with the exception of benzodiazepines, which may cause cleft lip during the first trimester, no other specific anesthetic agents have been implicated as having teratogenic potential. Certainly common sense would dictate that drugs that have been used for a long time in pregnant patients should be chosen rather than new or untested agents. Finally, elective surgery should be postponed until after the first trimester to avoid any risk of teratogenesis from either anesthetic agents or other medications that might be required perioperatively.

Maternal Considerations

It is frequently stated that maternal outcome is not influenced strongly by the anesthetic technique used for surgery other than delivery. However, extrapolation of maternal mortality data for anesthesia for cesarean section indicate that general anesthesia may be associated with increased risk because of airway difficulties and pulmonary aspiration. Whether a general anesthetic, regional anesthetic, or local anesthetic with sedation is anticipated, gastric chemoprophylaxis and airway maintenance and protection are the major maternal safety considerations. Increasing maternal gastric pH is an important measure since mortality rates are higher after acid aspiration with its associated severe pulmonary damage than after nonacid aspiration. Regardless of the anesthetic technique to be used, the operating room should be prepared for emergent maternal tracheal intubation and ventilation.

General Anesthesia

If general anesthesia is planned, the patient must either be intubated awake before induction or she must undergo rapid sequence induction. If preoperative assessment had revealed a possibly difficult airway, awake intubation using direct laryngoscopy or fiberoptic oral laryngoscopy should be performed. If rapid sequence induction is the technique chosen, attempts should be made to place the patient in the best possible sniffing position. Prior to induction, adequate preoxygenation and, ideally, denitrogenation should be accomplished, the latter usually requiring approximately 3 minutes of 100 percent oxygen delivery via a tight face mask. This will partially attenuate the rapid oxygen desaturation that occurs following cessation of maternal respirations due to the decrease in FRC and increased oxygen consumption associated with pregnancy. Maintenance of general anesthesia with inhalation agents should be conducted with consideration given to the possible decrease in MAC associated with pregnancy. Extubation should be performed after the patient is breathing adequately, awake, and judged able to protect her own airway.

Regional Anesthesia

Regional anesthesia is often chosen for peripheral surgery on the extremities and for lower abdominal and pelvic procedures. If epidural or spinal anesthesia are the techniques being considered, the former may be preferable, since pregnant patients are at relatively high risk for postlumbar puncture headaches. It should be noted that placement of a caudal rather than a lumbar epidural catheter may expose the patient to the least risk of postdural puncture headache since it is less likely that a wet tap will occur.

For epidural or spinal anesthetics, approximately two-thirds of the volume or mass of drug should be used for pregnant patients compared with what would be given to the same patient if she were not pregnant. With other regional anesthetics, such as upper extremity blocks, decreasing the dose is not as crucial, since adverse effects such as profound hypotension or total subarachnoid block are not likely to occur with these techniques.

Toxic dose ranges for local anesthetics are generally the same in pregnant and nonpregnant patients, with the possible exception of bupivacaine. Because there have been reports of intractable cardiac arrest in pregnant patients who have received presumed therapeutic doses of 0.75 percent bupivacaine, the use of 0.75 percent bupivacaine is not recommended for these patients. Lower concentrations of bupivacaine are frequently used in pregnant patients, with the total milligram dosage kept at less than 3 mg per kilogram.

POSTOPERATIVE MANAGEMENT

The main issues in the postoperative management of the pregnant patient include maternal comfort, documentation of postoperative fetal viability, and perhaps most importantly, detection and treatment of preterm labor.

A potential advantage of epidural anesthesia is that the catheter can be used postoperatively for narcotic infusions with or without patient-controlled analgesia (PCA). If epidural anesthesia is not used, the patient can receive postoperative intravenous narcotic infusions with or without PCA.

Documentation of postoperative fetal viability usually involves identification of the fetal heartbeat using a Doppler technique. If difficulty is encountered with this technique, ultrasonography may be necessary to locate the fetal heart and document fetal heart motion.

Because there is a high risk of preterm labor during the immediate postoperative period, pregnant patients should be carefully monitored in the recovery room for the occurrence of contractions. Depending on the recommendations of an obstetrician, the patient may require admission for an extended period of monitoring with tocodynamometry. Tocolytic agents such as terbutaline may be used to treat detected contractions. Terbutaline is also often used prophylactically in patients thought to be at high risk for preterm labor.

Postoperative management of the pregnant surgical patient should otherwise be identical to that of nonpregnant patients, with the exception that pregnant patients past 20 weeks' gestation should not be allowed to lie supine during recovery, but rather should be kept in left uterine displacement.

SUGGESTED READING

Duncan PG, Pope WDB, Cohen MM, Greer N. Fetal risk of anesthesia and surgery during pregnancy. Anesthesiology 1986; 64:790–794.

Malinow AM, Ostheimer GW. Anesthesia for the high risk parturient. Obstet Gynecol 1987; 69:951–964.

Niebyl JR. Drugs in pregnancy and lactation. In: Gabbe SG, Niebyl JR, Simpson JL, eds. Obstetrics: normal and problem pregnancies. New York: Churchill Livingstone, 1986.

PREGNANCY-INDUCED HYPERTENSION

LAUREN A. PLANTE, M.D.
GERTIE F. MARX, M.D.

The hypertensive disorders of pregnancy complicate 7 to 10 percent of all pregnancies and are the leading cause of both maternal and perinatal morbidity. The American College of Obstetricians and Gynecologists provides the following generally accepted classification of these disorders.

Pre-eclampsia, also called pregnancy-induced hypertension (PIH), is defined as the triad of hypertension, proteinuria, and generalized edema, developing after the 20th week of gestation. In this chapter, the terms *pre-eclampsia* and *PIH* will be used interchangeably. The term "*toxemia of pregnancy*" has fallen into disfavor as there is no evidence of a "toxin."

Hypertension may be defined by any of the following criteria:

1. A sustained increase in systolic pressure of at least 30 mm Hg or in diastolic pressure of at least 15 mm Hg over the gravida's normal values.
2. A sustained systolic pressure of 140 mm Hg or more or a diastolic pressure of 90 mm Hg or more in a previously normotensive gravida.
3. A sustained mean arterial pressure of 105 mm Hg or higher.

Hypertensive changes can be diagnosed by both arm and leg blood pressure measurements (Fig. 1). An increase in diastolic pressure is a more reliable diagnostic and prognostic sign than an increase in systolic pressure.

Proteinuria is defined as the presence of more than 300 mg of protein per liter of urine in a 24-hour collection (or more than 100 mg per liter in a random specimen). Generalized edema is recognizable by swelling of the upper body, hands, and face; dependent edema is common in normal pregnancies.

Eclampsia is the development of a generalized tonic-clonic seizure in a pre-eclamptic woman, provided that other causes of convulsions have been ruled out. Eclamptic seizures may occur before, during, or after labor and delivery—either suddenly or preceded by

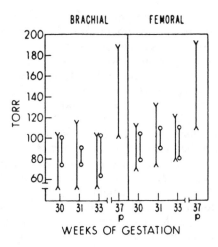

Figure 1 Brachial and femoral arterial pressures of a 17-year-old primigravida during four prenatal clinic visits. Position-related changes in both systolic and diastolic pressures were evident in both upper and lower extremities. In the supine position, consequent to aortocaval compression, systolic pressures declined while diastolic pressures increased. At 37 weeks, the patient developed pre-eclampsia, and measurements of blood pressure in the supine position were omitted.

V = systolic and diastolic values in the left lateral recumbent position; o = systolic and diastolic values in the supine position. (Republished with permission from Marx GF, Husain FJ, Shiau HF. Brachial and femoral blood pressures during the prenatalperiod. Am J Obstet Gynecol 1980; 136:11–13.)

apprehension, excitability, headache, and epigastric pain.

Chronic hypertension is the presence of sustained hypertension (140/90 mm Hg) both before and during pregnancy. Generally speaking, the presence of hypertension before the 20th week of gestation suggests that it antedates the pregnancy.

Superimposed pre-eclampsia is diagnosed when a gravida with chronic hypertension develops proteinuria, edema, or an increase in systolic blood pressure of 30 mm Hg or in diastolic blood pressure of 15 mm Hg.

Transient gestational hypertension refers to the development of hypertension without proteinuria or edema in a previously normotensive gravida whose blood pressure returns to normal within 10 days postpartum.

There is no single diagnostic test for pre-eclampsia, and it can be difficult to differentiate this disorder from chronic hypertension or from underlying renal disease. Although general statements can be made—it is predominantly a disease of first pregnancy and is most common in young teenagers, in gravidae older than 35 years of age, and in women with diabetes, renal disease, or multigravity—exceptions are easily found. Notwithstanding these vagaries, it is clear that there is a pathologic process specific to pregnancy that encompasses the spectrum from mild, asymptomatic elevations of blood pressure to hypertensive crisis, convulsions, and multisystem organ failure.

ETIOLOGY

The etiology of PIH is enigmatic, but two theories are under serious consideration: that of uteroplacental ischemia and that of immunologic injury. There are observations in support of both. The prevalence of the disease in primigravidae can be explained by insufficient development of the uterine vasculature as well as by lack of effective immunization to factors inherent in the pregnant state. Similarly, increased receptor sensitivity to endogenous and exogenous vasoconstrictor drugs or the well-established imbalance between the vasoactive prostaglandins thromboxane and prostacyclin may be a sequela to impaired uteroplacental blood flow rather than a primary event.

Recent observations support the premise of immunologic mechanisms. Histologic examination of products of conception collected from induced first trimester terminations showed, in certain cases, placental and decidual vasculitis (i.e., the pathologic findings typical of PIH), yet these were seen weeks before the onset of clinical signs of the disease. Tracheobronchial washings of 40 parturient women revealed a significantly greater incidence of epithelial multinucleation in the smears of the 12 women suffering from PIH than in those of non–pre-eclamptic women. High degrees of multinucleation occur in other disease states characterized by immune mechanism disturbances. The immunologic disorder may arise from an abnormal maternal-fetal antibody-antigen response or from the contents of seminal fluid; spermatozoa may produce antibody formation or prostaglandins may initiate uterine vasoconstriction. The concept of a sexually related origin has been brought to the forefront by the results of two epidemiologic investigations. A large-scale case-controlled study revealed that women who previously used barrier contraceptives were more than twice as likely as women who used other methods of contraception to develop pre-eclampsia, and that the risk of the disease was greater with fewer episodes of sperm exposure. A study of 72 unselected teenage parturients showed a statistically significant difference in the incidence of PIH between those having sexual activity after conception and those who did not. All 22 gravidae who developed PIH admitted to postconceptual sexual activity; of the 50 women who did not develop the disease, 37 had sexual activity and 13 did not. In addition, there appears to be a higher incidence of PIH in women whose mothers or sisters had the disease. And an analysis of the association between PIH and consanguinity of the gravida and her sexual partner suggested that women who developed PIH were less frequently related to the sexual partner than those with no signs of the disease. Finally, this concept would explain the occurrence of PIH in secundiparae who had a normal first pregnancy from a different sexual partner and might clarify the well-known fact that animals do not develop the disease spontaneously. Sexual receptivity among female animals is rigidly dependent on their hormonal state so that pregnant animals do not accept a male.

SIGNS AND SYMPTOMS

The syndrome of PIH is characterized by diffuse vasospasm, reduced intravascular volume despite edema, and decreased colloid pressure. In more severe forms, there is evidence of widespread endothelial cell damage. The pre-eclamptic woman loses the normal pregnancy-induced refractoriness to vasopressor substances perhaps as early as at 20 weeks' gestation. Long before any clinical signs develop, she may manifest a sensitivity to angiotensin infusion that is as much as three times that of gravidae who will not become pre-eclamptic.

PIH is a protean disease featuring a wide array of symptoms. Visual symptoms include diplopia, scotomata, blurred vision, and even cortical blindness. Other symptoms may refer to the central nervous system with headache, drowsiness, dizziness, or tinnitus, or they may be gastrointestinal, with nausea, vomiting, or pain over the epigastrium or right upper quadrant. Complaints of constant nasal stuffiness or other symptoms of upper respiratory infection may actually reflect mucosal engorgement.

Cardiac output may be normal, decreased, or increased. Increased cardiac output, together with the elevated peripheral resistance and elevated blood viscosity (secondary to the high hematocrit), increases the cardiac demand, which may progress to cardiac failure.

Vasospasm may be seen on retinal examination, particularly segmental vascular narrowing and a reduced arteriolar-to-venous diameter. Hyperreflexia signifies increased central nervous system irritability. Hepatic tenderness, which is believed to represent distention of Glisson's capsule, is especially ominous. Signs of pleural effusion, ascites, or coagulopathy may also be seen in severe forms of the disease.

Laboratory findings are helpful in confirming the disease and recognizing its severity. Serum creatinine and blood urea nitrogen may be elevated above the normal value for pregnancy (0.7 and 10 mg per deciliter, respectively), and creatinine clearance may be decreased below the normal value for pregnancy (125 ml per minute). A serum uric acid level of 5 mg per deciliter is abnormal and may, in fact, represent the first indication of developing or worsening PIH. Transaminase may be elevated. Disseminated intravascular coagulopathy (DIC) is manifested by thrombocytopenia or increased fibrin split products in 20 percent of severe pre-eclamptics. More sensitive laboratory tests show that the hemostatic system is also deranged in mild cases: levels of antithrombin III and alpha$_2$ antiplasmin are significantly reduced, implying an increase in both clotting and fibrinolysis.

Pre-eclampsia is considered "severe" when any of the following criteria are met:

1. The systolic pressure is 160 mm Hg or the diastolic pressure is 110 mm Hg, sustained, measured at rest.
2. Proteinuria is greater than 5 g per 24 hours.
3. Oliguria (400 ml per 24 hours) is present.
4. Cerebral or visual disturbances are present.
5. Pulmonary edema or cyanosis is present.

Acute pulmonary edema is uncommon prior to delivery, even in severe pre-eclampsia. It is a risk, however, up to 3 days later when excess third-space fluid is mobilized.

The so-called HELLP syndrome is considered a variant of severe pre-eclampsia. The acronym refers to the constellation of *h*emolysis, *e*levated *l*iver enzymes, and *l*ow *p*latelets. Of patients with the HELLP syndrome, 80 percent have DIC, and many are likely to develop potentially life-threatening complications such as subscapular hepatic hematoma, acute hepatic or renal failure, or refractory postpartum hemorrhage.

TREATMENT

The only definitive treatment of PIH is termination of pregnancy—that is delivery of the fetus and placenta. If the disease is mild and the fetus preterm, the gravida is treated with bedrest, lying on either side to prevent compression of the renal arteries by the enlarged uterus, until maturation of the fetal lungs has taken place. There is, however, no place for temporization in severe pre-eclampsia, which calls for delivery regardless of gestational age, and therefore is associated with a high rate of cesarean section.

Three issues are pertinent in the treatment of pre-eclamptic women: (1) control of hypertension; (2) management of volume status; and (3) seizure prophylaxis. In the United States, magnesium sulfate is the preferred and specific drug for therapy of moderate and severe pre-eclampsia and eclampsia. It may be administered by continuous intravenous infusion or by intermittent intramuscular injection. A bivalent cation, magnesium is a competitive antagonist of calcium. As such, it blocks the neuromuscular junction by inhibiting acetylcholine release, which depends on a certain concentration of calcium at the presynaptic level. It also inhibits release of catecholamines from the adrenal gland and peripheral nerves and reduces the sensitivity of alpha-adrenergic receptors, thus minimizing autonomic instability. Clinically, its primary effect is dilation of the vasculature and reduction in uterine contractility. In turn, blood pressure is lowered and uterine blood flow improved. However, it is not a potent antihypertensive agent. The cerebral effects of magnesium are twofold. First, it raises the seizure threshold, as shown in animal models, but is not an anticonvulsant drug. Second, it has a salutory effect on cerebral vasospasm, which is especially relevant in this disease process. Increased cerebral concentration of calcium promotes constriction of the cerebral arteries, an effect that can be reversed by calcium channel blockade (e.g., nimodipine) or by increased concentration of magnesium. Finally, the drug promotes production of prostacyclin by vascular endothelium.

Magnesium sulfate therapy is commonly initiated with a bolus of 3 to 4 g given intravenously over 15 minutes and is maintained as an infusion of 1.5 to 3 g per hour titrated to serum levels of 4 to 6 mEq per liter. Respiratory depression is seen at levels of 15 mEq per liter, and cardiac arrest at 25 mEq per liter. Fortunately, the loss of deep tendon reflexes occurs at approximately 10 mEq per liter, providing an important clinical clue to overdosage. Because the drug is cleared by the kidney, the dosage must be reduced in the presence of renal insufficiency. Transient neonatal hypotonia is to be expected. Administration of magnesium should be continued for 24 hours postpartum. The treatment for magnesium overdose is calcium gluconate, given as 10 ml of a 10 percent solution.

Antihypertensive therapy in pre-eclampsia is directed at preventing intracranial bleeding or hypertensive encephalopathy. It should therefore generally be reserved for those gravidae with a diastolic pressure greater than 110 mm Hg or a systolic pressure higher than 180 mm Hg. Too dramatic a decrease in blood pressure compromises both cerebral and uterine perfusion; thus no attempt should be made to normalize blood pressure. The desired endpoint is a diastolic pressure between 95 and 100 mm Hg.

Since the effective circulating volume is reduced in pre-eclampsia, adequate hydration must be established before the initiation of any antihypertensive therapy. This is accomplished by fluid loading with 500 to 1,000 ml of a balanced salt solution. The first-line antihypertensive drug is usually hydralazine hydrochloride, which is given intravenously in increments of 5 to 10 mg or intramuscularly in slightly higher doses. Treatment can be continued with the same dose every 6 hours, or a continuous infusion may be established. If no response is seen after the total initial dose of 30 mg has been given, adjuvant therapy should be initiated. Traditionally, the second-choice drugs were either alpha-methyldopa or diazoxide. They have been replaced by the beta-adrenergic–blocking agents propranolol and esmolol hydrochloride as well as by the mixed alpha- and beta-blocker labetalol. The latter may be given in increments of 10 to 30 mg titrated to effect (cumulative dose not to exceed 300 mg), followed by a continuous infusion of 1 to 2 mg per minute. Labetalol, which is potentiated by the inhalation anesthetics, should be given in smaller doses intraoperatively and postoperatively.

Most pre-eclamptic patients can be managed without a Swan-Ganz catheter. The only real indications for insertion of a pulmonary artery catheter are pulmonary edema (to differentiate between cardiogenic and noncardiogenic types) and oliguria unresponsive to a fluid challenge. After receiving a fluid challenge of 500 ml of balanced salt solution, pre-eclamptics who remain oliguric (urine output less than 30 ml per hour) can be stratified into the three following subsets:

1. Roughly 60 percent have hemodynamics consistent with hypovolemia: low pulmonary capillary wedge pressure, slightly elevated systemic vascular resistance, and hyperdynamic left ventricular function. These patients respond to further volume loading with improvement in cardiac output and resolution of oliguria.
2. Another 30 percent have essentially normal hemodynamic parameters, and their oliguria is attributed to specific renal artery vasospasm, which may be treated either with renal-dose dopamine or with a combination of fluids and vasodilators.
3. The remaining 10 percent have markedly elevated systemic vascular resistance and depressed cardiac output, requiring aggressive afterload reduction.

Aspirin in daily low doses (60 to 100 mg) taken during the last trimester has recently been shown to reduce the incidence of pre-eclampsia significantly in women at risk for the disease. This effect is attributed to correction of an imbalance between prostacyclin and thromboxane.

Preanesthetic considerations are summarized in Table 1.

ANESTHETIC MANAGEMENT

Pain relief during labor is a necessary part of good obstetric care. Well-chosen analgesia mitigates the parturient's physiologic responses to the pain of contractions, and well-managed anesthesia promotes the safe completion of complicated deliveries. Although this statement applies to all parturients, it is the sine qua non for the pre-eclamptic woman. Early consultation between obstetrician and anesthesiologist is essential, because the disease and its treatment pose special problems for preanesthetic and anesthetic management. Anemia is masked by the rising hematocrit. Contraction of the intravascular space produces exaggerated sensitivity to blood loss as well as to overhydration. Compensation for the effects of sympathetic blockade following regional anesthesia is hampered by hypovolemia, electrolyte imbalance, and the action of antihypertensive drugs and magnesium sulfate. Edema of the face and neck may extend into the tissues of the pharynx and larynx, causing respiratory embarrassment and difficulty in endotracheal intubation. Depolarizing and nondepolarizing muscle relaxants are potentiated by magnesium sulfate.

Specific anesthetic considerations are primarily (1)

Table 1 Preanesthetic Considerations in Pre-eclampsia

Physiologic	Pharmacologic
Hypertension	Magnesium sulfate
Hypovolemia, hypoproteinemia	Antihypertensives
Electrolyte imbalance	Low-dose aspirin
Anemia, coagulopathy	
Central nervous system irritability	
Hepatic involvement	
Renal involvement	
Cardiac involvement	

fluctuations in blood pressure; (2) decreased compensation for effects of sympathetic blockade; (3) edema-induced anatomic alterations; (4) potentiation of muscle relaxants; (5) drugs causing cerebral dysfunction; and (6) drugs excreted by the kidney.

Continuous monitoring of the patient's volume status and urine output along with serial determinations of hematocrit, coagulation factors, blood urea nitrogen, creatinine, and hepatocellular enzyme levels are mandatory during the entire peripartum period. Since circulating plasma volume deficit and electrolyte imbalances must be corrected before anesthesia is initiated, it is customary for the anesthesiologist to insert a central venous pressure (CVP) catheter or, in severe cases, a pulmonary artery catheter. In general, electrolyte-containing intravenous solutions suffice to raise the CVP to a normal level, but patients with severe hypoproteinemia or very low oncotic pressure should receive a limited amount of colloid. CVP readings of 4 to 6 cm H_2O are sufficient for labor and vaginal delivery; values of 6 to 8 cm H_2O are sufficient for abdominal delivery.

The presence of normal blood clotting must be established before selection of the method of anesthetization. Although platelet counts should exceed 100,000 platelets per milliliter, a recent report described 14 women with unrecognized peripartal thrombocytopenia of 15,000 to 99,000 platelets per milliliter who received regional anesthesia without excessive bleeding or neurologic sequelae. However, a platelet count of more than 100,000 platelets per milliliter does not guarantee normal function. It is therefore advisable to judge coagulation clinically and, in doubtful cases, resort to determination of the bleeding time. The use of low-dose aspirin during the last trimester has not been associated with hemorrhagic complications in either mothers or newborns.

Marked elevations or decreases in blood pressure should be prevented, the former by emotional support or mild sedation, the latter by judicious methodology. With the low levels of sensory blockade required for labor and vaginal delivery (T10-L1 and S2-4), significant postblock hypotension is not a problem, provided that the uterus has been adequately displaced. For cesarean section, by contrast, strict adherence to precautionary measures (normalization of circulating blood volume, uterine displacement) and to proper anesthetic dosage is mandatory to prevent hypotensive complications. Finally, drugs that tend to cause cerebral dysfunction or impair renal function should be avoided. Therefore, administration of anesthetic concentrations or prolonged use of analgesic concentrations of diethyl ether, methoxyflurane, or enflurane is not advocated. Hepatic involvement may slow drug metabolism, but administering low doses of the currently employed drugs should not be a cause for concern.

Regional Anesthesia

Regional blockade is the optimal anesthetic method for both vaginal and abdominal delivery, provided that normal blood clotting has been established and CVP has reached an acceptable level. Regional anesthesia has been administered successfully not only for pain relief, but also for treatment of the disease. Both single injection and continuous "high" (T8-6 sensory level) spinal and extradural blocks have been employed with excellent results in severe pre-eclampsia and after eclamptic seizures. Benefits include the ability to lower blood pressure gradually (so that the dose of antihypertensive drug can be reduced), a decrease in the level of circulating catecholamines, a reduction in the development of eclamptic seizures, and a shortening of the duration of postictal coma. The earliest evidence of the value of conduction anesthesia in managing pre-eclampsia/eclampsia was noted by Lund, who presented his preliminary observations before the Pittsburgh Society of Anesthesiologists in 1949 and published his experiences with 22 pre-eclamptic or eclamptic women in 1951. Figure 2 depicts his record of a spinal block administered after a postpartum eclamptic seizure. Lund emphasized that the segmental level of analgesia should be "sufficiently high to relieve renal ischemia," and that blockade of the sympathetic and sensory nerves is "more important" than blockade of the motor nerves. Whether the beneficial effects are due to improved perfusion of the kidneys or uterus, to blockade of the adrenals, or to more than one of these factors is as yet unknown.

For labor and vaginal delivery, regional analgesia offers specific advantages to both mother and infant. The degree of circulatory and intracranial pressure responses to the pain of contractions is minimized, and the hazard of a hypertensive crisis is reduced. Uteroplacental blood flow is significantly improved. Consequently, the incidence of neonatal depression is notably lower than after pudendal block or local perineal infiltration. Continuous segmental lumbar extradural analgesia has evolved as the method of choice, unless labor progresses so rapidly as to favor a single-injection extradural or low spinal block. (Paracervical block is not recommended because, in the presence of placental insufficiency, the incidence of untoward fetal effects is increased). While any of the currently popular local anesthetic drugs may be used, 2-chloroprocaine hydrochloride has minimal or no depressant effects on the infant and bupivacaine is potentiated more effectively than the other agents by added narcotics. Epinephrine should not be incorporated in the anesthetic solution for two reasons: (1) pre-eclamptic women are particularly sensitive to its chronotropic properties, and (2) uteroplacental blood flow tends to be decreased with its use. With either extradural or spinal analgesia, maternal oxygen inhalation during the second stage of labor is beneficial for the fetus.

Regional anesthesia is also preferable for cesarean section, provided that the previously mentioned precautionary measures (normalization of circulating blood volume, adequate uterine displacement) have been taken. If the blood pressure decreases despite these measures, a small dose of ephedrine (5 to 10 mg) should

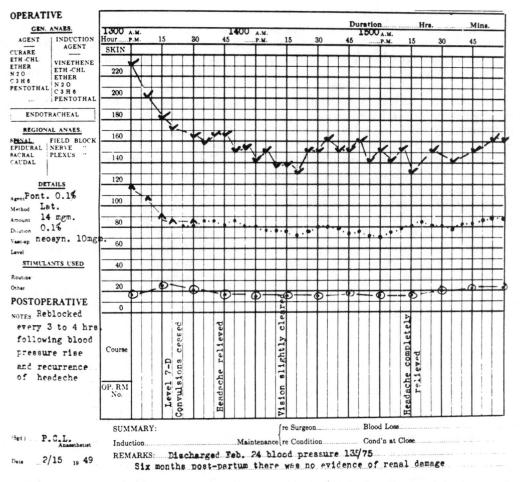

Figure 2 Anesthesia record of a spinal block administered following the development of an eclamptic seizure in a postpartum woman whose delivery had been accomplished with nitrous oxide anesthesia. According to Lund, although the usual treatment for eclampsia was instituted, the symptoms increased in severity. The beneficial results obtained from the spinal block are shown in the record. (Republished with permission from Lund PC. The role of conduction anesthesia in the management of eclampsia. Anesthesiology 1951; 12:693–707.)

be injected intravenously and may be repeated once. If the action of previously administered antihypertensive drugs (methyldopa) renders ephedrine ineffective, a dilute phenylephrine hydrochloride infusion is helpful. Extradural block without epinephrine produces less of a cardiovascular response in the mother than spinal block. The latter, however, requires only a minimal dose of anesthetic drug that neither taxes the maternal degradative processes nor significantly crosses the placenta. Oxygen inhalation is indicated until after the infant is delivered. Administration by face mask is preferable to the use of nasal cannulae, because a higher maternal oxygen tension delivers more oxygen to the fetus.

General Anesthesia

Inhalational analgesia with 40 percent nitrous oxide and 60 percent oxygen may be useful during labor when regional blockade cannot be employed. For vaginal delivery, this may be combined with a pudendal block. Ketamine in a dose of 5 mg given once or twice is not contraindicated in women whose hypertension has been controlled. It may in fact be advantageous in view of the resultant increase in uterine blood flow.

General anesthesia for cesarean section requires intravenous hydration with a balanced electrolyte solution. Pretreatment with an antacid is mandatory. Induction of anesthesia may be accomplished with a thiobarbiturate (up to 4 mg per kilogram) or a ketamine-thiobarbiturate sequence (ketamine, 0.4 to 0.5 mg per kilogram, followed 30 seconds later by thiobarbiturate, 2 mg per kilogram). With this combination, a ketamine-induced increase in blood pressure is minimized, the problem of "awareness" is obviated, and neonatal neurobehavioral scores have been higher than after a full-sleep dose of thiobarbiturate. Ketamine is contraindicated in patients with severe hypertension. When the blood pressure is hazardously high, additional elevations during laryngoscopy and endotracheal intubation must be prevented. This may be accomplished by pretreatment with an intravenous injection of fentanyl and droperidol or the infusion of trimethaphan camsylate (Arfonad) or nitroglycerin. We prefer trimethaphan because of its minimal tendency to increase maternal intracranial pressure, its relatively high molecular weight limiting placental transfer (597 versus 227 for nitroglycerin), and its lack of potentially fetotoxic breakdown products. Trimethaphan also reduces cardiac afterload, whereas nitroglycerin predominantly decreases preload. (The use of nitroprusside is controversial because of the possible accumulation of thiocyanate and cyanide in the fetus.) The inhaled oxygen concentration should be high, preferably 60 percent with 40 percent nitrous oxide or 100 percent with 0.5 to 0.75 percent isoflurane or 0.5 percent halothane. Use of a peripheral nerve stimulator is recommended for assessing the degree of neuromuscular blockade because of the potentiation of muscle relaxants by magnesium sulfate.

Ergot preparations cause peripheral vasoconstriction, which leads to an elevation in blood pressure and an increase in the work of the heart. They are therefore contraindicated in women with PIH. By contrast, synthetic oxytocins produce vasodilation, with an often precipitous decrease in blood pressure followed by reflex-induced tachycardia and increased cardiac output. They should be administered only in a dilute solution.

SUGGESTED READING

Chalon J, Marx GF, Katz JS. Tracheobronchial epithelial multinucleation in preeclampsia. Arch Pathol Lab Med 1976; 100:427–428.
Heller PJ, Schneider EP, Marx GF. Pharyngo-laryngeal edema as a presenting symptom in preeclampsia. Obstet Gynecol 1983; 62:523–525.
Klonoff-Cohen MS, Savitz DA, Cefalo RC, et al. An epidemiologic study of contraception and preeclampsia. JAMA 1989; 262:3143–3147.
Lund PC. The role of conduction anesthesia in the management of eclampsia. Anesthesiology 1951; 12:693–707.
Marx GF, Habib NS, Schulman H. Is pre-eclampsia a disease of the sexually active gravida? Med Hypotheses 1981; 7:1397–1399.
Marx GF, Husain FJ, Shiau HF. Brachial and femoral blood pressures during the prenatal period. Am J Obstet Gynecol 1980; 136:11–13.
Rasmus KT, Rottman RL, Kotelko DM, et al. Unrecognized thrombocytopenia and regional anesthesia in parturients: a retrospective review. Obstet Gynecol 1989; 73:943–946.
Schiff E, Peleg E, Goldenberg M, et al. The use of aspirin to prevent pregnancy-induced hypertension and lower the ratio of thromboxane A$_2$ to prostacyclin in relatively high-risk pregnancies. N Engl J Med 1989; 321:351–356.

VAGINAL DELIVERY

JEFFREY A. GRASS, M.D.
ANDREW P. HARRIS, M.D.

Anesthesia for obstetric patients has become a routine part of anesthesia care. Parturients are assuming a more active role in the management of their pregnancy and labor, including decisions regarding anesthesia. The trend has been away from "twilight sleep" and systemic medications during labor toward regional anesthetic techniques that are not only safer for both mother and infant, but allow the mother to participate fully in the delivery process. Because of this shift in emphasis, anesthesiologists have become increasingly involved in the care of patients during labor and vaginal delivery, as well as those undergoing cesarean section.

In order to provide safe obstetric anesthesia care one needs to be familiar with all aspects of obstetric physiology and anesthesia management, not only for the low-risk patient but also for the high-risk parturient. Ultimately, providing obstetric anesthesia coverage entails screening all parturients upon hospital admission, initiating and maintaining regional anesthetics for labor and vaginal delivery when appropriate, ensuring around-the-clock availability for performing anesthesia for emergency cesarean section, and providing expertise in newborn airway management and resuscitation.

When one is providing anesthesia for labor, all decisions must be made with consideration of the effect the intervention will have on (1) the safety of both mother and infant, and (2) the progress of labor, with the primary obstetric objective being a safe and expedient vaginal delivery. Obstetric anesthesia is unique among the subspecialty areas of anesthesia in that the anesthetic techniques, or interventions, that we employ are often misconstrued by our surgical colleagues as having a counterproductive effect on the accomplishment of their primary objective. It must always be remembered that labor and delivery can frequently be conducted without pharmacologic intervention, and that any anesthetic administered may have potential effects on two patients, the mother and her infant.

PREOPERATIVE EVALUATION

Patient evaluation prior to the initiation of labor analgesia should be as complete and thorough as a preoperative evaluation prior to surgery. The history and physical examination, as well as the anesthetic management, must be conducted with a clear understanding of how physiology and anatomy differ in pregnant and nonpregnant women, and the anesthetic implications of these physiologic alterations of pregnancy. Specifically, one must consider the hormonal changes that begin in the first trimester of pregnancy; the mechanical pressure from the expanding uterus causing other physiologic changes; the increased metabolic demand imposed by the growing fetus, uterus, and placenta; and the hemodynamic consequences and fetal implications of uteroplacental circulation. The parturient will often relate signs and symptoms associated with the normal increased demand placed on both the cardiovascular and pulmonary systems during pregnancy. One must specifically inquire about symptoms associated with the supine hypotension syndrome. In patients with significant underlying medical disease prior to pregnancy, one must carefully consider the physiologic implications of the normal alterations of pregnancy superimposed on already compromised baseline function. Epidural analgesia during labor and vaginal delivery is often recommended and provided for patients in whom additional cardiac workload would be detrimental. Similarly, one must carefully evaluate and consider the physiologic changes in blood constituents and hematologic function, renal function, hepatic function, gastrointestinal system function, with delayed gastric emptying and a combination of other factors increasing the risk of aspiration, and changes in the endocrine and nervous systems. Special consideration must be paid to the increased likelihood of difficult airway management, and such difficulty must be anticipated and preparations made before endotracheal intubation becomes emergently necessary.

PREPARATION AND MONITORING

Prior to the initiation of labor analgesia in a labor room, one must assure the immediate availability of all equipment necessary to provide full airway management, including laryngoscope, appropriate-sized endotracheal tubes with stylets, pharmacologic agents for rapid sequence induction, oxygen with equipment necessary for mask delivery, and a full set of cardiovascular resuscitation drugs. Most importantly, an obstetrician capable of performing an emergency cesarean section must be readily available.

The fetal heart rate (FHR) monitor should be considered the most important monitor in obstetric anesthesia. The FHR tracing provides the best available minute-to-minute monitor of the adequacy of uteroplacental blood flow and oxygen transfer and should be examined with vigilance by the anesthesiologist before, during, and after the administration of anesthesia. Anesthesiologists must learn to interpret normal FHR tracings and recognize signs of fetal distress in order to know when to withhold anesthetics, when to modify anesthetic plans, and when to apply treatment aimed at improving fetal oxygenation. Other monitors that should be routinely used during vaginal delivery include a blood pressure cuff, pulse oximeter, and electrocardiography. Supplemental oxygen should be administered to the mother routinely during delivery and with signs of increased risk of fetal distress during labor in order to improve fetal oxygen delivery and provide an added buffer against desaturation.

ANATOMY OF THE PAIN OF LABOR

Familiarity with the normal progression of labor and an understanding of the pain pathways of labor are important.

Labor is classically divided into three stages. The first stage begins at the onset of uterine contractions and ends with full dilation of the cervix. Pain during the first stage originates both from uterine contractions and more predominantly from stretching of the lower uterine segment and the relatively noncompliant cervix. Pain impulses from both the uterus and the cervix pass together through the paracervical uterine plexus, pelvic plexus, hypogastric nerve, superior hypogastric plexus, and sympathetic chain, and finally enter the central nervous system via the T10 to L1 spinal roots. They ascend via the medial and lateral systems of the spinal cord, through the brain stem, and ultimately travel to the cerebral cortex, where extensive and complex modulation of pain perception occurs. The second stage of labor begins with full dilation of the cervix and continues until delivery of the infant. Pain during the second stage originates predominately from stretching of the lower vagina and the perineum. Pain impulses from these areas are transmitted along the pudendal nerve and enter the spinal cord at the S2 to S4 level, ultimately ascending to the cortex. The distinction in pain pathway stimulus between the first and second stages of labor may vary to a significant degree depending on the rapidity of the progression of labor and the fetal presentation and head position. The third stage of labor extends from delivery of the infant to delivery of the placenta. During this stage and the ensuing episiotomy repair, pain originates from both the tetanically contracting uterus and the lower birth canal and involves the pathways for both the first and second stages of labor.

NONPHARMACOLOGIC METHODS OF PAIN RELIEF

The nonpharmacologic methods of pain relief during labor take advantage of the extensive modulation of noxious impulses that occurs in the central nervous system. Such methods of pain relief include psychoprophylaxis, hypnosis, acupuncture, and transcutaneous electrical nerve stimulation (TENS), all of which attenuate the perception of pain by altering levels of anxiety, diffusing attention away from painful stimuli, or interrupting pain impulses as they are conducted at various levels of the central nervous system (e.g., by enhancing the activity of descending inhibitory pathways or utilizing the gait theory of pain).

The most commonly used psychoprophylactic techniques are natural and prepared childbirth. These methods involve educating women about childbirth and hospital procedures and teaching techniques of distraction (e.g., breathing protocols during contractions). Antepartum instruction should lessen anxiety, and since the presence of anxiety reduces pain tolerance, perception of pain may be lessened as well. In this respect, efforts should be made to educate all pregnant women about childbirth, including obstetric anesthesia options and concerns. Similarly, distraction techniques during painful experiences such as labor may be useful in decreasing pain perception. Although psychoprophylaxis can be effective in reducing the pain of labor for selected patients, these techniques often involve lengthy prenatal preparation, and the supplemental use of pharmacologic analgesia is frequently required. When natural or prepared childbirth is attempted as the sole method of pain relief during labor, it is essential that the parturient not view the potential need for the use of supplemental pharmacologic methods of pain relief or cesarean section as representative of "failure" on her part.

Hypnosis has been reported to be effective in the minority of parturients who can achieve a hypnotic trance, but also requires many hours of antepartum preparation and shares the same disadvantages of psychoprophylaxis. Although acupuncture had been reported to be effective for cesarean section in some women, it has generally been found to be unsuccessful for labor, vaginal delivery, and cesarean section, and is rarely attempted by skilled acupuncturists. TENS can provide partial effective analgesia when applied over the dermatomes to which the pain of labor is referred. However, it requires specialized equipment, which may interfere with FHR monitoring, and does not offer complete pain relief, especially for the second stage of labor and episiotomy repair.

SYSTEMIC MEDICATION

Several different types of drugs are administered for the relief of pain during labor and vaginal delivery. These include narcotics, sedatives and tranquilizers, inhalation anesthetics, and ketamine. As our understanding of placental transfer of drugs and their effect on neonatal neurobehavior has improved, systemic medications for labor have been scrutinized more closely. Combined with the more widespread availability of safe and more effective regional anesthesia techniques for childbirth, and the maternal desire to remember the experiences surrounding childbirth, systemic medications are being used much less frequently during labor and vaginal delivery.

Narcotics

Narcotics that have been administered systemically to patients in labor include morphine, meperidine, fentanyl, pentazocine, nalbuphine, and butorphanol. All have essentially similar side-effect profiles in equianalgesic doses. In the mother, all narcotics produce dose-dependent analgesia and respiratory depression. Other undesirable narcotic-associated effects include nausea and vomiting, pruritus, sedation, and in some cases vasodilatation. Of significant concern is the further prolongation of maternal gastric emptying. Most importantly, the potential for causing fetal depression ultimately limits the use of systemic narcotics as delivery approaches, when analgesia is usually most required. Meperidine has been the most commonly used narcotic for labor and is typically administered intravenously (0.3 to 0.7 mg per kilogram) or intramuscularly (0.7 to 1.5 mg per kilogram). Meperidine and its active metabolites, including normeperidine, readily cross the placenta. The drug and its metabolites have long half-lives in the fetus and cause significant neonatal depression if given in high doses or multiple doses over the course of a long labor. Butorphanol has gained popularity among obstetricians for systemic administration during labor because it has no active metabolites that accumulate in the fetus and has been reported to have a "ceiling" of respiratory depressant effect. In clinically administered doses, however, the respiratory depressant effect of butorphanol is similar to an equianalgesic dose of morphine, and the sedative effect of butorphanol may be even greater owing to its kappa receptor agonist effect. Also, ominous sinusoidal FHR patterns (a sign of severe fetal distress) have been associated with butorphanol, confounding FHR interpretation. Fentanyl administered intravenously in doses limited to 50 or 100 μg per hour may provide effective analgesia during labor with less fetal depression than that associated with meperidine in equianalgesic doses.

Self-administration of intravenous fentanyl using patient-controlled analgesia (PCA) may provide more satisfactory pain relief during labor with less total drug requirement because serum drug levels are maintained at the minimal effective analgesic concentration necessary to relieve pain while avoiding "overshoot" into higher serum concentrations, which cause more sedation but provide no additional analgesic benefit. The psychological advantages of self-control of pain relief and the associated decrease in anxiety also may attenuate the perception of pain in the central nervous system, further reducing intravenous narcotic requirement with the PCA mode of delivery. Nonetheless, PCA still suffers from the same drawbacks of intravenous narcotic administration during labor: most important, the potential for causing neonatal respiratory depression. Whenever narcotics are used to relieve labor pain, the specific narcotic antagonist naloxone should be readily available for administration to the infant at delivery.

Sedatives and Tranquilizers

Sedatives and tranquilizers include barbiturates, phenothiazines, hydroxyzine, and benzodiazepines. Barbiturates are now used infrequently because they are antianalgesic and cause sedation. Benzodiazepines, although anxiolytic, are quite sedative and amnestic, which may be a particularly undesirable effect in patients who wish to recall the childbirth experience. On the other hand, hydroxyzine or phenothiazines (especially promethazine, 0.7 mg per kilogram intramuscularly, or 0.3 to 0.7 mg per kilogram intravenously) are more useful and can be administered more safely during labor. These drugs are less sedative in effect and are relatively anxiolytic and antiemetic, and they do not cause amnesia. In addition, because they enhance the analgesic properties of narcotics, the dose of narcotic and associated undesirable effects can be decreased when they are administered concurrently.

Inhalation Anesthetics

There has been a marked decline in the use of inhalation general anesthesia for vaginal delivery for three reasons: (1) the increased risk of aspiration during general anesthesia in pregnant patients, (2) the desire of mothers to be awake during routine delivery, and (3) the increased use of alternative techniques of pain relief, particularly lumbar epidural analgesia. General anesthesia using a halogenated agent may still be emergently necessary to provide the analgesia and perineal relaxation necessary for an unforeseen emergency forceps delivery, or when prompt uterine relaxation is indicated, such as in a difficult breech delivery with head entrapment, replacement of an acutely inverted uterus, or manual extraction of a retained placenta. Whenever general anesthesia is required, after oral administration of a nonparticulate antacid (sodium citrate, 30 ml), awake intubation or a rapid sequence induction with endotracheal intubation is mandated because of the increased risk of aspiration of gastric contents.

Nonetheless, "conscious inhalation analgesia" may still be useful in certain circumstances, such as during the second stage of labor for difficult spontaneous or instrument-assisted deliveries. Inhalation analgesics such as methoxyflurane (or other halogenated anesthetics) can be rapidly administered by face mask to provide safe levels of analgesia as long as consciousness and airway reflexes are being constantly monitored and maintained. The halogenated agents have a distinct advantage over nitrous oxide because a high concentration of oxygen can be administered along with analgesic concentrations of anesthetic. Methoxyflurane is unique in that it does not cause significant uterine relaxation at analgesic concentrations. Potential fluoride toxicity following methoxyflurane administration during labor is usually not of concern because exposure is limited to low doses over a relatively short cumulative time period. Inhalation analgesia during labor has now been mostly replaced by the use of other systemic medications and regional anesthetic techniques.

Ketamine

During difficult deliveries, intravenous ketamine may be particularly useful and safe both alone and as an adjuvant to other analgesic techniques. The incremental dose is 0.1 to 0.15 mg per kilogram, which may be repeated every 3 to 5 minutes as necessary. If the total dose is kept under 1 mg per kilogram, potential neonatal depression and uterine hypertonicity should not occur. Similarly, postoperative maternal dysphoria or subsequent nightmares should occur very infrequently. As with the inhalation agents, the level of consciousness must be constantly monitored to avoid oversedation with resultant loss of airway reflexes.

PERIPHERAL NERVE BLOCKS

Several peripheral block techniques have been found to be effective for specific stages of labor and delivery. These blocks have been traditionally administered by obstetricians and include the paracervical block in the first stage of labor, and in the second stage of labor the pudendal nerve block, perineal field block, and local infiltration.

Paracervical Block

The paracervical block anesthetizes the sensory fibers from the uterus, cervix, and upper vagina as they pass through the paracervical–uterine plexus (Frankenhauser's ganglion). It is effective in attentuating the discomfort associated with cervical dilation during the first stage of labor. A transvaginal approach is used to inject local anesthetic at the 2:30 and 9:30 o'clock positions in the cervical fornices. Although the paracervical block can provide excellent pain relief for the first stage of labor, it has been associated with a 10 to 30 percent incidence of fetal bradycardia and thus has become much less popular. Fetal bradycardia can be caused by high fetal drug levels (with a direct toxic fetal effect), but is more commonly related to uterine artery vasospasm and uterine muscle hypertonus, both of which decrease uteroplacental perfusion, producing fetal hypoxia and acidosis. The paracervical block can be modified in ways that reduce the incidence of fetal bradycardia, including (1) limiting the mass of local anesthetic administered by decreasing the volume and/or concentration of local anesthetic, (2) waiting 5 to 10 minutes (or two contractions) between the injections on each side, so that early signs of fetal distress will not be missed, (3) injecting no deeper than submucosally, thereby avoiding perivascular penetration, (4) injecting in more than one location on each side, and (5) using an ester local anesthetic such as 2-chloroprocaine, which is rapidly metabolized by the fetus as well as the mother. Unfortunately, although effective in reducing the incidence of fetal bradycardia, all of these modifications shorten the duration of effect and increase the need to repeat the block more frequently. Finally, the paracervical block is useful for only the first stage of labor and therefore must be supplemented with some other technique in the second stage.

Pudendal Block

For the second stage of labor and episiotomy repair, bilateral pudendal nerve block can provide safe and effective analgesia. The pudendal nerve is a branch of the sacral plexus with contributions from S2 to S4, which innervates the external rectal sphincter and skin and muscles of the perineum. This block is most commonly performed using the transvaginal approach with the fingers inserted in the vagina. The ischial spine and the sacrospinous ligament, which extends from the ischial spine to the sacrum, are palpated and a specialized 20-gauge, 6-inch needle with a "trumpet" guide assembly is inserted into the vagina with the trumpet positioned over the sacrospinous ligament at its attachment to the ischial spine. The needle is then advanced through the guide until it is felt to pop through the ligament. The pudendal nerve, artery, and vein all lie just deep to the sacrospinous ligament at this point. Following aspiration, 5 to 10 ml of local anesthetic, usually 1 percent lidocaine, is injected and the procedure is then repeated on the other side. Pudendal nerve block presents very little risk for mother and infant, and it can be repeated as necessary provided local anesthetic dosing limits are not exceeded. Perineal field block and local infiltration of the perineum are less effective but are as safe as the pudendal nerve block. The main caveats are to use larger volumes of more dilute local anesthetic and to allow adequate time for penetration.

Lumbar Sympathetic Chain Block

The lumbar sympathetic chain block is primarily of anatomic interest. It is performed bilaterally with a paramedian approach at the L2 level and interrupts pain pathways from the uterus and cervix. However, this block is not widely taught or performed because it is very painful for the patient, technically difficult to perform, carries the risk of causing significant hypotension, and requires supplementation by another technique for the second stage of labor. Simpler and more effective alternate regional anesthesia techniques exist.

MAJOR REGIONAL ANESTHESIA

Major regional anesthesia techniques for labor and delivery include epidural block (both lumbar and caudal approaches) for the first and second stages of labor and subarachnoid block for the second stage of labor. Recent innovations of these techniques also will be discussed.

As previously discussed, proper preparation for major regional anesthetic blockade during labor and delivery must include the ready availability of all equipment necessary for emergency airway management and intubation and full resuscitation drugs. Once the decision has been made to use a regional anesthetic, an intravenous line must be established and 10 to 15 ml per kilogram of a balanced salt solution should be administered to minimize the incidence of hypotension associated with the expected sympathectomy. Dextrose-containing solutions should be avoided because of the potential for neonatal rebound hypoglycemia after birth. Continuous uterine displacement to the left side to avoid aortocaval compression and FHR monitoring should be maintained throughout labor.

Caudal Epidural Block

Although once widely used for labor and delivery, caudal epidural block is now rarely used. When initiated early in the course of labor it may cause premature weakness of the pelvic floor musculature and interfere with fetal descent and rotation. Landmarks for the location of the caudal canal and placement of the block are not uniform; therefore, the caudal block is technically more difficult to perform than the lumbar epidural block. For these reasons, its use has been mostly replaced by lumbar epidural analgesia and subarachnoid block. Nonetheless, in selected thin, multiparous patients who present rapidly approaching the second stage of labor, the caudal approach to the epidural space may still be the anesthetic technique of choice to provide prompt and effective regional analgesia for the remainder of labor and vaginal delivery.

After appropriate topical sterilization and local anesthetic infiltration over the sacral hiatus, an epidural needle may be advanced with a distinct "loss of resistance" or "pop" as it penetrates the sacrococcygeal ligament into the caudal canal. A continuous epidural catheter may then be inserted 3 to 5 cm into the caudal canal and the needle removed. Prior to injection of medication or placement of a catheter, a rectal examination should be performed to rule out inadvertent puncture of the rectum or fetal head. Following a test dose, an analgesic dose of 0.125 to 0.25 percent bupivacaine, often in conjunction with a lipid-soluble opiate agent, is administered incrementally through the catheter. The level of block achieved with a given volume of local anesthetic is more variable than with lumbar epidural analgesia. Typically 15 to 20 ml of local anesthetic solution are necessary to achieve a T-10 level block. Because the drug is delivered in more concentrated fashion to the sacral nerve roots than with the lumbar epidural block, very effective analgesia for the second stage of labor is reliably achieved. Although the caudal catheter can be used to provide regional anesthesia for cesarean section, the volume of local anesthetic necessary to provide an adequate level of block is quite unpredictable and often approaches a toxic local anesthetic dose range.

Lumbar Epidural Block

The placement of a local anesthetic in the epidural space via the lumbar approach has become the regional technique of choice for obstetrics. Pain relief for both the first and second stages of labor can be conveniently achieved, and the continuous lumbar epidural catheter technique may be readily adapted to provide surgical anesthesia for obstetric procedures such as cesarean section or forceps delivery.

After identifying the epidural space using a "loss of resistance" technique, a flexible catheter is typically threaded approximately 3 cm into the epidural space.

(The "hanging drop" technique may not be as reliable during labor because transient positive pressures have been measured in the epidural space during contractions.) It is essential to administer an *epidural test dose* to rule out intravascular and especially intrathecal placement prior to the administration of the larger therapeutic dose of local anesthetic. The initial placement or migration of the epidural catheter into two potentially dangerous locations, the cerebrospinal fluid or a blood vessel, is not always revealed by aspiration of cerebrospinal fluid or blood through the catheter. Unintended intrathecal catheter placement can be reliably detected by injecting lidocaine, 30 to 45 mg; bupivacaine, 12.5 mg; or 2-chloroprocaine, 40 mg through the catheter and observing the patient for the rapid onset of sensory block following the injection. We use 2 ml of hyperbaric lidocaine 1.5 percent to test for intrathecal catheter placement because we find it to be reliable in providing a detectable sensory block 2 to 3 minutes after injection, whereas the hyperbaric solution minimizes the risk of excessive cephalad spread, which can result in a total spinal block during labor. The incidence of vascular catheter placement is much higher in pregnant than in nonpregnant patients (5 to 15 percent vs. 2.8 percent) owing to the increased engorgement of the epidural venous plexus during pregnancy. Aspiration can fail to detect as many as 50 percent of intravenously located epidural catheters. Although controversy exists over the safest, most efficacious way to detect unintentional vascular catheter placement, test doses containing epinephrine 15 μcg are most commonly used in obstetric epidural anesthesia. The efficacy of this test dose relies on a transient chronotropic effect on maternal heart rate, with the detection of a 10 to 20 beat per minute increase if the catheter is indeed located in a blood vessel and the epinephrine is hence administered systemically. Although probably the most reliable and commonly used test dose available, intravenous epinephrine does not always produce tachycardia and is therefore not 100 percent sensitive; in actively laboring women, maternal heart rate variability may exceed 20 to 30 beats per minute, making this test dose technique not 100 percent specific either. Ultimately, proper vigilance must be maintained in the subsequent administration of all local anesthetic even after a negative test dose, because any test dose is not 100 percent sensitive and because intravascular and subarachnoid migration can occur after initial successful placement of the catheter in the epidural space.

Once intravascular or intrathecal catheter placement has been ruled out, a dose of low concentration local anesthetic (Table 1) is administered to establish a T-10 segmental block for the first stage of labor. Bupivacaine, 0.25 percent, in a volume of 8 to 10 ml is most commonly administered to establish analgesia at our institution. Low concentrations of bupivacaine seem to provide the most differential sensory versus motor block with the longest duration of effect in comparison to other local anesthetics. The addition of 50 μg of fentanyl decreases the latency of onset of analgesia and increases the median duration of analgesia from 90 to 180 minutes. Increasing the fentanyl dose to 100 μg does not provide additional benefit. Sufentanil, 5 to 10 μg, and butorphanol, 1 to 3 mg, similarly improve the onset, quality, and duration of bupivacaine analgesia, but butorphanol results in greater maternal somnolence, and transient ominous sinusoidal FHR patterns have been reported even with the epidural route of administration. Epidural morphine, 2 mg, has also been shown to improve the duration and quality of analgesia with bupivacaine 0.25 percent; however, the risk of delayed respiratory depression associated with this more hydrophilic opiate makes this regimen less attractive. The addition of the aforementioned lipid-soluble opiates to local anesthetics has become commonplace, because these agents have revolutionized obstetric epidural analgesia by increasing the duration of local anesthetic effect and permitting the use of lower concentrations of local anesthetic so that motor power can be better preserved. Similarly, although analgesic doses can be repeated intermittently as necessary throughout the first and second stages of labor, the continuous infusion of lower concentrations of local anesthetic in conjunction with extremely low concentrations of opiates can provide more stable analgesia and avoid the transient periods of increased motor block associated with intermittent dosing regimens (Table 2). The overall goal is to achieve a more selective sensory block with less associated motor block while maintaining a sensory level of T-10 during the first stage of labor, with the block spreading to the sacral nerves for the second stage of labor and episiotomy repair. For example, continuous epidural infusion of 0.0625 percent bupivacaine with 0.0002% fentanyl (2 μg per milliliter) provides less intense motor block with analgesia similar to that provided by infusion of 0.125% bupivacaine alone. The epidural administration of the above-mentioned opiates to healthy full-term parturients during labor has been shown not to have any

Table 1 Labor Epidural Dose Guidelines: Intermittent Bolus Technique

Agent*	Labor Dose (ml)	Interval (min)	Delivery Dose (ml)
Bupivacaine 0.25%	6–10†	75–120	–
Lidocaine 1.0–1.5%	6–10	60–90	10–15 (1.5%)
2-Chloroprocaine 2%	8–12	30–45	10–15 (2 or 3%)†

*Fentanyl 50 μcg or sufentanil 10 μcg is usually added to initial dose.
†Most commonly used at Johns Hopkins Hospital.

adverse effects on APGAR scores, neurobehavioral scores, and the FHR pattern during labor (except as described with butorphanol). Caution should be exercised in generalizing these results to the administration of epidural opiates to parturients with preterm infants or high-risk obstetric complications.

Once epidural analgesia has been established, the analgesic infusion should be continued through the time of delivery. Intrinsic uterine activity has never been shown to be diminished by the epidural administration of nonepinephrine-containing local anesthetic solutions.

Even with the use of a continuous infusion technique, toward the end of the second stage of labor, a "delivery dose" of local anesthetic may be required to produce a sacral block for delivery and episiotomy repair (see Table 1). We typically administer 10 to 14 ml of 2-chloroprocaine (2 or 3 percent) as a delivery dose because it has a rapid onset and short duration of action.

Patient-controlled epidural analgesia (PCEA) using the same local anesthetic solutions as described earlier shows promise as a way to provide more satisfactory labor analgesia in selected patients and to decrease the number of personnel required to administer anesthesia and demands for epidural "top-up" injections (Table 3). Self-administered incremental doses as opposed to a continuous infusion technique may also lead to better sacral spread of the block and less need for delivery doses.

With any continuous epidural technique, including both epidural infusion and PCEA, the same vigilance for signs of intrathecal or intravenous catheter migration with hourly documentation of sensory block level and blood pressure must be maintained. On the initiation of lumbar epidural analgesia or with "top-up" doses, we always monitor the patient's blood pressure, onset of local anesthetic blockade, and FHR for at least 20 minutes, with subsequent hourly follow-up.

The potential complications of lumbar epidural anesthesia are similar in many instances to the side effects and complications associated with subarachnoid block. The placement of the epidural or spinal needle may involve such risk as postpartum back pain, postdural puncture headache (PDPH), and in extremely rare cases, neurologic damage associated with direct trauma, infection, or hematoma. Hypotension from sympathetic blockade is one of the most common side effects of both epidural and spinal anesthesia. As previously discussed, the prophylactic administration of an adequate volume preload prior to the injection of any local anesthetic and avoidance of aortocaval compression after placement of the block are mandatory. Nonetheless, hypotension still sometimes occurs, and one must be readily prepared to administer additional volume, and if necessary, vasopressors. Intravenous ephedrine (5 to 10 mg) is the vasopressor of choice in obstetric patients because it alone is not thought to cause a decrease in uterine blood flow. Unintentional intravascular injection of large volumes of local anesthetic is a potentially serious complication of epidural analgesia because it may result in maternal sedation, generalized seizures, and cardiovascular compromise, as well as fetal toxicity. Patients should be monitored constantly for signs and symptoms of intravascular injection, including sedation, tinnitus, metallic taste, and circumoral numbness. One must always be prepared to protect and manage the airway and provide treatment for seizures and cardiovascular collapse.

Table 2 Labor Epidural Dose Guidelines: Continuous Infusion Technique

Initial Load or "Top-up" Agent*	Dose (ml)	Maintenance Infusion Concentration	Rate (ml/hr)
Bupivacaine 0.25%	6–10	Bupivacaine 0.125%	8–14
Bupivacaine 0.25% + fentanyl 50 μg	6–10	Bupivacaine 0.125% + fentanyl 0.0002%	8–12
Bupivacaine 0.25% + fentanyl 50 μg	6–10	Bupivacaine 0.0625% + fentanyl 0.0002%	10–20†
Bupivacaine 0.25% + sufentanil 10 μg	6–10	Bupivacaine 0.0625% + sufentanil 0.00003%	10–16

*Bupivacaine 0.125% may be substituted for 0.25%.
†Most commonly used at Johns Hopkins Hospital.

Table 3 Labor Epidural Dose Guidelines: Patient-Controlled Epidural Analgesia

Initial Load or "Top-up" Agent	Dose (ml)	PCEA Administered Concentration	Basal Rate (ml/hr)	Self-Dose (ml)	Lockout Interval (min)	1-HR Limit (ml)
Bupivacaine 0.25% + fentanyl 50 μcg	6–10	Bupivacaine 0.125% + fentanyl 0.0002%	4	4	10	20
Bupivacaine 0.25% + fentanyl 50 μcg or sufentanil 10 μcg	6–10	Bupivacaine 0.0625% + fentanyl 0.0002% or sufentanil 0.00003%	8	4	10	24
			6	2	6	24

Subarachnoid Block

The modified saddle block (T-10 to S-5) is most useful at the end of the second stage of labor, particularly for instrument deliveries, episiotomy repair, or manual removal of the placenta. Spinal anesthesia has a more rapid onset and requires much less local anesthetic drug for a given level of block as compared with the lumbar epidural block. However, it cannot provide nearly the selectivity of sensory block and is not really feasible for prolonged analgesia during the first stage of labor unless a continuous subarachnoid catheter technique is employed, which typically requires a larger dural puncture and the associated increased risk of PDPH. A safe and effective saddle block for the second stage of labor can be provided by the subarachnoid administration of 2 ml of hyperbaric 1.5 percent lidocaine (30 mg), with a duration of action that closely matches the length of most delivery room procedures. Epinephrine may be added, or a longer-acting agent such as tetracaine or bupivacaine may be used if a prolonged procedure is anticipated. The risk of PDPH can be minimized by using a 26- or 27-gauge spinal needle with an acute angle of insertion (paramedian approach) and with the bevel inserted parallel to the dural fibers. The recently developed Sprotte and Whitacre needles may both be associated with a lower incidence of postdural puncture headache because they tend to separate the dural fibers as opposed to severing them. Although the incidence of PDPH tends to be decreased when a spinal catheter for continuous spinal anesthesia is used in nonpregnant patients, the insertion of a catheter has not been shown to decrease the incidence of PDPH in obstetric patients.

Intrathecal Opiate Labor Analgesia

With the advent of epidural opiate administration, there was great enthusiasm with regard to the administration of epidural opiates as sole regional anesthetic agents to provide analgesia while avoiding the motor, sensory, and sympathetic nerve block associated with local anesthetic administration. However, epidural opiate administration (without local anesthetic) has not proved to be clinically useful for relief of labor pain. In patients in whom epidural local anesthetics may not be well-tolerated (e.g., a cardiac patient who may not tolerate sympathectomy), intrathecal opiates administered either intermittently or continuously may provide satisfactory analgesia during the first stage of labor until perineal distension occurs. Intrathecal fentanyl, 25 µg, provides approximately 2 hours of rapid onset analgesia with few side effects. Adding 0.25 mg of morphine may further lengthen the duration of analgesia. Intrathecal sufentanil, 3 to 15 µg as a single dose, can provide up to 3 hours of effective analgesia with minimal side effects, and subsequent intrathecal infusion of 1 to 3 µg per hour via a microspinal catheter allows for sustained analgesia. The lack of motor and sympathetic nerve block makes intrathecal opiate analgesia potentially quite attractive for certain high-risk patients.

ANESTHESIA CONSIDERATIONS FOR HIGH-RISK DELIVERIES

High-risk parturients require specialized obstetric and anesthesia care. A basic understanding of how the specific pathophysiology of obstetric disease and associated pharmacologic therapy influence and interact with anesthetic care and techniques employed is essential for both the obstetrician and anesthesiologist. High-risk parturients often require special monitoring and represent a group of patients in which analgesic intervention is often specifically indicated to avoid decompensation from the increased stress associated with the cardiovascular and pulmonary demands imposed by painful labor and vaginal delivery. Some of the more common high-risk obstetric situations and implications with respect to anesthesia management for labor and vaginal delivery are discussed in the next section.

Preeclampsia/Eclampsia

Preeclampsia is a systemic disease process occurring after the first trimester of pregnancy that is characterized by hypertension, nondependent edema, and proteinuria. Neuronal irritability can progress to grand mal seizures, thereby defining eclampsia. The pertinent pathophysiology of preeclampsia includes generalized arteriolar vasospasm, retention of sodium and water, and altered coagulation processes. The patient's coagulation profile, liver and renal function, and volume status should be carefully evaluated. The cardiovascular system of the pre-eclamptic patient reflects the effects of increased arteriolar resistance and decreased circulating volume, with a hyperdynamic increase in cardiac output and an increase in left ventricular work. Although pulmonary capillary wedge pressure is usually not increased, injudicious intravenous fluid replacement or exacerbation of the hyperdynamic state may precipitate left ventricular failure and pulmonary edema. Nevertheless, restoring blood volume with crystalloid or colloid infusion prior to initiating epidural block is essential because these patients are frequently intravascularly volume depleted and at increased risk of precipitous drops in blood pressure associated with an increased risk of fetal distress due to baseline compromise of uteroplacental profusion. The amount of fluid needed varies and should be based on assessments of volume status, including blood pressure, physical examination, and urine output as measured with a Foley catheter. Invasive hemodynamic monitoring is typically reserved for the patient with severe preeclampsia who does not respond to initial pharmacologic treatment. Patients with oliguria unresponsive to fluid challenges of 500 ml may be better managed with a central venous pressure catheter. Patients with signs of obvious cardiorespiratory compromise, including pulmonary edema, are often best managed with a pulmonary artery catheter and arterial line. All patients with preeclampsia should be maintained on anticonvulsant therapy throughout the period of labor and delivery and for approximately 24 hours postpartum to protect against the development of eclampsia, which is a serious, life-threatening illness with significant morbidity and mortality. Antihypertensive medications (typically hydralazine or labetalol) should be administered as necessary to control hypertension (i.e., to ≤ 110 diastolic) prior to the initiation of regional anesthesia. Cerebrovascular accident related to extreme hypertension remains the leading cause of death in preeclampsia. A platelet count below 100,000 should prompt one to obtain a bleeding time, the prolongation of which might preclude the use of regional anesthesia. To avoid further uteroplacental compromise and ensuing fetal distress, blood pressure should be monitored closely, and a fall of greater than 15 to 20 percent following initiation of epidural anesthesia should be treated promptly with increased intravenous fluids, exaggerated left uterine displacement, and intravenous ephedrine in 5-mg increments as necessary, recognizing the potential for exaggerated response to vasopressor agents. For reasons mentioned previously, we use 100 mg of 2-chloroprocaine and avoid the use of epinephrine for our epidural test dose in preeclamptic patients. Ultimately, lumbar epidural anesthesia for labor can not only be safely administered in patients with preeclampsia, but may actually improve uteroplacental perfusion and fetal oxygen delivery owing to effects on the sympathetic nervous system and attenuation of catecholamine levels, thereby making it the analgesic regimen of choice in preeclampsia.

Preterm Delivery

The goals of anesthesia in preterm delivery should be to minimize fetal drug exposure, and to provide optimal conditions for a controlled second stage of delivery. Therefore, in the first stage of labor large quantities of systemic medications should be avoided, making regional techniques most desirable. Similarly, one may wish to limit or avoid the use of epidural opiate agents in conjunction with local anesthetics because the preterm infant is more sensitive to narcotic-associated respiratory depression, perhaps even with the low serum levels typically achieved with low-dose epidural opiate administration; there are very little clinical data available regarding this issue. A controlled second stage of labor to avoid head trauma in the preterm infant requires good perineal anesthesia to block the reflex urge to push while maintaining the patient's ability to cooperate with voluntary expulsive efforts. Saddle block, pudendal block, and epidural block are all effective methods for preterm delivery and result in low fetal drug levels.

Breech Delivery

When vaginal breech delivery is anticipated, the anesthetic technique chosen should provide good perineal anesthesia for the second stage of labor and yet preserve the ability to push. Saddle block or epidural block confined to a T-10 level and pudendal block can provide good conditions for delivery of the breech. Whenever a breech delivery is attempted vaginally, the anesthesiologist must be prepared to pharmacologically relax the lower uterine segment in the event that the fetal head becomes trapped after delivery of the body. Traditionally, halogenated general inhalation anesthetics such as halothane have been used to provide reliable immediate relaxation of the lower uterine segment. However, as always in the obstetric patient, the transition to general anesthesia with attendant loss of airway reflexes requires either awake intubation or rapid sequence induction with endotracheal intubation.

Manual Removal of the Placenta

In the past, general anesthesia has been administered to provide uterine muscle relaxation in patients who require manual removal of a retained placenta within a firmly contracted uterus. More recently, intravenous nitroglycerine administered in a dose as low as 50 μg intravenously has been reported to provide uterine relaxation sufficient to permit placental extraction within 30 to 40 seconds after administration, thereby avoiding unnecessarily exposing the mother to the risk of aspiration pneumonitis associated with the induction of general anesthesia.

Multiple Gestations

Multiple gestations are associated with an increased risk of obstetric complications, as evidenced by increased fetal morbidity and mortality, most often associated with prematurity and malpresentation. Supine hypotension is more common with multiple gestations, and the parturient often demonstrates severe aortocaval compression because of the excessively enlarged uterus. Similarly, excessive displacement of the diaphragm cephalad by the enlarged uterus further decreases the functional residual capacity of the lungs beyond the normal physiologic changes of pregnancy, rendering the parturient with multiple gestations more susceptible to hypoxemia and dyspnea. Maintaining the patient in the left lateral decubitus position at all times is essential. Continuous lumbar epidural analgesia is the preferred technique to manage labor and delivery in the patient with multiple gestations because it allows better control of the delivery with a relaxed perineum, decreases the excessive work of the maternal cardiovascular system, and minimizes the exposure of possibly premature fetuses to depressant systemic medications while providing excellent pain relief. As the number of infants to be delivered increases, the need for version or extraction increases. One must be prepared to provide effective analgesia for these interventions as well as cesarean section after one or more of the infants has already been delivered by the vaginal route. Spinal anesthesia is usually avoided because of the increased incidence of maternal hypotension with multiple gestations. Both subarachnoid spread and epidural spread of local anesthetic are less predictable with multiple than with single gestations, and motor block may rapidly reach the high thoracic or cervical dermatomes with relatively lower doses or volumes of local anesthetic. The maintenance of a functioning epidural catheter during vaginal delivery for multiple gestations serves as a reassuring standby route to provide regional anesthesia for cesarean section, avoiding the need to administer a subarachnoid block or a general anesthetic.

SUGGESTED READING

Chestnut DH, et al. Continuous infusion during labor: a randomized, double-blind comparison of 0.0625% bupivacaine/0.0002% fentanyl versus 0.125% bupivacaine. Anesthesiology 1988; 68:754–759.

Gibbs CP, Krischer J, Peckham BM, et al. Obstetric anesthesia: a national survey. Anesthesiology 1986; 65:298–306.
Malinow AM, Ostheimer GW. Anesthesia for the high-risk parturient. Obstet Gynecol 1987; 69:951–964.
Ostheimer GW, ed. Obstetric analgesia and anaesthesia. Clin Anaesthesiol 1986.
Ralston DH, Schnider SM. The fetal and neonatal effects of regional anesthesia in obstetrics. Anesthesiology 1978; 48:34–64.

ELECTIVE CESAREAN SECTION

ROBERT A. ABRAHAM, M.D., F.A.C.A.

Cesarean section is the most frequently performed major obstetrical procedure, with an incidence of 10 to 25 percent in general, and as high as 30 percent in some high-risk perinatal centers and highly affluent parts of the United States. With present-day birth rates in this country approaching 4 million annually, this amounts to approximately 650,000 cesarean sections performed each year. This three- to fivefold increase in frequency over the past 30 years is the result of (1) previous cesarean sections; (2) the trend to avoid potentially harmful midforceps, breech, or twin vaginal deliveries; (3) the availability of modern biophysical and biochemical methods to detect fetuses at risk; (4) the prompt availability of safer anesthetic and surgical techniques; and (5) the ever-increasing threat of medical litigation.

Public health statistics reveal the risk of death due to delivery by cesarean section is two to ten times greater than with vaginal delivery, with the common causes of death being severe sepsis, thromboembolic episodes, and anesthesia. In general, rather than undergoing decreases similar to those achieved with other causes of obstetrical death, fatalities related to the administration of anesthesia have simply paralleled the overall reduction in pregnancy-related mortality. Here and abroad, this has resulted in raising anesthesia into the number three position of the most frequent causes of maternal mortality.

CHOICE OF ANESTHESIA

Since there is no one ideal method of anesthesia for elective cesarean section, the anesthesiologist must choose the method believed to be the safest and most comfortable for the patient, to be the least depressant to her infant, and to provide the optimum working conditions for the obstetrician. This choice, in turn, depends on the skill and experience of the anesthesiologist, the wishes of the patient and the infant's father, the indication for the operation, and the experience of the obstetrician in working with various anesthetic techniques.

The process begins with the preoperative visit by the anesthesiologist, wherein he has the opportunity to review the patient's chart, perform a cursory physical examination, and familiarize himself or herself with pertinent laboratory data. From this, the anesthesiologist becomes aware of any important illnesses, injuries, previous anesthetic mishaps or unpleasant experiences, the presence of drug sensitivities, or familial disorders that would have a bearing on the choice of anesthesia. Likewise, the physical examination should rule out not only significant cardiorespiratory disease, but also upper airway or spinal disorders that would pose a problem for either inhalation or conduction anesthesia. It is at this time that the patient and the infant's father should be allowed to express any special feelings with regard to the anesthesia and to ask pertinent questions. They should be given proper explanations in order to understand fully the procedure that is to take place, in order that they may give a better informed consent. Possible untoward reactions and complications should be discussed, along with the probability of blood transfusion and the patient's spouse being asked to leave the operating theater due to a failed regional block requiring general endotracheal anesthesia. It is an ideal time to emphasize the importance of fasting after midnight, the necessity for taking an antacid for premedication, and the value of the left lateral position to both herself and her unborn child when leaving her room for the operating theater. This close, direct physical and verbal contact before surgery can only lead to a better physician-patient relationship, both during the operation and afterward, should a misunderstanding or complication occur.

PERTINENT PHYSIOLOGIC CHANGES OF PREGNANCY

Because the many, subtle maternal physiologic changes occurring during pregnancy are beyond the scope of this chapter, only the more important changes that have a direct bearing on the anesthesia for cesarean section are discussed.

Cardiovascular

The three most important changes in the maternal cardiovascular system during pregnancy are (1) the increase in blood volume; (2) an increased cardiac output; and (3) aortocaval obstruction by the gravid uterus.

Maternal Blood Volume

Maternal blood volume increases progressively throughout pregnancy, commencing at approximately 12 weeks' gestation. The early rapid expansion of the plasma volume of 45 percent combined with a slower increase in the red cell mass by 20 percent leads to a near-term (28 to 32 weeks) total blood volume increase of 35 to 40 percent. The preponderant increase in plasma volume over red cell mass leads to a dilutional effect termed the "physiologic anemia of pregnancy." Even though this dilution is responsible for a decrease in maternal hematocrit at term of 10 percent or more (a hematocrit of 42 decreasing to 37 percent or less), the pregnant patient has more red cell mass to oxygenate and more blood volume for tissue perfusion and protection against hemorrhagic shock than the nonpregnant patient. The gradual increase of this blood volume and/or its sudden translocation from the periphery to the central circulation immediately postpartum can lead to either early or late cardiac decompensation in the pregnant patient with limited or decreased myocardial reserve. Likewise, careless overhydration and/or the indiscriminate use of the ecbolic agent methylergonovine maleate (Methergine) could have serious consequences on the circulation due to a sudden increase in either preload and/or afterload.

Increased Cardiac Output

An increase in cardiac output of some 30 to 40 percent is a reflection of the increased myocardial demand from the growing and highly metabolically active maternal, fetal, and uteroplacental tissues. Because uteroplacental perfusion is pressure dependent, any decrease in cardiac output brought about by depressant drugs or decreased venous return leading to a secondary decrease in blood pressure results in poor intervillous perfusion, thus putting the fetus in jeopardy.

Obviously, any moderate-to-severe lowering of maternal blood pressure poses a threat to her well-being and must be corrected immediately by restoring the cardiac output toward normal. This is accomplished by the judicious use of the proper intravenous fluids, left uterine displacement (LUD), and the intravenous administration of a mixed-type vasopressor, such as ephedrine sulfate.

Aortocaval Compression

Aortocaval compression by the enlarging gravid uterus takes place from 20 weeks' gestation up until the time of delivery, whenever the patient assumes the supine position. This obstruction to flow from the pelvis and lower extremities results in a decrease in venous return, stroke volume, and cardiac output. If compensation takes place via reflex vasoconstriction, there is little or no change in maternal blood pressure (concealed-type) and the patient remains asymptomatic (90 percent of cases), but uteroplacental perfusion suffers. If reflex vasoconstriction is short-lived or absent (10 percent of patients), profound hypotension ensues—manifested by a shocklike state (revealed-type) and is known as the *supine hypotensive syndrome*. Both concealed and revealed types of caval syndromes result in decreased uterine blood flow and are prevented or reversed by the left lateral tilt of the pelvis by 15 degrees or more or by a full left lateral decubitus position. A more subtle condition is that of lumbar aortic compression, which is believed by some authorities to be more common and important than caval obstruction. This leads to impaired uteroplacental perfusion and variable degrees of fetal acidosis that may result in fetal distress. Patients with large babies, twin gestations, and polyhydramnios are most at risk. Sympathetic denervation blocks the compensatory reflex vasoconstriction mechanism of the concealed-type patient, and therefore any pregnant woman who undergoes this procedure is at risk when the supine position is assumed during the latter half of pregnancy.

Respiratory

The enlarging uterus pushes upward on the diaphragm and outward on the lower thoracic rib cage, thus compressing the dependent lung tissue resulting in a decrease in both expiratory reserve volume and residual volume. A 20 percent decrease in functional residual capacity (FRC) places the pregnant patient at greater risk for hypoxemia because of a smaller reserve space for oxygen storage and leads to a more rapid induction when the patient is exposed to inhalation anesthetic agents, due to a smaller dilutional residual gas volume. Oxygen consumption increases by approximately 20 percent. At term, minute ventilation increases by 50 percent to meet the oxygen demands of the increased work of breathing. The oxygen requirements of both the mother and fetus can best be provided during elective cesarean section by ensuring an FIO_2 of 0.5 or more.

Gastrointestinal

These changes consist of decreased gastric motility, decreased gastric absorption and secretion, and decreased lower gastroesophageal sphincter tone. There is an increase in gastric acidity as well as intragastric pressure. This increase puts the pregnant patient at added risk for vomiting, regurgitation, and possible pulmonary aspiration, and demands the routine use of oral antacids, cricoid pressure, and a cuffed endotracheal tube whenever she is rendered unconscious. This serious situation should be circumvented by the use of regional or local anesthesia whenever possible. Chronic gastrointestinal disorders such as peptic ulcer, gastroesophageal reflux, and prolonged gastric emptying syndrome require special drug therapy such as treatment with ranitidine or cimetidine, and/or metoclopramide.

Central Nervous System

Progesterone and endorphins have been cited as having some neurotransmitter-like function, which may be responsible for such phenomena as (1) the decrease in minimal alveolar concentration (MAC) of inhalation anesthetics during pregnancy, as well as (2) the increased susceptibility of nerve tissue to local anesthetics, which makes the pregnant patient analgesic with lower doses of drug than her nonpregnant counterpart.

BASIC PREPARATORY STEPS FOR CESAREAN SECTION

Seven preparatory steps should be completed before each elective cesarean section.

1. Preoperative order check.
2. Prehydration.
3. Preoxygenation.
4. Proper positioning.
5. Proper monitoring.
6. Availability of proper drugs, solutions, and equipment ensured.
7. An experienced assistant is present.

The *preoperative order check* should prohibit oral intake after midnight; 30 ml of 0.3 molar sodium citrate should be given orally on-call to the delivery suite, and an additional 15 ml should be administered on entering the operating theater. The patient should assume the left lateral position en route to the delivery suite and thereafter until delivery. A large-bore 16-gauge plastic intravenous cannula should be inserted on the floor with 5 percent dextrose in lactated Ringer's solution to run at 150 ml per hour for daily hydration and energy purposes. Sedatives and tranquilizers are not routinely prescribed. A completed type and screen procedure from the blood bank and a properly signed consent form should be confirmed.

Prehydration should be carried out 15 to 20 minutes before induction of anesthesia by the intravenous administration of 20 ml per kilogram (1,200 to 2,000 ml) of plain lactated Ringer's solution to offset the decrease in cardiac output from sympathetic blockade or secondary to caval obstruction by the gravid uterus. This decrease in cardiac output, if not reversed promptly, will lead to moderate-to-severe maternal hypotension, decreased uterine blood flow, and fetal acidosis. Glucose-containing solutions are not to be used for rapid hydration, because of the resultant hypoglycemia it causes in the newborn secondary to a hyperinsulinemic state from excessive maternal-fetal glucose levels.

Preoxygenation should be carried out routinely upon arrival of the patient in the operating room by the administration of an 8- to 10-L flow of oxygen using a plastic mask–reservoir bag and nonrebreathing valve system. This provides for both a high-inspired oxygen concentration and a high maternal arterial oxygen pressure (PaO_2) with little chance of gastric distention. Fetal partial pressure of oxygen (PO_2) can be increased substantially by this maneuver, and at the same time, can lead to a decrease in the time to sustained respiration (TSR) of the infant at the time of delivery (Table 1).

Proper positioning requires a left lateral pelvic tilt of at least 15 degrees by the insertion of a wedge (two rolled bedsheets) under the patient's right hip and shoulder in an effort to displace the gravid uterus and its contents (weighing approximately 6.5 kg) from the lumbar portion of the inferior vena cava and aorta. Failure to do so leads to the previously described aortocaval syndrome with resultant fetal acidosis.

Proper monitoring requires a blood pressure cuff, precordial stethoscope, 4-lead electrocardiogram, and pulse oximeter for patients receiving a regional block. Patients undergoing general endotracheal anesthesia additionally require a nerve stimulator, an in-line oxygen meter, and an end-tidal carbon dioxide monitoring. Precordial Doppler monitoring for possible air embolism is not routinely carried out at present; however, continuous fetal heart rate monitoring is performed up until the abdominal preparation is begun.

Proper drugs, solutions, and equipment must be available at all times in the operative delivery room (the isolated obstetric anesthesiologist has no time to be searching for emergency items in the midst of a crisis). Each operating room should be stocked (so as to be

Table 1 The Clinical Condition of Newborn Infants Improved with Increasing Inspired Oxygen Concentration

F_{IO_2}	T.S.R. (sec)	1-Minute Apgar ≤ 7
Low (0.28-0.33)	57 ± 8	12/25
Medium (0.66)	19 ± 3*	4/25
High (0.93-0.87)	12 ± 3*	2/25

*$p < 0.001$ vs low.
Mean ± S.E.M.
Modified with permission from Marx GF, et al. Can Anaesth Soc J 1971; 18:587.

self-sufficient) with special drugs such as diazepam, ketamine, droperidol, fentanyl, mephentermine, phenylephrine, and methylergonovine maleate, as well as the standard items such as ephedrine, atropine, succinylcholine chloride, curare, pancuronium, thiopental sodium, oxytocin (Pitocin), and anticholinesterases. All items should be clearly labeled and kept in their individual places. Special solutions should include 5 and 25 percent albumin solutions, artificial colloid solution (hetastarch) and 50 percent glucose solution, as well as routine fluids such as lactated Ringer's solution, 5 percent dextrose in water, and normal saline. A properly working anesthesia machine, suction apparatus, and six-way tilt operating table should be accompanied by a self-inflating bag-mask system and a ready-assembled emergency transtracheal jet ventilation kit stored in the operating room. A blood warming and pressure infusor system should likewise be readily available. A fiberoptic bronchoscope, tracheotomy set, and a cardiac defibrillator should be kept close by (although not necessarily in the operating room).

An experienced assistant should be present at every cesarean section to assist in the routine set-up, monitoring, and support of the patient during a block, applying cricoid pressure during tracheal intubation and lending psychological and moral support to the patient as required. Preferably, this should be an anesthetist, although it may also be a nursing personnel staff member, if properly trained and supervised by the obstetric anesthesiologist.

METHODS OF ANESTHESIA

Subarachnoid Block

According to a recent survey by the American College of Obstetrics and Gynecology, the subarachnoid block (spinal) is the most frequently performed method of anesthesia for cesarean section, despite the increasing popularity of epidural anesthesia worldwide. The large experience gained over the past 40 years has attested to the safety of this technique for both mother and infant. The improved methods of prophylaxis and/or treatment of significant hypotension following sympathetic denervation and aortocaval obstruction, along with the high success rate of an epidural blood patch in the treatment of postdural puncture headache, have led to a greater appreciation and the continued utilization of this valuable method of anesthesia.

Advantages of subarachnoid block include the following:

1. The patient is conscious with protective reflexes.
2. Mother and father may enjoy the birthing process together.
3. There is minimal fetal drug exposure.
4. It is simple to perform.
5. Induction of anesthesia is moderately rapid.
6. The technique is reliable.

7. Postpartum morbidity is usually less than with general anesthesia.

Disadvantages of subarachnoid block are as follows:

1. Moderate-to-severe hypotension is common.
2. Postspinal headache is possible.
3. The technique is not easily repeated if deficient.

Contraindications include the following:

1. Patient refusal.
2. Hypovolemia, dehydration, or severe anemia.
3. Coagulation disorders.
4. Local sepsis in lower lumbar area or generalized sepsis not covered by systemic antibiotics.
5. Active neurologic disease.
6. Severe orthopedic deformity.
7. Proven sensitivity to all local anesthetic agents.

Outline of Method for Subarachnoid Block

1. Carry out the previously outlined seven basic preparatory steps in the operating room while monitoring fetal heart rate.

2. Using a small 25- to 27-gauge spinal needle, perform a spinal tap with the patient under local anesthesia in the lateral decubitus position at L2-3 or L3-4 interspace with the aid of a 20-gauge introducer. A puncture parallel to the dural fibers is emphasized.

3. Hyperbaric tetracaine, 6 to 10 mg, or hyperbaric lidocaine, 50 to 80 mg, in dextrose solution with 0.2 mg of fresh epinephrine should be mixed thoroughly and injected over 12 seconds. For additional postoperative analgesia of 18 to 24 hours' duration, add 0.2 to 0.3 mg of preservative-free morphine sulfate to the above-mentioned local anesthetic solution.

4. Immediately after the injection has been completed the patient should be assisted onto her back and a wedge placed under the right hip and shoulder. Blood pressure should be checked every minute and oxygen administered until delivery or longer.

5. The sensory level is checked every 30 seconds to needle prick until a solid T-10 block occurs (usually within 2 to 3 minutes). Flex table into the reverse jackknife position with the patient flexed at the hips with the head and feet *slightly* elevated. This preserves the blood pressure by maintaining the venous return and at the same time limits the spread of the local anesthetic agent to the T4-6 level; this has been found to be most satisfactory for cesarean section.

6. For a decrease in blood pressure to 100 mm Hg, treat with an increased fluid load, more left uterine displacement, and repeated 10-mg doses of intravenous ephedrine sulfate. Bradycardia (heart rate <60 beats per minute) is treated with intravenous atropine. A blood pressure not responding to a second intravenous dose of ephedrine sulfate is treated with 100-μg doses of phenylephrine (Neo-Synephrine) intravenously.

7. After the delivery of the infant and placenta,

uterine bleeding is controlled by vigorous uterine massage and by adding 20 U of oxytocin to 500 ml of lactated Ringer's solution which is run in rapidly until efective. Administration of bolus intravenous oxytocin is to be condemned because of its marked vasodilating properties, which may cause a severe drop in blood pressure. Methylergonovine maleate (Methergine) is used only when absolutely necessary due to its generalized, intense vasoconstrictive action, which can cause severe hypertension, coronary spasm, or congestive heart failure.

8. Substernal and/or epigastric discomfort from peritoneal traction following delivery is treated with intravenous diazepam or droperidol combined with a narcotic (fentanyl), as well as oxygen inhalation. Close electrocardiographic monitoring at this time is mandatory in order to detect any ischemic changes.

9. Blood loss is replaced with lactated Ringer's solution at a ratio of 2:1. Losses approaching 4 U are treated with colloid and/or whole blood.

10. Bladder catheter remains in place until the block wears off.

11. Handle the patient gently in moving her from the operating table after surgery. To avoid sudden drops in blood pressure that cause nausea and vomiting, elevate the foot of the patient's bed before transfer.

12. Any additional postoperative pain relief can be obtained by enrolling the patient in the department's *intravenous* Patient-Controlled Analgesia (PCA) program.

Complications

The high incidence of hypotension (80 percent) can be reduced to approximately 25 percent by the liberal use of fluids preoperatively (20 ml per kilogram), proper positioning, and small, 10-mg doses of ephedrine sulfate administered intravenously along with preoxygenation. Persistent hypotension is usually caused by caval obstruction and/or bradycardia from sympathetic interruption and responds to repositioning and/or intravenous atropine and leg elevation. Any hypotension persisting after these added maneuvers requires 100-µg doses of phenylephrine administered intravenously for immediate correction. This has been shown to have no deleterious fetal effects in humans. The prompt, aggressive treatment of a lowered blood pressure (i.e., a systolic blood pressure <100 mm Hg) practically eliminates nausea and vomiting.

Postspinal headache is caused by the lowering of cerebrospinal fluid pressure from leakage of spinal fluid through the dural puncture site and is related to such factors as needle size, number of dural punctures, angle of dural rent, and state of hydration. The high incidence during pregnancy (22 percent using a 22-gauge spinal needle) can be reduced dramatically (to 3 to 6 percent) by the use of a 25- or 26-gauge spinal needle, liberal hydration, and prophylactic use of abdominal binders. Definite diagnosis is made by a history of a dural tap, a postural-type headache, and a positive "SEPT" sign (*sitting epigastric pressure test*). Headaches last an average of 5 to 7 days and respond readily to mild analgesics, forced fluids, and proper application of two firm abdominal binders applied from the xiphoid to the pubic bone for duration of symptoms. Ambulation is encouraged. If symptoms do not improve by Day 4 following a negative neurologic examination to rule out other serious causes of persistent headache, the afebrile patient is offered an epidural blood patch, which invariably provides prompt relief.

Excessively high or total spinal block is an uncommon but highly serious complication of subarachnoid anesthesia. The most common cause by far is an excessive amount of solute and/or volume of local anesthetic drug for the term pregnant state. Early diagnosis is made by detecting sensory loss in the upper extremities spreading to the deltoid area, followed by loss of hand grip strength. Later, difficulty in speaking and coughing, as well as restricted spontaneous breathing supervenes due to a markedly diminished vital capacity as measured by the machine's ventilometer and/or decreased bag movement during spontaneous respiration. Emergency treatment requires immediate cricoid pressure, followed by oxygenation and positive-pressure ventilation via cuffed endotracheal tube under light thiopental sodium/succinylcholine chloride anesthesia. Adequate perfusion pressure necessary for mother and fetus is maintained by administering intravenous ephedrine and more fluids and by placing the mother in the Trendelenburg position with LUD to ensure an adequate venous return and effective cardiac output. Prompt delivery is essential.

Epidural Block

This method of anesthesia has become increasingly popular for elective cesarean sections because of the introduction of more potent anesthetic agents with effect of varying duration, the in-depth study of the physiologic effects of epidural blocks, the possibility of redosing, the marked reduction in the occurrence of postspinal headache, and the use of epidural PCA for postoperative pain relief. Patients seem to be attracted to the long-lasting effects of a catheter technique and the strange, new name that does not remind them of the word "spinal" or of the possible complication of headache.

Advantages of epidural block include the following:

1. Less maternal hypotension.
2. Dural puncture headache is practically eliminated.
3. Greater versatility because of use of continuous catheter technique for pain relief, both during surgery and postoperatively.
4. Less motor weakness initially, and thus preservation of respiratory activity.
5. The patient is conscious with protective reflexes.
6. Mother and father may enjoy the birthing process together.
7. Postpartum morbidity is usually less than with general anesthesia.

8. The technique allows epidural PCA postoperatively.

Disadvantages of epidural block are as follows:

1. The technique is more complex to perform and maintain.
2. Onset is slower.
3. Large doses of local anesthetic agent are required, with possible adverse fetal effects.
4. There is a constant threat of a massive accidental intravenous or intrathecal injection of local anesthetic.

Contraindications include the following:

1. Patient refusal.
2. Local sepsis at injection site or generalized sepsis if not covered by systemic antibiotics.
3. Coagulation disorders.
4. Active neurologic disease.
5. Severe orthopedic deformities
6. Hypovolemia, severe dehydration, or marked anemia
7. Proven sensitivity to all local anesthetic agents

Outline of Technique

1. Follow the seven preparatory steps previously presented for elective cesarean section.

2. Use stronger concentrations of local anesthetic drugs for more dense analgesia and muscle relaxation: 2 percent lidocaine with 1:200,000 fresh epinephrine (preferred agent), 3 percent 2-chloroprocaine hydrochloride, or 0.5 percent bupivacaine without epinephrine.

3. After placement of a 17-gauge Tuohy epidural needle in the epidural space at the L3-4 interspace via a loss of resistance technique, inject 3 ml of the chosen local anesthetic agent through the needle and observe its effects for 3 minutes. Observe possible sudden onset of an increased heart rate (i.e., a heart rate increase >20 beats per minute), and/or a sudden increase in blood pressure (i.e., >20 mm Hg), both indicating an intravascular needle. An abrupt sensory loss in the lower extremities indicates intrathecal trespass.

4. If no such response occurs, inject an additional 15 to 20 ml of a local anesthetic slowly in 5-ml divided doses, pausing for 30 seconds between each injection in order to detect any untoward reaction.

5. Without delay, insert a Teflon radiopaque epidural catheter 2 cm cephalad into the epidural space and tape securely in place (after catheter patency is verified by the injection of 1 ml of sterile preservative-free saline solution through the catheter).

6. Turn the patient supine on the operating table with a wedge under the right hip and shoulder. Administer oxygen by a mask-reservoir bag at 8 to 10 L per minute.

7. Promptly verify epidural catheter position by administering a test dose, such as 2 ml of a *Hopkins hyperbaric epidural test dose solution* (1.5 percent lidocaine in 7.5 percent dextrose) with 15 μg of fresh epinephrine. This solution will detect an intravenous catheter by producing within 1 minute an increase in heart rate of more than 20 beats per minute and/or a simultaneous increase in systolic blood pressure of more than 20 mm Hg. The accidental placement of an intrathecal catheter will be detected by the rapid onset of analgesia to pinprick at the S_2 dermatome within 2 minutes, due to the marked hyperbaricity of this special test dose solution.

8. Check vital signs and monitors every minute for 20 minutes or until delivery. Treat decreases in blood pressure to 100 mm Hg promptly with bolus intravenous fluids, 10-mg doses of intravenous ephedrine, and increased LUD.

9. A sensory level to T4-6 is desirable. After 20 minutes, levels below this can be driven higher by injecting an additional 2 ml of local anesthetic solution per segment difference.

10. Administer reinforcing doses of 10 to 12 ml of additional local agent every 40 minutes for 2-chloroprocaine hydrochloride and every 80 minutes for lidocaine and bupivacaine.

11. After delivery of the infant and placenta, administer oxytocin rapidly via an intravenous infusion by adding 20 U of oxytocin to 500 ml of lactated Ringer's solution. The use of bolus oxytocin is to be condemned since it can cause a precipitous decrease in blood pressure, leading to sudden cardiovascular collapse, especially during a high regional block.

12. After cord clamping, add 100 μg of fentanyl (2 ml) via epidural catheter to smooth out the analgesia during abdominal closure.

13. Administer intravenous diazepam, droperidol, and/or fentanyl for traction pain or anxiety (observe electro-cardiogram closely for any ischemic changes after the paient's complaint of traction pain).

14. Blood loss is replaced at a ratio of 2:1 with lactated Ringer's solution. Losses approaching 4 U or more are treated with colloid and/or whole blood.

15. Move the patient gently to her bed from the operating table at the conclusion of the operation to avoid hypotension, nausea, and vomiting. To preserve blood pressure, elevate the foot of the bed in transporting the patient to the recovery room.

16. Retain epidural catheter in place postoperatively for administration of narcotics via a PCA program.

Complications

Hypotension following epidural anesthesia occurs less frequently but just as severely as with subarachnoid block; however, the blood pressure decrease with the patient under epidural block responds to routine treatment more readily. Treatment must still be prompt and relies on the "basic three": liberal use of intravenous fluids; LUD; and intravenous ephedrine sulfate and/or phenylephrine.

The incidence of *postdural puncture headache* following dural puncture with a 17-gauge epidural needle runs as high as 75 percent without prophylactic treatment. This can be reduced to 10 to 25 percent by the injection through the epidural catheter of preservative-free sterile saline solution, 30 to 60 ml every 6 hours for 24 hours, along with ensuring adequate hydration. In addition, we advocate firm abdominal binding for 48 hours to maintain cerebrospinal fluid pressure, and for its *antidiuretic effect*. Patients whose headaches get worse or do not improve by the fourth postpartum day are offered an epidural blood patch, which promptly relieves the headache.

An accidental intravenous injection of a large amount of local anesthetic can be avoided if, prior to any injection of the drug, a test dose containing 15 µg epinephrine is properly administered. An exception would be a patient treated with beta-blockers, but even then, an elevated blood pressure should be detected. Signs and symptoms of local anesthetic toxicity are dose dependent and can range from mild excitement to convulsions and/or total cardiovascular collapse with cardiac arrest.

Accidental intrathecal injection should occur only after misplacement of an epidural catheter or one that has migrated with postural change. Proper use of a special test-dose solution that is *hyperbaric* to cerebral spinal fluid will detect an intrathecal catheter within 2 minutes by producing prompt, perineal analgesia at the S_2 dermatome, which the usual, relatively isobaric test dose solutions do not do consistently (i.e., they are not heavy enough in cerebrospinal fluid to "fall" to the sacral roots within 2 minutes). Signs and symptoms of subarachnoid injection are volume/solute-dependent and may result in high or even total spinal anesthesia.

General Anesthesia

General anesthesia for cesarean delivery has changed over the past 30 years because of (1) the advent of newer inhalation anesthetic agents (halothane, enflurane, and isoflurane), and ultra short-acting induction agents (thiopental and ketamine); (2) the introduction of light, balanced anesthesia; and (3) reliable research studies showing little difference in fetal outcome between the use of general and regional anesthesia if performed in a meticulous, regimented manner utilizing adequate prehydration, preoxygenation, LUD, restricted drug doses, and liberal inhaled oxygen concentrations of at least 50 percent or more (Tables 2 and 3).

The advantages of general anesthesia include the following:

1. Rapid induction.
2. Cardiovascular depression (hypotension) is uncommon.
3. Greater controllability.
4. High reliability.
5. The technique can be used in cases of active

Table 2 Maternal and Fetal Blood PO_2 Analysis During Anesthesia (1977)

	Epidural Anesthesia (mm Hg)	General Anesthesia (mm Hg)
Maternal control PaO_2	92 ± 10	92 ± 9
Maternal delivery PO_2	326 ± 84	249 ± 51*
Umbilical vein PO_2	38 ± 7	42 ± 7
Umbilical artery PO_2	22 ± 5	26 ± 8

*$p < 0.001$ vs epidural anesthesia.
Mean ± S.D.
Modified with permission from Fox GS, et al. AM J Obstet Gynecol 1979; 133:15-19.

Table 3 Comparison of Fetal Blood Gas Analysis Following General Anesthesia for Elective Cesarean Section (1977 vs 1971)

	1977	1971
Umbilical vein		
PO_2 (mm Hg)	42.0 ± 7.0*	24.0 ± 11.0
pH	7.35 ± 0.03*	7.28 ± 0.01
PCO_2 (mm Hg)	40.0 ± 4.0†	45.0 ± 7.0
Base deficit (mEq/L)	3.4 ± 1.6*	6.8 ± 3.0
Umbilical artery		
PO_2 (mm Hg)	26.0 ± 8.0*	14.0 ± 8.0
pH	7.31 ± 0.03*	7.22 ± 0.07
PCO_2 (mm Hg)	46.0 ± 5.0‡	51.0 ± 9.0
Base deficit (mEq/L)	3.9 ± 1.5*	8.1 ± 3.4

*$p < 0.001$ vs 1971
†$p < 0.01$ vs 1971
‡$p < 0.05$ vs 1971
Mean ± S.D.
Modified with permission from Fox G.S., et al. AM J Obstet Gynecol 1979; 133:15-19.

bleeding, neurologic disease, and increased intracranial pressure.

The disadvantages of general anesthesia are as follows:

1. The patient is unconscious without protective reflexes.
2. Pulmonary aspiration is possible.
3. It is associated with airway problems of failed intubation and poor airway.
4. Drug-induced fetal depression is possible.
5. Maternal awareness is possible.

Outline of Technique

1. Carry out previously mentioned seven basic preparatory steps for elective cesarean section.
2. Administer 0.2 mg of glycopyrrolate or 0.4 mg of atropine, and 3 mg of curare or 1 mg of pancuronium intravenously within 5 minutes of induction.
3. Perform preoxygenation 3 to 4 minutes at high flow rates (i.e., 8 to 10 L per minute with expiratory valve open full).
4. An assistant should be available to apply cricoid

pressure just before induction until the trachea is sealed by a cuffed endotracheal tube.

5. When the surgeon is ready, administer 4 mg per kilogram of thiopental (or 1 mg per kilogram of ketamine) along with 1.5 mg per kilogram of succinylcholine chloride intravenously for induction of anesthesia and intubation.

6. Avoid positive-pressure ventilation until the trachea is securely sealed by a cuffed endotracheal tube.

7. Administer nitrous oxide (5 L per minute) plus oxygen (5 L per minute) plus halothane 0.5 percent (or enflurane 1 percent or 0.75 percent isoflurane) via a semi-closed circle system.

8. Avoid excessive maternal hyperventilation.

9. Monitor maternal vital signs regularly.

10. After the umbilical cord is clamped, deepen anesthesia with 70 percent nitrous oxide in oxygen, narcotics, or barbiturates; volatile agents are usually discontinued unless uterine relaxation is deemed necessary. Further abdominal relaxation is obtained by a continuous infusion of 0.05 percent succinylcholine chloride or 4 mg of pancuronium administered intravenously.

11. Administer oxytocic drugs by intravenous infusion, not by bolus injection.

12. After relaxant reversal, extubate patient awake with protective reflexes present and an adequate measured vital capacity.

13. Place patient in an *intravenous* PCA program for 24-hour postoperative pain relief.

Complications

Maternal aspiration syndrome is avoided or lessened by (1) NPO status 8 hours before induction of anesthesia; (2) administering clear antacids in order to raise the gastric pH above 2.5 (15 to 30 ml of 0.3 molar sodium citrate administered 1 hour before induction and upon entering the operating theater); (3) administering anticholinergic drugs (atropine, glycopyrolate) to decrease gastric secretion and increase gastric pH; (4) in special situations (hiatus hernia, severe heartburn, peptic ulcer), administer histamine$_2$-receptor antagonists (cimetidine or ranitidine) to inhibit gastric secretion and increase gastric pH, along with metoclopramide to facilitate gastric emptying and to increase the tone of the lower esophageal sphincter; and (5) an assistant applying constant cricoid pressure during each attempt at intubation.

Difficult airway management manifests itself as either failure to intubate or inability to ventilate the patient. During an elective procedure, the inability to intubate the trachea requires that the patient be awakened and the procedure be performed at a later time through the use of an awake intubation or a regional block. On the other hand, impaired ventilation and oxygenation during induction requires immediate attention. One must not wait until cyanosis, bradycardia, and cardiac arrest occur. If the anesthesia is light, the patient should be awakened and the problem evaluated further. On the

other hand, if anesthesia is deeper and recovery would be prolonged, an improved airway must be secured via the use of a fiberoptic bronchoscope, or through the application of transtracheal jet ventilation through a cricoid stick or an emergency tracheotomy.

Neonatal depression can be caused by maternal ventilation abnormalities and reduced placental perfusion caused by aortocaval compression. Both of these situations can be relieved by moderate hyperventilation of the mother and by assuring LUD at all times. Pharmacologic causes of neonatal depression include the use of excessive amounts of induction agents, neuromuscular blockers, nitrous oxide, volatile inhalation agents, as well as low-oxygen concentrations. This can be prevented by a meticulous technique using rigid control of induction agents, intermittent muscle relaxants, oxygen concentrations of 50 percent or better, no more than 50 percent nitrous oxide at any one time, and two-thirds MAC of any potent volatile inhalation agent. The effect of prolonged induction and delivery times can be minimized by delivering the infant within 90 seconds of the uterine incision and avoiding excessive hyperventilation.

Maternal awareness is a major problem if moderate concentrations of weak anesthetic agents (e.g., nitrous oxide) are used to minimize neonatal effects. The incidence of recall has been reported to range from 6 to 27 percent. Use of low concentrations of potent volatile anesthetic agents successfully prevents awareness and recall without ill effects to mother or fetus, as do small doses of diazepam or scopolamine used (although less effectively) as premedicants.

Local Infiltration

This almost forgotten method of anesthesia is presented last but not least in order to (1) stress its importance in the armamentarium of both the anesthesiologist and the obstetrician; and (2) advocate its increased use and application during elective cesarean section in those special situations of maternal and/or fetal deterioration in which time and immediate surgery are of the utmost importance and yet in which, by every reasonable assessment, both general and regional anesthesia are relatively contraindicated or impossible. Most obstetricians have had little or no experience with this technique since they have rarely, if ever, been called upon to use it. Consequently, when it is indicated, local infiltration anesthesia is often done improperly and the patient experiences undue pain, becoming uncooperative during the operation and eventually requiring general endotracheal anesthesia, or develops a systemic toxic reaction from too large a volume and/or concentration of a local anesthetic. This technique is recommended for only those who have had previous instruction or experience in its proper use. The obstetrician must be cautioned to use the more dilute solutions of local anesthetics, such as 1 percent 2-chloroprocaine hydrochloride, 0.5 percent lidocaine, or 0.25 percent bupivacaine. These concentrations produce prompt and adequate analgesia and permit the use of as much as 100 ml of solution with little or no risk of maternal systemic reaction or fetal depression.

The advantages of local infiltration include the following:

1. A "clutch" anesthetic technique (lifesaving).
2. A conscious patient with protective reflexes.
3. Minimal fetal drug effect.
4. The technique is simple to perform.
5. The technique is easily mastered.
6. Relative safety in use.
7. Little equipment is required.
8. The technique may be repeated.
9. Reliability when properly performed.

The disadvantages of local infiltration are as follows:

1. It is not appreciated.
2. It is not properly mastered.
3. Incomplete analgesia for the patient.
4. Onset is too slow for obstetricians.
5. Little or no muscle relaxation is provided.
6. Toxic overdose is possible.
7. Supplemental general anesthesia may be required.

Contraindications include the following:

1. Proven sensitivity to all local anesthetic agents.
2. Wild, disoriented, or mentally retarded patient.
3. Uncooperative obstetrician.

Outline of Technique

1. As time permits, explain the reason for and the course of action of the technique to the patient.

2. Recheck the security of the intravenous line, whether oral antacids have been administered recently, whether there is uterine displacement, and whether an experienced assistant is present.

3. Constantly reassure patient as the procedure progresses. Apply oxygen mask.

4. Administer a sedative-analgesic mixture of 2.5 mg of droperidol and 50 µg of fentanyl intravenously. Repeat dose if necessary.

5. Caution obstetrician on the use of limited quantities of dilute local anesthetic solutions.

6. To ensure relative patient comfort (only pressure should be felt), advise obstetrician to place a linear bead of local anesthetic drug wherever he plans to incise the skin and the subcutaneous, fascial, peritoneal, and myometrial tissues.

7. If pain is still intense, administer 10 to 15 mg of ketamine intravenously every 3 to 5 minutes to a total dose of 50 mg. Reassure patient constantly to minimize unpleasant dreams and maintain voice contact.

8. Following delivery of infant and placenta, and after control of bleeding, a more potent analgesic may be administered or general endotracheal anesthesia may be induced in a more calm, controlled manner, if not contraindicated.

Complications

Toxic overdose of a local anesthetic agent is manifested early by restlessness, excitability, and somnolence, and later by muscular twitching, seizures, and/or coma. Treatment is directed early toward seizure prevention and control with small doses of diazepam intravenously and later with cardiorespiratory support through positive-pressure oxygenation via a cuffed endotracheal tube and the use of intravenous ephedrine, especially if bupivacaine has been used.

Medicolegal action is sometimes taken by a disgruntled mother who claims undue suffering from excessive pain or being too amnestic to enjoy the birthing process. Full disclosure of the facts to the patient before the planned procedure and reasonableness should prevail, especially in light of obtaining a healthy infant. As so appropriately stated by the late J. Selwyn Crawford of Great Britain (1984), "the mother is undoubtedly likely to feel some discomfort during the entire operative procedure, but that is a small price to pay for the life of herself and her baby. The technique was in common use among obstetricians three to four decades ago before the availability of reasonably safe general anesthesia became widespread. *The technique must be relearned by the new generation of obstetricians because it is a life-saving method.* Just as no trainee anesthetist can be deemed worthy of undertaking full responsibility for the care of patients without being able to cope promptly and correctly with a failed intubation, so no trainee obstetrician can be deemed worthy of achieving similar status without demonstrating the capacity to perform, expediously and successfully, local infiltration analgesia for cesarean section."

SUGGESTED READING

Abraham RA, Harris AP, et al. The efficacy of 1.5 lidocaine with 7.5 dextrose and epinephrine as an epidural test dose for obstetrics. Anesthesiology 1986; 64:116–119.

Albright GA, et al. Anesthesia in obstetrics. 2nd ed. Boston: Butterworth, 1986.

Crawford JS. Obstetric analgesia and anaesthesia. 2nd ed. New York: Churchill-Livingstone, 1984.

Datta S, Alper MH. Anesthesia for cesarean section. Anesthesiology 1980; 50:142–160.

Ferrante FM, Ostheimer GW, Covino BG. Patient-controlled analgesia. Boston: Blackwell Scientific Publications, 1990.

Handler JS, Bromage PR. Venous air embolism during cesarean delivery. Reg Anaesth 1990; 15:170–171.

Ostheimer G.W. Manual of obstetric anesthesia. New York: Churchill-Livingstone, 1984.

Palmer CM, et al. Incidence of electrocardiographic changes during cesarean delivery under regional anesthesia. Anesth Analg 1990; 70:36–43.

Ralston DH, Shnider SM. The fetal and neonatal effects of regional anesthesia in obstetrics. Anesthesiology 1978; 48:34–64.

Zuckerman RL. Options in post-cesarean section pain relief. Anesth Rep 1989; 2:44–51.

EMERGENCY CESAREAN SECTION

ANDREW P. HARRIS, M.D.

According to studies of perinatal maternal mortality, anesthesia is a leading cause of death, and the majority of maternal deaths attributable to anesthesia occur during emergency cesarean sections. This is true even though emergency cesarean sections account for only a very small percentage of the total number of deliveries. The magnitude of the increased risk involved makes it incumbent that the practicing anesthesiologist understand the indications and the underlying physiology and pathophysiology, and master the anesthetic management of emergency cesarean section patients as well as the basic principles of resuscitating depressed newborns.

CATEGORIES OF EMERGENCY CESAREAN SECTION

For the purpose of this chapter, emergency cesarean sections will be defined as all cesarean sections that are not performed on a scheduled elective basis. Patients undergoing emergency cesarean section should be considered different from those undergoing elective cesarean section in that they may not have been NPO for a long period of time, they may not have had a comprehensive preanesthesia evaluation, and they may have unstable maternal and/or fetal physiology.

Before one can begin any discussion of appropriate anesthesia management, emergency cesarean section itself needs to be defined. The umbrella term *emergency cesarean section* can actually be subdivided into several categories. As will be shown, the distinctions among categories become extremely important when one is formulating anesthetic plans. The categories of emergency cesarean section include *stable* emergency cesarean sections, *urgent* emergency cesarean sections, and finally, *stat* emergency cesarean sections. The critical choice of the lowest-risk anesthetic plan consistent with the needs of the patient rests on this categorization of the urgency of the cesarean section (Table 1).

Stable Emergency Cesarean Section

The first category, stable emergency cesarean section, includes those situations in which the underlying maternal and fetal physiology is stable but in which a cesarean section nonetheless needs to be performed before destabilization occurs. Examples include patients presenting to the Labor and Delivery Suite after a nonreactive nonstress test (NST), a positive oxytocin challenge test (OCT) or contraction stress test (CST), or a low biophysical profile score. Although these tests do not indicate that a fetus is at *immediate* risk, such patients usually undergo cesarean section on the same day that these tests are performed. Another example might be the patient who presents with a fetus in the breech presentation and with ruptured membranes but who is not in active labor. Although the fetus is stable, cord prolapse or labor leading to entrapment of the fetal head during vaginal delivery might occur. Likewise, the patient who has undergone a previous lower segment transverse cesarean section and who now presents to the labor and delivery suite with ruptured membranes and/or in active labor is considered a stable emergency cesarean section.

Urgent Emergency Cesarean Section

The second category of emergency cesarean sections are those termed urgent. These are performed in

Table 1 Categories of Emergency Cesarean Section

Category	Examples	Preferred Anesthetic
Stable	Chronic uteroplacental insufficiency Malpresentation with ruptured membranes (not in labor) Previous lower segment cesarean section even in labor	Epidural, spinal
Urgent	Failure to progress Active herpes with rupture of membranes Nonbleeding placenta previa in labor Placental abruption without fetal distress Severe pre-eclampsia Chorioamnionitis Previous classical cesarean section in active labor Cord prolapse without fetal distress	Epidural (extended from labor), spinal
Stat	Agonal fetal distress Cord prolapse with fetal distress Massive hemorrhage Ruptured uterus	General, local, epidural (if T10 or higher level is present)

situations in which the underlying physiology is unstable but not immediately life-threatening to the mother or fetus (i.e., there is no fetal distress). Examples of indications for urgent cesarean section would include failure to progress, failed forceps delivery, ruptured membranes with active vaginal herpes, nonbleeding placenta previa in labor, placental abruption without fetal distress, severe worsening pre-eclampsia, chorio-amnionitis, or previous classical cesarean section in active labor. However, as long as neither fetal distress nor an immediate threat to maternal well-being are present, these situations do not fall into the next, highest priority category—stat cesarean sections. However, urgent cesarean sections need to be performed in a more timely manner than stable emergency cesarean sections.

Stat Emergency Cesarean Sections

Finally and rarely, there are true *stat* emergency cesarean sections. These are performed in situations in which continued in utero pregnancy would be immediately life-threatening for the mother and/or fetus. Such situations include severe agonal fetal distress, cord prolapse with any signs of fetal distress, massive maternal hemorrhage (whether from a placenta previa or a placental abruption), or a ruptured uterus. In such circumstances, operative delivery must be accomplished as soon as safely possible.

PREOPERATIVE PREPARATION

Because one can never predict in which patient an emergency cesarean section will need to be performed, there are certain basic preparations and precautions that need to be taken for all patients in the labor and delivery suite. Such preparations include a fully equipped cesarean section room immediately available at all times, prior placement of intravenous access, preoperative anesthesia assessment, and a blood specimen in the blood bank for blood typing and antibody screening.

Operating Room Set-Up

The anesthesiologist should equip the cesarean section operating room in such a way that an emergency anesthetic could be delivered within minutes. This means that drugs, airway equipment, suction, regional anesthesia trays, and emergency equipment (e.g., blood-warming devices, pressure infusion systems) must be ready for use. Drugs that should be available (and preferably drawn up) include a short-acting barbiturate, ketamine, succinylcholine chloride, atropine, and ephedrine. Phenylephrine, lidocaine, and an intermediate-duration nondepolarizing agent (atracurium besylate or vecuronium bromide) should be readily available but need not necessarily be drawn up. Sodium citrate (or another antacid) should be stocked in the operating room for oral administration just prior to anesthesia. The postpartum oxytocin infusion, if prepared before-

hand, should be well labeled. Methylergonovine maleate and prostaglandin methyl-$F_{2\alpha}$ may become necessary if uterine atony that is unresponsive to oxytocin occurs after delivery of the placenta. Otherwise, drugs should be available as in any other operating room in which general and major regional anesthesia are administered. For spinal and epidural anesthetics, trays and a variety of spinal needles should be stocked in the operating room, as well as a variety of local anesthetics appropriate for both spinal and epidural anesthesia.

Airway equipment in the operating room should include a checked functioning anesthesia machine, a variety of laryngoscope handles and blades, oropharyngeal and nasopharyngeal airways, bronchodilators (and the equipment to administer them), and transtracheal ventilation equipment as well as a back-up Ambu bag system. The anesthesia machine should be checked daily and after the use of every anesthetic. The machine should be similar to the anesthesia machine used elsewhere in the hospital, so that no confusion regarding the machine and its workings occur in an emergency. A short laryngoscope handle (Fig. 1) might be very useful in intubating pregnant patients, particularly those with large breasts. A variety of blades (including a No. 2 and No. 3 Miller, and a No. 3 and No. 4 MacIntosh blade), nasal and oral airways, and an assortment of masks of different sizes should be stocked in the operating room. Since the risk of vomiting and aspiration is higher in pregnant patients, it may be preferable to use clear face masks instead of black opaque masks, so that vomiting can be detected more easily if it occurs. A cuffed stiletted 6.5- or 7-mm tube should be checked and ready, and even smaller tubes should be kept nearby. Finally, equipment for emergency cricothyrotomy and transtracheal ventilation should be conveniently available in the

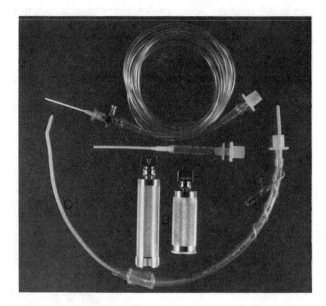

Figure 1 Emergency airway equipment available for wse in the obstetric operating room. *A*, cricothyrotomy ventilation sets; *B*, assorted laryngoscope handeles, including a short handle; *C*, a flexible intubating stylet.

operating room. A simple device would include a No. 14 gauge or larger cannula, a 3-cc syringe with the plunger removed, and a 7-mm endo-tracheal tube adapter (see Fig. 1).

Preoperative Evaluation

Whenever possible, patients should be evaluated for anesthetic risk immediately upon admission to the labor and delivery suite. If this cannot be done by a member of the anesthesia staff, then a short questionnaire targeted to specific areas of the medical history and physical relevant to anesthesia practice should be completed by either the admitting obstetric or nursing staff. When a patient at relatively high risk for anesthetic management (such as a patient with asthma or massive obesity) is admitted, this questionnaire will trigger contact with the anesthesiology staff to make them aware of the potential for the administration of a high-risk anesthetic. Further appropriate work-up and optimization of a medical condition can then be undertaken before the anesthetic is administered.

A blood specimen should be sent to the blood bank as part of the routine preoperative evaluation.

If possible, patients should be kept NPO in the labor and delivery suite whenever the potential for an emergency cesarean section exists. A rule of thumb is that if a fetal monitor is being used and a tracing consistent with fetal distress would result in a cesarean section, the patient should be kept NPO. No studies have been performed in pregnant patients to document the safety of oral intake (e.g., ice chips) during labor, but many studies have demonstrated delayed gastric emptying during labor.

Intravenous Access

All patients in labor and delivery should have intravenous access established. At the very least, a heparinized and capped angiocatheter should be placed in the case of an emergency if patients object to continuous intravenous fluids. A No. 16 gauge or larger intravenous line is preferred for emergency cesarean section, although a smaller gauge will suffice for induction, with placement of a larger intravenous line as necessary intra-operatively, for rapid fluid or blood administration. It is important to realize that without a secure intravenous line present, emergency regional or general endotracheal anesthesia is exceedingly hazardous or impossible.

CHOICE OF ANESTHETIC METHODS

Stable Emergency Cesarean Section

Since patients presenting for this operation are not different from patients presenting for elective cesarean section (with the exception of perhaps not being NPO for as long a period of time), the anesthetic management is identical to that of patients presenting for elective cesarean section with one exception: there should be an appropriate NPO period before the cesarean section is undertaken. Although the period of this required NPO will differ from institution to institution, at least the same criteria should be met as in the case of elective surgery (i.e., 8 hours after ingestion of solid food, 4 hours after ingestion of liquids). While these patients are awaiting surgery, usually in the labor and delivery suite, monitoring of the fetal and maternal status is conducted at regular intervals to ascertain that the need for an urgent cesarean section does not arise.

Anesthetic options for stable emergency cesarean section include epidural and spinal anesthesia. General anesthesia is reserved for only those patients for whom major regional anesthesia is contraindicated, such as patients with a documented coagulopathy. If doubt exists, coagulation studies should be done preoperatively, since time will permit such evaluation in almost all circumstances for patients who fall into this category. Epidural and spinal anesthesia in this circumstance should be performed in a manner similar to that used for elective cesarean sections.

Urgent Emergency Cesarean Section

Anesthesia for urgent cesarean section presents unique problems. Accurate categorization of the urgency of the procedure is essential. Patients with physiologic criteria that would more accurately place them in the stable emergency cesarean section category may frequently be placed into the urgent category by the posting surgeon. The indication for an urgent cesarean section is a basic underlying fetal or maternal physiologic abnormality which is *not* immediately life-threatening to the mother or fetus. Since the anesthetic plan undertaken is highly dependent on the correct categorization of emergency cesarean sections, the need for cooperation between the obstetrician and the anesthesiologist with regard to decision-making processes cannot be overstated. On the other hand, although such an occurrence is rare, an occasional patient will be presented to the anesthesiologist for an urgent cesarean section when it is actually a stat cesarean section that is necessary. Before deciding to undertake an anesthetic plan that may require at least 15 to 20 minutes until the delivery of the infant, the anesthesiologist should be certain that life-threatening fetal distress or maternal instability is *not* present. For this reason, the anesthesiologist should become familiar with the diagnosis of fetal distress and the interpretation of fetal heart rate traces. Assessment of the maternal condition is likewise an important part of the preoperative evaluation of urgency.

Rapidly conducted regional anesthesia or general anesthesia are the anesthetic options for patients who require urgent cesarean section. Epidural anesthesia should be used only in those patients in whom a pre-existing epidural catheter is in place and believed to be functioning. If an epidural catheter is in place and functioning (i.e., an effective labor epidural), the patient should be brought back to the operating room, a test dose given, and the epidural topped off with 12 to 15 ml of 1.5 percent or 2 percent lidocaine with 1:200,000 epinephrine. Two or three percent 2-chloroprocaine hydrochloride can be used as well. The use of bupivacaine in this circumstance is unwarranted since the latency to onset may be of an unacceptably long duration. While the top-up epidural dose is being injected, intravenous fluid is given rapidly so that the patient will have received a total of approximately 15 to 20 ml per kilogram by the time the epidural level is established for cesarean section.

Spinal anesthesia is appropriate in patients who have no contraindications to the technique and in whom delivery within less than 5 minutes is not necessary. Once it has been decided that spinal anesthesia will be used in the patient who is to undergo an urgent cesarean section, the intravenous fluid rate is increased so that 15 to 20 ml per kilogram of non-dextrose–containing crystalloid is administered before the onset of spinal anesthesia. The patient is brought into the operating room and placed immediately into the left or right lateral decubitus position in preparation for the spinal anesthetic. Monitors are placed on the patient, baseline vital signs are obtained, and the spinal anesthetic is administered. An agent should be chosen that provides good analgesia and that has a relatively rapid onset and a duration of action long enough to match the proposed maximum operative time for the particular surgeon. In many cases, tetracaine with or without epinephrine has a latency that may be too long for an urgent cesarean section, and a duration far exceeding the proposed surgical time. Lidocaine, although an anesthetic with a very short latency, may not have an adequate duration of anesthesia. For this reason, the combination of 40 mg of lidocaine, 4 mg of tetracaine, 200 μg of epinephrine, and 10 μg of fentanyl can be a more useful agent for spinal anesthesia for urgent cesarean section. To confine the spinal block to no higher than the high thoracic dermatomes, the surgical spinal dose should be administered at the L2-L3 or L3-4 interspace, with the cervicothoracic spine slightly elevated above the lumbar spine. The patient is then quickly turned into a left lateral tilt position with a wedge placed under the right hip. Blood pressure is measured every minute until the infant is delivered. Hypotension, or even impending hypotension, to a systolic blood pressure of less than 100 mm Hg should be immediately treated with 10 mg of intravenous ephedrine every 30 to 60 seconds until the systolic blood pressure is once again greater than 100 mm Hg. Blood pressures not responding satisfactorily to ephedrine should be treated with 50 μg doses of intravenous phenylephrine (Neo-Synephrine). The level of sensory block should also be checked every minute for the first 20 minutes of the block. This is accomplished by first testing for appearance of sensory block at the umbilicus (T10). Once a T10 level is established, the patient's abdomen can be prepped and draped. Sensory level can then be checked at the xiphoid (T5) or in the axilla (T2). Motor block can be assessed by evaluating hand grip strength. If the ma-

ternal and/or fetal conditions suddenly deteriorate, and the spinal sensory block is at T10 and rising, a low transverse incision cesarean section can be started. Supplemental doses of 10 mg of ketamine may be given intravenously as indicated. Using the ketamine supplementation technique, there is no need to delay incision and delivery until the final level of spinal anesthesia has been reached.

General anesthesia should be used in urgent cesarean section in cases in which regional anesthesia is either contraindicated or so technically difficult to perform that it would require a greater time frame than could be justified under the clinical circumstances. In such cases, the general anesthesia protocol for stat cesarean section (outlined below) should be followed.

Stat Emergency Cesarean Section

For emergency cesarean sections in which there is immediate maternal or fetal life-threatening danger, general anesthesia or local infiltration are the anesthetics of choice unless a working epidural catheter is in place with a T10 or higher sensory level. If such an epidural is in place and functioning, the cesarean section can be started with ketamine sedation, as outlined above. Additional lidocaine or chloroprocaine hydrochloride is administered to bring the level of block up, as described earlier in this chapter for urgent emergency cesarean sections.

Spinal anesthesia is usually avoided, because positioning for and attempting spinal anesthesia may delay delivery by one or two additional minutes, which may not be tolerated by the mother or fetus.

The technique of rapid-sequence induction of general anesthesia for emergency cesarean delivery is outlined in Table 2. The patient is brought into the operating room, where a final fetal heart rate trace is obtained if the cesarean section is being performed for the diagnosis of fetal distress. While that fetal heart rate trace is being obtained, anesthetic monitors are placed. Antacid, if not recently administered, should be given at this time.

When an awake intubation is indicated, topical anesthesia of the tongue and hypopharynx is begun. While the patient is being draped for surgery, laryngos-

Table 2 Outline of Technique for General Anesthesia for Stat Emergency Cesarean Section

1. Administer oxygen and ensure left uterine displacement.
2. Confirm administration of sodium citrate.
3. Review preanesthetic evaluation, especially airway consideration.
4. Place maternal and fetal monitors, as appropriate.
5. Preoxygenate by four vital capacity breaths.
6. Apply cricoid pressure.
7. Administer intravenous induction agent and succinylcholine chloride.
8. Administer ⅔ MAC potent inhalation agent in 100% oxygen until delivery.
9. Use N_2O/narcotic/amnestic/relaxant anesthesia after delivery.
10. Extubate patient awake.

copy is performed with a blade that is coated with local anesthetic jelly, so that the base of the tongue is anesthetized. When the surgeons are ready, awake intubation is attempted, and thiobarbiturate or ketamine is administered after the trachea has been secured by a cuffed endotracheal tube. If awake intubation is unsuccessful or impossible, rapid sequence induction is carried out as follows. In those rare instances in which rapid-sequence induction under general anesthesia is contraindicated (e.g., serious difficult airway problem, persistent vomiting) the obstetrician is advised to proceed immediately with the patient under local anesthesia. This must be suggested without delay to save time and prevent any further maternal-fetal damage.

For a rapid sequence intravenous induction, preoxygenation with four vital capacity breaths is carried out

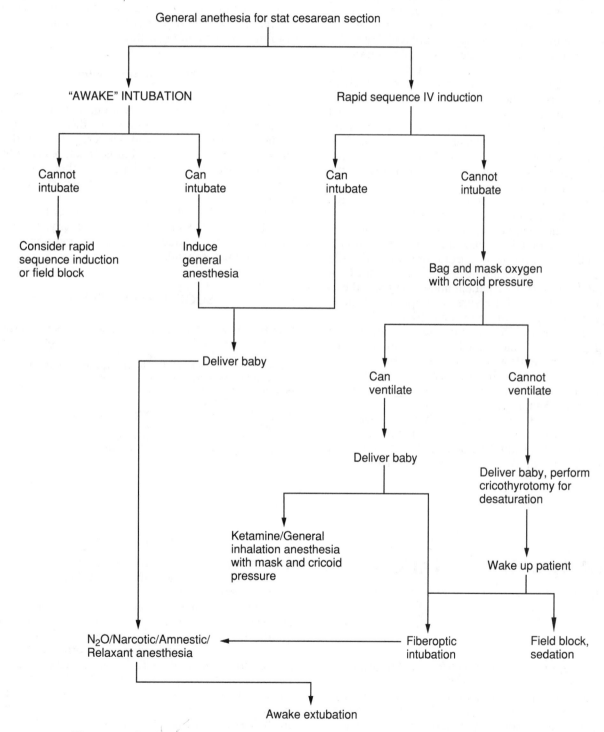

Figure 2 Algorithm for conducting general anesthesia for stat emergency cesarean sections.

when the surgery is ready to begin. Cricoid pressure by an experienced person is essential. Thiobarbiturate or ketamine is used to induce anesthesia, and 1 mg per kilogram of succinylcholine chloride is given to facilitate intubation. The succinylcholine can be flushed in with either intravenous fluid or with the last 2 to 3 ml of anesthetic. If intubation is accomplished, bilateral breath sounds should be heard and end-tidal carbon dioxide is detected; surgery may then begin. Low concentrations of potent inhalational agents (approximately two-thirds minimum alveolar concentration) are administered in 100 percent oxygen until delivery of the infant. The use of nitrous oxide is avoided to maximize the amount of oxygen delivered to the mother and therefore to the fetus. Although one study was unable to demonstrate any further increases in umbilical venous partial pressure of oxygen (PO_2) when maternal arterial PO_2 was increased above 300 mm Hg, there is no currently available method to measure the maternal PO_2 instantaneously and ensure that it is indeed greater than 300 mm Hg in a given patient. After delivery of the infant, nitrous oxide/oxygen/narcotic/amnestic/relaxant (as necessary) anesthesia is given. At the end of the operation, the patient is extubated awake.

If intubation cannot be accomplished during the rapid sequence induction, bag and mask ventilation is attempted with continued cricoid pressure (Fig. 2). Ventilation may or may not be possible. If it is, the baby can be delivered with the patient under mask anesthesia with continued cricoid pressure. The operation can be completed with the patient under mask anesthesia, or fiberoptic intubation can be attempted. In either case, cricoid pressure is maintained, and the surgeons are asked to be very gentle and avoid any epigastric pressure. This is especially important at the end of the procedure, when the contents of the uterus are normally expressed by abdominal compression.

If ventilation by mask is impossible, cricothyrotomy should be performed to achieve oxygenation. Simultaneously, the fetus should be delivered surgically if the indication for stat cesarean section was agonal fetal distress or a maternal condition that would be improved by emptying the uterus (e.g., placental abruption). At this point, the surgery can be halted, local anesthetic infiltrated, and the patient awakened so that other means of intubation can be attempted (such as fiberoptic intubation or tracheostomy), or the procedure can continue with the patient under local anesthesia with ketamine sedation.

Whatever algorithm is chosen for the failed intubation, it should be considered ahead of time. A stat emergency cesarean section is neither the time nor place to formulate such an algorithm.

Neonatal Resuscitation

During an emergency cesarean section, events can occur so rapidly in the delivery room that the attention of the anesthesiologist should not be diverted from the mother unless the infant is born severely depressed and no one else present is trained in neonatal resuscitation. For this reason, a pediatrician or another anesthetist should be called whenever an emergency cesarean section is performed.

Neonatal resuscitation is discussed elsewhere in this text. If neonatal resuscitation is necessary, the steps outlined in the protocols should be developed and considered beforehand.

SUGGESTED READING

Endler GC, Mariona FG, Sokol RJ, Stevenson LB. Anesthesia-related maternal mortality in Michigan, 1972 to 1984. Am J Obstet Gynecol 1988; 159:187–193.

Gibbs CP, Spohr L, Schmidt D. The effectiveness of sodium citrate as an antacid. Anesthesiology 1982; 57:44–46.

Morgan M. Anaesthetic contribution to maternal mortality. Br J Anaesth 1987; 59:849–855.

Norris MC, Dewan DM. Preoxygenation for cesarean section: a comparison of two techniques. Anesthesiology 1985; 62:827–829.

Tunstall ME, Sheikh A. Failed intubation protocol: oxygenation without aspiration. Clin Anaesthes 1986; 4:171–187.

NEONATAL RESUSCITATION

BRIAN K. TABATA, M.D.

Birth represents an extremely stressful transition for the fetus as it assumes an existence outside the uterus. The success or failure of that transition determines the difference between an infant who is healthy and one who may face serious morbidity or mortality. The goal of resuscitation is simple: *the recognition and treatment of neonatal asphyxia*. This process, if left untreated, can result in brain damage; myocardial, hepatic, or renal failure; pulmonary edema; and death.

The techniques of neonatal resuscitation have not changed much over the past several years, but there is a greater appreciation by all members of the delivery room medical team to provide every newborn with the best chance for quality survival. Ninety percent of all live deliveries occur uneventfully. It is therefore imperative to identify the remaining 10 percent who will have perinatal complications and to tailor the medical therapy to their specific needs. In the past, such responsibility was held by the anesthesiologist, pediatrician, or obstetrician. However, the new emphasis today is on the team approach. Resuscitation cannot be performed well by a single individual. It must be conducted by at least two people who are familiar with infant assessment as well as the techniques of resuscitation. This may not be a problem in tertiary medical centers where all the principal specialties are represented, but in community hospitals there may be a greater dependence on fewer individuals. Part of the problem for hospital personnel is the small size of the patient, but an understanding of the physiologic changes and basic approach to the neonate will help to make the resuscitation proceed more smoothly.

PHYSIOLOGY

The major neonatal changes occur in the cardiovascular and respiratory systems. The fetal circulation is characterized by two major shunts (foramen ovale and ductus arteriosus) and the placenta, the in utero organ of respiration that provides oxygenated blood into the inferior vena cava by way of the ductus venosus. This enriched blood is preferentially directed through the right atrium into the left atrium via the foramen ovale, then up the ascending aorta via the left ventricle, while the lower saturated blood from the superior vena cava is moved through the right ventricle and primarily shunted away from the lungs to the descending aorta via the ductus arteriosus. This arrangement ensures maximal oxygenation of the fetal brain via the carotid arteries that originate from the ascending aorta. The lungs are filled with fetal lung fluid (40 percent of total lung capacity), and because of their compressed size, pulmonary vascular resistance (PVR) is high—as high as or higher than systemic vascular resistance (SVR), which accounts for the preferential flow of blood from the pulmonary artery to the aorta via the ductus arteriosus.

At birth, several important events occur. With the first few breaths (spontaneous transpulmonary pressures of 40 to 80 mm Hg), the fetal lung fluid is removed from pulmonary airways and alveoli. The combination of increased lung expansion (less tension on pulmonary vessels), increasing arterial PO_2, and decreasing PCO_2 decrease PVR to one half of SVR, allowing for increased flow of pulmonary artery blood through the lungs. The increased blood return to the left atrium elevates left atrial pressure to physiologically close the foramen ovale, creating separation of right and left atrial blood flow. Increasing oxygen tension causes the ductus arteriosus to constrict, thereby completing the transformation to a completely "series circuit" circulation. Anatomic closure of the two shunts by creation of fibrotic tissue takes approximately 1 week. Hence, recurrence of shunting can occur as is commonly noted in the healthy crying infant who may intermittently turn cyanotic, while showing no evidence of cardiac disease. Persistent fetal circulation (PFC), or the more accurate term persistent pulmonary hypertension (PPH), can occur in neonates who are severely acidotic and hypoxic.

Retained fetal lung fluid is presumed to be the etiology of *transient tachypnia* of the newborn.

The physiologic events of asphyxia have been studied in the neonatal rhesus monkey. The fetus had a cesarean delivery with the head wrapped in a plastic bag. Before delivery, catheters were placed in major vessels through fetal surgery.

During the first minute after delivery, there were rapid gasping efforts with thrashing movements of the arms and legs. This was followed by 1 minute of *primary apnea,* during which spontaneous respirations could be induced by tactile stimuli. The heart rate dropped from initial values of 150 to 180 beats per minute (bpm) but remained above 100 bpm. For the next 5 minutes there were spontaneous deep gasps, which gradually weakened to the final agonal breath approximately 8 minutes after the onset of anoxia. Secondary apnea (no spontaneous breathing induced by tactile stimuli) then began, with death shortly thereafter if resuscitation was not begun. For every minute of delayed resuscitation after the final breath, there was an additional 2-minute period from the time of resuscitation to first spontaneous breath, and a further 4-minute period to onset of rhythmic breathing. During the first 10 minutes of total asphyxia, pH dropped from 7.3 to 6.8, PO_2 decreased from 25 to 0 mm Hg, PCO_2 increased from 45 to 150 mm Hg, and blood lactate levels rapidly elevated.

Compared with its simian counterpart, the human fetus and newborn may be able to tolerate higher degrees of asphyxia with less brain damage because of the latter's greater immaturity. However, there is great variability of duration from primary apnea to last gasp, so that it is extremely difficult to predict the occurrence of brain damage based on the duration of asphyxia. The studies in monkeys also began with a normal fetus, stressed at the time of cesarean birth. In the delivery room the human fetus may have already undergone perinatal stresses, inducing predelivery asphyxia. As a result, resuscitation efforts must be instituted as rapidly as possible for the neonate in distress.

GENERAL CONCEPTS

Once the child is born, there must be a rapid means to assess its needs and to gauge the ongoing success or failure of medical therapy. The Apgar scoring system (Table 1) provides a relatively simple way to assess the status of the infant and is based on five observed clinical parameters. Traditionally, the scores at 1 minute and at 5 minutes of age are recorded. The 1-minute score identifies the child in need of attention and the relative degree of asphyxia. The 5-minute score correlates less well with long-term morbidity and mortality. Extremely premature infants (<32 weeks' gestation) have lower Apgar scores because of their immature central nervous and muscular systems. Rapid assistance of their individual needs will ensure a successful outcome. Multiple scores at successive minutes of age can be an ongoing indication of the effectiveness of medical therapy.

Table 1 Apgar Scoring System

Clinical Parameter	Points		
	0	*1*	*2*
Heart rate	Absent	<100	>100
Respiratory effort	Absent	Irregular, slow, shallow, or gasping respirations	Robust, crying
Color	Cyanotic	Acrocyanotic; trunk pink, extremities blue	Pink
Muscle tone	Absent, limp	Some flexion of extremities	Active movement
Reflex irritability (nasal catheter, pharyngeal suctioning)	No response	Grimace	Active coughing and sneezing

The newborn infant should always be placed under a radiant warmer to prevent significant heat loss. A wet, naked infant exposed to ambient temperatures of 25°C will drop its core temperature by 2°C after 20 minutes. The hypothermic stress will add to the oxygen demand and deplete glucose stores, which may already be low in an asphyxiated child. A dry infant under a radiant warmer loses no significant heat.

The most important focus of resuscitative efforts is adequate ventilation: providing oxygen and removing carbon dioxide. In most situations, this is the only necessary condition to reverse the cardiorespiratory depression of asphyxia. Correction of hypoxemia and respiratory acidosis usually results in return of autoregulation and stabilization of metabolic function. Pharmacologic intervention is usually reserved for the most severely compromised infants.

The neonatal airway is characterized by relative macroglossia and micrognathia, which explains why masked ventilation and intubation are more difficult in this population than in older patients. Particular attention is given to the use of forward mandibular thrust and oral airway insertion to facilitate masked ventilation. Good visualization with a straight laryngoscopic blade helps intubation.

Moderately asphyxiated infants (Apgar scores of 3 to 6) are usually in primary apnea and often breathe in response to pharyngeal (suctioning, masked ventilation, or laryngoscopy) or tactile (drying of skin with a towel—avoid slapping of the body or extremities) stimulation. Severe asphyxia (Apgar scores of 0 to 2) requires endotracheal positive-pressure ventilation with initial inspiratory pressures of 40 to 50 cm H_2O to expand the compressed lungs. While there is concern about high airway pressures (greater than 55cm H_2O) leading to pneumothorax and stomach distention , manometry has some potential sources of error: all pressures are external to the infant's lungs, thereby possibly reflecting upper airway resistance rather than true transpulmonary pressure. The only clinically reliable method is the observation of chest movement and auscultation for breath sounds. Improvement of truncal skin color and a rising heart rate (if bradycardia

was present) are evidence of increased oxygen saturation.

Cardiac output in the fetus and neonate is primarily rate dependent. The fetal myocardium functions on the high end of the Frank-Starling curve and has little capacity for further positive inotropic changes. Furthermore, the autonomic nervous system has parasympathetic dominance, which can result in marked bradycardia in response to pharyngeal stimulation during ventilatory management. The normal neonatal heart rate is 120 to 150 per minute. Rates below 60 result in inadequate perfusion, and external cardiac massage becomes necessary. Fingers of both hands are wrapped around the infant's chest, meeting in the back, with both thumbs placed over the midsternum. Rates of 120 per minute should be maintained, with ventilation rates of 40 per minute. The easiest way to determine heart rate is to palpate the base of the umbilical cord. For the first few minutes, the arterial vessels pulsate strongly. Apical palpation and auscultation are less effective alternatives.

Maintenance of an adequate circulating volume is crucial to neonatal resuscitation. Hypovolemia may be absolute (secondary to blood loss) or functional (vascular sequestration due to asphyxia). For acute blood loss, blood is the most desirable volume expander because the addition of hemoglobin adds to the oxygen-carrying capacity of the infant's circulation. If no specifically cross-matched blood is available, low-antibody level, O negative blood, cross-matched with the mother's plasma should be available in the delivery room. The use of placental blood (drawn from the umbilical vein) is usually avoided except in dire situations because of the risk of bacterial contamination and the introduction of clots. In functional hypovolemia, plasma (colloid) preparations and crystalloid solutions are reasonable alternatives, although the former is associated with maintaining or increasing plasma oncotic pressure, while the latter decreases it. Umbilical venous catheterization offers the fastest and easiest intravenous access to the infant, although catheter insertion should be limited to no more than 4 to 5 cm from the base of the umbilicus to prevent insertion into the liver parynchyma, with resultant necrosis (ruptured ductus venosus). Initial infusions range from 10 to 20 ml per kilogram body weight, with additional increments of 5 to 10 ml per kilogram. After each infusion, the neonate's circulation should be assessed (e.g., color, capillary filling, blood pressure, blood gases, hematocrit) before additional volume expansion.

Unresponsiveness to proper ventilation, external cardiac massage, and intravascular volume expansion may result from severe hypoxemia, acidosis, and hypovolemia. Pharmacologic intervention may then become necessary. Administration of $NaHCO_3$ (1–2 mEq per kilogram) through the umbilical vein must be accompanied by good ventilation to be effective in treating metabolic acidosis. It is markedly hypertonic, serving as a volume expander as well as an alkali, and is usually diluted 1:1 with water to decrease the osmotic load. Epinephrine (0.1 ml per kilogram of 1:10,000) and atropine (0.01 mg per kilogram) may be given intravenously or through the endotracheal tube.

TECHNIQUE

Risk Identification

The first step is to identify the infant at high risk for perinatal complications. Table 2 summarizes the factors, separated into maternal and fetal causes. Maternal factors influence the adequacy of the uterine environ-

Table 2 Factors Associated with the High-Risk Neonate

Maternal
Maternal age <16 and >35 yr
Low socioeconomic class
Diabetes
Alcohol and drug abuse
High blood pressure
Toxemia of pregnancy
Premature rupture of membranes
Abnormal fetal growth
Previous cesarean delivery
Previous infant with jaundice, respiratory distress, or anomalies

Labor and Delivery
Premature (<37 wks' gestation) or postmature (>40 wks' gestation) onset of labor
Rapid or prolonged labor
Breech and other abnormal presentations
Prolapsed cord
Cesarean delivery
Maternal hypotension
Anesthesia and analgesics

Fetal
Multiple gestation
Meconium-stained amniotic fluid
Fetal asphyxia
Abnormality of fetal heart rate and rhythm

Neonatal
Low Apgar scores
Neonatal infection
Cardiopulmonary distress

ment in providing the fetus with oxygen and nutrients. Fetal factors may involve qualitative or quantitative maldevelopment that prevents a successful transition at birth.

Equipment

The next step is to check for the availability of proper equipment and medications (Table 3). The laryngoscope should be tested for light brightness. Several patent endotracheal tubes (2.5, 3.0, 3.5) and an obturator should be available. The oxygen flow meter should be working and the resuscitation bag checked for proper operation. Appropriately sized masks should be available. The suction equipment should be functional. Resuscitation efforts must be performed in an infant bed equipped with an overhead radiant warmer. All necessary needles, syringes, catheters, and medications should be present.

Apgar Scores 8–10

Diagnosis. No asphyxia.
Clinical Presentation. Responsive, crying, and active infant; pink to acrocyanotic; heart rate greater than 100 per minute.
Actions. Use the suction bulb to gently remove any oral secretions. Maintain under the radiant heater, dry the body thoroughly, and remove any wet towels from under the infant. Perform a brief physical examination to assess well-being and the presence of any physical abnormalities. Record 5-minute Apgar score and unite with the parents.

Apgar Scores 5–7

Diagnosis. Mild asphyxia.
Clinical Presentation. Mild hypotonia; less active;

Table 3 Equipment Needed for Neonatal Resuscitation

1. Well-lighted, flat area with overhead radiant warmer for assessment and treatment of infant
2. Supply of oxygen regulated by a calibrated flow meter, preferably heated and humidified
3. Suction equipment with appropriate hoses; Nos. 8, 10, and 12 French regulated suction catheters; pliable bulb syringe
4. Mapleson B or D anesthesia bag (allows for 100% O_2 administration and regulation of inspiratory pressures); assorted face mask sizes
5. Endotracheal tubes: 2.5, 3.0, 3.5 mm ID
6. Pediatric laryngoscopic handles with Miller Nos. 0 and 1 blade sizes
7. Assorted syringes and needles
8. Umbilical catheters: Nos. 3.5, 5.0, and 8.0 French sizes
9. Medications:

	Dose
$NaHCO_3$ (0.5 mEq/ml)	1–2 mEq/kg
Epinephrine (1:10,000)	0.1 ml/kg
Atropine (0.4 mg/ml)	0.01 mg/kg
Calcium gluconate (100 mg/kg)	100–200 mg/kg
Naloxone (0.02 mg/ml)	0.01 mg/kg
Albumin solutions; 0.9 NS; lactated Ringer's	10–20 ml/kg

slightly cyanotic with heart rate greater than 100 beats per minute; rapid shallow or periodic breathing.

Actions. Rapidly clear secretions from the airway with the bulb. Dry the infant thoroughly and maintain body temperature. Provide added tactile stimulation (rubbing the body or lower extremities) to stimulate spontaneous respirations while blowing low-flow oxygen over the face by means of the resuscitation bag and mask. If there is improvement, perform the physical examination and unite with the parents. If the heart rate falls below 100 beats per minute, proceed to "actions" for moderate asphyxia. Administer naloxone, 0.01 mg per kilogram intramuscularly, if the mother received narcotic analgesics more than 30 to 60 minutes but less than 4 hours before the delivery.

Apgar Scores 3–4

Diagnosis. Moderate asphyxia.

Clinical Presentation. Weak; minimally active; cyanotic; heart rate less than 100 per minute.

Actions. Call for additional personnel to monitor the circulation and help with airway management and ventilation, etc. Quickly clear secretions from the airway, dry the infant, and maintain body temperature. Attempt ventilation with a resuscitation bag and mask using 100 percent O_2. Initially inflate using 40 to 50 cm H_2O pressures for the first few breaths, while observing chest wall movement for adequacy of ventilation. Subsequent breaths can be achieved with approximately 20 to 30 cm H_2O provided there is good chest motion and/or breath sounds. If there is no chest movement, check for tightness of mask fit over the face and adequacy of O_2 flow rate, and insert an oral airway to help alleviate airway obstruction. If there is still no chest motion, proceed to intubation. Provide external cardiac massage if the heart rate falls below 60 per minute. If ventilation is adequate, observe for increasing heart rate and pink coloration over the next minute. Continue ventilation until the heart rate is greater than 100 beats per minute. Observe for return of spontaneous respirations with sufficient ventilatory exchange. Reinstitute controlled masked ventilation if the heart rate falls below 100 beats per minute. Consider administering naloxone if the mother received antenatal narcotics.

Apgar Scores 0–2

Diagnosis. Severe asphyxia.

Clinical Presentation. Limp; inactive; cyanotic; apneic or periodic gasping; heart rate less than 80 per minute or absent.

Actions. Suction the airway for secretions (less than 15 seconds) and rapidly proceed to intubation. Ventilate with positive pressure and 100 percent O_2 at rates of 40 to 50 per minute. The most common reason for failed ventilation is a misplaced endotracheal tube. Provide external cardiac massage at 120 to 140 compressions per minute, synchronized with ventilation (three to four compressions per breath). If the heart rate remains below 100 beats per minute after 2 minutes of aggressive ventilation and external cardiac massage, insert No. 3.5 or 5 French umbilical catheter in the umbilical vein (star-shaped vessel on the umbilical cord cross-section compared with the beadlike appearance of the two umbilical arteries). Restrict insertion to 3 cm to minimize the risk of hepatic parenchymal damage from direct infusion of hypertonic solutions into the liver.

Drug therapy begins with $NaHCO_3$ (1 to 2 mEq per kilogram) to correct for metabolic acidosis. Epinephrine or atropine can be administered intravenously or via the endotracheal tube to help support the heart rate. Cardiac output may also be enhanced by the infusion of calcium gluconate (100 to 200 mg per kilogram) over 2 to 3 minutes. If there has been acute blood loss, proceed to volume expansion with O negative blood or plasma preparations (10 to 20 ml per kilogram) with additional volumes of 5 to 10 ml per kilogram. Continuous assessment of circulation will indicate the infant's responsiveness to medical therapy. Try to obtain blood gas sampling and serum electrolyte, calcium, and glucose levels to help guide further therapy, although because of the somewhat long turn-around time in obtaining the results, their usefulness can be limited. It cannot be emphasized too strongly that without adequate ventilation and oxygenation, pharmacologic intervention will fail.

MECONIUM-STAINED FLUIDS

Meconium-stained fluid at the time of delivery should heighten concerns for meconium aspiration. The resultant airway obstruction, chemical pneumonitis, and possible pulmonary vascular abnormalities in the presence of long-standing fetal hypoxemia lead to marked ventilation-perfusion mismatch. A concerted effort is made to clear the airway early. At the time of delivery the obstetrician should use the bulb syringe to remove as much of the oral secretion as possible after the head is delivered prior to shoulder presentation. After complete delivery the infant is carried to the heated bed. If the child still remains depressed, immediately intubate the patient and apply suction to the endotracheal tube as it is removed to facilitate the removal of any material below the level of the vocal cords. If nothing is aspirated, proceed to mask ventilate the neonate with 100 percent O_2, and monitor for adequacy of ventilation. If there is no chest movement after 20 to 30 seconds, immediately reintubate and ventilate with 100 percent oxygen and positive-pressure ventilation until the heart rate is greater than 100 per minute and the patient begins to have spontaneous respirations. If meconium-stained fluid is aspirated from the endotracheal tube, quickly reintubate and suction again. The purpose is to clear the airway of debris completely, but this must be weighed against delaying the delivery of oxygen to an already compromised infant who may not tolerate any further prolongation of hypoxemia. A rough guide is to proceed with ventilation after 1 to 2 minutes of suctioning efforts. If the heart rate is greater than 100, 2 minutes may not be intolerable. If the heart rate at birth was less than 100, the 1-minute limit may be more reasonable. In either case, the most experienced person performing the intubation will ensure maximal success in clearing the airway with minimal stress to the infant. If the meconium staining was thin (not pea-soup consistency) and the infant was actively crying at birth, observe the child for upper airway obstruction. The risks of a difficult intubation attempt in an active child must be weighed against the questionable benefits of suctioning any material from the upper airways that may have already been drawn farther down by spontaneous ventilation.

LOW-BIRTHWEIGHT INFANTS

Premature infants (less than 32 weeks' gestation) have poor autoregulation of blood pressure, a higher incidence of respiratory distress secondary to pulmonary immaturity, and fragile intracerebral blood vessels that place them at higher risk for intraventricular hemorrhage. Failure to rapidly correct neonatal hypoxemia and respiratory acidosis, coupled with indiscriminate use of volume expanders and hyperosmolar intravenous agents causing wide swings in blood pressure, place these infants at higher risk for intracerebral bleeding and neurologic sequelae. Treatment is focused on rapid intubation to secure the airway and control ventilation, while trying to avoid fluid administration to correct hypotension except in cases of acute blood loss. Because of their higher surface area to body weight ratio and lower subcutaneous fat content, these infants suffer higher evaporative heat losses and can become more rapidly hypothermic than their full-term counterparts. Glycogen stores are smaller, and they can become hypoglycemic in a shorter amount of time. They require higher glucose infusions, but their pancreatic immaturity can lead to poor glucose control and occasional high elevations, which, in the presence of brain ischemia, can exacerbate neurologic recovery.

ANESTHESIA FOR TRAUMA

HEAD TRAUMA

ELIZABETH A. M. FROST, M.D.

Head injury is both a major medical emergency and a serious socioeconomic problem. It is the leading cause of death and disability in young adults today; every 5 minutes one American dies and another is permanently disabled (Interagency Head Injury Task Force Report, 1989). Largely because it affects the young, the total economic cost of traumatic brain injury (TBI) has been estimated at more than $25 billion per year. The incidence of TBI requiring hospitalization is approximately 200 in 100,000.

As part of the trauma team, the anesthesiologist must be able to provide initial resuscitation, appropriate care during neurodiagnostic testing, identification of an optimal anesthetic technique, and management of all aspects of intensive care.

Brain injury is a dynamic process. Not only does the pathologic process continue to evolve over the first few hours and days after trauma, often with devastating secondary injury, but the physiologic and clinical aspects of the recovery process can continue for years. The multiple poorly understood variables involved include changes in nutrition, intracranial dynamics, cardiopulmonary status, circulating catecholamines, and coagulation. Outcome prediction remains as much an art as a science. Thus, the notion of a "dynamic prognosis" requiring intermittent revision is especially relevant.

Although the initial brain damage resulting from the impact is not amenable to treatment, subsequent neurologic deterioration and systemic complications leading to a poor outcome or death should be preventable. In a group of patients known to have talked before dying as a result of head injury (i.e., the initial injury was not enough to cause death immediately), the most common extracranial causes of death were hypoxia and shock, and the most frequent intracranial complications were misdiagnosis, seizures, and delays in the initiation of therapy for intracranial hematomas.

DEFINITIONS

The National Head Injury Data Bank in the United States has defined severe head injuries as those head injuries occurring in patients who score 8 or less on the Glasgow Coma Scale (GCS) (Table 1) following neurosurgical resuscitation (volume resuscitation and correction of ventilatory failure).

Three types of patients with severe head injuries are considered:

1. Patients in whom death or a severely damaged state is inevitable (e.g., those with brain stem injuries on admission), patients with severe multisystem injuries, or critically injured elderly patients.
2. Patients in whom survival or good recovery is expected, even if no intervention is performed.
3. Severely injured patients not amenable to surgical therapy.

Nonsurgical care influences outcome in only approximately 50 percent of patients. However, the improvement in outcome appears to be substantial, and the degree of improvement appears to be increasing in all groups of patients.

Although head injury is diagnosed in 400,000 of the patients admitted to hospitals each year in the United States, 75 to 90 percent of these head injuries are not severe. Moderate head injuries are seen in patients with a GCS score of 9 to 12, and minor head injuries are associated with a GCS score of 13 to 15.

INITIAL RESUSCITATION

The anesthesiologist contributes to the emergency care of the head injury victim in several areas: establishment and maintenance of the airway, normalization of cardiovascular status, and control of intracranial pressure (ICP).

Respiratory Care

Several respiratory abnormalities have been documented after cranial trauma; these are generally

Table 1 The Glasgow Coma Scale*

	Score
Best verbal response:	
None	1
Incomprehensible sound	2
Inappropriate words	3
Confused	4
Oriented	5
Eyes open:	
No	1
To pain	2
To speech	3
Spontaneously	4
Best motor response:	
None	1
Abnormal extensor	2
Abnormal flexion	3
Withdraws	4
Localizes	5
Obeys	6
Total coma scale	15-3

*The Glasgow coma scale, first described as a prognostic indicator of outcome in head injury, is also used as an indicator of progress. Motor response is the most sensitive component and correlates best with extent and outcome of severe injury (i.e., category 3 above).

Table 2 Causes of Respiratory Abnormalities After Head Injury

Central	Peripheral
Apnea	Aspiration
Hypoxia	Multiple trauma
Hypercarbia	Fat embolism
Pulmonary edema	Diffuse intravascular coagulation
	Iatrogenic

classified as having either central or peripheral causes (Table 2).

The absence of spontaneous ventilation on admission to the hospital is associated with an extremely poor prognosis unless the patient is seen within minutes post-trauma, when the apnea may be part of early traumatic unconsciousness, a finding that applies also to children.

Both hypoxia and hypercapnia correlate directly with a poor outcome. Although hypoxic episodes are more common during the period immediately after head injury is sustained, they occur frequently for up to 2 weeks after injury. Both brief and prolonged episodes of hypoxia have been documented in equal numbers in the early and late monitoring stages. Hypoxia ($PaO_2 < 70$ mm Hg on room air) may occur in as many as 70 percent of severely head-injured patients. Hypoventilation and central neurogenic hyperventilation are common. In this latter ventilatory abnormality, minute ventilation increases, and hypoxia is caused by the increased work of breathing and the shift of the oxygen dissociation curve to the left.

The most common peripheral cause of respiratory difficulties after head injury is aspiration. Gastric dilatation and loss of protective pharyngeal and laryngeal reflexes caused by brain stem injury, alcohol ingestion, or concomitant spinal cord injury make aspiration an ever-present hazard. Videofluoroscopy has demonstrated a 50 percent incidence of aspiration, with less than half of these cases being identified by bedside clinical assessment.

Abnormalities of clotting parameters can be iden-

tified in most patients after major head injury. The brain is a rich source of tissue thromboplastin that may be released after cranial injury, causing both hemorrhagic and thrombotic events. Disseminated intravascular coagulopathy and adult respiratory distress syndrome may result.

Ventilatory problems exist if one or more of the criteria listed in Table 3 are present. Although clinically specific abnormalities of respiratory pattern have been correlated with the level of the central nervous system lesion, such changes are more consistently related to extent and bilaterality. In general, an eupneic pattern of breathing indicates a small, unilateral lesion, and the outcome is good. The presence of Cheyne-Stokes respiration indicates a bilateral lesion. Mortality rates exceed 50 percent. Apneustic patterns may indicate pontine infarction or drug intoxication, hypoglycemia, or severe anemia. Prognosis is poor. Ataxic respiration usually results from a posterior fossa lesion with medullary compression, and outcome is fatal.

Therapy aims to achieve arterial oxygen pressure (PaO_2) levels greater than 100 mm Hg and appropriate arterial carbon dioxide pressure ($PaCO_2$) levels. Frequently, adequate respiration may be achieved simply by tilting the head back, clearing the mouth, and inserting an airway. Supplemental oxygen should always be given. Because of the high related incidence of narcotic overdose in head injury, naloxone hydrochloride is often indicated. If these measures do not suffice, intubation should be performed and ventilation supported quickly. The mortality rate is significantly decreased if intubation and ventilation are established within 1 hour of trauma.

The sequence for intubation should be (1) application of cricoid pressure to diminish chances of aspiration; (2) administration of a primary dose of a nondepolarizing muscle relaxant; (3) ventilation with 100 percent oxygen and Ambu bag; (4) intravenous administration of sodium pentothal (2 to 3 mg per kilogram), lidocaine (1 mg per kilogram), and atracurium besylate (3 to 4 mg per kilogram) or vecuronium bromide (0.1 mg per kilogram); (5) continued ventilation; and (6) oral intubation. Any period of apnea may be accompanied by an increase in ICP, even though the $PaCO_2$ may remain within a relatively hypocapnic range (e.g., 27 to 33 mm Hg over 1 minute). Similarly, suctioning, if it is not preceded by hyperventilation and sodium pentothal injection, increases ICP. Bucking caused by inadequate respiratory control or insufficient sedation increases ICP and may initiate pressure waves. Orotracheal intubation is preferred even if a cervical lesion is suspected, as complications are less than with nasotracheal intubation. Manual in-line axial traction should be applied.

Hyperventilation has been shown to be effective in reducing ICP. However, if cerebral blood flow is already reduced because of brain edema, such a maneuver, by further reducing cerebral blood flow, may be deleterious. Arteriovenous oxygen saturation differences ($AJDO_2$) across the brain may be used to monitor critical cerebral oxygen delivery and cerebral blood flow (i.e., systemic arterial oxygen content minus jugular venous bulb [JVB] oxygen content).

An $AJDO_2$ of less than 10 volume percent indicates that cerebral blood flow is probably adequate and that intracranial hypertension can be treated by hyperventilation, as is commonly the case in children. Increased oxygen extraction indicates reduced flow, and diuretic therapy is indicated with maintenance of normocarbia. This situation is more frequently encountered in adults after blunt trauma. If normal arterial oxygen saturation and hemoglobin concentration exist, JVB oxygen tension may be used alone. Mechanical passive hyperventilation should be adjusted to levels of JVB oxygen tension of 28 to 30 mm Hg.

Although intubation secures the airway, assisted ventilation is usually necessary to ensure adequate tissue oxygenation and carbon dioxide removal. The current ventilatory modes of choice are continuous positive airway pressure (CPAP) in combination with intermittent mandatory ventilation (IMV).

Treatment of hypoxia that is caused by coagulopathies requires prompt administration of fresh-frozen plasma, cryoprecipitate, and platelets. Therapy for pulmonary complications associated with fat embolism includes cardio-respiratory support and infusion of aminophylline, narcotics, steroids, and low–molecular weight dextran. The use of alcohol and heparin is controversial.

Cardiovascular Support

Normovolemic hypotension after closed head injury is rare and is usually caused by brain stem injury with destruction of the vasomotor center in the medulla. Death is imminent. More commonly, hypotension is associated with major scalp lacerations and multiple trauma (usually splenic rupture). Only in infants may a cerebral hematoma be large enough to cause shock. Theoretically, hypotension could occur in hypertensive patients maintained on catecholamine-depleting antihypertensive medications.

The most frequently observed hemodynamic abnormalities are hypertension and tachycardia. Increases in mean arterial pressure of almost 30 percent and a heart rate of more than 50 percent are common. Less consistent increases in pulmonary artery pressure, pulmonary capillary wedge pressure, and peripheral vascular resistance occur. Cardiac output is usually increased, as is venous oxygen consumption, unlike the situation seen in essential hypertension, when these two param-

eters are usually normal. Several electrocardiographic changes have been described (see Table 3).

Autoregulation is disrupted by cerebral injury. At both ends of the autoregulatory curve, penumbral areas exist that are highly sensitive to hypotension. Hypotension increases cerebral blood flow (CBF), especially in the parietal cortex, which may worsen edema. All attempts should be made to maintain normal cerebral perfusion pressure (CPP = mean arterial blood pressure − ICP).

Beta-blockade has been proven effective in improving cerebral perfusion pressure. Propranolol may be infused at a rate of 1 mg per 15 minutes until the systolic blood pressure is less than 160 mm Hg and the diastolic pressure is less than 90 mm Hg. Sodium nitroprusside, nitroglycerine, and hydralazine all increase CBF by a cerebral vasodilatory action and should not be used in the patient with head injury before the skull is opened.

Control of Intracranial Pressure

Intracranial pressure (ICP) refers to cerebrospinal pressure within the cranial cavity. The normal range is 5 to 15 mm Hg. An ICP of more than 40 mm Hg is considered to be severely increased. Elevations in ICP result from changes in cerebrospinal fluid (CSF) absorption, cerebral circulation, and intracranial abnormalities. The deleterious effect of increased ICP is based on the reduction in perfusion pressure and CBF below the critical level (60 mm Hg), resulting in brain ischemia. Once a critical compensatory point is reached, rapid elevation in ICP occurs with minimal provocation.

The advantages and disadvantages of several techniques of monitoring ICP are listed in Table 4. Therapy of intracranial hypertension is outlined in Table 5.

Although "brain swelling" and "brain edema" are terms that are often used interchangeably to indicate a cause for an increased ICP, these terms can be more precisely applied to two distinct processes that occur after head injury. Brain swelling is an increase in cerebral blood volume, caused by cerebral vasoparalysis

Table 3 Abnormal Electrocardiography Findings in Head-Injured Patients Listed in Order of Frequency

Findings	Percentage
QTc (> 440 msec)	60
Tachycardai (> 100)	45
ST segment depression	20
QRS prolongation	15
Large U waves	15
ST-segment elevation	15
Ventricular extrasystoles	10
Heart block	8
Peaked T waves	8
PR interval prolongation	5
Bradycardia	2

Adapted from Miner ME, Allen SJ. Cardiovascular effects of severe head injury. In: Clinical Anesthesia in Neurosurgery, 2nd ed. Boston; Butterworth, 1990.

with resulting hyperemia. Prolonged hyperemia leads to vasogenic edema and increased ICP. The computed tomographic scan characteristic of cerebral hyperemia shows slightly increased brain density and compressed ventricles. This condition is more commonly seen in children immediately after injury. Appropriate therapy includes hyperventilation or other means of increasing vasoconstriction (e.g., use of barbiturates). Brain edema refers to increased water content of the extravascular spaces of the brain. Diuretic therapy is indicated. This condition is usually not an immediate consequence of head injury.

Steroid administration does not improve outcome after head injury and may have a detrimental effect, especially in children, by potentiation of a post-traumatic catabolic response and increased protein breakdown.

Both mannitol and furosemide decrease ICP. Although a bolus of mannitol may initially aggravate intracranial hypertension, the time of elevation of ICP is short and there are apparently no ill effects. Nevertheless, in infants or elderly patients with cardiac disease, the hyperosmolar effect of mannitol may precipitate cardiac failure.

Mannitol also decreases blood viscosity, which increases oxygen delivery to the brain and causes reflex vasoconstriction. Furosemide lowers ICP and brain water content, both alone and in combination with mannitol. It does not appear to increase ICP or blood volume and exerts little effect on electrolyte balance. In large doses, furosemide reduces CSF formation and may reduce water and ion penetration across the blood-brain barrier. Furosemide prolongs the effectiveness of mannitol. Administration of mannitol (0.5 g per kilogram) followed after 15 minutes by furosemide (0.5 mg per kilogram) is most effective in causing prompt and adequate brain shrinkage. Careful monitoring of electrolyte balance, especially sodium, is necessary.

Although bolus injections of barbiturates reduce increased ICP, long-term improvement in survival after global head injury has not been demonstrated. In laboratory studies, barbiturates have improved outcome after focal injuries.

FLUID RESUSCITATION

Appropriate fluid therapy is critical for optimal neurologic outcome after cerebral damage. As mentioned earlier, the maintenance of adequate cerebral perfusion and, thus, tissue oxygenation are of primary importance. Conflicting factors often make this state difficult to maintain. Hypovolemia caused by blood loss or diuretic administration with or without vasospasm may coexist with regional areas of hyperemia and cerebral edema caused by dysautoregulation.

A further goal is maintenance of the intravascular and extracellular electrolyte composition on which normal neuronal and glial function depend. These two functions are physiologically interrelated cellular functions that are subject to fluctuations or malfunction of the homeostatic mechanisms caused by disease or therapy.

The functional integrity of the blood-brain barrier, which has its structural basis in tight junctions between the endothelial cells of the cerebral capillary walls, is damaged by head injury, and ionic and molecular matter that is normally excluded passes across readily. Whether this is due to a "loosening" of the tight junctions or the increased vesicular transport across the cell or pinocytosis is unknown. Water moves rapidly across the blood-brain barrier, depending on the osmotic gradient between plasma and the brain.

One of the mechanisms of edema formation after cerebral ischemia is the production of excessive quantities of lactate. Increased intracellular osmolarity in the brain attracts water. Cerebral edema increases intercapillary distance, thereby making the cells furthest from the

Table 5 Reduction of Intracranial Hypertension

Pharmacologic Reduction	Mechanical Reduction
Diuretics	Release of hematoma
	Drainage of cerebrospinal fluid
Barbiturates	Craniectomy
Mannitol	Hyperventilation
Furosemide	"Head-up" position

Table 4 Methods of Measuring Intracranial Pressure

Method	Advantages	Disadvantages
Subarachnoid bolt	Simple	Cannot drain CSF
		Compliance measurement difficult
Intraventricular catheter	CSF drainage possible	Difficult if edema present
	Compliance measurements more accurate	
Implanted epidureal transducer	Infection unlikely	Cannot drain CSF
	Simple	Calibration more difficult to maintain
CT scan	Simple, noninvasive	One-time measurement only

capillaries more hypoxic and producing further lactic acidosis, a higher osmolality, and increased edema. Also, when the blood-brain barrier is disrupted, increases in intraluminal pressure force fluid out of the capillaries and into the surrounding brain. Dysautoregulation permits a higher intracapillary pressure and therefore enhances the formation of cerebral edema.

Glucose crosses the blood-brain barrier via bidirectional, energy-requiring active transport systems that permit the rapid equilibration of infused glucose between the blood and the cerebral intercellular fluid. Thus, the infusion of large quantities of 5 percent glucose significantly elevates ICP. Hypertonic glucose solutions act osmotically to decrease ICP initially, but a rebound increase in ICP occurs. Much experimental and clinical data point to the deleterious effects of glucose in the postischemic brain. Under hypoxic conditions, when blood glucose is elevated, high blood glucose levels correlate significantly with the severity of neurologic deficits in cerebral ischemia, perhaps secondary to a higher production of lactate. Causes of focal ischemia after head injury include vasoconstriction secondary to hyperventilation, hypotension, surgical brain retraction, and the initial injury. Further contributing factors include cerebral vasospasm secondary to subarachnoid hemorrhage and cerebral edema. Hyperglycemia in neurosurgical patients is increased by steroid administration.

Because the intact blood-brain barrier excludes molecules that have a molecular weight of more than 8,000, albumin (molecular weight of 69,000) is excluded. However, if the blood-brain barrier is disrupted, not only does albumin enter the brain, but it remains after the plasma levels decrease, thus considerably increasing cerebral edema. Plasmanate, which consists primarily of albumin, may also be hazardous in the patient with severe brain injury.

Trauma patients may have lost a significant percentage of circulating blood volume. Fever, which may be high in the presence of thalamic injury or of blood in the subarachnoid space, increases water loss from the skin. Prolonged ventilation with nonhumidified gases increases airway losses. Other factors influencing urinary fluid excretion include iatrogenic diuresis, a catabolic response with protein breakdown and excretion of nitrogen and water after major trauma, and the tendency of patients with severe intracranial disease to develop diabetes insipidus.

The rationale for maintaining hypovolemia, ostensibly to decrease the formation of cerebral edema, has been questioned for the following reasons:

1. Under experimental conditions, cerebral water content decreases minimally, despite complete fluid restriction.
2. Hypotension associated with hypovolemia may decrease regional CBF and increase hypoxia.
3. Hypovolemia may decrease oxygen transport to areas of the brain with normal autoregulation and cause a reflex vasodilatation and increased ICP.

4. Preoperative hypovolemia increases the risk of an unstable anesthetic course.

The primary goal of fluid therapy is to maintain the balance between overhydration with the risk of cerebral edema, and dehydration contributing to cardiovascular instability, respiratory complications, and further neurologic damage.

Resuscitation is usually initially performed with isotonic lactated Ringer's solution, albumin, or plasmanate, followed by whole blood, if needed, once type-specific blood becomes available. Hypertonic solutions have not been found to be beneficial. The least increase in ICP has been demonstrated when colloid solutions are used. However, administration of more than 3 U of this solution has been associated with abnormalities of clotting factors.

NEURODIAGNOSTIC TESTING

Increased ICP, hypoxia, and hypercapnia cause patients to become restless, agitated, or belligerent, often making neurodiagnostic studies difficult or the results equivocal. Cooperation is especially difficult to obtain from young children. Patients should be sedated only after the cause of the restlessness has been established and appropriate therapy initiated. Administration of narcotics or barbiturates to a hypoxic patient breathing spontaneously may be fatal. If there is any doubt as to the adequacy of the airway in restless patients, they must be managed with a general endotracheal anesthetic technique for the duration of the study.

ANESTHETIC MANAGEMENT

Only approximately 20 percent of head-injured patients have lesions amenable to surgical intervention. In the operative management of patients with head injury, the key aims are the establishment and maintenance of an impeccable airway, cardiovascular stability, and optimization of intracranial dynamics.

Choice of Anesthetic Agents

Controversy continues over what constitutes the preferred anesthetic technique for patients with head injury.

Routine administration of preoperative medication is not indicated. Pain is rarely a major complaint, and therefore the use of narcotics, which depress respiration, is not justified. Barbiturates and tranquilizers obscure changing neurologic status, and tachycardia caused by belladonna alkaloids may mask excessive blood loss. Phenytoin is the initial drug of choice for seizure control, as it causes less sedation. Side effects (hypotension, cardiac dysrhythmias, and central nervous system depression) are minimized if the drug is given at an intravenous rate of no more than 50 mg per minute.

In a review of outcome of patients with head injury

in our institution, in patients who had sustained blunt trauma, we obtained better results when inhalation agents were used. As the pathology of head injury is often one of decreased flow, maintenance of excess flow in relation to metabolic demands may provide better conditions for recovery (i.e., the uncoupling of flow and metabolism provided by isoflurane). Administration of nitrous oxide alone (i.e., 70 percent with muscle relaxation) yielded uniformly poor results. For patients with injuries characterized by diffuse vasodilation (patients with gunshot wounds and small children), outcome was slightly better after barbiturate anesthesia. Laboratory studies have confirmed these findings. Isoflurane alone improved neurologic outcome compared with nitrous oxide alone. However, the addition of lesser amounts of nitrous oxide to the inhalation agent did not worsen outcome.

The use of nitrous oxide is probably not justified. Its addition decreases the amount of inspired oxygen and increases the risks of tension situations developing if pneumothorax (e.g., in cases of multiple trauma) or pneumocephalus (e.g., fractured skull) exists. Also, the analgesic action of nitrous oxide may be easily provided by replacement with an infusion of low-dose fentanyl (1 to 2 μg per kilogram per hour).

Although satisfactory control of otherwise refractory intracranial hypertension may be achieved in 25 percent of patients by barbiturate infusion, outcome is not improved. Moreover, considerable patient variability exists in clearance of pentobarbital after head injury, and daily monitoring of barbiturate levels is indicated.

Succinylcholine chloride is often incorporated in rapid sequence intubation. At least one case of hyperkalemia has been reported after use of this muscle relaxant given to a nonparetic comatose patient. Also succinylcholine chloride may increase ICP by central and peripheral actions. The availability of other agents suggests that succinylcholine chloride should not be used in patients with cerebral damage. Vecuronium bromide, while generally effective, may be required in much higher doses in patients who have been maintained on antiseizure medications such as phenytoin (Dilantin) or phenobarbital because of rapid breakdown by microenzymes induced in the liver. While the breakdown product of atracurium besylate, laudanosine, has been implicated as a seizure-provoking agent in animals, the dose of atracurium besylate necessary to produce such toxic levels greatly exceeds that required in neurosurgical procedures. If the dose of atracurium besylate is limited to 0.5 mg per kilogram, problems with histamine-induced hypotension are more theoretical than actual. Until an ultra short-acting nondepolarizing agent becomes available, either atracurium besylate or vecuronium bromide can be used to aid intubation in patients with head injury.

Monitoring

Appropriate intraoperative monitoring includes continuous electrocardiography with the capability of strip recording. Pulse oximetry, capnography, and temperature recording are invaluable and mass spectrometry or infrared analyses are highly desirable. Arterial cannulation is essential to allow frequent blood gas and serum electrolyte analyses and continuous systemic arterial blood pressure monitoring. Trend recordings with availability of a final hard copy of all parameters provide indications of continued adequate cerebral perfusion. Urinary output and fluid balance must be monitored, both to balance the enormous fluid shifts caused by blood loss and diuresis and to provide early warning of the development of diabetes insipidus.

If the operation is performed in a "head-up" position or if the injury involves a venous sinus, Doppler monitoring and prior placement of a right atrial catheter are recommended. However, the patient should not be placed in a Trendelenburg position for this maneuver (this pertains also to the insertion of a pulmonary artery catheter). In addition, a subclavian approach interferes less with cerebral venous drainage than the internal jugular approach.

In patients with acute, arterial epidural hematomas, preanesthetic time should not be devoted to cannulation of vessels other than peripheral veins because of the potential for complete survival if the clot is released promptly. Rather, anesthesia should be induced and invasive monitoring established later.

After surgery has commenced, an arterial route can be established. In the interim, continuous assessment of blood pressure may be obtained by the use of a finger plethysmography, and pulse oximetry can monitor the adequacy of arterial flow.

POSTOPERATIVE CARE

Careful monitoring, attention to maintenance of cardio-respiratory stability, and frequent neurologic assessment in an intensive care setting are essential for all but the most minor head injuries.

If the patient was conscious or semiconscious preoperatively, the same state or better should be achieved at the conclusion of surgery. If at all possible, reversal of the anesthetic state and early extubation are desirable, as they allow the best conditions for neurologic examination. Early extubation decreases the likelihood of developing pneumonic complications and improves the patient's ability to cough. Patients in whom considerable cerebral edema was demonstrated preoperatively must be carefully observed for the development of hypercapnia, alteration in the sensorium, and further increase in ICP. If any of these conditions occur, reintubation and assisted ventilation must be performed immediately. Communication with the surgeon is essential. Operative findings may dictate continued ventilatory support.

Several complications of fluid balance may contribute to postoperative coma or seizure activity. Damage to the hypothalamus—either directly or in association with increased ICP—may manifest itself, usually postoperatively, as diabetes insipidus. Urinary output increases to as much as 1 L per hour, urinary osmolality decreases, and hypernatremia develops. Muscle irritability, seizures, and loss of consciousness occur at serum sodium levels of 160 mEq per liter. Urinary output should be replaced hourly with hypotonic solutions such as 0.25 to 0.5 percent sodium chloride with additional potassium chloride. If the polyuria exceeds 150 ml per hour, vasopressin tannate in peanut oil (Pitressin tannate in oil) 5 U subcutaneously, should be given. In cooperative patients, control can be obtained in minutes by nasal insufflation of 1-deamino-(8-D-arginine)-vasopressin (DDAVP). This drug is also available as a subcutaneous preparation. Parenteral Pitressin should be given slowly and the electrocardiogram monitored carefully, as dysrhythmias may occur. The syndrome usually resolves spontaneously in 72 hours. If it has been diagnosed after severe hypernatremia has developed, correction of the hyperosmolar state that is too rapid may cause fatal cerebral edema or brain damage. Half of the calculated free water deficit should be replaced with-in the first 24 hours, and the rest should be replaced over the next 1 to 3 days (in addition to the normal daily requirements).

Replacement with sugar-containing solutions should be avoided to prevent the development of nonketotic, hyperglycemic coma, a syndrome characterized by loss of consciousness, seizures, and even respiratory arrest. Laboratory values show a serum sodium level of 145 to 155 mEq per liter, serum osmolality of 350 to 380 mOsm per kilogram, and a serum glucose level of approximately 1,000 mg per deciliter. Therapy includes the use of Pitressin, withdrawal of sugar solutions, and administration of small doses of regular insulin. Occasionally, excessive administration of fluids may be given, especially if more than one vein has been cannulated. Generally, if the fluid balance exceeds 1 L, some degree of overhydration exists. A delayed return to consciousness and dilutional hyponatremia may result. Furosemide (20 mg) should be given.

Acute hypokalemia may occur after the combined administration of mannitol and furosemide. Complications include potentiation of neuromuscular blockade, cardiac dysrhythmias, and even respiratory arrest. Mineralocorticoids, glycosuria, and metabolic alkalosis enhance renal potassium excretion. Careful monitoring and addition of potassium to the infusion, as necessary, are required.

Multimodality-evoked potential and electroencephalographic (EEG) monitoring may reliably be used during the postoperative period or in the intensive care unit to follow the course of patients with head injury. Evoked potential techniques allow differentiation between patients with drug-induced EEG changes and those with brain injury, as well as allow evaluation of functional states and prognosis. Patients with raised intracranial pressure undergo characteristic alterations in flash- and brain stem–evoked potentials.

It is critical to evaluate coagulation factors preoperatively and postoperatively. An indicator of the development of complications after head injury is the activation of the complement system by enzymes that cleave clotting factors. Disseminated intravascular coagulopathy and adult respiratory distress syndrome may result. Early diagnosis is suggested by elevation of prothrombin and partial thromboplastin time. Therapy with fresh-frozen plasma or other appropriate blood products should be initiated.

Recent studies suggest that brain injury may be diminished and recovery accelerated by early parenteral hyperalimentation.

SUGGESTED READING

Bruce DA. Management of severe head injury. In: Cottrell J, Turndorf H, eds. Anesthesia and neurosurgery. 2nd ed. St. Louis: CV Mosby, 150–172.

Grande GM, Stene JK, Berhnard WN. Airway management: considerations in the trauma patient. Crit Care Clin 1990; 6:11–12.

Paly D, Wolf A, Matjasko J. Management of severe head injury: the anesthesiologist's role. Problems in Anesthesia 1990; 4:172–187.

Rockswald GL, Leonard PR, Nagib MG. Analysis of management in thirty-three closed head injury patients who "talked and deteriorated." Neurosurgery 1978; 21:51–55.

SPINAL CORD INJURY

ROSEMARY HICKEY, M.D.
TOD SLOAN, M.D., Ph.D.
MAURICE S. ALBIN, M.D., M.Sc.(Anes.)

EPIDEMIOLOGY

The incidence of spinal cord injuries (SCIs) ranges from 12.4 to 53.4 per one million individuals in the United States. Injuries sustained in vehicular accidents account for approximately half of all spinal cord injuries.

In 1982, the National Head and Spinal Cord Injury Survey indicated that roughly 10,000 new acute spinal cord injuries resulting in paraplegia and quadriplegia will occur each year. Approximately 4,000 of these patients die before reaching a hospital, and 1,000 die during hospitalization. In the United States, approximately 4,000 traumatic quadriplegics are added to the national pool each year, and it is estimated that in 1981, approximately 170,000 persons in the United States suffered from complete or partial paralysis resulting from trauma.

Epidemiologic data from many countries seem to indicate that the etiologic factors causing SCI are (in order of decreasing incidence) vehicular accidents, falls (both on the job or outside work), and sports injuries (particularly diving injuries). The incidence of SCI appears to be much higher among men, with the age of most patients ranging from 15 to 35 years. Not surprisingly, younger and middle-aged persons suffer from occupational injuries, while older persons are more likely to suffer SCI after falls at home. Within the group of patients older than 50 years of age, there appears to be a high percentage of cervical SCI without bone injury.

PATHOPHYSIOLOGY OF INJURY

A basic knowledge of the mechanism of injury is essential for understanding SCI. External loading of the spine can produce flexion, extension, compression, tension, rotation, and shear stresses; these forces can result in spinal injuries. The complexity of spinal deformation often involves various combinations of these biomechanical stresses, making it extremely difficult to classify the injuries. Spinal injuries may also be associated with impacts that transmit inertial forces to the column. The cervical column is particularly susceptible to injuries such as those caused by sudden and rapid acceleration or deceleration.

Acute impact injury to the cord causes mechanical destruction of neuronal elements, hemorrhage, decreased vascular perfusion, and attendant lowering of tissue partial pressure of oxygen (PO_2), edema, and necrosis. The acute trauma causes an immediate increase in spinal cord blood flow (SCBF). However, disruption of small blood vessels, edema, and the effects of vasoactive substances promote vasospasm and thrombosis. This may lead to further ischemia, infarction, edema, and extension of the neurologic deficit. The SCBF may be severely reduced for up to 24 hours after injury.

Autoregulation of SCBF is impaired after an SCI has been sustained. In the noninjured state, autoregulation maintains SCBF over a wide blood pressure range. In animal studies, it has been demonstrated that spinal cord autoregulation closely parallels that of the brain and occurs between spinal cord perfusion pressures of approximately 60 and 120 mm Hg. Below the lower limits and above the upper limits, SCBF becomes directly dependent on perfusion pressure. After SCI, loss of the autoregulatory response is particularly important, considering the tenuous blood supply to the spinal cord. Rudimentary development of the radicular arteries supplying the spinal cord (derived from vertebral, costocervical, and lumbar arteries) render it vulnerable to ischemia. The radicular branches are few in number and their wide spacing leaves large "watershed" areas along the course of the anterior spinal artery. In these watershed areas, the arterial inflow is precarious and interruption of blood flow can have serious ischemic consequences. The tenous blood supply to the cord, its interruption after injury, and alterations in autoregulation all point out the potential adverse vascular conse-

quences of SCI. They also emphasize the danger of deliberate anesthetic hypotensive techniques in patients with SCI.

CLINICAL PATTERNS

Depending on the degree of severity and type of injury, the resultant SCI may produce several syndromes relating to neurologic damage. Aside from bony injury without neurologic injury (intact), classification of injury patterns is based on the degree and distribution of neurologic dysfunction.

In complete SCI, total paralysis and loss of sensation result from a complete interruption of the ascending and descending pathways below the level of the lesion. High cervical lesions with damage to the brainstem to Cl are termed pentaplegia. These patients have paralysis of the lower cranial nerves and accessory muscles as well as sensory and motor loss to the arms and legs. Respiratory quadriplegics have functional levels at C2–3, leaving the face, neck, sternocleidomastoid, and accessory muscles intact. These patients require ventilatory support as diaphragmatic control is lost. Quadriplegia involves motor loss to the arms and legs (injury C4–8), while paraplegia involves motor loss to the legs only (injury T1–S1). Perineal paraplegia involves loss of sacral roots S2–5 and causes bowel, bladder, and sexual dysfunction.

In an incomplete injury, there is preservation of some of the sensory and/or motor fibers below the lesion. Incomplete injuries can be delineated according to the anatomic damage sustained and include the following symptom complexes: anterior SCI syndrome, Brown-Séquard's syndrome, central cord syndrome, thoracic anterior spinal artery syndrome, and the cauda equina syndrome.

Anterior SCI syndrome is characterized by immediate motor paralysis of the upper and lower extremities, hypoasthesia, and hypalgesia, but with preservation of position sense, vibration sense, and light touch. Anterior compression of the spinal cord by a ruptured disc or dislocation of vertebrae affect the lateral corticospinal tract and spinothalamic tract but preserve posterior column function.

Brown-Séquard's syndrome is caused by a lesion of the lateral half of the spinal cord and is manifested by ipsilateral paresis and contralateral loss of pain and temperature one or more levels below the lesion. This entity is commonly seen in patients with stab wounds and occasionally in those with blunt trauma.

Central cervical cord syndrome occurs when there is more cellular destruction in the center of the cord than in the periphery, causing there to be a disproportionate degree of motor paralysis in the upper extremities as compared with the lower. This is accompanied by varying degrees of sensory loss. One finds central destruction of the spinal cord due to hemorrhage or necrosis, with sparing of the peripheral leg area in the lateral corticospinal tract.

Thoracic anterior spinal artery syndrome is characterized by fracture or dislocation in the lower thoracolumbar area with sensory and motor loss that appears at a higher level than the lesion itself, because of ischemia and edema occurring after vascular compromise to the midthoracic cord.

The *cauda equina syndrome* involves peripheral nerves instead of the spinal cord directly. When complete, it is signaled by paralysis of the lower extremities, sensory loss, and bowel and bladder dysfunction. When it is incomplete, symptoms may include sciata, numbness, and patchy sensation, or bowel and bladder dysfunction with saddle anesthesia. Since peripheral nerves possess the ability to regenerate compared with the spinal cord, there appears to be a better prognosis for recovery.

One specialized form of incomplete lesion is the patient with sacral sparing. In these patients, the lesion appears to be complete except for the presence of function in the sacral area, such as rectal tone, perianal sensation, or deep touch. The identification of this condition as well as differentiation of other incomplete lesions from complete lesions is important in that the prognosis is often better than that with complete lesions if aggressive early care is provided.

PHYSIOLOGIC DISTURBANCES

Multiple system dysfunction may occur following SCI (Table 1). Dysfunction of the pulmonary and cardiovascular systems is especially important. Fluid and electrolyte imbalance, loss of temperature control, and associated injuries also complicate SCI.

Pulmonary System

Pulmonary complications are a major cause of morbidity and mortality after acute SCI. An epidemiologic study of 5,131 patients sustaining spinal cord injuries between 1973 and 1980 determined that pneumonia was the overall leading cause of death following SCI.

With SCI, dysfunction of any or all of the muscles of respiration may occur, depending on the level of injury. Damage to cord segments C-3 to C-5 involve the phrenic nerve nuclei, and when the lesion is above C-4, voluntary diaphragmatic respiration mediated by the phrenic nerve is not possible. Low-level cervical quadriplegic patients whose phrenic nerve nuclei are intact also have respiratory impairment. They lack the proper intercostal muscle activity necessary to stabilize the rib cage, and diaphragmatic contraction may result in a paradoxical inward motion of the upper thorax during inspiration. Abdominal muscle dysfunction also occurs, leading to the inability to achieve normal residual volumes during expiration. Hemorrhage and edema may extend the level of neurologic dysfunction above the initial level of injury, leading to deterioration in respiratory function.

A reduction in vital capacity (VC) occurs between 1 and 5 days after cervical SCI and gradually improves over time. Other alterations in pulmonary mechanics seen in

Table 1 Physiologic Disturbances Associated with Acute SCI

Pulmonary
  Respiratory muscle dysfunction
    ($\downarrow$ VC, $\downarrow$ TLC, $\downarrow$ ERV, $\uparrow$ RV, $\uparrow$ work of breathing)
  Chest trauma
  Aspiration
  Pulmonary edema
  Pulmonary embolism

Cardiovascular
  Loss of sympathetics to heart (T1-T4)
  Loss of vascular tone
  Myocardial injury
  Blood loss with trauma

Fluid and electrolyte
  Respiratory acidosis
  Hypercalcemia
  Altered response to succinylcholine chloride

Loss of temperature control
  Poikilothermia

Associated injuries
  Head injury
  Chest trauma
  Intra-abdominal injuries
  Musculoskeletal injuries
  Fat emboli

Spinal shock

quadriplegic patients include a reduction in total lung capacity (TLC), expiratory reserve volume (ERV), and forced expiratory flow rates with an increase in residual volume (RV) and the work of breathing. As a result of these alterations, these patients are subject to retention of secretions, atelectasis, increased $\dot{V}/\dot{Q}$ mismatch, and poor ability to sigh and cough. Retention of secretions may require nasotracheal suctioning or fiberoptic bronchoscopy. An abdominal push maneuver in which the patient's expiratory effort is assisted by posterior and cephalad abdominal pressure has been shown to improve peak expiratory flow rates during attempts to cough. In contrast to noninjured patients, a change in body position from the upright to supine position may improve ventilatory function in quadriplegic patients. This results from an improvement in vital capacity due to a reduction in RV (RV is abnormally elevated in the quadriplegic patient) from the effect of gravity on the abdominal contents.

In addition to the altered ventilatory function intrinsic to the patient with SCI, other insults may also compromise ventilation. Associated chest trauma at the time of injury may result in a pneumothorax, hemothorax, or pulmonary contusion. Gastric atony secondary to spinal shock may cause a large gastric air bubble that limits diaphragmatic excursion and increases the risk of aspiration. Patients who have depressed consciousness from associated head injury are at particular risk for aspiration. Pulmonary embolism secondary to deep venous thrombosis may occur as a consequence of bed rest, immobilization, and muscular paralysis.

The incidence of pulmonary edema is increased in the patient with acute SCI. In animal studies, after cervical cord transection, an increase in extravascular lung water has been demonstrated, suggesting alterations in pulmonary permeability following SCI. Pulmonary edema attributed to autonomic dysfunction at the time of injury (neurogenic pulmonary edema) has been noted in humans. Although the exact mechanisms leading to pulmonary edema are not fully understood, patients with cervical SCI are particularly vulnerable to this complication and require meticulous management of volume status.

Pulmonary therapy emphasizing the prevention, recognition, and treatment of secretion retention is valuable in the quadriplegic patient. This includes frequent repositioning, deep-breathing exercises, incentive spirometry, chest percussion, assisted coughing, and serial pulmonary function testing. When secretion retention is noted, intermittent positive-pressure breathing (IPPB), bronchodilators, and in some instances, fiberoptic bronchoscopy may be used to clear secretions.

Cardiovascular System

SCI is characterized by autonomic dysfunction that interferes with the maintenance of cardiovascular stability. Experimental studies in animals have shown that there is an initial increase in mean arterial pressure (MAP) following injury that may be accompanied by cardiac ectopic beats and blocked by alpha-adrenergic–blocking agents. This initial hypertensive response documented in animals has not been detected in humans, probably because the delay from the time of injury to the time of examination. After the initial period of hypertension, hemodynamic changes consistent with sympathetic denervation occur. Loss of sympathetic innervation to the heart at T-1 through T-4 cord levels leaves the parasympathetic cardiac innervation via the vagus unopposed, resulting in bradycardia. Elimination of sympathetic arterial tone results in hypotension. Cellular damage to the myocardium may also contribute to cardiovascular instability.

Bradycardia associated with SCI occurs most frequently in patients who have a complete injury at the cervical level. It generally resolves by 3 to 5 weeks after injury and does not require permanent pacemaker therapy. It occurs frequently with suctioning or changes in body position. Vagal stimulation that cannot be compensated for by an integrated sympathetic response is believed to be the mechanism underlying bradycardia associated with these events. Hypoxemia also plays a role during tracheal suctioning. Bradycardic episodes are treated with vagolytic therapy (atropine, propantheline bromide) and, if associated with tracheal suctioning, increased ventilation and oxygenation.

Hypotension associated with SCI may present a difficult management problem. The use of a pulmonary artery catheter is helpful in guiding management of hypotension and volume replacement in these patients. Fluid infusion is given until pulmonary capillary wedge pressure (PCWP) is approximately 18 mm Hg, and if hypotension persists, vasoconstrictors are added.

Fluid and Electrolytes

Electrolyte balance may be affected by pH alterations such as respiratory acidosis from alveolar hypoventilation. Metabolic alkalosis due to loss of gastric hydrochloric acid from nasogastric suction may occur, as may hypochloremia due to vomiting, gastric suction, or loss into dilated gut. Alterations in calcium balance may also be encountered. Immobility leads to increased mobilization of calcium from bone, hypercalciuria, and in some instances, hypercalcemia. This occurs as early as 10 days after injury and peaks at 10 weeks. Hypercalcuria leads to the formation of renal calculi and renal parenchymal damage.

Temperature Control

Body temperature may approach the temperature of the environment (poikilothermia). This is caused by the loss of the ability to sweat in hot environments or to vasoconstrict in cooler environments. These patients are prone to excessive heat loss during surgical procedures and easily become hypothermic.

Associated Injuries

Twenty-five to 65 percent of all patients with traumatic SCI also sustain other injuries. The possibility of concomitant head injury and SCI should always be considered, necessitating immobilization of the head and neck until SCI can be excluded in head trauma patients. Chest trauma may also occur, resulting in fractured ribs, pulmonary contusions, hemothorax, or pneumothorax. The diagnosis of intra-abdominal injuries, which occur in approximately 5 percent of patients sustaining blunt cervical SCI, may be particularly difficult. The loss of abdominal muscle tone and sensation as well as the hypotension that may be associated with acute cervical SCI mask the typical signs of blood loss due to abdominal injury. Musculoskeletal injuries including long bone fractures (with the possibility of fat emboli) as well as pelvic fractures and hip fractures/dislocation may also occur. In blunt spinal cord trauma, the majority of abdominal and other injuries follow motor vehicle accidents. Fewer associated injuries occur following blunt SCI due to falls, diving accidents, or other causes. In penetrating SCI such as that due to gunshot wounds or stab wounds, there is a high incidence of associated injuries to the esophagus, trachea, bronchi, and bowel.

Spinal Shock

The syndrome of spinal shock is characterized by the absence of all cutaneous and tendon reflexes below the level of the lesion. The patient exhibits flaccid paralysis and evidence of interruption of sympathetic pathways including bradycardia, hypotension, and decreased systemic vascular resistance. Sympathetic interruption associated with spinal shock also leads to gastric atony, dilation, and ileus that require nasogastric suctioning, and bladder atony that requires indwelling or intermittent catheterization. The duration of areflexia is variable but is usually 3 to 6 weeks in adults. Reappearance of the anal and bulbocavernous reflexes herald the return of spinal reflex activity, which generally occurs in a distal to cephalad direction.

ANESTHETIC MANAGEMENT

A major focus of SCI treatment is the period immediately following the actual injury. The basic life measures of airway, adequate ventilation, and maintenance of normal circulation are of primary concern to prevent secondary injury to the cord. Bony realignment by traction of the spine to place the spinal cord in an optimal environment for recovery is also of primary concern. The various physiologic disturbances associated with SCI discussed above must be considered. During this period, surgery is often reserved for correction of the associated injuries or for realignment of the spine to remove bone impingement on the spinal cord when traction is insufficient to cause realignment.

After the acute injury period, the focus of care becomes stabilization of associated medical problems. These medical problems may be underlying disorders, consequences of the trauma, or secondary to the neural dysfunction of injury. As the patient enters into the chronic phase of SCI, care revolves around rehabilitation. Surgery during this time is usually for correction of the long-term consequences of debilitation such as treatment of decubitus ulcers, renal stones, and release of muscle contractures.

Preoperative Assessment

As with any patient, a thorough preoperative evaluation is important. In addition to the usual concerns for allergies and medical problems, special focus in the spinally injured patient should be directed at the SCI and its consequences as well as associated injuries. The SCI and its consequences may be assessed by considering four basic aspects: spinal column stability, time since injury, degree of neurologic injury, and the spinal level injured.

Spinal Column Stability

Identifying preoperatively the patient who has an unstable spine is critical in planning patient intubation and positioning, as neurologic injury may be aggravated by improper management. Of particular concern are the patients who are unstable as a result of malfusion (when corrective surgery was not done or stabilization procedures were ineffective), since their instability may be overlooked. In some patients with acute SCI, muscle spasms may partially splint the bony instability, protecting the patient until anesthesia or muscle relaxants eliminate that effect.

Time Since Injury

Patients go through three basic phases after sustaining SCI, and each phase has different anesthetic concerns. During the acute phase immediately following injury, associated injuries sustained with the trauma and the presence of a full stomach warrant attention in addition to the SCI. In evaluating associated injuries, the frequent occurrence of head injury and chest trauma is notable, as both impact heavily on anesthetic care. Abdominal trauma is also extremely important, as neurologic injury may mask patient complaints and major abdominal bleeding may go undetected.

In patients with severe SCI and denervated muscle, the possibility of excessive potassium release after the administration of succinylcholine chloride must be considered when used more than 24 hours postinjury. Hyperkalemia following the use of succinylcholine chloride has been demonstrated as early as 3 days and as late as 6 months postinjury and may reach lethal levels; levels as high as 14 mEq per liter have been reported. It appears prudent to avoid the use of succinylcholine between 1 day and 1 year postinjury when denervation of muscle has occurred.

As the time postinjury progresses into the phase of chronic SCI, uncontrolled spinal reflexes may pose problems. Two hyperreflexic syndromes are identifiable. First, muscle spasms may occur due to hyperactive spinal reflexes controlling muscle tone. This "mass reflex" results from the loss of cerebellar and cortical coordinating activity and may make management of the unanesthetized patient difficult. The second syndrome of hyperreflexia is that caused by uncontrolled autonomic vascular reflexes. Usually beginning 2 to 3 weeks after injury, afferent impulses from manipulation of the bowel or bladder or other sensory input may elicit a spinal reflex that results in sympathetically mediated vasoconstriction. This causes an influx of blood into the circulation proportionate to the volume of contracted vasculature. Hypertension results if more blood volume is introduced into the circulation than can be accommodated by vasodilation in the unaffected vasculature. For complete neurological injuries above T-7, hypertension is observed in 65 to 85 percent of patients despite upper extremity vasodilation. Baroreceptor-mediated bradycardia usually accompanies the hypertension. Patients with lesions above T-4, however, may have tachycardia if the sympathetic innervation of the heart is included in the autonomic efferent activity. Autonomic hypertension should be treated promptly, as life-threatening sequalae may occur. Spinal, epidural, and general anesthesia are generally sufficient to prevent the reflex. If it does occur, usually during surgery attempted under local anesthesia, a vasodilator such as sodium nitroprusside or trimethaphan camsylate may be used to control the hypertension.

The patient with chronic SCI has many of the other problems of chronically debilitated patients. These may include gastric erosions, osteoporosis, hypercalcemia, hypercalcuria, renal calculi, and renal failure, as well as difficulties with emotional stability and substance abuse.

Degree of Neurologic Injury and Spinal Level Injured

The issue of neurologic dysfunction can be considered by examining the problems of a complete SCI, as the injury level varies with the anatomic level. Clearly the patient who is intact will have few problems related to neural dysfunction. Patients with severe injuries will share the consequences of the problems at all lower levels (Table 2).

The patient with a cauda equina lesion is often overlooked, but loss of bladder function results in urinary tract infections and renal insufficiency. These as well as other chronic infections such as decubitus ulcers may lead to amyloidosis and its attendant problems. Loss of bowel control may result in fluid and electrolyte disorders if not properly managed.

In patients with injury of the lumbar cord, there are further considerations as a result of the loss of neural control of the legs. Hyperkalemia associated with succinylcholine chloride may occur. Loss of sympathetic tone allows passive heat loss and heat gain through the skin surface and limits the ability of the vascular system to compensate for alterations in vascular volume. Chronically, the problem of reflex muscle spasms and contractures may make management difficult.

With injury in the thoracic column, the loss of abdominal and intercostal musculature results in the loss of pulmonary function necessary for efficient coughing and clearing of secretions. Acutely, bowel and gastric distention limits diaphragmatic excursion and also contributes to reduced pulmonary function. When the level ascends above T-7, autonomic reflexes in the chronically injured patient may lead to hypertensive episodes. In the high thoracic region (T1–4), the loss of sympathetic tone to the heart may cause bradycardia because of the relative imbalance of sympathetic and vagal influences. Some acutely injured patients experience severe bradycardia and even asystole when maneuvers such as airway manipulation increase vagal tone. Except for patients with heart disease who require pacemakers, atropine is usually sufficient treatment for bradycardia until spontaneous resolution occurs.

Injuries to the cervical region may make airway management difficult because of neck instability or devices applied for stabilization (such as a halo brace). In the midcervical region, loss of arm musculature causes further loss of tone in the vascular beds, leading to increased heat exchange with the environment and further inability to compensate for changes in vascular volume. Pulmonary artery catheters may be necessary in the acute phase or operating room to manage volume replacement in these patients. Excessive fluid infusion

Table 2 Problems Associated with Severe SCI at Different Levels

Level	Disorder
High cervical	Ventilation
Low cervical	Intubation Limited cardiovascular reserves
High thoracic	Reduced alveolar ventilation Loss of cardiac sympathetics (T-1 to T-4) Autonomic hypertension (T-7) (chronic phase)
Low thoracic	Loss of abodminal muscle function Reduced expiratory reserves Bowel and gastric distention (acute phase)
Lumbar	Hypercalciuria Poor vascular reserves Decubitus (chronic phase) Loss of temperature regulation Mass reflex (chronic phase) Deep venous thrombosis, pulmonary embolism Hyperkalemia associated with succinylcholine (1 day to 1 year)
Sacral	Loss of bowel function Alteration in fluid and electrolyte function Loss of bladder function Infection, renal failure Amyloidosis

*A lesion at any level shares the problems of all lower level injuries.

may result in congestive heart failure, and insufficient fluids may not allow optimal cardiac performance. Hypotension and cardiac arrest have been reported with position changes. Lesions in the high cervical region cause marked impairment of ventilation, as the innervation of the diaphragm via the phrenic nerve (C3–5) is impaired by injury or by edema from lower levels.

Several other factors must be considered, including problems of unusual positions (sitting, prone, lateral), invasive procedures (thoracotomy, transoral procedures), procedures with large blood losses, or other special considerations (e.g., large skin flaps). A discussion of these problems is beyond the scope of this chapter.

Preoperative Laboratory Studies and Premedication

Appropriate laboratory studies in severely injured patients should include electrocardiography, chest x-ray examination, measurements of glucose, creatinine, blood urea nitrogen, electrolytes, and liver function studies. In addition, assessment of the cardiovascular status and pulmonary reserves (arterial blood gases and basic pulmonary function tests including forced vital capacity [FVC] and negative inspiratory force) should be obtained in patients with high thoracic or cervical lesions. The preoperative visit should include a discussion of procedures that may be conducted while the patient is awake (such as intubation and positioning) and the possibility of intraoperative awareness, particularly if techniques such as a wake-up test are likely. After the patient has been assessed, the perioperative plan can be formulated. Premedication should be chosen cautiously in an attempt to allay anxiety without producing undue side effects such as ventilatory compromise. The drying action of anticholinergics such as atropine or glycopyrrolate is useful in patients for whom awake intubation with a fiberoptic is planned. Corticosteroids may be needed in patients who have received adrenally suppressive doses preoperatively.

Perioperative Monitoring

General Monitors

Basic monitoring that should be used for all patients is needed (e.g., electrocardiography and monitoring of blood pressure, oxygenation, ventilation, and body temperature). In addition, an arterial line is often used to provide continuous monitoring of arterial blood pressure and assess ventilation. Depending on the patient's injury and underlying physical status, a pulmonary artery catheter may be beneficial in assessing cardiovascular parameters and response to fluid therapy. If it is planned that these latter invasive monitors are to be used intraoperatively, their insertion before surgery may allow optimal preoperative preparation. The surgical position and procedure itself may also mandate the use of certain monitors, such as a central venous catheter for procedures performed with the patient in the sitting position or when excessive blood loss is likely to occur.

Monitoring of the Nervous System

Specialized monitoring of the nervous system is useful in procedures that may provoke neurologic injury in patients in whom neurologic function remains. Current methodology allows three forms of neurologic monitoring: testing in a conscious patient, sensory-evoked potentials, and motor-evoked potentials. Testing in a conscious patient may involve performing intubation and positioning while the patient is awake as well as awakening the patient after critical points in the procedure to ascertain that neurologic function is unchanged.

Somatosensory-evoked potentials (SSEPs) have been widely applied to assess neurologic function. The classic technique of SSEP measurement involves repetitive electrical stimulation of a peripheral nerve and recording of the resultant nervous signal as it traverses the nervous system into the sensory cortex. The SSEP signal travels the spinal cord primarily via the posterior columns that mediate proprioception and vibration. Several variations of the classic technique (e.g., recording or stimulating through paraspinal, epidural, or spinal electrodes) have also been used. Although good results

have been obtained with the use of SSEPs during spinal surgery, it should be kept in mind that only posterior column function is monitored. The potential for a motor cord deficit exists, therefore, even in the presence of preserved SSEPs.

Motor tract monitoring by stimulation of the cerebral cortex via electrical or magnetic means is currently receiving attention. With this technique, stimulation of the motor cortex elicits measurable responses in peripheral nerves and electromyogenic (EMG) activity in peripheral muscles. The major advantage of motor evoked potentials (MEPs) is the ability to assess anterior spinal cord pathways associated with motor function. Their use for patients with SCI is currently under investigation.

Choice of Anesthetic Agent

At present, no specific anesthetic agent or technique appears superior for either induction or maintenance of anesthesia. Inhalational anesthesia may be associated with less postoperative respiratory depression. A narcotic-based technique, however, offers a better opportunity to conduct an intraoperative wake-up test and is also preferred if intraoperative evoked potentials are to be utilized, because of the lesser effect of narcotics compared with inhalational agents on alteration of SSEPs. If EMG recordings are to be made as a component of motor tract monitoring, careful titration of muscle relaxants will be necessary to maintain the EMG response.

Key Points of Intraoperative Management

Patients who are acutely traumatized or have cervical lesions at a high level require careful continuation of the critical care management as they are moved to the operating room. Monitoring modalities should be established before induction of anesthesia and intubation so that baseline values can be known and preinduction adjustments made if necessary.

For patients with cervical SCI, performing intubation while the patient is awake is preferred so that neurologic status can be verified after intubation. Blind nasal or fiberoptic techniques are preferred so that neck manipulation can be minimized. Nasal intubation should be avoided, however, in patients with concomitant basilar skull fractures. Topical anesthesia, transtracheal local anesthesia injection, superior laryngeal nerve block, and judicious intravenous sedation are techniques often used singly or in combination to facilitate the intubation. After intubation, performing positioning while the patient is awake may often be desired to re-verify the adequacy of spinal alignment. Anesthesia is induced after positioning, generally with intravenous agents.

Maintenance of the anesthetic is similar to that for other patients, but attention must be focused on avoiding exacerbation of the pathophysiologic derangements of the SCI. Intubation and controlled ventilation should be used in the operating room to help avoid the problems of hypoxemia and hypercarbia, which are particularly prone to occur in patients with spinal injury because of reduced pulmonary reserves.

Fluid replacement must be carefully managed. The injudicious use of fluids may cause hypotension due to inadequate preload, or it may cause pulmonary edema due to excessive circulating volume. Fluid deficits should be corrected early (preoperatively if possible), and response to therapy should be monitored (urine output, central venous pressure, and/or PCWP). High ventilatory pressures that impede venous return should be avoided, and anesthetic agents must be carefully titrated to minimize cardiovascular depression. Sudden position changes may also alter cardiovascular dynamics and should be avoided. Because these patients are prone to excessive temperature swings due to limitations in thermal regulation, temperature monitoring and methods to avoid hypothermia should be used routinely in the cool operating room environment. These methods include appropriate ambient temperature control, heating and humidifying of inspired gases, warming of intravenous and irrigation fluids, and heating blankets.

As discussed above, SCBF autoregulation may be altered or lost after SCI, making SCBF pressure dependent. Deliberate hypotension, therefore, may compromise SCBF and is not advisable. This may be most critical when the injury is in the watershed regions of the spinal cord, such as between C-5 and T-2.

Deliberate hemodilution may also be deleterious. Reduction of the hematocrit to 30 to 33 percent may improve microcirculatory blood flow by reducing viscosity, but further reductions may compromise oxygen carrying capacity and oxygen delivery. Hemodilution with crystalloid solutions may aggravate spinal cord edema in the acute injury patient. The actual significance of this latter effect, however, is not well documented.

Ventilation is kept in the normal range as hypercarbia may cause a "steal" of blood from the injured area to adjacent dilated normal areas, and hypocarbia may further reduce flow. Thus, ventilation in the normal range, adequate blood pressure, and good oxygenation are used to provide an optimal spinal cord tissue environment.

As with other spinal procedures, blood loss may be massive. Treatment for excessive blood loss, such as transfusions, warming of fluids and the patients, and cell-salvaging techniques should be applied. Occasionally, fresh frozen plasma and platelet transfusions may also be needed.

During the surgery, a wake-up test may be used after critical spinal manipulations. This requires that anesthetic agents be reduced or eliminated. Partial reversal of the muscle relaxants or opioids used for maintenance may be needed at this time. When the patient is sufficiently awake, he or she is asked to acknowledge by hand grasp or head motion that he can understand the command, and then is asked to move his hands or legs. After the test, intravenous agents are added to reinduce anesthesia, and the maintenance agent is re-employed.

At the conclusion of the procedure, the anesthetic agents are eliminated and the patient awakened for reverification of neurologic status.

Postoperative Care

The patient is moved with all monitoring lines in place to the recovery room or to a special care unit. Extubation should be cautiously delayed, particularly in patients with cervical SCI. Residual effects of the anesthetic agents together with a preoperative neurologic deficit may markedly depress alveolar ventilation. Even in patients with cervical SCI who present without significant neurologic injury, edema of the spinal cord and associated cord dysfunction may attend the surgical procedure and make an adequate pulmonary reserve marginal. In addition, reintubation may be difficult or hazardous, as the urgency to ventilate is complicated by the recent neck surgery.

After surgery, a 12-lead electrocardiogram should be obtained as cardiac function may be compromised either primarily in the patient with underlying heart disease, or secondarily as a result of the SCI. A radiograph of the chest is taken to visualize the state of the pulmonary parenchyma and vasculature, as acute pulmonary edema can be a significant cause of morbidity and mortality in the postoperative quadriplegic patient.

Throughout all of the phases following spinal injury, these patients can present numerous anesthetic challenges. With good perioperative care, many of the potentially life-threatening complications of SCI can be acutely managed, assisting the patient through an often long and difficult hospitalization. Major advances in patient care, such as those available in specialized spinal care trauma centers, have improved the outlook for acute management and rehabilitation of these patients. Perhaps the best hope for long-term improvement in outcome rests in prevention. When good care is provided, many of these patients live highly productive lives.

SUGGESTED READING

Albin MS. Acute spinal cord injury. Crit Care Clin 1987; 3:441–697.
Albin MS, Bunegin L, Gilbert J, Babinski MF. Anesthesia for spinal cord injury. Problems in Anesthesia 1990; 4:138–154.
Hickey R, Albin M, Bunegin L, Gelineau J. Autoregulation of spinal cord and cerebral blood flow: is the cord a microcosm of the brain? Stroke 1987; 17:1183–1189.
Mackenzie CF, Ducker TB. Cervical spinal cord injury. In: Matjesko J, Katz J, eds. Clinical controversies in neuroanesthesia and neurosurgery. New York; Grune & Stratton, 1986:77.
Newer MR. Evoked potential monitoring in the operating room. New York: Raven Press, 1986.

CHEST AND CARDIAC TRAUMA

JEFFREY C. ELMORE, M.D.
ADOLPH H. GIESECKE, Jr., M.D.

The anesthesiologist who is responsible for a patient with thoracic injuries must heed all of the usual guidelines for the care of the traumatized patient and, in addition, attend to some unique problems presented by thoracic injuries.

Thoracic trauma is both common and lethal. In deaths due to trauma, thoracic injury is the major mechanism in 25 percent and contributes to an additional 25 percent. Immediate fatalities are the result of cardiac or major vascular disruption with rapid exsanguination. Early fatalities occurring within hours of injury involve airway obstruction, aspiration, dysrhythmia, and tamponade. Respiratory insufficiency, infection, and multiorgan failure are common causes of death during the postoperative phase. Anesthesiologists must be able to recognize obstruction in upper and lower airways, tension pneumothorax, open pneumothorax, massive hemothorax, flail chest, pericardial tamponade, pulmonary contusion, aortic disruption, tracheobronchial disruption, esophageal disruption, traumatic diaphragmatic hernia, and myocardial contusion.

Thoracic trauma is a disease of young men. In 1988, 110 patients underwent operative procedures at Parkland Memorial Hospital for traumatic injuries involving the chest. Eighty-five percent of these were men, and 81 percent were younger than 40 years old. Fourteen patients were dead upon arrival in the operating room or died intraoperatively. An additional six patients died within 24 hours of operation. Several deaths involved direct cardiac, aortic, and caval injuries. Injuries to the main pulmonary artery or its proximal branches were also particularly lethal. Isolated penetrating injuries to the heart were not usually fatal. Severe head injuries or multiple abdominal organ injury in association with thoracic injury were predictably morbid. Shock of more than 30 minutes' duration carried a grave prognosis, but was a rare phenomena. The mechanism of death was usually exsanguination accompanied by hypothermia, acidosis, and coagulopathy. Hypoxemia was generally a premorbid occurrence. Less commonly, myocardial failure from contusion, dysrhythmia, or prolonged ischemia resulted in death.

The purpose of this chapter is to present the unique anesthetic problems imposed by patients with simple and complex thoracic injuries.

EVALUATION AND PREPARATION

Centers receiving major trauma patients on a regular basis should have a mechanism for their orderly evaluation and treatment. This means that anesthesia personnel should be present in the hospital at all times, and an operating room equipped and designated for major trauma should be available. Severely injured patients require maximal and well-directed efforts. A team consisting of three or more anesthesiologists is often required. All too often, major resuscitation turns into "Brownian Motion" with an unsatisfactory result. In general, one person should be given the responsibility of airway management, one person should be designated record keeper, and one should be given the responsibility to direct the efforts. In many cases, all three will be pumping blood.

All anesthesiologists are aware of the ABCs of basic life support: airway, breathing, and circulation. In the evaluation of the traumatized patient, the abbreviations assume a slightly expanded meaning and the letters D and E are commonly added. "A" must include an evaluation for obstruction and integrity of the upper and lower airways. "B" must include a search for depressed ventilation, pneumothorax, flail chest, and hypoxemia. "C" must include hemorrhage control and a search for hidden blood loss. "D" refers to an evaluation of disability, especially with regard to neurologic and musculoskeletal systems. Finally, "E" involves exposing or completely undressing and examining the entire patient. Every traumatologist has had some young patient who died of a suspected medical illness, only to find on closer inspection a small bullet entry wound at the base of the skull or an ice pick entry wound on the back.

A badly injured patient's only hope for survival may be immediate surgical intervention with no time for set up and little time for evaluation. A room should be designated and equipped for emergencies at all times. Trauma rooms should be large enough to accommodate the anesthesia team, multiple surgical teams, and their attendant equipment (Table 1). These rooms should have individual thermostats capable of warming the air to temperatures of more than 24°C. The anesthesiologist should have in this room an electrocardiographic monitor, noninvasive blood pressure monitor, a two-channel pressure monitor, a temperature monitor, a stethoscope with the ability for transesophageal and unilateral auscultation, an end-tidal carbon dioxide monitor, a pulse oximeter, a warming blanket, a heated humidifier, and devices for warming fluids. Intravenous catheters and kits for central venous, pulmonary artery, and arterial cannulation are essential. A full complement of resuscitation drugs, muscle relaxants, and anesthetic agents should be updated daily. An anesthesia machine with standard alarm systems and a ventilator capable of positive end-expiration pressure (PEEP) and high airway pressures are necessary. The common adjuncts to airway management, including oral and nasal airways, endotracheal tubes, masks, laryngoscope, and blades in a wide array of sizes, should be available. A device for transtracheal jet ventilation should be at hand. Additional equipment that should be in the hospital and easily summoned to the operating room include a fiberoptic bronchoscope, double-lumen endotracheal tubes, transvenous cardiac pacer, defibrillator, an extra-

Table 1 Room Supplies for Trauma Operating Room

Fluids:
 Balanced salt solutions
 Colloids including albumin, plasma protein fraction, Hespan, and
  high molecular weight dextran
 D5W for dilution and drips
Warmers:
 Fluid warmers
 Warming blanket
 Heated humidifier
 Room thermostat
 Warmed fluids for irrigation
Monitors:
 Noninvasive blood pressure
 Electrocardiography
 Double-channel pressure monitor
 Esophageal and flat precordial stethoscopes
 End-tidal CO_2
 Pulse oximeter
 Temperature
 Oxygen analyzer
 Pressure alarm
Airway:
 Laryngoscope and blades in a wide array of styles and sizes
 Nasal and oral airway devices
 Transtracheal jet ventilation system
 Ventilator capable of positive end-expiratory pressure and high
  airway pressures
Circulation:
 Intravenous catheters
 Central venous cannulation kits
 Arterial cannulation kits
 Pulmonary artery cannulation kits
Cardiac:
 Transvenous pacemaker
 Defibrillator
Other:
 Anesthesia machine with standard alarms
Available equipment:
 Fiberoptic bronchoscope, double-lumen endotracheal tubes,
  cardiopulmonary bypass machine, echocardiogram

corporeal bypass machine, and an echocardiogram, preferably transesophageal.

Having a perfusionist in the hospital 24 hours per day and having a cardiopulmonary bypass (CPB) machine primed and ready around the clock is not the practice at Parkland Memorial Hospital. During the past year, we have used CPB on two chest trauma patients; one survived. With the exception of isolated penetrating injuries that require work on the back of the heart, CPB does not usually contribute to improved outcome and sufficient time exists to summon a perfusionist to prepare a pump.

MONITORING

The extent of monitoring should be based on the severity of injury and pre-existing disease. When any doubt exists, one should use an invasive approach. Sometimes patients will appear in the operating room with resuscitation in progress after having undergone little or no evaluation. These patients are dead or in that gray area between life and death. Priorities must be established. Adequacy of ventilation and intravenous access must be ensured before or during the pursuit of invasive monitors.

In hemodynamically stable patients, the usual monitors for intrathoracic procedures should be instituted before surgery. These include a 5-lead electrocardiogram, an intra-arterial catheter, a central venous or pulmonary artery catheter, a pulse oximeter, and automated noninvasive blood pressure monitor. End-tidal carbon dioxide monitoring, an oxygen analyzer, an esophageal stethoscope, temperature probes, a peripheral nerve stimulator, and a urinary catheter should be placed. If esophageal injury is suspected, nothing should be placed in or through the esophagus before surgical exploration. If the patient is to be turned laterally, a flat stethoscope should be placed under the dependent hemithorax to ensure selective auscultation. Meters for airway pressures are essential as high airway pressures, PEEP, and frequent adjustments of minute ventilation will be necessary.

The value of central venous cannulation is clear. These lines provide reliable routes for resuscitative fluids and drugs, as well as an estimate of intravascular volume. The internal and external jugular veins have long been favored by anesthesiologists. During thoracic surgery, neck lines can be placed and managed more easily than subclavian or antecubital lines. Unrecognized carotid cannulation is a more common event in hypotensive, hypovolemic patients. Successful placement requires a knowledge of anatomy and the confidence born of experience. Impedance to jugular venous drainage may be dangerous in patients with head injury and should be considered when one is placing these lines and positioning for surgery. In most instances of thoracic trauma, central venous catheters may be preferable to pulmonary artery catheters. Central venous pressure catheters are superior for fluid administration and usually provide an adequate estimate of intravascular volume. For trauma victims, the first answer to hypotension is volume replacement. Rare patients may have serious myocardial compromise superimposed on trauma; others may have acute dysfunction from myocardial contusion. These patients will benefit from the better estimates of left ventricular end-diastolic volume provided by a pulmonary artery catheter. Oximetric technology for continuous measurement of mixed venous oxygen saturation has been incorporated into the design of several pulmonary artery catheters. These provide a continuous estimate of the adequacy of perfusion, can be utilized to calculate shunt fractions, and guide respiratory interventions.

Transesophageal echocardiography (TEE) may soon find a place in thoracic trauma. TEE certainly demonstrates left ventricular volume and dysfunction. In addition, intraoperative echocardiography is occasionally mandatory to diagnose valvular lesions or confirm myocardial dysfunction in unexplained hypotension. In the past, this was done with a sterile probe applied to the surface of the heart. With more experience, it will be done through the esophagus. Mediastinal injury and esophageal injury will contraindicate the esophageal probe.

As surgery progresses, serial monitoring of arterial blood gases, hemoglobin, adequacy of coagulation, and serum electrolytes are necessary. Because thoracic trauma may compromise cerebral or spinal cord function, monitoring for ischemia in these areas is sometimes desirable. Sometimes the operative procedure involves interruption of thoracic aortic blood flow with the potential for central nervous system (CNS) damage, and commonly chest trauma is associated with head injury. Unfortunately, spinal cord– and brain stem–evoked potentials are not applicable in the setting of an unstable, blood-drenched patient. Spectral analysis electroencephalographic monitoring is more reliable but difficult to interpret without a baseline in some settings. All patients with coma, increased intracranial pressure, and mass lesions should undergo ventriculostomy before surgery outside the head. Evaluation of CNS function during general anesthesia is difficult. A ventriculostomy provides an early warning of increased intracranial pressure and permits treatment by withdrawal of cerebrospinal fluid (CSF).

ANESTHETIC TECHNIQUE

Chest trauma encompasses a wide variety of clinical presentations. All cases should be individualized. A few constant presentations deserve mention.

The patient should be considered to be at high risk for aspiration of stomach contents. Nonparticulate antacids should be given within 30 minutes of induction of anesthesia. In the setting of suspected injury to the stomach, esophagus, or small bowel, the risk of additional contamination is small and should not preclude administration of sodium citrate and citric acid (Bicitra). Patients without cervical spine injury and examination indicating adequate airways for direct oral intubation should be intubated in rapid sequence fashion with bimanual cricoesophageal compression. One hand applies pressure on the cricoid cartilage while the other hand supports the back of the neck. The cricoid pressure provided by two hands is more specific and uniform and results in a better "sniffing position," which facilitates laryngoscopy and intubation (Fig. 1).

When tamponade is present or suspected, or in the setting of hemodynamic instability, the patient should be prepped and draped for median sternotomy before induction of anesthesia. In this situation, blood should be ordered and be readily available. Special consideration must be given to patients with associated head and spinal injuries, thoracic aortic injury, bronchial disruption, pericardial tamponade, and pulmonary and myocardial contusions.

Associated Head Injuries

The care of the head injury patient with chest trauma follows the same physiologic principles as iso-

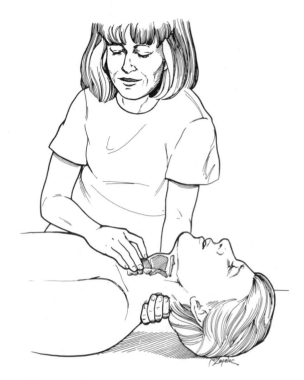

Figure 1 Bimanual cricoesophageal compression.

lated head injury. Subtle changes in neurologic function should be aggressively investigated. Tachypnea is common in chest trauma, but it is also an early sign of neurologic deterioration. Increases in respiratory rate therefore necessitate detailed physical evaluation, with any detectable neurologic change indicating computed tomography (CT). Changes in heart rate are also common in chest trauma and are an early sign of CNS change. These should also be meticulously investigated. Complaints of headache are specific for increased intracranial pressure (ICP) and cannot under any circumstances be dismissed.

If evidence of increased ICP is present, CT scanning is indicated before thoracic surgery, and consultation from a neurosurgeon should be sought. In general, mass lesions with a midline shift of less than 5 mm are not decompressed. This will vary from neurosurgeon to neurosurgeon, with temporal lobe clots receiving more aggressive therapy. In the case of increased ICP with no mass or with a mass causing a midline shift of less than 5 mm, interventricular catheters should be placed before surgery for diagnostic and therapeutic purposes. Intraoperatively, ICP must be continuously monitored with increases of more than 20 mm Hg being treated and the surgeons notified of the gravity of the situation. When one is positioning for surgery, care must be taken to facilitate venous drainage by elevating the head. An inspection for venous obstruction should be the first maneuver in response to increasing ICP.

Cervical spine injuries should be suspected in all trauma patients. When any uncertainty exists, injury to the cervical spine should be assumed. Management of these difficult situations is discussed in another section of this book. In-line traction with skull tongs is the preferred method for neck stabilization before intubation. Thoracic spine injuries are usually more obvious and less difficult to manage. The syndrome of spinal shock is common in patients with thoracic and cervical spine injuries and should be anticipated if it is not present in patients with spine injury.

Aortic Injuries

Aortic injuries following trauma have several causes and presentations. The most common sites of rupture are in the proximal aorta just distal to the left subclavian artery and at the ascending aorta just beyond the valve. Aortic tears are usually transverse and may result in complete disruption with rapid death or a small intimal tear with subtle symptoms before disruption or dissection. This diagnosis must be entertained in every patient with chest trauma. Symptoms of injury include chest and back pain, asymmetric pulses in the upper extremity, cervical hematoma, paralyzed left vocal cord, and tracheal deviation. The chest radiograph may show a blurred aortic knob or widened mediastinum.

Aortic root or proximal injuries require cardiopulmonary bypass for repair. It may be necessary to initiate CPB in the femoral vessels with hypothermic arrest before approaching some proximal aortic tears that involve the arch vessels. Unfortunately, uneven cooling, hepatic congestion, renal impairment, and coagulopathy are more common with this type of bypass circuit. Aortic repair distal to the left subclavian artery is usually performed in the lateral position with left atrium to left femoral artery partial bypass. Under these circumstances, oxygenated blood from the patient's lungs is partially bypassed from the left atrium to the vital organs distal to the aortic cross-clamp by a single roller pump into the femoral artery. The flow across the pump is regulated to maintain pressure in the lower limbs above a mean arterial pressure of 60 mm Hg. The bypass circuit typically flows 1,500 to 2,000 ml per minute to maintain this perfusion. This setup simultaneously decompresses the areas proximal to the aortic cross-clamp, eliminating the need for vasodilator therapy. In most clinical settings, a modest fluid bolus with the institution of this partial bypass provides improved blood flow on both sides of the cross-clamp. Placement of a double-lumen endotracheal tube facilitates the surgical approach but may be poorly tolerated if the patient has concomitant injury in the right lung.

Bronchopleural Fistulae

Abnormal communications between the lung and pleural space are common after trauma. The most frequent cause is parenchymal laceration from a broken rib. Rarely, a disruption in a bronchiole or larger airway results from blunt or penetrating trauma. Pneumothorax and/or hemothorax is a consequence of these injuries. Tension pneumothorax causes severe hemodynamic

compromise and must be treated quickly. This possibility must always be kept in mind when one is anesthetizing traumatized patients. Simple pneumothorax may be converted to tension pneumothorax by positive-pressure respirations or by the use of nitrous oxide.

In many instances of parenchymal tear, conservative therapy will suffice. With more severe injuries, blood vessel disruption accompanies airway injury, mandating surgical exploration. These patients can be very sick and require immediate surgery. Ventilation is difficult and may become worse with positive-pressure ventilation before chest tube placement. Once chest tubes are appropriately placed, ventilation should improve, but it may continue to be inadequate if a large pleural leak is present. The flexibility of double-lumen intubation is rarely afforded under these circumstances, necessitating other means of separating the lungs. Selective mainstem intubation with a regular endotracheal tube can temporize until the surgeon gains control of the air leak. With the guidance of a fiberoptic bronchoscope, this can be accomplished intraoperatively, if necessary, with the patient in the lateral position. The scope is used as a stylet after it has been passed into the appropriate airway. Right mainstem intubation is particularly hazardous because the right upper lobe bronchus frequently is obstructed, leaving only two lobes to accomplish ventilation and resulting in a large anatomic shunt. Endobronchial blockers may provide superior separation but are not always as readily available or as easily manipulated. Endotracheal tubes are commonly cut before intubation to reduce the risk of endobronchial intubation or kinking at the teeth. Uncut tubes should always be used in thoracic trauma because manipulation into a broncus may be beneficial.

Pericardial Tamponade

Pericardial tamponade can be deceptive. Young, otherwise healthy patients can appear stable in the presence of moderate or severe tamponade. The pericardium is a closed space normally containing 20 to 30 ml of fluid with a limited ability to accommodate acute changes in volume. As fluid fills the pericardial sac, ventricular filling is decreased with resultant diminished stroke volume. The body compensates by increasing the chronotropic and inotropic state of the heart. Endogenous catecholamine surge also enhances ventricular filling. Because the pericardial sac has a limited ability to dilate acutely, chest roentgenography may fail to suggest this condition. Fortunately, tamponade is rarely subtle and is revealed by clear clinical signs. Tachycardia, tachypnea, decreased pulse pressure, and pulsus paradoxus are present. Jugular venous distention and muffled heart sounds are frequent. In more severe cases, bluish discoloration of the skin on the face, neck, and chest may be present. Pericardiocentesis is diagnostic and temporarily therapeutic. Echocardiography can be helpful in establishing the diagnosis in less obvious cases.

The anesthetic approach to surgical decompression of the pericardial sac varies with the severity of hemodynamic compromise. The safest approach is local anesthesia for a subxiphoid pericardial window. If more extensive surgical manipulation is required, general anesthesia can be induced after pericardial decompression. Positive pressure ventilation with decreased venous return and general anesthetics with sympatholysis, vasodilatation, and direct myocardial depression are sometimes poorly tolerated in this setting. Many patients tolerate general anesthesia with ketamine and succinylcholine chloride for these brief procedures. High filling pressures, atrial contribution to cardiac output, systemic vascular resistance, and tachycardia should be maintained. An arterial line is mandatory before induction of anesthesia or surgical exploration with the patient under local anesthesia. Central lines demonstrate high venous pressures and are useful for volume replacement. Pulmonary artery catheters show right atrial, right ventricular, diastolic, and pulmonary artery wedge pressures approaching unity with more severe tamponade but rarely contribute to improved outcomes.

Pulmonary Contusion

Pulmonary contusion is a serious and persistent complication of chest trauma. Decreased functional residual capacity, airway collapse, bronchorrhea, and capillary leak lead to regional increases in vascular resistance and ventilation/perfusion mismatches. Mechanical compromises in ventilation from thoracotomy tubes, rib fractures, muscle dysfunction, intrathoracic fluid, and air collections also contribute to the pathophysiology of pulmonary contusion. Management under anesthesia includes positive-pressure ventilation with PEEP as required to maintain arterial oxygen pressure (PaO_2) above 60 mm Hg with a fractional inspired oxygen (FIO_2) below 0.5 mm Hg. Aggressive pulmonary toilet should be pursued. Careful attention to fluid balance is critical, with the patient being kept normovolemic with isotonic salt solutions. Although proponents of colloidal solution are many, no convincing evidence exists in the medical literature that colloidal solutions have any advantage over balanced salt solutions. In the setting of capillary injury, colloidal solutions may in fact increase lung water. Forced diuresis or volume depletion is ill advised in a normovolemic or hypovolemic patient and can aggravate hypoxia by compromising cardiac output. Pulmonary contusions are usually unilateral. With severe contusion, separation of the lungs with selective ventilation can improve oxygenation as the patient recovers. PEEP in the injured lung will help expand the alveoli and shunt blood to the less impaired lung being ventilated without PEEP. This results in a better match of perfusion and ventilation with improved oxygenation. Some patients with contusions can be managed without positive-pressure ventilation in the postoperative intensive care unit setting. This group should have a PaO_2 of more than 60 mm Hg while breathing FIO_2 less than 0.5 mm Hg. Bedside respiratory measurements must demonstrate tidal volumes greater than 5 ml per kilogram and a vital capacity of more than 10 ml per kilogram, and the respiratory rate should not exceed 30 breaths per minute. An intra-arterial line facilitates frequent blood gas analysis. The value of adequate analgesia cannot be overstated. Lumbar epidural opiates or a combination of dilute local anesthetic and opiate via a thoracic epidural catheter are the preferred methods for achieving pain relief.

Myocardial Contusion

Myocardial contusion is a specific entity marked by cellular injury. Cell wall disruption results in the release of creatinine phosphokinase (CPK) and other markers of myocardial cell necrosis. Red blood cell extravasation, polymorphonuclear leukocyte infiltration, and muscle cell necrosis are the histologic findings. Cardiac injury can occur with minimal signs of external trauma. The most commonly associated problems include rib fractures (53 percent), pulmonary contusions (43 percent), pneumothorax (33 percent), hemothorax (30 percent), and sternal fractures (7 percent). Clinical signs and symptoms are nonspecific. Chest pain typical of angina and tachypnea may be present. If the contusion results in septal, free-wall, or valvular disruption, characteristic murmurs will be heard. Because of its anatomic relationship with the sternum, the right ventricle is most susceptible to injury. The left-sided heart valves are probably at greater risk because of the higher pressures in these chambers. Pre-existing valve disease has been found to predispose to injury.

The mass relationships between the right and left ventricles can result in false-negative electrocardiograms with right ventricular contusion. However, ST segment changes compatible with ischemia are common. T-wave abnormalities encountered in the order of frequency include peaked T-waves (75 percent), inverted T-waves (44 percent), and flattened T-waves (24 percent). Mild QT interval prolongation is also common. Dysrhythmias frequently accompany contusion, with their severity and duration correlating with the extent of injury in animal models. Many types of rhythm disturbances have been seen in patients with cardiac contusions, with tachycardia being most frequent, followed by premature atrial contraction (PAC) or premature ventricular contraction (PVC) in as many as 50 percent of patients with contusion. Rarely, couplets, bigeminy, ventricular tachycardia, or fibrillation will occur. Metabolic derangements from associated injuries can be severe, resulting in electrocardiographic changes compatible with contusion. The frequency of this occurrence is unknown, but it is probably common with states of hypoxia and acidosis. The lack of sensitivity and specificity limit the usefulness of electrocardiography in diagnosing myocardial contusion.

Testing of serum enzymes is more sensitive and specific. Creatinine phosphokinase myocardial bands (CPK-MB) above 5 percent of the total CPK indicate myocardial cell necrosis. Rare causes of false-positive CPK-MB are tongue injuries and muscular dystrophies. Negative CPK-MB probably rules out significant cell death but may mask cellular injury and dysfunction, short of death. This less severe condition of concussion can lead to dysrhythmia. Chest x-ray examinations are nonspecific but identify injuries frequently seen in the presence of myocardial contusion. Pulmonary contusion and fractured clavicle, sternum, or upper ribs should all lead one to suspect myocardial injury.

Echocardiography can provide quantitative and qualitative information concerning contusions. The existence of valve dysfunction, wall or septal injuries, tamponade, thrombus, and the presence of intracardiac shunts can all be simultaneously ascertained. For these reasons, echocardiography remains the most valuable clinical tool in the evaluation of myocardial performance following trauma.

Airway management with the establishment of adequate ventilation is followed by ensuring circulation in the initial step in the treatment of cardiac contusion. A baseline electrocardiogram should be obtained for future reference and as an initial screen, keeping its low specificity and sensitivity in mind. Continuous monitoring for the occurrence of dysrhythmias is instituted, and initial CPK-MB isoenzyme is drawn. These are repeated at 8-hour intervals for the first 24 hours. If myocardial contusion is suspected on clinical grounds, from the initial electrocardiogram, CPK-MB, or associated injuries, a two-dimensional echocardiogram should be obtained. The reduction in pump function caused by a contusion correlates with the amount of myocardium affected. Cardiac failure may result and is best managed by invasive monitoring with a pulmonary artery catheter. At times, inotropic support, vasodilators, and fluids are necessary to increase the cardiac index to acceptable levels. An intra-aortic balloon pump must be considered a heroic measure in patients with chest trauma and is used in highly individualized situations. Multiply traumatized patients in cardiogenic shock on ionotropes pose many logistical challenges to intra-aortic counterpulsation. Generally, patients on balloon pumps are heparinized, a procedure ill-advised in trauma. In addition, the technical problems in placing the balloon in an unstable trauma patients can be prohibitive.

COMMENTARY

Trauma is a leading cause of death. Maximizing outcome requires well directed and early intervention. The majority of patients with chest trauma will arrive in the operating room after an initial period of evaluation and stabilization. If problems with oral intubation are not anticipated, a rapid-sequence intubation with bimanual cricoesophageal compression is performed. Ketamine 1 mg/kg IV with succinylcholine 1.5 mg/kg IV are the most common induction agents. We usually do not "pre-block" with nondeporalizing agents, preferring to have obvious faciculations as an indication of the onset of neuromuscular blockade. If the interoperative course is stable the patient is maintained on moderate-dose sufentanyl (0.25-2 μg/kg) and forane in air and oxygen. If patients are to have a thoracotomy in the lateral position the anesthetic would be maintained with a ketamine infusion or higher dose sufentanyl (2-3 μg/kg). This would be supplemented with a volatile anesthetic to control blood pressure. Inhibition of hypoxic pulmonary vasoconstriction by volatile agents is a real but usually inconsequential phenomenon.

Too often a patient will arrive in the operating room hemodynamically unstable, resuscitation in progress. These patients are usually intubated in the field or emergency room. The first priority is to assure the adequacy of ventilation and IV access. We paralyze these patients with vecuronium and administer small doses of midazolam (1 mg increments) or ketamine (10 mg increments) until the patients stabilizes. Pavulon will increase heart rate and cardiac output, but we prefer vecuronium, which preserves heart rate as an indication of intravascular volume. We use more specific agents to augment cardiac output if necessary. Early administration of blood and coagulation products is critical. If rapid transfusion will be necessary to restore adequate hemodynamics a dilutional and consumptive coagulapathy may result, and we prepare to give platelets and plasma early and often. Hypothermia is frequently present due to shock, exposure, and infusion of cold fluids. Every effort should be made to maintain the patients' temperature. This includes warming and humidifying inspired gases, warming fluids, a warming blanket under the patient, warmed prep solutions, and warming the room to at least 24° C. Fortunately, chest trauma usually occurs in young men able to survive a substantial insult. Meticulous attention to detail and vigilance, with early and aggressive intervention, are essential for good outcomes.

SUGGESTED READING

Birkell WH, Shaftan GW, Mattox KL. Intravenous fluid administration and uncontrolled hemorrhage (editorial). J Trauma 1989; 29:409.
Marshall BE, Longnecker DE, Fairley HB, eds. Anesthesia for thoracic procedures. Boston: Blackwell Scientific Publications, 1988.
Mattox KL. And the beat goes on (editorial). J Trauma 1989; 29:1452.
Mattox KL. The debate goes on (editorial). J Trauma 1989; 29:1298.
Mattox KL, Moore EE, Feliciano DV, eds. Trauma. Norwalk, CT: Appleton & Lange, 1988.
Shires GT, ed. Principles of trauma care. 3rd ed. New York: McGraw-Hill, 1979.
Tenzer M. The spectrum of myocardial contusion: a review. J Trauma 1985; 25:620–627.

ABDOMINAL TRAUMA

CHRISTOPHER M. GRANDE, M.D.
JOHN K. STENE, Jr., M.D., Ph.D.

The early involvement of the well-trained trauma anesthesiologist/critical care specialist (TA/CCS) in the protocol-based, necessarily concurrent assessment and care of a trauma patient affords several advantages, both for the patient and the TA/CCS. First, it precludes duplication of efforts at defining the patient's condition and injuries, thereby saving critical moments of the "golden hour." It also ensures rapid institution of appropriate interventions for the management of the airways, ventilation, intravenous fluids, sedation, analgesia, and anesthesia, and it familiarizes the TA/CCS with the patient on an emergent basis, avoiding the disadvantage of anesthetically managing an unfamiliar patient in the operating room. It ensures that the appropriate personnel, pharmacologic agents, and equipment are prepared and ready for the patient when he or she enters the operating room, and finally, it should reduce the incidence of emergency tracheostomies by presenting the opportunity to control ventilation via endotracheal intubation. These advantages have particular relevance to the patient with abdominal injuries (which are often a diagnosis of exclusion), the patient who requires emergency thoracotomy (ET), or the patient whose overall status is affected by the spinal shock, coincident disease, the use of drugs or alcohol, or the need for transport.

ABDOMINAL INJURIES

Because intra-abdominal injury usually mandates surgical intervention, the diagnosis of the actual type or degree of injury is far less important than diagnosis of its presence. To appreciate the anesthetic implications of diagnosis and resultant intervention, it is necessary for the TA/CCS to have a thorough understanding of abdominal anatomy, the mechanisms of injury involved, and the methods of diagnosis, in addition to knowledge of anesthetic concerns.

Anatomy

The TA/CCS will primarily be concerned with three general areas of the abdomen: (1) the peritoneal cavity, (2) the retroperitoneal space, and (3) the pelvis.

Peritoneal Cavity. The peritoneal cavity consists of an abdominal and an intrathoracic section. Because the latter (contained within the rib cage and consisting of the diaphragm, spleen, stomach, liver, and transverse colon) can ascend to the fourth intercostal space when the diaphragm fully exhales, penetrating trauma to the lower chest or rib fractures of the lower ribs may be associated with intra-abdominal injuries (Fig. 1).

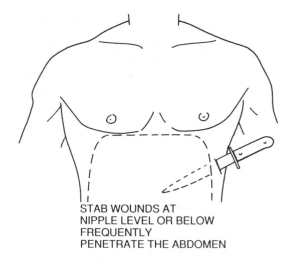

STAB WOUNDS AT
NIPPLE LEVEL OR BELOW
FREQUENTLY
PENETRATE THE ABDOMEN

Figure 1 All penetrating chest wounds below the fifth intercostal space are potentially associated with intra-abdominal and diaphragmatic injury. (Republished with permission from Campbell JE. BTLS: Basic prehospital trauma care. Englewood Cliffs, NJ: Prentice Hall, 1988:20.)

Retroperitoneal Space. Within this space are the aorta, vena cava, pancreas, kidneys, and ureters, as well as portions of the colon and duodenum. Diagnosis of retroperitoneal injuries is difficult but important because this space can harbor life-threatening hemorrhage.

Pelvis. The bony structure of the pelvis houses the rectum, bladder, iliac vessels, and female reproductive organs. As with the peritoneum, the pelvis can obscure internal injuries and make diagnosis difficult.

Mechanisms of Injury

The abdomen can be injured by blunt, penetrating, and/or combined trauma, although injuries from the first two mechanisms have differing indications for exploratory celiotomy. Because the anatomic structure of the abdomen may conceal significant, even life-threatening, hemorrhage before exhibiting signs of distention (Fig. 2), the initial diagnosis must be made based on the mechanism of injury.

Blunt trauma, as from motor vehicle accidents, usually causes significant hemorrhage secondary to injured solid organs (e.g., liver, spleen, and kidneys). In addition, the improper use of seat belts can result in entrapped bowel-loop rupture and/or lumbar-spine injury.

Penetrating trauma inflicts both direct and indirect injuries—for example, organs or soft tissue injured by the passage of a knife blade or by the widespread effects of blast injuries, respectively. In the presence of contamination, penetrating trauma also predisposes to peritonitis. If penetration of the superficial fascia cannot be ruled out, all penetrating wounds to the lower torso should be surgically explored. Injury patterns (commonly the liver, small bowel, colon, and stomach)

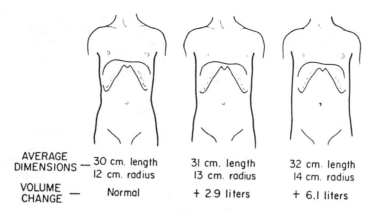

AVERAGE
DIMENSIONS — 30 cm. length   31 cm. length   32 cm. length
                12 cm. radius   13 cm. radius   14 cm. radius

VOLUME
CHANGE   —   Normal   + 2.9 liters   + 6.1 liters

Figure 2 The abdomen can contain a significant amount of hemorrhaged blood with minimal changes in external dimensions. (Republished with permission from Trunkey DD, Sheldon GF, Collins JA. The treatment of shock. In: Zuidema GD, Rutherford RB, Ballinger WF, eds. The management of trauma. 4th ed. Philadelphia: WB Saunders, 1985; 105–125.)

depend on the location and size of the specific abdominal organs relative to the entrance site, path, and size of the wounding object. The examining clinician must remember that the path of a bullet, and thus the "line" of structures at risk, may sometimes be traced in the patient between the entrance and exit wounds, *but only in the position at moment of impact.* Since positioning the patient on the examining table can distort the wound tract, and since the path taken by a bullet once it enters the body is often not a straight line, careful exploration is mandatory.

Diagnosis

Since a normal abdominal examination does not guarantee the absence of significant hemoperitoneum (it can occur in as many as 20 percent of trauma patients), the clinician must *suspect* intra-abdominal injury based on a knowledge and conceptual understanding of the mechanisms of injury and the patient's cardiovascular stability. Methods for confirming the suspected abdominal injuries include serial physical examinations of the abdomen, laboratory studies (serial hematocrit determinations), minimally invasive measures (diagnostic peritoneal lavage, or DPL, contrast-enhanced computed tomography, or CT), and/or exploratory celiotomy.

Serial Examinations

For most blunt trauma patients who are cardiovascularly stable, clinicians use observation, repeat physical examinations, and repeat hematocrit values to diagnose intra-abdominal injuries. Delayed peritonitis (without other causes for peritoneal signs), a progressive decrease in hematocrit, or a slow change in abdominal examination indicates the need for celiotomy and repair of injuries in these patients.

Diagnostic Peritoneal Lavage

Repeat diagnostic peritoneal lavages (DPLs) can screen patients for hemoperitoneum (sensitivity of 96 percent and a specificity of 99 percent) and is especially useful in mass casualty situations involving large numbers of patients. A positive DPL indicates the need for immediate celiotomy. When DPL is performed, the returned lavage fluid is examined for red blood cells, white blood cells, amylase, bile, and Gram stain (Table 1).

A properly trained TA/CCS or emergency physician may perform the DPL; however, a positive result indicates that a surgical consultation is imperative. Most centers consider more than 100,000 red blood cells per cubic millimeter as a positive result but, depending on the particular trauma center and the surgeon's evaluation of an individual patient's overall status (i.e., an elevated index of suspicion), a much smaller ratio (50,000, 10,000, or even 1,000 red blood cells per cubic millimeter) may mandate surgical intervention. A negative result suggests that the peritoneal cavity has not been contaminated by either blood or bowel contents, but retroperitoneal bleeding or inadequate lavage of the peritoneal cavity can cause false-negative results. It should be understood that a single DPL may, in fact, impose a higher false-positive rate on subsequent diagnostic procedures.

The main drawback to using DPL is that it alters subsequent abdominal examinations by introducing both intra-abdominal and free intraperitoneal air and by causing pain and abdominal tenderness. Thus, the consulting surgeon must choose to accept the reports of a patient's signs, symptoms, and DPL results or to repeat the DPL because of altered signs and symptoms on physical examination.

Again, although the TA/CCS or emergency physician can easily, safely, and correctly perform a DPL, he

Table 1 Diagnostic Peritoneal Lavage Fluid Results:
Indications for Operating

Aspirate > 10 ml free blood after catheter insertion
Red blood cell count of returned lavage fluid > 100,000/mm^3
Red blood cell count of returned lavage fluid > 50,000/mm^3 with
   other indicators of intra-abdominal injury, especially with
   penetrating trauma
White blood cell count of returned lavage fluid > 500/mm^3
Amylase concentration of returned lavage fluid > 175 IU/L
Vegetable fibers, bacteria
Loss of lavage fluid through chest suggests a diaphragmatic rupture

or she should probably do so only if patient transfer
depends on the results, as the TA/CCS is not the one
who makes the final decision to operate based on the
results obtained.

Contrast-Enhanced Computed Tomography

The CT scan enhanced with 100 ml of an intravenous
contrast agent and 400 ml of an intragastric contrast
agent offers several advantages for abdominal examination: (1) good sensitivity for intra-abdominal hematoma, solid organ injuries, free intraperitoneal fluid,
and free intraperitoneal air; (2) lack of interference with
the abdominal physical examination; (3) disadvantage-
free repeatability (as opposed to DPL); and (4) superiority to DPL in precluding frequent abdominal examinations, especially important for blunt trauma patients with
multiple injuries requiring immediate and/or prolonged
surgery (e.g., closed-head injury, extensive orthopedic
injuries) and for defining retroperitoneal injury. Its main
disadvantage is that it defines the diaphragm poorly.

Exploratory Celiotomy

Celiotomy, indicated for penetrating wounds to the
lower rib cage and/or abdomen, allows evaluation of
injuries to the diaphragm, solid organs, bowel, and retroperitoneal space and is required for their definitive repair. Some authors recommend a limited celiotomy incision in blunt trauma patients with serious injuries that
have a high probability of causing multiorgan failure.

Traumatic Diaphragmatic Hernia

Although the initial assessment and examination at
the trauma center may identify a traumatic diaphragmatic hernia (TDH), often TDH is found incidentally
during thoracotomy, laparotomy, or other procedures.
The decision to surgically correct the TDH depends in
part on the time of its discovery (preoperatively or
intraoperatively). Transdiaphragmatically herniated organs (most often the stomach, omentum, transverse
colon, and small bowel) can induce cardiopulmonary
compromise by compressing the lung and thus causing
changes in pulmonary compliance and airway resistance,
as well as mediastinal shift. Sequelae of trauma, such as
pulmonary contusion, hypovolemia, and tension pneu-

mothorax, can intensify this compromise. A TDH may
also remain hidden until years after the traumatic
incident, when the initially small, asymptomatic defect
entraps adjacent viscera, leading to visceral infarct or
obstruction.

Incidence and Etiology

Although reports in the literature indicate that the
incidence of TDH is low, if the incidence of TDH found
at autopsy were included, that percentage would increase substantially. TDH can occur secondary to either
blunt or penetrating trauma.

Historically, blunt trauma–induced TDH was believed to occur primarily (in 90 to 95 percent of cases) in
the left diaphragm because the right hemidiaphragm is
relatively protected by the liver and because cadaver
studies indicated a predisposition of the left hemidiaphragm to congenital weaknesses. However, recent
studies indicate that left-sided TDH from blunt trauma
occurs only slightly more frequently than on the right
hemidiaphragm. The location of TDH from penetrating
trauma varies: TDH secondary to stabbings occur
predominantly on the left because most stab wounds are
inflicted by right-handed assailants facing their victims;
TDH secondary to gunshot wounds occur equally in both
hemidiaphragms.

Blunt trauma can cause a TDH by creating excessive
abdominothoracic pressure (> 100 cm H$_2$O) if the victim
gasps against a closed glottis (Mueller's maneuver)
simultaneously as external forces increase the intra-
abdominal pressure; diaphragmatic distortion of and/or
shearing injury secondary to thoracic compression; and
diaphragmatic injury through congenital weakness.

Diagnosis

The TA/CCS must have a high degree of suspicion
for TDH in the presence of injuries caudad to the fifth
intercostal space, and/or injuries associated with high-
energy impact (e.g., fractures of the clavicles, upper ribs,
scapulae, sternum, pelvis, or thoracolumbar spine). If
the TA/CCS suspects a TDH, clinical symptoms of
dizziness, cyanosis, lower chest pain, or upper abdominal
discomfort (especially referred to the shoulder) and/or
clinical signs of diminished/absent breath sounds, bowel
sounds in the chest, tracheal shift, abdominal distention,
respiratory distress, or shock can reinforce that suspicion.

Preoperative diagnosis of TDH is usually made by
chest x-ray examination, which some clinicians believe
requires prior placement of a nasogastric tube (if not
contraindicated in the individual trauma patient) for
stomach decompression. Table 2 lists the radiographic
findings that may indicate a TDH. The diagnostician
must guard against interpreting the "pseudodiaphragm"
(caused by abdominal viscera mimicking the diaphragmatic contour) or the elevated hemidiaphragm (caused
by phrenic-nerve injury) as TDH indications. Equivocal
findings on the chest radiograph mandate additional

Table 2 Radiographic Indications of Traumatic Diaphragmatic Hernia

Gass-filled loops of bowel in chest
Unilaterally elevated hemidiaphragm
Abnormal diaphragmatic contours
Nasogastric tube coiled in stomach above diaphragm
Platelike atelectasis above indistinct diaphragm
Mediastinal shift away from injured side
Gas bubbles or air-fluid levels above diaphragm
Pleural effusion*

*In the presence of a pleural effusion, thoracoscopy is an alternative to thoracentesis to avoid iatrogenic penetration of entrapped viscera.

analysis, such as other radio-graphic studies (inspiration, expiration, and changed-position films); measurement of external abdominal pressure; fluoroscopy; or contrast studies. Contrast studies (which can demonstrate contrast-filled viscera above the diaphragm, abrupt obstruction to flow of contrast media, or failure of media to progress in serial films) may increase the risk of regurgitation, pulmonary aspiration, and perforation of strangulated or necrotically obstructed organs. The use of water-soluble contrast media decreases those risks.

Several other methods have been proposed to be diagnostic for the presence of TDH. DPL and diagnostic pneumoperitoneum both have a 20 percent false-negative rate, possibly because of the isolation of the hemorrhaging viscera above the diaphragm without contamination of the intraperitoneal space; the latter is also associated with a risk of air embolism, which can be decreased by using carbon dioxide as the insufflation gas. Thoracoscopy is currently under investigation, and CT has been shown to be nondefinitive.

Anesthetic Concerns

The TA/CCS managing a patient with abdominal trauma faces several potential problems: (1) significant hemorrhage (associated with injuries to solid organs, liver, spleen, and kidney as well as vascular injuries and pelvic fractures); (2) frequent hypothermia (as a result of surgery-induced increased heat loss through the open mesentery and reduced heat production from shock and anesthesia); (3) sepsis; and (4) interference with ventilation. Such a patient will usually require the insertion of at least two large-bore intravenous cannulae prior to draping for surgery; the TA/CCS should also seriously consider establishing an intra-arterial catheter in the unstable patient with abdominal trauma to dose-monitor blood pressure and provide a route for serial blood sampling for laboratory evaluation (blood gases, hematology, and chemistry).

Priorities in Multitrauma

Blunt trauma that produces intra-abdominal injuries also frequently causes transection of the thoracic aorta, giving rise to the therapeutic dilemma of priori-

tizing angiography, laparotomy, and thoracotomy. There is currently little consensus as to the correct order of procedures, except that it depends on multiple, individual factors. On the one hand, the aortic injury is repaired first because initial survivors have a high mortality rate within the first few hours after injury, but the cause of death has not been definitively identified as aortic rupture and exsanguination or associated injuries. On the other hand, in the absence of aortic rupture and large external blood loss, intra-abdominal injury is the most likely cause of persistent shock, and laparotomy should therefore be performed first; the literature reports successful laparotomies for patients with traumatic aortic aneurysms but no rupture. For patients who are stable after fluid resuscitation, one current recommendation is angiography followed sequentially by thoracotomy and laparotomy, but for unstable trauma patients, laparotomy first, followed by angiography and thoracotomy is recommended. Another possibility is simultaneous surgical procedures for the thoracic and abdominal injuries; however, such a scenario creates a problem relative to optimal patient positioning.

OTHER CONSIDERATIONS

If common, major injuries have been ruled out as the cause of a trauma patient's unresponsiveness to appropriate resuscitation maneuvers, the clinician must consider spinal shock, coincident disease, chronic or current use of drugs or alcohol, and the effect of transfer.

Spinal Shock. In the presence of low blood volume, a high spinal cord injury, which can cause maximal vasodilation, may cause profound hypotension. Spinal shock, which differs from traumatic shock, has been described elsewhere.

Coincident (Pre-existing) Disease. Diseases such as myocardial infarction or adrenal apoplexy can precipitate the initial traumatic event as well as complicate resuscitation and repair of injuries. In the latter case, the condition may also have resulted from bilateral injury or hemorrhage into the adrenal glands. Adrenal insufficiency, either chronic or acute, will aggravate hemorrhagic shock.

Drugs and Alcohol. Several studies have shown that many trauma patients are chronic drug and/or alcohol abusers and that most have one or more illicit substances "on board" on admission. However, the patient may also have "legitimately" taken over-the-counter or prescribed medication that can interact and interfere with resuscitative and interventional pharmacology and anesthesia (e.g., meperidine and monoamine oxidase inhibitors).

Effect of Transport. Physiologic stress caused by the rigors of transport, which may interfere with adequate shock resuscitation, has been described elsewhere.

EMERGENCY THORACOTOMY

The continuing debate between surgeons and nonsurgeons about emergency surgery (ET) focuses largely not on who *can* or *should* perform this procedure but, rather, on who is to be *allowed* to perform it. Although institutional solutions to this debate vary, depending on the organization of the medical staff, it would seem logical to permit a responsible, licensed physician with special interest and advanced training in traumatology to perform a *lifesaving* procedure on *appropriate* patients. Therefore, instead of wasting time on nonproductive medicopolitical arguments, one should focus efforts on the selection, training, qualification, and utilization of physicians to perform ET.

However, before the physician begins the ET procedure, he or she must consider the following points:

1. The presence of one or more indications for the control/repair of cardiac wounds with or without tamponade; the control/repair of the great vessel rupture; relief of internal cardiac compression in hypovolemic arrest, as from inadequate closed chest cardiac massage; open cardiac massage and cross-clamping of the pulmonary hilum (in air embolism); control of distal hemorrhage and maximization of cardiocerebral perfusion by cross-clamping the descending aorta.
2. The presence of any contraindication (prolonged cardiac arrest with no electrical activity of the heart of signs of neurologic death).
3. Whether the proposed operator is qualified.
4. Whether the necessary equipment is available.
5. Whether the institution has the equipment and personnel to provide postresuscitative critical care.

SUGGESTED READING

Ayella RJ. The chest. In: Ayella RG, ed. Radiologic management of the massively traumatized patient. Baltimore: Williams & Wilkins, 1978; 85–143.

Cowley RA, Turney SZ. Blunt thoracic injuries: the ruptured aorta. In: Cowley RA, Conn A, Dunham CM, eds. Trauma care: surgical management. Philadelphia: JB Lippincott, 1987; 1:172–181.

Estrera AS, Landay MJ, McClelland RN. Blunt traumatic rupture of the right hemidiaphragm: experience in 12 patients. Ann Thorac Surg 1985; 39:525–530.

Estrera AS, Platt MR, Mills LJ. Traumatic injuries of the diaphragm. Chest 1979; 75:306–313.

Grande CM, McCauley M, Williams D. Critical care transport: mobile management of the trauma patient inside and outside of the trauma center. In: Stene JK, Grande CM, eds. Trauma anesthesia. Baltimore: Williams & Wilkins, 1991; 407–439.

Jarrett F, Bernhardt LC. Right-sided diaphragmatic injury: rarity or overlooked diagnosis? Arch Surg 1978; 113:737–739.

Kanowitz A, Marx JA. Delayed traumatic diaphragmatic hernia simulating acute tension pneumothorax. J Emerg Med 1989; 7:619–622.

Kearney PA, Roubana SW, Burney RE. Blunt rupture of the diaphragm: mechanism, diagnosis, and treatment. Ann Emerg Med 1989; 18:1326–1330.

Madden MR, Paull DE, Finkelstein JL, et al. Occult diaphragmatic injury from stab wounds to the lower chest and abdomen. J Trauma 1989; 29:292–298.

Rodriguez-Morales G, Rodriguez A, Shatney CH. Acute rupture of the diaphragm in blunt trauma: analysis of 60 patients. J Trauma 1986; 26:438–444.

Soderstrom C, Carson SL. Update: alcohol and other drug use among vehicular crash victims. MD Med J 1988; 37:541–545.

Stene JK, Grande CM, Giesecke AH. Shock resuscitation. In: Stene JK, Grande CM, eds. Trauma anesthesia. Baltimore: Williams & Wilkins, 1991; 100–132.

ACUTE ANESTHETIC MANAGEMENT OF BURNS

WILLIAM R. FURMAN, M.D.

Burn-injured patients pose challenging physiologic and technical problems for the anesthesiologist. During the immediate postburn period, patients may require urgent endotracheal intubation to treat respiratory failure. Operative anesthesia may be necessary for an emergency surgical procedure, such as a fasciotomy or escharotomy, and débridement and grafting operations must be undertaken despite severe metabolic derangements. This chapter discusses the acute anesthetic care of burn victims, with particular attention to the management of respiratory failure due to inhalational injury and to operative anesthetic care during the first week after burn injury.

Burns are categorized according to the extent and depth of the destruction they cause. The extent of injury is the percentage of the body surface area (BSA) that is burned. This is usually estimated using a formula such as the Lund and Browder chart (Fig. 1). The depth is classified as first, second, third, or fourth degree for superficial, partial-thickness, or full-thickness burns or full-thickness burns with destruction of underlying structures, respectively (Table 1). Surgical intervention is required for deep partial-thickness and all full-thickness burns, because they do not heal spontaneously or they heal with poor functional and cosmetic results. Mortality is directly related to the extent and depth of injury, the age of the victim, and the presence of

AREA	PERCENT OF BURN					SEVERITY OF BURN		TOTAL PERCENT
	0-1 Year	1-4 Years	5-9 Years	10-15 Years	ADULT	2°	3°	
Head	19	17	13	10	7			
Neck	2	2	2	2	2			
Ant. Trunk	13	17	13	13	13			
Post. Trunk	13	13	13	13	13			
R. Buttock	2½	2½	2½	2½	2½			
L. Buttock	2½	2½	2½	2½	2½			
Genitalia	1	1	1	1	1			
R.U. Arm	4	4	4	4	4			
L.U. Arm	4	4	4	4	4			
R.L Arm	3	3	3	3	3			
L.L. Arm	3	3	3	3	3			
R. Hand	2½	2½	2½	2½	2½			
L Hand	2½	2½	2½	2½	2½			
R. Thigh	5½	6½	8½	8½	9½			
L Thigh	5½	6½	8½	8½	9½			
R. Leg	5	5	5½	6	7			
L Leg	5	5	5½	6	7			
R. Foot	3½	3½	3½	3½	3½			
L Foot	3½	3½	3½	3½	3½			
				Total				

Figure 1 A common method of calculating the extent of burn injury is to use the Lund and Browder Chart. Second- and third-degree burns are catalogued according to location, and the chart is consulted to determine the percentage of the total body surface area represented by each area burned. The extent of the burn is defined as the sum of the areas involved by second- and third-degree injury.

Table 1 Estimating the Depth of Burn Wounds

Burn Wound	Appearance	Sensation	Causes
First-degree	Warm and erythematous	Sensitive	Sunburn
Second-degree	Mottled, pink, with bullae	Very sensitive	Flash burns, scald (spilled)
Third-degree	Dry, white, or charred	Anesthetic	Flame, scald (immersion), electrical
Fourth-degree	Dry, white, or charred	Anesthetic	Electrical

high-voltage electrical injury. Associated smoke inhalation increases mortality by an average of 40 percent. Major burns are generally defined as those with second-degree depth in excess of 15 to 20 percent of the BSA, and those with associated inhalational injury.

RESPIRATORY FAILURE

Respiratory failure during the first few hours to days after inhalational injury is usually caused by one of three problems: (1) asphyxia due to carbon monoxide poisoning; (2) upper airway obstruction due to edema of the tissues of the pharynx or larynx; and (3) lower airway damage in the form of tracheobronchitis and parenchy-

mal damage. The pattern and severity of the injury is determined by the type, temperature, and concentration of gases inhaled, the solubility of the gases, the presence or absence of super-heated particulates in the inhaled smoke, and the duration of exposure. The most severe inhalational injuries occur when victims are trapped in an enclosed space and when the fire involves burning plastics.

Asphyxia

When victims are trapped in burning buildings or vehicles, they become hypoxic from breathing a gas mixture that contains carbon monoxide and is deficient in oxygen. Although the low inspired oxygen concentration contributes to tissue hypoxia, the effect of carbon monoxide poisoning is far more important. Carbon monoxide binds to hemoglobin 200 times more readily than oxygen, decreasing the amount of hemoglobin available for oxygen transport. In addition to decreasing the arterial content of oxygen, carbon monoxide increases the stability of the oxyhemoglobin molecule, inhibiting release of oxygen to the tissues and ultimately causing hypoxic organ dysfunction and cell death in the brain, heart, and abdominal viscera.

Because the consequences are so dire, carbon monoxide poisoning must be suspected in any fire victim who has been trapped in a confined space, and it must be treated promptly. The principal signs and symptoms are complaints of headache, nausea, angina pectoris, or shortness of breath, and tachypnea, irritability, or delirium, but not cyanosis. The degree of carbon monoxide poisoning can be quantified by measuring the carboxyhemoglobin level, expressed as the percent saturation of hemoglobin in arterial blood (SaCO). Saturations greater than 15 percent are usually toxic, and those greater than 50 percent are nearly always lethal.

The treatment for carbon monoxide poisoning is removal of the victim from the fire and administration of 100 percent oxygen. The half-life of elimination of carbon monoxide is 4 hours breathing room air, but the time is reduced to 40 minutes if 100 percent oxygen is administered. Consequently, any patient with a suspected (or documented) elevation of SaCO should receive as high an inspired concentration as possible. Intubation of the trachea is the surest way to accomplish this.

Neuromuscular blocking agents are generally not required during airway management of *comatose* burn victims. However, patients who are stuporous or delirious tend to resist manipulation and may therefore require muscle relaxation during intubation. The use of a depolarizing muscle relaxant (succinylcholine chloride) is not contraindicated during the first few hours after a burn. Rather, it is the preferred agent because of the need to perform a "rapid sequence" type intubation using cricoesophageal pressure to resist aspiration of gastric contents. Since gastric emptying ceases at the time of significant injury, it should be assumed that every burn victim has a full stomach and is at risk for active or passive regurgitation during intubation.

Although delirious patients almost invariably suffer memory loss, many anesthesiologists prefer to administer a sedative/hypnotic agent when a muscle relaxant is given to an awake but confused patient during intubation. Although thiobarbiturates (thiamylal sodium, thiopental sodium) are suitable, they possess myocardial depressant properties and are usually best used in reduced doses or avoided in favor of the benzodiazepines (midazolam, diazepam) or ketamine.

Upper Airway Obstruction

Upper airway injury (above the true vocal cords) may result from inhaling hot air, flames, and toxic chemicals. This problem occurs in 20 to 30 percent of the burn victims who suffer inhalation injury. It must be recognized and treated early, as swelling may rapidly become so extreme that successful laryngoscopy and intubation become impossible, thus necessitating emergency tracheostomy.

The possibility of upper airway obstruction should be anticipated in all victims of closed-space fires, particularly when the patient has facial burns, an injected tongue, sooty oral or nasal secretions, or hoarseness. The development of upper airway edema parallels the generalized extravascular fluid deposition that occurs during volume resuscitation of the burn patient. There is often erythema, blistering, and necrosis

of the surface epithelium, with edema becoming significant after a latent period of 4 to 48 hours. The mucosa over the false cords, the aryepiglottic folds, and the arytenoid eminences may become so edematous that they prolapse and produce partial or complete airway occlusion.

Early intubation is recommended for any patient with significant intraoral or pharyngeal burns, because progressive edema may make later intubation extremely hazardous or impossible. This conservative approach leads to endotracheal intubation of some patients who would not have progressed to significant airway compromise. An alternative approach is to evaluate these patients with either pulmonary flow-volume curves or nasopharyngoscopy. Both techniques require a cooperative patient, and serial evaluations are often necessary. Evaluations should be performed at frequent intervals, for the upper airway may become impaired gradually, provoking little or no change in the patient's clinical appearance until nearly complete obstruction occurs.

Early intubation reduces the risk that advanced swelling will be present when intubation is ultimately attempted. It also allows the use of succinylcholine, which is contraindicated later on. Patients with major burns are hypersensitive to depolarizing muscle relaxants and can respond to their administration with an exaggerated and potentially life-threatening increase in serum potassium, especially if the burn exceeds 10 percent of the BSA. The onset of this effect occurs 24 to 72 hours after a burn, with a peak effect between 15 and 60 days. This response is most likely to occur from 5 days to 3 months after a burn. It certainly appears to be safe to use succinylcholine chloride during the first 8 to 12 hours. However, when exactly this drug becomes unsafe (probably 24 to 72 hours afterburn) and when it is once again safe to use remain controversial. It is generally believed that the drug may be used after 6 months if all the burn wounds have healed.

Pulmonary Insufficiency

Respiratory failure due to inhalational injury to the lower respiratory tract may develop at any time from 3 hours to 3 days after smoke exposure. The inciting injury is chemical in nature, as true thermal damage to the lower respiratory tract does not occur unless steam or burning gases have been inhaled. This is because the heat associated with inhalation of hot air is dissipated in the pharynx and supraglottic areas, and because the heat involved evokes reflex closure of the epiglottis. Bacterial infection is a common complicating factor in the development of postburn respiratory failure.

When pulmonary insufficiency develops after the first 8 to 12 hours, a nondepolarizing muscle relaxant (NDMR) is generally used to facilitate intubation, because of the uncertainty about exactly when succinylcholine chloride becomes unsafe. Burn victims develop resistance to NDMRs as they become sensitive to depolarizing agents, especially if the burn exceeds 40 percent of the BSA. Accordingly, during the first 2 days, which is when upper airway obstruction usually develops, resistance to NDMRs should not be expected and the standard dosages for rapid sequence induction may be used. Later (5 days to 3 months after a burn), when pneumonia and the adult respiratory distress syndrome usually occur, the doses often have to be increased to two to five times what would ordinarily be required to achieve relaxation in a patient of the same age and size. This is especially true for patients with larger burns. The cause of this insensitivity to NDMRs is under investigation. The classical theory of an increase in receptor number has recently been disputed by studies showing that the serum of burn victims is able to inhibit the effect of muscle relaxants in nonburned animals.

OPERATIVE ANESTHESIA

Preoperative Approach

The preoperative approach to the patient with a major burn is directed toward three areas: (1) determination of the severity of the physiologic compromise caused by the burn injury and its therapy; (2) identification of potential sites for intravascular access and application of monitoring devices; (3) and delineation of associated nonburn injuries.

Physiologic Compromise

The most common area of physiologic compromise is the intravascular volume. Burn patients require and receive aggressive fluid resuscitation, especially during the first 2 days after a burn. Up to 4 ml per kilogram of crystalloid for each 1 percent of BSA burned is needed during the first 24 hours. Several formulas have been

designed to calculate this need (Table 2). During this period, these patients become catabolic and their plasma protein levels decrease. This decrease in plasma oncotic pressure reduces the intravascular volume and causes prerenal azotemia. Despite the development of hypoproteinemia and a demonstrable capillary leak, the role of colloid administration remains controversial, and not all resuscitation formulas include it. When there is doubt about the adequacy of the intravascular volume, central venous or pulmonary artery pressure monitoring is required.

The ability to secure the airway is always an important concern in the preoperative evaluation of a burn patient, especially if smoke inhalation has occurred. Upper airway edema can make intubation difficult and ventilation by mask and resuscitator bag nearly impossible. In addition, topical antibiotics and skin grafts on the face may preclude effective application of a mask. The preoperative evaluation of the airway must therefore give special consideration to the safest approach to intubation, which may require an awake technique.

Renal, hepatic, cardiovascular, and pulmonary dysfunction and coagulopathies are frequent complications of major burns and burn-wound sepsis. Although these are potentially reversible problems, aggressive surgical débridement and grafting are viewed as the preeminent means of controlling infection, often making it necessary to anesthetize a compromised patient. In such instances, the role of the anesthesiologist is to identify the abnormalities and adapt the anesthetic plan to meet the exigencies they impose. Critically ill burn patients routinely undergo frequent measurements of serum electrolytes, glucose, urea nitrogen, arterial blood gases, and hematocrit. Anemia and chemical abnormalities can usually be satisfactorily managed before and during

Table 2 Standard Fluid Resuscitation Formulas for Burn Patients

Formula	First 24 Hrs	Second 24 Hrs
PARKLAND		
Crystalloid	4 ml LR/% burn/kilogram ½ during first 8 hr ½ during next 16 hr	D$_5$W maintenance
Colloid	None	0.5 ml/% burn/kilogram
BROOKE		
Crystalloid	2 ml LR/% burn/kilogram ½ during first 8 hr ½ during next 16 hr	D$_5$W maintenance
Colloid	None	0.5 ml/% burn/kilogram
MGH		
Crystalloid	1.5 ml LR/% burn/kilogram ½ during first 8 hr ½ during next 16 hr	Not specified
Colloid	0.5 ml/% burn/kilogram None during first 4 hr ½ during 2nd 4 hr ½ during next 16 hr	Not specified

D$_5$W = 5 percent dextrose in water.

surgery if anticipated and recognized at the time of the preoperative visit.

Coagulopathy may lead to an increased requirement for blood and blood products. Renal dysfunction, which is common in burn patients, may be caused by chemicals associated with burns, prerenal azotemia due to hypoproteinemia or inadequate fluid resuscitation, antibiotic toxicity, or acute tubular necrosis related to myoglobinuria. Metabolism of pharmacologic agents, most notably antibiotics, theophylline, and histamine-blocking agents, is commonly compromised in burn patients because of renal and hepatic dysfunction.

Burn injury is reported to cause the release of a myocardial depressant. However, the most common cause of a low cardiac output is a reduced circulating volume. Myocardial ischemia occurs in patients who have pre-existing coronary artery disease, especially if they have suffered inhalational injury. If not already in use, cardiac failure may require the introduction of inotropic or vasoactive agents before surgery.

For the patient with respiratory failure, the anesthesiologist must identify the parameters of mechanical ventilatory support in use (level of inspired oxygen, tidal volume and rate, and level of positive end-expiratory pressure, if any), and consider bronchodilator therapy. A plan for continuing this support during transport to the operating room and during surgery should be made at this time.

Monitoring and Access

Routine monitoring of blood pressure, electrocardiography (ECG), and oxygen saturation are complicated by burns of the limbs and trunk. If a sphygmomanometer cannot be located on an unburned extremity that will not be used as a skin graft donor site, an arterial line may be required. Nonstandard ECG electrode placements may be necessitated by the location of the burns or donor sites, making it difficult to interpret the shape of the QRS complex. Ordinary adhesive gel electrodes cannot be used in patients with nearly total burns. Alternative methods for achieving electrical contact are to use needle electrodes or skin staples, which are connected to the oscilloscope by "alligator" clips. Pulse oximetry probes may have to be applied to the ear or nose when the fingers and toes are not accessible.

Secure vascular access is needed during burn surgery because of the magnitude of blood loss that occurs. The preoperative visit should therefore include an inventory of existing peripheral and central venous lines and an assessment of their adequacy in the context of the surgery being planned.

Associated Injuries

The final step in the preoperative evaluation of a burn patient is to review other traumatic injuries associated with the burn. Fractures sustained jumping from a burning building or in an automobile collision may require attention during positioning for surgery. Injuries that involve the neck may complicate intubation.

Intraoperative Approach

The intraoperative care of the burn patient requires special attention to (1) pharmacology of muscle relaxants and other drugs; (2) blood transfusion requirements; (3) prevention of heat loss; and (4) the occasional need to provide operative anesthetic care in a location outside the operating room, such as the tub room or admitting area of the burn unit.

Pharmacology

In contrast to the strikingly abnormal responses of burn patients to muscle relaxants, the clinical effects of the anesthetic agents (barbiturates, benzodiazepines, ketamine, narcotics, and the inhalational agents) are not greatly altered by burn injury. All of these agents can be used safely if the intravascular volume of the patient is maintained. Because of the predictably large volume of blood lost during débridement procedures, an anesthetic plan that minimizes myocardial depression and vasodilatation is desirable.

Blood Loss

For every 1 percent of BSA excised and débrided, the patient can be expected to lose about 3 percent of the total estimated blood volume. This means that a typical skin grafting procedure in which 10 percent of the BSA is excised and grafted results in a blood loss of approximately 30 percent of the blood volume. For an average, 70-kg male patient, this estimate is equal to 30 percent of 5,250 ml (1,575 ml), or about 3 units of blood. This blood loss can take place very rapidly, sometimes over a period of 30 to 60 minutes. It is therefore helpful to estimate the amount of blood loss expected during the procedure and predict whether the patient can sustain that loss without transfusion. If not, blood administration can be started at the time of induction of anesthesia, and blood can be infused throughout the procedure at a slower rate than would be required to replete a 3-unit loss over 30 minutes.

Heat Loss

Burn patients are hypermetabolic and have large amounts of skin and subcutaneous tissue exposed to the dry ambient conditions of the operating room. Thus they are especially susceptible to intraoperative hypothermia. Every available method of conserving body heat should be employed, including heating the environment above 25°C (77°F); warming all administered solutions; using heating lamps and a heating pad on the operating table; and insulating the patient by covering the head and limbs if they are not part of the operative field. All of the operative field should be covered when it is not being actively operated on. To reduce evaporative heat loss through the respiratory tract, the patient should be ventilated either with heated, humidified gases or at low fresh gas flows.

Anesthetic Care Outside the Operating Room

It is sometimes necessary to provide anesthetic care in the burn intensive care unit. Urgent initial débridements (such as after hot tar burns incurred in roofing accidents), fasciotomies, or escharotomies may be required when access to the operating room is limited by the existing caseload. There should be a pre-established protocol for safely anesthetizing, monitoring, and if necessary, resuscitating patients at the level of current operating room standards.

Although most anesthetic agents can be tailored for use in the burn unit, ketamine is particularly valuable because it ordinarily provides hemodynamic support and requires neither an anesthesia machine nor scavenging from the environment. Hallucinations are a recognized side effect of ketamine, but they can be minimized by the use of small doses of benzodiazepines or droperidol.

Postoperative Care

During the postoperative period, two issues receive the greatest amount of attention: the timing of extubation, and the method of treating postoperative pain.

Extubation

The decision to wean from mechanical support and extubate burn patients is based on the same criteria applied in any other intensive care setting. The cause of respiratory failure should be resolved, and the patient should not have cardiovascular instability, hypothermia, significant metabolic derangement, or worsening sepsis. Extubation requires that the patient be alert enough to protect the upper airway from obstruction or aspiration. The metabolic derangement that results from major burn surgery may be significant enough to warrant postoperative mechanical support for several hours to ensure adequate oxygenation and ventilation. This is especially true if the patient is hypothermic at the conclusion of the procedure. Extubation may have to be delayed when a skin graft has been applied to the patient's back and the surgical plan requires that the patient remain in the prone position after surgery. In this situation, reintubation to correct postoperative ventilatory failure would require turning the patient supine, thereby compromising the grafts. Delaying extubation for several hours would be the more prudent course.

Analgesia

Because first- and second-degree burns and skin graft donor sites are intensely painful, all burn victims require analgesia. Narcotic analgesics are widely used; there is no evidence to indicate that repeated doses result in addiction. Although studies have not revealed burn patients to be resistant to the effects of morphine, they do require larger and more frequent doses over a long period of recovery. These large doses may be appropriate due to the great degree of pain they experience. After débridement and grafting, the patient inevitably has pain that lasts for many hours. Accordingly, administration of a long-acting narcotic such as morphine, meperidine, or buprenorphine is indicated as soon as the patient's condition is stable, either during or after surgery. The amount of drug required must be titrated to the level of pain, which can only be gauged by the patient's verbal report, as there are no reliable objective measures of chronic pain.

SUGGESTED READING

Boswick JA Jr, ed. The art and science of burn care. Rockville MD: Aspen Publishers, 1987.

Haponik EF, Munster AM, eds. Respiratory injury: smoke inhalation and burns. New York: McGraw-Hill, 1990.

Martyn JAJ, ed. Acute management of the burned patient. Philadelphia: WB Saunders, 1990.

COMMON TECHNIQUES OF REGIONAL ANESTHESIA

EPIDURAL ANESTHESIA AND ANALGESIA

WILLIAM F. ECKHARDT, M.D.
J. KENNETH DAVISON, M.D.

Epidural and spinal anesthesia have been in existence since the late 1800s. Corning and Bier performed the first spinal anesthetic, and Cathelin is given credit for the first caudal epidural in 1901. Before the advent of adequate neuromuscular blocking drugs in the 1940s, both techniques enjoyed great popularity because they offered a degree of muscle relaxation. During the past 10 to 15 years, epidural anesthesia has enjoyed renewed popularity in primarily three respects: (1) as an alternative to general anesthesia for surgery of the lower abdomen and extremities; (2) as the major technique for obstetric anesthesia and analgesia; and (3) as a major part of the burgeoning interest in postoperative pain management.

ANATOMY

The epidural space is a potential space filled with loose connective tissue, fat, and blood vessels. Although no free fluid exists in the epidural space, local anesthetic solutions, when injected into the space, spread in all directions, bound only by the anatomic borders of the space. At the cephalad end, the epidural space ends at the foramen magnum. At the caudal end, the epidural space terminates at the level of the fourth sacral vertebra. The anterior boundary of the epidural space is the posterior longitudinal ligament, which connects the posterior surface of each vertebral body. The posterior border of the epidural space is defined by the laminae and the ligamentum flavum. The ligamentum flavum is a continuous connective tissue band, 3 to 5 mm thick, lying 3.5 to 5 cm from the skin. In addition, a structure known as the dorsomedian connective tissue band holds the dura to the ligamentum flavum. This structure has been visualized with both contrast computed tomography and epidurography, and it has been hypothesized to be a potential cause of unilateral epidural blocks as well as a cause of difficulty in passage of epidural catheters via a midline approach.

The size of the epidural space varies depending on its location along the vertebral spinal. In general, the epidural space has a depth of 3 to 4 mm in thoracic segments, and of 5 to 6 mm in lumbar regions. However, at the two areas of spinal cord enlargement corresponding to the brachial and lumbar plexuses—C-7–T-2 and T-9–T-12—the size of the epidural space may be smaller.

EQUIPMENT/TECHNIQUES

This review will not describe the different techniques for epidural blockade, but will refer the reader to excellent summaries by Bromage, Mulroy, and Miller. Since epidural blockade lends itself so well to continuous catheter techniques, the question of how far to thread these becomes important. Recent radiologic studies of epidural placement by Sanchez and Muneyuki reveal a high percentage (up to 75 percent) of catheter malpositions when long lengths (6 to 20 cm) of catheter were passed. Their studies revealed that thoracic epidural blockade was associated with the highest rate of straight catheter placement (69 percent), even when up to 10.2 cm of catheter were passed. They found no improvement in ability to thread straight epidural catheters when 15 ml of normal saline was injected before attempted cannulation in the lumbar space.

To avoid this, it is currently suggested that catheters be threaded only 2 to 5 cm into the epidural space, and that stylets be used only to aid in initial passage into the space. Each of these maneuvers should minimize the potential risk of passing the catheter into an epidural vein or through the dura. Although their use may increase the likelihood of catheter malposition, the incidence of straight catheter placements may be higher with the use of styletted catheters.

With the increasing popularity of using continuous epidural infusion for postoperative analgesia, several studies have examined the potential problem of catheter migration. Slappendel et al examined final catheter position and correlation of dye spread versus extent of anesthesia in patients in whom thoracic epidural catheters were inserted at T3-4 or T4-5 via the paramedian approach. Two catheter malpositions were noted (in the paravertebral space); in both, there was difficulty with catheter insertion (paresthesia in one and lack of catheter advancement beyond 1.5 cm in the other). In three other cases, contrast dye was not visible on chest radiograph, despite an adequate level of anesthesia.

Mourisse et al examined the migration of thoracic epidural catheters placed via a paramedian approach at T3-4 or T4-5 over a 3- or 4-day infusion for postoperative analgesia. Twenty-five epidural catheters were evaluated: four for 3 days, and 21 for 4 days. Nine, or 36 percent, of catheters had *not* changed from their initial positions, whereas 13 or 56 percent had demonstrated an inward migration (range of 0.5 to 2.5 cm). This correlated with an increase in mean height of the sensory block by one segment in eight, or 34 percent, with no change noted in 11 or 47 percent. In no case was there migration into the subdural space, epidural blood vessel, or through an intervertebral foramen. The cause of this inward catheter migration is unclear, but current theories include that the ligamentum flavum may exert a gripping action on the catheter or that potential subatmospheric epidural pressure may draw the catheter inward.

Finally, the increasing popularity of using epidural catheters for postoperative analgesia has focused attention on the problem of how best to protect such catheters if they are left in place for 2 to 7 days. Hord has recently described a simple method of using a 16 gauge 2-inch catheter (Angiocath) and a No. 11 scalpel blade to facilitate passage of an epidural catheter through a subcutaneous tunnel to exit at a distant site. One may wish to tunnel such catheters to the anterior abdominal wall in a debilitated cancer patient, as it may facilitate dressing care. In addition, for patients undergoing thoracotomy, it may be useful to tunnel such catheters away from the site of surgery, as the epidural dressing might interfere with the surgical field. Potential advantages to tunneling such catheters may be a decreased epidural infection rate, as the skin exit site is far removed from the epidural space, and decreased catheter migration. This method appears to be simpler, less expensive, and creates a smaller tunnel than previous reports using either malleable metal tunneling tools or plastic sheath-trocar units.

PHYSIOLOGY OF EPIDURAL BLOCKADE

Epidural administration of local anesthetics causes inhibition of neuronal activity in dorsal and ventral spinal nerve roots. In addition, Bromage has demonstrated that such agents are also able to cross the dura and cause neural blockade in the spinal cord, although local anesthetic concentrations at this location are much lower than in spinal nerve roots. Onset of blockade begins with small, unmyelinated sensory fibers followed by preganglionic autonomic, and finally, larger, heavily myelinated motor fibers. Sacral anesthesia is considerably slower in onset after injection of local anesthetic in either the thoracic or lumbar epidural space, owing to the relatively large size of the S-1 nerve roots, which act as a barrier to diffusion.

The clinical implications of testing for the onset of thoracic or lumbar epidural anesthesia begin with flushing and warming of the extremity, followed by the inability to distinguish cold (temperature) and pain, a lost sense of position, diminished touch and pressure sensation, and finally, motor paresis and paralysis. Epidural anesthetics have a variety of effects, which depend on the location of the block (i.e., caudal, lumbar, thoracic, or cervical) as well as on the uppermost dermatomal extent.

Pulmonary

The pulmonary effects of epidural anesthesia depend on the highest thoracic level blocked. Wahba studied pulmonary function in patients with T-4 sensory level block and noted no effect on functional residual capacity (FRC), vital capacity (VC), forced expiratory volume in one second, or alveolar ventilation (VA). They believed that this occurred because the level of motor block would have been approximately T-8 or T-9, thus allowing normal function of the diaphragm and intercostal muscles. McCarthy examined the effect of T-5 epidural blockade on pulmonary function where the uppermost level of anesthesia extended to T-2. He was unable to show any significant effects on FRC, VC, closing capacity, or oxygenation. Sundberg noted a decrease in pulmonary function following epidural block at T-4. He noted that the upper level of sensory block extended to T-1, and measured a significant decrease in total lung capacity (TLC), VC, inspiratory capacity (IC), and maximal inspiratory flow at 50 percent (MIF50) secondary to intercostal nerve block. Expiratory function (e.g., expiratory reserve volume [ERV]), maximal expiratory flow from 25 to 75 percent (MEF25-75) was unaffected, as the diaphragm and abdominal muscles were intact.

Takasaki studied the effect of cervical and thoracic epidural blockade performed at C-7–T-1 or T-12–L-1. Levels of sensory block in the cervical groups extended from C-4–T-7 in the cervical groups, and from T-5– L-4 in the thoracic groups, respectively. Both groups demonstrated a significant effect on pulmonary function. In the cevical block group, significant depression of IC, VC, TLC, tidal volume (VT), minute ventilation (VE), FEV, MEF25–75, and partial pressure of oxygen (Po$_2$). Their differences may have been related to blockade of motor fibers to both the intercostal and abdominal musculature in the thoracic block group, and phrenic nerve blockade in the cervical group. This demonstrated that diminished expiratory reserve may lead to decreased ability to cough and clear bronchial secretions.

Cardiovascular

The hemodynamic effects of epidural anesthesia also vary and depend on the level of blockade, the cardiovascular status of the patient, and whether or not the patient is hypovolemic. With high dermatomal level blocks, sympathetic blockade may lead to hypotension, in addition to bradycardia if the sympathetic cardioaccelerator fibers are blocked from T1-4. Sundberg has studied the effect of T-4 epidural blockade on hemodynamics. He noted significant decreases in heart rate, mean arterial blood pressure, cardiac output, and stroke volume. This was believed to be secondary to partial blockade of cardiac sympathetic fibers. Otton and Wilson described the effect of C-7–T-1 epidural blockade, and reported significant decreases in cardiac output, heart rate, and mean blood pressure, with increased central venous pressure and systemic vascular resistance, and no change in stroke volume. They believed the effects were secondary to cardiac sympathetic blockade accompanied by decreased myocardial contractility, as there was no change in stroke volume.

In our experience, a thoracic or lumbar epidural that results in analgesia from T-4 to L4-5 would be expected to cause the following: decreased heart rate and blood pressure; a minimal decrease in central venous pressure, pulmonary artery pressure, and pulmonary capillary wedge pressure; and a minimal-to-modest decrease in cardiac output. Each of these changes can usually be remedied with infusion of a pressor and volume.

Finally, two animal studies suggest a beneficial effect of epidural blockade-induced sympathectomy on distribution of myocardial blood flow during ischemia and infarction. Klassen studied the effect of high thoracic epidural block (C-7–T-1) on the distribution of myocardial blood flow as measured by radioactive microspheres in dogs undergoing both coronary ischemia and infarction. He noted increased endocardial blood flow (the area most at risk for ischemic damage) and increased endocardial/epicardial flow ratios. Davis also studied the effect of T1-2 thoracic epidural blockade on hemodynamics after coronary artery ischemia. One hour after coronary artery occlusion, either saline or local anesthetic was injected through the epidural catheter, and this was continued hourly for the next 6 hours. In animals treated with thoracic epidural anesthesia, cardiac index, heart rate, mean blood pressure, and LV dp/dT decreased significantly, and endocardial/

epicardial flow ratios and regional endocardial blood flow increased. Myocardial infarct size was significantly smaller in the epidural group, and the overall area of ischemic tissue (as defined by ST segment elevation mapping) was decreased in the epidural group.

The effect of epidural blockade on regional organ blood flow appears to be dependent on the level of mean blood pressure. When an epidural block affects high dermatomal levels, the ensuing sympathetic nervous system inhibition and loss of vasomotor tone will result in decreased renal blood flow, hepatic blood flow, and possibly cerebral blood flow (if the lower limit of autoregulation is passed). In addition, epidural blockade has a salutory effect on peripheral blood flow, demonstrating peripheral vasodilatation, decreased peripheral vascular resistance, and increased graft blood flow in patients undergoing arterial revascularization of the lower extremities.

STRESS HORMONE RESPONSE

Both surgery and anesthesia exert a profound effect on endocrine balance and stress response, both of which may affect the postoperative complication rate and overall outcome. Both humoral and neural stimuli play a part in the stress response, as do activation of the complement pathway, clotting cascade, and fibrinolytic systems. In addition, these are affected by local metabolites such as prostaglandins, histamine, serotonin, leukotrienes, substance P, and peptides (e.g., interleukin 1 and tumor necrosis factor) (Fig. 1).

Regional anesthesia, either alone or as part of a combined technique with general anesthesia, is able to prevent many of these stress hormonal responses. For patients undergoing lower abdominal or lower extremity surgery, regional anesthesia is able to blunt the cortisol, aldosterone, and renin response, in addition to blunting the stress-induced increases in norepinephrine (NE), epipinephrine (epi), adrenocorticotropic hormone (ACTH), antidiuretic hormone (ADH), beta-endorphin, and thyroid-stimulating hormone (TSH). Regional anesthesia can stabilize glucose and lipid metabolism, so that inhibition of lipolysis and

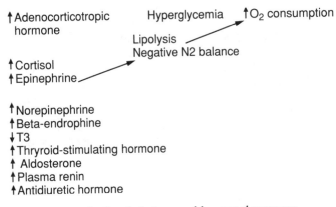

Figure 1 Surgical stress and hormonal response

hepatic glycogenolysis results. Thus, the usual stress-induced increase in oxygen consumption is prevented, and positive nitrogen balance occurs for at least the first 3 postoperative days.

Neumark has studied the effect of regional anesthesia on stress hormone response during labor. Normally, one finds high levels of plasma cortisol, epinephrine, and norepinephrine during labor. These may be potentially harmful if they lead to decreased uterine blood flow, fetal hypoxemia, or uterine hypertonus. Lumbar epidural anesthesia with bupivicaine hydrochloride 0.25 percent results in significant decreases in epinephrine and cortisol, but not norepinephrine.

Interestingly, these beneficial changes in hormonal stress response have not been borne out by studies on patients undergoing thoracic or upper abdominal surgery. Kehlet suggests that there may be many reasons for these observations: (1) variable degrees of sensory analgesia; (2) relatively brief duration of neural blockade; (3) varied surgical procedures and need for perioperative fluid therapy; and (4) the nature of the block itself—were vagal afferents blocked, afferents blocked, did sympathetic and somatic afferent blocks occur, and finally, did release of humoral factors occur?

In summary, there are data to suggest a beneficial effect of regional anesthesia in lower abdominal and lower extremity surgery. There are data that suggest that this beneficial effect may also extend to thoracic and upper abdominal surgery, although there are certain factors which may affect this. Epidural opioids are *not* as effective as local anesthetics in preventing the surgical stress response, although a study by Tsuji suggests an improvement in postoperative nitrogen balance and reduced stress response by epidural morphine in patients undergoing gastrectomy. It would appear that ensuring an adequate efferent and afferent sympathetic block in addition to an afferent somatic block may improve the effectiveness of epidural techniques in alleviating stress hormonal responses to major thoracic and abdominal surgery.

COMPLICATIONS

Although many of the complications related to epidural anesthesia are the same as for spinal anesthesia, the more common use of continuous epidural catheter techniques brings with it unique problems.

Hypotension

Epidural blockade frequently results in inhibition of sympathetic nervous system tone, and consequently, diminished venous return can cause arterial hypotension. The onset of hypotension is generally gradual, but may be rapid. Typical high-risk patients for epidural-induced hypotension include hypertensive patients, dehydrated patients, and those who are bleeding. Volume loading with 500 to 1,000 ml of crystalloid or the use of an alpha-adrenergic agonist is an integral part of the management.

High Spinal Block

This is a more serious problem when it occurs during an epidural block rather than a spinal, because the larger volume of local anesthetic used in an epidural block leads to the rapid onset of a long-lasting spinal. Patients may be at risk for this complication both during initial catheter placement as well as because of the migration of epidural catheters being used for postoperative analgesia. Clinically, one might find loss of consciousness, hypotension, bradycardia, and respiratory arrest. The treatment protocol is simply the ABCs of resuscitation: airway intubation; ventilation; circulatory support with fluid, atropine, and pressors.

Prevention and recognition of this complication are the most useful ways to avoid the problem. Likewise, injection of a test dose, slow titration of incremental doses, followed by careful assessment of sensory and motor blockade are the best ways to detect this complication.

The reported incidence of subarachnoid puncture during performance of an epidural block ranges from 0.2 to 3 percent, and many investigators have studied this problem. What are the options if this occurs? One may simply convert this to a continuous spinal catheter technique, if appropriate for the surgery. Some advocate pulling the needle back several millimeters into the epidural space and then passing a catheter, whereas others would simply replace the epidural at a different interspace.

Review of several large studies of epidural blockade suggest that this is a very rare complication, with 520 cases occurring among 25,000 epidurals placed, and with only one resulting in a total spinal. A recent report by Hodgkinson detailed three total spinal complications from a series of 2,603 cesarean sections (during which 58 inadvertent dural punctures occurred). Each of these cases involved an inadvertent dural puncture, followed by successful epidural catheterization one interspace more cephalad. Each case resulted in respiratory arrest requiring endotracheal intubation and pressors. I suggested that it might be reasonable to replace the epidural catheter at a different level and then to inject a reduced dose of local anesthetic while observing the patient for the potential onset of spinal block.

Intravascular Injection

This is one of the most serious complications of epidural anesthesia, given that large volumes of local anesthetics are often injected via indwelling plastic catheters. Inadvertent intravascular injection results in high systemic blood levels of local anesthetics, with the attendant hazards of cardiac (arrhythmias and hypotension) and central nervous system toxicity (seizures). It is often difficult to detect this problem, given that epidural venous pressure is very low or even negative, thus causing such veins to collapse easily. Patients at high risk for this complication include those with epidural venous engorgement (as in pregnancy, portal hypertension, and extensive intra-abdominal or retroperitoneal malignancy) and those patients in whom great lengths (> 5 cm) of epidural catheter have been inserted. One may prevent this hazard by administering test doses containing epinephrine, as well as by administering intermittent small-volume injections when establishing a level of neural blockade. In addition, one must be highly suspicious of this possibility any time a catheter is used postoperatively, as catheters may migrate into blood vessels over time. Finally, this risk once again underscores the importance of allowing only individuals trained in such techniques to monitor and adjust their use.

Back Pain

Although it is unusual, epidural blockade may result in local back pain. Causes may include muscle spasm, ligamentous injury, muscular hematoma formation, or periosteal injury. These problems are usually very mild and are treated with rest, local heat, and analgesics.

Inadequate Blockade

Occasionally, unilateral or patchy epidural blocks occur in the setting of appropriate placement of local anesthetic in the epidural space. Several explanations for this have been suggested. It has become clear that within the epidural space, dorsomedian connective tissue bands may potentially affect compartmental diffusion. This is also the explanation for potential problems in the extent of anesthesia in patients who have undergone back surgery, or who may have had a previous epidural catheter leading to the formation of adhesions.

Advancing the catheter far into the epidural space (> 5 cm) may lead to catheter tip egress through the intervertebral foramen, and resultant dense but patchy blockade.

Insertion techniques where large quantities of air or saline are used to locate the epidural space have been postulated to prevent free diffusion or cause significant dilution of local anesthetic.

Fractured Catheter

During difficult epidural catheter placement, it is possible to sheer the tip of a catheter when withdrawing it via an angled bevel introducer needle. For this reason, it is important that one simultaneously remove a catheter and needle en bloc when a catheter will not thread. If the tip of the catheter *is* sheered, it would *not* be harmful to the patient, as these catheter materials are nonirritating and tissue-implantable; however, it is possible that an avenue for the introduction of infection could be established. Surgical removal should be considered for the latter complication, and all patients should be informed of this, as future radiographs will reveal such radiopaque fragments.

Neurologic Injury

Neurologic injury following epidural anesthesia is very rare. A recent review by Kane discovered that only three of 50,000 patients who were administered epidural anesthetics have suffered persistent paralysis or paresis of the lower extremities. Possible mechanisms of injury include cord compression secondary to epidural hematoma; spinal cord ischemia or infarction from prolonged hypotension; aseptic meningitis; cauda equina syndrome; adhesive arachnoiditis; anterior spinal artery occlusion (caused by spasm, trauma, arteriosclerosis, thrombosis, or syphilis); or trauma to the spinal cord or nerve roots.

Epidural Hematoma

Spontaneous epidural hematomas (SEH) have been rarely described in the neurology literature, and most often occur in anticoagulated patients. There are no reports of SEH in the anesthesia literature. Neurologic injury following epidural anesthesia is a very rare phenomenon, estimated by Usubiaga to have an incidence of one in 11,000 patients. Potential causes include ischemia, infection, anesthetic toxicity, toxicity of preservative agents, spinal stenosis, patient position, prolonged hypotension, and epidural hematoma.

In unanesthetized patients, the hallmark of epidural hematoma is severe back pain, often with a radicular component. Pain is usually followed by the development of progressive neurologic deficits. This may be difficult to recognize in the anesthetized patient, but one should be suspicious of a motor and sensory block that exceeds the expected duration for the drug used. In addition, such patients may complain of low back pain as the block recedes. Diagnostic studies should include myelography or CT, and definitive therapy involves an emergent decompressive laminectomy.

Generally accepted contraindications to epidural catheter placement are patients with pre-existing coagulopathies, either medical or pharmacologic in origin.

There are two studies that have examined the relationship between regional anesthesia and subsequent heparinization, and postoperative outcome. Matthews et al performed lumbar puncture with 20- to 25-gauge spinal needles in order to administer intrathecal morphine 50 minutes prior to going on cardiopulmonary bypass in patients having coronary artery surgery. They reported no cases of epidural hematoma or neurologic dysfunction. Rao and El-Etr studied 3,164 patients having epidural anesthesia and 847 having continuous spinal anesthesia for lower extremity vascular surgery. None of these patients received anticoagulants before anesthesia, and no patient developed evidence of subarachnoid or epidural hematoma.

Finally, Odoom et al reported on the use of 1,000 epidural anesthetics in 950 patients who took oral anticoagulants prior to anesthesia. Each patient was subsequently heparinized for vascular surgery, and no patient developed neurologic dysfunction or epidural hematoma. Although the insertion of an epidural catheter in patients to be heparinized may be controversial at some centers, clinical experience supports this as acceptable practice.

Occasionally during placement of an epidural needle or catheter, an epidural vein is cannulated. At some institutions, anesthesiologists might advocate stopping the procedure if it is to involve anticoagulation, and they might cancel surgery for that day. They will then bring the patient back for general anesthesia on a subsequent day. It has been our practice to remove the epidural needle or catheter, and replace it at a different interspace, even in patients who will be anticoagulated for noncardiac vascular surgery. Our patients have had no neurologic complications as a result of this practice, and there are currently no reports in the literature of such complications.

Postdural Puncture Headache

The incidence of postdural puncture headache (PDPH) varies from 1 percent (in patients having spinal anesthetics with 25-gauge needles) to more than 30 percent in pregnant patients after accidental dural puncture with 17- or 18-gauge epidural needles. Postdural headache occurring within 5 days of epidural or spinal block is diagnostic. The headache is worse when the patient is sitting or standing and is relieved when the patient is supine. Headache duration is usually 2 to 3 days, rarely more than 1 week. Location varies; 50 percent are frontal, 25 percent are occipital, and 25 percent are diffuse, with a small number also involving the neck. Association symptoms may include auditory changes (e.g., dizziness, tinnitus, decreased hearing acuity) and visual problems (e.g., blurred or double vision, and abducens or cranial nerve VI palsies).

Treatment of accidental dural puncture during epidural block includes the following: conversion to a continuous spinal catheter technique; replacing the epidural at a different interspace; pulling the needle back until free cerebrospinal fluid (CSF) flow stops, then attempting to thread an epidural catheter; placing a prophylactic blood patch and continuing with epidural anesthesia at a different interspace; or conversion to a general anesthetic. Please refer to Table 1 for information on prevention of postdural puncture headache.

Currently controversy exists in obstetric anesthesia regarding the role of prophylactic epidural blood patch after accidental dural puncture. Colonna-Romano have recently reported an 80-percent incidence of PDPH in

obstetric patients, which was decreased to 21 percent following placement of a prophylactic epidural blood patch (injection of 15 ml blood via the epidural catheter). However, others take issue with this practice, arguing that it is difficult to predict who will develop a PDPH, and that complications can occur from epidural blood patches (e.g., failure to provide analgesia; dural puncture; backache; radiculopathy; infection; arachnoiditis; and neck stiffness).

Suggested therapy for PDPH includes bedrest (85 percent of cases are mild to moderate in nature); epidural saline infusion (15 to 25 ml per hour); or intravenous caffeine (500 mg caffeine solution benzoate in 500 ml saline over 2 hours) to act as a cerebral vasoconstrictor. Epidural blood patch may be performed if the headache is refractory.

PERIOPERATIVE PAIN MANAGEMENT WITH EPIDURAL NARCOTICS

The use of epidural narcotics for postoperative analgesia has become increasingly popular since its inception by Behar in 1979. Spinal axis opioids act on the substantia gelatinosa of the dorsal horn of the spinal cord, where they affect interneurons that modulate pain perception from peripheral sensory neurons. Thus, they offer a selective block of pain conduction, but have no effect on sympathetic nervous system tone or motor function. Once in the epidural space, narcotics are distributed by several mechanisms:

1. Systemic absorption by epidural veins.
2. Uptake by radicular arteries which directly penetrate the spinal cord.
3. Diffusion across the dura: (a) one portion remains in the CSF and may be responsible for delayed respiratory depression; (b) a second portion diffuses into the dorsal horn of the spinal cord.

Different narcotics have a variable affinity for spinal cord receptors, and thus the speed of onset, duration, potency, and incidence of side effects may be related to the agent's lipid solubility (Table 3). For example, morphine (which is the least lipid-soluble) is slow to

---

Table 1 Prevention of Postdural Puncture Headache

1. Needle size: use small-gauge needles (25- to 30-gauge). Not practical for epidurals.
2. Age: less of a problem over 50 yrs of age.
3. Sex: twofold greater incidence in women.
4. Hydration: volume loading to prevent to treat PDPH has no benefit.
5. Position: recumbency will not prevent PDPH.
6. Needle type: Greene, Sprotte, and Whitacre may be preferable to the Quinke.
7. Needle orientation: lowest headache incidence occurs with a 30° needle approach versus 60 or 90°; and needle insertion parallel to the longitudinal dural fibers.
8. Conversion of an epidural to continuous spinal technique: the reported low PDPH rate (0.86%) is probably due to inflammatory reaction with fibrosis around the catheter.

Table 2 Factors Influencing Extent of Epidural Block

Drug:
  Total milligram dose
  Concentration
  Volume of injectate
  Addition of vasoconstrictor: epipinephrine or neopinephrine

Patient:
  Old age
  Obesity
  Pregnancy
  Tall stature

Technique:
  Gravity +/−
  Site of block: caudal, lumbar, thoracic, or cervical

Table 3 Epidural Narcotics

Agent	Dose	Onset	Duration	Lipid Solubility
Morphine (Duramorph)	5 mg	30–60 min	12–24 hr	1.42
Fentanyl	100 μg	4–20 min	4–8 hr	813.0
Sufentanil	50–75 μg	10–15 min	2–5 hr	1,778.0
Meperidine hydrochloride	30–100 μg	5–20 min	5–7 hr	38.8
Methadone	5 mg	12–18 min	7–15 hr	116.0
Hydromorphone	1 mg	12–25 min	10–15 hr	NA
Alfentanil hydrochloride	1,000 μg	12–16 min	2–4 hr	NA

Table 4 Epidural Morphine and Potential Complications

Complication	Incidence
Nausea, vomiting	34%
Pruritus	11%
Urinary retention	42%
Dysphoria/sedation	1%
Respiratory depression	0.9%

penetrate the spinal cord and tends to diffuse more readily into the CSF. Lipid-soluble drugs, such as fentanyl and sufentanil, readily penetrate the spinal cord but are of shorter duration and result in lower CSF concentrations. Thus, one is left with two approaches to analgesia: use of a long- acting agent such as morphine, or use of a short-acting agent such as fentanyl or sufentanil, the latter often administered by constant infusion.

Additional factors that may affect the adequacy of postoperative analgesia with the use of epidural narcotics include (1) drug diluent volume (e.g., increased volume > 5 to 10 ml may facilitate spread); (2) site of epidural catheter (e.g., lumbar epidural blockade may not provide adequate analgesia for high thoracic or cervical pain); and (3) addition of vasoconstrictors.

The complication rate seen with 6,000 cases of epidural morphine (Duramorph) administration in Gustafsson and Stenseth's report is displayed in Table 4.

The main factor that has limited general acceptance of epidural narcotic analgesia for postoperative pain management is the potential for respiratory depression. Epidural narcotics gain access to the CSF, where they then circulate along the normal flow pathway for CSF secretion from the chorionic villi in the lateral and third ventricles to absorption by the venous system at the arachnoid granulations. Bromage has reported that bolus doses of contrast agent (metrizamide) introduced in the lumbar subarachnoid space can reach the basal cisterns within 0.5 to 3 hours. In pregnancy with increased epidural venous pressure or straining (e.g., vomiting), faster CSF transit time may occur. When lipid-insoluble drugs such as morphine enter the CSF, they can circulate to the midbrain and potentially depress the function of cardiorespiratory control centers in the pons and medulla. Bromage has examined the rostral spread of epidural morphine in patients receiving

10 mg of morphine via lumbar epidural catheters. He noted the onset time of different symp-toms to be pruritus at Hour 3, nausea at Hour 4, and vomiting at Hour 6. He believes that this represents cephalad spread of morphine in the CSF ascending past the medulla and pons.

Based on the results of five studies, the incidence of side effects attributed to epidural fentanyl are shown in Table 5. Of these five studies, all but one studied analgesia following cesarean section. Torda reported analgesia after abdominal aortic aneurysm repair, thoracotomy, and major genitourinary procedures. Madej is the only investigator to report respiratory depression, and this was described as a respiratory rate of less than 8 breaths per minute within 20 minutes of drug administration, but with no other clinical sequelae.

Several investigators have described a biphasic respiratory depression that accompanies the use of epidural narcotics. Kafer et al studied the effect of lumbar epidural morphine on the control of ventilation. Their mean dose was 7.9 mg diluted in a 16-ml volume. They noted a rightward shift of the ventilatory response curve to carbon dioxide and a decreased respiratory rate, tidal volume, and minute ventilation. These patients were followed for 24 hours after receiving injection of epidural morphine. It was noted that maximal respiratory depression occurred 2 hours after injection and that peak plasma morphine levels were measured 15 minutes after injection. It was concluded that biphasic respiratory depression may accompany the use of epidural morphine and that early depression may result from systemic narcotic absorption from the epidural venous plexus, while late depression may be caused by cephalad distribution of morphine within the CSF.

Negre et al performed a similar study assessing the effect of lumbar epidural fentanyl (200 μg per 10 ml) on ventilatory response to 7 percent carbon dioxide. This group was compared with a control group that received 200 μg fentanyl via an intramuscular route. There were no differences in respiratory rate, minute ventilation, or end-tidal carbon dioxide between groups. The epidural fentanyl group had significantly smaller slope values (VE/PET CO$_2$) at 30, 60, and 120 minutes after drug administration, suggesting respiratory depression. Plasma fentanyl levels were significantly lower in the epidural group. These authors suggest that epidural fentanyl may have a different mechanism of action or

Table 5 Side Effects of Epidural Fentanyl

Study	Dose	Nausea	Vomiting	Pruritus	Hypotension
Ellis, 1990	1.5 μg/kg	61%	NA	42%	NA
Madej, 1987	100 μg	20%	10%	40%	NA
Reynolds, 1989	100 μg	7%	6%	50%	7%
Fischer, 1988	50 μg	3.4%	NA	22%	NA
Torda, 1982	60 μg	0	0	0	0

distribution than morphine and that direct rostral spread of fentanyl via a perimedullary vascular channel may be the mechanism. This hypothesis needs further investigation.

Ahuja et al have also reported the effect of epidural fentanyl on ventilatory response after bolus injection and constant infusion. They examined the effect of fentanyl (1.5 μg per kilogram) injected via a thoracic epidural catheter at T4-10 on two groups: a control group receiving no narcotic premedication and a study group receiving intramuscular morphine, 0.1 to 0.2 mg per kilogram, before administration of epidural fentanyl. One hour after a bolus dose of epidural fentanyl, a continuous epidural fentanyl infusion was started at 0.5 μg per kilogram per hour (dose 10 μg per milliliter). These infusions were continued for 3 days in postsurgical patients and for 5 days for post-trauma patients. Their data revealed a significant decrease in respiratory rate within 10 minutes of injection of the epidural catheter, with the respiratory rate remaining depressed for the next 16 hours. Patients who received narcotic premedication before receiving epidural narcotic had lower respiratory rates and higher end-tidal carbon dioxide values, which persisted for up to 5 hours. Plasma fentanyl levels were measured throughout the study and ranged from 0.65 ng per milliliter within minutes of bolus injection; 0.3 ng per milliliter at 60 minutes after injection; 0.45 ng per milliliter at 12 hours; and 0.6 ng per milliliter at 18 hours during the constant infusion. There were no reported complications, although the authors did describe the development of tolerance to epidural fentanyl occurring in 75 percent of patients at 36 to 48 hours into the infusion.

It might be helpful to analyze some of the case reports of delayed respiratory depression following the use of epidural narcotics to determine if there are any identifiable factors that might place a patient at greater risk. Ready et al reported their experience with the establishment of a postoperative pain service at the University of Washington. They reported their experience with 820 patients—623 of whom received epidural narcotics, 167 of whom received patient-controlled analgesia, and 30 of whom received a mix of pain blocks, nitrous oxide, and other techniques. Patients who received epidural opiates were evaluated hourly for 48 hours (during the first 24-hour period, respiratory rate, sedation level, and ventilation were followed, whereas during the second 24-hour period only the level of sedation was followed). Four cases of marked respiratory depression occurred, and their

unifying characteristics were as follows: all were elderly; all were high-risk patients who underwent lengthy procedures (e.g., Whipple's operation, esophagogastrectomy, ileal loop, colectomy); 75 percent had received parenteral narcotics as part of their anesthetic management (e.g., fentanyl 600 μg, fentanyl 750 μg, and sufentanil 225 μg); and the epidural morphine dose was 4 to 5 mg in catheter locations from T-7–L-3. Although no patient became apneic, the lowest recorded respiratory rates were 8, 8, 11, and 12 breaths per minute; 75 percent had adequate oxygen saturation (O_2 of 95, 97, 99, and 89); peak carbon dioxide partial pressure (PCO_2) levels were high (66, 95, 85, and 63 mm Hg); and each patient demonstrated a profound level of sedation. All patients had been alert and responsive at the time of epidural morphine injection. The time interval between initial morphine injection and peak respiratory depression varied from 2.75 hours to 8.75 hours, 9.5 hours, and 13.5 hours. All episodes of respiratory depression were rapidly reversed with naloxone 0.2 mg, and no further complications were reported.

Naloxone has proved useful not only in the management of epidural opiate-induced respiratory depression, but also in the management of accidental epidural opiate overdose and in the prophylactic treatment of people at high risk for delayed respiratory depression. In the former case, Dahl et al reported a healthy woman who underwent minor orthopedic surgery under epidural blockade. Postoperative analgesia was provided by epidural morphine, until she was given an accidental epidural injection of 400 mg of morphine (10 ml of a solution of morphine 40 mg per milliliter). This was not immediately recognized, and 25 minutes later she became very somnolent with marked cyanosis and respiratory depression. She was ventilated with 100 percent oxygen via a face mask and was given naloxone, 0.2 mg, which restored her level of awareness and respiratory efforts. Over the next 26 hours, she was treated with a naloxone infusion, titrated to maintain blood gases, level of consciousness, and respiratory rate. Plasma morphine levels drawn at 1, 8, 19, and 27 hours after injection revealed concentrations of 1,988, 183, 39, and 42 ng per milliliter, respectively. During the first 24-hour period after overdose, her level of consciousness varied, although she was generally drowsy. PCO_2 levels drawn at 1, 7, 10, 13, and 28 hours after injection were 49, 72, 65, 54, and 43 mm Hg, respectively. Naloxone infusion was stopped after 26 hours, and she was discharged 4 days later, without complication. The total naloxone dose that she received was 4 mg, which she tolerated without any complications such as pulmonary edema.

Rawal has reported the use of prophylactic naloxone infusion to minimize the risk of delayed respiratory depression after administration epidural narcotics while it still preserves analgesia. Naloxone infusion at 5 μg per kilogram per hour prevented the reduction of minute ventilation and decreased the elevation of end-tidal carbon dioxide seen after the use of epidural morphine, whereas an infusion of 10 μg per kilogram per hour appeared to reduce the duration of analgesia by approximately 25 percent.

Clearly an element of caution must be taken when one is using epidural morphine, so that patients are monitored for increasing level of sedation, which may signal the onset of respiratory depression. Despite these concerns, it is interesting that many reports exist suggesting the efficacy of cervical epidural narcotics for the management of pain from malignancies of the upper body.

Waldman et al have reported the use of cervical epidural morphine to manage intractable cancer pain from the neck, shoulder, upper extremity, and thorax. Twelve patients with severe pain unresponsive to oral narcotics, adjunctive medications, chemotherapy, and radiation were first evaluated by their response to a test injection of lumbar epidural morphine (10 mg). This was not successful, so all were evaluated with a test dose of cervical epidural morphine (1 mg per 6 ml). Eleven patients experienced excellent analgesia without respiratory depression for 10 to 24 hours, and one was excluded because of inability to assess his degree of analgesia secondary to mental confusion. An implantable narcotic delivery system attached to a subcutaneous reservoir was placed via hemilaminectomy at C5-6. Patients were initially managed by a single daily injection of 1 to 2 mg morphine diluted in 6 ml of normal saline solution. As tolerance developed over the ensuing 6 to 8 weeks, the analgesic regimen was altered to include a slightly larger dose and twice-daily dosing, up to a maximum of 2.5 mg morphine twice daily. These patients were managed in this fashion for 3 to 17 months, with excellent analgesia reported up to the time of their death (N = 6) or publication of their report. No patient developed any side effects, although tolerance continued to bother four patients. This was treated by injection of a combination of cervical epidural morphine, local anesthetic, and methylprednisolone, with good analgesia reported. There were no complications reported for this subgroup, and further studies will need to be done addressing the pharmacokinetics and physiology of cervical epidural narcotics.

ANALGESIC MIXTURES FOR EPIDURAL USE

Combinations of narcotic and local anesthetic have become popular for epidural administration to provide analgesia and anesthesia. Potential advantages include an ability to provide analgesia superior to that provided by epidural local anesthetics or narcotics alone, while avoiding deleterious side effects such as motor blockade and hypotension from sympathetic blockade. This therapeutic option has been studied most extensively in obstetric patients having epidural analgesia for labor and anesthesia for cesarean section. Both Chestnut and Preston have evaluated the effect of epidural fentanyl/local anesthesia versus epidural local anesthesia on the progress of labor, the adequacy of anesthesia for cesarean section, and neonatal transition to extrauterine life. They noted improved intraoperative anesthesia, as well as postoperative analgesia, and no effect on the duration of the second stage of labor, on the delivery method, and on the complication rate in patients who were treated with combinations of epidural fentanyl and local anesthetic. In addition, there was no evidence of neonatal respiratory depression or neurologic abnormalities, as evidenced by normal Apgar scores, neonatal blood gases, and Neurologic and Adaptive Capacity scores. A recent study of epidural analgesia for labor reported by Cohen et al demonstrated the impressive potentiation of neural blockade from dilute bupivicaine hydrochloride solutions (0.205 and 0.068 percent) by the addition of fentanyl 100 μg. The mechanism behind this interaction is unclear at the current time.

The potentiation of neural blockade by narcotics has also been demonstrated for spinal blockade and intrathecal narcotic administration. Hunt et al studied the effect of different intrathecal fentanyl concentrations when mixed with spinal bupivicaine for cesarean section. She noted that the addition of 6.25 μg of fentanyl prolonged the period of effective analgesia from 72 minutes to 192 minutes, and that higher dosage did not increase this duration but only increased the incidence of side effects such as pruritus, nausea, and somnolence.

MODULATION OF ANALGESIA BY EPIDURAL CLONIDINE

Alpha-adrenergic agonists, such as clonidine, have been shown to produce analgesia in both animals and humans. This effect is believed to be mediated by postsynaptic alpha$_2$-adrenergic receptors located in the dorsal horn of the spinal cord.

Drasner et al have demonstrated potentiation of analgesia for the combination of intrathecal clonidine and systemic morphine in an animal model. Intrathecal alpha agonists alone in doses necessary to cause analgesia (2 to 4 μg per kilogram) may be impractical given the increased incidence of side effects such as hypotension, bradycardia, and disturbed motor function. Presumably, the use of epidural alpha$_2$-agonists also has analgesic effects, as has been demonstrated by Vercauteren et al. They compared the combination of epidural sufentanil, 25 μg, plus clonidine, 1 μg per kilogram, with epidural sufentanil, 50 μg, for postoperative analgesia following abdominal surgery. The onset of analgesia was significantly faster (5.8 versus 8.8 minutes) in the group that received sufentanil alone, although the period of complete analgesia (Visual Analog Pain Score <1) was significantly longer in the sufentanil-clonidine group (251 versus 144 minutes). In addition, there appeared to be less respiratory depression in the sufentanil-clonidine group, as oxygen saturation was significantly lower than control in the sufentanil alone group (O_2 saturation of 96 at control versus 90 at 10 minutes and 93 at 20 minutes after injection). In addition, 65 percent of the group that received sufentanil alone required supplemental oxygen to maintain adequate saturation, compared with 20 percent in the sufentanil-clonidine group. Finally, the sufentanil-clonidine group demonstrated significantly lower blood pressure for up to 3 hours after injection in 12 patients versus five in the combination group.

In the future, it is hoped that other agents will be developed to aid in the modulation of analgesia while minimizing adverse side effects.

COMBINED ANESTHETIC TECHNIQUES FOR INTRAOPERATIVE MANAGEMENT AND POSTOPERATIVE ANALGESIA

The initial operative use of combined anesthetic techniques (spinal or epidural with general anesthesia) probably predated the development of muscle relaxants, and most recently, their use has stemmed from the need for improved postoperative analgesia. For a time, it was popular to place epidural catheters preoperatively to be used for postoperative analgesia after injection of local anesthetic, narcotics, or a combination of the two at the end of the case. Recently, different groups have advocated a "combined anesthetic" technique, especially for high-risk patients or procedures (thoracic, vascular, and major abdominal), stressing the potential benefits of shortened intensive care unit and overall hospital admission, decreased postoperative morbidity and mortality, and improved analgesia.

Drasner et al have demonstrated that intrathecal narcotic use can decrease minimum alveolar concentration (MAC) for halothane by 40 percent in women undergoing gynecologic surgery. Presumably, this relationship would exist in the case of other inhalation anesthetics, as well as in the case of epidural narcotics, although this remains to be proven. However, clinical experience suggests that this relationship would exist given the minimal need for supplemental inhalation anesthetics or intravenous narcotics in patients undergoing abdominal surgery under combined anesthesia and receiving both epidural local anesthetics and narcotics.

With this in mind, a natural evolution has occurred in the use of epidural anesthetics to decrease intraoperative anesthetic requirements, while providing excellent postoperative analgesia. Some of the potential benefits are shown in Table 6.

Epidural anesthesia has been reported to reduce blood loss in patients undergoing total hip arthroplasty, but this remains to be examined in patients under combined anesthesia. Combined anesthetic technique has proven useful in the management of morbidly obese patients undergoing gastroplasty for weight reduction. Such patients had improved analgesia, fewer pulmonary complications, shorter time to mobilization and ambulation, shorter overall hospitalization, and a trend toward a decreased incidence of deep venous thrombosis.

Cousins et al have reported initial increased graft blood flow in patients undergoing peripheral vascular surgery under epidural blockade. Combined anesthetic techniques have also been commonly used in gastrointestinal surgery for postoperative analgesia and to decrease the incidence of pulmonary complications following upper abdominal surgery. However, a recent study suggests that combined anesthesia may pose certain problems for patients undergoing colon surgery. Bredtmann et al have reported complications after colon surgery using a combined anesthetic technique (GA with T8-9 thoracic epidural). They reported that the combined anesthetic group had improved analgesia and shorter time to recovery of bowel motility, while also demonstrating a slight trend toward a higher rate of rectal anastomosis breakdown (although this was not proven through use of contrast radiographs or CT). One result of such an anesthetic may be a small contracted bowel with shortened gastrointestinal transit time, all of which may make the creation of bowel anastomoses more difficult.

Table 6 Combined Anesthetic Technique

Advantages	Disadvantages
Excellent anesthesia	Hypotension
Muscle relaxation	Contracted bowel in
Hormonal stress response	gastrointestinal surgery
Normal heart rate	Fluid management
Excellent postoperative analgesia	dilemmas
Rapid emergence	
Improved postoperative morbidity and mortality in high-risk patients	
Reduced incidence of deep venous thrombosis	
Improved pulmonary function	
Shorter ICU admission	
Shorter hospital admission	
Decreased cost of hospitalization	

In 1987, Yeager reported significantly decreased morbidity and mortality data for a group of high-risk surgical patients treated with a combined anesthetic technique (epidural with general anesthesia). Yeager's high-risk patients included those undergoing major vascular, thoracic, and intra-abdominal procedures requiring postoperative intensive care. They noted significantly lower morbidity and mortality statistics for the group receiving combined anesthesia, with an overall complication rate of 32 percent for the combined group versus 76 percent for the group receiving general anesthesia alone. In addition, the combined technique group had decreased cortisol secretion consistent with blunted hormonal stress response, decreased duration of postoperative ventilation, decreased overall physician and hospital expenses, and no mortality, compared with a 16 percent mortality rate in the group that received general anesthesia alone.

There were several problems with Yeager's study: (1) small study size; (2) inadequate clinical information with which to compare the two groups; (3) inadequate information about the epidural technique—i.e., what level, what drugs were administered, what was the ultimate block distribution; and finally (4) the study was discontinued prematurely as the weight of their information suggested a clear benefit for the combined technique group. Although Yeager's data were suggestive, the definitive study to analyze overall outcome following the use of combined anesthetics for high-risk patients remains to be done.

POSTOPERATIVE ANALGESIA

Whether or not one uses an epidural catheter for intraoperative anesthetic management, there seem to be clear indications for their use in analgesia, whether for chronic pain, for postoperative use, or for post-trauma use.

Clearly both epidural and intraspinal narcotics play a useful role in the management of chronic pain secondary to malignancy, as demonstrated in reports by Wang et al for pain of prostate cancer metastatic to lumbosacral plexus, and Waldman et al for upper body pain from malignancies of the lung, breast, and kidney.

Bach et al have reported on the use of preoperative and intraoperative lumbar epidural anesthesia to decrease the incidence of phantom limb pain following amputation. In patients given a continuous preoperative lumbar epidural block for 3 days with bupivicaine hydrochloride 0.25 percent and morphine, the incidence of phantom limb pain was 27 percent 7 days postoperatively versus 64 percent in the control group. This trend continued, as patients in the preoperative epidural block group were pain free at 6 and 12 months postoperatively, compared with the control group, which had an incidence of phantom limb pain of 38 percent at 6 months and 27 percent at 12 months. The authors suggest that lumbar epidural blockade may block the afferent limb of abnormal reflexes as well as block sympathetic fibers whose hyperreactivity may have sensitized peripheral nociceptors.

Many studies suggest the benefit of epidural blockade for both the intraoperative and postoperative management of major vascular cases. Her et al have recently reported a study of outcome following infra-renal abdominal aortic aneurysm repair in which they compared the use of combined general and epidural anesthesia with that of general anesthesia alone. The general anesthesia group demonstrated greater intraoperative hemodynamic instability, manifested by a postinduction need for vasodilators; increased pulmonary capillary wedge pressure and decreased cardiac index after aortic cross-clamping; and a higher postoperative complication rate (63 percent incidence of continued mechanical ventilation, 37 percent incidence of respiratory failure, 47 percent incidence of hemodynamic instability, and prolonged ICU admission). This study suggested that combined anesthetic techniques might offer more stable intraoperative and postoperative hemodynamics, a decreased incidence of postoperative respiratory failure, and reduced postoperative morbidity, with overall improved outcome.

Bonnet et al have reported on the use of cervical epidural anesthesia for carotid endarterectomy. They suggest that cervical epidural blockade may be advantageous, as it allows reliable monitoring of cerebral function, is a technically easy block to perform with a low failure rate and carries an acceptable postoperative cardiovascular complication rate (0.75 percent incidence of postoperative myocardial infarction). Their complication rate included hypotension, 11 percent; bradycardia, 2.8 percent; epidural venipuncture, 1.5 percent; generalized seizure, 0.25 percent; dural puncture, 0.51 percent; and respiratory failure, 0.76 percent (the latter occurring in patients with chronic obstructive pulmonary disease who developed phrenic nerve blockade). Postoperative complications included hemiplegia, 3 percent; myocardial infarction, 0.75 percent; and death, 2.3 percent (with causes of the latter ranging from myocardial infarction in one patient, cervical hematoma in two, and severe neurologic deficit in six).

Epidural and intrathecal analgesia has also been used to control the pain of myocardial infarction as well as unstable angina. In addition, both methods have been used to provide analgesia after coronary artery surgery, where the potential advantages include excellent analgesia; increased forced vital capacity; increased peak expiratory flow rate; and reduced postoperative stress (as determined by a diminished need for sodium nitroprusside to control blood pressure and a decreased secretion of cortisol and beta-endorphin).

Both epidural and caudal block techniques have been used for postoperative analgesia in pediatric patients. Tyler has described the dramatic effect of inadequate analgesia in a 14-month old child following thoracotomy. They reported that as the effect of caudal morphine wore off after thoracotomy, the child became agitated and respiratory distress developed with splinting, accessory muscle use, and respiratory acidosis (pH

7.21, PCO$_2$ 64). She was given bupivacaine hydrochloride 0.25 percent followed by preservative-free morphine, and quickly became comfortable. A pinprick level was detected at T-6, and arterial blood gases were improved at pH 7.31, PCO$_2$ 47. Thereafter, her caudal catheter was injected with morphine every 8 to 12 hours for the first 3 postoperative days to maintain her excellent analgesia.

Many other investigators have compared different analgesic regimens (local anesthetic versus narcotic) as well as different methods of administration (epidural versus caudal) in pediatric patients. Although the most common nerve block for postoperative pediatric analgesia is probably a continuous caudal catheter, some patients have absolute or relative contraindications to their use (e.g., perianal infection, open wounds, burns, and neurologic abnormalities such as meningomyelocele).

Although the epidural space is more limited in a child and poses increased technical risks during catheter placement, Meignier et al have reported the use of T-7 thoracic epidural analgesia in six children who ranged in age from 6 months (4.5 kg) to 15 years (15 kg). All patients underwent Nissen fundoplication to correct hiatal hernia with reflux or stenosis, and each had underlying respiratory risk factors (such as kyphoscoliosis, trisomy 21 with ventricular septal defect, mucoviscidosis, and neonatal anoxic encephalopathy), for which excellent postoperative analgesia was desired. There were no complications, and each child had excellent analgesia supplied by an infusion of bupivacaine hydrochloride 0.25 percent, 4 mg per kilogram per day.

Finally, Krane et al have reported on the use of caudal morphine for postoperative analgesia after orthopedic and urologic procedures in pediatric patients. They used 0.1 mg per kilogram of preservative-free morphine and noted (1) a longer duration of analgesia (9.9 hours) versus parenteral narcotics (2 hours) and caudal bupivacaine (6.7 hours); (2) a longer time interval to supplementation with intravenous narcotic (12 hours for caudal morphine versus 45 minutes for intravenous morphine and 5 hours for caudal bupivacaine); and (3) a trend toward a slightly increased complication rate that was not significant for the caudal narcotic group. There were no cases of respiratory depression.

A variety of analgesic techniques have been studied in patients after thoracotomy or chest trauma. These include operative and postoperative intercostal blockade; intrapleural blockade; cryoanalgesia; trancutaneous electrical nerve stimulator; epidural and caudal blockade; as well as patient-controlled analgesia. Of these different methods, patient-controlled analgesia and caudal or epidural blockade would seem to offer the greatest advantage in terms of quality of analgesia and lack of potential side effects. Extreme pain and inadequate pulmonary function frequently accompany rib and chest wall trauma, and if untreated, atelectasis, decreased compliance, increased A-a gradient, and respiratory failure may occur. Johnston, MacKersie, and Dittmann have all reported on the beneficial effect of epidural narcotics in the management of patients after

chest trauma. They reported excellent analgesia, improved arterial blood gases, improved vital capacity, improved dynamic lung compliance, and increased FRC.

After thoracotomy and upper abdominal surgery, there is a tendency toward progressive alveolar collapse, as total lung capacity, FRC, and residual volume significantly decrease, and ventilation-perfusion mismatching may result with shunting, further atelectasis, and finally, pneumonia or respiratory failure. James, Shulman, and El-Baz et al have all studied the effect of epidural analgesia on pain and pulmonary function after thoracotomy. Their reported benefits include: improved analgesia; long duration of analgesia; and significantly less depression of pulmonary function as measured by FVC, FEV, and PEFR (peak expiratory flow rate).

Gough et al compared the effect of cryoanalgesia and thoracic epidural analgesia with fentanyl on post-thoracotomy pain and found the latter to offer significantly better analgesia that was of longer duration.

Intrapleural administration of local anesthetics offers incomplete pain relief after thoracotomy, despite temporary clamping of the pleural drainage system, compared with a control group receiving intercostal nerve blocks during wound closure and parenteral narcotics thereafter.

Brodsky et al have reported the use of combined general and caudal anesthesia for the management of a patient undergoing thoracotomy. Interestingly, the patient had undergone L3-4 laminectomy 7 days earlier. Analgesia was maintained without complication with intermittent caudal morphine injections (10 mg in 10 to 20 ml saline) every 6 to 12 hours for the first 3 postoperative days.

Logas et al and Hasenbos et al have reported improved analgesia with continuous administration epidural narcotic or a combination of epidural narcotic and local anesthetic compared with intercostal blockade or parenteral narcotics. In addition, Hasenbos et al have suggested the potential advantages of high thoracic (T3-4) epidural blockade, which are as follows:

1. Limited zone of analgesia, T1-10. One might avoid block of the resistance and capacitance vessels of the splanchnic and lower extremity vascular beds.
2. Decreased incidence of hypotension.
3. Possible decreased incidence of bronchospasm secondary to blockade of afferent nerve input.
4. Excellent analgesia which promotes endobronchial toilet.
5. Specific blockade of afferent neural input from the airways and lungs, and from the sympathetic nerves to the upper four thoracic segments.

Finally, a definitive prospective study comparing continuous epidural narcotic infusion with patient-controlled analgesia for post-thoracotomy analgesia remains to be done. However, a study by Rosenberg et al comparing preoperative epidural morphine (4 mg), intercostal block, standard parenteral narcotics, and on-demand intravenous fentanyl for control of pain following gastrectomy and cholecystectomy revealed that none of these techniques had any significant analgesic advantage, although the trend was toward decreased pain and increased patient satisfaction with the level of analgesia in the epidural narcotic and patient-controlled analgesia groups. No significant changes in blood gases, peak expiratory flow, or chest radiograph abnormalities were seen, although there was a very large variation in fentanyl administration (maximum 24-hour dose of 814–2,233 μg) and need for supplementation (additional boluses ranged from 3–155). Unfortunately, the epidural narcotic group involved a single injection of morphine (4 mg) before the induction of general anesthesia. Many studies suggest that a higher morphine dose might be required for adequate analgesia, and it would also be interesting to compare the level of analgesia provided by a continuous infusion of epidural fentanyl with that of patient-controlled analgesia.

Epidural anesthetic techniques will continue to advance in the future, with improved modulation of pain and other modalities. We look forward to the development of new agents that will provide analgesia with little toxicity, in addition to the more widespread use of such techniques for postsurgical pain management.

SUGGESTED READING

Blomberg RG. The dorsomedian connective tissue band in the lumbar epidural space of humans: an anatomical study using epiduroscopy in autopsy cases. Anesth Analg 1986; 65:747–752.

Blomberg RG. Technical advantages of the paramedian approach for lumbar epidural puncture and catheter introduction. Anaesthesia 1988; 43:837–843.

Bromage PR. Epidural analgesia. Philadelphia: WB Saunders, 1978.

Cathelin MF. Une Nouvelle Voie d'injection rachidienne. Methode des Injections Epidurales Par Le Procede Du Canal Sacre. Application a L'homme. C R Soc Bios (Paris) 1901; 53:452.

Corning JL. Spinal anesthesia and local medication of the cord. NY J Med 1855; 42:483.

Miller RD. Anesthesia. 2nd ed. New York: Churchill Livingstone, 1986.

Mulroy MF. Regional anesthesia. Boston: Little & Brown, 1989.

Muneyuki M, Shirai K, Inamoto A. Roentgenographic analysis of the positions of catheters placed in the epidural space. Anesthesiology 1970; 33:19–24.

Sanchez R, Acuna L, Rocha F. An analysis of the radiological visualization of catheters placed in the epidural space. Br J Anaesth 1967; 39:485–489.

Slappendel R, Gielen M, Haenbos M, Haystraten F. Migration of thoracic epidural catheters. Anaesthesia 1988; 43:939–942.

INTRAVENOUS REGIONAL ANESTHESIA

BRADLEY E. SMITH, M.D.

TECHNIQUE

Materials

The following materials are needed for intravenous regional anesthesia (IVRA): (1) 0.5 percent lidocaine or 0.5 percent prilocaine without preservative; (2) a 60-ml syringe; (3) a double-lumen thin tourniquet (cuff) or two narrow orthopedic cuffs (these devices should have a reliable mechanism for maintenance of constant pressure and should be rechecked for perfect function before each use); (4) suitable flexible intravenous catheters of almost any size; (5) intravenous extension tubing, or scalp vein infusion sets, 500 or 1,000 milliliters of intravenous solution; and (6) one Esmarch bandage.

Resuscitation Equipment

The following resuscitation equipment should be immediately available before each IVRA procedure: (1) diazepam, midazolam, or a short-acting barbiturate (according to the choice of the physician); and (2) equipment for positive pressure breathing—an Ambu bag or other IPPB device, an IPPB mask of suitable size, and an oxygen source; (3) equipment for establishment of an airway—oral and nasal airways of the proper size, a laryngoscope of the proper size, an endotracheal tube of the proper size, and succinyldicholine (in case of need for intubation of the trachea).

Preparation of Patient

History and Physical Examination. Obtain suitable history, physical examination, and laboratory evaluations. Look for contraindications such as allergy to local anesthetics, peripheral infection, peripheral vascular disease, peripheral neuropathy, and blood dyscrasia, particularly sickle cell anemia.

Informed Consent. Obtain suitable informed consent. Mention convulsions and death as known, but very rare, complications.

Oral Premedication. Administer suitable premedication, usually oral (followed later by intravenous supplement). Oral diazepam in the sedative dose is frequently used.

Methods

Start an intravenous infusion in an extremity other than the one which is to be anesthetized for the instillation of sedatives and/or emergency medications. Establish the intravenous line with a flexible plastic catheter, placing the catheter close to the proposed area of surgery but well below the antecubital fossa, and carefully tape the catheter flat in place. Wrap the limb with cotton or gauze at the intended site of placement of the pneumatic cuff. (Use upper arm or thigh, not forearm or calf.) Check the patient's blood pressure. Place a wide, double pneumatic cuff with pressure gauges and *secure* stop cocks or strong clamps. Check all working parts for proper function. (Wider cuffs will be necessary on the thigh.)

Administer a light intravenous sedative dose of midazolam or diazepam (i.e., 1 to 5 mg of diazepam or 0 to 3 mg midazolam). Elevate the arm for 3 minutes; apply pressure on the brachial artery. Continue brachial artery compression and limb elevation while firmly wrapping the limb from the distal to the proximal end with a latex bandage (Esmarch bandage). Warn the patient that this maneuver may be painful, particularly in the presence of a wound or fracture. (If this procedure is too painful, other methods may be substituted, including the use of a pneumatic splint, which is less painful.) The success rate of this block is closely correlated with the degree of exsanguination. Inflate the proximal cuff to 50 mm Hg above to the highest observed systolic pressure. Warn the patient of initial discomfort. Remove the latex bandage and discontinue brachial artery pressure.

The calculated volume of local anesthetic is now injected into the intravenous site at a slow rate (complete in no less than 1 minute). Take care not to unduly elevate venous pressure distal to the cuff. A waiting period of 3 to 20 minutes may be required for the complete onset of analgesia, but surgical preparations and draping can continue during this period. Lidocaine, 1.5 mg per kilogram, made up to a total volume of saline of 40 to 60 ml depending on the bulk of the arm is recommended. A similar procedure and dose for prilocaine (up to 2.0 mg per kg) is preferred by some authors. For the leg, 2.0 mg per kg may be used in a total volume of 60 to 100 ml, with a similar dose of prilocaine if desired. Bupivacaine is not recommended for IVRA because of its potential toxicity.

Wait to inflate the distal of the two pressure cuffs until the first cuff begins to cause pain. (In some patients the second cuff may never be needed.) After the distal cuff is securely inflated to the same pressure, the proximal cuff is released. Elevated systemic concentrations of anesthetic are often found 2 to 3 minutes after injection. Tourniquet (cuff) pressure should not be maintained for longer than 2 hours or until the end of the surgical procedure, but never less than 20 minutes.

At the end of the surgery, or no later than 2 hours, deflate the cuff only for 5 to 10 seconds at a time, then reinflate the cuff for a period of time to allow for systemic recirculation of any residual local anesthetic, which may be returned in systemic circulation. The patient should be observed for the onset of complications due to the local anesthetic agent or the sedative drugs for at least 15 minutes after the last deflation of the upper cuff.

HISTORY

Although August Bier reported its use from 1908 through 1910, it apparently was not until 1970 that the name "Bier block" was applied to the use of IVRA. Bier was also largely responsible for the introduction of intrathecal anesthesia with local anesthetics. Of interest is the observation that Bier injected methylene blue along with local anesthetic solution prior to amputation. He thus showed on postamputation dissection that the dye penetrated through all the tissues, including the perineurium and the periosteum. Despite an immediate flood of acceptance, Bier's technique was used only sporadically over the next 50 years. Originally described with intravenous surgical cut-down, the procedure was simplified in 1931 by use of percutaneous needle venipuncture for IVRA. However, it was not until the virtual reintroduction of the technique in 1963 that it almost instantly achieved its present level of popularity.

Various controversies over dose, drug, and volume arose in the 1960s, particularly in light of an early editorial in the *Journal of the American Medical Association* in response to the first reported cardiac arrest due to IVRA. Although the procedure survived, a call for the ban of bupivacaine for IVRA was strongly voiced in the 1980s in response to several deaths, usually associated with accidents.

INDICATIONS

Indications for use of IVRA include limb surgery lasting 1.75 hours or less; soft tissue surgical or orthopedic procedures such as ganglionectomy, repair of Dupuytren's contracture, reduction of Colles' fracture, reduction or manipulation of some other simple fractures (however, periosteal pain may prove unmanageable with this block), "hammer toe" procedures, tenotomy, simple tenodesis, release of carpal tunnel; and sequential operations in different extremities. IVRA may be used in selected children with suitable dose reduction.

PREMEDICATION

Because placement of the cuff may cause discomfort, a relatively heavy sedative and analgesic regimen is often recommended for surgery or cleansing of a wound. Many, if not most, other procedures for which IVRA is suitable can and often are performed on an ambulatory surgery basis and, therefore, evanescent action of the premedication is usually desirable. Nausea and vomiting are frequent concomitants of opioid analgesics, and here again the benefits should be weighed against the incidence of postoperative complications. The use of restricted doses of midazolam (1 to 5 mg given intravenously) combined with intravenous butorphanol (0.5 to 1.5 mg given intravenously) has been found to be satisfactory in many cases; however, an almost limitless variety of drugs is appropriate for presurgical or intraoperative sedation when used judiciously.

Inclusion of diazepine has been found to be very effective in reducing the incidence of systemic neurologic reactions to intravenous local anesthetics, and the barbiturates share some degree of this same protective effect. However, concern with the "antianalgesic" effects of these drugs has reduced the popularity of barbiturates in recent years. Several authors do not premedicate patients about to receive IVRA because of the general absence of discomfort. Others advocate premedication with papaveretrum and/or hyoscine.

CHARACTERISTICS OF IVRA

Onset of Action

Onset of analgesia takes place within 5 minutes, but 20 minutes may be necessary for the maximal analgesic effect to be reached. Duration is up to the maximum permissible cuff time, which is 2 hours. Sensory anesthesia is usually more profound than motor anesthesia. Both motor and sensory functions return to normal usually within 5 to 10 minutes, but no more than 15 minutes. The degree and character of muscle relaxation has remained controversial even though most experimental results both by clinical observation and also by more elaborate electromyography techniques have demonstrated good muscle relaxation.

Muscle Relaxation

The degree and character of muscle relaxation have remained controversial. However, most experimental results, both clinical and by electromyography, have demonstrated good relaxation. Various authors have felt that muscle relaxation with IVRA was insufficient for resetting of some fractures or when there was need for profound muscle relaxation. Clinically, this argument can be obviated by inclusion in the original injected solution of 3 mg of D-tubocurare, which will ensure good muscle relaxation. Other authors found adequate relaxation with all local anesthetics but with some variation in the onset of action and return of motor activity. This was recently verified by a clinical study.

Site of Action

The site of action of the local anesthetic in IVRA is still controversial. Evidence that the site of action may be peripheral includes the observation that fingers with injured vascularity often remain sensitive to pain during IVRA. It has been reported that during IVRA the local anesthetic rapidly concentrates in the region of the elbow, where large venous channels are in proximity to the median and ulnar nerves. These nerves commonly achieve anesthesia before the radial nerve.

Volunteers allowed two cuffs to be placed, one on the upper arm and one on the forearm, to prevent en-

trance of the local anesthetic solution to the wrist and hand. After injection of the local anesthetic solution, they developed complete anesthesia of the arm and the hand distal to the cuff. On a separate occasion, inflating both cuffs without injection of the anesthetic *did,* after 40 minutes, produce a less profound sensory and motor blockade beginning at the fingers and progressing upward. Nerve stimulation in both circumstances showed distinctly different characteristics, demonstrating that ischemia may contribute to but is not responsible for the nerve block.

Through injection studies, Bier showed that the medication is distributed to the nerve trunks. Injection of radioactive lidocaine in dogs by the technique of IVRA has shown accumulation along nerve trunks but not in skin and muscle. Similarly, motor nerve conduction studies have suggested a significant peripheral site of action in the neuromuscular blockade, which is not reversed by neostigmine.

Nerve conduction studies have been performed both with ischemia and during IVRA. Nerve transmission recordings during IVRA based on single muscle fiber action potentials were studied with lidocaine, prilocaine, and procaine and showed that, electrically speaking, IVRA gives complete relaxation of the muscles if sufficient time is allowed for the block to develop. These studies excluded the motor endplate and the terminal nerve twig peripheral to its branching point as possible sites of this action. They concluded that the local anesthetic was most likely exerting its effect on the nerve at the terminal branching point.

CHOICE OF ANESTHETIC AGENT

Procaine, 0.5 percent, was initially used by Bier and by most authors until 1963, when lidocaine, 0.5 percent, was proposed for this technique. Lidocaine, 0.5 percent, subsequently achieved the most frequent use of all local anesthetics for this purpose, but the use of 1 percent lidocaine, 0.25 percent lidocaine, and 0.5 percent mepivacaine has also been reported. Prilocaine in concentrations between 0.5 percent and 2 percent has been recommended by many authors. Chloprocaine was briefly used, but owing to its evanescent action and the possibility of thrombophlebitis from its usual preservatives, it has been unpopular in the United States for IVRA.

Dose

Lidocaine

Authors have used from 0.5 to 2.0 percent lidocaine, injecting a volume of 10 to 40 ml. It has been demonstrated that a natural peak plasma concentration after cuff release is 40 percent lower if the same total dose is injected in the form of 0.5 percent lidocaine rather than 1 percent lidocaine. An effective dose has been calculated by various authors; however, no consensus exists as to the best dose. Some authors use the relation of volume of anesthesia to the total volume of muscle mass to be anesthetized, whereas others have calculated the dose in milligrams per kilogram of body weight. Others have stated unvarying arbitrary dosages (e.g., 1.5 mg per kilogram of lidocaine for the upper extremity, and 2 mg per kg for the lower extremity) and mixed the calculated dose with a volume of normal saline to fill a volume of 40 to 60 ml for arms and 60 to 100 ml for legs.

It has been demonstrated that a natural peak plasma concentration after cuff release is 40 percent lower if the same total dose is injected in the form of 0.5 percent lidocaine rather than 1 percent lidocaine.

Prilocaine

Prilocaine, 0.5 percent, 40 ml (200 mg) has been favorably compared with lidocaine, 0.5 percent, 40 ml (200 mg) for IVRA in several studies. In no report has more than 3 mg per kg body weight been advocated; 2 mg per kg is the most common dose used.

Bupivacaine

The use of bupivacaine has been advocated by some, most often in the dose of 40 ml of 0.2 percent bupivacaine without adrenaline. Its advocates suggest that it has long-acting properties because it becomes fixed to the tissues and on release of the cuff, analgesia is not lost as rapidly as in the case of lidocaine. This is useful in cases in which hemostasis must be achieved by the surgeon after release of the cuff. However, the use of bupivacaine for IVRA has been soundly denounced because at least seven deaths have occurred during IVRA when, due to accident, high plasma concentrations of bupivacaine led to cardiac arrest that was refractory to resuscitation. Not only is cardiac arrest less frequent during similar accidents with lidocaine or prilocaine, but resuscitation for arrest appears to be much less difficult with either of these two agents.

It has been suggested that as much as 50 percent of the full dose is still bound to the tissues or in the extracellular fluid as long as 30 minutes after the cuff is released, and therefore, for re-establishment of an IVRA after a recent previous IVRA, it has been suggested that half the initial dose is sufficient.

Injection Volume

Volume of injection of the local anesthetic clearly has an effect on venous pressure reached in the occluded limb and will depend on (1) the volume of blood left in the veins at the time of cuff inflation and (2) the speed of the injection. Several reports indicate volume insufficient to fill the vascular space leads to inadequate anesthesia even if a corresponding increase in the concentration of the local anesthetic is substituted.

Although the temperature of the injected local anesthetic does not affect the character of the analgesia, solutions at body temperature cause the least discomfort.

Needle Placement Site

It is essential not to place the needle inadvertently in either the brachial or radial artery. Injection of the local anesthetic may not be dangerous if no preservatives are present, but this complication should be avoided. Placement of the needle near the antecubital fossa greatly increases the danger of "leak" and consequent toxic effects of the injected anesthetic owing to high venous pressure caused by the generally competent venous valves, which effectively reduce the volume of the injection compartment. This is not the case when the injection site is distal in the isolated limb compartment because the valves are competent only to back flow.

CUFF TECHNIQUE

Number of Cuffs

Several authors report the use of only a single cuff and do not infiltrate the skin proximal to the cuff. However, with only one cuff, the patient frequently experiences an ischemic-type pain from 30 to 45 minutes after inflation of the single cuff. One report states that only 3 percent of 564 patients experienced severe pain from the single cuff technique; however, the majority of more recent authorities advocate the two cuff technique to avoid ischemic cuff pain.

Cuff Position

Although the position of the cuff on upper arm or mid thigh is most frequently reported, placement of the distal cuff around the forearm rather than the upper arm also has been advocated and is said to reduce complications due to toxicity. On the lower limb, the distal cuff has also been applied to the calf without reported complications.

Cuff Inflation Pressure

Nerve damage (the radial nerve appears to be most susceptible) has been reported from nerve ischemia due to excessive cuff pressure. Pressures as low as 40 mm Hg above the patient's systolic pressure at the time of injection, and as high as 300 mm Hg in the arm and 450 mm Hg in the leg have been advocated. There is some evidence of correlation of "leak" and toxicity with the cuff pressure, but the pressure in the venous component of the limb compartment during injection is also a consideration and should be kept to a minimum. Convulsions have been reported during both arm IVRA and leg IVRA in cases in which the cuff has remained fully inflated.

When using the inflatable arm splint technique, the inflation pressure of the inflatable splint must be at least

40 mm higher than the systolic arterial pressure, and it is less effective if the arm cannot be straightened owing to a fracture or deformity.

A patient who experienced cyanosis, bradycardia, and cardiac arrest during bupivacaine IVRA was resuscitated and made a complete recovery. During resuscitation, it was noted that the cuff was still inflated to 300 mm Hg. Two days later, using the same cuff, phlebography revealed leakage under the cuff. This was shown to occur with this cuff in four of six patients and volunteers. The cuff pressures were always at least 80 mm above the systolic pressure. Venous pressures during simulated IVRA have been measured in the forearm and exceeded systolic pressure by 50 mm in three of four subjects.

Cuff Time

The total permissible duration of cuff arterial occlusion of the extremity is still in doubt. Cuff occlusion of only 30 minutes causes evidence of damage to motor endplates. Several authors demonstrated that the duration of anesthesia following the release of the cuff was greater in direct proportion to the duration of cuff occlusion, indicating a component of ischemia. Membrane and action potentials diminish progressively under ischemic conditions even without the presence of local anesthetics. In fact, after 1 hour of total ischemia the action potential of muscle fibers equals the membrane potential. It appears that structural changes in the muscle fiber cell membrane account for this diminution.

Where the cuff fails prematurely, analgesia is lost very quickly. Even more important, however, are the many reports of systemic hypotension, convulsions, or even respiratory or cardiac arrest after premature cuff release. These complications may be the result of the rapid elevation in systemic local anesthetic concentration caused by the flushing of local anesthetic solutions from the limb.

Many investigators have voiced the opinion that the longer the duration before releasing cuff pressure, the greater the safety to the patient, and they have variously recommended a minimum interval between injection and release of the cuff of from 20 minutes to 1 hour. However, some authors have reported no side effects even when the cuff was inadvertently deflated early in the anesthetic procedure.

Cuff Release

Another safety factor on which a consensus has not yet been reached is the relative importance of cyclic or intermittent release of the cuff when discontinuing the anesthetic. Many authors contend that cyclic or intermittent release is essential for safety. Nonetheless, others recommend slow, steady release of the cuff. Even with intermittent cuff release and reinflation, transient neurologic symptoms such as dizziness, drowsiness, or faintness may appear in as many as 12 percent of patients. Plasma concentration in the venous circulation

after release of the cuff has been studied with lidocaine, prilocaine, and bupivacaine. It has been calculated that 30 percent of the injected dose is still in the vessels when the cuff is released 30 minutes after injection. Fortunately, 60 to 80 percent of the local anesthetic enters the substance of the lungs, delaying its appearance in the arterial blood. In general, these studies have shown that the peak concentration occurs in the first 30 seconds after the release of the cuff. Prilocaine and lidocaine appear to have similar distribution characteristics, and both show a second maximum peak in venous blood local anesthetic concentrations exiting the anesthetized limb between 150 and 240 seconds after release of the cuff.

After doses of 3 mg per kilogram of lidocaine for IVRA the maximum venous plasma level was 1.2 μg per ml either during IVRA or after cuff release. However, others have found venous plasma levels to be from 0.9 μg per milliliter to 4.3 μg per milliliter, usually with little apparent relationship to the total dose administered. Inspection of all available literature indicates little direct relationship between venous plasma concentration in the opposite limb and the time after release of the cuff up to 15 minutes. Even though maximum plasma concentration generally is reported to be less with intermittent release, not all studies have confirmed this.

Cuff Pain

The incidence of cuff pain may be significantly lessened by the use of the double cuff technique and particularly by delay of inflation of the distal cuff and release of the proximal cuff until pain appears under the proximal cuff. Other authors emphasize that the degree of pain may be related to positioning of the cuff. Subcutaneous infiltration of a local anesthetic ring above the cuff margin is also effective in reducing ischemic pain. Pain has been reported following the injection of prilocaine to establish IVRA. However, in these cases pain may have been due to a preservative such as methylhydroxybenzoate.

Exsanguination of Limb Technique

The function of exsanguination is not completely understood. It may represent prevention of dilution of the intravenous agent, thus retaining a higher concentration of a local anesthetic. However, some authors indicate that higher concentrations of injected anesthetic agents are not more reliable in establishing a block. Another theory holds that draining of the blood from the vascular space is necessary to make space for the injected volume of anesthetic.

The use of brachial artery occlusion, limb elevation, and elastic bandages have all been studied comparatively. The use of each component has generally reduced failures. Furthermore, proper exsanguination of the limb prior to cuff inflation will greatly reduce the venous pressure achieved during injection of the local anesthetic, thus increasing safety.

COMPLICATIONS

The most important and frequent complications of IVRA are acute local anesthetic toxicity (this can occur before or after cuff release), local tissue reaction, and venous thrombosis in the injected limb.

Cardiovascular Complications

In one large study, 9 percent of patients became drowsy within 30 seconds of the release of the cuff and two lost consciousness without twitching or convulsions. A fallen pulse rate of over 10 beats per minute was noted in 15 percent of cases. Twenty-one percent of patients experienced a decrease in blood pressure. Fifteen percent of patients experienced electrocardiographic abnormalities. Three demonstrated ventricular extrasystole and one demonstrated atrial extrasystole. One transient S-T sigmoid depression and one transient nodal rhythm were seen. In another study, cardiovascular complications occurred in fewer than 0.5 percent of 514 patients; yet another author reported a 30 percent overall combined incidence of cardiovascular complications in a large study of lidocaine IVRA. However, one report noted a 31 percent incidence of bradycardia following release of the cuff when 200 mg of lidocaine were used.

Local anesthetics, in sufficient plasma concentrations, commonly are mild depressants of cardiac contractility, and in greatly elevated concentrations, these agents may depress ventricular automaticity. The peripheral vascular system is often dilated. Electrocardiographic evidence of bradycardia and occasional "wandering pacemaker" were found after doses of 3 mg per kilogram of lidocaine for IVRA. However, these changes are not consistently identified by all authorities. One of the earliest reports showed electrocardiographic deviations from baseline values in 15 to 24 percent of 77 patients studied with lidocaine IVRA, and reported a nonfatal case of cardiac arrest in the 78th patient. Continuous electrocardiographic tracings also have been studied with prilocaine IVRA and have shown similar findings.

Disturbing reports of cardiac arrest with bupivacaine IVRA began to appear in 1981, and eventually at least eight cases were reported. It appears that the cardiac toxicity of bupivacaine in higher concentrations causes a type of conduction defect that is much harder to reverse than that caused by either lidocaine or prilocaine, and therefore numerous appeals have been made to ban its use in IVRA, although these have not been unanimous.

Central Nervous System Complications

Central nervous system signs and symptoms that may occur either during the initial injection or because of a leak in the cuff or at the end of the procedure include drowsiness, nystagmus, ataxia, tinnitus, lightheadedness, giddiness, and a feeling of detachment or apprehension, and these may progress to more serious signs such as twitching and finally convulsions. Some of these central nervous system signs and symptoms have been reported in as many as 50 percent of patients after the use of 0.5 percent lidocaine, but have been reported in far fewer numbers by most other authors. The incidence of minor neurologic signs and symptoms with lidocaine has been reported to be as low as 0.5 percent, and is usually less than 3 percent.

Prilocaine at 0.5 percent appears to result in even fewer central nervous system symptoms than 0.5 percent lidocaine. Some twitching and mild central nervous system symptoms have even been seen after the use of chloroprocaine for IVRA.

Convulsions

Generalized convulsions are not infrequently reported. An early clinical series of 1,400 IVRA procedures reported three patients with generalized convulsions and five with symptoms of serious cortical stimulation, all necessitating treatment with barbiturates. Another series of 514 IVRAs with lidocaine produced only one convulsion. Convulsions during IVRA are usually the result of elevated local anesthetic concentrations. Early investigations indicate that blood concentrations as great as 5 μg per milliliter plasma lidocaine concentrations could be tolerated after rapid infusion of lidocaine, and perhaps as much as 10 μg per milliliter of lidocaine plasma concentration could be tolerated when lower build-up rates of infusion were used. Concentrations of lidocaine in plasma following release of the cuff at the planned interval have generally measured 1 to 2 μg per milliliter. In general, intravenous plasma concentrations of lidocaine after IVRA (1.5 μg per milliliter) have been demonstrated to be less than after axillary block (2.5 μg per milliliter) or even lumbar epidural block (3.1 μg per milliliter). The total plasma concentration level during or after IVRA with lidocaine almost never reaches the levels that would have been achieved after direct intravenous administration. In fact, it has been estimated that only about 30 percent of the initially injected dose eventually reaches the circulation after the cuff is released.

Thrombophlebitis

Thrombophlebitis has sometimes occurred, particularly following the now nearly extinct use of chloroprocaine. The low pH of the anesthetic stabilizers such as para-aminobenzoic acid, sodium bisulfite, and benzol alcohol have been suggested to be possible factors in initiating thrombophlebitis. These preservatives should be avoided.

Methemoglobinemia

Methemoglobinemia was associated with the use of prilocaine IVRA; nonetheless, some advocate the use of this agent. These advocates contend that the degree of methemoglobinemia caused by prilocaine is not significant in IVRA owing to the limited total dose administered.

Hematoma

Hematoma formation at the site of the needle puncture has been reported as a complication but is rarely a significant problem.

Failure to Produce Anesthesia

Few series report 100 percent success in attempted IVRA. A 3 percent failure rate is common. However, one group reported an overall failure incidence of 20 percent of 206 attempted IVRAs. Errors contributing to failure include (1) failure to exsanguinate the arm adequately prior to injection; (2) failure to prevent clot formation in the needle, resulting in blockage of the needle; (3) dislodgment of the needle during placement of the Esmarch bandage with tissue infiltration of the injectate; (4) loss of pressure in the constricting cuff leading to a loss of local anesthetic; and (5) unexplained failures.

Fatalities

No fatalities were reported in the first 10,000 documented uses of this technique in its first 68 years of its existence. However, at least 10 deaths are now known, owing to cardiac arrest. Anaphylaxis has not been reported.

CONTRAINDICATIONS

A history of adverse reactions to the local anesthetic is, of course, the most important contraindication. Most authors also list infection in the limb to be blocked, peripheral vascular disease, and hemolytic diseases such as sickle cell anemia and thalassemia as contraindications to IVRA. Some authors also include conditions including peripheral neuropathy and epilepsy, pronounced arterial atheromatous disease, and Monkeberg's calcinosis in their list of contraindications. Some authors include heart block as a possible contraindication. A preponderance of opinion totally contraindicates the use of bupivacaine for IVRA.

SUGGESTED READING

Eckstedt J, Stålberg E, Thorn-Alquist AM. Impulse transmission to muscle fibres during intravenous regional anaesthesia in man. Acta Anaesthesiol Scand 1971; 15:1–21.

Heath ML. Bupivacaine toxicity and Bier blocks (letter). Anesthesiology 1983; 59:481.

Lawes EG, Johnson T, Pritchard P, et al. Venous pressures during simulated Bier's block. Anaesthesia 1984; 39:147–149.

Rosenberg PH, Kalso EA, Tuominen MK, et al. Acute bupivacaine toxicity as a result of venous leakage under the tourniquet cuff during a Bier block. Anesthesiology 1983; 58:95–98.

Sorbie C, Chacha P. Regional anaesthesia by the intravenous route. Br Med J 1965; 1:957–960.

PAIN MANAGEMENT

SYMPATHETICALLY MAINTAINED PAIN

SRINIVASA N. RAJA, M.D.
NELSON HENDLER, M.D., M.S.

The syndrome of causalgia, characterized by burning pain, vasomotor instability, and trophic changes in an extremity following major peripheral nerve injury, was first described by Mitchell and co-workers in 1864. It was not until the early part of the 20th century, when Leriche reported his observations that denudation and excision of the periarteriolar sympathetic plexus resulted in relief of causalgic pain, that the role of sympathetic nervous system in this pain state was known. Over the past five decades, several other clinical pain syndromes, such as reflex sympathetic dystrophy, Sudeck's atrophy, minor causalgia, reflex neurovascular dystrophy, and shoulder-hand syndrome have been described. These chronic pain states share the following common clinical characteristics: (1) pain and hyperalgesia that are often exacerbated by stimuli that evoke sympathetic responses (e.g., stress or emotional disturbance); (2) signs of increased sympathetic tone such as vasomotor, sudomotor, and trophic changes; and (3) the immediate and often dramatic relief of pain and hyperalgesia following blockade of the sympathetic innervation to the affected extremity. This observation has led to the concept that in this subset of chronic pain patients pain and hyperalgesia is maintained by the sympathetic nervous system; the term *sympathetically maintained pain* has been used to describe this clinical condition.

CLINICAL FEATURES

Sympathetically maintained pain has been reported to follow a variety of traumatic, postoperative, neurologic, and other conditions (Table 1). While the majority of the injuries have involved the extremities, sympathetically maintained pain following injuries to the spinal cord or even following cerebrovascular accidents has been reported.

Table 1 Precipitating Factors and Diseases Associated with Reflex Sympathetic Dystrophy

Peripheral	Central
Soft-tissue injury	Brain tumor
Arthritides	Severe head injury
Infection	Cerebral infarction
Fascitis, tendonitis, bursitis	Subarachnoid hemorrhage
Venous or arterial thrombosis	Cervical cord injury
Fractures, sprains, dislocations	Subacute combined
Operative procedures	degeneration
Malignancy	Syringomyelia
Aortic injury	Poliomyelitis
Myelography, spinal anesthesia	Amyotrophic lateral sclerosis
Paravertebral alcohol injection	Other
Postherpetic	Idiopathic
Brachial plexopathy, scalenus	Prolonged bedrest
anticus syndrome	Familial
Radiculopathy	
Immobilization with cast or	
splint	
Vasculitis	
Myocardial infarction	
Weber-Christian disease	
Polymyalgia rheumatica	
Pulmonary fibrosis	

Adapted from Schwartzman RJ, McLellan TL. Reflex sympathetic dystrophy: a review. Arch Neurol 1987; 44:555–561. Copyright 1987, American Medical Association.

Sympathetically maintained pain is characterized by the triad of sensory, autonomic, and motor changes. The symptoms may be gradual in onset, beginning days to weeks after the injury. In some instances, however, especially in the case of peripheral nerve injury, pain may be present immediately after the injury has been sustained.

Depending on the stage of the disease, the sensory, autonomic, and motor signs and symptoms may be present to varying degrees (Table 2). Classically, three different stages of the disease have been described. The first stage is the acute phase in which patients present with pain and hyperalgesia that is disproportionate to the injury and is often in a peripheral nerve distribution. Initially, the skin is often warm and dry, but may later become cold. Trophic changes such as localized edema and increased growth of hair and nail may be seen. This stage usually lasts several weeks. During the *second (dystrophic) stage*, the pain and hyperalgesia is not localized to a single nerve but is in more of a "glove and

Table 2 Clinical Staging of Sympathetically
Maintained Pain

Stage I (acute)
  Pain: Pain and hyperalgesia disproportionate to injury.
  Localized to the distribution of a peripheral nerve initially. Later,
    pain spreads.
  Skin: warm, dry, and red during initial stages.
  Later, cyanotic, cold, and sweating.
  Localized edema, muscle spasm.
  No radiographic changes.
  Increased growth of hair and nails.
  Duration: Several weeks.
Stage II (dystrophic)(3–6 months if untreated)
  Pain: Pain and hyperalgesia not localized to single nerve.
  Skin: Cool and hyperhidrotic.
  Glove and stocking distribution.
  Edema: spreads; from soft to brawny with glazed overlying skin.
  Scant hair, nails brittle, cracked and heavily grooved.
  Spotty to diffuse osteoporosis.
  Passive motion intact, limited range of motion secondary to pain.
  Increased thickness of joint.
  Muscle spasms and wasting.
Stage III (atrophic):
  Marked trophic changes that become irreversible.
  Hair coarse. Skin cool, smooth, glossy, drawn and pale or
    cyanotic.
  Decrease in fat pads; digits thin and pointed.
  Muscle atrophy, decreased active and passive range of motion,
    muscle spasms.
  Scarring, contractures, subluxations.
  Diffuse and marked bone atrophy, pathologic fractures.
  Paralyzed, useless extremity.
  Resistant to any therapy.
  May spread to other extremities.

stocking" distribution. The skin is usually cool, hyperhidrotic, and glazed. Characteristic soft tissue edema associated with changes in hair and nails are often observed in the affected extremity. This stage, which lasts from 3 to 6 months, may be associated with radiologic changes of diffuse osteoporosis. During this stage, patients often guard the affected hand or foot and wear a protective glove or stocking. During the *third, or atrophic, stage*, marked hyperalgesia to mechanical and cooling stimuli is observed. This late stage of the disease is often associated with minimal therapeutic success. Diffuse osteoporosis and marked changes in skin digits and joint stiffness are observed.

We recently reported the results of sensory testing in patients with sympathetically maintained pain and sympathetically independent pain. Patients were tested for pain to mechanical stimuli, vibratory stimuli, movement of hair follicle, and cooling stimuli which consisted of a drop of acetone or alcohol in the hyperalgesic region. The pain and hyperalgesia to mechanical stimuli was marked, but was similar in the sympathetically maintained pain and sympathetically independent pain groups. The results of sensory testing to cooling stimuli was, however, markedly different in the sympathetically maintained pain and sympathetically independent pain groups. All patients with sympathetically maintained pain had hyperalgesia to cooling stimuli. By contrast, only 40 percent of patients with sympathetically inde-

pendent pain had hyperalgesia to cold stimuli. Thus, hyperalgesia to cooling stimuli is a sensitive, although not specific, test for sympathetically maintained pain.

In summary, the commonly observed clinical features of sympathetically maintained pain are spontaneous pain, hyperalgesia to mechanical and to cooling stimuli, soft tissue swelling, vasomotor and sudomotor disturbances, trophic skin changes, diminished motor functions, and pain relief after sympathetic blockade.

DIAGNOSIS

It is important that sympathetically maintained pain be diagnosed early, as the degree of ultimate therapeutic success is often dependent on early treatment. An early diagnosis can be made by a heightened awareness of the clinical spectrum and through knowledge of the wide array of predisposing or precipitating events that may trigger this syndrome.

The diagnosis of sympathetically maintained pain is predominantly based on its characteristic clinical features. There are some early clinical signs that should lead the physician to suspect the presence of sympathetically maintained pain. These include (1) pain and hyperalgesia that are disproportionate to the injury; (2) pain persisting long beyond the expected healing period; and (3) pain that does not follow classical dermatomal or peripheral nerve distribution.

Other diagnostic tests have been suggested to be useful in the diagnosis of sympathetically maintained pain. These include thermography, radiography, and scintigraphy. Thermography appears to be fairly nonspecific in its role as a diagnostic test for sympathetically maintained pain. Depending on the phase or stage of sympathetically maintained pain, the affected extremity may be warmer or cooler than the normal extremity. While thermography is a highly sensitive test, it is not specific, since some sympathetically independent pain states associated with nerve injury may present with a similar decrease in temperature in the affected extremity. Because pain is a subjective symptom, however, thermography is useful for documenting organic pathology in a patient thought to have "psychogenic" pain. Also, if performed before and after the block, thermography may be useful in confirming the adequacy of sympathetic ganglionic blockade. There are some characteristic radiographic abnormalities in patients with sympathetically maintained pain. These may be in the form of patchy, local, or diffuse demineralization or osteopenia. In particular, osteopenia in a periarticular distribution is believed to be characteristic of this syndrome. However, radiography also lacks specificity, as other diseases associated with osteoporosis may have similar features. In addition, detectible osteopenia rarely occurs before 6 weeks. Ideally, an x-ray examination of both hands or both feet should be performed on the same plate to facilitate comparison.

Several recent reports have indicated that three-phase bone scintigraphy using technetium-labeled phosphates are useful in the diagnosis of sympathetically maintained pain. The three phases in the study involve an early phase immediately after the injection of the labeled phosphates that is indicative of blood flow; a second, blood-pool phase, which occurs 1 to 5 minutes after the injection; and the delayed or bone phase, which occurs 2 to 3 hours after the initial injection. Studies have shown that the delayed bone phase characteristically shows a generalized increase in uptake especially marked in the periarticular region. The sensitivity of bone scans ranges from 60 to 90 percent in different studies, while the specificity is usually more than 90 percent. An interesting clinical aspect of scintigraphy is that a couple of patients have been reported who had characteristic abnormal scans before the appearance of clinical symptoms. It has been suggested that the scintigraphic changes may precede the development of clinical symptoms and could therefore be useful as an early diagnostic tool.

The relief of pain and hyperalgesia after sympathetic blockade is still considered the gold standard in the diagnosis of sympathetically maintained pain. In fact, Bonica has stated that if there is no relief of pain after sympathetic blockade, the diagnosis of causalgia should not be made. Since adequate sympathetic blockade of the affected extremity plays such a crucial role in the diagnosis of sympathetically maintained pain, appropriate care should be taken in the performance and interpretation of sympathetic blocks. Traditionally, the

diagnosis of sympathetically maintained pain is made by assessing pain relief after local anesthetic blocks of the stellate ganglion in the neck or the lumbar sympathetic ganglia, depending on whether the upper or lower extremity is involved. The goal in sympathetic blockade is a selective blockade of the sympathetic ganglia that does not block the somatic nerves. A potential pitfall of the diagnostic local anesthetic sympathetic ganglion blocks is a conduction block of the adjacent somatic nerve roots leading to false-positive results. This is particularly true when the pain and hyperalgesia are in the distribution of L2 that is around the knee. Thus, it is very important to perform sensory testing before and after the block to rule out inadvertent somatic blockade. False-negative results are usually a consequence of inadequate blockade of the sympathetic efferent fibers. This can be avoided by looking for objective evidence of sympathetic blockade, such as warming of the limb, a sine qua non of an adequate block.

Various tests of sympathetic function or regional blood flow have been used to demonstrate the adequacy of sympathetic blockade. We have generally used the tests of blood flow, such as measurements of change of skin temperature, thermography, or laser Doppler for assessment of adequacy of sympathetic blockade. Additional tests are discussed elsewhere in this text.

Figure 1 shows the results of a lumbar sympathetic block in a patient with sympathetically maintained pain. After the local anesthetic sympathetic block, there is a

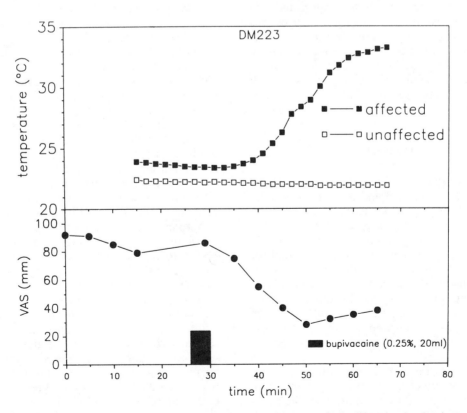

Figure 1 Lumbar sympathetic block in a patient with sympathetically maintained pain. Ongoing pain was rated by patient on a 100-mm Visual Analog Scale (VAS).

characteristic increase in the cutaneous temperature of the affected extremity and a dramatic decrease in the intensity of ongoing (stimulus-independent) and stimulus-evoked pain.

There are several potential complications associated with the local anesthetic sympathetic ganglion blocks, such as recurrent laryngeal nerve block leading to hoarseness, phrenic nerve block causing diaphragmatic paralysis, and intravascular and epidural injections.

More recently, a new diagnostic test for sympathetically maintained pain using systemic administration of the alpha-adrenergic antagonist phentolamine has been recommended as a specific, sensitive test for sympathetically maintained pain. This test is less invasive, has fewer potential side effects, avoids false-positive results (including placebo responses), and is preferred by patients.

DIFFERENTIAL DIAGNOSIS

Many other chronic pain disorders may be mistakenly diagnosed as sympathetically maintained pain because of similarities in clinical presentations. A common disorder that mimics sympathetically maintained pain is peripheral nerve entrapment, which can be diagnosed by (1) electromyographic and nerve conduction velocity studies; (2) pain relief with local anesthetic blocks of the nerve proximal to the site of entrapment; (3) absence of pain relief from appropriate sympathetic ganglion blocks; (4) negative bone scans; and (5) thermography demonstrating temperature changes only in the distribution of a single peripheral nerve. Other sympathetically independent pain states resulting from peripheral nerve injury, peripheral neuropathies, myofascial pain, and Raynaud's disease may present with clinical features similar to those of sympathetically maintained pain.

TREATMENT

The course of treatment for sympathetically maintained pain is of long duration and is often frustrating, especially if proper therapy is not started early on in the course of the disease. Transient relief of pain is often followed by recurrence of symptoms. Although a variety of therapeutic modalities have been recommended for sympathetically maintained pain, the most effective therapies are aimed at interrupting the sympathetic innervation to the affected region. In some instances, especially those of sympathetically maintained pain following nerve injury, treatment of the underlying cause such as a neuroma is also important in improving the success of therapy.

Sympathetic ganglionic blockade with local anesthetics is the most effective therapy in patients with sympathetically maintained pain. Blockade of the cervicothoracic (stellate) ganglia is indicated in patients with pain in the upper extremity, while a lumbar sympathetic block at the level of the L2 or L3 vertebra is effective in relieving pain in the lower extremity. A series of five to ten blocks is indicated. The first few blocks are usually done at frequent intervals, two to three times per week. The subsequent blocks may be performed at weekly intervals. Raj and co-workers have reported good results in hospitalized patients after the use of continuous local anesthetic sympathetic blockade with indwelling catheters near the sympathetic chain.

Hannington-Kiff has popularized the use of intravenous regional sympathetic blocks with guanethidine in the treatment of sympathetically maintained pain. Although this form of treatment is popular in Europe, parenteral preparations of guanethidine are not readily available in the United States. Intravenous regional guanethidine (10 to 20 mg) results in prolonged temperature increases, indicating pharmacologic sympathetic blockade. Guanethidine displaces noradrenaline from its storage sites in the sympathetic nerve endings and prevents the re-uptake of the neurotransmitter resulting in prolonged sympathetic block. Other drugs such as reserpine (1.5 to 2 mg of reserpine to 35 to 45 ml of 0.5 percent lidocaine) and bretylium tosylate have been administered using the Bier block technique. Onset of action of reserpine is relatively slow, and depletion is maximal after 24 hours. The results with these latter drugs have not been as encouraging as with guanethidine.

A subset of patients achieve good pain relief with repeated local anesthetic sympathetic blocks, but the effects are transient. In these patients, surgical sympathectomy often provides long-lasting pain relief.

Physical therapy directed toward improving the mobility of the affected extremity should be an important part of the overall management of these patients. However, patients do not usually tolerate physical therapy unless adequate pain relief is achieved. Thus, it is important to coordinate physical therapy with the nerve blocks such that the patient can undergo physical therapy during the pain-free periods that immediately follow the use of the sympathetic blocks. In some cases, pain relief may be achieved for extended periods, with continuous catheter techniques facilitating aggressive physiotherapy during this time. In most cases, immobilization of the affected limb has led to worsening of symptoms rather than improvement.

Several different drug regimens have been suggested to be useful in the treatment of sympathetically maintained pain. These include corticosteroids, calcium channel blockers such as nifedipine; alpha-adrenergic–blocking agents such as phentolamine, phenoxybenzamine, and prazosin hydrochloride; tricyclic antidepressants; and anticonvulsants. Of these agents, corticosteroids and alpha-adrenergic–blocking agents seem to be most promising. Beta-adrenergic–blocking agents are not effective. Prednisone in doses ranging from 20 to 200 mg per day has been reported to provide good pain relief in approximately 60 percent of patients. Treatment with steroids is indicated only in the group of patients who refuse or cannot tolerate treatments aimed at blocking the sympathetic efferent fibers. Ghostine et al have reported resolution of pain in patients with causalgia secondary to battlefield injuries following 6- to 12-week therapy with phenoxybenzamine in doses ranging from 40 to 120 mg per day. Side effects included ejaculatory dysfunction and orthostatic hypotension. These patients were acute cases (less than 6 weeks in duration), and the study was not a controlled one. Whether similar results can be obtained in chronic sympathetically maintained pain patients still remains to be proven.

Electrical stimulation techniques such as transcutaneous nerve stimulation (TENS) or epidural stimulation have been reported to relieve pain in some patients with sympathetically maintained pain. We have not found the stimulation techniques a useful treatment in our patient population, which consists mostly of patients who have had pain for more than 1 year.

SUGGESTED READING

Abram SE. Pain of sympathetic origin. In: Raj PP, ed. Practical management of pain. Chicago: Year Book Publishers, 1986:451.

Bonica JJ. Causalgia and other reflex sympathetic dystrophies. In: Bonica JJ, ed. The management of pain. Philadelphia: Lea & Febiger, 1990:220.

Ghostine SY, Comair YG, Turner DM, et al. Phenoxybenzamine in the treatment of causalgia: report of 40 cases. J Neurosurg 1984; 60; 1263–1268.

Hannington-Kiff JG. Relief of causalgia in limbs by regional intravenous guanethidine. Br Med J 1979; 72:367–368.

Hendler N. Reflex sympathetic dystrophy and causalgia. In: Tollison DC, ed. Handbook of chronic pain management. Baltimore: Williams & Wilkins, 1989:444.

Payne R. Reflex sympathetic dystrophy syndrome: diagnosis and treatment. In: Fields HL, ed. Pain syndromes in neurology. London: Butterworths, 1990:107–130.

Raja SN, Treede RD, Davis KD, et al. Systemic alpha-adrenergic blockade with phentolamine: a diagnostic test for sympathetially maintained pain. Anesthesiology 1991; 74:691–698.

Stanton-Hicks M. Pain and the sympathetic nervous system. Boston: Kluwer Academic, 1989.

Stanton-Hicks M, Jänig W, Boas RA. Reflex sympathetic dystrophy. Boston: Kluwer Academic, 1989.

Treede R-D, Raja SN, Davis KD, et al. Evidence that alpha-adrenergic receptors mediate sympathetically maintained pain. In: Bond MR, ed. Pain research and clinical management. Amsterdam: Elsevier, 1991:373.

DRUGS FOR CHRONIC PAIN

WARREN R. McKAY, M.D.
BENJAMIN G. COVINO, M.D., Ph.D.
LINDA CAMERON, M.D.

Patients who suffer with chronic pain can present one of the most difficult challenges in clinical medicine. These patients typically have complex symptom presentations and have been given a wide range of diagnoses that may or may not reflect the true pathologic process. Successful pharmacologic management of these patients depends on adherence to a few basic principles. These principles are oriented more toward the management of the patient with nonmalignant pain, but the approach is sound for management of cancer pain also.

There is no substitute for establishing an accurate picture of the pathophysiologic and psychological processes that are present in a patient with chronic pain. A good place to start is a detailed history and physical examination. Diagnostic studies, when indicated, contribute to the determination of an anatomic differential diagnosis. Drug choices can be made in a more salient fashion if the site and nature of the lesion are defined. Associated issues such as depression, insomnia, appetite loss, degree of disability, and general psychological profile must be considered for successful pharmacologic trials regardless of the cause of the pain.

The second essential principle for successful pharmacologic management of pain is a broad working knowledge of the different classes of drugs and their most appropriate use. Clinicians must be aware of the pharmacologic profile of each drug and choose a particular agent based on its mechanism of action, need for titration, side effects, and risks. These choices should be made based on the results of sound clinical studies that document effectiveness of the agent. Each agent should be given an appropriate trial both in dosage and duration before additional medications are added to the regimen or the original agent is stopped.

Finally, a third essential element of successful pain management is patient education. Patients should understand the rationale behind the choice of a particular drug, and be informed of potential side effects and risks. If titration is planned and immediate effects of the medication may not be apparent, an informed patient is more likely to comply with the treatment plan. Other, nonpharmacologic options for treatment such as physical therapy, TENS, epidural stimulation, and psychologically oriented treatments should be explored with the patient if appropriate.

The rest of this chapter provides an overview of the types of drugs used in the treatment of chronic pain. Common pain syndromes that often respond to logical pharmacologic management include low back pain, rheumatoid and osteoarthritis, postherpetic neuralgia, painful polyneuropathies, and post-traumatic pain. Cancer pain can be especially difficult to treat in some patients, but once again, a rational approach provides best results. The scope of this chapter is limited to descriptions of the various types of medications used in treating chronic pain syndromes.

NON-NARCOTIC ANALGESIC AGENTS

The NSAIDs (nonsteroidal, anti-inflammatory drugs) are the most common agents employed for mild to moderate pain. Their primary mode of action is believed to be the inhibition of the enzyme prostaglandin synthetase. This enzyme is involved in the conversion of arachidonic acid to prostaglandin E_2 (PGE_2), which sensitizes certain tissues to the painful effects of bradykinin, e.g., the pain from bone metastases. Thus, the analgesic action of most NSAIDs is believed to be peripheral in origin, although certain agents such as aspirin also exert a central effect on the thalamic ventrobasilar nuclei.

The NSAIDs are orally effective but vary in terms of their duration of action and required frequency of administration (Table 1). Aspirin, acetaminophen, and ibuprofen have a relatively short half-life and must be taken at 4- to 6-hour intervals for maximum effectiveness. On the other hand, piroxicam has a long half-life and is suitable for once daily therapy. Although these agents are particularly useful for chronic pain due to arthritis, some agents such as ibuprofen have also proved useful for pain related to bone metastases. Ketoprofen, 50 to 75 mg by mouth, has been shown to relieve pain in cancer patients with an efficacy comparable to that of 10 mg morphine sulfate. This pain-relieving quality of ketoprofen may be due in part to this drug's ability to block leukotriene production and its antibradykinin activity. Ketorolac tromethamine is an NSAID that can be given intramuscularly and will soon be available in an intravenous formulation. The pain-relieving properties of this drug in clinical trials via the intramuscular route approach levels achieved with morphine.

Gastrointestinal complaints are the most common side effects reported with NSAIDs. Gastric bleeding may occur with prolonged aspirin therapy. In such situations acetaminophen may be substituted, although its analgesic potency is lower in inflammatory conditions. Melena and hematemesis have been reported with indomethacin, and rashes can be caused by all of these drugs. The NSAIDs have also been reported to occasionally produce allergic rhinitis, bronchospasm, and angioneurotic edema. In general, however, the frequency of adverse reactions associated with the NSAIDs is relatively low.

NARCOTIC ANALGESICS

Narcotics bind to specific opiate receptors in the central nervous system to inhibit the conduction of nociceptive impulses. Narcotics also stimulate descending systems in the brain stem to further inhibit pain at the spinal cord level. These drugs are useful for the treatment of chronic pain from malignant or nonmalignant causes. The narcotic analgesics vary in potency and are useful for the treatment of moderate to severe pain (Table 2). These agents may be administered intravenously, intramuscularly, or orally. In addition, in recent years, some of these drugs have been injected into the epidural or subarachnoid space for the treatment of severe pain. Morphine is the only narcotic officially approved by the Federal Drug Administration for epidural or intrathecal use. It provides prolonged analgesia of 12 to 24 hours' duration. Fentanyl and meperidine have also been employed epidurally and produce a duration of analgesia of 4 to 6 hours.

With regard to orally administered narcotics, three agents are available for mild to moderate pain: codeine, oxycodone, and propoxyphene. These agents are less potent than morphine but have the same pharmacologic profile. They possess a higher analgesic potential than the non-narcotics but lack the antipyretic and anti-inflammatory properties of the NSAIDs. The peak and duration of analgesia for oxycodone are shorter than those of aspirin, whereas codeine and propoxyphene have a pharmacologic profile similar to that of aspirin. Side effects include sedation and constipation. Physical dependence and tolerance can also occur.

The potent narcotic analgesics, such as morphine, should be employed when the weaker narcotics are ineffective. The intensity of pain, not the life expectancy of the patient, should determine the use of potent narcotics. For severe pain, morphine is usually the initial choice and can be given intravenously, intramuscularly, subcutaneously, orally, or rectally. Although the majority of patients experiencing severe pain can be controlled with oral morphine, some become refractory to it and require intramuscular or continuous intravenous or

Table 1 Non-narcotic Analgesia

Agent	Oral Dose (mg)	Plasma Half-Life (hr)	Duration (hr)	Comments
Aspirin	650–1000	3–5	4–6	GI and hematologic side effects
Acetaminophen	650–1000	3–5	4–6	Safer than aspirin
Ibuprofen	200–400	3–5	4–6	Higher analgesic ceiling than aspirin
Ketoprofen	50–75	2	6–8	tid
Ketorolac tromethamine	15–60	4–6	4–8	qid, can be given IM
Naproxen	250–500	14	8–12	bid
Piroxicam	10–20	45	24	qd morning or night

subcutaneous morphine. Intravenous or subcutaneous morphine can be given by the patient via one of the patient-controlled analgesia devices available today. In certain severe pain states such as failed back syndrome or widespread metastatic disease, direct central nervous system application via the epidural or subarachnoid space can be employed.

Morphine given orally or parenterally has a duration of action of 4 to 6 hours; this can be increased by using a sustained-release preparation. The two sustained-release tablets available are MS contin (12 hours, twice a day) and Roxanol SR (8 hours, three times a day).

Two other commonly used narcotics deserve mention. Methadone is a long-acting orally effective narcotic with a plasma half-life of 18 to 24 hours but a duration of action of 6 to 8 hours. Meperidine is not very effective by the oral route and has a short duration of action. An active metabolite of meperidine, normeperidine, has been associated with central nervous system hyperirritability and seizures. Normeperidine accumulates with continued administration of meperidine and limits meperidine's role in chronic pain treatment.

In recent years, mixed agonist-antagonist opioids such as nalbuphine and butorphanol have been employed for the treatment of acute pain (Table 3). However, these agents appear to have limited use in the treatment of chronic pain. They produce psychotomimetic effects with chronic administration and can precipitate acute withdrawal symptoms in opiate-tolerant patients. Only pentazocine is available orally; nalbuphine and butorphanol require parenteral administration. Buprenorphine, a partial agonist, was recently approved by the Federal Drug Administration. It is available in parenteral or intramuscular form.

Patients should be chosen carefully for narcotic analgesic trials to treat nonmalignant pain. The clinician should be satisfied that all other reasonable attempts at alternative analgesia have been exhausted. Patients with a history of substance abuse are not good candidates for long-term narcotic therapy. The successful use of narcotics in nonmalignant pain is enhanced when a single practitioner has primary responsibility for the drug management and a well-planned treatment regimen is followed.

Failure to achieve at least partial pain relief on low to moderate doses of narcotics and rapid dose escalations while on maintenance dosages suggest the patient's pain may not be well controlled by this method. Prior to starting chronic narcotic therapy, the patient has to be fully informed of the risks involved. These risks include low likelihood of psychological dependence, potential cognitive impairment, and, in pregnant patients, the chance that children born while the mother is receiving narcotic maintenance therapy will be physically dependant at birth.

Patients with nonmalignant pain have been managed for years without escalation of their narcotic doses. Tolerance may be a problem, however. Cross tolerance between narcotic analgesics may be incomplete. Therefore, if opiate tolerance develops, changing to an alternate opiate and starting with half the equianalgesic dose is recommended.

The most common side effects of opiate analgesics are sedation, nausea and vomiting, and constipation.

Table 2 Narcotic Analgesics

Agent	Starting Oral Dose (mg)	Equianalgesic Dose		Plasma Half-Life (hr)	Duration (hr)	Comments
		IM	PO			
Codeine	30–65	130	200	3	4–6	Useful initial narcotic analgesic; biotransformed in part to morphine
Oxycodone	5–10	15	30	—	3–5	Shorter acting; use in combination with non-narcotics (oxycodone hydrochloride and acetaminophen), which limits dose escalation
Meperidine	50–100	75	300	3–4	4–6	Short-acting; poor oral potency, toxic metabolite normeperidine
Propoxyphene hydrochloride	65–130	—	65–130	4–6	3.5–15	Weak narcotic, used in combinations with non-narcotic analgesics; potentially toxic metabolite (norpropoxyphene) accumulates with repetitive dosing
Morphine	30–60	10	60	2–3.5	4–7	Slow release tablets available
Hydromorphone	4–8	1.5	7.5	2–3	4–6	Slightly shorter acting than morphine
Methadone	10–20	10	20	15–30	6–8	Good oral potency; long plasma half-life does not equal analgesic duration
Levorphanol	2–4	2	4	12–16	4–6	Good oral potency; caution with initial dosing to avoid drug accumulation

Table 3 Narcotic Agonist-Antagonist

Drug	Equianalgesic IM Dose (mg) (10 mg Morphine Equivalent)	Plasma Half-Life (hr)	Duration (hr)	Comments
Pentazocine (PO)	60	2–3	4–6	May precipitate withdrawal in narcotic-tolerant individuals. May produce psychotomimetic effects
	150		4–7	
Nalbuphine	10	5	4–6	No oral form, fewer psychotomimetic effects than pentazocine; may precipitate withdrawal in narcotic-tolerant individuals
Butorphanol	2	2.5–3.5	4–6	Same as nalbuphine
Buprenorphine	0.3	—	4–6	Similar side effects as agonist-antagonist

Respiratory depression is the dose-limiting side effect. Sedation may be avoided by reducing total dose, increasing the interval between doses, changing from oral or parenteral administration to the epidural route, or switching to an opiate with a shorter half-life. Fortunately, tolerance to the sedative effects of narcotics develops before the analgesic activity declines.

Tolerance to nausea and vomiting also develops, but if this side effect persists, an antiemetic agent may be useful. In addition, substitution of an equianalgesic dose of another narcotic may be helpful. Cathartics and stool softeners should be employed whenever chronic narcotic therapy is initiated.

Tolerance to the respiratory depressant effect of the narcotic analgesics also develops. In general, central nervous system depression is not a major problem with chronic narcotic administration. Respiratory depression secondary to epidural or intrathecal narcotics may occur when this route is employed for the treatment of acute pain, but it is rarely seen in chronic pain patients. Naloxone can be used to reverse the respiratory depression, but care must be taken to prevent withdrawal symptoms.

The pruritus seen with epidural narcotics used for acute pain is rarely a problem when narcotics are used intraspinally for chronic pain in opiate-tolerant patients.

Although patient-controlled analgesia (PCA) has enjoyed widespread use for acute postoperative pain, its usefulness in the chronic pain arena is still controversial. Psychological issues centering on control in relation to narcotic analgesics can make the decision to initiate PCA in patients with chronic pain difficult. PCA should be considered in place of oral narcotics if the management of severe pain from cancer or chronic benign pain has failed, if tolerance develops, or if side effects such as nausea or vomiting limit their usefulness. PCA can be administered by either the intravenous or subcutaneous routes with equal efficacy; and although PCA injection doses of morphine sulfate of 1 to 3 mg per hour are commonly administered for acute pain, the chronic pain or opiate-tolerant individual may require much larger doses. Generally, a continuous background infusion of 1 to 2 mg morphine sulfate is used along with the PCA injection dose. Patients may also be discharged home with one of the many compact PCA devices available today to be monitored by home therapy nurses. To convert a patient from oral opiates to intravenous or subcutaneous opiates, the conversion ration is 3 to 6:1 (e.g., 3 to 6 mg oral MSO_4 = 1 mg intravenous/subcutaneous MSO_4).

Reduction of side effects and additional analgesia are possible through the use of narcotic and non-narcotic combinations. Combinations of drugs provide additive analgesic effects without escalation of the narcotic dose. Agents employed with narcotics include an antihistamine (hydroxyzine), tricyclic antidepressants (amitriptyline), or non-narcotic analgesics (aspirin, acetaminophen, or ibuprofen).

ANTIDEPRESSANTS

Tricyclic antidepressants are used to treat pain that results from injury or chronic changes in central or peripheral somatosensory pathways that cause abnormal afferent activity to reach the dorsal horn and central structures (neuropathic pain) (Table 4). Some examples include diabetic neuropathy, postherpetic neuralgia, and phantom limb pain. Tricyclic antidepressants also alleviate tension and may prevent migraine headaches. The analgesic effects are independent of the antidepressant effects, and analgesia occurs early in the course of therapy. These drugs are also helpful in reducing insomnia caused by chronic pain.

Tricyclic antidepressants are believed to potentiate the descending analgesic pathways that arise in the brainstem. Serotonin and norepinephrine are the important neurotransmitters in the descending pathways, and the tricyclic antidepressants appear to facilitate monoamine transmission by inhibition of the reuptake of these neurotransmitters. The tricyclic antidepressants can potentiate the analgesic effect of the opiates.

Table 4 Miscellaneous Drugs for Chronic Pain

Drug	Daily PO Dose Range	Comments
Antidepressants		
Amitryptyline	10–300 mg	Use lower dose for elderly; escalate dose slowly over several weeks; onset of action usually 3–5 days; amitryptyline and imipramine produce more side effects than nortriptyline, trazodone, or desipramine. Fluoxetine is taken in the morning; may cause weight loss and has minimal side effects.
Imipramine	20–300 mg	
Nortriptyline hydrochloride	10–150 mg	
Trazodone hydrochloride	50–600 mg	
Desipramine hydrochloride	20–300 mg	
Fluoxetine	20–80 mg	
Anticonvulsants		
Carbamazepine	Initial 100–200 mg tid Average 400–600 mg tid (as high as 1,800 mg/day)	Effective within 24 hours; lower dose to decrease side effects.
Phenytoin	300–600 mg/day Divided doses	Slowly increase dose. Plasma drug concentration increases disproportionately as dosage is increased; effective in 3 days.
Clonazepam	Initial 1.5 mg/day	Drowsiness, fatigue, ataxia. Fewer side effects than carbamazepine or phenytoin. Increase dose every 3 to 7 days to total 20 mg/day.
Valproic acid	100–300 mg/day Divided doses	Anorexia, nausea, vomiting, sedation, ataxia, and tremor usually respond to dosage; rash and alopecia, rarely; elevation of hepatic enzymes.
Psychotropics		
Haloperidol	2–30 mg Divided doses	Coanalgesic doses lower than doses for psychiatric symptoms, potent antiemetic.
Methotrimeprazine (IM)	10–20 mg qid	Tolerance to sedation; postural hypotension develops; tardive dyskinesia and extrapyramidal reactions possible with long-term use.

The anticholinergic or cardiovascular side effects of the tricyclic antidepressants can be dose-limiting. These include dry mouth, constipation, urinary retention, blurred vision, orthostatic hypotension, and cardiac arrhythmias. Nortriptyline, trazodone, and desipramine have minimal anticholinergic properties and should be considered in patients at risk of developing toxicity, such as those with glaucoma or benign prostatic hypertrophy. Also, fluoxetine, a nontricyclic compound that inhibits the presynaptic uptake of serotonin, is useful for the treatment of chronic pain and has minimal side effects.

ANTICONVULSANTS

Anticonvulsants can be used to treat neuropathic pain caused by trigeminal neuralgia, diabetic neuropathy, herpetic neuralgia, deafferentation states, or pain from multiple sclerosis and scleroderma (see Table 4). Carbamazepine, phenytoin, valproic acid, and clonazepam suppress spontaneous neuronal firing and inhibit transynaptic spread. Clonazepam and valproic acid also increase gammaaminobutyric acid activity at the receptor level. The anticonvulsants may also have a central effect on pain, as evidenced by their effect on multiple sclerosis.

Carbamazepine is chemically related to imipramine, and its antidepressant activity may contribute to its usefulness in chronic pain syndromes. Adverse reactions to carbamazepine include drowsiness, ataxia, confusion, and hematopoietic disorders (leukopenia, thrombocytopenia, aplastic anemia, agranulocytosis). During the first month of therapy, patients should have blood drawn weekly to assess possible white blood cell suppression; thereafter they should be checked monthly. Anticonvulsant drug therapy should be stopped every 3 months, since some patients do not have a recurrence of pain.

Phenytoin may also be useful for the treatment of chronic pain. Side effects of this agent include ataxia, nystagmus, gingival hyperplasia, and hematopoietic disorders.

PSYCHOTROPIC AGENTS

Psychotropic agents such as fluphenazine, haloperidol, and methotrimeprazine have been used to treat chronic neuropathic pain refractory to more traditional medications. These agents may be effective in severe pain associated with delerium or nausea.

Haloperidol, a butyrophenone, has a high binding affinity for opiate receptors, which suggests it may act as an opiate agonist. It can be useful as a coanalgesic and to treat side effects of narcotics. Compared with the phenothiazines, haloperidol causes less sedation and fewer anticholinergic and cardiovascular effects, and it is a more potent antiemetic.

Methotrimeprazine, a phenothiazine, has analgesic properties that are not related to the opiate receptor mechanism. This drug is particularly useful in the opiate-tolerant individual. Side effects such as sedation and postural hypotension may occur, but repeated administration results in tolerance to them.

These agents should not be used as first-line therapy because they have definite associated toxicities and primarily anecdotal support of their effectiveness. Chronic use of these agents has been associated with tardive dyskinesias and other extrapyramidal side effects.

SYMPATHETIC BLOCKING AGENTS

Clinical presentations of the sympathetic-mediated pain syndromes are extremely varied. Usually the pain is described as burning and confined to a single limb, and it does not correspond to segmental or peripheral nerve distribution. Associated changes include vasomotor instability and pseudomotor disturbances. The etiology of the pain is believed to be related to excessive or abnormal sympathetic activity.

Guanethidine displaces norepinephrine and prevents reuptake in storage sites for hours or days to produce a chemical sympathectomy. If pain is present in a single limb, guanethidine may be administered intravenously following tourniquet occlusion of the limb, in a fashion similar to the use of intravenous regional anesthesia. The drug may also be administered orally for chronic therapy. Postural hypotension, weakness, and diarrhea are common side effects.

Reserpine produces depletion of catecholamines by preventing the uptake of norepinephrine in chromaffin granules. The sympathectomy produced by intravenous regional administration of reserpine seems to be shorter acting than that produced by intravenous regional guanethidine. Diarrhea, fatigue, and even depression are side effects with this drug. It should not be used in depressed patients.

Both guanethidine and reserpine are difficult to obtain; guanethidine is not approved by the Food and Drug Administration for intravenous use and reserpine is no longer manufactured in the United States. For these reasons, another sympathetic blocking agent, bretylium tosylate, is fast becoming a widely used drug for intravenous regional sympathetic block. In a dose of 1 mg per kilogram added to 50 ml 0.57 percent lidocaine, no adverse reactions have been observed.

Other agents used for sympathetic-mediated pain include intravenous phentolamine, oral phenoxybenzamine hydrochloride, an alpha$_1$-receptor antagonist, or prazosin hydrochloride, an alpha antagonist. Propranolol, a beta-receptor—blocking agent, also can provide relief for certain sympathetic-mediated pain syndromes.

ANTIHISTAMINICS

The antihistaminics may be of limited use in the treatment of chronic pain, although the analgesic mechanism of action is not clear. Antihistaminics are sometimes useful in the management of headache, insomnia, trigeminal neuralgia, atypical facial pain, low back pain, and dysmenorrhea.

The side effects of the antihistaminics are minimal, with little or no respiratory or gastrointestinal effects. Hydroxyzine is probably the most commonly prescribed antihistaminic for analgesia. The half-life of hydroxyzine is 6 to 24 hours. The combination of hydroxyzine and morphine may be a useful analgesic regimen that allows a reduction in the dose of both drugs.

INTRAVENOUS LOCAL ANESTHETICS

Local anesthetics such as procaine, chloroprocaine, and lidocaine have been administered intravenously for the treatment of certain chronic pain syndromes. Lidocaine has been used for low back pain with radiculopathy, atypical facial pain, diabetic or ischemic neuropathies, and certain sympathetic-mediated pains. These agents must be administered slowly over 30 minutes to avoid central nervous system toxicity.

The duration of response to systemically administered lidocaine varies from hours to weeks. The analgesic action of the local anesthetics is speculative but may involve antagonism of chemical mediators such as substance P or modulation of nociceptive information along afferent nerves within the spinal cord. Monitoring for local anesthetic toxicity is important during infusion of these relatively high doses of local anesthetics. Signs of central nervous system toxic effects are those of excitation, such as tinnitus, circumoral numbness, confusion, lightheadedness, hypertension, tachycardia, and convulsions. Signs of cardiovascular toxicity include decreased cardiac output, hypotension, and bradycardia. The use of intravenous local anesthesia for the treatment of chronic pain should probably be reserved for patients in whom conventional analgesic therapy is no longer effective.

Mexiletine, an oral analogue of lidocaine, has been tried with some success in the treatment of neuropathic pain. Definitive studies documenting the effectiveness of this agent are needed.

SUGGESTED READING

Benedetti C, Butler SH. Systemic analgesics. In: Bonica JJ, ed. The management of chronic pain. Malvern, PA: Lea & Febiger, 1990: 1637–1675.

Edwards WT, Habib F, Burney RG, Begin G. Intravenous lidocaine in the management of various chronic pain states. Reg Anesth 1985; 10:1-6.

Ford SR, Forrest WH, Eltherington L. The treatment of reflex sympathetic dystrophy with intravenous regional bretylium. Anesthesiology 1988; 68:137-140.

Portenoy RK. Pharmacologic management of chronic pain. In: Fields HL, ed. Pain syndromes in neurology. London: Butterworths, 1990: 257–277.

Portenoy RK, Foley KM. Chronic use of opioid analgesics in nonmalignant pain: report of 38 cases. Pain 1986; 25:171–186.

Rumore MM, Schlichting DA. Clinical efficacy of antihistaminics as analgesics. Clinical efficacy of antihistaminics. Pain 1986; 25:7–22.

Sunshine A, Olsen NZ. Non-narcotic analgesics. In: Wall P, Melzack R, eds. The textbook of pain. New York: Churchill Livingstone, 1989:670–723.

Weiss OF, Sriwatanakul K. Methotrimeprazine analgesia. Drug Ther 1982; Sept.:145–147.

DRUG ADMINISTRATION ROUTES FOR ACUTE AND CHRONIC PAIN MANAGEMENT

LINDA CAMERON, M.D.
P. PRITHVI RAJ, M.B.B.S., F.F.A.R.C.S.

Choosing the proper route for the administration of drugs in the treatment of pain entails a rational approach that synthesizes an understanding of the basic pathophysiology of the pain syndrome with a good working knowledge of drug administration techniques. Resorting to long-term epidural infusions in a cancer patient who could be managed with a proper oral regimen creates unnecessary hardship for the patient and is certainly not cost effective.

The goal of this chapter is to provide an overview of drug administration techniques that are useful in the management of various pain states. These techniques provide an armamentarium from which we can choose treatment options for patients in the acute postoperative setting, obstetrical suite, chronic pain clinic, and oncology ward.

A prelude to this discussion should stress the need for a multimodality approach to many types of pain problems (Table 1). In the chronic pain setting, physical therapy, relaxation techniques, stimulation-produced analgesia, and psychological support can be valuable adjuncts to pharmacologic management. At the other end of the spectrum are neurolytic blocks and neuroablative procedures that can provide relief for the cancer patient with intractable pain that has not been well controlled with pharmacologic agents. An understanding of the pathophysiology and natural history of the pain syndrome is imperative in order to develop a rational treatment plan that incorporates risk-benefit issues.

ORAL ROUTE

The oral route for the administration of drugs to treat pain offers many advantages, including widespread availability, ease of administration, relative lack of expense, and a high degree of effectiveness. Unfortunately, many patients do not get proper relief of pain from oral regimens. The problem usually lies not with the lack of effectiveness of the agent, but rather with a misunderstanding by the clinician of the appropriate use and limitations of the medications. Many practitioners underestimate dosage requirements, overestimate duration of action, or have irrational fears of producing psychological or physical addiction and respiratory depression.

In addition, with some types of medication, careful titration is needed so that unpleasant side effects do not undermine the pain-relief potential of a drug. An

Table 1 Treatment Modalities

Pharmacologic routes
  Oral
  Rectal
  Transcutaneous
  Subcutaneous
  Intravenous
  Neuroaxis

Nerve blocks
  Central
  Peripheral
  Sympathetic

Stimulation-induced analgesia
  Transcutaneous electrical nerve stimulation
  Acupuncture
  Dorsal column

Ablative neurosurgery
  Cordotomy
  Dorsal root entry zone
  Myelotomy

Psychological techniques
  Biofeedback
  Relaxation therapy
  Hypnosis
  Operant conditioning

Physical therapy
  Mobilization and exercise
  Heat and cold

effective medication trial requires a compliant patient who has been informed of the risks and side effects of the medication. If the pain-relieving effects of a medication may not be immediate, an educated patient will be much more likely to adhere to the treatment plan.

The preceding chapter ("Drugs for Chronic Pain") presents various oral medications used for the treatment of chronic pain. In cancer pain management, a "ladder" approach to the use of oral narcotic agents is used in hopes of preventing the rapid development of tolerance to potent narcotics as well as achieving the best analgesia with the fewest side effects (Table 2).

Some narcotics can be given rectally in the form of a suppository if oral medications cause nausea and vomiting.

TRANSDERMAL ROUTE

Recently a transdermal fentanyl patch (Duragesic) has been introduced. Fentanyl is a highly lipophilic narcotic analgesic with a potency 75 to 100 times that of morphine. The structure of the patch includes an outer backing membrane, which is in contact with the drug reservoir, and a microporous membrane with a specific permeability that allows for controlled release of the drug onto the skin. The patches are designed to release fentanyl at a controlled rate for up to 72 hours and are available in five dose forms: 25, 50, 75, 100, and 200 μg per hour.

Although few clinical studies to date have documented the effectiveness of the fentanyl patches, the

Table 2 Stepladder Approach to Analgesic Tailoring

Step 1	Aspirin-type drugs	Acetylsalicylic acid (ASA) Acetaminophen (Tylenol) Nonsteroidal anti- inflammatory drugs
Step 2	Aspirin-type drugs and/or mild narcotics	ASA + codeine Acetaminophen + codeine Propoxyphene (Darvon) Pentazocine (Talwin)
Step 3	Moderately potent narcotics	Oxycodone (Percodan) Hydrocodone (Vicodin)
Step 4	Highly potent narcotics	Meperidine (Demerol) Hydromorphone (Dilaudid) Methadone (Dolophine) Levorphanol (Levo- Dromoran) Oxymorphone (Numorphan) Heroin

From Ferrer and Brechner. Cancer. In: Raj PP, ed. Practical management of pain. Chicago: Year Book, 1986:312–328, with permission.

transdermal route has some promise in the management of postoperative and cancer pain. This route of administration is especially useful if the patient is unable to take medications by the oral route.

The clinical work that has been done demonstrates that stable blood levels of fentanyl can be achieved after administration of the patch. In surgical patients the patch should be applied several hours early (usually at the beginning of surgery), in order to achieve adequate blood levels in the postoperative period. Usually the patch alone cannot provide total analgesia in the immediate postoperative period, but it can significantly reduce the amount of supplemental parenteral analgesic required.

The obvious advantages of this route of drug administration are the avoidance of needles and the high degree of patient acceptance (Table 3). Stable blood levels of the drug can be obtained in a sustained fashion, and the gastrointestinal tract is avoided. This route also circumvents the first-pass metabolism of the liver and gastrointestinal tract. The transdermal approach can be invaluable in pediatric patients and has been demonstrated to be a relatively safe method of narcotic administration for all ages.

One of the disadvantages of the fentanyl patch is the persistence of high levels of drug after the patch is removed. This effect is probably due to the accumulation of the highly lipophilic drug in the body's fat stores. Therefore, if the patient has an overdosage of the medication or is suffering unpleasant side effects, there may be some lingering effect of the drug after removal of the patch. Other disadvantages include easy dislodgement of the patch and an inability to titrate the drug to effect.

The introduction of the transdermal route for the administration of a narcotic analgesic offers one more option for the clinician treating tough pain problems. Understanding the limitations of the pharmacokinetics

Table 3 Advantages and Disadvantages of the Transdermal Fentanyl Patch

Advantages	Disadvantages
Convenient drug administration	Slow onset of effect
No needles	Easy to remove or dislodge

Gastrointestinal tract not
  required
	Difficult to reverse toxic
	  side effects

Can be used in pediatric patients	Cannot be titrated

Long-lasting drug reservoir
  (3 days)
	Cannot be applied to
	  abnormal skin

with this method is important when choosing this approach.

SUBCUTANEOUS ROUTE

Continuous Subcutaneous Infusions

Continuous infusions via a subcutaneous (SQ) route have been used effectively in the management of pain not responsive to the oral route. This method is most commonly used for administration of narcotics in cancer patients. Studies have been done that compare the SQ route with intravenous (IV) infusions in postoperative and cancer patients. The narcotic blood levels and pain relief were comparable with each route. In a comparison of SQ infusions with intramuscular (IM) injections in the postoperative patient, one study demonstrated less nausea in the SQ group.

Continuous SQ narcotic infusions require the use of a pump similar to those used in the administration of chemotherapy. The pump should have a syringe or bag reservoir and should have the capacity to pump at low hourly volumes.

Benefits of this method of narcotic administration

include patient comfort, the avoidance of painful IM injections, and the preservation of veins in a cancer patient who probably has poor IV access. As with continuous IV administration, peaks and troughs of the medications are avoided, and better pain relief can be obtained.

One limitation of this route of administration is that the SQ space has limited absorptive capabilities. If the drug requirements of a patient are high, the concentration of the drug rather than the infusion rate is increased. When the infusion rate is greater than 1 cc per hour there is increased skin irritation and probably diminished absorption of the drug. Standard pharmaceutical preparations of some narcotics can be reconstituted to yield a higher concentration.

Complications cited with SQ administration include skin irritation at the needle site, dislodgement of the needle during the infusion, local tissue infections, and bleeding (seen in an anticoagulated patient). These infusions require monitoring in a hospital setting or supervision by trained medical personnel in the home. Patients and their families must be able to learn how to operate a pump and be able to recognize and deal with potential complications. Since this method of drug administration requires home supervision and the purchase or rental of an infusion pump, the cost of the treatment must be considered.

Subcutaneous Injections

Subcutaneous infiltration of local anesthetics has been used as a therapeutic intervention in postherpetic neuralgia, neuroma, painful subcutaneous fibrotic nodules, and spermalgia and labial pain. For herpetic pain, a solution of 0.2 percent triamcinolone in 0.25 percent bupivacaine or of dexamethasone (16 mg per 50 ml) in 0.125 percent bupivacaine is prepared. The solution (10 to 50 ml) is injected subcutaneously throughout the area of intense pain or in the vesicular distribution. The injections are tailored to the acute or chronic nature of the process, but the total number ranges from one to ten. In each patient, a finite trial of injections is undertaken, the patient is reassessed, and a decision is made whether to try an alternative form of therapy.

INTRAMUSCULAR ROUTE

Despite ubiquitous use of the IM route for drug administration in the postoperative setting and for other acute pain problems, the disadvantages of this route outweigh the advantages in most instances. The advantages include ease of administration, low cost, and established safety.

IM injections are painful and often anxiety producing for the patient. Blood levels of a medication administered IM are unpredictable because intramuscular absorption can be irregular and dosing intervals are often variable. Studies have documented a poor correlation between maximum blood levels achieved and body mass. Thus, the basis on which we typically derive a dose for a particular patient is also inaccurate. Often large doses of IM analgesics are prescribed in order to make the effects of the injection "last." This produces an unpleasant cycle of pain alternating with sedation and nausea. Wide swings in the blood levels of the analgesic are the norm.

In addition, there are some inherent problems with the administration of IM medications in the postoperative setting. Usually, a surgeon will write a standing "as needed" IM medication order. The typical patient will wait until he is in some degree of pain before calling the nurse to request pain medication. Some patients dread the needle so much that they suffer as long as possible before requesting medication. The nurse must then check the medication orders, prepare the injection, and administer the drug. This process routinely may take 30 minutes or more on a typical understaffed ward. The drug must then be absorbed into the blood stream, which may take an additional 20 minutes or more.

INTRAVENOUS ROUTE

The IV route of drug administration is important for effective drug administration in the diagnostic and therapeutic management of pain. This route of access provides a means by which drugs can be administered in a controlled fashion and titrated as needed to achieve target blood levels. As the complex physiology of pain is unraveled, diagnostic tests of various pharmacologic agents can be administered IV to sort out characteristics of a particular pain syndrome. An example of an IV diagnostic test is a phentolamine trial, which can assess the sympathetically mediated component of a pain syndrome.

Intravenous Local Anesthetics

Intravenous local anesthetics have been used in the chronic pain clinic for diagnostic and therapeutic purposes. This technique has been beneficial in managing such painful conditions as burns, postsurgical pain, central pain, deafferentation syndrome, Raynaud's disease, phantom limb pain, causalgia, neuritis, and myofascial pain.

Various theories have been proposed to describe the effects of IV local anesthetics on pain. Leriche proposed that injury to tissue caused reflex vasoconstriction, resulting in anoxia, capillary dysfunction, and increased permeability. This process would lead to the accumulation of nociceptive metabolites and to the irritation of peripheral nerve endings. He believed that procaine, by acting directly on the arteriolar, meta-arteriolar, and capillary endothelia, produced widespread vasodilation, thereby anesthetizing the irritated endothelial nerve endings and breaking the reflex arc.

Lundy observed 4 hours of analgesia in several jaundiced patients with pruritus after the slow injection of 20 ml of 0.1 percent procaine solution. His results supported Leriche's theory that peripheral irritation is accompanied by capillary hyperpermeability, allowing the transudation of procaine into the tissues, anesthetizing the nerve endings.

Choice of Drug

Procaine has been the classic local anesthetic agent for IV administration because of its potency and low toxicity; however, its short action, even at maximum doses, has been its major disadvantage. Since 1940 other local anesthetics have been utilized in an attempt to increase analgesic effects without compromising potency and low toxicity; such anesthetic agents are tetracaine, lidocaine, and chloroprocaine.

Many authors have shown an interest in the efficacy of IV lidocaine in managing painful conditions such as neuralgia, deafferentation syndrome, and paroxysmal attacks associated with postherpetic neuralgia. Hatangdi and associates used IV lidocaine, 1.0 to 1.5 mg per kilogram. In general, there was complete relief of lancinating pain within seconds after the injection. In addition, the degree of success with IV lidocaine often indicated patient response to oral antiepileptic drugs. Boas used this local anesthetic agent in patients with deafferentation syndrome and noted significant pain relief within 15 to 20 minutes after starting the infusion. Atkinson advocated IV lidocaine for the management of intractable pain from adiposa dolorosa, administering 0.1 percent solution of lidocaine IV until a total dose of 200 mg had been delivered over a 35-minute period. Significant pain relief lasted for 2 to 12 months or more.

Administration

Infusions of lidocaine are usually performed over 20 to 30 minutes at a dose of 1 to 5 mg per kilogram, depending on the author. The patient must be monitored for an IV local anesthetic infusion with electrocardiogram, blood pressure checks, and frequent questioning for symptoms of toxicity. Early signs of toxicity include metallic taste, tinnitus, lightheadedness, drowsiness, and agitation. Moderate toxicity may be manifest by perioral numbness, nystagmus, slurred speech, and a sense of heaviness in the legs. Seizures, cardiac arrhythmias, and cardiovascular instability are late signs of local anesthetic toxicity.

Intravenous Patient-Controlled Analgesia

The concept of patient-controlled analgesia (PCA) has evolved as a result of attempts to improve on the postoperative analgesia achieved by the IM and IV routes. PCA allows the patient to administer small doses of narcotics at a set time interval. PCA bolus dosing can be used alone or superimposed on a low-dose basal infusion. This method of dosing provides an opportunity to achieve steady-state drug levels comparable to those resulting from more traditional IV infusion techniques, but individualized to each patient's needs.

PCA as a safe method of providing analgesia is based on two concepts. The first is that analgesia can be produced at blood levels lower than those that produce sedation and respiratory depression. The second safety aspect is the mandatory bolus dose lock-out time interval that allows the patient to receive the benefit of a bolus dose before he can receive a second dose. The rare reports of respiratory depression related to IV PCA have been a result of human error in programming the pumps or in drug concentration. Thus, PCA combines the advantages of continuous IV infusions with the safety of "as needed" dosing.

The optimal administration of PCA requires a relatively light-weight, portable, computerized volumetric pump that allows individualized programming. These pumps have features that enhance patient safety, including lockable security doors that prevent tampering by unauthorized individuals and display features that indicate operational status, total cumulative dose, number of boluses administered per hour, as well as other alarm messages. Lock-out intervals prevent too-frequent bolusing of the narcotics.

PCA is becoming increasingly popular in the management of the postsurgical patient. In addition, PCA in the IV route can play a role in the cancer pain patient who has been unrelieved by oral medications. Often a cancer patient in an acute pain crisis can be controlled by an appropriate PCA regimen, which in turn provides valuable information about the patient's drug dosing requirements. Once the patient has stabilized, the information gained can be converted into a more effective oral regimen.

In addition to the IV route for PCA, epidural PCA has also been shown to be effective. Most of the studies that have evaluated these two routes of administration have been in post–cesearean section patients. The theoretical advantage of epidural PCA in the postoperative setting is that a segmental analgesia of the spinal cord can be obtained, minimizing the systemic side effects that are mediated via more central pathways. Clinical studies have not been done to verify these claims.

Most postoperative patients should be started on a routine set of orders specifying PCA settings (Table 4). These orders are modified to the patient's individual requirements as needed. PCA orders should also include monitoring parameters and provisions for the treatment of common side effects that may occur (e.g., nausea, pruritus).

NEUROAXIS ROUTE

The administration of both opiates and local anesthetics into the epidural and subarachnoid space has gained a definite role in the treatment of both acute postoperative pain and intractable cancer pain. In addition, valuable information about the nature of chronic pain syndromes and their development, as well as the introduction of new treatment modalities, have

Table 4 Examples of Initial PCA Pump Settings

Orders	Intravenous	Epidural
Volume	250 ml in pump	250 ml in pump
Drug	Morphine 250 mg in normal saline	Fentanyl 5,000 μg in normal saline
Concentration	Morphine 1 mg/ml	Fentanyl 20 μg/ml
Bolus dose	1 mg	40 μg
Delay (lock-out)	10 min	10 min
Basal rate	1 mg/hr	60 μg/hr
One-hour limit	10 mg	300 μg

been a result of the use of pharmacologic agents in the neuroaxis.

Prolonged Analgesia with Epidural Infusions

The object of producing prolonged epidural analgesia for chronic pain is both prognostic and therapeutic. The volume and concentration of the local anesthetic agent is determined by how many segments need to be blocked. The bolus injections then maintain that quality of analgesia for a period of time, usually days, so that the physician can evaluate the beneficial effect of pain relief and its side effects. This state of prolonged analgesia allows the patient to experience the accompanying feeling of numbness or weakness. The patient can then determine whether a proposed neurolytic block in that region would be tolerable. When prolonged analgesia is used for a therapeutic regimen, the benefits of prolonged sympathetic block, an exercise program during the pain-free period, and the benefits of reducing the nociceptive impulses on the reflex mechanisms are evaluated.

Infusion Technique

A bolus of 3 percent 2-chloroprocaine or 2 percent lidocaine is initially injected via a well-anchored catheter in the epidural space to provide analgesia in the affected pain dermatomes. The volume of the local anesthetic is determined by the site of catheter placement. The maximum volume injected is similar to that used in the bolus technique (caudal, 25 ml; lumbar, 20 ml; thoracic, 10 ml; cervical, 5 ml). After confirming that the epidural is functioning, infusion of bupivacaine is started via a volumetric infusion pump. Generally, 10 ml of 0.25 percent bupivacaine is needed for a 5 foot, 10 inch, 70-kg man when the catheter is placed in the lumbar space. Volume or concentration is changed by 12 hours if more than necessary segments are blocked (volume change) or motor and sensory block is intense (concentration change). In the thoracic space, 5 to 10 ml is infused with similar concentrations. For the success of this technique, nursing monitoring is mandatory, with ready availability of physician personnel when required.

Adequate pain relief is usually obtained in 75 percent of patients with this technique. The other 25 percent may have less than 50 percent pain relief and can be administered further bolus doses of 5 to 10 ml of 1 percent lidocaine once or twice a day. The initial concentration of infusion is 0.25 percent bupivacaine in patients with A-delta-fiber pain, and 0.125 to 0.625 percent bupivacaine in patients with C-fiber pain. The patients can be infused for 7 or more days. Concentrations of bupivacaine are decreased in the patient who has adequate relief but shows signs of motor paresis or numbness in other areas or urinary retention. In our series, 69 percent of patients with an initial 0.25 percent concentration had their concentrations lowered (0.125 percent) after 24 hours. The volume of infusion per hour is determined by assessing the number of segments to be blocked. Usually 12 ml per hour is infused for blocking of segments greater than six, 10 ml per hour for segments between four and six, and 5 ml per hour for segments less than four. The dose is reduced when there is increasing quality of block and adequate analgesia is still present. Tachyphylaxis has not been observed with prolonged infusion up to days or weeks.

Long-Term Analgesia with Spinal Opiates

Repeated epidural injections of opiates can provide sustained analgesia for several months in patients with cancer. A logical extension of this technique is to use a method of continuously infusing opiate solution via a catheter in the epidural space. The continuous infusion techniques avoid the peak and trough concentration pattern arising from repeated injections. At dose rates ranging from 2 to 30 mg of morphine sulfate per day, there was no evidence of respiratory depression, pruritus, nausea, or urinary retention in the small group of patients studied.

In analyzing the usefulness of the intraspinal route of administration, several points are pertinent. The choice of opiate is important. Preservative-free solutions are essential, although the use of sodium metabisulfite does not appear to be contraindicated. Morphine, a water-soluble pure agonist, may not be the most appropriate choice. Its prolonged sojourn in the cerebrospinal fluid increases the duration of action in an unpredictable fashion. In contrast, the more lipid-soluble agents are more rapidly removed from cerebrospinal fluid and are less likely to cause late-onset adverse effects. In terms of "patient preference" for lipid-soluble agents given epidurally, a decreasing progression from methadone to meperidine to fentanyl was reported. Although each of these agents has merits, methadone clearance from plasma is slow, and while this can augment the spinally mediated analgesia, it may lead to centrally mediated adverse effects after several days of continuous or repeated dosing. Meperidine, like morphine, is rapidly absorbed systemically, may also produce peripheral effects, and does not cause histamine release. The duration of action is not necessarily a problem, since epidural catheter techniques can be used to control this. The partial agonist buprenorphine was reported to cause fewer side effects than morphine.

Techniques of Delivery of Spinal Opiates

Three basic approaches have been in use: (1) implantation of an intraspinal catheter exiting percutaneously, (2) implantation of a subcutaneous reservoir with or without a valve mechanism in series with an intraspinal catheter, and (3) implantation of a continuous infusion device in series with an intraspinal catheter.

In all three approaches, the intraspinal catheter placement involves standard percutaneous techniques. Tunneling the catheter to reduce the hazard of infection is essential for prolonged use. Optimal kits and materials have not been identified as yet. Long experience and study in lumbo- and ventriculoperitoneal shunts confirm the essential acceptability of Silastic catheters.

Prior to any such procedure, preparations for a surgical aseptic technique should be complete. Prophylactic antibiotics such as Cephadyl (sterile cephapirin sodium) should be administered. Anesthesia can be provided via general or regional anesthesia at the operative site. The procedure should be done in the operating room and under fluoroscopy.

Intraspinal Cannulation. Actual epidural cannulation is performed with a modified epidural needle and using standard techniques, except that a small incision must be made. Epidural placement is accomplished using a standard loss-of-resistance technique. If morphine is used, thoracic or cervical epidural cannulation may be avoided. However, for more lipid-soluble drugs demonstrating regional localization such as fentanyl, placement adjacent to the afferent input may be required. Again, catheter placement is guided by fluoroscopy. The final position of epidural catheters is best defined by water-soluble radiopaque contrast injection if possible (5 to 7 ml of 190 to 200 mg per deciliter of metrizamide).

Tunneling. In order to tunnel the catheters laterally from the intraspinal area, a small incision about 1 inch long is made down to the posterior spinous ligament prior to needle insertion. The catheter must be anchored to prevent dislodgement. Placement of the stitch is best accomplished at this point, prior to needle insertion. Actual lateral tunneling is done through the incision following intraspinal cannulation by passing a shunt tunneling instrument or blunt clamp laterally from the incision. If an infusion device or reservoir is to be connected to the intraspinal catheter, it is done at this point over a straight metal titanium or stainless steel connector.

Once an intraspinal catheter is implanted and tunneled, it is a simple matter to convert the procedure from a percutaneously exiting lateral flank catheter to an implanted reservoir. Infusaport and Port-A-Cath are the currently used reservoirs.

Implanted Infusion Devices. A device such as the Infusaid 400 can be attached to the intrathecal conduit to deliver 1.5 to 5 ml per day. Driven by a fluorocarbon generating 428 mm Hg of pressure at body temperature, the device reliably delivers a fixed flow of agent from a bellows drug chamber. Refill of the 30- or 50-ml reservoir is accomplished by percutaneous injection. The refill cycle is dependent on the flow rate. Flow rates vary with temperature, viscosity, and barometric pressure. The device is implanted on the abdominal or chest wall through a 3- to 4-inch incision. A subcutaneous pocket is formed by blunt dissection, with cautery used to prevent hematoma formation. The device is anchored to the bed of the wound (fascia) with four-quadrant single Prolene ligatures. The initial dosage range is 0.5 to 2 mg per day intrathecally or 4 to 10 mg per day epidurally. This dose may have to be increased to as much as 60 mg per day epidurally as patients develop tolerance.

Choice of Route

The choice between the intrathecal and the epidural route is made on the basis of several issues. For infectious reasons, long-term intrathecal catheters must be attached to a subcutaneous infusion device to obtain a "closed" system. This greatly enhances the cost of drug administration and is more appropriate for chronic benign pain or for a cancer patient with a life expectancy greater than 6 months. Tunneled epidural catheters can be exteriorized for intermittent bolus injection or attached to a subcutaneous infusion port.

Finally, when making the decision to choose the neuroaxis route for the administration of analgesia in a pain patient, the risks of the method must be considered. DuPen recently published his results of 350 patients with cancer and the acquired immunodeficiency syndrome who received analgesia through a tunneled epidural catheter. He cites a 5 percent infection rate in his patients, including local skin exit-site infections as well as deep track and epidural infections.

NERVE BLOCKS AND INDWELLING CATHETERS

Drugs for neural blockade can be administered by a number of routes, including intravenously, subcutaneously, via an indwelling catheter, and directly via a needle next to the nerve. Injection of local anesthetics and/or steroid preparations on peripheral nerves plays a valuable role in both diagnosing and treating patients with select pain syndromes.

Myofascial Trigger Point Injections

Myofascial trigger point injections of local anesthetics are the simplest and most frequently used analgesic block in the treatment of pain. Simplicity and apparent lack of risk make this a first-line treatment in certain types of musculoskeletal pain.

Dry needling of trigger points without injecting any solution may be effective but does not equal the therapeutic effectiveness of injecting a local anesthetic. Krause noted that postinjection pain followed dry needling. Sola and Kuitert treated a series of 100 patients by injecting normal saline into their trigger points. They found saline to be effective in relieving the pain. Hameroff and colleagues, on the other hand, found that long-acting local anesthetics, i.e., bupivacaine and etidocaine, produced better and longer pain relief for up to 7 days after injection.

Travell and Simons advocate mixing corticosteroids with a local anesthetic for trigger point injections in two groups of patients: (1) patients with soft tissue inflammation (adhesive capsulitis) and (2) those with postinjection muscle soreness. Steroid may be responsible for a burning sensation in the area of injection 24 to 48 hours later, but this subsides, and patients continue to have prolonged pain relief for 7 to 10 days afterward.

Diagnostic Blocks

In the patient who has chronic pain of unclear etiology, a series of diagnostic local anesthetic nerve blocks can often help sort out anatomical issues. An example is a patient who has severe pain of a radicular nature in the leg. Radiologic studies show that the patient has severe, multilevel degenerative spine disease, and it is unclear which lumbosacral level is the source of the pain. A series of diagnostic nerve root blocks can be performed on the basis of the examination. If the patient's pain is entirely relieved by an S1 nerve root block (for example), this information can be valuable in making therapeutic decisions.

Epidural Steroids

An example of the usefulness of nerve blocks in the acute setting is the epidural steroid injection. The value of this procedure is in the treatment of discogenic pain of relatively recent onset (3 months or less) that has not responded to conservative management. Even though some claim superior results with subarachnoid injection, most believe that epidural steroids are safer and produce equally good results. Since the nerve root compression is extradural in discogenic disease, it is rational to introduce the steroid epidurally at the site of compression rather than intradurally, where it will be subject to dilution, dispersion, and precipitation.

Epidural puncture should be done at the level of the nerve root lesion, with the patient's painful side down in the lateral decubitus position. When the epidural space has been identified by standard techniques, 80 mg of methylprednisolone acetate or 50 mg of triamcinolone diacetate is suspended in 10 ml of 0.25 or 0.125 percent bupivacaine and injected slowly into the epidural space. If the patient has had previous back surgery, identification of the epidural space may be difficult. Initial administration of local anesthetic makes identification of the epidural space easier in this circumstance.

After epidural steroid injection, a catheter can be introduced to inject another dose of steroid and local anesthetic if needed to reach the appropriate nerve root. This is determined objectively by measuring improvement in the straight leg test and the absence of radicular pain during the performance of the test. The patient remains in the lateral position for 10 minutes to keep the injected solution on the dependent side.

Two weeks after the epidural steroid injection, the patient is re-evaluated. If there is significant improvement in function and subjective pain relief, no further epidural injection is administered. However, if the initial improvement is not maintained after the first injection, the injection can be repeated, up to a maximum of three. Similarly, if there is no change in the patient's condition after the first injection, alternative measures are sought.

Many workers have reported impressive results with epidural steroid injections. Winnie reported subjective total pain relief in 80 percent of patients with either epidural or subarachnoid injections. Brown reported "excellent to good" results in 100 percent of patients with acute discogenic disease of less than 3 months' duration but in only 15 percent of those with pain that had lasted more than 3 months. Erdemir studied 122 patients with postlaminectomy syndrome after treatment with intradural and extradural steroids. Fifty-three percent of patients reported satisfactory results, i.e., 70 to 100 percent pain relief. Unfortunately, good prospective, double-blind studies have not been performed to document the effectiveness of the technique.

When considering epidural steroid administration, keep the following points in mind:

1. Histologic and biochemical evidence supports its use in the 30- to 50-year-old group; with low back pain or cervical pain with a radicular component, the pain is primarily discogenic.
2. Features of this syndrome are shooting pain in the distribution of the brachial plexus, sciatic or femoral distribution with sensory and/or motor deficits, reflex change, and straight leg raising positive at 30 degrees.
3. Epidural and subarachnoid injections have proponents on both sides. The subarachnoid approach carries the risk of arachnoiditis and meningitis without appreciable advantages over the epidural group.
4. Bupivacaine 0.125 to 0.25 percent with either methylprednisolone (Depo-Medrol) 80 mg, or triamcinolone (Aristocort) 50 mg, in 8 to 10 ml, is commonly used.

Interpleural Catheters

A variety of techniques may have a role in the management of acute pain, including interpleural, brachial plexus, and lumbar plexus catheters with a continuous infusion of local anesthetic. Several published reports have suggested that a continuous interpleural infusion of a local anesthetic may provide good analgesia for post-thoracotomy and postcholecystectomy pain, as well as the severe pain related to multiple rib fractures from trauma.

The mechanism of action with local anesthetics in the interpleural space is thought to be a diffusion process resulting in blockade of the intercostal nerves. This technique is useful in unilateral pain and provides a mechanism for continuous infusion of a local anesthetic for upper abdominal and thoracic pain. The blind placement of these catheters is not without risk. One study found a high percentage of interpleural catheters embedded in the lung and a significant incidence of pneumothorax. In selected patients (for example, a patient with a flail chest) an interpleural catheter may be the ideal method of providing analgesia.

SUGGESTED READING

Benzon HT. Epidural steroid injections for low back pain and lumbosacral radiculopathy. Pain 1986; 24:277-295.

Cousins MJ, Bridenbaugh, eds: Acute and chronic pain: use of spinal opioids in neural blockade.

Covino BG. Inteplevin regional analgesia. Anesth Analg 1988; 67:427–429.

DuPen SL. Infection during chronic epidural catheterization: diagnosis and treatment. Anesthesiology 1990; 73:905–909.

Edwards WT. Intravenous lidocaine in the management of various chronic pain states. Reg Anesth, January-March 1985.

Miser AW, et al. Transdermal fentanyl for pain control in patients with cancer. Pain 1989; 37:15–21.

Penn RD, et al. Intrathecal analgesia applied by pumps. In: Advances in pain research and therapy. Vol 13. New York: Raven Press, 1990.

Plezia PM, et al. Transdermal fentanyl: Pharmacokinetics and preliminary clinical evaluation. Pharmacotherapy 1989; 9(1):2–9.

Sheidker VR. New methods in analgesic delivery. In: Cancer pain management. Orlando: Grune & Stratton, 1987.

White PF. Patient controlled analgesia: an update on its use in the treatment of postoperative pain. Anesth Clin North Am 1989; 7:63–78.

STELLATE GANGLION BLOCK

DENIS L. BOURKE, M.D.

The stellate ganglion block is one of the most useful and practical nerve blocks the anesthesiologist can perform. In addition to being a valuable therapeutic modality, it is relatively free of complications and can provide a wealth of diagnostic information. Stellate ganglion blocks are extremely useful in discriminating the cause of pain in the head, meninges, face, neck, shoulder, chest, arm, and hand. As a therapeutic modality, the stellate ganglion block is the first-line treatment for sympathetically maintained pain syndromes of the upper extremity. The term *sympathetically maintained pain syndrome* is now the preferred nomenclature for a variety of problems that include those previously called *causalgia* or *sympathetic dystrophies*. The stellate ganglion block can be a valuable adjunct in treating ischemia of the upper extremity from a variety of causes. The block is also useful in treating the pain associated with herpes zoster, in both the acute and chronic phases. The stellate ganglion block can usually be performed safely on an outpatient basis.

By far the most common use of the stellate ganglion block is in diagnosing and treating sympathetically maintained pain syndromes of the upper extremity. It is unfortunate that despite the well-known history, symptom complex, and diagnostic signs associated with sympathetically maintained pain of the upper extremity, many patients remain undiagnosed or misdiagnosed for long periods of time. These patients are frequently treated by numerous other techniques such as oral and parenteral narcotic analgesics and surgical intervention before the diagnosis becomes obvious. This is particularly unfortunate because although the devastating effects of sympathetically maintained pain can be effectively treated with stellate ganglion blocks, the success of treatment is directly related to early diagnosis and aggressive treatment.

ANATOMY

The stellate ganglion is so named because of its multipointed star-like appearance. It consists of the fused first thoracic and inferior cervical sympathetic ganglia and is part of the paravertebral sympathetic nervous system. Preganglionic sympathetic fibers from T-1 to T-4, or occasionally as low as T-6, converge and ascend to form and pass through the stellate ganglion. Some fibers exit at the stellate ganglion to the periphery, whereas others continue cephalad to the cervical sympathetic ganglia. Sympathetic fibers that exit at the stellate ganglion continue onward to provide sympathetic innervation to the lung, heart, neck structures, face, scalp, brain, and ipsilateral upper extremity.

The stellate ganglion is approximately 2.5 cm long, 1 cm wide, and approximately 0.3 cm thick. It lies near the lateral borders of the bodies of C-7 and T-1. In cross-section the stellate ganglion lies just anterior to the longus colli muscle. The longus colli muscle is a longitudinal muscle that runs on the anterior lateral aspect of the vertebral bodies and is 2 to 5 mm thick. On the anterior surface of the longus colli muscle, the stellate ganglion lies just posterior and medial to the carotid sheath. Other nearby structures include the vertebral artery, the subclavian artery, and the inferior thyroid artery. The recurrent laryngeal nerve courses just anterior to the stellate ganglion.

BLOCK TECHNIQUE

Because the stellate ganglion block technique is quite simple to perform and is relatively painless, premedication with analgesics or sedatives is seldom needed or indicated. In fact, as a general rule, the use of analgesics and sedatives for diagnostic blocks tends to obscure the diagnostic precision of the block.

The key technical maneuver in performing a successful stellate ganglion block is to place the block needle on the anterior aspect of the transverse process of C-7 medially where it joins the body of C-7. The patient is positioned in a semirecumbent position with a pillow or roll under the shoulders to extend the neck. The head is turned slightly away from the side to be blocked. The following anatomic landmarks are identified and indicated with a skin marking pen:

1. The cricoid cartilage is palpated and marked, indicating the level of C-6. Palpation medially from just posterior to the sternocleidomastoid muscle to identify Chassaignac's tubercle also helps to identify the tip of the transverse process of C-6.
2. A mark is placed overlying Chassaignac's tubercle, approximately 3.0 to 3.5 cm lateral from the midline.
3. The transverse process of C-7 should be 1.0 to 1.5 cm below the mark indicating the tip of the transverse process of C-6. A skin mark is placed at this point, indicating the location for insertion of the block needle. A more convenient way of locating the point over the transverse process of C-7 in most adult patients is to measure 2 fingerbreadths lateral and 2 fingerbreadths cephalad to the sternal notch.

Fluoroscopy can be helpful in locating and identifying landmarks, but it is seldom necessary to the performance of a successful stellate ganglion block.

To perform the block, a skin wheal is raised with a 25-gauge needle at the point overlying the transverse process of C-7. The block is performed with a 10-ml syringe full of local anesthetic attached to a 3.8-cm or a 5-cm 22-gauge needle. The needle is inserted through the point over the transverse process of C-7 perpendicular to the plane of the skin and is advanced until either the transverse process of C-7 is encountered or a paresthesia is elicited. If a paresthesia is elicited, the needle is withdrawn slightly and redirected either cephalad or caudad, depending on the dermatome of the paresthesia. The needle is again advanced to impinge on the transverse process of C-7. Once the needle rests firmly on the transverse process of C-7, and with the operator's hand braced firmly against the patient, the needle is withdrawn approximately 3 mm so that the tip lies just anterior to the longus colli muscle in the loose areolar tissue. After careful aspiration for blood and cerebrospinal fluid, several milliliters of local anesthetic are injected. If there is no evidence of intravascular or subarachnoid injection after 30 to 45 seconds, the remaining contents of the syringe are injected and the needle withdrawn. Some clinicians advocate retracting the sternocleidomastoid and the carotid sheath laterally during the block procedure. This usually prevents a carotid puncture; however, the maneuver is not necessary because puncture of the carotid artery with a 22-gauge needle is of little consequence.

The drug and dose to be used are best determined by the purpose of the block. For purely diagnostic blocks, 6 to 8 ml of 0.5 percent lidocaine is usually sufficient. If a somatic nerve is accidentally blocked using this regimen, the diagnostic stellate block can be repeated within several hours. After the diagnosis is certain and the stellate block becomes part of a therapeutic series of blocks, a somatic block is of much less consequence, and the goal is a more certain, profound, and prolonged sympathetic block. In the latter case, 10 to 15 ml of 0.25 to 0.375 percent bupivacaine with epinephrine 1:200,000 is a better choice. For neurolytic blocks, 2 to 3 ml of 50 percent alcohol can be used. Because an alcohol block is painful, the physician will be immediately warned if a somatic nerve is being blocked. The neurolytic block may have to be repeated, however, because a low volume of alcohol (2 to 3 ml) must be used to ensure safety.

ASSESSMENT OF THE BLOCK

The signs and symptoms of a successful sympathetic nerve block are the unilateral findings of ptosis (drooping of the eyelid), myosis (small pupil), and enophthalmos (sinking inward of the eyeball). These three symptoms constitute the classic Horner's syndrome. Other signs and symptoms may include anhydrosis of the face, neck, and ipsilateral arm; flushing of the skin; conjunctival injection; lacrimation; stuffiness of the nose; engorgement of the veins; and increased skin temperature. The annoying symptoms of lacrimation and nasal stuffiness can be treated easily with the topical alpha-agonist, Neo-synephrine. Although these signs and symptoms indicate a sympathetic blockade, they do not guarantee that a successful sympathetic blockade of the upper extremity has occurred. The appropriate signs and symptoms must be observed on the upper extremity as well as the face and neck. In addition, several tests can confirm specific sympathetic blockade of the upper extremity. These tests include skin conductance response (SCR), skin potential response (SPR), plethysmography, thermography, any one of the several sweat tests, and the psychogalvanic reflex (PGR) test. It is also particularly important during diagnostic stellate ganglion blocks to perform a careful and thorough neurologic examination of the upper extremity to rule out the possibility of an inadvertent somatic nerve blockade. Unnoticed somatic blockade during a diagnostic stellate ganglion block may easily relieve pain and falsely imply that the cause of the pain is a sympathetically maintained pain syndrome.

APPLICATIONS

Sympathetically Maintained Pain

Sympathetically maintained pain, formerly called either *reflex sympathetic dystrophy* or *causalgia,* usually begins insidiously as a diffuse burning type of pain that frequently follows a relatively minor injury. Often the injury may have been so minor as to have gone unnoticed or been forgotten. As the syndrome progresses, the skin becomes exquisitely sensitive to touch. It is also typical for cold to provoke pain. In the early stages of disease, the skin frequently is warm and dry and may appear flushed. As the disease progresses, edema may appear. Increasing pain limits activity, and prolonged limitation of activity results in atrophic changes that include the skin, the muscle, and eventually the bony structure (Sudeck's atrophy). Finally, in addition to atrophy, inactivity may cause limitation of motion due to muscle, tendon, and joint fibrosis. In its most dramatic manifestation, the shoulder-hand syndrome, immobilization of the shoulder joint eventually results in extensive fibrosis and, ultimately, a permanent bony fusion. In the last stages of a sympathetically maintained pain syndrome, the skin may become cool and pale; sweating may also be a prominent feature. Pain and profuse sweating of the affected limb may be provoked by touch, temperature changes, or even emotional stress.

The essential ingredients in treating a sympathetically maintained pain syndrome are early diagnosis and aggressive treatment. Classically, a sympathetically maintained pain syndrome of the upper extremity is diagnosed by the virtual complete relief of pain and other symptoms following a stellate ganglion block. New evidence suggests that intravenous phentolamine may be as specific and sensitive as the stellate ganglion block in diagnosing sympathetically maintained pain syndromes. It may have the further advantage, due to the intravenous mode of therapy, of permitting the physician to differentiate the malingering patient from the patient with real pain.

Treatment of the sympathetically maintained pain syndrome consists of sympathetic blockade. Stellate ganglion blocks should be repeated as often as daily until relief from successive blocks becomes progressively longer. Results are best in patients whose diagnosis and treatment are initiated in the first 6 months of their disease. After 2 years, the results of treatment are

disappointing even with aggressive therapy. Some authors advocate continuous sympathetic blockade for a period of several days. Although this is technically more feasible for the lower extremity, it has also been used successfully in treating the upper extremity pain syndrome. An important aspect of treating sympathetically maintained pain syndromes is the inclusion of physical therapy. Early in the treatment phase, physical therapy and stellate ganglion blocks should be coordinated so that the benefits of physical therapy can be achieved during the peak period of pain relief immediately following the sympathetic nerve block.

Herpes Zoster and Postherpetic Neuralgia

Sympathetic nerve blocks are valuable adjuncts in treating acute herpes zoster. Results indicate that sympathetic blocks effect prompt pain relief, may decrease the severity and duration of the eruptions, and may actually accelerate healing. These results can be particularly dramatic in cases of herpes zoster ophthalmicus.

Although less effective than in the acute phase, sympathetic blockade can also be effective in treating postherpetic neuralgia. Sympathetic blocks done daily or every other day for a total of 6 to 10 blocks can produce long-lasting pain relief. Results appear to be better when the time period from the acute phase until the onset of the postherpetic symptoms is relatively short.

Postamputation Phantom Pain

Symptoms of postamputation pain syndromes have a wide variety of manifestations. In cases in which the predominant symptom is a burning, aching type of pain that is associated with vasomotor and sudomotor changes in the stump, sympathetic blockade is most likely to be effective. Sympathetic blocks should be repeated daily or on alternate days for as long as progressively longer pain relief occurs. Other types of postamputation pain, such as the sensation of an extremely abnormal position or lancinating paroxysms of pain, are less likely to respond to sympathetic blockade. However, a trial of sympathetic blockade is warranted in any postamputation pain syndrome that is refractory to other forms of treatment. Mounting evidence indicates that preoperative regional anesthesia and intraoperative regional anesthesia have a positive effect in attenuating or preventing the postamputation pain syndromes.

Vascular Diseases

A variety of acute and chronic vascular disorders are amenable to treatment with stellate ganglion blockade. Acute posttraumatic segmentary vasospasm may benefit from sympathetic blockade. Likewise, ischemia and pain due to acute phases of chronic occlusive arterial disease are frequently improved by sympathetic nerve blocks. Generalized arterial vasospasms resulting from a variety of causes, including accidental intra-arterial injections of such drugs as the thiobarbiturates, respond to sympathetic blockade. Acute pain caused by Raynaud's disease also responds to the sympathetic blockade. Likewise, chronic occlusive diseases can benefit from sympathetic blockade during the acute phases. Since sympathetic efferents, after leaving the ganglia, travel distally with the blood vessels, extended continuous treatment of vascular disorders of the upper extremity, using either a continuous axillary block or continuous subclavian block as described by Winnie, may be technically more effective by blocking sympathetic nerves where they lie in company with the blood vessels.

Acute Myocardial Infarction

When the pain of acute myocardial infarction is severe and refractory to conventional analgesic therapy such as morphine, stellate ganglion blocks may be effective in reducing pain. An added benefit is prevention of sympathetically induced reflex coronary vasoconstriction.

Angina Pectoris

In patients with severe intractable angina who are not a candidates for coronary artery bypass surgery, stellate ganglion block may relieve the pain. After an initial trial with local anesthetics, successful long-term relief of anginal pain in these patients may be accomplished with a stellate ganglion neurolytic blockade.

Status Asthmaticus

If all other therapy has failed, a stellate ganglion block may be effective in terminating status asthmaticus. This treatment is indicated only in extreme cases in which conventional therapy has failed.

Miscellaneous Complaints

In experienced hands, several other symptoms may be worthy of an attempt at treatment with a stellate ganglion blockade. These symptoms include unexplained edema, unhealed ulcers, bursitis-like pains, and miscellaneous joint stiffness.

COMPLICATIONS

The large number of vital structures in the neck can lead to various complications of the stellate ganglion block. Prompt recognition of a complication and skill in airway management and general resuscitative measures are therefore essential for anyone performing stellate ganglion blocks.

A common minor complication is inadvertent block of the recurrent laryngeal nerve. Patients need only be reassured that the hoarseness will subside and warned not to eat or drink while the hoarseness persists. Inadvertent somatic nerve block of the upper extremity is also a fairly common minor complication. Again the patient need only be reassured that the symptom is temporary. Care, however, should be taken to note a possible somatic block so that it does not confuse the diagnostic process. Block of the vagus nerve is not uncommon but is of little consequence.

More serious complications of the stellate ganglion block include unintentional injection of local anesthetic into the intravascular or subarachnoid spaces. Injection of local anesthetic into the subarachnoid space at this level of the spinal cord almost invariably results in an immediate total spinal anesthetic. The patient will require immediate airway and cardiovascular support. Intravascular injection of local anesthetic into the vertebral artery, which lies just anterior to the stellate ganglion, or into the carotid artery, which lies somewhat further anterior and slightly lateral to the stellate ganglion, can introduce a relatively high dose of local anesthetic into the central nervous system and lead to respiratory arrest or convulsions. Again, immediate expert airway management and cardiovascular support are the mainstays of treatment. Convulsions should be promptly treated with small doses of short-acting barbiturates or benzodiazepines. Occasionally, violation of the pleura can result in a pneumothorax. If any symptoms or signs of a pneumothorax are observed oxygen should be administered and a chest radiograph should be obtained immediately. If the approach to the stellate ganglion is too near the midline, perforation of the esophagus can occur, possibly leading to an infection that must be treated vigorously with antibiotics.

Neurolytic blocks of the stellate ganglion should be performed by experienced clinicians only and preferably with fluoroscopic guidance.

SUGGESTED READING

Bonica JJ, Buckley FP. Regional analgesia with local anesthetics. In: Bonica JJ, ed. The management of pain. 2nd ed. Philadelphia: Lea & Febiger, 1990:1883–1966.

Lofstrom JB, Cousins MJ. Sympathetic neural blockade of upper and lower extremity. In: Cousins MJ, Bridenbaugh PO, eds. Neural blockade in clinical anesthesia and management of pain. 2nd ed. Philadelphia: JB Lippincott, 1988:461–500.

Moore DC. Anterior (paratracheal) approach for block of the stellate ganglion. In: Moore DC, ed. Regional block: a handbook for use in the clinical practice of medicine and surgery. 4th ed. Springfield, IL: Charles C Thomas, 1975:123–137.

Verril P. Sympathetic ganglion lesions. In: Wall PD, Melzack R, ed. Textbook of pain. 2nd ed. New York: Churchill Livingstone, 1989:773–783.

Winnie AP. Plexus anesthesia. Volume I. Perivascular techniques of brachial plexus block. Philadelphia: WB Saunders, 1983:117–188.

CELIAC PLEXUS BLOCK

ROBERT SPRAGUE, M.D.
SOMAYAJI RAMAMURTHY, M.D.

Celiac plexus block is an extremely valuable and often underutilized tool in the anesthetic armamentarium. It is used most frequently in patients with terminal cancer, although there are many other areas in which this relatively simple block can be of benefit.

This chapter reviews the anatomy of the celiac plexus and discusses the various indications for celiac block, the possible approaches for performing this procedure, agents for use in celiac blockade, the "blind" versus radiologically guided block controversy, celiac versus splanchnic block, and finally the possible side effects of this technique.

AUTONOMIC INNERVATION OF THE ABDOMEN

The celiac plexus is a diffuse, weblike system of nerve fibers woven about the aorta and periaortic space. These fibers are derived from the thoracic sympathetic chain, parasympathetic contributions from the vagus nerve and visceral afferent origins. The visceral afferent components that travel with the sympathetic fibers have their cell bodies in the dorsal root ganglion. The plexus innervates most of the abdominal viscera, with main contributions to the pancreas, kidneys, biliary tract, liver, stomach, spleen, adrenal glands, small and large bowel, and the "watch dog" of the abdomen, the omentum.

Two splanchic nerves, the great and lesser splanchnic nerves, contribute to the formation of the celiac ganglia. The great splanchnic nerve originates from the roots of either the fifth or sixth thoracic segments to the ninth or tenth thoracic level. The nerve forms a distinct cord and travels in a paravertebral gutter to pierce the crus of the diaphragm bilaterally to enter into the abdominal cavity. The nerve then ends in the semilunar, or celiac, ganglion on its respective side. Most of these fibers in the greater and lesser splanchnic nerves are classified as preganglionic sympathetics, but visceral afferent fibers travel in the bundles as well. The lesser splanchnic nerve has its origin from the ninth through the eleventh thoracic levels and arrives in the celiac ganglion by travelling with the greater nerve in the thorax and entering the abdomen with, or lateral to, the crural entry point of the great nerve. From this celiac central station, postganglionic fibers are given off to various other abdominal ganglia, to include the aortic, renal, and hypogastric plexuses. The abdominal viscera receive their innervation from these "substations." A key point to remember is that the celiac plexus is not a distinct anatomic entity, but a diffuse network of autonomic fibers of which the celiac ganglia are a major part. The visceral pathways to the gut and related structures can be blocked at the splanchnic level or at the level of the celiac plexus. Approaches for both the celiac and splanchnic blocks as well as reasons for separate blocks are discussed later.

Upon cadaveric study, the location of the celiac plexus in humans has shown numerous anatomic variations. The celiac ganglia are paired organs that lie immediately above the pancreas in the midline and are in close approximation to the adrenals. The first lumbar vertebra lies immediately posterior. The aorta is surrounded by the plexus, while the vena cava lies to the right and anterior. Both of these large vascular structures are important landmarks in performing the block, and transgression of either structure has been used in identifying needle placement. As mentioned earlier, the plexus itself consists of sympathetic, parasympathetic, and visceral afferent elements that intertwine around the base of the celiac and superior mesenteric arteries. In a cadaver study in 1979, Ward et al dissected the celiac plexus in 20 adult cadavers and found the location of the celiac plexus to be quite varied. They found the celiac ganglia to number from one to five and vary in size from 0.5 to 4.5 cm in diameter, as well as in location from the intervertebral disc of T-12 L-1 to the midbody of L-2. The ganglia on the left were consistently lower than those on the right, and were from 0.6 to 0.9 cm below the origin of the celiac artery. These anatomic considerations, discussed in the procedural section of this chapter, are of import in performing the technique of celiac block.

INDICATIONS

There is a generally held, although incorrect, belief that blockade of the celiac plexus is to be used only for the relief of terminal cancer pain. Although this area of treatment of intractable cancer pain is the primary use for this block, there are numerous other diagnostic and therapeutic uses for this modality.

Perhaps the most rewarding use of celiac block is in the treatment of cancer pain, most often in terminal pancreatic cancer. This type of cancer, as well as other types of upper abdominal visceral malignancies, are often poorly responsive to oral or parenteral narcotic analgesics. If narcotics are able to control the pain, the patient is often left in a stuporous existence, unable to function meaningfully. Constipation secondary to the narcotic is also problematic. With a celiac plexus block, the patient can often reduce or stop taking narcotic analgesics and can be relatively pain free for the remaining days. Patients should be placed on a tapering scale of narcotics postblock to prevent acute withdrawal symptoms. The side effect of increased peristalsis with celiac blockade will often ameliorate the constipation symptoms. As is mentioned later in this chapter, a diagnostic local anesthetic block is usually undertaken before neurolytic blockade, although some clinicians proceed directly to neurolytic block once the diagnosis of terminal cancer is made. Cancer patients with metastatic lesions may have body wall involvement as the primary source of pain, which celiac blockade will not relieve.

Celiac blockade is also helpful in the treatment of acute pancreatitis. As is the case with pancreatic cancer, the pain of acute pancreatitis is often resistant to the analgesic effects of narcotics. The pain of this malady is greatly relieved with a celiac plexus block. The course of the disease may also be altered by this block. The spasm of the ducts and sphincters is believed to be the basis of pain in acute pancreatitis, and the addition of methylprednisolone to the local anesthetic solution used in the block has been shown to decrease the severity of the attack. The use of neurolytic celiac blockade in patients with chronic pancreatitis is controversial. The patients are not terminally ill, and the neurolytic agents used in celiac block afford 4- to 6-month blockade, obviously necessitating repeat blocks with all the associated complications of the block. Other reasons to avoid using the block in chronic pancreatitis patients include the patient population and the creation of a "silent abdomen." The group of patients most likely to suffer from chronic pancreatitis is the alcoholic population, who may interpret pain relief as an opportunity to imbibe once more. The second problem stems form the total lack of visceral sensation postblock and its obvious consequences in masking pain from intra-abdominal emergencies. Some studies, however, have shown dramatic improvement in the management of chronic pancreatitis pain with neurolytic blocks. In these cases, it is of the utmost importance to obtain adequate psychological support in reference to further substance abuse. The use of steroids with celiac plexus block for chronic pancreatitis has also been studied and has met with some success.

Celiac plexus block is also a useful diagnostic tool in determining whether the source of chronic pain is visceral or autonomic. Combined with the use of intercostal blocks placed over the correct dermatomes of the patient's reported pain, celiac block can delineate a visceral source from a body wall source of the pain nidus.

Perhaps the areas in which celiac plexus blocks are used least are the operating room and the radiology suite. The combination of intercostal blocks and a celiac plexus block provides excellent operating conditions for procedures on the upper abdomen. Additionally, as is the case with subarachnoid block, the gut is constricted secondary to vagal preponderance after sympathetic blockade, leaving the surgeon with compacted intestine away from the operative field. Interventional radiology is an area in which celiac block is perhaps the technique of choice. Biliary tract procedures, including stent placement, stone removal, dilation, transhepatic cholangiography, and liver biopsy, have all been easily accomplished under celiac plexus block, rendering the patient pain free and cooperative. A recent study comparing celiac plexus block with thoracic epidural anesthesia for biliary procedures reflects more favorably on celiac block. Radiologists themselves have been performing celiac blocks for biliary procedures. Other radiologic

procedures, such as removal of renal calculi, have been accomplished with the aid of celiac block.

TECHNIQUES

The patient should not take anything by mouth for 8 hours if possible and should give consent for the block in usual fashion. The patient should be questioned about iodine allergy, as iodine-containing contrast medium is frequently used. Nonionic contrast is available for allergic patients. It is advisable to have an electrocardiographic display available and to obtain blood pressure measurements with the patient in both the sitting and supine positions, as hypotension may occur postblock and baseline values will aid in treatment. Because of the aforementioned hypotension, it is also necessary to have a functioning intravenous catheter in place to allow for fluid boluses. To prevent the patient from being disappointed postblock, it is helpful to inform him or her that the block may not relieve all of the pain. The patient should not be overly sedated, as verbal communications with the patient is extremely valuable in evaluating any possible complications during the execution of the block. It is also important that the patient not be given his or her usual narcotic dose preblock, as the patient must be able to assess pain relief for proper diagnostic and neurolytic therapy.

As with most nerve blocks in anesthesia, there are several approaches to the celiac plexus block, each with its proponents and each with different complications. For the purpose of this discussion, conventional approaches to include the posterior, anterior, transaortic, and the loss of resistance techniques are examined.

The technique employed at our facility is one originally defined by Kappis with refinement by Moore, with our refinement of the use of fluoroscopy (Fig. 1). This posterolateral approach is the most practiced and proven route used clinically. The patient is placed prone on either a stretcher or on the table of the fluoroscopy unit. It is helpful to place a pillow or support under the patient's abdomen not only for the patient's comfort, but also to straighten out the natural lumbar lordosis. The patient's arms are either left to hang over the sides of the table or tucked beneath the head. Pancreatic or other visceral cancer patients may not be able to tolerate the prone position secondary to pain and may require the judicious use of sedation or the use of the lateral decubitus position.

The next step in performing the block is the identification of several important anatomic landmarks and marking them on the skin. It is highly preferable to mark the skin with ink to prevent misdirection of the needle later in the block. The landmarks for this approach are the twelfth ribs bilaterally and the inferior aspects of the T-12 and L-1 spinous processes. These landmarks should be delineated for every block and connected to form a shallow isosceles triangle (see Fig. 1). The points where the line from the inferior aspect of the L-1 spinous process intersects with the twelfth rib

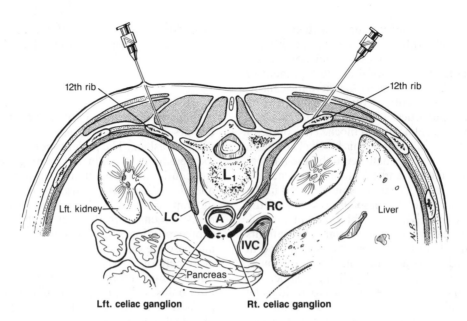

Figure 1 Kappis-Moore technique.

should lie 7 to 8 cm from the midline. This point usually corresponds to the junction of the paraspinal muscles and the twelfth rib. It is extremely important to insert the needle no farther laterally than 8 cm, as it has been shown that more lateral insertion endangers the kidneys. The whole area is prepared and draped in a sterile fashion, and skin wheals with local anesthetic are then raised at the intersection points.

Needle selection should be based on the size of the patient. For most patients, a 6- to 7-inch, 20- to 22-gauge spinal needle is adequate and provides excellent tactile sensation for the operator. Obese patients may require longer needles to allow proper placement. The first needle pass should be angulated at 45 degrees from the horizontal plane of the patient's back (see Fig. 1). The direction should be at the body of the first lumbar vertebra, which should be encountered as bony contact at an average depth of 6 to 9 cm; earlier bony contact is indicative of touching the transverse process. After contact with the body of the vertebrae has been achieved, the needle should be grasped at skin level to give the operator the depth of the pass on subsequent insertions. The angle of the needle is then increased to approximately 60 degrees and readvanced. The second advance should meet bone at a depth 2 to 3 cm deeper than the previous attempt. The needle is then progressively "walked off" the lumbar body. Correct needle placement on the left can often be confirmed by the observation of needle pulsation transmitted from the aorta and the tactile sense of needle movement. The insertion of the right-sided needle should progress in a similar fashion, using the depth knowledge gained through the left placement. Placement of both needles should be 1 to 1.5 cm anterior to the anterior vertebral margin. Aspiration tests should then be performed in four quadrants and a test dose of local anesthetic given.

Epinephrine in a 1:200,000 concentration may be added to signal unintentional intravascular injection. Using epinephrine containing local anesthetic for the skin wheal and muscle infiltration may also help in preventing painful hematomas in these areas during the postblock period. The introduction of the local anesthetic should have little resistance and may approximate the sense of an intravascular injection, given the loose areolar tissue surrounding the plexus. One may then proceed with placement of further local anesthetic or neurolytic solutions. Considerable argument takes place in the literature on the issues of single injection versus bilateral injection, radiologic guidance, and the volumes of anesthetics. These controversies will be discussed later in this chapter.

Two other techniques of celiac plexus block have recently been espoused in the anesthetic literature. These are the transaortic and the transaortic loss of resistance techniques. Landmarks are the same as those for the posterolateral approach, and the needle is advanced until a characteristic sense of aortic wall penetration occurs and free-flowing blood is aspirated. The needle is advanced through the anterior wall of the aorta until either no blood is aspirated or a 5 ml loss of resistance syringe with saline meets an increased resistance to injection, indicative of aortic wall penetration, followed by loss of resistance of the anterior periaortic space. This method virtually guarantees spread of solutions on the celiac plexus, although dilution of the agent by leaking blood may be problematic. No significant complications have been reported with this approach.

The anterior percutaneous approach was first described by Wendling in 1917. His technique involved infiltrating the abdominal wall with local anesthetic and inserting a needle just below and to the left of the xiphoid process until meeting bony contact o the vertebral column. He then blindly placed between 50 and 80 ml of local anesthetic through the needle. Authors and reviews of the day felt this approach to be inherently risky and this technique was abandoned. The radiologic community has recently begun to use this technique once more, both with good results and with low complication rates. Lieberman et al recently used an anterior approach with 20-gauge needles and fluoroscopic control to place local anesthetic at the first lumbar vertebral level. Despite the fact that this approach may easily allow puncture of the colon and other intra-abdominal organs, none of their patients suffered any ill consequences; specifically no occurrences of retroperitoneal hematoma or abscess, peritonitis, pancreatitis, or biliary problems were noted. The radiologic literature abounds with reports on transabdominal biopsies of pelvic lymph nodes in which intestine and vascular structures are probably violated, all with extremely low complication rates. Radiologists also perform translumbar aortic puncture for aortography with needles 20 gauge and larger, with a complication rate of 0.6 percent. Although more clinical data and trials on this technique need to be accumulated, it may very well become a standard approach in the future because of its ease of employment.

In almost all of the major studies on celiac plexus block, the two-needle approach is used. With this technique, good to excellent pain relief is achieved in 90 to 94 percent of patients with visceral cancer pain. Although originally this two-needle approach was based on anecdotal clinical results, recent studies have confirmed the anatomic basis for the success of the technique. These reports show that unilateral injection has very inconsistent spread to the contralateral side and that the aiming point for the left-sided needle should be at the upper third of L-1, with the right-sided needle aimed 1 cm higher. In a recent study of Ischia et al using the transaortic approach in cancer patients, one needle was used, and a success rate of 93 percent was achieved. Computed tomographic (CT) scans confirmed circumferential aortic spread of the neurolytic solution. Until this technique of transaortic needle placement has been studied on a larger scale, the two-needle technique will remain the standard approach.

The volume, concentration, and types of neurolytic solutions used in celiac plexus block are also varied. For diagnostic blocks, the local anesthetic should be chosen on the basis of its potency and the likelihood of systemic toxicity. Lidocaine, 0.5 to 1 percent in 10 to 15 ml volumes per side, is effective in diagnostic block and can provide 1 to 2 hours of pain relief. Epinephrine in a 1:200,000 concentration should be added to the local anesthetic to signal intravascular injection. Tetracaine 0.1 percent or bupivacaine 0.25 percent can be added after the lidocaine to give longer-lasting pain relief, again in 10 to 15 ml volumes per side blocked. When celiac plexus blockade is used in the operating room, the postoperative side effect of postural hypotension should dictate the type of local anesthetic used, i.e., long-acting

agents provide long-acting hypotension. In our experience, diagnostic blocks have occasionally provided long-term pain relief.

Phenol and absolute alcohol, the two most common neurolytic solutions used in long-term celiac plexus block, have histologically identical effects on nervous tissue. Obviously, the incorrect placement of either solution can have disastrous consequences. The unintentional intravascular injection of alcohol produces inebriation, while phenol may cause tinnitus and central nervous system symptoms, including seizures. In general, most large studies have used alcohol in concentrations of 50 to 100 percent. We use 50 percent alcohol mixed with 1 percent lidocaine, as alcohol injection may be associated with exquisite pain. Some clinicians prefer not to mix local anesthetic with alcohol because they use this feeling of deep visceral reproduction of pain as a confirmation of needle placement. The volume of this agent to be used is 20 to 25 ml per side. Alcohol has the disadvantage of not being compatible with radiographic contrast media, while phenol is miscible with contrast medium. If phenol is selected, 15 to 20 ml of 6 percent solution per side is adequate. Some question also arises as to whether the block may be repeated at frequent intervals as both alcohol and phenol are not permanent blocks. If the patient survives long enough to require a second or third block, these may be safely performed at 2- to 6-month intervals with success rates of more than 90 percent.

Perhaps the most frequently discussed topic in anesthetic pain management today is that of the debate over the use of radiologic techniques in identifying needle placement. Some authors believe that there should be no x-ray guidance, while others advocated CT for celiac blocks. In a large retrospective study on celiac blocks for patients with pancreatic cancer pain, Brown found that radiologically guided needle placement did not affect the quality of pain relief nor the incidence of complications. Other authors, however, recommend CT for all celiac plexus blocks. CT does not, however, prevent complications from occurring, despite the claims of its proponents, as case reports in the literature prove. The prudent approach seems to be one that takes the middle ground. Fluoroscopy, although exposing the clinician to radiation, allows accurate placement of block needles without undue expense or involvement of very complicated equipment. Fluoroscopy also allows visualization of injection of contrast before neurolytic injection. It has been our clinical experience that, even with negative aspiration of the block needles, rapid disappearance of dye, indicative of intravascular injection, has occurred. Fluoroscopy also allows the operator to see muscle fascicles and respiratory variation of the dye injection, representing intradiaphragmatic placement of the block needle tip. One can also easily obtain "hard copies" of the block placement for patient files. CT is most likely to be of use in the patient who is massively obese, has evidence of metastasis with distortion of anatomy, or in the previously blocked patient with incomplete relief.

SPLANCHNIC BLOCK

Some authors make a distinction between celiac plexus block and splanchnic block. Although the end result is the same blockade of the sympathetic and visceral contributions, little or no parasympathetic blockade occurs with splanchnic block. The difference between celiac and splanchnic block lies in the final location of the block needle, since the target for celiac block is the L-1 body, while in splanchnic block, the target is the T-12 anterolateral margin. The needle tip in splanchnic block therefore lies posterior or cephalad to the diaphragm, while the needle in the classic Kappis-Moore technique described earlier lies anterior or caudad to the diaphragm. Purported advantages in splanchnic block are that less volume is needed for successful blockade and that there is less hypotension because the lumbar sympathetics are not blocked by this route. Definite disadvantages include that there is a considerable risk of pneumothorax compared with celiac block as well as endangerment of the thoracic duct.

COMPLICATIONS

The complications related to celiac block can be divided into three areas: (1) hypotension secondary to the sympatholytic nature of the block; (2) structures unintentionally transgressed along the way; and (3) those related to incorrect placement of the needle with injection of neurolytic or local anesthetic solutions. The family of the patient with terminal cancer should also be counseled that the patient may die within a few days of receiving the block. It is our clinical experience that the patient with terminal cancer is often driven by the pain, and death is not uncommon shortly after the relief of pain.

Hypotension is by far the most common complication encountered. Decreases in systolic blood pressure of 30 to 40 mm Hg are not uncommon and are usually seen when the patient assumes the upright or sitting position postblock. These orthostatic changes usually disappear after 24 to 48 hours and are often ameliorated by volume loading preblock. Severe hypotension with 80 mm Hg pressure swings are encountered in fewer than 20 percent of patients. The hypotension is caused by pooling of blood in the gut after the loss of vasoconstrictor activity secondary to the block.

Pneumothorax has been reported in celiac plexus blockade, but occurs in less than 1 percent of patients. Similarly, there is risk of renal perforation, especially if the needles are placed more than 7.5 cm from the midline. When they are inserted more laterally, renal impalement can be expected to occur in approximately 10 percent of cases. Other structures, such as the thoracic duct, have been reported to be punctured in extremely rare instances. An interesting case report revealed that, subsequent to receiving a celiac plexus block, a patient became paraplegic; this was believed to be secondary to injury to the artery of Adamkiewicz occurring during the block. The authors of the above report suggest a single-needle approach on the right to avoid the artery, but the rarity of this complication, combined with the overall better results with the two-needle approach, seems to warrant the continued application of the latter technique.

Violation of the vena cava or the aorta would not seem prudent because of the theoretical risk of retroperitoneal hematoma; however, the risk of bleeding after puncture has proved to be nonexistent. The intentional perforation of these vascular structures in the techniques of Ischia and Feldstein reported earlier has led to no serious complications in patients followed for appropriate time intervals. Patients who are anticoagulated are not candidates for deliberate transgression of the aorta or vena cava. Obviously, intravascular injections are to be avoided and should be prevented by careful aspiration techniques along with the use of fluoroscopy.

Incorrect placement of the needle in the subarachnoid or epidural space has been reported. It is most likely caused by striking the transverse process of either T-12 or L-1 and mistakenly identifying this depth as the body of the corresponding vertebrae. Use of radiologic guidance should preclude this event.

Permanent neurologic damage can obviously occur with the placement of phenol or alcohol near motor fibers. Paralysis, sexual dysfunction, and dysesthetic changes in the lower extremity due to spread to the lumbar plexus or centrally have been reported. Interestingly, in a large retrospective study, radiologic technique has not been proven to reduce the incidence of these complications. It would seem prudent, however, to employ either fluoroscopy or CT when performing neurolytic blocks. An additional insurance against nerve damage is to clear the needle of neurolytic solution by injection of local anesthetic or saline before removal of the needle to prevent against deposition on nerves during withdrawal. Pleural effusion has also been reported with alcohol blocks of the celiac plexus, presumably secondary to diaphragmatic irritation with exudation of fluid.

SUGGESTED READING

Adriani JD. Regional anesthesia techniques and applications. St. Louis: Wilt Green Inc, 1985.

Brown DL, Bulley K, Quiel EL. Neurolytic celiac plexus block for pancreatic cancer pain. Anesth Analg 1987; 66:869–873.

Cousins MJ, Bridenbaugh PO. Neural blockade in clinical anesthesia and management of pain. Philadelphia: JB Lippincott, 1988.

Ischia S, Luzzani A, Ischia A, Faggion S. A new approach to the neurolytic block of the celiac plexus: the transaortic technique. Pain 1983; 16:333–341.

Lieberman RP, Nance PN, Cuka DJ. Anterior approach to celiac plexus block during interventional biliary procedures. Radiology 1988; 167:562–564.

Moore DC. Regional block. A handbook for use in the clinical practice of medicine and surgery. 4th ed. Springfield IL: Charles C. Thomas, 1965:145.

Raj PP. Practical pain management. Chicago: Year Book, 1986.

Ward EM, Rorie DK, Nauss LE, Bahn RC. The celiac ganglion in man: normal anatomic variations. Anesth Analg 1979; 58:461–465.

ORGANIZATION OF A PAIN CLINIC

P. PRITHVI RAJ, M.B.B.S., F.F.A.R.C.S.

Although Bonica introduced the idea of team approach to the treatment of pain as early as the 1950s, it was much later, in the 1960s, that the first multidisciplinary pain center was developed at the University of Washington in Seattle. In 1976, Medical World News listed only 17 pain clinics across the country, but the number mushroomed to 278 by 1979. A directory recently published by the American Pain Society and the American Academy of Pain Medicine lists among its members 240 pain clinics in the United States. How many more are functioning outside these Societies is unknown.

Early unidisciplinary pain clinics offered mainly anesthetic and surgical methods for pain relief. Their outcomes were generally poor, due to the lack of knowledge of pain mechanisms and limited technical resources. Today there is a much broader knowledge of pain mechanisms and a variety of improved techniques along with a desire on the part of clinicians to work together as an interdisciplinary team. This bodes well for future success in the management of patients with chronic pain.

ORGANIZATION OF A UNIVERSITY-BASED PAIN CENTER

There is no standard approach to developing a pain center in a university hospital. Opening even a modest pain center involves an incredible amount of planning, writing, negotiating, and public relations.

Initial Phase

One or two physicians actively engaged in the care of chronic pain patients should become leaders and form an ad hoc committee to investigate the feasibility of establishing a pain center. The first issues that this committee must deal with are the scope of pain center and the documentations of a present and potential pool of eligible patients.

The conclusions of the ad hoc committee on the establishment of the pain center should be presented to the executive body of the institution, which should include the chairpersons of various departments, the dean of the medical school, and the chief administrator of the hospital. Once these proposals pass the executive committee, the dean or the chairman of the department should actively engage in appointing a director, encouraging existing pain clinic activities, and publicizing the work of its members.

The selection of an appropriate director is crucial to the development and success of a pain center. The director must demonstrate the qualities of a scientist, clinician, teacher, and administrator. He or she must be interested in the formation of a center for the multifaceted study of pain. First and foremost, he should have considerable experience in managing patients with chronic pain and must actively participate in pain clinic activities. His academic background should document his deliberate attempts to obtain experience in basic researches in pain.

The director must be able to integrate ideas related to the role of the pain center. He must carefully monitor the quality and quantity of research to be conducted by the center. He must also be a good personnel manager and be able to define the roles of the clinical and nonclinical faculty associated with the center. Responsibilities of the pain director are listed in Table 1.

Although there are advantages to appointing the director through the department, the pain center is best served if the director is directly responsible to the dean of the medical school. This arrangement gives the director independence from departmental pressures and allows him to function more efficiently.

Formation of the Pain Team

Clinical Staff

Depending on the results of a needs assessment by the ad hoc committee, the director should be empowered to recruit as assistant professors at least two nontenured clinicians with an interest in pain to provide 5-day per week coverage of the pain clinic. Other qualified and interested physicians already in the institution should be drawn into the clinic. Generally, anesthesiologists, neurologists, neurosurgeons, psychiatrists, and psychologists form the nucleus of the team (Table 2).

Not all staff specialists need to work as primary

Table 1 Responsibilities of the Pain Center Director

Administrative
- Overall operation of the center
- Developing policies and procedures according to accepted medical standards
- Developing short-term and long-term goals of the center
- Preparing annual operating budget
- Selecting and appointing appropriate motivated staff in the pain center

Clinical
- Personally providing clinical care; being identifiable to patients
- Coordinating the multidisciplinary input to develop patient pain management program
- Assuring quality care for all patients treated at the center
- Directing the pain conference

Research and Education
- Initiating and coordinating all research and educational activities of the center

physicians; they can also play an important role as consultants. For example, a team pharmacologist can fulfill a key role in the drug detoxification program. The functions of the nonphysician clinical staff is delineated in Table 3.

Secretary

The secretary is vital to the smooth functioning of a pain center. He or she functions as an appointment secretary, receptionist, and telephone operator. Through careful scheduling, the secretary can avoid embarrassing delays and inconvenience to everyone. He or she can save the physician a great deal of time and screen out patients who will not have better outcome from the pain center management. The secretary also coordinates patient admissions to the hospital. His or her feedback regarding the patient's feelings and reaction to the therapy can be valuable.

Administrative Manager

From its beginning, the center needs an administrative manager. He or she should be familiar with the medical center and the medical faculty billing practices, policies, and procedures of the hospital and medical school. The manager is helpful in the early planning phase and can later serve as the financial officer of the pain center.

The administrative manager should be committed to planning and carrying out a cost-center approach to the financial management of the Center. During the early phase, he or she must develop a formula for the participation of all members of the interdisciplinary team. It must be understood that a high patient volume will be required for the center to achieve self-sufficiency, which assumes a substantial time commitment from the clinical faculty. Individual arrangements must be negotiated with departmental chairpersons, as well as with the hospital, for the nonphysician employees of the center. Until the center is operating to capacity, a contract or other mechanism to cover overhead must be negotiated with the hospital and/or the medical school. The contract with the hospital should cover space, equipment, and salaries for nonmedical pain center personnel.

The administrative manager should study the relative advantages of billing and collection systems. In most centers, the best approach is likely to be a negotiated contract with the medical faculty practice system because of the pain center's interdisciplinary personnel, the variety of patients served, and the need for outside consultants.

Physical Facilities

The need for and type of facilities may vary from one center to another, depending on the patient load, the

Table 2 Functions of Pain Center Physicians

Psychiatrist
- Performs psychiatric evaluation and develops behavioral program
- Treats psychopathic conditions
- Monitors drug abuse and drug withdrawal symptoms

Orthopedist
- Serves as a consultant for low back pain, arthritis, reflex sympathetic dystrophy, and sports injuries
- Assesses the functional disability of patients and their prognosis

Physiatrist
- Assesses functional disability
- Conducts active rehabilitation and work hardening program

Neurologist
- Performs a full neurological consultation and investigation
- Has special expertise in treating headaches, facial pain, neuropathies, and central pain syndromes

Neurosurgeon
- Serves as a consultant for radiculopathies, spinal stenosis, peripheral nerve injuries, cranial and spinal cord lesions, and cancer pain.

Anesthesiologist
- Offers a diagnostic and therapeutic nerve block service
- Objectively assesses the mechanism underlying the pain
- Diagnoses pain pathways
- Performs neurolytic therapeutic nerve blocks for visceral and cancer pain
- Performs therapeutic invasive procedures for low back pain, myofascial pain, herpes zoster, reflex sympathetic dystrophy, and cancer pain

Table 3 Functions of the Nonphysician Clinical Staff

Nurse
- Plans and organizes the patient flow in the pain center
- Assists in procedures at the center
- Monitors patients
- Orders supplies and equipment
- Facilitates communication between staff and the patient
- Coordinates medical care in case of emergencies

Psychologist
- Does structured interview and psychometric testing
- Teaches appropriate coping skills
- Offers operant conditioning and group therapy programs

Physical therapist
- Educates patients regarding their functional goals
- Assesses patient progress by objective measurements of their functions
- Provides physical therapy program

Vocational counselor
- Performs vocational assessment to determine whether a patient can return to a former job or requires retraining

Social worker
- Performs psychosocial evaluations of the patient
- Provides follow-up psychosocial counseling
- Provides the center with valuable feedback of home environment of the patient
- Encourages family participation in the program

expertise of the individual consultants, and the nature of the clinical program. The planning for space should begin long before the director is hired. Only by early and direct intervention at the level of the dean and or chief hospital administrator to consolidate relevant ambulatory clinics can the director hope to acquire the space needed by the pain center.

The facilities should be easily accessible to a patient from the patient parking lot. It should be centrally located to the general flow of ambulatory patients. The design of the pain center should permit a neat and orderly flow of patient traffic from the reception and waiting area to the consultation office, the treatment room, and the billing clerk. There should be ample room for transport of patients who arrive in wheelchairs and on stretchers.

Sharing space with other clinics (e.g., oncology, neurology, or orthopedics) can be hectic if not properly organized. Specifically, shared space is usually not conducive to the psychiatric interview of patients. Assignment of temporary space should not be tolerated for long, since the process of relocation can drain enthusiasm of the clinic's leaders, and moving offices disrupts patients.

Outpatient facilities should consist of a waiting room, the secretary or receptionist's office, several examination rooms, a minor operating or nerve-block room, proper rooms for psychiatric interventions, and adequate storage for patient records, equipment, research materials, and maintenance supplies. In addition to patient care facilities, the pain center director and staff require office space for patient consultation as well as for study and teaching. A large conference room is needed for weekly conferences, which can house a library.

Scope of the Pain Center

The initial scope of the center should be limited, and realistic service limits may be necessary. It may be advantageous to have a research focus which may bring participants together. Too rapid growth into a large, undifferentiated pain center may overwhelm and fragment staff efforts and diminish accomplishments. A modest, well-focused start may be preferable. Initial patient referrals can be acquired through informal chats with colleagues, formal presentation at departmental meetings, and communications with referring physicians and physicians in various other specialty clinics. Ethical techniques to increase the number of patients include radio, television, and newspaper interviews. A brochure that describes the pain center and its services in some detail is useful for both patients and referring physicians.

One particularly delicate matter is the formation of pain teams through which the consultants work. Their composition and member contributions reflect the team's philosophy of treatment, which varies according to the discipline of the team leader. Since all members of the pain team are involved either directly or indirectly in the evaluation and treatment of each patient, and as evaluations and interviews are done routinely by indi-

vidual members, a working relationship must allow debate about specific management under the umbrella of conceptual consensus. The team accumulates all information on each individual patient and collects it to form a coherent evaluation and treatment plan. The patient perceives this system as helpful. The patient is encouraged to experience the program as a supportive environment in which all staff members are genuinely involved.

DAY-TO-DAY ACTIVITIES AT THE PAIN CENTER

Preadmission Patient Screening

Since patients are referred by a private physician or workmen's compensation board, every effort should be made to obtain and review patient records before an appointment is made. The patient's referring physician is requested to send a complete resume of previous treatment and consultations, a comprehensive summary of the patient's current condition and diagnosis, laboratory results, and radiographs. This summary is carefully reviewed by the medical director and/or screening committee to determine whether or not a patient should be admitted to the pain center.

Making an Appointment

All appointments should be made by the secretary and confirmed in writing. New patients should receive a letter indicating the date, time, and precise location of the appointment. A descriptive brochure of the pain center is enclosed with the letter that describes its operation in some detail, including instructions on how to reach the center, how to make an appointment, what is needed for consultation, and what to expect during the first visit.

Fees and Payments

The patient should be made aware of the professional fee structure when he makes the first appointment. The initial consultation fee should be competitive with similar fees charged by other specialists in the community.

Initial Visit

The director admits each patient and assigns a physician (patient manager) to him or her. The manager is responsible for the initial examination of the patient, for requesting and coordinating consultants, and for liaison between the patient, his or her personal physician, and other members of the pain team.

Medical Evaluation

Appropriate therapy depends on an accurate physical and psychological diagnosis. Nothing can replace a good history and a thorough physical examination including appropriate investigations. The medical evaluation includes selected radiographic and laboratory studies as well as electromyography and thermography when indicated.

Psychological Evaluation

All patients should have a psychological interview and should undergo psychological testing by a clinical psychologist or a psychiatrist designed to assess pain levels, personality, and attitudes toward health, and to screen for anxiety, depression, and hypochondrias.

The Pain Conference

The pain conference is essential for the patients in whom the diagnosis or therapy are uncertain. It must be attended by the medical director, pain consultants, pain staff (including the nurses), and administrative manager. The frequency of the meetings varies with patient volume, but they should be held at least once per week. At these meetings, the patient's manager makes a formal case presentation to the group. Members of the pain group who have not seen the patient are given an opportunity to ask questions and make comments. After the conference, the patient's manager relays the recommendation of the team to the patient and to the referring physician. The referring physician can then decide whether the therapy can be carried out in the pain center or by him. If treatment is to be done at the pain center, the manager helps coordinate the treatment plan. The patient's manager is responsible for writing progress reports and providing follow-up.

Most of these patients can be seen as outpatients. They must occasionally be admitted to the hospital for intensive or specialized evaluation or therapy. Patients who require admissions include the following:

1. Those at risk for psychosis or suicide.
2. Those requiring a well-monitored drug withdrawal program.
   Emergency admission for potential serious sequelae (e.g., pneumothorax or hypotension) to drugs or techniques.
3. Those who will benefit over the long term from an initial intensive rehabilitation therapy.
4. Those with complex problems that require multidisciplinary invasive work-up and/or a surgical procedure for pain relief.

It is preferable that the patients be admitted to a separate unit where the nursing staff can be trained to observe their responses to diagnostic and therapeutic procedures, to run drug profiles, and to watch patients during withdrawal.

On-Call Coverage

Night and weekend inpatient care and telephone coverage for outpatients must be provided. In the university set up, residents and fellows assume this responsibility under the guidance of the pain faculty on-call.

Record Keeping

The history and physical examination, review of the facts pertinent to the pain syndrome, diagnosis, plan of management, and treatment must be recorded in the patient's chart. Letters are dictated promptly to the referring physician insurance carriers, workmen's compensation bureau, and if necessary, to employers and lawyers. Follow-up visits and patient response to the treatment program is recorded in a standardized manner by the multidisciplinary team and communicated to responsible parties promptly.

Follow-Up

Patient follow-up visits allow periodic monitoring to assure team members and patients that gains made are maintained in their home environment. New problems are identified, medications are adjusted, and education and cognitive awareness are promoted.

Research

Clinical research can usually start soon after the establishment of the center without additional funding. As specialties are brought together through activities of the developing center, interaction and communication increase and collaborative research projects ensue.

Teaching

Since pain centers require extensive resources and facilities, they are usually located in major medical centers. They therefore should become more responsible for developing effective teaching programs for undergraduate, graduate, and postgraduate health care professionals. Medical students should be offered an elective in the pain center. Residents in anesthesiology, neurosciences, physical medicine, and psychiatry should spend 1 to 2 months in the center. A pain fellowship program of 6 months to 1 year should be offered.

ORGANIZATION OF A FREE-STANDING PRIVATE PRACTICE PAIN CLINIC

A private practice pain center is organized by individuals, hospitals, or various health and medical organizations. It generally consists of medical, surgical, psychiatric, and support personnel working in a cost-effective environment that has its own budget autonomy. Various consultants share responsibility in such a clinic, based on mutual agreements and following well-defined guidelines.

Most private pain centers are located in or immediately adjacent to a hospital. The advantages of such a location are (1) the proximity of the operating rooms; (2) the availability of specialized personnel in other medical disciplines; and (3) the availability of ancillary care, such as critical care and emergency care units.

The operations of private pain centers involve the integration of multiple specialties and health care personnel into a team for treating patients with complex chronic pain syndromes, using a novel constellation of techniques. The successful management of such an endeavor requires a strong center director.

A private pain center may satisfy many significant needs of a community that otherwise can provide no solution for such problems as industrial injuries, back pain, arthritis, and pain due to cancer. Pain centers can also provide relief to local physicians who must treat an escalating population of patients with chronic pain. Physicians in the community welcome the availability of highly specialized and comprehensive pain managers who were otherwise available in only a few major metropolitan medical centers.

SUGGESTED READING

Bonica JJ. Importance of the problem in evaluation and treatment of chronic pain. In: Aronoff GM, ed. Evaluation and treatment of chronic pain. Baltimore, Munich: Urban and Schwarzenberg, 1985.

Carron H, Rolwingson JG. Coordinated outpatient management of chronic pain at the University of Virginia Pain Clinics. In: New approaches to treatment of chronic pain: a review of multi-disciplinary pain clinics and pain centers. Rockville, MD: NIDA Research Monograph 36, 1981:84.

Ghia JN, ed. The multidisciplinary pain center: organization and personnel function for pain management. Boston: Kluwer Academic Publishers, 1988.

Maya F, Mayne GE. Organization of a pain clinic. In: Raj PP, ed. Practical management of pain. Chicago: Year Book Publishers, 1986:20.

Simmons JW, Avant WS Jr, Demski J, Parishen D. Determining successful pain clinic treatment through ventilation of cost effectiveness. Spine 1988; 13:342–344.

OUTPATIENT ANESTHESIA

ADULT OUTPATIENT ANESTHESIA

L. REUVEN PASTERNAK, M.D., M.P.H.

Ambulatory surgery remains the fastest growing and, to a large extent, the least explored area of anesthesia practice to date. Unlike other advances in health care which arose in response to new technologies or breakthroughs in research, ambulatory surgery has developed largely as a response to financial and social concerns from nonmedical groups. Both private and government third-party payors have mandated that procedures be performed on an outpatient basis to control the rising costs of health care. As a result, this area has sustained the greatest expansion of any surgical program, growing from less than three million to more than eight million procedures from 1980 to 1988. It is anticipated that by the mid-1990s, out-patient surgery will account for more than 50 percent of all surgical procedures, with an even greater proportion among pediatric patients. These figures do not include same-day admission patients. The equally impressive growth of this group has also contributed to a precipitous decline in preoperative admissions.

In addition to its growth in volume, ambulatory surgery is changing in the medical acuity of patients and nature of procedures performed in this setting. At the beginning of its explosive growth in the early 1980s, ambulatory surgery tended to consist of relatively minor procedures performed in healthy patients. During the last several years, however, performance of ambulatory surgery on ASA Class III and IV patients has become commonplace. Furthermore, the list of procedures has expanded to include such operations as tonsillectomies and major laser surgery of the airway. New surgical techniques, especially the performance of abdominal surgery through the laparoscope, are opening up the prospect of performing such major procedures as cholecystectomies and resection of uterine fibroids on an outpatient basis. These and other developments are moving ambulatory surgery from the realm of minor procedures in ancillary operating rooms to the forefront of major changes and challenges in anesthesia practice.

PREOPERATIVE EVALUATION

Philosophy

Decisions regarding procedure and patient selection have usually been based on the presumed complexity of the surgery without consideration of the medical condition of the patient and the associated risk of anesthesia. Although anesthetic technique is being modified for this patient population, it is increasingly apparent to clinicians that even the most diligently administered anesthetic often carries a greater risk for the patient than the surgical procedure itself. This concern is especially true for patients undergoing general anesthesia and for those with significant medical disease. However, little information is available concerning risk assessment with no agreement on appropriate risk stratification or morbidity measures. Consequently, one of the areas of greatest concern to anesthesiologists is that of the preoperative evaluation. While surgeons have retained the ability to assess their patients fully before surgery, the anesthesia staff often find that they must evaluate their patients in a hurried fashion immediately before surgery.

The philosophy of the preoperative history and physical examination is to address those issues relevant for the safe administration of anesthesia. As such, the rule is to do what is reasonable rather than to engage in preparation for every remote circumstance. The preoperative examination is not an appropriate time or place to engage in primary care or general health care screening. Histories, physical examinations, and laboratory tests should be obtained on the basis of their utility to the anesthesia staff and not as a general overall medical screening. The goals include identifying risk factors that may affect the patient's clinical management, obtaining appropriate laboratory work in a timely fashion, and educating the patient regarding issues relevant to his or her anesthesia. When previously undiagnosed or inadequately controlled medical conditions are encountered, the patient should be referred back to the surgeon or primary care provider, where appropriate and consistent care may be instituted.

452

Agreement among the anesthesia staff regarding the content and conduct of appropriate preoperative assessments is very important, especially when performed by ancillary staff under their supervision. While there is sufficient art in the practice of anesthesiology to allow for individual variation in practice, it is imperative that the anesthesia group reach a consensus on major issues. These concern such matters as required laboratory tests, accepted values for these tests, and causes for cancellation, such as NPO violations, upper respiratory infections, and significant abnormalities on physical examination.

A major issue in this area is the timing of the preoperative evaluation. There is a clear advantage for both the patient and anesthesiologist in having a preoperative evaluation before the day of surgery. In addition to educating the patient about his or her anesthesia, there is greater assurance that avoidable cancellations or delays can be averted. However, appropriate patient preparation must be balanced against the inconvenience of taking additional time off from work and home responsibilities to make a visit to the surgical facility. There are clearly circumstances in which the scope of surgery and risk of anesthesia are sufficiently minor to allow for evaluation by anesthesia staff on the day of surgery on the basis of information provided by their primary care provider or surgeon. In such a system, it must be made clear that the evaluation by other physicians does not constitute a clearance for surgery. This decision is the province of the anesthesiologist on the basis of the available data in consideration of his or her unique knowledge about anesthetic techniques and agents.

Nonetheless, there are several medical conditions of sufficient concern to the anesthesiologist because of potential perioperative and postoperative morbidity (Table 1). It is strongly advised that patients with these medical conditions be evaluated by the anesthesia staff before the day of surgery to allow appropriate preparation for their procedure. Patients who are otherwise healthy but who are undergoing more complex procedures, such as intra-abdominal resections or explorations, are also best evaluated by the anesthesia staff before surgery. Objections by surgeons or patients to such a visit should be answered with an explanation that the special risks associated with these circumstances can only be appropriately assessed by a trained anesthesia staff.

History and Physical Examination

The history and physical examination should be directed to specific anesthesia concerns. A patient questionnaire filled out before the history will help direct the examiner's attention to appropriate organ systems. Auscultation of the heart and lungs and examination of the airway are of course routine, as well as any observation of gross neurologic or other abnormalities. As with any preoperative assessment, careful documentation of findings is important. At our institution, the history and

Table 1 Conditions for Which Preanesthesia Evaluation is Recommended Before the Day of Surgery

Cardiocirculatory
History of angina
History of coronary artery disease
History of myocardial infarction
Past cardiac surgery
Symptomatic arrhythmias (atrial and/or ventricular)
Hypertension (diastolic > 110 mg Hg, systolic > 160 mm Hg)
History of congestive heart failure

Hematopoeitic
Sickle cell disease or other hemoglobinopathy, coagulopathy
Coagulation disorder

Respiratory
Asthma: patient is taking chronic bronchodilator or is steroid dependent and/or has had an acute episode within 1 month
Significant chronic obstructive pulmonary disease
Past major airway surgery
Other significant respiratory disease or history
Upper and/or lower airway tumor or obstruction

Endocrine
Diabetes mellitus controlled with insulin or oral agents
Adrenal disorders
Active thyroid disease

Neuromuscular
History of seizure disorders
History of significant central nervous syndrome
History of myopathy or other muscle disorders

Hepatic
Ascites
Other active hepatobiliary disease or compromise

Musculoskeletal
Kyphosis and/or scoliosis causing functional compromise
Temporomandibular joint disorder
Cervical or thoracic spine injury or surgery

Oncologic
Patients receiving chemotherapy
Other oncology process with significant physiologic residual

Gastrointestinal
Massive obesity (> 140 percent ideal body weight)
Hiatal hernia
Symptomatic gastroesophageal reflux

physical examination are entered on a standardized form that is also provided to primary care providers to maintain consistency of documentation.

Patients likely to receive regional anesthesia should also receive an examination of the back, extremity, or other area where anesthetic may be administered and/or surgical intervention may occur.

Laboratory

While the physical examination is somewhat standard, the nature of appropriate laboratory testing remains ambiguous. Protocol testing has evolved as a convenient means of relieving the examiner of the responsibility of decision making and to ensure the availability of all required tests on the day of surgery. Such an approach has found greatest utility in circumstances where anesthesia staff have delegated this responsibility to other physicians or ancillary staff.

Such a practice has a strong tendency to result in excessive testing, however, subjecting the patient to potential invasive procedures and added costs. In a review by Kaplan et al of 2,000 patients undergoing elective surgery who received a routine battery of complete blood cell count, differential cell count, prothrombin time (PT), partial thromboplastin time (PTT), platelet count, glucose level, and six channel chemistries, it was found that 60 percent of these tests would not have been performed had they been done only on the basis of clinical indications. Of these, only 0.22 percent revealed abnormalities that might have affected perioperative management. Interestingly, none of these were acted upon or affected surgical or anesthetic management. Similarly, Wyatt's study of ambulatory patients over a 1-year period was done with one group receiving selective work on the basis of demonstrated need and another undergoing protocol bio-chemical profile, complete blood count, and urinalysis. In both groups, patients older than 40 years of age underwent electrocardiography, those older than 50 years of age underwent chest radiography, and those receiving anticoagulant therapy were tested for PT and PTT. Cancellation rates for the two groups were virtually unchanged (6.9 percent versus 6.4 percent). In the group undergoing routine laboratory tests, 99 percent of the 4,058 tests were normal, with only 1 percent resulting in an abnormality requiring cancellation. Of the electrocardiograms, 99.93 percent were normal, as were 99.97 percent of the chest films. While this patient population was likely quite healthy, it does note the limited benefit and increased costs of automated laboratory profiles.

Clearly, the performance of laboratory tests beyond those ordered by the surgeon should be considered on the basis of their potential utility to the anesthesiologist. The patient's medical condition and likely form of anesthesia for the procedure should be taken into consideration. While appropriate data need to be available, numbers should not be generated solely on the basis of obscure possibilities or curiosity. In this area more than any other, the anesthesia staff must arrive at a consensus to provide direction for surgeons, their own assistants, and primary care providers. Our protocol represents an evolution that is a combination of observation and consensus.

At present the only universally required test is a hematocrit (Table 2), although the utility of even this test in a young, healthy patient is debatable. Although routine urinalyses were standard in the past, they have been discontinued due to the very limited yield of information in patients without problems obtained from the history and physical examination. Urinalyses are now performed only in individuals with a positive history of genitourinary disease, metabolic disorders (e.g., those with diabetes mellitus) or who are undergoing surgery in this organ system. Similarly, chest films are now obtained only in individuals with a history or physical examination positive for respiratory or cardiac disease.

A review of preoperative laboratory requirements at our institution by a consensus group of anesthesiologists, surgeons, and internal medicine specialists has produced a re-evaluation of the need for routine electrocardiography in patients older than 40 years of age, for serum anticonvulsant levels in patients receiving anticonvulsive

Table 2 Preoperative Laboratory Testing

Laboratory Test*	Patient Group
Hematocrit	All patients
WBC, Platelets, PT, PTT	Oncology patients
	Patients receiving anticoagulant therapy
Type and screen	As per surgery
Sickle cell test	At-risk patients without prior documented results
Na, K	Patients receiving diuretic therapy who do not have renal compromise
Na, K, Cl, BUN, creatinine, glucose	Patients with renal compromise
	Diabetes mellitus
	Hepatic dysfunction
Urinalysis	Patients with renal compromise
	Genitourinary infection
	Urologic procedure
Electrocardiography	Patients with any history of cardiac disease or arrhythmia
	Age > 50 years
Chest x-ray examination	Patients with acute/chronic respiratory condition
	Patients undergoing thoracic procedure
Theophylline, Anticonvulsant Levels for patients on these drugs.	

*These are recommended laboratory tests and are not comprehensive. Testing should be individualized based on the patient's medical condition and needs.

medication, and for serum theophylline levels in patients taking bronchodilators. Cardiologists and internists believed that patients who were under the regular care of a physician and who had no indication of cardiac disease on the basis of the history and physical examination need not undergo this test until the age of 50 to 60 years. Similarly, anesthesia staff indicated that their principal concern for patients receiving anticonvulsants and bronchodilators was not the serum level but their clinical presentation. Internists concurred in this assessment, noting that these levels were guidelines titrated to clinical improvement. Thus, patients who are symptom free may, in the future, be considered under adequate management regardless of serum medication levels. Subsequently, these routine tests will likely be deleted in the near future; decisions in this regard should await further studies. However, the significant reduction in testing likely to emerge from these groups indicates the need for continual review of these practices. The recommended tests in Table 2 may thus be considered highly sensitive, with future parings enhancing specificity.

PATIENT SELECTION

Although the patients and procedures in the ambulatory setting are increasingly diverse, it must be remembered that these procedures are elective and should be undertaken only in patients who are appropriate candidates and adequately prepared for surgery. Patients should be medically stable; those with systemic illnesses must be under the care of a primary care physician or appropriate specialist and compliant with prescribed therapy. The procedure should be brief in duration (preferably <3 hours) and with little likelihood of significant postoperative complications for both surgery and anesthesia, such as respiratory distress or bleeding from the operative site. Patients in whom major fluid shifts are anticipated, especially those requiring transfusion, or who are likely to experience postoperative respiratory, cardiac, or other system compromise should be admitted postoperatively for observation. The assignment of a patient to ASA class III or IV should not in itself preclude performance of surgery on an outpatient basis. However, this practice is dependent on adequate preoperative evaluation, appropriate patient selection, and judicious management as indicated by the availability of appropriate preoperative information in a timely fashion.

Finally, but not least in importance, patients must expect to be ready for discharge within 4 hours of completion of the procedure and be assured that appropriate care is available at their discharge location to assist with any problems. This requires that a responsible adult accompany the patient to that location and be available immediately if necessary. Absence of such assistance is a contraindication to continuing with the procedure unless the surgical service is prepared to admit the patient postoperatively.

Decisions regarding preoperative or postoperative

admission must often be made without the guidance of definitive clinical studies or protocols. When one is faced with this circumstance, it is appropriate to apply a common sense approach that requires that several conditions be met. Indications for preoperative admission include the need to perform further preoperative diagnostic tests, therapeutic preparation (e.g., hydration, pulmonary toilet), or preparation for special anesthetic techniques that cannot be done on an outpatient basis. Admission for elective consultations, rapid correction of chronic conditions, or for physician or patient convenience to preserve the elective surgical schedule is inappropriate. When time is of the essence for performance of the surgical procedure and the risk of delay is greater than the potential risk of anesthesia, the surgeon should note in the record the reasons why surgery cannot be delayed, and arrange admission to minimize the risk from anesthesia.

Age

There is no inherent limit to the age at which ambulatory surgery procedures may be performed in the geriatric population. We have routinely done outpatient procedures in patients older than 80 years of age without complications. The limiting factor in these individuals is not age but by the medical condition of the patient and anticipated problems with surgery or anesthesia.

Cardiocirculatory Disease

Cardiocirculatory disease is one of the most common medical conditions encountered in ambulatory surgery for adults. Outpatient procedures in patients with cardiocirculatory disease is dependent on the extent of the lesion and physiologic compromise. A patient whose cardiac disease, whether corrected or not, leaves him or her in a debilitated state should not be considered for outpatient surgery and is best observed overnight and discharged the following day.

Hypertension is the most commonly encountered cardiocirculatory condition. In general, it is desirable that systolic blood pressure be below 160 mm Hg and the diastolic pressure below 110 mm Hg. Compliance with medical therapy is imperative, with referral for appropriate medical management in instances of poor control or compliance. Sometimes, even with maximal medical management, optimal control is not achieved. In these cases, patients are allowed to arrive the day of surgery with admission indicated postoperatively in those cases where they experience significant perioperative changes that persist through the recovery period.

Because hypertension is associated with cardiac, renal, and cerebrovascular compromise, thorough evaluation and laboratory tests, including electrocardiography, are indicated. Measurements of serum sodium and potassium are mandatory for patients on diuretic therapy and, like the electrocardiogram (ECG), should be obtained within a week of surgery. Hypokalemia (K<3.5) is a relative contraindication to surgery due to the enhanced risk of arrhythmias, although further assessment may change this level to 3.0. Normalization of serum potassium by intravenous pushes on the evening before or the day of surgery is inappropriate, since it does not address the need to re-establish intracellular stores.

Patients with documented carotid artery disease or episodes of altered mental status must also have these problems addressed before surgery can be considered. If surgical correction or further medical therapy is not indicated, postoperative observation overnight should be considered if general anesthesia has been administered.

Patients should take their regular medication on the morning of surgery to ensure appropriate control through the perioperative period. Due to the NPO status of these patients, diuretic therapy may be withheld to avoid intravascular depletion. It is better to have patients bring their medication with them and take it in the ambulatory surgery center where fluid intake can be controlled. Otherwise, they should be instructed to take their medications with sips of water at the usual time.

Angina pectoris is the other entity frequently encountered among the adult population. Patients who have had coronary artery bypass grafts with subsequent relief from all symptoms and no evidence of change on the ECG are managed in a routine fashion. At our institution, unstable angina, defined as angina at rest or episodes of changing frequency or severity, is treated as an absolute contraindication to outpatient management, and patients are admitted postoperatively. In those patients with stable angina, a visit with their cardiologist or internist is required before their anesthesia evaluation, including an ECG within 1 week of the procedure. A change in the ECG within the past 6 months or an abnormality in a patient who has no known cardiac disease is an indication for consultation with an internist or cardiologist before consideration for outpatient management. In these instances, clearance for ambulatory management is contingent on the determination that the change does not represent evidence of recent infarct or ischemia.

As with patients receiving antihypertensive medication, established drug regimens for this condition should be continued through the day of surgery, including beta-blocking agents, calcium channel blockers, and nitroglycerin patches. Anesthetic management for these patients requires scrupulous attention to avoid hypertension, tachycardia, and hypoxia. Administration of short-acting beta-blocking agents, such as esmolol or labetalol, immediately before induction of anesthesia have been demonstrated to blunt undesired physiologic responses to laryngoscopy and intubation.

Asthma

Asthma is the most common chronic respiratory disease encountered in the ambulatory setting. It can vary from mild, easily controlled episodes of bronchospasm to fatal episodes of respiratory failure. Intraoperative events such as endotracheal intubation or surgical stimulation may provoke bronchospasm; therefore, the patient with asthma should be optimally treated preoperatively. All chronic bronchodilator medications are continued throughout the perioperative period.

If theophylline preparations are given, administration of a serum theophylline concentration within 24 hours of surgery may be helpful. In the past, a documented therapeutic level before surgery was considered mandatory. However, because of the significant variation in response to this class of drugs, it has been decided that one should proceed with surgery on the basis of clinical presentation rather than on the basis of pharmacologic levels. Patients who are not experiencing distress and who have been symptom free for several months are accepted for surgery without the need to obtain theophylline levels. On the other hand, those patients who have demonstrated a proclivity to reactive airways are required to have demonstrated therapeutic levels before surgery can be begun.

Patients receiving inhalation nebulized bronchodilator therapy should receive treatment immediately before coming to the operating room. Individuals who are steroid dependent should also receive their medication as scheduled on the day of surgery, with additional "stress" doses of 100 mg of hydrocortisone administered immediately preoperatively and 4 hours after surgery, even in instances where steroids have been discontinued within the past 12 months. A chest x-ray examination is indicated for patients with a history of recurrent episodes of respiratory distress.

Pulmonary function studies are indicated for patients with evidence of major reactive airway disease who, despite appropriate medical treatment, have indications of respiratory compromise. These tests are then repeated after administration of bronchodilator therapy, with a 15-percent improvement indicating the presence of reversible disease for which further medical therapy should be instituted before surgery is performed.

Chronic Obstructive Pulmonary Disease

Patients with chronic obstructive pulmonary disease are managed in a fashion similar to that of asthmatics in that they must be under the continuing care of a physician with appropriate medical management to optimize their condition. A chest x-ray examination and pulmonary function studies are advised, especially if general anesthesia is likely. While preoperative admission for pulmonary toilet is rarely indicated, patients experiencing dyspnea at rest or with minimal activity are inappropriate candidates for ambulatory surgery for other than minor procedures with sedation or regional anesthesia. When general anesthesia is planned or likely, it is best to ensure the availability of a postoperative bed for observation.

Diabetes Mellitus

Diabetes mellitus is the most common endocrine problem managed in the ambulatory surgical setting.

Given the high incidence of end-organ disease, especially in adults with long-standing insulin-dependent diabetes mellitus, attention must be directed to determining the extent of such conditions as renal or cardiocirculatory compromise.

A principal concern in managing these individuals is the avoidance of hyperglycemia and hypoglycemia. Insulin-dependent diabetics should have their cases scheduled in the morning at a time that alows adequate preoperative preparation and postoperative recovery. In our unit, they are instructed to arrive at the preoperative preparation site no later than 8:00 AM with their insulin, which is administered after obtaining a Dextrostix and the starting of an intravenous solution containing glucose, usually D5 lactated Ringer's. The usual dose is half of the normal dose if the glucose is above 150 and one-third of the normal dose for values of 90 to 150.

Patients taking oral hypoglycemic agents are instructed not to take their medication on the day of surgery, as the extended half-life of these medications is greater than 24 hours. The balance of appropriate management is difficult for diabetics. The stress of surgery is known to increase serum glucose through several mechanisms, and careful attention to this issue should include a test of the patient's glucose level during the perioperative and recovery periods. Based on Dextrostix obtained during the perioperative and postoperative period, sliding-scale insulin is used as necessary for these and insulin-dependent diabetics. In fact, we have generally not needed to administer insulin to these patients.

Seizures and Mental Retardation

Patients with seizure disorders should have optimal control of seizures before outpatient surgery or any elective surgery is considered. Patients with intractable seizures or seizures based on metabolic derangements, or those who require extensive continual nursing care are not appropriate candidates for outpatient surgery and should be admitted postoperatively. As with asthmatics, we are tending to rely more on clinical presentation than on pharmacologic data. Patients whose seizures are well controlled generally do not need serum anticonvulsant levels. The exceptions to this rule are those with a history of seizures despite careful medical management and children who, because of their rapid rate of growth, need frequent adjustment of their dose of medication. These latter two groups of patients are best advised to have seen the physician managing their disorders immediately before surgery.

Patients with cerebral palsy and seizure disorders may be at risk for aspiration. Episodes of choking, cyanosis, or other related distress increase the risk for aspiration of stomach contents under anesthesia. A chest radiogaph should be obtained to determine the extent to which chronic aspiration and/or pneumonia may have resulted in residual damage, and as a baseline for further reference.

Sickle Cell Disease

Patients with sickle cell disease are at particular risk for crises when they experience dehydration, acidosis, or hypoxia. As such, prolonged NPO status can predispose these individuals to unnecessary risks. Initially, we had required that all patients with sickle cell disease be admitted preoperatively. However, as with the patients with diabetes mellitus and other chronic conditions, we have encountered a spectrum of presentation and have modified our approach. Those patients who are stable without a history of crisis within the previous 12 months and who are otherwise in good health are brought to the outpatient unit at 7:00 AM regardless of surgery start time. Intravenous access is established and hydration is initiated with maintenance plus one-quarter the calculated deficit per hour for a minimum of 2 hours before surgery. In our experience, these patients have done well without increased morbidity. Patients with a history of end-organ infarction or frequent crises are admitted preoperatively to ensure overnight hydration before surgery.

Patients requiring transfusion to decrease the sickle hemoglobin (Hbs) concentration to less than 40 percent do so the day before surgery as outpatients under the direction of their respective medical services. Because of the risks and questionable benefits of this practice for minor surgery, however, preoperative transfusion is being re-evaluated and is likely to be modified in the near future.

Upper Respiratory Infections

The viral upper respiratory tract infection (URI) is usually a mild, self-limiting disease that does not preclude routine activities. However, the URI is perceived to be a much more significant disease by the anesthesiologist, and considerable controversy persists about the advisability of anesthesia for patients with current or resolving upper respiratory infections. It is generally agreed that the presence of productive or "croupy" cough, fever, purulent nasal discharge, malaise, or an abnormal chest radiograph are indications for postponing the elective case. This approach is based on the observation that bronchial reactivity is markedly increased for up to 6 weeks after a URI and that, in animal studies, anesthetics have been associated with depressed lung bactericidal activity. Furthermore, arterial oxygen desaturation has been shown to be more prevalent in individuals with current URIs than in their healthy cohorts. We generally proceed with anesthesia in individuals with clear rhinorrhea who are afebrile without other evidence of distress. In clinical practice, many anesthesiologists anesthetize children who have recently recovered from a URI, because some children develop URIs with such frequency that it is nearly impossible to find periods between recovery and the "the next URI" during which to perform the operation. This situation is frequently encountered in children undergoing myringotomy for placement of tubes due to chronic otitis media. The difficult decision of whether to proceed with surgery is further compounded in patients who may have traveled significant distances for their surgery or for whom a delay in surgery poses a significant hardship.

Recently, there has been speculation that the presence of an URI does not constitute a contraindication to general anesthesia. However, two of these studies evaluated children undergoing mask anesthesia for myringotomy tube placement, while a third did not mention the nature of the procedures being assessed. More definitive studies will be needed to evaluate the response of these children to intubation and more prolonged anesthesia before adopting these guidelines, especially concerning bronchospasm as a phenomenon most often induced by mechanical forces in medically susceptible patients.

Under the circumstances, a rational approach to the patient with a URI or to the patient who is recovering from a URI is to reschedule for elective surgery at least 2 weeks—preferably 3 weeks—after the resolution of symptoms. Exceptions to this policy may be at the discretion of the anesthesiologist in consideration of the individual patient's medical history. Some may consider this an overly cautious recommendation; however, as these procedures are elective in nature, we believe that this conservative approach is warranted until well-controlled, prospective studies prove otherwise.

PATIENT INSTRUCTIONS

After the history and physical examination, written and verbal instructions are given to patients and their families, including NPO instructions, arrival times, and what to expect on the day of surgery. All patients are advised of the need to be escorted home by a responsible adult and of the advisability of having an adult available in their residence on the day of surgery. The possibility of unscheduled admission is also discussed, regardless of how minor the surgery or healthy the patient. Plans should be made for the possible care of children or dependent adults in the event that admission is required.

Preoperative Fasting

Preoperative fasting is aimed at reducing the risk of aspiration upon induction of anesthesia, with the duration of fasting balanced against the risk of hypoglycemia and dehydration. Although specific recommendations vary among centers, most are relatively similar. Interestingly, recent studies in adults demonstrate reduced gastric contents when patients are given 150 ml of clear fluid 2 hours before surgery. While new information may lead to changes in the practice of preoperative fasting, current guidelines at our center are consistent with the general practice of requiring NPO status after midnight. In anticipation of morning hunger, some patients may have a late dinner with large volumes of solids only 8 to 10 hours before general anesthesia. It is preferable that

they be advised not to have any solids after 9 PM to better ensure that these items have been adequately digested before induction of anesthesia.

Time of Arrival

Patients are instructed to arrive 2 hours before the scheduled start of the procedure to allow adequate time for preparation, with the patient ready in the event that the operating room is moving ahead of schedule. Discharge criteria (Table 3) are reviewed so that they know what they may have to expect postoperatively for discharge. As important, patients are specifically instructed to call the ambulatory surgery unit if an acute illness develops before the scheduled surgery. We have found this detailed approach to be of great value in minimizing delays, cancellations, and frustrations on the day of surgery.

PERIOPERATIVE MANAGEMENT

Ambulatory surgery is best performed with operating and recovery rooms and medical and nursing staffs dedicated to this purpose. Only in this circumstance can the specialized techniques and considerations unique to this specialty be appropriately employed. While having a dedicated area, patients undergoing anesthesia for ambulatory surgery procedures are nevertheless subject to the same risks as their inpatient counterparts and require the same intraoperative vigilance. This includes appropriate monitoring consisting of at least electrocardiography, blood pressure monitoring, and pulse oximetry/capnography.

Aspiration Prophylaxis

Several clinical conditions place patients at risk for aspiration. These include obesity, hiatal hernia, duodenal or gastric ulcers, or symptoms suggestive of esophageal reflux. As aspiration pneumonitis represents a potentially lethal complication, prophylaxis for these patients should routinely be given in the preparatory area, regardless of anticipated type of anesthesia. Ranitidine (150 mg) and metoclopramide (10 mg) taken orally with sips of water 1 hour or more before surgery have been demonstrated to reduce gastric contents significantly and to raise the pH of gastric fluids. Oral sodium citrate (25 ml) before induction, while increasing

Table 3 Discharge Criteria

1. Stable vital signs
2. No airway difficulties
3. No respiratory distress
4. Return to usual state of alertness
5. Return to usual ambulatory status (except as limited by surgery)
6. Stable wound site
7. Ability to retain fluids
8. Responsible adult caretaker to accompany patient and available at postdischarge site

the volume, will also increase gastric pH. Droperidol in doses of 10 to 20 μg per kilogram have also been demonstrated to decrease postoperative nausea and vomiting and the likelihood of complications during the postoperative period. Utilizing these measures, the anesthesia team can avoid placing itself in the position of having to perform rapid sequence inductions to avoid aspiration.

Preoperative Sedation

Preoperative sedation is used to produce a calm, cooperative patient and allow a smooth induction of anesthesia without prolonging the recovery period. Recommendations vary according to the preference of individual anesthesiologists and the specific needs of a given patient. In some centers, all patients receive preoperative sedation. However, we reserve preoperative sedation for those patients experiencing a heightened state of anxiety. In general, we have found the need for premedication to be minimal. Our approach is to establish good patient rapport and provide a gentle compassionate environment.

When sedation is needed, intramuscular injections should be avoided, with an oral agent administered with sips of water at least 1 hour before induction of anesthesia. Diazepam (5 to 10 mg by mouth) or midazolam (2 to 3 mg IV) are usually sufficient. In either case, preoperative sedation should be administered in a controlled setting and avoided when circumstances require transport of patients by nonmedical personnel from one distant location in the hospital to another. In addition, sedation is withheld from all patients experiencing respiratory compromise so as to prevent hypoventilation associated with sedation. Sedated patients should only be transported to the operating room with assistance and by stretcher or wheelchair. Finally, sedation administered immediately before induction in the operating room is usually "too little too late" in that it only prolongs the induction, enhances patient anxiety as he or she lies awake on the operating room table, and carries the greatest risk for postoperative sedation. If sedation is not accomplished before the patient enters the operating room, then the best course to pursue is that of an expedited but gentle induction.

Anesthesia Technique

As with any anesthetic, the primary concern is the provision of anesthesia in a fashion that allows for the performance of the procedure in a manner that is safe for the patient. However, the anesthesiologist must also be sensitive to concerns about efficiency and postoperative distress when selecting among techniques and agents. These include the time required for induction of anesthesia, emergence, and residual effects during the recovery period that may prolong the time to discharge. Anesthetic agents in ambulatory surgery should have a rapid onset, brief duration of action, and minimal side effects.

Intravenous Sedation, Regional Anesthesia

When surgical technique permits, sedation with local anesthesia provides the best guarantee of minimal postoperative distress. Individuals with significant respiratory and cardiac disease are especially good candidates for this management, as the potential risks of general anesthesia are avoided. Supplementation with regional anesthesia, such as axillary blocks, has been performed without difficulty in the ambulatory setting. Some of the traditional agents such as fentanyl and midazolam are currently being supplanted with shorter-acting narcotics such as alfentanil and the nonbarbiturate induction agent propofol.

Spinal and Epidural Anesthesia

"Central" regional anesthesia has a definite role in the ambulatory setting. Some procedures, such as arthroscopy of the knee, are especially suited to this method. In addition, procedures performed in the lower abdominal and perineal region or lower extremities in unstable patients, such as those with significant reactive airway disease, are appropriate for this management. However, in using epidural anesthesia, the increased induction time must be considered, and one must consider the potential for postoperative spinal headaches in the use of spinal anesthesia. The 20-minute period required for an epidural anesthetic to take effect may in fact prevent the performance of another brief procedure in that same room. More important, patients who sustain a spinal headache postoperatively are at risk for losing several days from duties at home or work. They may also potentially require admission and an equally invasive blood patch to remedy their condition. Patients receiving regional anesthesia must demonstrate a resolution of the block before discharge from the surgical facility. In those circumstances in which conductive anesthesia provides no definitive advantages over general anesthesia, the latter may be preferred for its rapid induction and emergence. The anesthesiologist must therefore weigh the relative risks and benefits of these techniques in making a decision.

General Anesthesia

General anesthesia, including endotracheal intubation, has been found to be a safe technique in the ambulatory setting. When possible, endotracheal intubation should be avoided so as to decrease the risks associated with intubation, including sore throat and other trauma to the airway. Of course, when airway compromise is likely, as with diagnostic laparoscopies with patient in the Trendelenburg position, intubation is indicated. The most common side effect of general anesthesia tends to be nausea and emesis. The best treatment for postoperative nausea and emesis is prevention in the operating room. Administration of droperidol (1.25 mg in adults, 25 to 50 μg per kilogram in children) at the time of induction of anesthesia and evacuation of all gastric contents immediately before extubation have proved successful in reducing this problem. The issue of whether narcotics or inhalational agents are more prone to induce nausea or emesis has yet to be resolved. In our experience, a balanced technique that permits lower concentrations of the volatile agents (less than ⅓ MAC) is also successful in preventing nausea and postoperative drowsiness. Data implicating nitrous oxide as a cause of nausea are still preliminary and are not sufficient to justify abandoning this agent.

POSTOPERATIVE CARE

As with inpatient procedures, transportation to the recovery area should be undertaken only after recovery from anesthesia with uncompromised ventilation and stable cardiocirculatory status have been demonstrated. Ambulatory surgery patients who undergo general anesthesia are as prone as their inpatient counterparts to develop transient hypoxia and should therefore receive supplemental oxygen during transport and initial recovery.

Despite the large number of procedures and techniques encountered in the ambulatory surgical setting, a common philosophy with regard to recovery is that no patient should be discharged whose physical function is significantly impaired and who will not have assistance readily available if needed. Previously, a mandatory recovery time of 4 hours for patients receiving general anesthesia and 2 hours for patients receiving sedation was strictly enforced. However, many of these patients, especially those receiving sedation, were clearly ready for discharge long before these times had been reached. Rather than using time guidelines, patients are discharged when they fulfill the physiologic discharge criteria.

Patients are held in the recovery room before discharge to the final stepdown unit contingent on stable vital signs, an alert mental status, and no respiratory distress. The stepdown unit should include private recovery areas and should have a quieter, more relaxed atmosphere than the recovery room. Patients should be placed in reclining chairs and encouraged to ambulate. Discharge criteria include stable vital signs, a return to preoperative mental and ambulatory status, a normal airway without signs of respiratory distress, a stable wound site, an ability to retain sips of fluid, and the assistance of a responsible individual who will be comfortable caring for the patient at home (see Table 3).

The problems most consistently delaying discharge

are postoperative pain and nausea with or without emesis, with the latter being the most frequent cause of unscheduled admission. A variety of analgesic regimens are appropriate for the postoperative pediatric and adult patient, but all should be used with the caveat that prolonged periods of drowsiness tolerated in the inpatient setting are not acceptable for the outpatient.

If discomfort is present but is mild in nature, acetaminophen is given if oral intake is tolerated. If narcotics are needed, small doses are titrated intravenously (e.g., morphine, 2 to 4 mg) as needed for analgesia. In a patient who is adequately relieved, these agents should be titrated to an endpoint to allow the patient to lie still while remaining alert and oriented. In those patients requiring postoperative analgesia, discharge orders from the surgeon should include medications for analgesia at home. Prior to discharge, written and verbal instructions are given. The written material should include clear instructions on how to reach a surgeon and anesthesiologist if a problem arises.

A frequently overlooked aspect of the ambulatory surgical system is that of follow-up. The discharge of the patient from the facility does not relieve the anesthesiologist of responsibility for the welfare of the patient during the postoperative period. Provisions for follow-up must be an integral portion of the performance of ambulatory surgery. As mailed questionnaires for follow-up have a notoriously poor record, telephone contact the day after surgery to detect postoperative complications and to address any questions is advised. At our institution, this system has provided a follow-up rate in excess of 90 percent.

SUGGESTED READING

Guay J, Santerre L, Gaudreault P, et al. Effects of oral cimetidine and ranitidine on gastric pH and residual volume in children. Anesthesiology 1989; 71:547–549.

Kaplan EB, Sheiner LB, Boeckman AJ, et al. The usefulness of preoperative laboratory screening. JAMA 1985; 253:3576–3581.

Kitz DS, Slusarz-Ladden C, Lecky JH. Hospital resources used for inpatient and ambulatory surgery. Anesthesiology 1988; 69:383–386.

Manchikanti L, Canella MG, Hohlbein LJ, Colliver JA. Assessment of effect of various modes of premedication on acid aspiration: risk factors in outpatient surgery. Anesth Analg 1987; 66:81–84.

Parnass S, Rothernberg D, Kerchberger J, Ivankovich A. Single dose esmolol for prevention of hemodynamic changes of intubation in an ambulatory surgery unit. Anesthesiology 1989; 71:A12.

Shott SR, Myer CM, Cotton RT. Efficacy of tonsillectomy and adenotonsillectomy as an outpatient procedure: a preliminary report. Int J Pediatr Otorhinolaryngol 1987; 13:157–163.

Wyatt WJ, Reed DN, Apelgren KN. Pitfalls in the role of standardized preadmission laboratory screening for ambulatory surgery. Am Surg 1989; 55:343–346.

PEDIATRIC OUTPATIENT ANESTHESIA

EUGENE K. BETTS, M.D.
ELIZABETH NICHOLAS, M.D.

Ambulatory anesthesia suits pediatric patients well because they usually lack systemic disease and convalesce rapidly, and because of the simplicity of many surgical procedures in young children as compared with adults. For example, congenital inguinal herniorrhaphies during infancy require only ligation and transection of the hernia sac at a high level, whereas acquired adult herniorrhaphies call for reconstruction of the inguinal canal.

Day surgery minimizes the length of the child's separation from the parents and decreases the incidence of nosocomial infections, a problem most common in the infant. In a 1968 study, the incidence of nosocomial infections was reduced from 17 percent to 5 percent by avoiding hospitalization. However, a study at The Children's Hospital of Philadelphia (CHOP) failed to demonstrate this advantage in a modern facility.

PATIENT SELECTION

The day surgery facility serves two classes of patients. The majority undergo admission, surgery, and discharge on the same day. Patients in the other group are hospitalized following surgery. Those expected to be ready for discharge the following morning stay overnight in a short-stay unit; those needing a longer postoperative hospitalization become inpatients. During fiscal year 1990 at CHOP, 51 percent of the 12,075 patients coming to the operating room were treated as straight day surgery patients. An additional 23 percent came to the operating room for day surgery but were then admitted as inpatients (48 percent) or short-stay patients (52 percent). In essence, any patient who does not need to be hospitalized for preoperative stabilization or evaluation is a candidate for admission to the operating room through day surgery.

Surgical or anesthetic considerations may require postoperative hospitalization. Prematurely born infants of less than 45 weeks' conceptual age frequently develop postanesthetic apnea and bradycardia. All the patients in Liu's study and 33 percent of the patients in Steward's study who developed postanesthetic apnea had a prior history of apnea. The authors of both studies conclude that prematurely born infants of less than 3 to 4 months postnatal age should receive inpatient apnea monitoring for 24 hours after anesthesia. More recent work by Kurth supports monitoring all prematurely born patients of less than 60 weeks' conceptual age for 12 to 24 hours postoperatively, but there are anecdotal reports of apnea occurring in these patients during their second year of life. Full-term (38 or more weeks postconception) infants become suitable candidates for day surgery after attaining 4 weeks of postnatal age *and* at least 44 weeks of postconceptual age.

PREANESTHETIC EVALUATION AND PREPARATION

Preanesthetic evaluations emphasize different areas in the child than in the adult. One- to two-year-olds are more prone to upper respiratory infections (URI), experiencing two to four colds a year. Secondary bacterial infections frequently prolong the disease beyond its usual 4-day course. Children with any two of the following have an URI: (1) mild sore or scratchy throat, (2) mild malaise, (3) sneezing, (4) rhinorrhea, (5) nasal congestion or stuffiness, (6) nonproductive cough, (7) mild fever (not greater than 38°C or 100.4°F). Combinations of 1 and 2, 3 and 4, or 5 and 6 require an additional symptom to make the diagnosis. The patient's mother is frequently a good judge of the presence or absence of an URI in her child.

Pulmonary mechanics return to normal about 5 weeks after an URI. However, URIs recur in many children during this interval. A large study by Cohen and Cameron of over 17,000 children demonstrated that patients with current or recent URIs were four- to sevenfold more likely to sustain a respiratory complication during or after general anesthesia than children without a history of URI. The relative risk of adverse respiratory events rose to 11 percent when the anesthetic management of the URI group included intubation.

More recent studies by Tait and co-workers in patients administered anesthesia by mask and by Betts and colleagues in intubated and nonintubated patients, using the criteria of Tait to define an URI, demonstrated no deleterious effects from anesthetizing *healthy* patients with an URI. Patients with signs and symptoms of lower airway disease (moist cough, rales, rhonchi, diminished breath sounds) are not healthy. At CHOP, most healthy patients with an URI are anesthetized.

Approximately 5 percent of our day surgery patients cancel before anesthesia is induced. Half of these patients cancel from home, and about half of the day surgery cancellations are for infectious processes, most commonly URI.

Loose deciduous teeth and dental appliances are common in children. Innocent (functional) heart murmurs need to be distinguished from organic lesions. The anesthetic implications of congenital syndromes must be determined. A prior history of infectious laryngotracheitis (croup) may indicate the presence of mild to moderate subglottic stenosis, as may the presence of a tracheostomy scar.

Recent exposure to an infectious disease may mean the patient is infectious, as many of the childhood exanthems are infectious during the prodromes. For example, varicella (chickenpox) is infectious from the onset of prodromal symptoms, about 24 hours before the appearance of the rash, until all of the lesions are crusted (usually 6 to 7 days after the eruption). As the incubation period varies from 11 to 21 days, we exclude from the day surgery unit children exposed to chickenpox 9 to 21 days earlier, as well as those with uncrusted lesions. The exception to this policy is roseola, which is relatively common and innocuous. These patients are not excluded.

Healthy patients do not require any routine preoperative laboratory determinations, but we feel it is prudent to obtain a hemoglobin or hematocrit determination within the 30 days before anesthesia if the patient is younger than 1 year old. The incidence of asymptomatic anemia in the general population is about 1 percent, and the physical examination lacks sensitivity in detecting anemia. If the patient has a microcytic anemia, surgery can usually be delayed until iron therapy has repaired the deficit. All postpubertal females are routinely screened for pregnancy as part of their blood work. Although we do make exceptions, we strongly prefer to do our preanesthetic evaluation within the 30 days prior to the day of surgery. This provides the opportunity to give written as well as verbal feeding instructions. Unfortunately, a major disadvantage of day surgery arises here, because the anesthesiologist who evaluates the patient only rarely anesthetizes the patient.

The preanesthetic visit also provides an opportunity for the child to become familiar with the hospital and some of the routines used during an anesthetic induction. This allays both their anxiety and that of the parents.

After the operating room schedule has been "finalized" for the next day, the patients are assigned times to arrive in the day surgery unit. The day surgery unit nurses call each family with these times and provide final feeding instructions as well as another opportunity to ask questions.

Preanesthetic Fasting

Recommendations for the duration of preanesthetic fasting in children are quite variable. Several recent studies suggest that traditional lengthy fasting practices may be overly restrictive. Sandhar and colleagues evaluated postintubation gastric volumes in children who had been fed 2 to 3 hours preoperatively with 5 ml per kilogram of pulp-free orange juice (maximum of 150 ml). They found no significant difference between these gastric volumes and those measured in unfed patients. Similarly, Schreiner and co-workers found no significant differences in gastric volume and pH when children permitted clear liquids *ad libitum* until 2 hours prior to induction were compared with those fasted in a conventional manner. The findings of these and other investigators have led us to modify our practice in recent years. We prohibit solid foods and milk products for 12 hours and offer clear fluids until up to 2 hours prior to the intended time of anesthetic induction. Breast milk is

treated as if it were a clear liquid. These guidelines hold for healthy children of all ages.

Despite careful planning and the use of verbal and written instructions, day surgery patients are frequently fasted longer than intended. The duration of fasting should be determined for each patient and, if prolonged, postoperative dehydration and hypoglycemia should be prevented by intraoperative intravenous 5 percent dextrose in lactated Ringer's solution. Half of the deficit may be repaired during the first hour and the balance during the succeeding 2 hours, in addition to the maintenance fluids required during this time.

Formerly, about 7 percent of our day surgery cancellations (0.3 percent of the total day surgery population) were because the feeding instructions were not followed and the child was fed on the morning of surgery. Permitting clear fluid oral intake until the patient leaves home for the hospital has reduced this cause of cancellations to nearly zero. In addition, if surgery is going to be delayed more than 2 hours, clear liquids can be offered, making the wait more easily tolerated by the young patient.

Premedication

The unallayed anxiety of unpremedicated children frequently prevents smooth anesthetic inductions. Stormy anesthetic inductions in children lead to an increased incidence of postoperative behavioral problems. The psychological advantages offered by premedication of a child can be negated by the battle and ensuing trauma associated with an intramuscular injection. An oral premedication using meperidine elixir, 1.5 mg per kilogram, diazepam, 0.2 mg per kilogram, and atropine, 0.02 mg per kilogram, provides postoperative analgesia (diminishing emergence delirium), mild relief of preoperative anxiety and tension, and diminishes the flow of saliva. The onset of action is rapid (10 to 20 minutes), and the premedication does not prolong emergence from anesthesia.

Midazolam given orally (0.5 to 0.75 mg per kilogram), rectally (0.5 to 1.0 mg per kilogram), or intranasally (0.2 mg per kilogram) effectively decreases preoperative separation anxiety and improves the quality of anesthetic induction. Emergence is not prolonged following operations of 1 to 2 hours' duration. Although intramuscular injections are usually avoided, the agitated and uncooperative child can be sedated with low-dose ketamine given intramuscularly. Hannallah has shown that a dose of 2 mg per kilogram facilitates intravenous cannulation or mask induction, without incurring the risk of postemergence hallucinations or nightmares.

We encourage young children to bring a security object (pacifier, doll, blanket) to the operating room with them. Some institutions allow the patient's parents to be present during the induction. The child is offered the mask and a story is told that includes the sensations the child is feeling, e.g., a rocket trip to the moon. After the anesthetic induction, monitors are applied. If the child declines the mask, anesthesia is induced intravenously. The global threat of being "suffocated" with a mask is psychologically much greater than the localized threat of a needle.

Of the three available approaches for anesthetic induction—rectal, intravenous, and inhalation—the last is the most commonly used. Halothane is an excellent inhalation induction agent; isoflurane is associated with a 5 percent incidence of coughing and breath holding during induction. We have seen laryngospasm with isoflurane inductions. Patient acceptance of inhalation inductions is increased by using masks "flavored" with an aromatic oil or solution (available in grocery stores).

Intravenous inductions using a 25- or 27-gauge needle can be used in the uncooperative child, or preferentially. A dose of barbiturate just sufficient to induce sleep (2 to 6 mg per kilogram), rather than anesthesia (5 to 7 mg per kilogram) may provide a more rapid emergence.

Rectal barbiturate or ketamine has also been used to induce anesthesia in patients 3 months to 5 years of age. Absorption of these agents is unpredictable, and their onset of action is variable owing to the presence of fecal material in the rectum and the first-pass effect of the liver. A dose of 25 mg per kilogram of methohexital does not prolong the emergence from anesthesia, when compared to 5 mg per kilogram of intravenous thiopental. However, rectal inductions are not as rapid as either inhalation or intravenous inductions (they add at least 10 to 20 minutes to the anesthetic).

Anesthetic Maintenance

The establishment of an intravenous infusion may not be necessary during an anesthetic if the superficial surgical procedure is short in duration (less than 20 minutes) and is not associated with a high incidence of postoperative nausea and vomiting. However, if the child has fasted for an unduly long time, an intravenous infusion should be started.

Oral or nasotracheal intubation does not contraindicate discharge home on the day of surgery. Postintubation croup is uncommon, especially when the diameter of the endotracheal tube permits a leak at less than 25 cm H_2O. The early signs of its development are usually present within an hour of tracheal extubation. If a barky cough or other sign of postintubation croup appears, our policy is to admit the patient for overnight hydration, humidification, and observation.

POSTOPERATIVE MANAGEMENT

Anesthesia

The anesthetic management should be designed to produce an awake patient at the conclusion of surgery who needs only a minimum of recovery room nursing. The need for postoperative pain relief should be met in the child as carefully as it would be in the adult. Simple wound infiltration with a long-acting local anesthetic such as bupivacaine can provide up to 3 to 5 hours of analgesia. Regional anesthetic techniques can provide excellent postoperative relief from the pain of many operations (circumcision, herniorrhaphy, orthopedic procedures).

Infants of 60 conceptual weeks of age or less are monitored for a minimum of 2 hours in the recovery room with a cardiorespiratory monitor equipped with an alarm. The following infants are monitored in this way for at least 18 hours after discharge from the recovery room (this obviously precludes their being discharged on the day of surgery): all infants of 44 conceptual weeks of age or less (both full-term and prematurely born); infants of less than 60 conceptual weeks of age with a preoperative history of apnea, bradycardia, or breathing abnormality; and infants who have apnea or bradycardia during the recovery room observation period.

Patients are discharged from the day surgery unit when they are medically fit for discharge, rather than being discharged according to a fixed time duration. Children who have had a myringotomy, with or without placement of a ventilating tube, are generally discharged 30 minutes after the conclusion of the anesthetic. Most other patients require at least 60 minutes.

We no longer require well-hydrated children to demonstrate their ability to tolerate oral intake prior to discharge. After repairing the preoperative fluid deficit intraoperatively, we take advantage of the recovery period to hydrate the patient with additional intravenous fluid equivalent to 8 hours at a maintenance rate. The parents are instructed to offer food or liquids only when the child expresses hunger (and not simply thirst). With this regimen, the incidence of vomiting is low.

Complications

Postanesthetic complications occur infrequently in these healthy patients. Approximately 2 percent of our straight day surgery patients are admitted postoperatively. Fifty percent are admitted because the operation performed was different than the one planned. The likelihood of emesis may be further reduced by intraoperative administration of an antiemetic such as droperidol, particularly during procedures notorious for eliciting vomiting such as strabismus repair or tonsillectomy. Inability to take fluids orally is the most common cause of admission after the patient has left the day surgery unit.

On the whole, the pediatric population is well suited to outpatient anesthesia and surgery. Although only 30 to 50 percent of surgery is done on outpatients today, it appears that the popularity of outpatient pediatric surgery will continue to increase. Diagnostic-related groups and prospective payment systems will also force reexamination of the need for preoperative inpatient admission the day prior to surgery. As long as patient safety can be maintained, this trend appears to be appropriate.

SUGGESTED READING

Broadman LM. Regional anesthesia for the pediatric outpatient. Anesthesiol Clin North Am 1987; 5:53–72.

Cote CJ. NPO after midnight for children: a reappraisal. Anesthesiology 1990; 72:589–591.

Epstein BJ, Hannallah RS. Outpatient anesthesia. In: Gregory GA, ed. Pediatric anesthesia. 2nd ed. New York: Churchill Livingstone, 1989: 729–766.

Kurth CD, Spitzer AR, Broennle AM, et al. Postoperative apnea in preterm infants. Anesthesiology 1987; 66:483–488.

MONITORING TECHNIQUES DURING ANESTHESIA

ELECTROCARDIOGRAPHIC MONITORING

DANIEL M. THYS, M.D.
JOLIE NARANG, M.D.

The intraoperative use of the electrocardiogram has developed markedly over the last several decades. Originally, this monitor was used during anesthesia for the detection of dysrhythmias in high-risk patients. In recent years, however, its importance as a standard monitor has been recognized, and its use during the conduct of any anesthetic is now recommended. Beyond its usefulness for the intraoperative recognition of dysrhythmias, one of the major indications for its use lies in the intraoperative diagnosis of myocardial ischemia.

THE NORMAL ELECTROCARDIOGRAM

Normal cardiac activity depends on the continuous transfer of electrically charged particles across cell membranes. As a result of this transfer, the electrical polarity in and around cardiac cells also changes continuously. Not all cells are depolarized at the same time, however, and electrical gradients are created. Along these gradients, small amounts of electrical current flow. The sum of all the currents flowing through the heart at any given moment represents the electrical potential of the heart. The electrocardiogram depicts a recording of the heart's electrical potential.

Normal Electrical Activity

The P wave

Under normal circumstances, the sinoatrial (SA) node has the most rapid spontaneous depolarization rate and is, therefore, the dominant cardiac pacemaker. From the SA node, the impulse spreads through the right and left atria. Conducting tracts can conduct the impulse to the atrioventricular (AV) node, but they are not essential. On the electrocardiogram (ECG), depolarization of the atria is represented by the P wave (Fig. 1). The initial depolarization involves primarily the right atrium and occurs predominantly in an anterior, inferior, and leftward direction. Subsequently, it proceeds to the left atrium, which is located in a more posterior position.

The PR Interval

Once the depolarization has reached the AV node, a delay is observed. The delay permits contraction of the atria and supplemental filling of the ventricular chambers. On the ECG, it is represented by the PR interval.

The QRS Complex

After passage through the AV node, the electrical impulse is conducted along the ventricular conduction pathways consisting of the common bundle of His, the left and right bundle branches, the distal bundle branches, and the Purkinje fibers. The QRS complex represents the progress of the depolarization wave through this conduction system. After terminal depolarization, the ECG normally returns to baseline.

The ST Segment and T Wave

Repolarization of the ventricles begins at the end of the QRS complex and consists of the ST segment and T

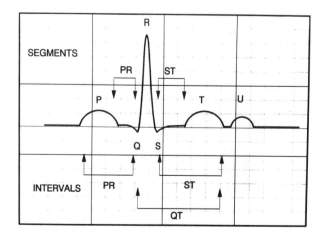

Figure 1 Segments and intervals of the normal ECG.

wave. While ventricular depolarization occurs along established conduction pathways, ventricular repolarization is a prolonged process occurring independently in every cell. The T wave represents the uncancelled potential differences of ventricular repolarization. The junction of the QRS and the ST segment is called the J-junction. The T wave is sometimes followed by a small "U" wave, the origin of which is unclear. An inverted "U" wave has been associated with several clinically significant conditions, such as hypertension, coronary artery disease, valvular heart disease, and certain metabolic disorders. There may be an association between exercise or rest-related "U" wave inversion and significant stenosis of the left anterior descending artery or the left main coronary artery.

Standard and Precordial Lead Systems

The small electric currents produced by the electrical activity of the heart spread throughout the body, which behaves as a volume conductor, allowing the surface ECG to be recorded at any site. The standard leads are **bipolar**, because they measure differences in potential between pairs of electrodes. The electrodes are placed on the right arm, the left arm, and the left leg. The leads are formed by the imaginary lines connecting the electrodes, and the polarities correspond to the conventions of Einthoven's triangle (Fig. 2). If each of the three standard leads is connected through a resistance of 5,000 ohms, a common central terminal with zero potential is obtained. When this common electrode is used with another active electrode, the potential difference between them represents the actual potential. On a standard 12-lead ECG, three unipolar limb leads are usually recorded: aVR, aVL, and aVF. The "a" indicates that they are augmented limb leads and were obtained using Goldberger's modification. In this modification, the resistors

are removed from the lead wires and the exploring electrode is disconnected from the central terminal, thus resulting in larger ECG deflections.

Additional information on the heart's electrical activity is obtained by placing electrodes closer to the heart or around the thorax. In the **precordial lead** system, the neutral electrode is formed by the standard leads and an exploring electrode is placed on the chest wall. The ECG is normally recorded with the exploring electrode in one or more of six precordial positions (Fig. 3). The positions are indicated by the letter "V" followed by a numeral from 1 to 6 indicating the location of the electrode on the chest wall.

INDICATIONS

Diagnosis of Dysrhythmias

Dysrhythmias are common during surgery, and their causes are numerous. They are most common during endotracheal intubation or extubation and occur more frequently in patients with pre-existing cardiac disease. The following are the major contributing factors to the development of perioperative dysrhythmias:

1. Anesthetic agents. Halogenated hydrocarbons, such as halothane or enflurane, are known to produce dysrhythmias, probably by a re-entrant mechanism. Halothane has also been shown to sensitize the myocardium to endogenous and exogenous catecholamines. Drugs that block the reuptake of norepinephrine, such as cocaine and ketamine, can facilitate the development of epinephrine-induced dysrhythmias.
2. Abnormal arterial blood gases or electrolytes. Hyperventilation is known to reduce serum

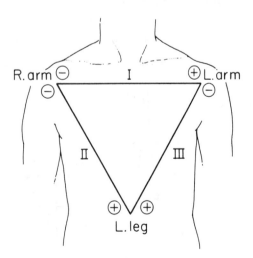

Figure 2 Einthoven's triangle. (Republished with permission from Thys DM, Kaplan JA. The ECG in anesthesia and critical care. New York: Churchill Livingstone, 1987.)

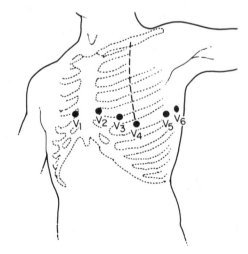

Figure 3 Standard precordial lead positions. (Republished with permission from Thys DM, Kaplan JA. The ECG in anesthesia and critical care. New York: Churchill Livingstone, 1987.)

potassium. If the preoperative potassium is low, it is possible to reduce serum potassium into the range of 2 mEq per liter and thus precipitate severe cardiac dysrhythmias.

3. Endotracheal intubation. This may be the most common cause of dysrhythmias during surgery and is often associated with hemodynamic alterations.
4. Reflexes. Vagal stimulation may produce sinus bradycardia and allow ventricular escape mechanisms to occur. In vascular surgery, these reflexes may be related to traction on the peritoneum or direct pressure on the vagus nerve during carotid surgery. Stimulation of the carotid sinus can also lead to dysrhythmias.
5. Central nervous system stimulation and dysfunction of the autonomic nervous system.
6. Pre-existing cardiac disease. It has been shown that patients with known cardiac disease have a much higher incidence of dysrhythmias during anesthesia than patients without known disease (60 percent versus 37 percent).
7. Central venous cannulation. The insertion of catheters or wires into the central circulation often leads to dysrhythmias.

Once a dysrhythmia is recognized, it is important to determine whether it produces a hemodynamic disturbance, whether treatment is required, and how urgently it should be applied. Treatment should be instituted promptly if the dysrhythmia results in marked hemodynamic impairment. Additionally, treatment should be instituted if the dysrhythmia is a precursor of a more severe dysrhythmia (frequent multiform PVCs, with R on T phenomenon) or when the dysrhythmia may be detrimental to the patient's underlying cardiac disease (tachycardia in a patient with mitral stenosis). For the detection of rhythm disturbances, the standard limb lead II is usually used, as it has a large P wave. (The detailed description and the management of dysrhythmias is dealt with elsewhere in this text.)

Diagnosis of Ischemia

Factors that predispose to the development of perioperative ischemia include the presence of pre-existing coronary artery disease, and perioperative events that affect the myocardial oxygen balance. Several perioperative clinical studies have found a high incidence of electrocardiographic evidence of ischemia (20 to 80 percent) in patients with coronary artery disease undergoing cardiac or noncardiac surgery. In the anesthetized patient, the detection of ischemia by ECG becomes even more important, because the hallmark symptom of angina is not available.

In recent years, it has also become evident that a significant number of patients suffer from asymptomatic or "silent ischemia." In these patients, ischemia is manifested by the characteristic ECG signs of myocardial ischemia in the absence of angina and is not necessarily associated with changes in hemodynamics or heart rate.

The ECG changes occurring during myocardial ischemia are often characteristic and can be detected with careful ECG monitoring. Although the ECG criteria for ischemia were established in patients undergoing exercise stress testing, they may also be applied to anesthetized patients (Table 1).

Although ST-segment analysis provides sensitive information about myocardial ischemia, it should be remembered that in approximately 10 percent of patients, underlying electrocardiographic abnormalities hinder the analysis. Such abnormalities include hypokalemia, digitalis administration, left bundle branch block, Wolff-Parkinson-White syndrome, and left ventricular hypertrophy with strain.

Diagnosis of Conduction Defects

Conduction defects occurring during surgery can result from the passage of the pulmonary artery catheter through the right ventricle, or they can be a manifestation of myocardial ischemia. Because high-grade (second- and third-degree AV blocks) conduction defects often have deleterious effects on hemodynamic performance, it is important that they be recognized intraoperatively.

ELECTROCARDIOGRAPHIC MONITORING SYSTEMS

The Three-Electrode System

As the name implies, this system utilizes only three electrodes to record the ECG. In such a system, the ECG is observed along one bipolar lead between two of the electrodes while the third electrode serves as a ground. A selector switch allows the user to alter the designation of the electrodes and, without changing the location of the electrodes, three ECG leads can be examined in sequence. While the main advantage of the three-electrode system is its simplicity, a major disadvantage is that for the diagnosis of ischemia it provides only a limited reflection of myocardial electrical activity.

Modified Three-Electrode Systems

Numerous modifications of the standard bipolar limb lead system have been developed, some of which are displayed in Figure 4. The modifications are used in

Table 1 ECG Criteria for Ischemia

Upsloping ST segment: 2 mm depression, 80 msec after J point
Horizontal ST segment: >1 mm depression, 60 msec after J point
Downsloping ST segment: >1 mm from top of curve to PQ junction
ST segment elevation
T wave inversion

an attempt to maximize P-wave height for the diagnosis of atrial dysrhythmias or to increase the sensitivity of the ECG for the detection of anterior myocardial ischemia. In clinical studies, these modified three-electrode systems have been shown to be as sensitive or more sensitive than the standard V_5 lead system for the intraoperative diagnosis of ischemia.

CS_5 Lead (Central Subclavicular)

The central subclavicular lead is particularly well suited for the detection of anterior wall ischemia. The right arm (RA) electrode is placed under the right clavicle, the left arm (LA) electrode is placed in the V_5 position, and the left leg electrode is placed in its usual position to serve as a ground. Lead I is selected to detect anterior wall ischemia, and lead II can be selected to monitor inferior wall ischemia and dysrhythmias. In the operating room, this CS_5 lead is the best and easiest alternative to the true V_5 lead for monitoring myocardial ischemia.

CB_5 Lead (Central Back Lead)

The CB_5 lead is efficacious for the detection of ischemia and supraventricular dysrhythmias, as demonstrated in a study comparing CB_5 and V_5 leads in patients with closed and open chests. The P wave was 90 percent larger than in lead V_5, and a good correlation between ventricular deflections of CB_5 and V_5 leads was noted. CB_5 is obtained by placing the RA electrode over the center of the right scapula and the LA electrode in the V_5 position. This lead may be used in certain patients with ischemic heart disease who may be susceptible to

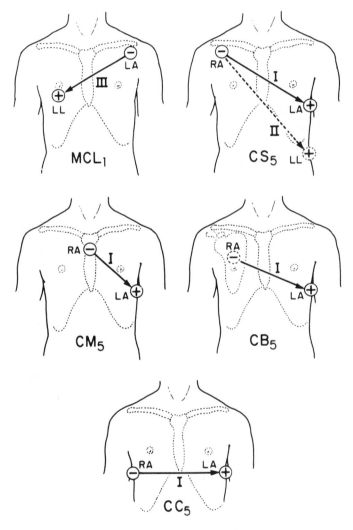

Figure 4 Modified precordial lead arrangements. (Republished with permission from Thys DM, Kaplan JA. The ECG in anesthesia and critical care. New York: Churchill Livingstone, 1987.)

the development of dysrhythmias during the perioperative period.

The differences between true unipolar precordial leads and the commonly utilized modified bipolar leads are well recognized. Bipolar precordial leads usually show a greater R-wave amplitude than standard precordial leads, and this can result in amplification of the ST-segment response. It has been shown that normalization of the degree of ST-segment depression to the height of the R wave increases the sensitivity and specificity of treadmill exercise testing. While similar corrections have not yet been tested during intraoperative monitoring, their possible importance should be kept in mind when one is examining intraoperative ECG recordings.

The Five-Electrode System

The use of five electrodes allows the recording of the six standard bipolar limb leads as well as one precordial unipolar lead. Generally, the unipolar lead is placed in the V_5 position, along the anterior axillary line in the fifth intercostal space. With the addition of only two electrodes to the ECG system, up to seven different leads can be monitored simultaneously. Thus, several areas of the myocardium can be monitored for ischemia or a differential diagnosis between atrial and ventricular dysrhythmias can be established.

In a recent study, patients were monitored with a 12-lead ECG system in an attempt to identify the leads, or combination of leads, that provide the maximal detection of intraoperative ischemia. Using a single lead, the greatest sensitivity was obtained with lead V_5 (75 percent), followed by lead V_4 (61 percent). Combining leads V_4 and V_5 increased the sensitivity to 90 percent, while with the standard lead II and V_5 combination, the sensitivity was only 80 percent.

Invasive Electrocardiography

The electrical potentials of the heart can be measured not only from a surface ECG, but also from body cavities adjacent to the heart (esophagus or trachea) or from within the heart itself.

Esophageal

The concept of esophageal electrocardiography is not new, and numerous studies have demonstrated the usefulness of this approach in diagnosing complicated dysrhythmias. A prominent P wave is usually displayed in the presence of atrial depolarization, and its relationship to the ventricular electrical activity can be examined. The esophageal electrodes are incorporated in an esophageal stethoscope and welded to conventional ECG wires. To observe a bipolar esophageal ECG, the electrodes are connected to the RA and LA terminals and lead I is selected on the monitor. In one study of 20 cardiac patients, 100 percent of atrial dysrhythmias were correctly diagnosed with the esophageal lead (using intracavitary ECG as the standard), while lead II led to a correct diagnosis in 54 percent of the cases and V_5 in 42 percent of the cases. Additionally, the esophageal ECG may help detect posterior wall ischemia due to its proximity to the posterior aspect of the left ventricle. With esophageal ECG, strict electrical safety precautions must be followed to minimize the risk of esophageal burn injury.

Endotracheal

The endotracheal ECG allows monitoring of the ECG when it is impractical or impossible to monitor the surface ECG. The endotracheal ECG consists of a standard endotracheal tube in which two electrodes have been embedded. This device may be most useful in pediatric patients for the diagnosis of atrial dysrhythmias.

Intracardiac

For many years, long central venous catheters filled with saline have been used to record intracardiac ECG. More recently, the use of a modified balloon-tipped flotation catheter for recording intracavitary electrograms was described. The multipurpose pulmonary artery catheter that is presently available has all the features of a standard pulmonary artery catheter. In addition, three atrial and two ventricular electrodes have been incorporated into the catheter. These electrodes allow the recording of intracavitary ECGs and the establishment of atrial or AV pacing. The diagnostic capabilities with this catheter are great since atrial, ventricular, or AV nodal dysrhythmias and conduction blocks can be demonstrated. The catheter is useful in the anesthetic management of many critically ill patients. The high-fidelity tracings obtained from the intracordial electrodes are relatively insensitive to electrocautery interference and are therefore useful for intra-aortic balloon pump triggering.

RECORDING AND INTERPRETATION

Basic Requirements

The function of the ECG monitor is to detect, amplify, display, and record the ECG signal. The ECG is usually displayed on an oscilloscope, and several monitors now offer nonfade storage oscilloscopes to facilitate wave recognition. These offer no advantages over direct-writing recorders, which enable accurate interpretation of difficult ECGs and provide a written record for the patient's chart. All ECG monitors for use in patients with cardiac disease should have paper recording capabilities. The recorder is needed to make accurate diagnoses of complex dysrhythmias and to allow careful analysis of all the ECG waveforms. In addition, the recorder allows one to differentiate real ECG changes from oscilloscope artifacts.

Standard ECG Recordings

The ECG is normally recorded on special paper consisting of grids of horizontal and vertical lines. Distances between vertical lines represent time intervals, while distances between horizontal lines represent voltages. The lines are 1 mm apart, with every fifth line intensified. The speed of the paper is standardized to 25 mm sec^{-1}. Therefore, on the horizontal axis, 1 mm = 0.04 sec and 0.5 cm = 0.20 sec. On the vertical axis, 10 mm represents 1 mV. On every recording, a 1 cm = 1 mV calibration mark should indicate that the ECG is appropriately callibrated.

Artifacts

The electrical signal that is generated by the heart and is monitored by the ECG is very weak, amounting to only 0.5 to 2 mV at the skin surface. To avoid signal loss at the skin-electrode interface, it is therefore imperative that the skin be prepared optimally. The skin should be clean and free of all dirt, and it is best to abrade the skin lightly to remove the part of the stratum corneum, which can be a source of high resistance to the measured voltages. To avoid the problem of muscle artifact, electrodes should be placed over bony prominences whenever possible. Muscle movement in the form of shivering can produce significant ECG artifact.

Electrodes and Leads

Loose electrodes and broken leads can produce a variety of artifacts that may simulate dysrhythmias, Q waves, or inverted T waves. Pre-gelled, disposable silver/silver chloride electrodes are usually used in the operating room. It is important that all of the electrodes be moist, uniform, and not out-dated. To ensure good contact between the electrode and the skin, the electrical resistance of the skin should be minimized (i.e., rubbed with alcohol) and excess body hair should be removed. Needle electrodes should be avoided because of the high risk of thermal injury. Some ECG monitors have built-in cable testers that enable a lead to be tested by connecting the cable's distal end to the monitor. A high resistance causes a large decrease in voltage, indicating that the lead is faulty. The main source of artifact from ECG leads is caused by the loss of the integrity of the lead insulation. This subsequently causes the lead to pick up other electric fields in the operating room such as the 60-Hz alternating current from lights or currents from an electrocautery device. Any damaged ECG lead should therefore be discarded. Lead movement can also lead to artifact.

Operating Room Environment

Many pieces of equipment found in the operating room emit electric fields that can interfere with the ECG: 60-Hz power lines for lights, electrosurgical equipment, cardiopulmonary equipment, and defribillator discharges. Most of this interference can be mini-mized by proper shielding of the cables and leads of the cardiogram, although at present the interference created by the electrosurgical equipment cannot be reliably filtered without distorting the ECG. Electrocautery is the most important source of interference on the ECG in the operating room, and it usually completely obliterates the ECG tracing. Analysis of the electrocautery has identified three component frequencies. The radio-frequency between 800 kHz and 2,000 kHz comprises most of the interference, coupled with 60 Hz AC frequency and 0.1 to 10 Hz low-frequency noise from intermittent contact of the electrosurgical unit with the patient's tissues. Preamplifiers may be modified to suppress radiofrequency interference, but these filter circuits are still not widely available in the operating room.

Monitoring System

Most ECG monitors have filters to decrease environmental artifacts. They can usually operate in two modes. The first is the monitoring mode operating in the frequency response range of 0.5 to 50 Hz. The monitoring mode eliminates artifacts, such as wandering baseline, but prevents clinical judgment about height of QRS or degree of ST-segment depression or elevation. Monitors also operate in diagnostic mode, which has a greater frequency response to 0.05 to 100 Hz. This mode should be used during cardiac surgery cases, because it allows the diagnosis of ischemia.

Automatic Recording

Holter monitoring has been used by a number of anesthesiologists to document the perioperative incidence of dysrhythmias and ischemia. In Holter monitoring, ECG information from one or two bipolar leads is recorded by a miniature magnetic tape recorder. Up to 48 hours of ECG signals can be collected. Subsequently, the tape is processed by a playback system and the ECG signals are analyzed. On most modern systems, the playback unit includes a dedicated computer for rapid analysis of the data and automatic recognition of dysrhythmias. The application of Holter monitoring is primarily limited to research. The Q-Med device is a small continuous ECG recorder that has been used in patients undergoing cardiac and noncardiac surgery. The device not only records the ECG signals, but also automatically analyzes the ECG tracing and sounds an alarm when ischemic changes are recognized. Abnormal events are selectively stored and are subsequently retrievable.

Computer-Assisted ECG Interpretation

There is little doubt that during prolonged visual observation of the ECG on the oscilloscope, certain dysrhythmias will go undetected. It was, for instance, clearly demonstrated that coronary care unit nurses failed to detect serious ventricular dysrhythmias in 84 percent of their patients. Various computers have therefore been designed for the automatic detection of dysrhythmias in an attempt to increase the detection of abnormal rhythms. In a prospective evaluation of such a system, it was found that the computer accurately detected 95.4 percent of ventricular premature beats but only 82.4 percent of supraventricular premature beats. Computer programs for on-line analysis of dysrhythmias and ischemia are now commercially available. Although they are used primarily in ambulatory care for the analysis of Holter monitor recordings, they can also be used intraoperatively. Recently, a system designed for continuous ST-segment analysis with display of trends in ST segment depression and elevation has been evaluated intraoperatively. The device monitored three selected leads and displayed the absolute values of the ST segment as a line. Upward deflection of the trend line indicated worsening ischemia, while a downward trend reflected a return of the ST segment toward the isoelectric line. It was suggested that once the device was clinically accepted, the awareness for ischemic changes was heightened among the participating anesthesiologists and therapeutic interventions were more rapidly instituted.

SUGGESTED READING

Clements FM, de Bruijn NP. Electrocardiography: monitoring for ischemia. In: Clinical monitoring. Lake CL, ed. Philadelphia: WB Saunders, 1990; 27.

McCloskey GF, Curling P. Electrocardiography. Anesth Clin North Am 1988; 6:903–916.

Thys DM, Kaplan JA. The ECG in anesthesia and critical care. New York: Churchill Livingstone, 1987.

CARDIOVASCULAR MONITORING

GREGG S. HARTMAN, M.D.
STEPHEN J. THOMAS, M.D.

In order to maintain cardiovascular homeostasis during the variable and often unpredictable stresses of surgery and anesthesia, the anesthesiologist must continually observe, quantify, integrate, and finally, act on all available data relevant to cardiovascular function. These include information from the patient's history, the surgical field, the conduct of the anesthetic as well as the continuous stream of numbers, pictures, and alarms from the impressive array of mechanical and electronic devices currently known as cardiovascular monitors. Each item of information must be interpreted in the context of the entire clinical picture; no specific piece of data is sacrosanct. Therapeutic decisions must be based on true, not erroneous, information.

It is useful to categorize cardiovascular monitoring in terms of either detection of myocardial ischemia or assessment of cardiac pump function. The former includes the electrocardiogram (ECG) (ST and T wave changes) and the echocardiogram (Echo) (changes in regional wall motion or systolic wall thickening). Measurement of pump function encompasses measurement of ventricular preload (central venous pressure, pulmonary artery pressure or left ventricular filling pressure, left ventricular volume as assessed by Echo), resistance to ventricular ejection (calculation of systemic vascular resistance, calculation of wall stress), contractility (ventricular function curves, end systolic pressure/volume relationships, ejection fraction), heart rate, and rhythm.

There is no difference of opinion as to whether to monitor or not; however, there is debate regarding whom and how much to monitor. Selection of monitors for a specific patient is based on the patient's preoperative medical condition and the physiologic trespasses anticipated from the proposed surgery. A precordial stethoscope, noninvasive arterial blood pressure determination, and ECG are sufficient monitors for the fit teenager undergoing a peripheral procedure. In contrast, the elderly cardiac cripple would merit direct blood pressure measurement and some or all of the equipment described above for evaluation of ischemia and pump function. The information or potential information gleaned from monitoring must be viewed in terms of the risk of complications directly attributable to the monitoring devices and the cost of the equipment versus the benefits derived from the data obtained (improved patient care and perhaps reduced hospital stay). This discussion focuses on monitoring devices currently available, the data they provide, indications for their use, and potential complications. Inspection, palpation, and auscultation, although crucial in complete evaluation of the patient, are not mentioned.

ELECTROCARDIOGRAPHY

The electrical activity of the heart (*not* its pumping function) is displayed on the ECG. Heart rate is easily calculated (R-R interval), and cardiac arrhythmias and myocardial ischemia are detected and diagnosed. The ECG is used for virtually all anesthetics.

ECG systems currently available employ three, four, or five electrodes that may be arranged in various configurations. Any arrangement should include either a true V5 (unipolar precordial) or modified V5 (bipolar frontal) lead for identification of anterolateral ischemia, a lead similar to the standard lead II for arrhythmia identification because P waves are usually of maximal amplitude in this lead, or both. Eighty-nine percent of the ST-T wave changes noted on a 12-lead ECG will be identified in lead V5, and the combination of V5 and lead II detects approximately 95 percent of these events. The most common set-up for three- or four-electrode systems is to place the left arm lead in the precordial V5 position with all others in their normal locations. Setting the selector switch to I permits monitoring of the modified V5 while lead II remains unchanged. The CB5 lead system also places the left arm lead in the V5 position but repositions the right arm lead over the right scapula to record P waves of larger amplitude. The CB5 system does not allow for assessment of ST segment changes from the inferior portion of the heart. The CB5 system places the right arm electrode inferior to the right clavicle and is most often used in exercise stress tests and continuous Holter recordings. This lead reportedly detects ST segment alterations more frequently than any other three-lead system. However, it is not as helpful for diagnosis of arrhythmia. Five-electrode systems allow monitoring of the six bipolar frontal leads and a true unipolar precordial V5.

Attention to certain details is also essential. Skin resistance should be minimized through abrasion and cleansing. Calibration (10 mm = 1 mV) of both the CRT display and the print-out device should be performed regularly. Most operating room monitors were originally designed primarily for rhythm analysis. To minimize noise and baseline drift secondary to movement artifact, filtering of all frequencies below 0.4 to 0.5 Hz is performed in this "monitoring" mode. Unfortunately, this method may lead to detection of spurious ST segment changes. Proper detection of myocardial ischemia is achieved when the monitor is set in the "diagnostic" mode, in which the filtering threshold is 0.14 to 0.15 Hz.

In addition to these commonly used systems, other techniques are available for special situations. Recordings from behind the left atrium are possible from electrodes incorporated into esophageal stethoscopes. Because P waves are very prominent, this technique can facilitate diagnosis of arrhythmias, especially in children, in whom rapid rates and the inability to identify P waves in routine leads may make arrhythmia diagnosis quite difficult. In addition, posterior wall ischemia is more easily identified when esophageal leads are used.

In many institutions epicardial leads are sutured directly to the heart prior to separation of the patient from cardiopulmonary bypass. In addition to pacing capabilities, these leads offer the advantage of providing direct atrial electrograms. These simplify the diagnosis of arrhythmias by augmenting atrial deflections. Electrograms also can be recorded from endocardial electrocardiographic leads available in multipurpose pulmonary artery catheters.

One can often diagnose ischemia or an arrhythmia from observation of the fleeting image on the oscilloscope. For more detailed examination, a calibrated print-out is required and ideally should be available in all ECG equipment. A permanent recording is necessary to evaluate subtle changes in ST segment position or T wave morphology and to analyze complex arrhythmias. It is likely that computer processing of the ECG will be available for arrhythmia detection in the near future.

Computer trending and summation of elevation and/or depression of ST segments is available. This may facilitate earlier diagnosis of ischemia, especially when ST changes are minimal and easily overlooked on visual scanning. Portable interactive equipment that detects ST segment changes and signals an alarm is available. If identification and treatment of postoperative ST segment changes prove efficacious, such devices may be invaluable.

The ECG also is useful for detection of electrolyte and drug effects, pericardial disease, chamber enlargement, axis deviation and chamber strain, and pacemaker function.

The ECG is extremely safe. The only complications are associated with the electrodes. Electrical burns can occur at the site of lead placement, usually secondary to the improper grounding of the electrocautery. The other complication is inaccurate ST data because of improper lead placement. To re-emphasize, V5 is positioned at the fifth intercostal space at the anterior axillary line.

ARTERIAL PRESSURE MONITORING

The monitoring of arterial blood pressure either invasively or noninvasively is indicated during all anesthetic procedures. Bear in mind that pressure is being measured, *not* total flow. Ohm's law as applied to the circulation, i.e., $BP = CO \times SVR$ (where BP = blood pressure, CO = cardiac output, and SVR = systemic vascular resistance) emphasizes that cardiac output *and* systemic resistance determine arterial pressure.

Three techniques are used for indirect blood pressure measurement: auscultation, oscillometry, and detection of either flow or arterial wall movement distal to a blood pressure cuff (palpation, photoelectric, ultrasound). Automatic devices currently available make use of each of these methods either alone or in combination. Newer electronic equipment can cycle quickly and also display arterial waveforms.

Auscultation of Korotkoff's sounds (Riva-Rocci method) is dependent on proper technique. The cuff width should be greater than approximately 30 percent of limb circumference. Readings are artificially low if the cuff is too wide or if deflation is too rapid. Speciously elevated pressures are recorded when the cuff is too narrow or wrapped too loosely. Calibration of aneroid manometers, frequently neglected, should be done periodically.

The oscillometric technique senses the pulsatile movement transmitted to the cuff itself as blood flow is gradually restored. After inflation to suprasystolic pressure, the cuff is then deflated until oscillations return. Systolic pressure is recorded at the pressure at which oscillations initially appear. The point of maximal oscillation reflects mean pressure, and the final minimal oscillation probably indicates diastolic pressure. The mean pressure is the most reproducible value. This technique is widely used in automatic, microprocessor-driven devices.

Techniques detecting flow distal to a blood pressure cuff provide accurate systolic blood pressure measurement by detecting the initial pulse of blood (Doppler sounds, changes in light transmission). The accurate determination of diastolic pressure is less reliable because it is difficult to detect "full pulsatility." The exquisitely sensitive Doppler ultrasonography method senses arterial flow after cuff pressure is reduced below the systolic pressure. It is often used in pediatric patients, in obese patients, and in those patients with weak or absent pulses. Finger plethysmographic–blood pressure devices are now available. These use light-emitting diodes and automated plethysmography to detect small changes in volume of the finger occurring with each systolic pressure wave. This permits analysis and display of pulse flow and blood pressure for each cardiac beat, thus approaching the beat-to-beat analysis of invasive arterial monitoring. Pulse oximetry is also useful as a monitor of circulation. The magnitude of the plethysmographic display on many oximeters correlates with the strength of the peripheral signal. Although many factors can interfere with signal transmission, one that must be addressed is that of low flow.

Direct invasive arterial pressure monitoring is used when one desires either beat-to-beat knowledge of blood pressure or a site for frequent arterial blood sampling. In addition, visualization of the arterial waveform can often provide useful clinical information. Hypovolemia is often manifested by pronounced swings in systolic pressure coincident with the phases of mechanical ventilation.

Unfortunately, despite earlier hopes to the contrary, the wave form provides little information regarding myocardial contractility, stroke volume, or systemic vascular resistance. The wave is altered during transmission through the vasculature and the "plumbing" linking the artery with the transducer. The wave recorded in the radial artery is a wave of energy transmitted from the heart and central aorta; it is not a "flow" wave. As pressure is recorded more distally, peak systolic pressure increases and the dicrotic notch appears later. Also, reflected waves from the narrow peripheral arterioles may augment true systolic pressure. It is important to note that mean pressure remains constant despite these changes.

In addition, there are the perturbations introduced by the electrical-mechanical coupling system. The transducer is the site of conversion of a mechanical signal (pressure) to an electrical signal and, although a potential source of interference, usually performs accurately. The major source of difficulty is in the pressure measuring tubing. The pressure measuring system and the arterial tree have a frequency response of approximately 20 Hz and 50 to 100 Hz, respectively. As the frequency response of the monitoring system approaches that of the arterial tree, accentuation of the systolic signal will occur ("ringing" or an underdamped system).

This is promoted by the use of excessive lengths of tubing, multiple stopcocks, and low compliance tubing.

The use of direct arterial pressure measurement has increased dramatically in recent years. This rise reflects increased numbers of high-risk surgical patients, the use of complex anesthetic and surgical techniques, and the paucity of complications associated with direct arterial cannulation. There are several specific indications for the use of direct arterial pressure measurement, including surgery in patients with severe cardiac and/or pulmonary disease; major cardiac, vascular, thoracic, or trauma surgery; intracranial procedures; and the induction of deliberate hypotension or hypothermia.

The most common site used for arterial cannulation is the radial artery. Other possible sites include the ulnar, brachial, femoral, dorsalis pedis, axillary, and superficial temporal arteries. Numerous studies have attempted to define optimal technique for radial cannulation. Currently, the "ideal" is a small-diameter (20-gauge or less), nontapered, Teflon catheter, flushed continuously with a dilute heparin solution, positioned in the artery the shortest possible time. Whether one uses direct cannulation or "through-and-through" technique is probably immaterial. Direct surgical exposure of the artery is associated with a higher infection rate.

Allen's test for assessment of ulnar collateral flow has been recommended prior to radial artery puncture. However, there is no evidence that this test is effective in either predicting or preventing (if one elects not to use the artery) vascular complications. Cannulation of the radial artery is contraindicated if the site appears infected.

Complications from arterial cannulation include thrombosis, embolization (clot, torn catheter, air), distal and/or proximal, skin or tissue ischemia, pain, hematoma formation, arterial trauma, and infection. Low flow states, injection of noxious drugs, and lack of careful observation and removal at the first sign of trouble likely account for the ischemic complications.

CENTRAL VENOUS PRESSURE

Central venous pressure (CVP), here used synonymously with right atrial pressure, is determined by intravascular volume, venous return, vascular smooth muscle tone (venous compliance), and right ventricular function. It is also influenced by ventilatory patterns and by variations in mediastinal and intrathoracic pressure, falling when intrathoracic pressure falls (spontaneous inspiration) and increasing with elevations in intrathoracic pressure Valsalva. The normal range for CVP is 0 to 8 mm Hg. Pressure measurement is only one of many indications for obtaining access to the central venous circulation. It is also necessary as a site for drug, fluid, or hyperalimentation infusions, as a route for placement of temporary pacemaker leads or a pulmonary artery catheter, and as a port for frequent sampling of venous blood.

The CVP is usually measured by observing changes

in the height of a water column. This method is easy, relatively inexpensive, and usually reliable. However, the fluid column does not respond rapidly to changes or follow the fluctuations in pressure that often occur with respiration. Transducing the pressure alleviates these problems and, in addition, displays the venous waveform, a valuable source of information. The wave is composed of three positive deflections and two negative troughs. The positive waves are the a, c, and v waves. The a wave represents venous distention secondary to atrial contraction, the c wave indicates bulging of the tricuspid valve into the right atrium during ventricular systole, and the v wave results from atrial filling during ventricular systole when the tricuspid valve is closed. The x and y descent represent atrial relaxation and rapid inflow of blood (rapid filling phase of ventricular diastole) into the ventricle, respectively. Analysis of the these waves is often of diagnostic value. The a wave is absent in atrial fibrillation, whereas it is enlarged (cannon a wave) when the atrium contracts against increased resistance as in tricuspid stenosis, junctional rhythm (closed arteriovenous valve), or right atrial myxoma. A large v wave is often present with tricuspid insufficiency.

The CVP aids in assessing right ventricular (RV) function because, as long as there is no obstruction across the tricuspid valve, CVP reflects RV filling pressure. This is of singular importance whenever there is RV failure or a potential for RV dysfunction, as is often the case in patients with mitral valve disease, pulmonary hypertension, or severe lung disease. CVP is almost uniformly elevated in cardiac tamponade, reflecting right atrial and/or RV compression.

There is controversy over the reliability of CVP measurements in evaluating left ventricular (LV) function. In general, it is a useful indicator of overall cardiac performance when LV structure and function are normal. It is less reflective of LV filling when the LV is poorly compliant (e.g., chronic hypertension, aortic stenosis) or has contractile abnormalities (e.g., acute ischemia, myocardial infarction). Nevertheless, the CVP is often very helpful in determining the adequacy of intravascular volume. Many clinicians feel that observing trends and noting the response to a rapidly administered volume challenge provides more information than any absolute number, especially when the CVP is in the normal range.

Complications from CVP measurement are usually related to central vein cannulation. The list of problems related to internal jugular vein catheterization is formidable and includes pneumothorax, carotid artery puncture, brachial plexus injury, air embolism, and thoracic duct injury (left internal jugular cannulation) among others. Many of these problems can be prevented with increased experience in catheter placement and meticulous attention to detail during catheter insertion. Other sites are often used. The external jugular approach eliminates the possibility of carotid artery puncture, but at the price of a much lower success rate for gaining central access. The same is true when the brachial or cephalic veins of the arm are used. The subclavian approach increases the risk of pneumothorax.

PULMONARY ARTERY CATHETER

The pulmonary artery catheter (PAC) allowed the clinician for the first time to have a measure of left heart function. Although there is still great disagreement over exactly which patients merit a PAC and even more over which patients benefit from one, there is little doubt that it has revolutionized hemodynamic management. The catheter allows measurement of RA, RV, PA, and pulmonary artery occluded pressure (PAOP). In most clinical conditions, PAOP reliably depicts left atrial (LA) pressure; pulmonary venous stenosis (admittedly, a rare condition) and the use of high levels of pulmonary end-expiratory pressure (PEEP) are the most notable exceptions. LA pressure in turn reflects left ventricular filling pressure, a measure of LV preload. PAOP may underestimate LV filling pressure if the ventricle is stiff and noncompliant or when there is any obstruction across the mitral valve as in mitral stenosis or atrial myxoma.

The PAOP can reflect acute changes in LV compliance (sudden increase in PAOP with little or no change in LV volume), although such changes are rare. The increases in PAOP that occasionally occur with ischemia probably reflect reduced systolic function rather than impaired diastolic compliance. In patients with chronically reduced LV compliance (e.g., aortic stenosis), PAOP may fluctuate widely, reflecting only minimal changes in LV volume. It is sometimes difficult to determine whether an increase in PAOP indicates a change in preload or compliance, especially after cardiac surgery. The echocardiogram should help resolve some of these problems because estimation of LV volume is possible.

Measurement of PA pressure is desirable in patients with pulmonary hypertension or impaired RV performance. Such patients often respond poorly to RV volume or pressure overload. Pharmacologic reduction of RV afterload requires knowledge of PA pressures, RV and LV filling pressures, and cardiac output (CO).

Cardiac output can be determined simply, reliably, and accurately by using the thermodilution method. To ensure reproducability, strict attention to detail with respect to injectate temperatures and volumes as well as speed and timing of injection is important. Derived hemodynamic variables such as pulmonary and systemic vascular resistance can be calculated after CO determination. This is of inestimable help in diagnosis and therapy of unexplained hypotension or the low output state. Inotropes and vasodilators can be administered while monitoring their effects on ventricular filling, forward flow, and systemic and pulmonary resistance. Therapy can be re-evaluated and, if necessary, altered rapidly.

The PA catheter provides a site for obtaining mixed venous blood samples from the pulmonary arterial (distal) port. Mixed venous oxygen tension is required for calculations of pulmonary shunt fraction, oxygen consumption, and the arterial-venous oxygen difference. Newer oximetry catheters provide continuous on-line display of mixed venous oxygen saturation (SVO_2). This may be of value in determining the adequacy of cardiac output since it helps to define the relation between oxygen delivery and peripheral oxygen utilization. SVO_2 is diminished when total oxygen supply is reduced (low output states, anemia, decreased arterial oxygen content) or when demand is increased (i.e., fever, increased metabolism). SVO_2 is increased (and serves as an early warning sign) when blood cyanide levels are elevated. Increases are also noted in the presence of sepsis, hypothermia, often after anesthetic induction, and when the catheter is "permanently wedged." Special PA catheters can be used therapeutically to pace the RA, RV, or both.

As stated earlier, indications for PA catheter placement vary. In many institutions, PA catheterization is routine for cardiac surgery, whereas in others it is performed sparingly. As a general guideline, a PA catheter is useful whenever the data derived would materially alter anesthetic or hemodynamic management. A key word in decision-making is "unstable"; if the patient has cardiac or pulmonary disease that is unstable preoperatively or likely to become so postoperatively, or if the planned surgery is unstable in terms of physiologic insult, knowledge of cardiac pressures and flow can greatly facilitate management.

Complications relating to pulmonary artery catheterization result from venous cannulation (discussed above), catheter insertion and from catheter location in situ. Mechanical stimulation of the cardiac conducting system during passage of the catheter may result in a variety of arrhythmias. Ectopic beats are frequent; more severe arrhythmias are rare. Patients with acute ongoing ischemia are at greatest risk of developing ventricular tachycardia or ventricular fibrillation. There is a risk of developing right bundle branch block. In the presence of pre-existing left bundle branch block, complete heart block can result, but this occurs very infrequently. Catheter knotting is also possible during catheter insertion. Many in situ complications such as injury to the tricuspid or pulmonary valve, endocarditis, jugular vein thrombosis, and pulmonary infarction have been reported but are usually of minimal clinical importance. The most catastrophic complication is pulmonary artery rupture. The frequency of this complication is estimated at 0.05 to 0.1 percent. The pulmonary artery may be perforated during catheter insertion or when manipulating the catheter while in place (i.e., flushing, balloon inflation). Perforation most commonly occurs in the distal pulmonary arterial tree; however, rupture may also occur in more proximal vessels. Studies indicate that pulmonary hypertension, old age, and hypothermia all predispose to pulmonary artery rupture, but inappropriate catheter manipulation also plays a major role. The risk of perforation is increased when the catheter is located too far distally, if the balloon remains inflated for an excessive amount of time, or if the catheter is flushed or balloon inflated when in a wedge position. Treatment of pulmonary artery rupture will vary with the severity of the injury. In some instances, positive airway pressure will control hemorrhage. It may be necessary to isolate the bleeding lung with a double-lumen endotracheal tube or a bronchial blocker and in some cases perform a lobectomy or pneumonectomy. Despite these emergency measures, mortality from PA perforation is high.

TWO-DIMENSIONAL TRANSESOPHAGEAL ECHOCARDIOGRAPHY

Echocardiography uses computer analysis of high-frequency sound above the audible range to form images of the heart and vascular structures. With the addition of pulsed wave Doppler color imaging, flow through the cardiac structures can be visualized and measured. Mechanical scanners are used in transthoracic echocardiograms. The transducer is held against the chest and is mechanically rotated to examine the entire sector. Continuous observation for long periods is difficult. Of more interest to the anesthesiologist is a phased array transducer, which electronically moves the beam. This transducer is mounted on a gastroscope and inserted into the esophagus, usually after anesthetic induction and endotracheal intubation, although it is now commonly used in the echocardiology laboratory in awake patients, with sedation and topical anesthesia. The gastroscope is then positioned to afford optimal echocardiographic images. Complications from insertion are few, and include patient discomfort, gagging and vomiting, oral-pharyngeal trauma, and extremely rarely, esophageal perforation. A wide variety of data is available from two-dimensional transesophageal echocardiology (2D-TEE). Early diagnosis of acute ischemia is possible by analysis of alterations in regional wall motion and/or systolic wall thickening. These are sensitive, early signs of ischemia and often precede ST segment abnormalities or changes in ventricular function. The specificity of these changes is still undergoing extensive evaluation. To the present time, evaluation of regional wall motion abnormalities has taken place off-line, by analysis of the recorded images. Currently, algorithms are being developed to facilitate on-line recognition of wall motion changes.

It is also possible to determine end systolic and end diastolic areas. This allows estimation of ventricular volume and may prove to be a much better index of preload than ventricular filling pressures. This eliminates many of the problems with pressure interpretation related to acute or chronic changes in ventricular compliance.

Color Doppler analysis permits recognition of valvular insufficiency and intercardiac shunts. Because of the ability to detect valvular insufficiency, this technique has become extraordinary helpful in evaluating the results of valvular repair. Also in the field of cardiac surgery, the detection of intracardiac air is facilitated with 2D-TEE. Correlations between echocardiographically visualized air and neurologic dysfunction following cardiac surgery has yet to be made, but such visualization is useful in the assessment of the adequacy of air removal maneuvers following open chamber cardiac procedures.

Two-dimensional transesophageal echocardiography is now routinely used in cardiac surgery, especially for the evaluation of valvular function. Its use as an ischemia monitor for the detection of regional wall motion abnormalities must await the development of procedures to allow on-line recognition of these changes, as mentioned above.

NEUROLOGIC MONITORING

SCOTT M. ELEFF, M.D.

For most operations, normal oxygenation as measured by pulse oximetry, normal ventilation as measured by capnography, and a normal cerebral perfusion pressure as estimated by the mean arterial blood pressure virtually guarantees that the results of the neurologic examination will be unchanged from the preoperative state. However, the existence of particular disease states (Table 1) regardless of proposed operation or certain operations regardless of coexisting diseases (Table 2) places the patient at increased risk of sustaining intraoperative neurologic damage. This risk can be reduced by a neurologic examination in the awake patient or electroencephalography (EEG) and evoked potential (EP) recordings to monitor neurologic function in the anesthetized state.

Many anesthesiologists have resisted using EEG and EP in the operating room because of the inherent complexities of electrophysiologic interpretation. The neurologist, after performing a neurologic examination and recording EEG and EP, must decide if the results deviate from normal values. The anesthesiologist has the luxury of a control value done on the patient prior to surgical positioning and need only decide if a deviation from this baseline occurs. This requires the ability to collect reproducible results and a knowledge of the effects of anesthetic depth on the electrophysiologic data. Having eliminated artifactual causes, a significant change from baseline signals an acute neurologic deficit in the same way that a significant change in the ST segment of the electrocardiogram reflects myocardial ischemia. This chapter concentrates on two commonly used intraoperative monitors, EEG and somatosensory evoked potentials (SSEP). It cannot be overstressed that a clinical examination of the awake or lightly sedated patient is cost effective and allows a more full assessment of the nervous system. For example, a patient with an unstable cervical vertebra can be intubated using topical anesthesia and nerve blocks and positioned while lightly sedated. This allows motor and sensory examinations to be conducted and repositioning accomplished with greater speed and certainty than is possible using SSEPs.

Carotid endarterectomy performed with the patient under regional anesthesia in the lightly sedated patient allows subtle neurologic deficits to be discovered before EEG changes would be obvious. However, many surgeries are better done, and many patients more easily hemodynamically controlled, with general anesthesia. In these circumstances SSEP and EEG monitoring may be invaluable.

ELECTROENCEPHALOGRAPHY

The EEG is simply the measurement of voltage variations with time from different areas of the scalp arising from excitatory and inhibitory postsynaptic potentials of the pyramidal cells of the cortex. This is analogous to electrocardiographic recordings measured over different areas of the chest, except that the chest voltage recorded from the heart is 1 to 5 mV and EEG amplitude is only 2 to 200 μV. Because the EEG signal is so small, careful attention must be used to ensure the electrodes are accurately placed, low impedances (less than 3,000 ohms) achieved, the cables well insulated, and the amplifier placed as close to the patient's head as

Table 1 Coexisting Diseases That Place the Patient At Increased Risk of Neurologic Deficit

Severe cervical or lumbar disc disease
Intracranial abnormalities—e.g., tumors, aneurysms
Severe carotid or vertebral artery disease
Peripheral nerve disease and brachial plexus abnormalities
Acute trauma presenting for emergent non-neurologic surgery with an abnormal neurologic examination
Medically intractable seizure disorders

Table 2 Surgical Procedures in Which EEG and EP Monitoring are Useful

Carotid endarterectomy
Intracranial vascular surgery—e.g., aneurysm, arteriovenous malformation
Removal of an intracranial mass especially involving the brainstem and cranial nerves
Major spine surgery, especially corpectomies and scoliosis surgical procedures
Thoracic aneurysmectomy
Partial lobectomy for removal of a seizure focus

possible. Simple attention to the details, and careful placement of the appropriate EEG electrodes allow reproducible tracings to be easily acquired.

Analysis of the EEG relies on assessing the relative amplitude in differing frequency bands at different electrode (scalp) sites. Tables 3 and 4 show that EEG is useful in diagnosing both hypoxic and ischemic insults to the cortex. These tables also show the profound effects anesthetics and physiologic changes have on the frequency composition of the EEG. Although these changes are predictable, it is crucial that anesthetic depth, blood gases, and body temperature be kept nearly

constant for at least 10 minutes before an anticipated neurologic event (e.g., clamping of the internal carotid artery during an endarterectomy) may occur. To the extent that the patient may be at risk throughout the procedure, maintenance of an anesthetic steady state is invaluable in eliminating false-positive EEG readings.

The gold standard for EEG monitoring is continuous recording of 16 channels using electrodes placed over the entire skull using the International 10–20 Electrode System. However, the ensuing 300 pages an hour of data, the vast majority of which contains no new information, has led to several different methods of computer-enhanced data reduction. All of these methods use a mathematical technique (usually the Fourier Transform) to change the EEG display from voltage versus time to voltage versus frequency. Characteristic changes in voltage versus frequency caused by ischemia or hypoxia warn the anesthesiologist and surgeon of impending neurologic damage at a time when the damage may be fully reversible (e.g., placing a shunt in a carotid endarterectomy).

Several EEG monitors are available from monitors where only one EEG lead is used and a single value derived (frequency information is lost) to power spectrum analysis (in which frequency information is maintained, but phase information is lost). Power spectrum analysis converts a small-time sample, or epoch (2 to 16 seconds) of EEG data into the square of the amplitude of its frequency components. This reduces a page of EEG data to 30 numbers. Two techniques used to

Table 3 EEG Frequency Bands

EEG Rhythm	Frequency (Hz)	Associations
Delta	0–4	Normal deep sleep; deep anesthesia; coma (metabolic or hypoxic)
Theta	4–8	Infants; normal light sleep; hyperventilation
Alpha	8–13	Relaxed with eyes closed recording over the occiput; deep anesthesia and coma recording anywhere over the entire cortex
Beta	13–30	Alert and attentive; also seen over frontal area for up to 2 weeks after taking barbiturates or benzodiazepines

Table 4 Anesthetic Effects on SSEP and EEG

Agent	EEG Frequency	EEG Power	SSEP Amplitude	SSEP Latency
Inhalational Agents:				
Halothane	Progressive slowing	↓	↓	↑
Isoflurane	Shift to 15–35 Hz	↓	↓	↑
Enflurane	Loss of high frequencies seizure activity possible	↓	↓	↑
Nitrous oxide	Shift to 20–35 Hz	↑	↓	—
Intravenous Agents				
Thiopental	Biphasic initially increase then slowing and burst suppression	↓	↓ –	↑
Fentanyl	Slowing	↑	– ↑	– ↑
Etomidate	4–8 Hz predominantly with underlying for activity	↑ ↑	↑	↑
Diazepam	Shift to 13-25 Hz	↓	↓	↑
Ketamine	Shift to 15-30 Hz High dose may cause seizures	↓	↑	↑
Blood Gases				
Hypocapnia	↓	↑	—	↓ –
Hypercapnia	↓	↑	—	—
Hypoxia (early)	↑	↓	↓	↓
Hypoxia (late)	↓ ↓	↓ ↓	↓	↓
Hypothermia	Slowing	↑	↓	↑ (~1 msec/°C)
Decreased cerebral flood flow	Slowing	↓	↓	↑

(↑ = increase; ↓ = decrease; — = no change).

display this information are the compressed spectral array (CSA) and density-modulated spectral array (DSA). CSA plots the amplitude of all frequencies and updates this every epoch, creating a pseudo-three-dimensional display of power per frequency band per epoch. In this way, almost all of the EEG data is maintained. Unfortunately, the small amplitude epoch from a transient episode of ischemia may be obscured. DSA uses dots of different densities to represent amplitude, doing away with the peaks and valleys of CSA. However, the range of plottable densities is only 1 to 10, whereas EEG power ranges from 1 to 100. Regardless of the technique employed, monitoring the unprocessed EEG is invaluable in eliminating errors caused by data reduction of artifacts such as muscle movement, electrocautery, and ECG breakthrough.

Somatosensory Evoked Potentials

SSEP is the average of EEG signals that are synchronized to a discrete electrical stimulus such as median or posterior tibial nerve stimulation. An EEG signal that is not related to this stimulus has random phase and quickly (1 to 2 minutes) averages to zero. The resultant small SSEP waves (1 to 2 μvolts) allow amplitude and latency (time from the stimulus) to be directly measured. The direct effect of ischemia and hypoxia (see Table 4) on these easily measured values is a major advantage of SSEP over EEG. Furthermore, since generation of the SSEP requires an intact pathway, function of peripheral nerve, spinal cord (posterior columns), and brain (brainstem, medial lemniscus, internal capsule, and contralateral somatosensory cortex) are continuously monitored.

Up to five recording electrodes and four stimulating needles are used in the typical SSEP study. Two electrodes are placed over C-4 and C-3 (right and left median nerve somatosensory cortex) and C_z' (the posterior tibial nerve somatosensory cortex is in the interhemispheric groove and monitored over the midline). Two additional electrodes are placed at FP_z (lower forehead) and the earlobe for use as reference and ground electrodes, respectively. Finally, paired 23-gauge stimulating needles are placed subcutaneously over the median and posterior tibial nerves. Stimulus site depends on the anticipated level of injury. Stimulating the

median nerve, which enters at the cervical cord level, would not be appropriate for a thoracic spinal cord tumor. However, the cortical signal from median nerve stimulation arises from a region fed by the middle cerebral artery (MCA) and would be appropriate when monitoring for an MCA aneurysmectomy. Stimulating the posterior tibial nerve stimulates an area of the brain fed by the anterior communicating artery and is more appropriate for surgery involving the frontal lobes. SSEP from any nerve stimulation is effected by global hypoxia or ischemia. The first positive and negative peaks, which have a latency of approximately 15 and 20 msecs, respectively, are particularly robust and useful for analysis in the operating room.

EEG Versus SSEP

SSEPs are easier to quantitate although slightly more difficult to obtain than an EEG. Sixteen-lead EEG is the monitor of choice when small areas of focal ischemia are anticipated, as might occur in a trauma patient with an altered level of consciousness presenting for emergent surgery (see Table 1). SSEP and EEG are equally useful when large areas of cortex are at risk (aneurysm clipping, carotid endarterectomy, or in patients with severe carotid artery disease). EEG becomes isoelectric at regional cerebral blood flow levels of 16 to 18 ml per 100 g per minute; SSEPs are abolished at 15 ml per 100 g per minute. Prolonged (>20 minute) exposure to flows below these levels often leads to permanent neurologic deficits. EEG is obviously not useful for spinal cord surgery or for positioning a patient with an unstable cervical cord. However, it should be appreciated that loss of the anterior spinal artery as can occur with thoracic aorta aneurysmectomy, or straightening of the spine in scoliosis surgery may spare the dorsal columns and result in a normal SSEP in a patient with a severely damaged spinal cord. Motor evoked potential recording may be useful in these situations.

SUGGESTED READING

Desmedt JE. Neuromonitoring in surgery. New York: Elsevier, 1989.
Niedermeyer E, Lopes da Silva F. Electroencephalography, basic principles, clinical applications and related fields. Baltimore: Urban & Schwarzenberg, 1987.

MONITORING THE NEONATE

JEFFREY N. DORNBUSCH, M.D.
MARK A. ROCKOFF, M.D.

Adequate monitoring of a newborn in the operating room is a challenge that can be frustrating. Most of the problems occur because of difficulties in collecting data that are simple to obtain in older patients. However, precision and accuracy of information are especially vital in the neonate. For example, a 10 mm Hg decrease in blood pressure may be insignificant in an adult, but represents a 20 percent decrease in a small premature infant with a baseline systolic pressure of 50 mm Hg. Furthermore, the rapid metabolic rate of children enables problems to progress rapidly.

Simple mechanical factors present an impediment to accurate monitoring. Breath and heart sounds may be faint, pulses difficult to palpate, respirations difficult to measure, and invasive monitoring catheters difficult to insert. These patients are small, and clinical assessment is difficult, since they tend to end up completely covered by the surgical drapes. There is no body part that is not close to the surgical field and potentially subject to movement or pressure during the operation. Thus, in these very patients in whom high-quality monitoring is critical, it is more difficult to obtain reliable data. This chapter outlines our approach to monitoring the neonatal surgical patient.

CARDIOVASCULAR MONITORING

In the newborn baby, several factors mandate careful cardiovascular monitoring in the operating room. Circulating blood volume is only about 300 ml for a term infant, so "small" errors in fluid administration or in estimation of blood loss can have major consequences. In addition, newborns (even "healthy" ones with normal cardiovascular anatomy) may have a sudden decrease in pulmonary blood flow because of blood shunting across the foramen ovale or ductus arteriosus, with many physiologic stresses. The neonatal myocardium also is more easily depressed by anesthetic agents. Cardiovascular monitoring in the neonate need not be complex but does require forethought and attention to detail.

Inspection and palpation can yield useful information. Coolness of the hands or feet is a useful sign of poor perfusion and is frequently due to hypovolemia. Slow capillary refill of a fingertip after blanching by light touch is also helpful in this regard. To check these simple signs, one needs access to the infant. At least one extremity is frequently available to the anesthetist. Usually the elbows can be flexed so that the hands are near the head. A flashlight can help one better see portions of the patient that are largely hidden by the drapes. One should always listen to the heart rate and strength of the heart sounds with an appropriately sized precordial or esophageal stethoscope. Small, lightweight, low-profile precordial stethoscopes work well in newborns because it is easy to hear through a thin chest wall, but esophageal monitors are subject to less interference by surgical manipulation.

The electrocardiogram is also an essential monitor. It is most helpful in diagnosing arrhythmias and for displaying the heart rate. In infants without cardiovascular disease, hypoxia or hypoventilation are the usual causes of arrhythmias. Small contact pads that are specially made for infants can be used, or those used for adults can be trimmed.

In spite of some mechanical difficulties, all neonates should have their blood pressures monitored in the operating room. For simple cases in relatively healthy infants, intermittent cuff pressure measurements are adequate. The cuff should be appropriate for the size of the patient and have a width about two thirds the length of the upper arm. If a perfectly sized cuff is not available, it is safer to choose a slightly larger one, since this will tend to underestimate the true blood pressure. Some manual methods of blood pressure determination (such as auscultation of Korotkoff's sounds or oscillometry) are difficult to perform accurately in small infants and are seldom used. Palpation of the distal pulse is usually feasible in an anesthetized baby but can be impossible if blood pressure or peripheral perfusion is low. A simple noninvasive method for determining blood pressure is with a small Doppler probe taped over an artery distal to the cuff. As the cuff deflates, Doppler sounds reappear at systolic pressure. Automated blood pressure monitors (using either the oscillometric or Doppler principle) are reliable, even in sick neonates. Appropriate units are designed and set (some have a switch) for infants; these employ lower cuff inflation pressures than do devices used for adults. Because of occasional problems in obtaining an automated pressure determination quickly and accurately (e.g., when the extremity is being jostled or blood pressure has dropped suddenly), it is good practice to have a manual cuff method available as a back-up.

Invasive arterial monitoring is frequently helpful during anesthesia for neonates because many of these patients require emergency surgery in which major volume shifts occur. Display scales should be appropriate for low pressures. Either umbilical or peripheral arteries can be used. Some sick newborns from neonatal intensive care units will already have umbilical arterial catheters in place. This is handy, but these lines have special risks and problems. An umbilical arterial catheter enters one of the umbilical arteries and loops down into an iliac artery and up into the aorta. The position of the tip should be confirmed by x-ray examination. Some neonatologists prefer placement "high" (about T7 to T10) and some "low" (below L3). Both positions avoid having the catheter tip near the renal or superior mesenteric arteries. This is important because thrombi may form at the distal end of the catheter. If either leg appears ischemic, the catheter must be removed promptly. Peripheral arterial catheters have fewer complications. They are sometimes difficult to insert but can usually be placed percutaneously (or by cutdown) using a 22- or 24-gauge plastic catheter. The most common sites are the radial, dorsalis pedis, or posterior tibial arteries. Major problems are rare at these sites because of good collateral circulation. Catheters in the femoral artery have more complications, particularly distal ischemia. Temporal arterial lines can be dangerous, since it is easy to flush retrograde into the internal carotid artery.

Because neonates are so small, all arterial catheter sites are close to the central circulation. A casual squirt of even 1 ml or less of flush solution into an arterial line can easily send fluid, and possibly air bubbles or clot, into the cerebral vessels. To avoid this, flushing of lines (especially after blood sampling) should be slow and with the minimal volume necessary. To keep the catheter patent, one can either flush it intermittently or use a pump to deliver a constant infusion at 2 to 3 ml per hour. The solution should usually be saline, containing heparin, 1 U per milliliter. One should keep track of the volume of flush solution used and of blood sampled: these amounts can be significant in a tiny baby. An arrangement that can reduce the volume of blood wasted during sampling and the volume of solution needed to flush the line uses a T connector with a rubber injection port attached to the end of the catheter and a syringe filled with heparized saline back near the transducer. To sample blood, first draw back on the syringe to fill the tubing with blood, then close the stopcock. Next, draw the sample from the T connector, and after sampling, slowly flush the dead space blood and a small volume of heparinized saline into the catheter. If the hub of the catheter is inaccessible under the drapes, arrange a system with a stopcock for sampling as close to the patient as possible, and be certain that attachments are secure in order to avoid disconnection. The goal is to discard the minimal blood needed before sampling and to use the minimal volume of flush solutions. It is not necessary to flush every trace of blood out of the line.

Excessive variation of blood pressure with controlled ventilation is an excellent sign of hypovolemia. Sometimes the pressure wave may have a slow upstroke, from cardiovascular impairment or damping of the tracing due to clot, vasospasm (common in small vessels), or a surgeon pressing on the extremity. Inspection of the limb and a small, slow flush may solve the problem.

Urinary output can be monitored using a small feeding tube in the bladder and a small collection bag. Although a low urinary output (less than 0.5 ml per kilogram per hour) often indicates decreased renal perfusion, urine sometimes will not drain through the tubing, and a sudden gush may appear once the infant is moved. If urinary output is high, this may be secondary to an osmotic diuresis from glycosuria, since the newborn has a low renal threshold for glucose.

We seldom monitor central venous pressure (CVP) in neonates because there are other good indicators of volume status, particularly respiratory variation in arterial line tracings. Furthermore, slipping in a CVP line may be a difficult task in such small patients. CVP catheters are most worthwhile when a large, secure line is necessary for infusion of fluids or medications. The easiest sites of entry are usually the external or internal jugular vein or the femoral vein. Those with experience may choose the subclavian vein, but this presents an increased risk of pneumothorax that can be particularly hazardous if not recognized during administration of anesthesia. In neonates during the first days of life, a catheter inserted into an umbilical vein sometimes passes through the ductus venosus and liver into the right atrium. Often, however, umbilical vein lines do not pass easily into the atrium but instead lodge in the liver. This makes them useless for CVP determination and dangerous for the administration of medications.

RESPIRATORY MONITORING

Monitoring the respiratory system in neonates is a prime concern of anesthesiologists. In fact, many circulatory changes (e.g., bradycardia) often result from abnormalities in gas exchange. The neonatal respiratory system, like the cardiovascular system, is also in a state of transition. Normal newborns have a striking increase in P_{AO_2} in the first hours after birth because of clearance of fluid from the lungs and opening of alveoli. Newborns with pneumonia or respiratory distress syndrome can have rapidly changing abnormalities in compliance and oxygenation. Continued attention to respiration is vital.

New sophisticated monitors do not replace the need for close clinical assessment. "Move the chest" is just as important a rule whether one is anesthetizing a newborn or an adult. A tunnel under the drapes, a flashlight, and an occasional palpating finger can allow visual or tactile estimation of chest movement in even the tiniest patient. Observation of skin, mucous membranes, and the surgical field is important for a clue to oxygenation, although it can occasionally be misleading. Auscultation is also important. Although either a precordial or an esophageal stethoscope can work well, it is sometimes easier to hear breath sounds with a precordial scope. This is because the sounds of air leaking around an endotracheal tube may obscure true breath sounds if an esophageal stethoscope is used. Careful placement of a precordial stethoscope can facilitate early detection of problems in special circumstances. For example, during a right thoracotomy for repair of a tracheoesophageal fistula, precordial monitoring near the left axilla gives immediate warning if the endotracheal tube slips into the right mainstem bronchus or into the fistula itself.

A manometer in the breathing circuit helps detect changes in compliance within the patient (e.g., pulmonary edema or secretions) or within the system (e.g., a kinked endotracheal tube). Infants with healthy lungs should have good chest excursion with inspiratory pressures of approximately 20 mm Hg. If it is necessary to use pressures much greater than this, compliance is abnormal. Sudden changes in pressure during a procedure (while delivering a constant tidal volume) should be cause for immediate concern. Spirometers generally are not useful in neonates because they are frequently inaccurate due to the very small volumes and fast rates found in infants.

The definitive test of adequacy of ventilation and oxygenation comes from arterial blood gas measurement. An arterial catheter enables one to obtain multiple samples without repeated arterial punctures. During less extensive procedures in healthier babies, blood gas monitoring may be unnecessary.

Arterial blood gases, although helpful, provide only an intermittent assessment of gas exchange. Continuous monitoring of oxygenation is so important that it has become a standard of care for neonates undergoing general anesthesia. This is best done with a pulse oximeter. These are easy to apply and give immediate and accurate readings of oxygen saturation. Monitoring with a pulse oximeter provides early warning of arterial desaturation. This is particularly important in neonates and should improve anesthetic care of these patients.

Pulse oximeters are accurate even in the presence of fetal hemoglobinemia or hyperbilirubinemia. There may be interference from overhead warming lights, but an opaque wrapper (such as that from an alcohol wipe) placed over the probe will solve this problem. Probe sizes are available to fit even the smallest premature infant. In addition to detecting hypoxia, oximetry allows adjustment of the oxygen saturation to desired levels in premature infants at risk for retrolental fibroplasia. It is important to recall that the PaO_2 is lower at a given saturation in a neonate than that of an adult, owing to the predominance of fetal hemoglobin.

Transcutaneous oxygen monitoring is much more cumbersome. Time for calibration and equilibration, the need to change electrode sites at intervals, and fluctuations due to changes in peripheral circulation all make transcutaneous monitoring a poor substitute for pulse oximetry in the operating room.

Transcutaneous electrodes can also estimate arterial carbon dioxide (PCO_2) but are cumbersome for the same reasons as for transcutaneous oxygen measurements. An indirect method is to analyze the amount of CO_2 in exhaled gases by either absorbance spectrometry (a standard CO_2 monitor) or mass spectrometry. If gases are withdrawn from the circuit for sampling (as in sidestream CO_2 analyzers and all mass spectrometers), there is inevitably some mixing of inspired and expired gases during the sampling process in newborns. This is because of small tidal volumes and high respiratory rates. Although the end-tidal CO_2 obtained may be lower than arterial CO_2, it may be useful for following trends. With mainstream CO_2 analyzers (which do not withdraw gases from the circuit for analysis), there is less mixing of inspiratory and expiratory gases. However, the sensing chamber adds dead space and involves extra connections that can be another source of airway disconnections.

TEMPERATURE MONITORING

Temperature should be monitored in all neonates. The large surface area to weight ratio, paucity of fat, inability to shiver, and impaired thermoregulation make hypothermia a much more common problem in infants than in older patients. Esophageal or rectal temperature probes give accurate readings and are simple to insert. One must be gentle, since it is possible to cause injury. A radiant warmer usually has a shielded skin temperature sensor as part of its thermostatic control. Monitoring airway temperature when using a heated humidifier helps to avoid overheating of inspired gases.

NEUROMUSCULAR MONITORING

Peripheral nerve stimulators are simple to use and require no special adaptations for small infants. They are helpful in neonates, since the response to fixed doses of relaxants may be variable and the clinical assessment of recovery is more difficult. Aside from sustained tetanus with nerve stimulation, other clinical signs correlate well with adequate strength after reversal of neuromuscular blockade. These include a negative inspiratory force of greater than 20 cm of water and the ability to flex the hips well against gravity.

ADDITIONAL MONITORING

Another important task in the operating room is to monitor blood loss. Although an experienced eye on the surgical field is helpful, there is no substitute for measurement. Small, graduated suction bottles should be used. In addition, a record should be kept of the volume of irrigation fluid used and the weight of sponges. Of course, blood tests can supplement clinical observations. Determinations of hematocrit and of ionized calcium, sodium, potassium, and glucose levels can be performed with less than 1 ml of blood. The indications for and interpretation of blood chemistries are beyond the scope of this review, and metabolic homeostasis is dealt with in many textbooks of neonatology. In general, neonates need careful attention paid to fluid and electrolyte levels. Hypoglycemia and hypocalcemia are common, especially in infants who are sick, premature, small for gestational age, or born to diabetic mothers.

SUGGESTED READING

Cote CJ, Goldstein EA, Cote MA, et al. A single-blind study of pulse oximetry in children. Anesthesiology 1988; 68:184–188.

Durand M, Ramanathan R. Pulse oximetry for continuous oxygen monitoring in sick newborn infants. J Pediatr 1986; 109:1052–1056.

Friesen RH, Lichtor JL. Indirect measurement of blood pressure in neonates and infants utilizing an automatic noninvasive oscillometric monitor. Anesth Analg 1981; 60:742–745.

Poppers PJ. Controlled evaluation of ultrasonic measurement of systolic and diastolic blood pressures in pediatric patients. Anesthesiology 1973; 38:187–191.

ACID-BASE BALANCE AND ARTERIAL BLOOD GAS MONITORING

JOANNE L. FLOYD, M.D.
ROBERT K. STOELTING, M.D.

Currently, available technology has radically altered the practice of anesthesiology. The greatest recent advance in anesthetic safety is the evolution from occasional sampling of arterial blood to continuous, noninvasive monitoring of blood oxygenation and end-tidal carbon dioxide. Despite the convenience and the rapidity of these determinations, analysis of arterial blood gases has not been entirely replaced. This chapter focuses on current utilization of acid-base and arterial gas monitoring during the perioperative period, and on interpretation of these readings.

PREOPERATIVE INDICATIONS FOR ACID-BASE OR ARTERIAL BLOOD GAS DETERMINATIONS

Because indiscriminant preoperative "screening" tests add little to an adequate history and physical examination, laboratory testing should be used selectively. Spirometry screening for the presence of and severity of pulmonary disease is limited to patients with risk factors for hypoxemia or with postoperative pulmonary complications (i.e., obesity, age > 60 years, history of smoking, prolonged hospitalization, ASA class > 2). The arterial blood gas analysis frequently done as part of screening spirometry is probably not indicated routinely.

If baseline oxygenation is the only concern, adequate information can be obtained noninvasively and less expensively by a single pulse oximetry reading. Suspected or expected respiratory acidosis requires investigation of pH and arterial carbon dioxide pressure ($PaCO_2$). If pulmonary resection is planned, the efficiency of ventilation should be documented preoperatively. Also, postoperative ventilation may be altered in patients undergoing thoracic or upper abdominal procedures. For routine surgery, arterial blood gas measurements should be reserved for suspicion of acid-base derangements.

The discovery of a previously unsuspected metabolic acidosis by serum chemistry screening requires further investigation by analysis of arterial blood gases. The etiology may have a significant effect on prognosis and management. Volume depletion is the most common cause of an incidental finding of metabolic alkalosis and a contraindication to major conduction anesthesia.

CURRENT INTRAOPERATIVE MONITORING

Of all of the procedures performed perioperatively, monitoring during surgery is the most dramatically changed by new technology. Monitors designed to increase safety by continuous data display have proved to be reliable, without risk, and affordable. The common employment of respiratory monitors (Table 1) have secondarily decreased utilization of arterial blood gases. Obviously, the best technology is only a supplement for continuous vigilant observation of the patient under anesthesia.

CUTANEOUS OXYGEN SATURATION MONITORING

Observation of nailbeds provides late and unreliable signs of hypoxia. Currently available cutaneous saturation monitors provide beat-to-beat assessment of oxygen saturation and a very high degree of correlation with directly measured arterial oxygen saturation. Although cost continues to be a factor (the price of these monitors is approximately $6,000 per unit), the early hypoxia warning provided is more than worth the investment as a patient safety issue. Current practice suggests that virtually all anesthetics and many patients on mechanical ventilatory support should be monitored with cutaneous oxygen saturation monitoring. The sensors must be shielded from bright light and the technique has limited usefulness with significant hypotension, hypothermia, and low cardiac output states. The beat-to-beat plethysmographic recording allows an assessment of the accuracy of the oxygen saturation obtained and pulse rate.

END-TIDAL CARBON DIOXIDE MONITORING

The ability to monitor end-tidal carbon dioxide has also become of increasing importance in the operating room and the intensive care unit. Real-time capnography has decreased the risk of undetected esophageal intubation and aided early detection of air embolism. Analysis of the tracing may assist in early recognition of residual muscle paralysis or airway obstruction. Although intermittent blood gas analysis is useful, capnography decreases the frequency of blood sampling required for carbon dioxide measurements. An initial equating analysis must be done when the absolute arterial value is important, such as when the intracranial

Table 1 Intraoperative Monitors Decreasing Arterial Blood Gas Utilization

Inspiratory oxygen analyzer
Breathing circuit manometry with low-pressure alarm
Spirometry with low minute-volume alarm
Pulse oximetry
Capnography

pressure is increased. Once the arterial to end-tidal carbon dioxide difference is ascertained, unless there is a change in dead space, this difference can be used to make an accurate estimation of $PaCO_2$.

The current major disadvantage to routine end-tidal carbon dioxide analysis is the cost of the technology. Although multiple patients can be assessed by a single mass spectrometer, it does not provide a breath-to-breath analysis of any individual patient unless individual units are employed. More recently, modified infrared technology has allowed the development of individual patient gas monitors that, for about $10,000 per patient, provide analysis of carbon dioxide, oxygen, and end-tidal anesthetic gas concentrations.

The noninvasive, safe, and accurate measurement of oxygen, ventilation, and anesthetic gases has become routine for the use of virtually all anesthetics.

TRANSCUTANEOUS BLOOD GAS ANALYSIS

A very close approximation of directly measured arterial oxygen pressure (PaO_2) and $PaCO_2$ can be obtained noninvasively and on a continuous basis by measurement of oxygen and carbon dioxide tension in the skin. This technology relies on local heating of the skin to create a vasodilated hyperemic area that will arterialize capillary blood. Employment of this technology has been limited to pediatric patients because accuracy is lost with increasing thickness of skin. The technique also fails in patients with edema, hypotension, cutaneous vasoconstriction, and concurrent electrocautery. For these reasons, transcutaneous blood gas analysis has few applications in intraoperative monitoring.

INTERMITTENT BLOOD GAS SAMPLING

Blood may be drawn for arterial blood gas determinations by percutaneous arterial puncture with a small-gauge needle or from an indwelling arterial line. Monitoring indications and complications of arterial line placement are discussed elsewhere in this text. Placement of an arterial line is also indicated if more than three arterial blood samples are to be obtained during a 24-hour period. In addition to analysis for pH, carbon dioxide partial pressure (PCO_2), and partial pressure of oxygen (PO_2), blood can also be analyzed by a co-oximeter for carboxyhemoglobin, methemoglobin, and directly measured arterial oxygen saturation.

Blood gas specimens must be heparinized, which is usually done by flushing the syringe with 1,000 U per milliliter of heparin. If higher-concentration heparin solutions are used or if the heparin is not completely evacuated from the syringe, the pH determination will be artifactually low. Blood should be drawn and transported anaerobically to prevent diffusion of carbon dioxide into the air, lowering the measured $PaCO_2$ and raising the pH. Samples should be placed immediately in

ice to inhibit oxygen consumption by blood neutrophils, especially if the granulocyte count is unusually high (e.g., in the case of leukemia) or if a delay is anticipated before the oxygen tension and pH can be measured.

Although clinical trials are under way for several devices for continuous blood gas analysis, none is yet in routine clinical use. As technologic advancements provide ever-smaller sensing electrodes, indwelling blood gas analyzers may provide continuous monitoring when pulse oximetry fails (hypothermia and low cardiac output states).

Acid-base monitoring is diagnostically important during the use of an anesthetic when hemodynamic instability occurs. Metabolic acidosis lowers the threshold for induction of arrythmias such as ventricular fibrillation. Acidemia interferes with catecholamine-receptor interaction and depresses cerebral sympathetic nervous system outflow, depressing ventricular performance. Respiratory or metabolic alkalosis decreases ventricular contractility, but is usually not clinically significant.

In those patients who have or are at risk of having untoward hemodynamic respiratory or metabolic events, the combination of continuous cutaneous oximetry and an end-tidal carbon dioxide monitor plus an intra-arterial catheter for intermittent sampling as needed currently provides the optimum combination of metabolic and respiratory assessment.

POSTOPERATIVE INDICATIONS FOR ACID-BASE OF ARTERIAL BLOOD GAS DETERMINATIONS

Respiratory acidosis is the most common acid-base disorder during the postoperative period. Table 2 lists the clinical findings that aid recognition in unmonitored patients. Monitoring an extubated patient in the post-anesthesia care unit for the onset of respiratory acidosis is a difficult problem. Because hypercapnia is often not associated with hypoxemia when supplemental oxygen is provided, pulse oximetry will fail to detect the problem. Capnography is insensitive in extubated patients because of dilution of samples. Respiratory acidosis must be confirmed by arterial blood gas monitoring.

Metabolic acidosis may be noted during the postoperative period because of pre-existing conditions such as diabetic ketoacidosis or renal failure. Those cases can be predicted and arterial blood gas monitoring instituted preoperatively. Also, pH should be monitored when inadequate oxygen delivery or utilization is suspected. Lactic acidosis explains the majority of cases of metabolic acidosis occurring de novo during the perioperative period. The etiologies include hypovolemia and other causes of low cardiac output, severe hypothermia, extreme anemia, and sepsis. Treatment requires slowing the rapid lactic acid generation (warming, volume and hemoglobin replacement, inotropes) until lactic acid metabolism and renal acid excretion restore the balance.

Respiratory alkalosis caused by hyperventilation

Table 2 Risk Factors of Postoperative Respiratory Acidosis

Risk Factors	Presentation	Treatment
Residual anesthetics	Agitation	Arousal
Residual muscle relaxants	Dyspnea	Reversal of muscle relaxants
Increased airway resistance	Tachypnea	Open upper airway
Decreased pulmonary compliance	Hypertension; tachycardia; dysrhythmias	Treat bronchospasm; positioning to facilitate chest expansion
Shivering	Increased sympathetic nervous system activity	Warming/cooling
Hyperthermia	Increased intracranial pressure in patients at risk	Warming/cooling

Table 3 Diagnosis of Acid-base Disorders

Acidosis	
Respiratory	$pH < 7.38$ and $PaCO_2$ is elevated.
Acute	The pH is decreased 0.08 U for each 10 mm Hg the $PaCO_2$ is above normal (no time for metabolic compensation).
Metabolic	The serum bicarbonate is less than normal.
	Anion gap acidosis refers to a metabolic acidosis with an elevated anion gap. The etiologies are limited. In mixed disorders, the gap will remain even when the pH is corrected by the respiratory component.
	Nongap Acidosis (also known as hyperchloremic acidosis) refers to a metabolic acidosis *with* an anion gap, but the gap is within the normal range.
Alkalosis	
Respiratory	Lowering of $PaCO_2$ resulting in an elevation in pH.
Acute	The pH is increased 0.08 U for every 10–mm Hg decrease in $PaCO_2$.
Chronic	Compensation for respiratory alkalosis occurs with suppression of renal tubular acid secretion, depleting bicarbonate over a course of several weeks. If the alkalosis is of fairlyrecently onset, compensation should not be complete: pH isgenerally increased 0.03 U for each 10–mm Hg decrease in $PaCO_2$ after 2 weeks.
Metabolic	Increase in the serum bicarbonate concentration.

may occur during recovery. Pain or anxiety may cause spontaneous hyperventilation, and mechanical ventilation may induce iatrogenic hyperventilation. When the clinical diagnosis is obvious and oxygenation has been evaluated by pulse oximetry, analgesics or sedatives are given without delaying for a blood gas determination. Mechanical ventilation of a sedated patient postoperatively requires arterial blood gas monitoring, as respiratory alkalosis may not be clinically apparent.

Postoperative metabolic alkalosis is nearly limited to two situations: pre-existing alkalosis from gastrointestinal and renal losses and the administration of bicarbonate intraoperatively. Both situations require continued arterial blood gas monitoring.

INTERPRETATION

Partial Pressures of Oxygen and Oximetry

Both partial pressure and oxygen saturation quantify *blood* oxygen, utilizing different units of measure. These two values can be interconverted through the familiar hemoglobin-oxygen dissociation curve. The ultimate goal of respiratory monitoring is tracking of the essential delivery of oxygen to tissues for utilization, which is a function of oxygen content of blood and cardiac output. Hemoglobin is essentially saturated at an oxygen partial pressure of 100 mm Hg. At any level of oxygen partial pressure, most blood oxygen content is bound to

Table 4 Acid-Base Disorders: Etiologies of Alkalosis

Respiratory alkalosis
  Major central nervous system disturbance: intracranial
    hemorrhage
  Drugs: salicylates, progesterone
  Pregnancy
  Reflex hyperventilation: interstitial fibrosis
  Anxiety and pain
  Hepatic cirrhosis
  Sepsis

Metabolic alkalosis
  Volume depletion; gastrointestinal, renal, skin, respiratory losses
  Intravascular volume depletion due to "third spacing": ascites,
    bowel edema, hemorrhage into body cavities
  Extraordinary causes: mineralocorticoid excess, Bartter's
  syndrome,   bicarbonate ingestion

Table 5 Acid-Base Disorders: Etiologies of Acidosis

Respiratory acidosis
  Central nervous system depression: drugs, central nervous system
    disease, obesity-hypoventilation syndrome
  Pleural disease: pneumothorax, pleural effusion
  Lung disease: COPD, ARDS, pneumonia, pulmonary emboli
  Musculoskeletal disease: kyphoscoliosis, Guillain-Barré syndrome,
    myasthenia gravis, botulism, polymyositis

Metabolic acidosis
  Nongap acidosis
    Gastrointestinal bicarbonate loss: bowel preparation
    Renal tubular losses
    Compensation for chronic respiratory alkalosis
    Carbonic anhydrase inhibitors
    Ureteral diversions
    Vasoactive peptide-producing tumors
    Drugs: carbonic anhydrase inhibitors, amphotericin B,
      cyclosporine

Increased gap acidosis
  Renal insufficiency
  Ketoacidosis
  Drugs or poisons: methanol, salicylates, paraldehyde, ethylene
    glycol
  Lactic acidosis

ARDS = adult respiratory distress syndrome; COPD = chronic obstructive pulmonary disease.

hemoglobin, so content decreases rapidly with hemoglobin concentration. Both arterial blood gas sampling and continuous oxygen saturation monitoring can give false security when acute hemorrhage suddenly lowers the carrying capacity, leaving the PaO_2 and saturation levels high but lowering content.

Capnography and Partial Pressures of Carbon Dioxide

Although capnography and blood gas determinations report familiar partial pressures of carbon dioxide, one quantifies *blood* carbon dioxide, one *expiratory gas* carbon dioxide. The end-tidal:arterial carbon dioxide ratio is primarily dependent on the dead space of the patient. In normal patients, the difference between end-tidal carbon dioxide and actual arterial carbon dioxide is rarely more than 3 or 4 mm Hg. However, in patients who have a significant dead-space component to their ventilatory physiology, the difference can be much higher.

The importance of blood carbon dioxide is reflected in the effect on acid-base balance.

Acid-Base

The concentration of hydrogen ion in serum is remarkably low in comparison with the concentrations of other measured electrolytes. It is usually expressed as a pH rather than as a concentration unit (e.g., milliequivalent liter^{-1}. Despite the diminutive values of hydrogen concentration, changes in pH cause shifting of other electrolytes effecting cardiac rhythm and altering hemoglobin binding of oxygen.

Metabolism results in the production of respiratory acid (carbon dioxide), which exists in equilibrium with bicarbonate radical (HCO_3^-) and hydrogen ion ($H+$) via carbonic acid. Aberrations in excretion of respiratory acid occur with changes in ventilation and result in respiratory acidosis or alkalosis. Nonvolatile end products of metabolism include "metabolic acids" (pyruvate,

lactate, acetoacetate, beta-hydroxybutyrate), and inorganic acids (phosphoric, sulfuric, uric). The normal conversion of metabolic acids to carbon dioxide and H_2O can be overwhelmed by rapid production. Excessive lactic acid is produced and accumulates from anaerobic metabolism with sepsis, hypoperfusion, aortic clamping, or tourniquets. Renal excretion is required for organic acids, and inadequate excretion of fixed acids in renal failure will also result in accumulation causing acidosis. pH is obtained by direct measurement with ion-sensitive electrodes. Bicarbonate is reported as a calculated value. Following direct measurement of pH and arterial carbon dioxide pressure ($PaCO_2$), bicarbonate concentration is calculated via the Henderson-Hasselbalch equation. While this method can be criticized for assuming a stable equilibrium, it provides a reasonable estimate of the serum bicarbonate concentration. The alternative is the direct measurement of total serum carbon dioxide, which is more affected by $PaCO_2$ and therefore provides less appropriate information.

INTERPRETATION OF ARTERIAL BLOOD GASES FOR DIAGNOSIS OF ACID-BASE DISORDERS

Blood gas results allow sorting of acid-base derangements into categories: acidosis, alkalosis, respiratory, metabolic. Calculating the anion gap for metabolic acidosis further defines the disorder and narrows the differential diagnosis. The anion gap is usually calculated as follows: $Na - (Cl + HCO_3)$. The normal range of an anion gap is 10 to 14 mEq per liter. The calculated gap is an index of unmeasured anions, which include negatively charged proteins (15 mEq per liter), phosphates (2 mEq per liter), sulfates (1 mEq per liter), and organic acids (5 mEq per liter). The discrepancy between the total unmeasured anions (23 mEq per liter) and the calculated anion gap is attributable to the "unmeasured" cations: potassium (4.5 mEq per liter), calcium (5 mEq per liter), and magnesium (1.5 mEq per liter) (Table 3). These categories are not academic. The etiology must be defined before the patient can be appropriately treated (Tables 4 and 5).

The indications and interpretation of arterial blood gases were discussed separately in this chapter for the sake of simplicity. Obviously, they cannot be separated in the practice of anesthesiology. Detection and treatment of abnormalities of acid-base balance, arterial PaO_2, or $PaCO_2$ is the purpose of blood gas monitoring.

CLOTTING STATUS

TODD DORMAN, M.D.
BRIAN A. ROSENFELD, M.D.

In anesthesiology, monitoring coagulation status requires the ability to evaluate the hemostatic system rapidly and objectively. This is necessary in order to diagnose and follow underlying preoperative bleeding disorders, acutely developing intraoperative bleeding problems, and pharmacologic interventions that alter the coagulation system. Monitoring may involve a specific test for a known or suspected deficiency or drug-induced abnormality, a generalized screening test of the coagulation system, or multiple screening tests for an unknown bleeding diathesis. The ability to obtain the results quickly can also influence the choice of testing. The anesthesiologist must have a basic understanding of platelet function, the coagulation cascade, and the clinical situation in which bleeding problems may develop in order to choose the right test.

HEMOSTASIS

Normal hemostasis occurs in three stages. Platelet aggregation, fibrin formation, and fibrinolysis function in a system of checks and balances in response to bleeding from a site of injury. The system promotes clot formation at the site of injury while preventing clot formation distant to the site of injury. In addition, the system functions to keep the clot at the site of injury from persisting longer than physiologically necessary. Abnormalities in any of the three components of this system can result in thrombotic or hemorrhagic disorders.

The first stage of clot formation involves platelet adherence and aggregation. Normal endothelial cells are resistant to platelet adherence because of several inhibitors synthesized by the endothelial cell. These inhibitors include prostacyclin, thrombomodulin, heparan and plasminogen activator. Injury to the endothelium causes platelets to adhere to collagen fibrils exposed by the disrupted endothelial cell lining. von Willebrand factor (vWF) is required in this stage as a bridge between the collagen fibrils and platelets. Once a basal layer of platelets has formed, additional platelets adhere to this layer, creating activated platelet aggregates. Activated platelets have surface receptors for fibrinogen and vWF. The conversion of fibrinogen to fibrin causes the aggregated platelets to bind to the vessel wall in a fibrin network.

The coagulation cascade represents the second stage of the hemostatic process. It is usually broken down into the intrinsic, extrinsic, and common pathways, culminating in cross-linked fibrin formation (Fig. 1). The common pathway is the terminal portion of the cascade, starting with factor X activation by either the intrinsic or extrinsic pathways. Activated factor X converts prothrombin to thrombin, with factor V serving as a cofactor. Thrombin then binds to fibrinogen, causing the liberation of fibrinopeptides A and B and resulting in the formation of fibrin monomers. The fibrin monomers polymerize and are cross-linked by the action of factor XIII.

Initiation of the common pathway by the extrinsic pathway starts with the activation of factor VII by tissue thromboplastin. The factor-VII thromboplastin complex activates factor X, triggering the common pathway. The intrinsic pathway begins with activation of Factor XII by disrupted endothelial surfaces and is facilitated by the action of high molecular-weight kininogen. Factor XII cleaves factor XI into its active form, which in turn activates factor IX and factor X, thereby triggering the common pathway. Activation of factor X by factor IX requires factor VIII, which exists in plasma noncovalently complexed with vWF.

Several inhibitors can help localize and control the coagulation cascade. These native anticoagulants include antithrombin III, protein C, and protein S. Antithrombin III serves to inhibit activated factors IX, X, and thrombin. This inhibition is potentiated by heparin, which binds to antithrombin III, causing a conformational change that increases the rate of thrombin inactivation. Protein C serves to inactivate factors V and VIII, with protein S functioning as a cofactor in this process. Insufficient quantities of these native anticoagulants predispose patients to thrombotic disorders.

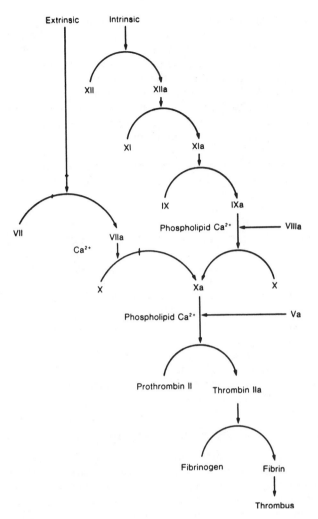

Figure 1 Coagulation cascade, including extrinsic, intrinsic, and common pathways.

Proteins C and S, prothrombin, and factors VII, IX, and X are vitamin K–dependent proteins. They share in common a residue at the N-terminal end that requires vitamin K for synthesis. Warfarin's action inhibits all of the vitamin K–dependent proteins and thus leads to a prolonged protime. Some antibiotics (cefamandole, cefoperazone, and moxalactam) used in surgical patients have a methylthiotetrazole (MTT) side chain. This side chain acts as a competitive inhibitor of the vitamin K–dependent postribosomal carboxylation of prothrombin. Without this modification, prothrombin's activity is altered by an inability to bind calcium or attach to phospholipid.

Fibrinolysis, the last stage of hemostasis, serves as a repair mechanism to enable recanalization to occur. Fibrinolysis begins with endothelial cell release of tissue plasminogen activators, which convert plasminogen to plasmin. Plasmin initiates the degradation of fibrinogen and cross-linked fibrin. The degradation of cross-linked fibrin causes the formation of D-dimers, which can be distinguished from fibrinogen degradation products by different assays.

ROUTINE CLOTTING TESTS

Platelet Count

The platelet count is routinely ordered because both thrombocytopenia and thrombocytosis produce hemostatic abnormalities. In the perioperative setting, platelet counts can be determined rapidly and accurately through the use of automated counters. These counts will vary within certain limits, depending on the counter and the laboratory. Platelet counts outside these limits require a more time-consuming manual count. The quantitative platelet count does not provide any information about the quality of platelet function.

Thrombocytosis occurs in three forms: physiologic, primary, and reactive. Physiologic thrombocytosis results from mobilization of platelets in response to exercise or epinephrine administration. Primary thrombocytosis reflects an elevated rate of platelet production and can lead to either hemorrhage or thrombosis. Usually caused by a myeloproliferative disorder, platelet numbers may require reduction with chemotherapeutic agents or plateletpheresis perioperatively. Reactive thrombocytosis also results from accelerated production but rarely requires therapeutic intervention. It usually occurs in response to hemorrhage, infection, carcinoma, or lymphoma. The large platelets seen in primary and reactive thrombocytosis can be misread by the automated counters as erythrocytes, resulting in factitiously low platelet counts.

Thrombocytopenia is more commonly encountered than thrombocytosis perioperatively. It occurs secondary to decreased production, decreased survival, splenic sequestration, or dilution. Platelet counts of less than 20,000 platelets per cubic millimeter can lead to spontaneous bleeding with central nervous system or gastrointestinal hemorrhage. Thrombocytopenia from decreased production, survival, or sequestration is usually recognized preoperatively from concomitant medical problems. Rarely, thrombocytopenia from decreased survival may occur during the intraoperative period. This may be caused by the development of disseminated intravascular coagulation (DIC) or the use of cardiopulmonary bypass equipment. Dilutional thrombocytopenia caused by blood loss, platelet consumption, and the administration of fluids lacking platelets is the most common cause of acquired intraoperative bleeding.

Qualitative platelet abnormalities may occur in patients with normal or abnormal platelet counts. These disorders are caused by congenital or acquired abnormalities of platelet function. von Willebrand's disease is the most common congenital disorder, leading to decreased platelet function. Patients with this disease lack a specific plasma protein necessary for platelet adherence to injured endothelial surfaces. Infusion of cryoprecipitate, which contains sufficient quantities of vWF, will usually correct this bleeding problem. The most frequently encountered acquired disorder of platelet function is uremia. This is believed to be secondary to an altered endothelial cell factor VIII-vWF-platelet interaction. This disorder is improved with dialysis (peritoneal > hemodialysis) or the administration of DDAVP. Some commonly used drugs including salicylates, nonsteroidal anti-inflammatory agents, and carbamazepine also inhibit platelet function and should be withheld preoperatively if possible. Qualitative platelet function can be assessed preoperatively by a bleeding time. This test is not performed intraoperatively, but platelet dysfunction should be considered in patients with normal coagulation tests and platelet numbers who are "oozing." The thromboelastograph (which will be discussed later) is another test that provides some assessment of platelet function and can be used intraoperatively.

The correction of thrombocytopenia or functional disorders of platelets may require platelet transfusions. Each random donor unit of platelets contains platelets, some white cells, and approximately 60 ml of plasma. This plasma fraction contains approximately 100 mg of fibrinogen and all of the factors normally found in fresh frozen plasma (FFP). The patient's platelet count can be expected to increase by 5,000 to 10,000 per milliliter per unit infused. In situations of increased platelet destruction or consumption, platelet transfusions are less effective. In patients refractory to infusion of random donor platelets, single-donor or HLA-matched platelets may be required.

Prothrombin Time and Partial Thromboplastin Time

Coagulation cascade disorders can involve any problem with concentration or function of coagulation factors (Table 1). Abnormalities of these factors are routinely screened by two tests: the prothrombin time (PT) and the activated partial thromboplastin time (aPTT). The PT test screens for abnormalities in the extrinsic pathway of coagulation. This test was originally believed to reflect the concentration of prothrombin

(factor II) in plasma, but was later found to be most sensitive for levels of factor VII. The test is performed by adding tissue factor (thromboplastin) and calcium to plasma and comparing the time to clot formation versus control. A prolongation of the PT time may be secondary to deficiencies or inhibitors of either extrinsic or common pathway proteins. Abnormalities of this test are seen most frequently in patients receiving warfarin and those with liver disease, fat malabsorption, or starvation, in conjunction with antibiotic therapy. Factor deficiencies from starvation, malabsorption, or warfarin use that lead to a prolongation of the PT can be corrected slowly with vitamin K or more rapidly with FFP. Specific factor deficiencies are corrected with FFP.

The aPTT test screens for protein factor abnormalities in the intrinsic pathway of coagulation. The test utilizes an efficient activating surface to maximize contact for factor XII. The activator substances kaolin or celite are added to a mixture of diluted phospholipid (partial thromboplastin) and calcium. The time to clot formation is then compared with control plasma. Prolongation of this test reflects deficiencies or inhibitors of either the intrinsic or common pathway. This test is most commonly used to monitor the effects of heparin therapy. Factor deficiencies leading to prolongation of the aPTT can be corrected with FFP, cryoprecipitate, or specific factor transfusions.

Activated Clotting Time

The use of extracorporeal circuits for surgery or cardiopulmonary assist devices requires anticoagulation to prevent clot formation. Before the advent of the activated clotting time (ACT), empiric protocols for heparin administration were used. Experience during this time demonstrated that the dose and clearance of heparin varied widely from patient to patient, and neither could be predicted on the basis of the patient's age, body weight, or body surface area. The ACT is a test that both rapidly and accurately monitors the degree of anticoagulation and protamine reversal needed. The

Table 1 Nomenclature and Concentration of Blood Coagulation Factors Required for Normal Hemostasis

Factor Designation	Common Name	Concentration Required for Normal Hemostasis
I	Fibrinogen	100 mg/dl
II	Prothrombin	30%–40%
V	Accelerator globulin, labile factor, proaccelerin	30%–40%
VII	Proconvertin, stable factor, serum prothrombin conversion accelerator	30%–40%
VIII	Antihemophilic globulin, antihemophilia A factor	30%–40%
IX	Christmas factor, antihemophilia B factor	30%–40%
X	Stuart-Prower factor	30%–40%
XI	Plasma thromboplastin antecedent	20%
XII	Hageman factor	None required
XIII	Fibrin-stabilizing factor	1%
Prekalikrein	Fletcher factor	None required
High molecular-weight kininogen	Williams-Fitzgerald-Flaujeac factor	None required

ACT was first introduced by Hattersley in 1966. The test is easily performed in the operating room or at the bedside. A linear dose-response curve is generated to determine the dosage of heparin and protamine required (Fig. 2).

To perform this test, a small amount of arterial blood (2 ml) is added to a tube containing diatomaceous earth (activator) and a magnetic stirbar. The tube is placed in a hemochron instrument and the timer is started. Clot formation stops the stirbar, which in turn stops the timer. A dose-response curve is plotted using the patient's ACT before heparinization and after 2 to 3 mg per kilogram (1 mg = 100 units) of heparin has been administered. Baseline values should be approxi-

mately 120 to 140 seconds, with adequate anticoagulation keeping the ACT greater than 480 seconds. Subsequent doses of heparin can be administered based on the previously constructed dose-response curve.

Protamine is the agent used to reverse the effects of heparin. The dose of protamine necessary to return patients to their initial ACT can be determined by checking an ACT at the conclusion of cardiopulmonary bypass. Plotting this time on the previously constructed dose-response curve enables the anesthesiologist to determine the amount of heparin remaining in the circulation. The neutralizing dose of protamine is then calculated by multiplying the circulating heparin dose by a factor of 1.3. After several minutes, another ACT is

Figure 2 Procedure for construction and the use of the activated coagulation time test.

Step 1: Construct graph axes.

Step 2: Determine initial ACT (A) and administer 2 mg per kilogram of heparin, then measure ACT (B) and plot both values. Extrapolate an imaginary line through "A" and "B" to intersect with 480 second line to find point "C." Example:3.5 mg per kilogram of heparin is needed to produce 480 second ACT or 1.5 mg per kilogram in addition to the 2 mg per kilogram heparin already given.

Step 3: After required heparin has been given, measure ACT. Plot point "D". If point "D" does not superimpose on point "C," then a dose-response curve is drawn from "A" to a point midway between "C" and "D."

Step 4: After 60 minutes, measure the ACT, determine amount of heparin in patient's circulation from the dose-response curve. Example: assume an ACT of 350 seconds. The heparin level would be 2.8 mg per kilogram. To return the ACT to 480 second, 1.2 mg per kilogram of heparin is needed.

Step 5: To reverse anticoagulation, determine circulating heparin level as in Step 4. The neutralizing dose of protamine is heparin level mg per kilogram × 1.3. Example: ACT of 325 seconds is measured. Heparin level is 2.6 mg per kilogram and 3.4 mg per kilogram protamine is required.

(From Bull BS, Hose WM, Brauer FS. Heparin therapy during extracorporeal circulation. J Thorac Cardiovasc Surg 1975; 69:686; used with permission.)

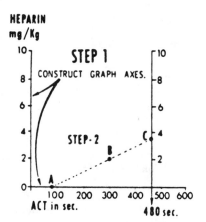
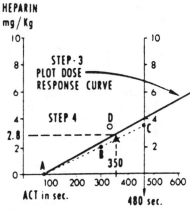
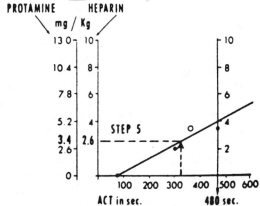

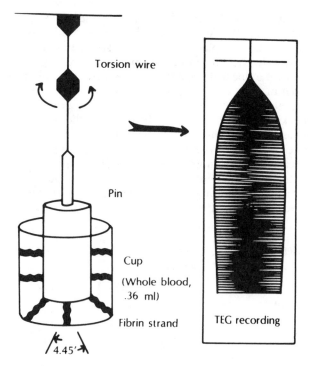

Figure 3 Thromboelastograph. (Reprinted with permission from the International Anesthesia Research Society; Anesthesia and Analgesia, 1985, 64:890.)

measured to determine the adequacy of neutralization, and additional protamine can be given as needed. The protamine must be administered carefully, however, because it is associated with an IgE-type allergic reaction that causes systemic hypotension and pulmonary vasoconstriction. Excess free protamine (not bound to heparin) also functions as an anticoagulant. Several studies have shown that protamine dosing has been more effective since the development of careful monitoring with the ACT. An alternative, simpler method for determining the neutralization dose of protamine utilizes the automated protamine dose assay. Bleeding noted after "normalization" of the ACT is secondary to surgical hemostasis, thrombocytopenia, or fibrinolysis.

Thromboelastograph

The thromboelastograph (TEG) was developed by Hartert in 1948 (Fig. 3). It monitors the presence and effects of clotting factors both quantitatively and qualitatively by testing the viscous and elastic properties of a fibrin clot. The test is reproducible and can be performed in the operating room. The entire TEG test takes approximately 5 to 6 hours, but the majority of information needed can be obtained within the first 60 to 90 minutes. Because of the time required to obtain information from this test, it is not suitable as an intraoperative routine screen, but is beneficial in surgical procedures of long duration (e.g., liver transplantation). In liver transplant procedures, the TEG is an ideal monitor because liver recipients frequently have abnormalities in the number and function of coagulation factors and

platelets. The addition of TEG to intraoperative monitoring of liver transplant patients has changed transfusion practices. These patients are now receiving fewer red blood cell and FFP transfusions and greater numbers of platelet and cryoprecipitate transfusions.

The test is performed by placing 0.36 ml of whole blood in a stainless steel cuvette (Fig. 4). The cuvette is kept at 37°C and oscillates at a 4-degree 45-minute angle. A piston attached to a torsion wire is lowered into the sample and the sample is covered by several drops of mineral oil to prevent evaporation. While the sample remains fluid, its motion will not effect the piston. However, when fibrin strands begin to form, they couple the cuvette to the piston. The elasticity of the forming, retracting, and lysing clot are then transmitted to the piston and recorded on thermal paper.

There are several variables routinely measured from this recorded graph (see Fig. 4). The *r-value* or reaction time is an indicator of the generation of plasma thromboplastin and is influenced by factors of the intrinsic pathway. Any quantitative or qualitative abnormality of these factors produces a prolonged r-value (normal = 6 to 8 minutes). The alpha-angle is determined by the speed at which a solid clot forms. Also known as the clot formation rate, it is a function of the quality of fibrinogen and platelets (normal >50 degrees). The *MA* or maximal amplitude is the largest amplitude attained and reflects the maximal elasticity of the clot. When the graph reaches MA, there is usually a slight diminution in the width of the graph caused by clot retraction. The MA is an indicator of both platelet number and function (normal = 60 to 70 mm). Finally, the whole blood clot lysis time or *F* represents fibrinolysis. When this time period is shortened (normal >5 hours), the process is accelerated. Determining these variables can diagnose abnormalities and help guide specific therapy (Fig. 5). If the r value is greater than 15 minutes, consider FFP; for an MA or less than 40 mm, consider platelets. If there is no improvement and the alpha-angle remains less than 40 degrees, consider cryoprecipitate, and if the F time is less than 120 minutes, consider epsilon-aminocaproic acid.

Physiologic homeostasis is also necessary when one is monitoring coagulation status. Hypothermia, acidosis, and hypocalcemia can all have detrimental effects on clot formation in the presence of normal clotting factors.

MONITORING FOR FIBRINOLYSIS

DIC remains a poorly understood syndrome that is initiated by multiple endogenous and exogenous factors. The syndrome manifests itself as a bleeding diathesis, diffuse clot formation, or a combination thereof. It can occur either acutely or chronically. The laboratory abnormalities associated with this syndrome vary from patient to patient and include hypofibrinogenemia, thrombocytopenia, prolonged PT, aPTT, thrombin time, and elevated levels of fibrinogen degradation products (FDP), and D-dimers. Anesthesiologists should be familiar with the syndrome and with which diagnostic

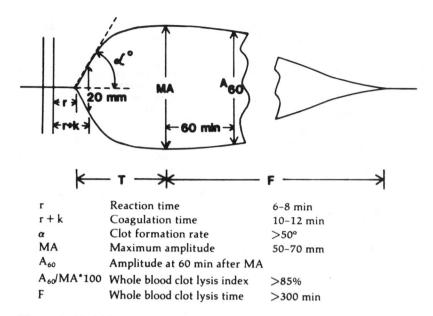

r	Reaction time	6–8 min
r + k	Coagulation time	10–12 min
α	Clot formation rate	>50°
MA	Maximum amplitude	50–70 mm
A_{60}	Amplitude at 60 min after MA	
A_{60}/MA*100	Whole blood clot lysis index	>85%
F	Whole blood clot lysis time	>300 min

Figure 4 Variables and normal values measured by the thromboelastograph. (Reprinted with permission from the International Anesthesia Research Society; Anesthesia and Analgesia, 1985, 64:891.)

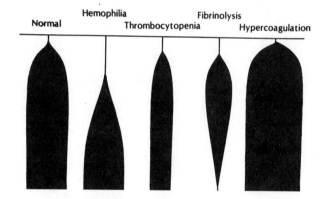

Figure 5 Thromboelastograph patterns of abnormal states.

tests to order. They may encounter its chronic form in some cancer patients, and its acute form in patients with amniotic fluid embolism, pre-eclampsia, transfusion reactions, hypothermia, heat stroke, trauma, and sepsis.

Fibrinogen (factor I) is exclusively synthesized by the liver, and levels are depressed in DIC (normal levels are 300 to 400 mg per deciliter). Although bleeding is more common when levels fall below 100 mg per deciliter, there is no direct correlation between fibrinogen levels and the risk of bleeding. In fact, patients with afibrinogenemia demonstrate that a second insult is required before bleeding will occur. When hypofibrinogenemia (< 50 mg per deciliter) is severe and associated with bleeding, cryoprecipitate transfusions should be administered. Each unit of cryoprecipitate contains approximately 200 to 300 mg of fibrinogen.

The thrombin time (TT) measures the formation of a fibrin clot in plasma by the action of thrombin on fibrinogen. Thrombin normally causes the conversion of fibrinogen to fibrin by catalyzing the cleavage of the alpha- and beta-chains from fibrinogen. This cleavage releases fibrinopeptides A and B. The resulting central fibrin monomer, now exposed, interacts with other monomers to form cross-linked fibrin. Normal TTs should be within 2 seconds of control (13 to 15 seconds). A prolonged TT indicates either an abnormality of fibrinogen (quantitative or qualitative) or the presence of thrombin inhibitors like heparin or FDPs.

FDPs, which are themselves anticoagulants, are detected by mixing diluted patient serum with latex particles that are coated with antibodies to fibrinogen fragment D. The agglutination of these particles demonstrates the presence in the serum of any molecule containing the D moiety, including fibrin and fibrinogen. For this reason, only serum (clotted plasma) can be tested, and it is important that all fibrinogen be clotted, or false-positives will occur. Dysfibrinogenemia, which can occur primarily, or in some patients with liver disease, will also produce false-positive results because all of the fibrinogen will not have clotted in the specimen. Therefore, although this test is highly sensitive as a screen for DIC (100 percent), its specificity is only 56 percent.

To improve the specificity of diagnosing DIC, a D-dimer test can be performed. When its results are positive, this test can help rule out false-positives FDPs. The test measures fibrin degradation products by mixing plasma with monoclonal antibody–coated latex particles directed against the D-dimer fragment of fibrin. The test is specific for the lysis of fibrin and is not affected by fibrinogen or its degradation products, and it has an 85 percent sensitivity and 97 percent specificity. False-positives can occur in patients who have tested positive for rheumatoid factor. Elevated levels of D-dimer are detected whenever the patient's condition is associated with fibrin deposition and subsequent lysis (i.e., venous thrombosis, pulmonary embolism, pre-eclampsia). At present, the role of the D-dimer test remains that of a confirmatory test in patients with positive FDPs. It is important to remember that these laboratory tests are merely suggestive of DIC, and the diagnosis remains one based on clinical findings.

Rapidly diagnosing and treating disorders of hemostasis in the perioperative setting is necessary to improve patient safety, to limit the exposure to foreign antigens from inappropriately transfused blood products, and to reduce the cost of medical care. It is incumbent on anesthesiologists to understand the coagulation system, its abnormalities, and the therapeutic options.

SUGGESTED READING

Bull BS, Korpman RA, Huse WM. Heparin therapy during extracorporeal circulation: Parts I and II. J Thorac Cardiovas Surg 1975; 69:674–689.

Carr JM, McKinney M, McDonagh J. Diagnosis of disseminated intravascular coagulation. Am J Clin Path 1989; 91:280–287.

Counts RC, et al. Hemostasis in massively transfused trauma patients. Ann Surg 1979; 190:91–99.

Kang YG, et al. Intraoperative changes in blood coagulation and thromboelastographic monitoring in liver transplantation. Anesth Analg 1985; 64:888–896.

Mannucci PM. Desmopressin: nontransfusional form of treatment of congenital and acquired bleeding disorders. Blood 1988; 72: 1449–1455.

Rivard DC, Thompson SJ. Demonstration of heparin reversal with protamine administration using an automated protamine dose assay: a comparison of two methods. Ject 26th International Conference Proceedings 1988; 56–61.

Winter PM, Kanger YG. Hepatic transplantation anesthetic and perioperative management. New York: Praeger Scientific, 1986.

POSTOPERATIVE CONSIDERATIONS AND ANESTHETIC COMPLICATIONS

PROLONGED NEUROMUSCULAR BLOCKADE

RONALD D. MILLER, M.D.

An unexpectedly prolonged neuromuscular blockade in the postoperative period can be caused by many pharmacologic and physiologic abnormalities, the most common of which will be discussed in this chapter. Of prime importance is determining whether a residual blockade exists and treating it accordingly. This chapter deals with the differential diagnosis, causes, and treatment of a prolonged neuromuscular blockade in the postoperative period.

DIAGNOSIS

Of prime importance is ensuring that a patient does not have an undetected subtle neuromuscular blockade with associated hypoventilation and hypocarbia that could lead to progressive weakness, hypoxia, and cardiac arrest. Equipment and personnel must be arranged properly to ensure that weakness and resultant hypoventilation are detected before the disastrous scenario described earlier occurs. When hypoventilation (e.g., decreased tidal volume and/or respiratory rate), hypoxia (e.g., as determined by pulse oximetry), or weakness (e.g., decreased hand grip strength) occurs, the differential diagnosis must be pursued. Inadequate ventilation may be caused by several factors other than a residual neuromuscular blockade.

Central respiratory depression as manifested by an inadequate respiratory drive can be caused by residual respiratory depression from intravenous or inhaled anesthetics. Narcotics are the prime culprit. In this regard, the administration of naloxone can sometimes be helpful. Poor respiratory muscle function is another cause of inadequate ventilation, which can occur from various types of surgery interfering with the patient's ability to take a large breath as measured by vital capacity. Nearly all patients have reductions in vital capacity that are the greatest on the day of surgery.

Patients undergoing upper-abdominal surgery have the greatest reduction in vital capacity, showing as much as 60 percent reduction on the day of surgery. This problem is also related to diaphragmatic impairment resulting in reduced carbon dioxide elimination and hypoxia. Certainly, other causes such as obesity, gastric dilation, tight dressings, and body casts also can inhibit respiratory function and predispose to hypercarbia and hypoxia.

When one is ascertaining the cause of hypoventilation or muscle weakness, a prolonged or inadequately reversed neuromuscular blockade should be considered. The most efficient way to monitor neuromuscular function is by the use of a peripheral nerve stimulator. Although there are a variety of approaches that can be used, I believe that subtle stimulation should be started initially with a gradual increase in the intensity of stimulation. For example, stimulation could be started by using the single twitch (e.g., 0.1 Hz every 2 to 3 seconds). If there is no response to this type of stimulation, train-of-four stimulation could be initiated. This type of stimulation is available in all peripheral nerve stimulators. If there is no response to train-of-four stimulation, then application of tetanic stimulus of 50 Hz to 100 Hz should be instituted. If there is no response to this form of stimulation, either a profound neuromuscular blockade or a malfunctioning stimulator exists. It is obviously more important to rule out a malfunctioning stimulator as the cause. An immediate approach to ruling out the latter cause is to apply the stimulator to yourself. The single twitch does not hurt and should evoke a contraction of the hand muscles. If such stimulation is not perceived by the clinician, a new stimulator should be sought. If the new stimulator appears to be functioning adequately and no response by the patient is observed, this is extremely strong evidence that a prolonged neuromuscular blockade is either totally or partially responsible for the inadequate ventilation and weakness.

What is more likely to occur in a patient who is not apneic but has inadequate spontaneous ventilation is partial response to peripheral nerve stimulation. Although there are many forms of stimulation that can be used, it is useful to use the train-of-four method of stimulation to ascertain whether the response of the thumb contraction is fading. If there is a fade, a neuromuscular blockade is probably present. If there is no fade, the clinician has preliminary evidence that a residual neuromuscular blockade does not exist. However, the clinician should not stop evaluating the patient for the possibility of a residual neuromuscular blockade at this point. Train-of-four stimulation will not detect-subtle degrees of neuromuscular blockade. When response to train-of-four stimulation is normal, then the clinician should take measures that are more precise and more stressful to the neuromuscular junction. For example, the head lift for 5 seconds is an extremely good test for assessing the presence of neuromuscular blockade. If the patient can lift his or her head for 5 seconds, it is reasonable to assume that a prolonged neuromuscular blockade is not present. Alternatively, using maximum inspiratory pressure can be very helpful; if the inspiratory pressure is more than -35 cm H_2O, then it is reasonable to assume that a residual neuromuscular blockade is not present. If one or more of these measures indicates the presence of a prolonged neuromuscular blockade, then the cause and treatment should be sought as described below.

CAUSES

There are several reasons why a neuromuscular blockade may be prolonged. They are usually related to altered pharmacokinetics, other concomitantly administered drugs, acid–base abnormalities, and hypothermia.

Pharmacokinetics

Renal Failure

Renal failure can profoundly affect the pharmacokinetics of neuromuscular blocking drugs. Table 1 summarizes the degree to which various neuromuscular blocking drugs are dependent on the kidney for their elimination. Gallamine and metocurine are virtually entirely dependent on the kidney for their elimination. Fortunately, these drugs are rarely used and are there-

Table 1 Dependence (Percentage of Injected Dose) of Neuromuscular Blocking Drugs on the Kidney for their Elimination

Drug	Percentage of Injected Dose
Gallamine	100
Metocurine	80–100
Doxacurium	60–90
Pipecuronium	60–90
Pancuronium	60–80
Alcuronium	70–90
D-tubocurarine	40–60
Rocuronium	10–25
Vecuronium	10–25
Atracurium	<5
Mivacurium	<10

Adapted from Miller RD, Savarese JJ. Pharmacology of muscle relaxants and their antagonist. In: Anesthesia. 3rd ed. New York; Churchill-Livingstone, 1990: 398.

fore rarely a cause of prolonged neuromuscular blockade. Pancuronium, fazadinium, and alcuronium are often used and are extensively dependent on the kidney for their elimination and, therefore, could easily be the cause of neuromuscular blockade in a patient with renal failure. Two drugs newly approved by the Food and Drug Administration, doxacurium and pipecuronium, are heavily dependent on the kidney for their elimination.

As depicted in Table 1, vecuronium, atracurium, and possibly mivacurium are dependent on the kidney for their elimination to a minor extent only. Only about 10 to 25 percent of an injected dose of vecuronium appears in the urine. The remaining vecuronium is probably excreted in the bile, both as the parent drug and as its 3-desacetyl metabolite. Although vecuronium depends little on the kidney for its elimination, administration of large doses (e.g., >0.1 mg per kilogram) or repetitive doses can result in a prolonged neuromuscular blockade in patients with impaired renal function. Because of its metabolism, atracurium appears not to be dependent on the kidney for its elimination and should, in theory, not cause prolonged neuromuscular blockade from impaired elimination.

Liver Dysfunction

Pancuronium is partially dependent on biliary excretion for its elimination and can therefore cause a prolonged neuromuscular blockade in patients with impaired hepatic function. Because vecuronium is predominantly dependent on biliary excretion for its elimination, initial predictions indicated that its duration of action would be prolonged in patients with liver disease. However, subsequent studies indicate that if the dose of vecuronium is less than 0.15 mg per kilogram, the duration of action is not prolonged (Table 2). Theoretically, the neuromuscular blockade of atracurium would not be prolonged in patients with liver disease. In fact, atracurium's duration of action with doses of 0.15 mg per kilogram or less is either unchanged or shorter in patients with impaired liver function as compared with that in patients with normal liver function.

Vecuronium and atracurium are increasingly being used; liver dysfunction should not be the cause of prolonged neuromuscular blockade unless unusually large doses of either one of these neuromuscular blocking drugs have been given.

Table 2 Pharmacokinetics of Vecuronium in Patients with Normal Hepatic Function and those with Cirrhosis

	Normal	Cirrhosis
Clearance (ml/kg/min)	4.5	4.4
Volume of distribution (L/kg)	0.18	0.22
Terminal elimination half-life (min)	57	51

Adapted from Miller RD, Savarese JJ. Pharmacology of muscle relaxants and their antagonists. In: Anesthesia. 3rd ed. New York: Churchill-Livingstone, 1990: 399.

Other Drugs

There are multiple other drugs that can either prolong the neuromuscular blockade from nondepolarizing muscle relaxants; separating those drug interactions that are of clinical importance from those of academic curiosity is crucially important. In my opinion, the antibiotics, local anesthetics, and magnesium are the drugs of prime importance.

Antibiotics

There are hundreds of reports regarding enhancing of neuromuscular block from nondepolarizing muscle relaxants by antibiotics. Most of the antibiotics are in the aminoglycoside category, including streptomycin, gentamicin, kanamycin, and the polymyxins. The penicillin type drugs are not known to interact with neuromuscular blocking drugs. Usually it is difficult to ascertain which component of the neuromuscular blockade is caused by the muscle relaxant and which is caused by the antibiotic. As a result, we have developed a rather arbitrary approach to dealing with this issue. We arbitrarily administer an antagonist such as neostigmine up to 5 mg per 70 kg. We do not give more neostigmine because that dose should be able to antagonize any neuromuscular blockade. More neostigmine will be ineffective. If this dose of neostigmine is ineffective, ventilation should be controlled until neuromuscular blockade terminates spontaneously. Although calcium will transiently antagonize an antibiotic-induced neuromuscular blockade, its antagonism is usually not sustained, and calcium may antagonize the antibacterial effect of the antibiotics.

Local Anesthetics

In large doses, most local anesthetics block neuromuscular transmission. In smaller doses, they enhance the neuromuscular blockade from both nondepolarizing and depolarizing muscle relaxants. Thus, local anesthetics given as part of regional anesthetic technique or to treat ventricular dysrhythmias in patients who have had nondepolarizing muscle relaxants may result in a prolonged neuromuscular blockade. It is impossible to determine which aspect of the neuromuscular blockade is caused by the local anesthetic and which aspect is caused by the muscle relaxant. Furthermore, the ability of neostigmine to antagonize a combined local anesthetic–muscle relaxant neuromuscular blockade has not been studied.

Magnesium

Magnesium enhances the neuromuscular blockade from both nondepolarizing and depolarizing neuromuscular blockers. Magnesium decreases the amount of acetylcholine released from the motor nerve terminal, decreases the depolarizing action of acetylcholine on the cholinergic receptor, and depresses the muscle membrane itself. Sometimes critically ill patients have ele-

vated levels of magnesium, depressed levels of calcium, or both. The more likely situation in which the interaction predominates is in obstetrical anesthesia in which an eclamptic toxemic woman may need magnesium therapy. This therapy could be reason for a prolonged neuromuscular blockade.

Acid-Base Balance

Although multiple acid-base abnormalities can influence a neuromuscular function, respiratory acidosis is the one that is the most troublesome. Respiratory acidosis may augment and prolong a nondepolarizing neuromuscular blockade. Furthermore, respiratory acidosis can interfere with antagonism of neuromuscular blockade. For example, it is often difficult to antagonize a neuromuscular blockade in the presence of a $PaCO_2$ greater than 50 mm Hg. This has many clinical ramifications. For example, if a patient hypoventilates in the recovery room, attempts to antagonize a residual neuromuscular blockade may fail. Administration of narcotics may increase the likelihood of this untoward event. Such a sequence contains an element of potential positive feedback in which a respiratory depressant produces more acidosis and augments a neuromuscular blockade and, therefore, more respiratory depression. Obviously, acid-base status should be determined in the presence of a prolonged neuromuscular blockade, and ventilation augmented if the $PaCO_2$ is elevated.

Body Temperature

Hypothermia can prolong and intensify a nondepolarizing neuromuscular blockade. Although there are differences between neuromuscular blocking drugs, usually a combination of delayed renal and biliary excretion and an increased sensitivity of the neuromuscular junction accounts for this intensified neuromuscular blockade. Hypothermia markedly prolongs that neuromuscular blockade from both vecuronium and atracurium, and to a lesser extent, from D-tubocurarine. The above-mentioned conclusions have been based on rather profound hypothermia (i.e., body temperature of 30°C). Obviously, body temperature of this magnitude is usually not a factor in the postoperative patient. However, more recent evidence has shown that with a body temperature of 34.5°C, a vecuronium or atracurium neuromuscular blockade could be markedly long. As a result, body temperature should be checked in the presence of a prolonged neuromuscular blockade.

TREATMENT

Acetylcholinesterase Inhibitors

Acetylcholinesterase inhibitors, such as edrophonium and neostigmine, are highly effective antagonists of nondepolarizing neuromuscular drugs. With a clear response to peripheral nerve stimulation, 2.5 to 5 mg per

70 kg of neostigmine or 0.5 to 1.0 mg per kilogram of edrophonium should effectively antagonize the neuromuscular blockade. If there is no response to peripheral nerve stimulation, these drugs should not be given. The presence of no response to peripheral nerve stimulation indicates that either the neuromuscular blockade is very profound or that the stimulator is itself not working. In the presence of a profound neuromuscular blockade, these acetycholinesterase inhibitors are not likely to be effective.

If the previously mentioned doses of neostigmine or edrophonium do not reverse the neuromuscular blockade, no more drugs should be given until the following questions have been answered.

1. Has enough time been allowed for neostigmine or edrophonium to antagonize the block, i.e., at least 10 to 15 minutes? (The clinician should recognize that edrophonium has a more rapid onset of action than neostigmine [Table 3]).
2. Is the neuromuscular blockade too intense to antagonize?
3. What is the patient's acid-base and electrolyte status?
4. What is the temperature?
5. Is the patient receiving any drugs that may make antagonism difficult?
6. Has excretion of the muscle relaxant been reduced?

Often, answers to these questions can provide the answer for failure of neostigmine or edrophonium to antagonize the nondepolarizing neuromuscular blockade.

Another reason for not giving more neostigmine is that larger doses may themselves cause a cholinergic block.

Controlled Ventilation

Obviously, if the neuromuscular blockade cannot be antagonized, ventilation must be controlled until the

Table 3 Time of Onset of Action (minutes) of Edrophonium and Neostigmine

Percent of Peak Antagonism	Edrophonium	Neostigmine
50%	0.4	3.2
100%	1.2	7.1

block terminates spontaneously. The question arises as to when controlled ventilation can be terminated. Obviously, the usual criteria for extubation of the trachea of any patient should be applied. However, the clinician should be well aware that the normal vital capacity can occur in the presence of a residual neuromuscular blockade. In other words, the patient may have a normal vital capacity but not enough strength (e.g., weak pharyngeal muscles) to maintain a patent airway. Therefore, more stringent criteria than the presence of a normal vital capacity need to be applied. These criteria are the same as described earlier, i.e., an inspiratory pressure that is at least -35 cm of H_2O and the ability to lift the head for at least 5 seconds. Once these criteria have been met, it is likely that the residual neuromuscular blockade has been terminated and, therefore, the patient will be able to sustain normal ventilation.

SUGGESTED READING

Miller RD, Savarese JJ. Pharmacology of muscle relaxants and their antagonists. In Miller RD, ed. Anesthesia. New York: Churchill-Livingstone, 1990:389.

Pavlin EG, Holle RH, Schoene RB. Recovery of airway protection compared with ventilation in humans after paralysis with curare. Anesthesiology 1989; 70:381.

Viby-Mogensen J, Jorgensen BC, Ording H. Residual curarization in the recovery room. Anesthesiology 1979; 50:539.

MALIGNANT HYPERTHERMIA

THOMAS J.J. BLANCK, M.D., Ph.D.

Malignant hyperthermia (MH) is a lethal inherited disorder of skeletal muscle that is triggered by all the volatile anesthetics and depolarizing muscle relaxants. The syndrome was first described by Denborough and Lovell in 1960. They reported the occurrence of marked elevation in temperature, cyanosis, hypotension, and tachycardia in a man who was given a halothane anesthetic. They note in their report that ten relatives of this patient had died after receiving ether anesthetics and that owing to this history, it was deemed safer to give their patient halothane anesthesia. It was not. Subsequent to this report, MH gradually became well-recognized as a syndrome, and it was observed that it often clusters in families and that once it is initiated it almost always results in death.

The syndrome most often occurs in the operating room after induction of anesthesia with succinylcholine chloride and halothane. The other two volatile anesthetics in common use, enflurane and isoflurane, have also been reported to trigger the syndrome. The incidence is said to be one in 50,000 in adults and one in 15,000 in children. Until 10 years ago, the mortality rate was 76 percent, most often due to cardiovascular collapse, a late consequence of the syndrome. However, 10 years ago, the drug dantrolene sodium was introduced, which can specifically reverse the MH syndrome if it is rapidly recognized. The availability of dantrolene sodium and the education of anesthesiologists regarding the recognition and treatment of this syndrome have resulted in a marked decline in the mortality rate to approximately 20 percent.

The premonitory signs of this syndrome are often tachycardia and arrhythmias. These are followed by an increase in the production of carbon dioxide, muscle rigidity, severe metabolic acidosis, and a marked elevation in body temperature. The temperature elevation (which can be in the range of 43 to 44° C if the patient has not been treated) should not be the symptom on which the diagnosis is based, because if one waits to observe the remarkable increase in temperature, the patient will soon be dead or severely damaged neurologically.

PATHOPHYSIOLOGY

The MH syndrome in humans is mirrored by an almost identical disorder in certain strains of swine. In swine, as in humans, the disorder can be triggered by volatile anesthetics and depolarizing muscle relaxants, but in swine stress alone can also initiate the syndrome. The similarity of syndromes has allowed in-depth investigation of the pathophysiology in swine which, for the most part, has been verified in less detail in humans. Four questions can be asked relating to the manifestations of this syndrome: (1) Why do anesthetics trigger MH? (2) Why does the muscle become rigid? (3) Why does the acidosis develop? and (4) Where does the heat come from? Unfortunately, although the syndrome can be successfully treated with dantrolene sodium, we have few answers at this time to the above questions. In skeletal muscle, three membranous systems are known to control Ca^{++} homeostasis: the outer cell membrane called the sarcolemma, which maintains low intracellular Ca^{++} levels in the face of high extracellular concentration; the sarcoplasmic reticulum (SR), which controls the thousandfold phasic increase and decrease of intracellular Ca^{++} during contraction and relaxation; and the mitochondrion, which produces adenosine triphosphate (ATP), the energy source of the cell, while buffering Ca^{++} concentration over a broad tonic range. Each of these membrane systems has been carefully examined, and it appears that the SR from MH-susceptible humans and swine is abnormal. Several investigators—Ohnishi, Nelson, Michelson, and their

co-workers—have noted that the volatile anesthetics enhance the release of Ca^{++} from isolated SR at lower concentrations in SR from MH swine than from normal SR. It has been suggested that this phenomenon is related to triggering of the syndrome and to the development of elevated intracellular Ca^{++} and rigidity. Lopez and colleagues have measured intracellular Ca^{++} levels in vivo using a Ca^{++} electrode and have observed an increase in the resting intracellular Ca^{++} concentration, which, upon exposure of the MH-susceptible animal to halothane, increased severalfold. This did not occur in the control animals. The elevated intracellular Ca^{++} in the triggered animal appears to explain the increase in rigidity noted in classical MH. However, little evidence is available to explain either the marked acidosis or the elevated temperatures satisfactorily. Studies of isolated mitochondria from MH muscle have not shown that the volatile anesthetics alter respiratory function any differently than they do in mitochondria from normal muscle.

The most recent data suggest that the Ca^{++} release channel, also known as the ryanodine receptor, of the sarcoplasmic reticulum is abnormal. An abnormality of this structure and an increased Ca^{++} conductance of the release channel when exposed to halothane could certainly explain several aspects of the continued muscle activation in MH muscle.

RECOGNITION AND TREATMENT

Appropriate and efficacious treatment of MH demands early recognition of the syndrome. As mentioned earlier, the initial symptoms are usually both atrial and ventricular tachycardia and arrhythmias. This is accompanied by an elevation in the end-tidal carbon dioxide, which in the spontaneously breathing anesthetized patient results in an increase in the respiratory rate. Other accompanying symptoms include muscle rigidity, which can occur despite the use of neuromuscular blockers, cyanosis, and mottling of the skin, poor peripheral perfusion evidenced by cold extremities, and elevated and rising core temperature. This symptom complex can appear with the induction of anesthesia, soon after induction, late in use of the anesthetic, or even, on rare occasions, in the recovery room. The rate of development of the syndrome is variable but can be virulent and rapid and, if not treated immediately, can be lethal.

Emergency Treatment

Once the diagnosis has been made, any triggering anesthetics must be discontinued if the patient is to survive. One hundred percent oxygen should be administered, hyperventilation should be instituted, all operating room (OR) personnel should be informed of the situation, and help should be called. For treatment to be effective, the institution should have considered and designed an approach to the syndrome before it has ever occurred in that institution. An OR dantrolene sodium supply (approximately four vials) should be immediately available; the entire 36-vial supply should be obtained from the hospital pharmacy. One person should be assigned to reconstituting the dantrolene sodium and administering it at an initial dose of 2 mg per kilogram. Each vial contains 20 mg and requires 60 ml of sterile water per vial. While the anesthesiologist is monitoring and ventilating the patient, the surgical team must complete the surgery as rapidly as possible. If further anesthesia is required, a combination of fentanyl, thiopental, and pancuronium bromide is recommended. Another member of the OR team should be assigned to assure that intravenous access is adequate, (i.e., at least one large-bore catheter is placed). If the situation is deemed precarious, an arterial catheter and central venous catheter should also be placed, but therapy must continue during this period. All anesthetic tubing should also be rapidly changed to remove any previously dissolved volatile anesthetics. Arterial blood gases should be obtained and appropriate sodium bicarbonate therapy given; in the absence of blood gas analysis, 1 to 2 mEq per kilogram of bicarbonate should be given. The patient should also be cooled by all available methods, including the administration of cold intravenous fluids, surface cooling with ice, and if necessary, nasogastric lavage. If arrhythmias persist despite the administration of dantrolene sodium, procaine amide hydrochloride should be given in repeated doses as needed. The aim of therapy is to gain control of the situation that is, to control arrhythmias, normalize temperature, normalize pH, decrease muscle rigidity, and maintain adequate oxygenation.

Intravenous therapy with dantrolene sodium should be continued until control of physiologic and metabolic functions is obtained. The average dosage of dantrolene for effective treatment of MH is 2.5 mg per kilogram. Other concerns during the course of therapy include hyperkalemia, decreased urine output, and late in the course of MH, clotting abnormalities. Dantrolene sodium therapy can be continued to increasing dosages. There are no apparent contraindications to giving more than 10 mg per kilogram of dantrolene sodium, as is necessitated by the clinical situation. In the disastrous situation in which control of the MH syndrome has not been obtained despite high doses of dantrolene sodium, and otherwise appropriate therapy, further administration of dantrolene might be associated with alterations in cardiac rhythm. Once control of the syndrome has been obtained, the patient should be monitored in the intensive care unit for at least 25 hours because the reappearance of MH has been reported. Conversion to oral dantrolene sodium therapy should begin once the patient's condition has stabilized; 4 mg per kilogram per day should be administered in divided doses for 48 hours after the operation.

The syndrome varies in its appearance and virulence. For example, it has been reported that 40 to 60 percent of patients who have developed masseter spasm subsequent to the use of succinylcholine chloride and in whom muscle was tested by contracture studies demonstrate contracture characteristics consistent with the diagnosis of MH. It is uncertain how many patients who have developed masseter spasm after the use of succinylcholine chloride would have gone on to have MH. Therefore, it is necessary to discontinue anesthesia and cancel surgery in any patient who demonstrates masseter spasm after succinylcholine chloride administration.

RECOMMENDATION TO THE PATIENT

Currently we consider what recommendations should be given to patients who have had MH episodes or whose relatives have had MH. Any patient who has had an unequivocal episode of MH must be informed of this and should wear a Medic Alert bracelet. Since the inheritance of MH is believed to be autosomal dominant, the patient's family should also be informed of the possibility that some of them are MH susceptible. Currently only one test is available for the diagnosis of MH, and it requires considerable inconvenience, time, and money. The test is the halothane-caffeine contracture examination of excised muscle bundles. A skilled, dedicated physiology laboratory along with a surgeon who can obtain a muscle specimen 1 cm by 3 cm without injuring the myofibrils are necessary to perform this test. A brief list of the biopsy centers in the United States is shown in Table 1, and a more complete list can be obtained from the Malignant Hyperthermia Association of the United States (MHAUS), P.O. Box 191, Westport, CT 06881-0191.

Recent advances in the biochemistry of MH and in the mapping of the human genome have indicated that the locus of the MH gene is on chromosome 19. MacLennan et al and McCarthy et al have suggested that the locus on chromosome 19 is region q13.1 and the ryanodine receptor is a likely candidate for the MH gene. This evidence gives hope that a noninvasive test for MH might result from recent biotechnology advances.

It is often asked who should be biopsied. In making this decision it is important to realize that not all biopsies give definitive results, and that anyone with a questionable episode of MH who has a negative biopsy would probably still be treated as if he or she were MH susceptible should he or she require an anesthetic. Considering the information that can be obtained from the muscle biopsy, it is recommended that biopsy be performed in patients who definitely want to know if they have MH; patients whose occupational status might be altered by the diagnosis (e.g, military personnel), and patients whose family history of MH is questionable and for whom a positive diagnosis would at least clarify the situation.

PREOPERATIVE PREPARATION

The patient who is suspected of having MH and who requires surgery should be informed that he or she can

Table 1 Malignant Hyperthermia Biopsy Centers

Physicians	Locations
Glenn E. DeBoer, M.D. Hiroshi Mitsumoto, M.D.	Cleveland Clinic Foundation Cleveland, OH
Gerald A. Gronert, M.D.	University of California-Davis Davis, CA
Lawrence Jacobson, M.D.	University of Washington Seattle, WA
Richard F. Kaplan, M.D.	University of South Florida Tampa, FL
Debra L. Kennamer, M.D.	University of Texas Medical Branch Galveston, TX
John F. Kreul, M.D.	University of Wisconsin Madison, WI
Dennis F. Landers, M.D., Ph.D.	University of Nebraska Medical Center Omaha, NE
Jordan D. Miller, M.D.	UCLA Medical Center Los Angeles, CA
Sheila M. Muldoon, M.D.	Uniformed Services University of the Health Sciences Bethesda, M.D.
Thomas E. Nelson, Ph.D.	University of Texas Health Sciences Center Houston, TX
Henry Rosenberg, M.D.	Hahnemann University Philadelphia, PA
Martin D. Sokoll, M.D.	University of Iowa Iowa City, IA
Peter Waterman, M.D.	University of Pittsburgh Pittsburgh, PA
Barbara E. Waud, M.D.	University of Massachusetts Worcester, MA
Denise Wedel, M.D.	Mayo Clinic Rochester, MN

be given a safe anesthetic. However, it should be pointed out that since MH is not completely understood, there is a small chance that it could occur when they undergo anesthesia. Dantrolene sodium should be administered preoperatively to the patient who has had a definite history of MH. The current recommendation is that 2.5 mg per kilogram be given intravenously approximately 15 minutes before the induction of anesthesia. This dose of intravenous dantrolene sodium is likely to result in significant muscle weakness, so respiratory status should be carefully and continuously assessed. The patient with an uncertain history of MH who does not have a personal history or whose family history is vague does not require pretreatment, provided the anesthesiologist foresees an uncomplicated anesthetic. Dantrolene sodium should be available in the OR. All volatile anesthetics should have been previously removed from the anesthesia machine and the machine should have been flushed overnight with 100 percent oxygen. Preferably the anesthetic for an MH patient should be the first in a particular OR so that it does not follow the use of volatile anesthetics in the same OR. All personnel in the OR involved in the care of an individual suspected of MH susceptibility should be made aware of the patient's disorder and should be oriented as to their role should MH crisis occur. Finally, intraoperative monitoring should include an electrocardiogram, end-tidal carbon dioxide, a transcutaneous oxygen monitor, and the continuous measurement of core temperature. Electrocardiographic and core temperature monitoring should be continued in the recovery room. One should also be aware that MHAUS maintains a 24-hour physician consultation that can be reached by calling the Medic Alert Foundation International at (209) 634-4917 and asking for Index Zero.

SUGGESTED READING

Blanck TJJ, Gruener RP. Commentary malignant hyperthermia. Biochem Pharmacol 1983; 32:2287–2289.

Denborough MA, Lovell RPH. Anaesthetic deaths in a family. Lancet 1960; 2:45.
Gronert GA. Malignant hyperthermia. Anesthesiology 1980; 53: 395–423.
MacLennan DH, Duff C, Zorzato F, et al. Ryanodine receptor gene is a candidate for predisposition to malignant hyperthermia. Nature 1990; 343:559–561.

FAILURE TO AWAKEN AFTER ANESTHESIA

STEPHEN DERRER, M.D.

Anyone practicing clinical anesthesia will periodically be confronted with a patient who does not regain consciousness promptly, or who is significantly less responsive than would have been anticipated. Failure to awaken, delayed awakening, and blunted responsiveness constitute a continuum which must be recognized, diagnosed accurately, and responded to appropriately.

AROUSAL AFTER ANESTHESIA

With few exceptions, practically any of the agents commonly used as anesthetics or adjunctive agents could be used to produce prolonged unresponsiveness, even if no other drugs or pathology are present. Most anesthetic plans aim to have the patient awake or responsive at the conclusion of the surgical procedure, and for good reasons (Table 1). There are certain occasions in which it is often desirable to leave the patient unresponsive at the end of a procedure, such as after cardiac surgery to facilitate mechanical ventilation or after some airway procedures to enable a patient to tolerate better an endotracheal tube. On those occasions in which the patient's responsiveness is much less than was anticipated, a host of possible etiologic factors, some usually

obvious, others quite obscure, must be considered quickly to provide the patient with the best care possible and to allay apprehension on the part of those caring for the patient and the patient's family.

DIFFERENTIAL DIAGNOSIS OF DIMINISHED RESPONSIVENESS POSTOPERATIVELY

Postoperatively it is often difficult to distinguish quickly the difference between a patient who is comatose and an individual who is paralyzed and therefore unable to respond. The accurate diagnosis of unresponsiveness should include consideration of both of these major categories. Diminished responsiveness is usually the result of a complex interaction between multiple factors (Table 2).

DRUG-INDUCED UNRESPONSIVENESS

As mentioned earlier, practically any of the agents used as a component of anesthetic can cause prolonged unresponsiveness. The possible exception might be nitrous oxide, which, because of its low blood:gas partition coefficient and consequent poor solubility in blood, is usually eliminated quickly from the body, even in the presence of advanced pulmonary and cardiac

Table 1 Advantages to Early Arousal After Anesthesia

Neurologic evaluation
Return of airway reflexes
Prevention of atelectasis
Early ambulation and prevention of deep venous thrombosis
Early ambulation and discharge
Efficient utilization of recovery facilities

Table 2 Factors Contributing to Postoperative Unresponsiveness

Agents used as a component of the anesthetic
Other intraoperative medications
Preoperative medications
Pre-existing medical anesthesia
Prolonged surgery and anesthesia
Major intraoperative events
 Cardiac arrest
 Cerebral hypoxia
 Stroke
Homeostatic disturbances
 Fluid and electrolyte imbalances
 Hypothermia
Extremes of age

disease which slow the elimination of nitrous oxide through the lungs. Even nitrous oxide alone, however, could conceivably cause prolonged unconsciousness in a patient with pneumocephalus after intracranial surgery, as tension pneumocephalus has been reported in this situation. For other agents used in anesthesia, prolonged unresponsiveness is an extension of the therapeutic effect of the agents.

Inhaled Agents

Recovery from the major inhaled agents (i.e., halothane, enflurane, and isoflurane) is usually smooth and predictable. During a surgical procedure, most clinicians are able to achieve a proper steady-state delivery based on the patient's sensitivity and the degree of surgical stimulation, and then are able to discontinue the delivery of the agent at an appropriate time to facilitate timely recovery. The clinician may err in his or her assessment of the patient's anesthetic requirement during maintenance. There is clearly considerable biologic variability in the response of an individual to an inhaled agent, as with any other drug. Some medical conditions may cause an overestimation of anesthetic requirement. This occurs in asthma, where high concentrations of major agent may be needed to suppress airway reactivity, and in hypertension, where blood pressure, usually an important source of information to the clinician about depth of anesthesia or anesthetic requirement, may be misleading.

Because these agents are eliminated largely through the lungs, waking time is dependent on fresh gas flow rate to the patient's breathing circuit during emergence and on the patient's minute ventilation, whether controlled or spontaneous. Use of low flows or closed circuit delivery may allow the inspiration of anesthetic concentrations long after a vaporizer is turned off. Hypoventilation will also slow the removal of the inhaled agent from the body. Because anesthetic concentrations of these agents depress ventilation, they may blunt their own elimination in a spontaneously breathing patient.

Narcotics

Large doses of any narcotic, even short-acting agents, can produce a characteristic form of postoperative depression. Profound respiratory depression, pinpoint pupils, and a rapid and complete response to narcotic antagonists are diagnostic of narcotic-induced unresponsiveness. Although this picture is most readily produced by the use of long-acting narcotics such as morphine, even alfentanil hydrochloride can produce postoperative unresponsiveness if given in sufficient doses near the end of a procedure.

A patient presenting with postoperative unresponsiveness in whom narcotic overdose is strongly suspected by the clinical picture (i.e., the agent used, size of the most recent dose and the time it was administered, pinpoint pupils, profound respiratory depression) when

given a short-acting narcotic antagonist such as naloxone should be observed carefully in a monitored setting for the reappearance of respiratory depression, as the duration of the narcotic agent often exceeds that of the antagonist. Rapid reversal of narcotic action has also produced lethal ventricular arrhythmias and congestive heart failure in susceptible individuals, as well as acute hyperalgesia. For these reasons, airway protection and supported ventilation are often a reasonable alternative to narcotic reversal if other more serious causes of unresponsiveness have been ruled out.

Muscle Relaxants

Residual neuromuscular blockade can produce profound unresponsiveness that is at first glance indistinguishable from coma. Hypertension and tachycardia may be present, and are certainly more common in residual paralysis than they are in anesthetic overdose. Diagnosis can usually be made with the use of a nerve stimulator.

Residual paralysis after the use of succinylcholine chloride is seen almost exclusively in individuals with abnormal pseudocholinesterase. Postoperative nerve stimulation in affected individuals may show either a depolarized blockade or nondepolarized pattern. Even when a depolarized blockade pattern is present, the response to anticholinesterase agents is unpredictable. Airway and ventilatory support and reassurance are indicated; sedation may be helpful until the succinylcholine chloride is eliminated.

Profound nondepolarized blockade can produce a degree of paralysis that is not completely or adequately reversible by cholinesterase inhibitors. Inadequate reversal of neuromuscular blockade can occur for a number of reasons. Some medical conditions, such as renal disease, slow the elimination of many muscle relaxants, particularly pancuronium bromide. Demyelinating diseases, myopathies (such as that seen in Cushing's syndrome), and similar entities may enhance an individual's sensitivity to nondepolarizing agents. Certain other drugs, particularly some antibiotics, may have effects on the neuromuscular junction that are synergistic to the muscle relaxants. Finally, there is considerable individual variation in the response to these agents. Much of the risk associated with the use of muscle relaxants can be avoided by conscientious use of a nerve stimulator intraoperatively and judicious dosing practices.

Other Intravenous Agents

Many other intravenous agents, including barbiturates, benzodiazepines, ketamine, the major tranquilizer droperidol, and the induction agents etomidate and propofol, are capable of producing postoperative unresponsiveness. The postoperative unresponsiveness due to short-acting barbiturates and that due to etomidate and propofol are usually seen only briefly if a bolus injection has been recently given, or may be prolonged if very large doses or a continuous infusion of long duration have been used. The diagnosis in either clinical circumstance is usually obvious.

Ketamine produces a unique state of unresponsiveness. Respiratory exchange is often adequate unless other depressant drugs are also present. Staring and REM-like eye movements are common, as are purposeless movements of the extremities. Vocalizations are also common. While many of these manifestations will diminish if sedatives or tranquilizers are administered, these agents will not hasten the return of consciousness. The usual practice is to allow the drug to wear off in quiet surroundings, but with appropriate monitoring.

Prolonged unresponsiveness due to benzodiazepines resembles that seen with the inhalation agents and barbiturates. The frequency of this phenomenon and the duration of unresponsiveness are quite agent-specific, and widespread use of midazolam maleate has largely eliminated this phenomenon, which may be quite common with the longer-acting drugs diazepam and lorazepam.

Droperidol can produce profound sedation, usually with preserved ventilatory drive. The patient may continue to be responsive to some tactile stimuli or even verbal commands despite the appearance of deep sedation. Atropine and scopolamine can produce a similar state, although scopolamine in particular can cause delirium. The effects of these anticholinergic agents can often be lessened at least temporarily with intravenous physostigmine. Physostigmine in this situation often produces enough clearing of the sensorium to facilitate a more thorough evaluation of the patient.

Antibiotics

Many antibiotics have been shown to potentiate the neuromuscular blockade produced by nondepolarizing neuromuscular blocking agents (Table 3). Notable for their lack of this effect are the cephalosporins, which have achieved very widespread use during the perioperative period. The risks associated with the structurally related penicillins are largely theoretical, based on their in vitro properties, and these drugs are usually quite safe when used perioperatively in conjunction with neuromuscular blocking agents. It has occasionally been reported, however, that with the use of the penicillins there have been complications related to exaggeration of neuromuscular blockage.

Most antibiotic-induced problems with neuromuscular transmission involve the use of aminoglycosides, whether used intravenously or intraperitoneally as an irrigant. When these drugs are used intraoperatively, a reduction in the relaxant requirement should be anticipated and a nerve stimulator should be used. When clinically practical, it is wise to avoid administration of aminoglycosides for several hours after adequate postoperative reversal of nondepolarizing blockade; recurarization can occur when aminoglycosides are given soon after an apparently complete reversal.

Table 3 Antibiotics Potentiating Neuromuscular Blockade

Aminoglycosides
  Streptomycin
  Gentamicin
  Tobramycin
  Kanamycin
  Amikacin
  Netilmicin
Beta-lactams
  Penicillin G
  Penicillin V
  Piperacillin
Others
  Polymyxin A and B
  Colistin
  Lincomycin
  Clindamycin
  Tetracycline

The response of an antibiotic-enhanced neuromuscular blockade to reversal agents is unpredictable and undependable. If residual muscle relaxation cannot be adequately reversed and neuromuscular blocking antibiotics have been used, intravenous calcium chloride may sometimes enhance reversal of the paralysis. While the benefit of calcium chloride in this setting may not prove therapeutic, it may help establish the diagnosis and facilitate more detailed evaluation of an otherwise unresponsive patient. As in other postoperative cases of drug-induced unresponsiveness, supportive care is the most beneficial therapy once other serious causes of unresponsiveness have been ruled out.

CHRONIC MEDICAL PROBLEMS

Several commonly encountered medical conditions enhance sensitivity to or decrease the elimination of anesthetic and sedative agents. Thus, even a patient with a clear sensorium preoperatively may exhibit prolonged unconsciousness postoperatively when given routine doses of anesthetics. The astute clinician will, of course, be aware of the medical condition and its impact on pharmacokinetics, and may limit dosing accordingly only to be faced with an anesthetic which is suboptimal or inadequate for the surgical procedure. The clinician balances conflicting concerns during anesthetic maintenance, and often, prolonged postanesthetic recovery is the price that must be paid. At other times, however, prolonged unconsciousness is unexpected.

Liver Disease

In liver disease, there are several major components that can contribute to postoperative unconsciousness. First, liver disease if often associated with decreased plasma protein levels. Drugs that are usually extensively bound to plasma proteins, such as barbiturates and benzodiazepines, are thus more readily available to the brain in the unbound form than when a comparable dose is given to a patient with a normal liver. Also, because plasma proteins have a considerable influence on plasma volume, the total circulatory volume may be lower, which will also tend to cause higher peak levels after a dose is given.

The liver takes part in the metabolism and elimination of many drugs to some extent; consequently, the duration of action of some drugs may be increased with liver disease. This mechanism is seldom of great consequence by itself, because the action of most intravenous agents is limited by redistribution rather than by elimination. There are many scenarios, of course, in which the prolonged residual effects of several drugs, in combination with other mechanisms, may play a role in producing prolonged unresponsiveness.

Finally, liver disease by itself can produce decreased levels of consciousness progressing to stupor and coma. An individual who appears reasonably well compensated preoperatively may be far more sensitive to residual levels of anesthetic and sedative agents.

Renal Disease

Several nondepolarizing blocking agents, particularly pancuronium bromide, gallamine, and metocurine iodide, are eliminated largely by the kidneys. Inability to achieve adequate reversal of paralysis after the use of these drugs can produce prolonged unresponsiveness.

These problems are best avoided by using short-acting muscle relaxants (i.e., succinylcholine chloride, vecuronium bromide, or atracurium besylate) in patients with renal disease. Advanced, untreated renal failure can also produce a generalized metabolic encephalopathy that will enhance the central nervous system (CNS) depression of anesthetic and sedative agents.

Respiratory Insufficiency

The lungs are the primary organs of elimination for nitrous oxide and the volatile anesthetic agents. Elimination of these agents can be substantially slowed by lung disease. Many individuals with chronic lung disease exhibit loss of ventilatory responsivity to carbon dioxide and may be highly sensitive to the sedative and respiratory depressant effects of residual anesthetics, narcotics, and sedatives.

Because respiratory depression and hypoventilation will further delay awakening by reducing the elimination of inhaled agents, attention to ventilation adequacy and providing support when needed are vital in the postoperative care of patients with lung disease.

Other Encephalopathic States

Any clinical entity that can produce a global decrease in cerebral function, such as hypothyroidism, congestive heart failure, hydrocephalus, and any encephalopathic state, can produce a heightened sensitivity to anesthetic drugs, so that residual levels of drugs that are usually well tolerated may produce profound postoperative unconsciousness. The likelihood of this phenomenon should be considered in any individual with a potentially encephalopathic disorder who exhibits postoperative coma, even if preoperative global function appeared nearly normal.

Extremes of Age

Age-related sensitivity to the anesthetics has been implicated in both the very young and very old. There are several possible explanations. Individuals in these age ranges, particularly the elderly, are more likely to have other significant clinical disorders. While the sensitivity of these populations to the central effects of anesthetics is probably different from normal, a greater difference is probably seen in the hemodynamic responsivity to stimuli, and a clinician is thus more likely to administer inappropriate doses of anesthetics based on misinterpreted data.

ACUTE HOMEOSTATIC DERANGEMENTS

A variety of metabolic changes can produce or contribute to postoperative unresponsiveness. These include changes in electrolyte, pH, and body temperature.

Electrolytes

Several common electrolyte abnormalities can impair postoperative responsiveness by potentiating neuromuscular blockade. These include hypokalemia, hyperkalemia, hypermagnesemia, and hypocalcemia.

Hypokalemia is commonly seen in patients receiving diuretics or undergoing intraoperative diuretics. Hypokalemia may also be precipitated by intraoperative hyperventilation. Hyperkalemia, most commonly seen in patients with renal failure, can occur after multiple transfusions. Both hypokalemia and hyperkalemia can occur paroxysmally in familial disorders.

Hypermagnesemia can also occur in renal failure, but is more commonly problematic in eclamptic or pre-eclamptic parturients who receive supplemental magnesium. In these individuals, the effects of nondepolarizing relaxants can be dramatically enhanced.

Acidosis alone can produce a decreased level of consciousness or coma, and can exacerbate the CNS depressant effects of anesthetics. Alkalosis is rarely severe enough by itself to produce mental status changes. Alkalosis, particulary respiratory alkalosis, is associated with decreased respiratory drive and consequently slows elimination of inhaled agents. Hyponatremia can cause profound mental depression, coma, and seizures. Hyponatremia is most commonly a problem during clinical anesthesia after transurethral resection, where nonionic solution under pressure are used to irrigate continuously the urinary outflow tract during surgery. Substantial volumes of irrigant can be absorbed. Altered mentation in this setting can occur from congestive heart failure or from hyponatremia. When glycine-containing solutions are used as irrigants, hyperammonemia can occur in susceptible individuals, usually patients with liver impairment.

Hypoglycemia

Because surgery, general anesthesia, and the associated stresses tend to elevate blood glucose levels, hypoglycemia is rarely a problem even in the fasted state unless hypoglycemic agents have been given either intraoperatively or preoperatively. In addition to insulin and the oral hypoglycemic agents, several substances can produce hypoglycemia as an idiosyncratic reaction; these include ethanol, salicylates, and sulfonamides. The diagnosis of hypoglycemia should be considered in any diabetic patient with depressed consciousness postoperatively.

Neonates are also susceptible to hypoglycemia, particularly infants born to diabetic mothers. The very young do not tolerate long fasts well, have diminished glycogen reserves, have a high metabolic rate, and often are unable to sustain adequate gluconeogenesis.

Hyperglycemia

Confined largely to diabetics, nonketotic hyperosmolar coma is another problem that can produce delayed postoperative awakening. Glucose levels are usually greater than 600 mg per deciliter in this setting. Hyperosmolar coma is often precipitated by pneumonia, sepsis, or another serious infectious process, and is usually associated with profound dehydration. Overly aggressive therapy of hyperglycemia can precipitate cerebral edema and produce further deterioration of mental status.

Hypoxia and Hypercarbia

Postoperative respiratory failure can produce delayed awakening. Carbon dioxide itself is a CNS depressant, and impaired ventilation of any etiology, whether pulmonary, airway, neuromuscular, or cerebral, can thus produce further mental depression.

Hypoxia usually produces an anxious, confused state. However, if autonomic responses to hypoxia are blunted, as occurs when residual CNS depressants are acting during emergence, the response will be further depression of mental state.

Body Temperature

Both hypothermia and hyperthermia can depress mentation. Hyperthermia is rarely of concern postoperatively, unless there is or has been a malignant hyperthermic reaction.

Hypothermia can slow awakening by several mechanisms. The metabolic depression produced by hypothermia will slow the elimination of many agents from the body. Hypothermia enhances the effects of neuromuscular blocking agents and can make adequate reversal of

paralysis impossible. Low body temperature increases the solubility of anesthetics and slows their elimination. Low body temperature can also directly depress mental state.

MAJOR INTRAOPERATIVE EVENTS

Intraoperative cardiac arrest or any of several different neurologic events can prevent postoperative waking. The appearance of postoperative coma after an intraoperative disaster is rarely perplexing, although there are some neurologic conditions, such as seizures, and some situations, such as after intracranial surgery, in which the problem may be more subtle.

Cardiac Arrest

Cessation of circulation produces serious cerebral hypoxia within seconds. After only a few minutes of cerebral hypoxia, permanent deterioration is likely. The encephalopathy present after cardiac arrest may clear within several hours or after several weeks, or it may be permanent with or without partial recovery. Although many agents have been investigated for their ability to salvage cerebral function after cardiac arrest, none can be recommended at this time.

Cerebral Embolism

Cerebral embolism of air, clot, or other intravascular debris can produce either focal or global neurologic deficits, or both. Cerebral embolism is a common cause of stroke after carotid endarterectomy or endovascular neuroradiologic procedures. Cerebral air embolism can occur during extracorporeal bypass. Small amounts of intravascular air, which are usually insignificant, can produce major injury in an individual with anatomic right-to-left shunts, as commonly occurs in patients with congenital heart disease.

Treatment of cerebral embolism is primarily supportive. It is important to maintain adequate oxygenation and ventilation. Cerebral circulation may be supported by most hypertension and may help improve circulation to marginally perfused brain areas.

Seizures

Postoperative seizures, or a postictal state postoperatively, can produce a failure to awake. Postoperative seizures need not be accompanied by tonic-clonic movements. There may be only subtle ocular muscle manifestations, or no motor signs at all. If the patient has no history of a seizure disorder, postoperative seizures may go unrecognized. Usually, however, there is a history of previous seizures, and the diagnosis can be made by electroencephalography (EEG). Anticonvulsive therapy is then appropriate. Perioperative factors that may contribute to the development of seizures include hyperventilation and electrolyte abnormalities, which should be corrected if present. The drugs enflurane and ketamine have been implicated as seizure-producing agents.

Cerebral Edema and Hemorrhage

Other major intracranial problems, including edema and hemorrhage, are unusual except in neurosurgery or in patients with previously defined intracranial pathology. Cerebral edema can occur as a result of sudden metabolic changes, such as changes in glucose, sodium, or volume status. Cerebral hemorrhage can occur in neonates, particularly premature infants, eclamptic parturients, or individuals with recent head trauma or coagulopathies. Diagnosis of major intracranial events is best established by computed tomography (CT).

EVALUATION AND TREATMENT OF UNRESPONSIVENESS

While a patient is being evaluated postoperatively for failure to awaken, it is vital to make certain that primary concern is directed to the support of the airway, ventilation, oxygenation, and circulation. With this fundamental support, most patients will recover with continued observation alone. Routine laboratory evaluation, including measurements of glucose and electrolytes, blood gas determination, chest x-ray examination, and electrocardiography, may be helpful to establish or exclude many causes of prolonged unconsciousness. A

review of the history may suggest or indicate additional specific diagnostic tests. CT and EEG may be indicated in prolonged unconsciousness after intracranial surgery, or if there is known CNS pathology. CT and EEG are routinely indicated if coma persists for more than several hours without adequate explanation.

Pharmacologic intervention may prove both diagnostic and therapeutic. Naloxone hydrochloride, physostigmine, cholinesterase inhibitors, and calcium chloride have important roles in specific circumstances to antagonize the effects of narcotics, anticholinergics, and muscle relaxants, respectively. The use of "shotgun therapy" is to be avoided, however, and there should be a reasonable expectation of success when an antagonist is used. The use of nonspecific analeptic agents is to be condemned, as these agents are often associated with considerable risks that are likely to be compounded if there has been a serious intracranial event.

SUGGESTED READING

Denlinger JK. Prolonged emergence and failure to regain consciousness. In: Orkin FK, Cooperman LH, ed. Complications in anesthesiology. Philadelphia: JB Lippincott, 1983:368.
Eger EI II. Anesthetic uptake and action. Baltimore: Williams & Wilkins, 1974.
Mackie K, Pavlin EG. Recurrent paralysis following piperacillin administration. Anesthesiology 1990; 72:561–563.
Plum F, Posner JB. Diagnosis of stupor and coma. 3rd ed. Philadelphia: Davis, 1980.
Sokoll MD, Gergis SD. Antibiotics and neuromuscular function. Anesthesiology 1981; 55:148–159.

PERIOPERATIVE ARRHYTHMIAS

JAMES R. ZAIDAN, M.D.

Intraoperative arrhythmias can range in severity from a simple junctional rhythm in an otherwise healthy athlete, resulting in minimal hemodynamic alteration, to one as complex as an atrioventricular nodal re-entrant tachycardia in a patient with critical aortic stenosis. In the latter case, the patient could suffer cardiovascular collapse unless the arrhythmia was quickly corrected.

While the decision to treat simple or complex arrhythmias should be based on their possible hemodynamic consequences, the form of treatment must be based on the underlying pathophysiologic mechanism. Treatment options include drug therapy, cardioversion or defibrillation, and pacing. Underlying mechanisms

include re-entry, changes in automaticity, and triggering. In this chapter, the therapies suggested will be based on the specific arrhythmia's mechanism.

ELECTROPHYSIOLOGIC MECHANISMS OF ARRHYTHMIAS

Several mechanisms are known to cause arrhythmias. These mechanisms include re-entry, changes in automaticity, and triggering. Each of these can be further subdivided.

Re-entry

For re-entry to occur, there must be a complete circuit around which an impulse can propagate, a unidirectional block in one area of the circuit, and a disparity in the conduction velocities of different limbs of the circuit. Several subtypes of re-entry exist, including the macroanatomic, functional, and reflection subtypes.

Macroanatomic Re-entry

First described by Mines in 1913, this subtype comprises a large, anatomically defined pathway composed of bundle branches, atria, ventricles, and the atrioventricular or sinoatrial nodes. In macroanatomic re-entry, the wavelength of the impulse, or the distance the impulse travels during the refractory period of one limb of the circuit, is shorter than the total length of the anatomic circuit. The disparity between the wavelength of the impulse and the length of the anatomic circuit permits a small area of tissue between the leading edge of the returning circuit and the trailing edge of the same impulse to be responsive. This responsive tissue can accept a second premature impulse, which makes it refractory to the leading edge of the impulse traveling around the circuit. The second impulse could arise from a pacemaker. For this reason, a pacemaker can be used to terminate macroanatomic re-entry.

Functional Re-entry

A second type of re-entry does not require a defined anatomic pathway to maintain the circuit. Functional re-entry implies that the pathway constantly changes, occurs on a cellular level, and has a very short wavelength. In fact, the wavelength is short enough to allow the leading edge of the impulse to follow the trailing edge closely. The leading edge of the impulse will follow any microscopic pathway that is not refractory. A clinical example is atrial or ventricular fibrillation. Functional re-entry does not have a responsive area of tissue that can accept a perfectly timed second impulse from a pacemaker, and therefore pacing techniques will not terminate functional re-entry. Only uniform, sudden depolarization of the involved area, such as that which occurs in defibrillatory shock, will stop functional re-entry.

Reflection

If a Purkinje cell in an electrolytic solution is electrically stimulated, the action potential will uniformly travel the length of the cell. A block occurring in an isolated segment of the cell will slow the conduction velocity of the impulse entering this area. Conduction could be slowed to the point at which the impulse can depolarize the area behind the impulse as well as the area ahead of the impulse. This reflection of the original impulse becomes available to excite other cells and, in fact, a second action potential can be recorded in the area proximal to the block. Clinically, reflection can occur in the ischemic myocardium in the border zone between the ischemic and normal areas. The block itself could be caused by potassium leaking out of the ischemic cell and bathing a small segment of tissue.

Automaticity

Enhanced normal and abnormal automaticity occur in the clinical setting to cause arrhythmias.

Enhanced Normal Automaticity

The Purkinje cell normally spontaneously depolarizes during Phase 4 of the action potential to the threshold level. The cell in which the rate of change is fastest during Phase 4 will control the patient's heart rate. The slope of Phase 4 can change depending on the control of the sympathetic nervous system. If the slope of Phase 4 of the action potential increases in atrioventricular nodal cells, then the atrioventricular (AV) node would be the fastest pacemaker, and the patient would have a junctional rhythm. Likewise, if the Purkinje cells in the sinoatrial (SA) node increased the slope of Phase 4, then the patient could develop a sinus tachycardia. Enhanced normal automaticity implies that the normal mechanisms that cause Phase 4 remain in effect; however, the location of the controlling pacemaker or the rate can change. Sinus tachycardia and sinus bradycardia are examples of changes in normal automaticity.

Abnormal Automaticity

Myocardial cells that do not experience spontaneous depolarization are located in the atrium and the ventricle. These cells do not normally control the heart rate. If they become ischemic, they will partially depolarize. Fewer sodium channels will be available to cause a rapid phase 0. It is thought that the slow inward current created by the movement of calcium ions spontaneously depolarizes the cell. Therefore, the cell that normally has a diastolic resting membrane potential now develops a maximal diastolic potential and can act as the controlling pacemaker cell. Clinically, atrial tachycardia is an example of an arrhythmia caused by this mechanism. Parasystole can be considered a type of abnormal automaticity with undirectional block of impulses into the abnormal area.

Triggered Arrhythmias

Once the myocardial cell has repolarized, it normally remains at the resting potential until stimulated to reach threshold again. Occasionally, the cell develops a spontaneous depolarization that can actually reach threshold and create another action potential. This spontaneous activity not related to Phase 4 is called an after-depolarization. If the after-depolarization occurs on the downslope of the action potential when the cell is repolarizing, the activity is called an *early* after-depolarization. When it clearly occurs after the cell has repolarized, the activity is called a *delayed* after-depolarization. An after-depolarization cannot occur without a preceding action potential or pacemaker impulse. Clinically, these after-depolarizations can trigger bursts of tachycardia and are thought to initiate the arrhythmias associated with cardiac glycosides. In contrast to the re-entrant arrhythmias, a pacemaker impulse could initiate a triggered arrhythmia, because a triggered arrhythmia must have an initiating stimulus.

SPECIFIC ARRHYTHMIAS

Supraventricular Arrhythmias (Table 1)

Sinus Bradycardia

Sinus bradycardia does not always require treatment in otherwise healthy patients. One should proceed with caution, however, because sinus bradycardia occurs when the patient is hypoxic or hypertensive. The underlying causes of these problems should be treated; for example, atropine should not be administered to a bradycardic hypertensive patient. A vasodilator such as sodium nitroprusside might be a more logical form of treatment. Reflex bradycardia is another cause of intraoperative sinus bradycardia, and atropine now becomes a reasonable treatment. Consider the possibility of elevated intra-cranial pressure in neurosurgical patients. Chronic drug therapy with the beta-blocking agents is another reason why a patient might be bradycardic. Volatile anesthetic agents depress the slope of Phase 4 of the action potential and, theoretically at least, slow the heart rate through this mechanism. Overall, sinus bradycardia is usually a benign arrhythmia; however, when it occurs acutely, one must quickly determine the cause and initiate therapy.

Sinus Tachycardia

Likely the most common intraoperative arrhythmia, sinus tachycardia has many causes. The primary considerations are hypoxia, hypercarbia, and hypovolemia. Lighter planes of anesthesia, another cause of sinus tachycardia, occur especially when the surgical stimulus waxes and wanes. During light anesthesia, the sympathetic nervous system increases the slope of Phase 4 of the action potential to increase the heart rate. Consider the possibility of hyperthermia and of drugs such as the antimuscarinics. Sinus tachycardia generally has a gradual onset. This finding, important in determining the proper treatment, should be compared with the sudden onset of SA nodal re-entrant tachycardia. When observing the electrocardiogram, one cannot distinguish between these two arrhythmias; nevertheless, they call for different therapies. (the re-entrant arrhythmia is discussed later in this chapter). One should always treat the underlying cause of sinus tachycardia rather than simply administer beta-blocking drugs. Assume that sinus tachycardia is caused by hypoxia and hypercarbia.

Atrial Fibrillation

The exact mechanism by which atrial fibrillation is initiated remains unknown. Maintenance of this arrhythmia is likely caused by multiple wave fronts traversing microcircuits at different velocities. There is no definite anatomic substrate; rather, the impulses themselves form the necessary blocks to maintain the microcircuits. Atrial fibrillation is generally associated with ischemic or valvular cardiac disease and a high incidence of stroke. Even patients without other overt evidence of cardiac disease will experience a fivefold increase in the incidence of stroke. Many of the patients with atrial fibrillation will be receiving anticoagulants and might therefore have a relative contraindication to some types of regional anesthesia. Although most clinicians associate atrial fibrillation with heart disease, other more obscure causes including occult thyrotoxicosis, acute alcoholic intoxication, hypovolemia, acute hypomagnesemia, and acute hypokalemia have been described. The most important goal of treating atrial fibrillation is control of the ventricular rate; conversion to sinus rhythm is secondary. Digoxin remains the mainstay of therapy, but the Class 1A and Class 1C antiarrhythmics will control the rate and convert the arrhythmia to sinus rhythm in a significant number of cases. Chronic atrial fibrillation that continues throughout the anesthetic course presents a problem only because of the underlying cardiac disease. The acute onset of atrial fibrillation causes major hemodynamic consequences because of the associated rapid ventricular rate. Rate control is of paramount importance. Consider administering an alpha-adrenergic agent to raise the blood pressure and reflexly decrease the heart rate. Administration of beta-blocking drugs will also help control the rate but not necessarily convert to sinus rhythm. Pacing techniques will not terminate atrial fibrillation. Cardioversion will convert this arrhythmia to sinus rhythm if the atrium is not enlarged. One should not hesitate to cardiovert an anesthetized patient who experiences extreme cardiovascular changes due to the acute onset of atrial fibrillation.

Atrial Flutter

Although atrial flutter may develop through automatic or re-entrant mechanisms, its most common cause is re-entry. The surface electrocardiogram cannot distinguish between these two mechanisms. Atrial flutter is electrocardiographically characterized by a saw-tooth baseline and inverted P waves. When atrial flutter develops acutely, the ventricular response is characteristically approximately 150 beats per minute. The atrial rate, however, is 250 to 350 beats per minute for type 1 atrial flutter and 340 to 450 beats per minute for type 2. Organic heart disease is a clinical cause of atrial flutter, especially if it is associated with atrial distention. The

Table 1 Supraventricular Arrhythmias

Arrhythmia	Mechanism
Sinus bradycardia	Decreased slope Phase 4
Sinus tachycardia	Increased slope Phase 4
Atrial fibrillation	Functional re–entry
Atrial flutter	Macro–re-entry
Atrioventricular nodal re-entrant tachycardia	Macro–re-entry within AV node
Pre-excitation	Macro–re-entry
Ectopic atrial tachycardia	Abnormal automaticity
Sinoatrial re-entrant tachycardia	Macro–re-entry within SA node

treatment includes administration of drugs, cardioversion, and rapid atrial pacing. Verapamil and beta-blocking drugs are successful in converting flutter to sinus rhythm. During the use of an anesthetic, these drugs could create a very high degree of atrioventricular block; they must therefore be used with caution. Class 1A antiarrhythmics, which also terminate this arrhythmia, decrease the atrial rate and decrease concealed conduction, thereby increasing the ventricular rate. For this reason, the Class 1A antiarrhythmic agents will likely require the simultaneous use of beta-blockade. Synchronized cardioversion starting with as little as 30 J and increasing to 200 J should convert this arrhythmia to sinus rhythm. Pacing techniques successfully terminate re-entrant atrial flutter because the wavelength of the re-entrant impulse is shorter than the anatomic circuit. The rapid pacing generator should be connected to the atrial electrodes and the output of the generator should be slowly increased until atrial capture occurs. The rate of the generator should be increased until the P wave changes configuration. The rate might have to be as high as 500 to 700 J on the generator. The generator's rate should then be slowly decreased to 80 to 100 impulses per minute and observed for the return of atrial flutter. If flutter recurs, the process should be begun over again until the pacemaker clearly paces the heart with an upright P wave. At this time, one should begin decreasing the pacemaker rate again and look for a normal electrocardiographic pattern with a rate faster than that of the pacemaker. The pacemaker can be turned off at this time. If the patient does not have a physiologic heart rate, atrial pacing should simply be continued. Occasionally, this kind of pacing will initiate atrial fibrillation, which should be terminated through the use of drugs and cardioversion. The advantage of pacing is that it is painless, requires minimal time, and will not further depress normal cardiac conduction. When atrial flutter is automatic in nature, pacing techniques generally will only reset the atrium to a slightly different rate but will not terminate the arrhythmia.

Atrioventricular Nodal Re-entrant Tachycardia

The circuit for this arrhythmia occurs in the AV node. Two forms exist. In the more common form, the antegrade limb conducts slowly and the retrograde limb conducts very rapidly. Since the returning impulse enters the atrium at the same time that the antegrade impulse enters the ventricle, the P wave is hidden inside the QRS complex. In the less common form, exactly the opposite takes place. The retrograde limb conducts slowly, so that the P wave is inverted just after the QRS complex. Since this arrhythmia is re-entrant and includes the AV node, other types of therapy are available. Standard therapy would include administration of verapamil as the drug of choice, with beta-blocking agents and cardiac glycosides as possibilities. Since the circuit includes the AV node innervated by the vagus nerve, any therapy aimed at increasing the vagal tone could terminate this arrhythmia. The therapy therefore also includes carotid mas-

sage and administration of edrophonium. Rapid atrial pacing and cardioversion are also successful. Therapy of acute onset of this arrhythmia during anesthesia should center around ventricular rate control. During anesthesia, all forms of therapy are reasonable, including drug administration, carotid massage, rapid atrial pacing, and cardioversion.

Pre-excitation

Pre-excitation is said to occur when impulses from the SA node bypass the AV node or Purkinje system. In the Wolff-Parkinson-White syndrome, the impulse travels from the atria to the ventricles through one of two pathways. In one of these pathways, the impulse goes through the AV node, bundle of His, and the Purkinje system to the ventricle. The second pathway bypasses the AV node by the bundle of Kent and proceeds directly to the ventricle. Since the impulse reaches the ventricle very quickly, the PR interval is shorter than normal. When the impulse reaches the ventricle, it is outside the conducting system and travels more slowly than usual. The result is a delta wave that is an initial slurring of the QRS complex. The delta wave widens the QRS complex at the expense of the PR interval. It is also possible to have negative delta waves that can be interpreted as Q waves. For the Q waves to be significant for myocardial infarction, they must be at least 25 percent of the voltage of the subsequent R wave or greater than 0.04 seconds in duration. The Lown-Ganong-Levine syndrome includes a short PR interval with a normal QRS complex, implying that the AV node is bypassed but that the ventricle is normally activated.

AV-reciprocating tachycardia and atrial fibrillation are two arrhythmias that occur in patients with bypass tracts. A common form of the reciprocating tachycardia is initiated by a precisely timed atrial premature beat that is blocked in the accessory pathway but is conducted through the AV node and the bundle of His. When the impulse reaches the ventricle it can now travel back in a retrograde fashion to the atrium by way of the accessory pathway and prematurely reactivate the AV node and bundle of His. The tachycardia is therefore initiated by the premature atrial beat. Although one should not avoid using central venous pressure catheters, caution should be exercise in their insertion, since they can create a premature atrial contraction.

Drug therapy centers around eliminating the dispersion between the conduction velocities and refractory periods of the normal and accessory pathways. Medical therapy generally includes one of the Class 1A antiarrhythmic agents, because they increase the effective refractory period (ERP) and decrease conduction velocity of the accessory pathway. Beta-blocking agents are useful in terminating the reciprocating tachycardia because they slow conduction velocity and increase the ERP in the AV node without affecting the accessory pathway. In this case, the AV node would be refractory to the premature impulse returning from the accessory pathway, but could accept the impulse from the SA node. If the patient is in atrial fibrillation, beta-blockade will not slow the ventricular rate, because the beta-blocking agents do not slow conduction or increase the ERP in the accessory pathway. Digoxin is a complex drug which is occasionally used in patients who have experienced the reciprocating tachycardia. Digoxin slows conduction in the AV node, but shortens the ERP of the accessory pathway. The overall effect widens the dispersion of the conduction characteristics of the two pathways. Do not administer digoxin to a patient with Wolff-Parkinson-White syndrome who is experiencing atrial fibrillation. This drug will allow impulses to enter the ventricle more frequently and could initiate ventricular fibrillation. Occasionally, a patient with pre-excitation will receive digoxin; however, this decision should be made only after electrophysiologic studies have been done is a very individual matter. In general, one should avoid the use of digoxin. Verapamil is used more safely, but it also can decrease the ERP of the accessory period and result in a rapid ventricular rate if atrial fibrillation develops. If the patient is experiencing atrial fibrillation, consider therapy with procainamide.

Patients with a rapid ventricular rate secondary to the reciprocating tachycardia or atrial fibrillation should be cardioverted. Underdrive pacing and dual chamber pacing are also successful in terminating the reciprocating arrhythmia. Underdrive pacing implies that the pacemaker rate is adjusted to a rate below the intrinsic rate. Eventually, one of the pacing impulses will enter the conducting system at the critical time and terminate the arrhythmia. Dual chamber pacing may stop the arrhythmia by critically timing one impulse on each end of the re-entrant circuit.

Ectopic Atrial Tachycardia

This arrhythmia, caused by changes in automaticity, is found in patients with acute myocardial infarctions, hypokalemia, digoxin toxicity, catecholamine excess, and chronic lung disease. Since the arrhythmia is not re-entrant, pacing techniques will not stop it. The fact that neither the SA nor the AV nodes are involved eliminates vagal stimulation as a therapeutic option. Occasionally, the Class 1A agents will convert this tachycardia to sinus rhythm. One should treat the underlying cause while using digoxin or beta-blockade to achieve ventricular rate control.

Sinoatrial Re-entrant Tachycardia

SA re-entrant tachycardia occurs when the re-entrant circuit is confined to the SA node. It is very difficult to distinguish from sinus tachycardia because, once the impulse exits the SA node, the atrium depolarizes in a normal manner. The onset of the re-entrant arrhythmia occurs very abruptly, while common sinus tachycardia has a more gradual onset. If the onset of the tachycardia is gradual, one should consider adjusting the anesthetic level. Therapy for SA nodal re-entry includes administration of verapamil or beta-blocking agents, rapid atrial pacing, vagal stimulation, and cardioversion. This arrhythmia should be easily terminated with the administration of verapamil.

JUNCTIONAL ARRHYTHMIAS

The junctional rhythms occur when the AV node or an area within the bundle of His increases its rate through enhanced automaticity. A block within the AV node will also result in the appearance of a junctional rhythm even though the atrial rate might be faster. These arrhythmias are named according to the intrinsic rate. A junctional rhythm implies that the ventricular rate is less than 70 beats per minute. A junctional tachycardia has a rate of 70 to 100 beats per minute and an accelerated junctional tachycardia has a rate greater than 100 beats per minute. Definitive treatment is based on finding the cause, usually myocardial ischemia, while temporizing measures depend on the functional status of the AV node. Medical therapy includes administration of atropine to increase the SA nodal rate. Some clinicians have used very low doses of beta-blocking agents theoretically to decrease the AV nodal rate and allow the SA node to control the heart rate. When the AV node is capable of conducting impulses, atrial pacing re-establishes a proper AV contraction sequence. If the AV node is blocked, then atrial pacing will not control the heart rate. Use AV sequential pacing to time atrial and ventricular contraction. Begin with a pacing rate of 80 to 85 beats per minute and a PR interval of 175 msec. Administering an antimuscarinic will do no more than increase the atrial rate and increase the block.

VENTRICULAR ARRHYTHMIAS

Ventricular arrhythmias occur as unifocal and multifocal PVCs, ventricular tachycardia, and ventricular fibrillation. Common causes are related to ischemic and valvular heart diseases. If the preoperative assessment reveals a history of ventricular arrhythmias in the absence of overt ischemic heart disease, then one should consider silent myocardial ischemia. Other causes of preoperative ventricular arrhythmias include dilated and hypertrophic cardiomyopathy, the idiopathic and drug-related prolonged QT syndromes, and mitral valve prolapse. Although usually associated with ischemic or valvular heart disease, ventricular arrhythmias also occur in patients with normal hearts who are hypoxemic or hypercarbic during anesthesia. Other considerations during anesthesia include acute myocardial ischemia and all of its antecedent causes; reflex bradycardia with ventricular escape beats; direct cardiac manipulation during thoracic procedures; acute electrolyte imbalance; and, rarely, stimulation from a pulmonary arterial catheter.

When ventricular arrhythmias develop, adequate oxygenation and ventilation should be ensured and the depth of anesthesia should be readjusted. If this

Table 2 Arrhythmia Treatment

Mechanism	Primary Treatment
Automaticity	
Change in normal automaticity	1. Adjust depth of anesthetic
	2. Atrial pacing
Abnormal automaticity	1. Treat myocardial ischemia
	2. Administer lidocaine
	if ventricular
Re-entry	
Macro–re-entry	
Including SA or AV node	1. Increase vagal tone
	2. Calcium channel blockade
	3. Cardioversion
	4. Pacing
Not including SA or AV node	1. Calcium channel blockade
	2. Cardioversion
	3. Pacing
Micro–re-entry (functional)	1. Cardioversion
Reflection	1. Treat ischemia
Triggering	1. Treat glycoside toxicity
	2. Diphenylhydantoin

management does not terminate multifocal PVCs, then more complex therapy is indicated. Lidocaine has been the mainstay of therapy, and bretylium tosylate is another reasonable first-line drug. Other forms of therapy include beta-blockade for tachycardic patients, and atropine or glycopyrrolate for bradycardic patients. If pacing electrodes are available, consider using atrial pacing to establish a physiologic heart rate, provided that AV nodal conduction is intact. Theoretically, verapamil could be used to terminate an abnormally automatic focus created by myocardial ischemia. In patients who develop ventricular tachycardia, lidocaine should be administered while cardiopulmonary resuscitation is continued and the defibrillator is prepared.

Torsade de pointes deserves special note. This type of ventricular tachycardia can develop in patients who receive the Class 1A antiarrhythmics and in patients with idiopathic prolonged QT syndrome. Lidocaine will not necessarily reverse the arrhythmia and could prolong its duration. Patients with the congenital type of torsade des pointes could require a permanent atrial pacemaker.

It is difficult to distinguish ventricular tachycardia from supraventricular tachycardia with aberrant conduction. Generally, a QRS duration greater than 0.12 seconds, full compensation, dissociation from atrial activity, and prematurity in relation to the sinus beat indicate that a QRS complex is ventricular in origin. When in doubt, treat the case as a ventricular arrhythmia.

SUGGESTED READING

Atlee JL, Bosnjak ZJ. Mechanisms for cardiac dysrhythmias during anesthesia. Anesthesiology 1990; 72:347–374.

Damiano BP, Rosen MR. Effects of pacing on triggered activity induced by early after-depolarizations. Circulation 1984; 69: 1013–1025.

Rozanski GJ, Jalife J, Moe GK. Reflected re-entry in nonhomogeneous ventricular muscle as a mechanism of cardiac arrhythmias. Circulation 1984; 69:163–173.

Zaidan JR. Pacemakers. Anesthesiology 1984; 60:319–334.

Zaidan JR. Electrical treatment of arrhythmias. Anesthesiol Clin North Am 1989; 7:459–481.

CARDIOPULMONARY RESUSCITATION

CHARLES W. OTTO, M.D., F.C.C.M.

In cardiac arrest, time is of the essence. Brain adenosine triphosphate (ATP) is depleted after 4 to 6 minutes if there is no blood flow, although it returns nearly to normal within 6 minutes of starting cardiopulmonary resuscitation (CPR). Recent animal studies have suggested that good neurologic recovery may be possible after 10 to 15 minutes of normothermic arrest if good circulation is promptly restored. In clinical practice, survival is dependent on the rapid institution of resuscitation attempts. Optimum outcome is obtained only when basic life support (BLS) is begun within 4 minutes *and* advanced cardiac life support (ACLS) is available within 8 minutes. The longer a heart fibrillates, the more difficult is defibrillation. This factor is so important that defibrillation should take precedence over all other resuscitative efforts if the diagnosis of ventricular fibrillation can be made and a defibrillator is available. Acid-base status is probably not important during most resuscitations lasting only a few minutes. However, with prolonged cardiac arrest, the judicious use of sodium bicarbonate may help resuscitation. Therefore, finding out how long the victim has been arrested may be important to resuscitative efforts. In spite of the occasional success of prolonged resuscitation, standard closed chest CPR is able to sustain most victims for only 15 to 30 minutes. If restoration of spontaneous circulation has not occurred in that time, the results are dismal. Consequently, it is important to optimize resuscitative measures quickly. In order to efficiently participate in CPR efforts, the anesthesiologist must be fully trained in the skills of BLS and ACLS.

BASIC LIFE SUPPORT

BLS encompasses the skills necessary to support the circulatory and ventilatory functions of a victim in cardiac arrest. The standard sequence of procedures for BLS are shown in Table 1.

Airway Management and Ventilation

The head tilt/chin lift maneuver and jaw thrust are the methods usually recommended for opening the airway during CPR. In the absence of an endotracheal tube, the distribution of gas to the lungs and stomach during mouth-to-mouth or bag-valve-mask ventilation will be determined by the relative impedance to flow into each compartment. Since esophageal opening pressure is relatively low, gastric insufflation can be avoided only by keeping inspiratory airway pressures low. A major cause of gastric insufflation is partial airway obstruction by the tongue and pharyngeal tissues. Many individuals cannot manage effectively a self-inflating resuscitation bag and mask. Larger volumes at lower pressures are usually delivered by mouth-to-mouth or mouth-to-mask ventilation. If the bag and mask are used, two individuals should manage the airway: one to hold the mask and maintain the airway and one to squeeze the bag.

Even with an open airway, a relatively long inspiratory time is necessary to provide significant tidal volumes at low pressures. One to 1.5 seconds should be taken for each ventilation. If a single rescuer is performing CPR, two breaths should be given initially and following every 15 chest compressions. If multiple rescuers are available, two breaths are given initially and one during a 1.5 second pause following every fifth chest compression. If an additional rescuer is available, pressure on the arch of the cricoid cartilage (Sellick maneuver) is a useful adjunct to help prevent gastric insufflation. The best way to ensure adequate ventilation without gastric distention is endotracheal intubation. It should be performed whenever a resuscitation attempt lasts longer than a few minutes and an individual trained in intubation is available. Supplemental oxygen (100 percent) should be administered as soon as possible. Defibrillation should not be delayed for intubation. Following intubation, ventilation should proceed at 12 breaths per minute without regard to chest compression cycle, and no pause in compressions should be made for ventilation.

Table 1 Basic Life Support Sequence of Procedures

1. Determine unresponsiveness
2. Call for help
3. Position victim supine on firm surface
4. Open airway
5. Determine absence of breathing
6. Perform mouth-to-mouth ventilation; two breaths
7. Determine absence of pulse
8. Activate emergency medical services or code team
9. Initiate chest compression
10. Alternate 15 compressions with two breaths

Chest Compressions

Two theories have arisen to explain the mechanism of blood flow during closed chest compression. The cardiac pump theory proposes that the heart is compressed between the sternum and the spine, resulting in ejection of blood from the heart into the aorta, with the atrioventricular valves preventing backward blood flow. The thoracic pump theory proposes that chest compression raises intrathoracic pressure, forcing blood out of the chest, with venous valves and dynamic venous compression preventing backward blood flow and with the heart acting as a passive conduit. Studies have been done in animals and humans to support both theories; they are not mutually exclusive. Undoubtedly, fluctuations in intrathoracic pressure play a significant role in blood flow during CPR and it is likely that the cardiac pump mechanism contributes under some circumstances. Which mechanism predominates likely varies from victim to victim and even during the resuscitation of the same victim.

Introduction of the thoracic pump theory suggested several changes in or alterntives to the standard chest compression technique, including abdominal binding, military antishock trousers, simultaneous ventilation and compression (also called "new CPR"), interposed abdominal compressions, pneumatic vest compression, and "high impulse" compressions. Despite promising early studies with these alternatives, none has proven better than the standard technique, although some modifications have been adopted. Emphasis is now placed on maintaining compression for a period equal to that of relaxation, since this improves blood flow. A faster rate of compression makes it easier to keep this ratio and may also improve flow. It is currently recommended that the lower half of the sternum be compressed 1.5 to 2 inches at a rate of 80 to 100 per minute with a compression: relaxation ratio of 1:1. With multiple rescuers and before intubation, a pause is made after every fifth compression to allow ventilation. After intubation, no pause should occur in compressions for any reason except to check for return of spontaneous circulation.

ADVANCED CARDIAC LIFE SUPPORT

ACLS encompasses those cognitive and technical skills that are necessary to restore spontaneous circulatory function when simple support does not result in resuscitation.

Defibrillation

The longer ventricular fibrillation continues, the more difficult it is to defibrillate and the less likely it is to resuscitate successfully. The amplitude of the fibrillatory waves on electrocardiography reflect the severity and duration of the myocardial insult. As the myocardium becomes more ischemic, the electrocardiographic pattern becomes finer and defibrillation becomes more difficult. Although epinephrine makes the electrocardiographic pattern more coarse, it does not influence the success of defibrillation. Thus, defibrillation should not be postponed for any other therapy but should be carried out as soon as fibrillation is diagnosed and the equipment available. The precordial thump, although rarely successful, can be tried while one is awaiting a defibrillator in monitored fibrillation or a witnessed arrest.

Defibrillation is accomplished by the electrical current causing simultaneous depolarization of a critical mass of myocardium. The output of currently available defibrillators is indicated in energy units (joules [J]) that will be delivered when discharged into a 50-ohm load. As impedence increases, the delivered energy is reduced and, even at a constant delivered energy, the delivered current will decrease. Transthoracic impedance during human defibrillation varies from 15 to 150 ohms among victims. Optimum success of defibrillation is obtained only by keeping this impedance as low as possible. Factors that reduce impedance include large paddle size (> 8 cm diameter), use of defibrillation paste and firm paddle pressure (at least 11 kg) to improve electrode-skin contact, and defibrillation during the exhalation phase of ventilation. Transthoracic impedance also decreases with successive shocks. In animals, high-energy shocks repeated at close intervals result in myocardial necrosis. The amount of damage occurring in human defibrillation is not clear, but it would seem prudent to keep energy levels as low as possible. Current evidence suggests that most adults can be defibrillated with energy levels of 200 J or less if transthoracic impedence is kept low. The first defibrillation should be attempted at 200 J, the second should be attempted at 200 to 300 Joules, and subsequent defibrillations should be attempted at 300 to 360 J.

Pharmacologic Therapy (Table 2)

Routes of Administration

The preferred route of administration of drugs during CPR is intravenous. The most rapid and highest drug levels occur with administration into a central vein through a central venous catheter, although peripheral intravenous administration is also effective. A central line should be used for drug administration if it is available in the arrest victim. However, if no intravenous access is available at the time of arrest, an antecubital peripheral line should be the site of choice because of the low complication rate and lack of interference with other resuscitation efforts. Response time to peripheral

injection may be improved by following the drug with a bolus of fluid. Epinephrine, lidocaine, and atropine (but *not* sodium bicarbonate) do not injure the lungs and can be absorbed from the tracheal mucosa. However, the time to effect and drug levels achieved are inconsistent during CPR. Therefore, administration via the endotracheal tube is reserved for those times when no intravenous access is available. Intracardiac epinephrine should be used only if neither the intravenous route nor the endotracheal route can be used.

Epinephrine

The only drug universally accepted as being useful in helping resuscitation from cardiac arrest is epinephrine. Its efficacy lies entirely in its alpha-adrenergic agonism, which causes vasoconstriction, elevating aortic diastolic pressure and increasing coronary and cerebral perfusion. Animal studies have shown that epinephrine's beta-adrenergic effects are unnecessary for successful resuscitation and are potentially harmful because they increase myocardial oxygen consumption. Although other vasopressors with strong alpha-adrenergic agonism have been as successful as epinephrine in the laboratory, none has been shown to be superior. Epinephrine remains the drug of choice. The standard dose is 1 mg administered intravenously every 5 to 10 minutes during arrest. However, there is a wide range of individual responses and it has been suggested that this dose is too low. Studies of higher doses in human CPR are being conducted.

Lidocaine and Bretylium Tosylate

Lidocaine is primarily an antiectopic with few hemodynamic side effects. It tends to raise the ventricular fibrillation threshold caused by ischemia or infarction. It is useful during CPR to treat ventricular ectopy and to help suppress recurrent fibrillation following successful defibrillation. The initial dose of lidocaine is 1 mg per kilogram, followed by 0.5 mg per kilogram every 8 to 10 minutes as needed, up to a total dose of 3 mg per kilogram. Bretylium tosylate has theoretic electrophysiologic advantages over lidocaine in the cardiac arrest setting. However, bretylium tosylate can be associated with delayed hypotension. Clinical studies have shown no difference in survival when the two drugs are compared. Currently, bretylium tosylate is reserved for use in ventricular fibrillation refractory to defibrillation and lidocaine. The dose is 5 mg per kilogram and can be increased to 10 mg per kilogram, if necessary, and repeated at 10- to 15-minute intervals up to a total dose of 30 mg.

Sodium Bicarbonate

Although it used to be recommended that sodium bicarbonate be given during CPR, there is little evidence that it is needed during most resuscitations. Metabolic (lactic) acidosis develops slowly during CPR. If severe

Table 2 Advanced Cardiac Life Support Drug Doses

	Adult	Infant + Child
Epinephrine	1 mg	0.01 mg/kg
Lidocaine	1 mg/kg	1 mg/kg
Atropine	1 mg	0.02 mg/kg
Sodium Bicarbonate	1 mEq/kg	1 mEq/kg
Bretylium tosylate	5-10 mg/kg	5-10 mg/kg

acidosis does not precede cardiac arrest and there is no prolonged arrest before CPR, acidosis severe enough to require treatment is unlikely before 20 to 30 minutes of CPR. Although a few animal studies have shown improved results, most outcome studies have shown no better survival or neurologic status after CPR when sodium bicarbonate is used. As compared with metabolic acidosis, tissue respiratory acidosis occurs very quickly during cardiac arrest. Whenever blood flow is reduced, the products of metabolism (primarily carbon dioxide) begin to accumulate in the tissue. Consequently, in the no-flow state of cardiac arrest or the low-flow state of CPR, tissue acidosis is caused primarily by the accumulation of carbon dioxide because blood flow is inadequate to remove it. Bolus sodium bicarbonate administration results in the liberation of carbon dioxide, causing a transient increase in arterial carbon dioxide pressure ($PaCO_2$). Because carbon dioxide easily crosses cell membranes and the bicarbonate ion does not, sodium bicarbonate administration could cause a further increase in intracellular carbon dioxide and a paradoxical worsening of intracellular or intracerebral acidosis. Studies of brain intracellular and cerebral spinal fluid pH during CPR have been unable to confirm this potential adverse effect. However, the adverse effects of severe hypernatremia, hyperosmolality, and metabolic alkalosis after aggressive bicarbonate therapy during CPR are well known and associated with poor survival. Therefore, current knowledge suggests that sodium bicarbonate should be used judiciously during CPR. It may be useful if a known pre-existing severe metabolic acidosis is present or if the cardiac arrest is prolonged. If possible, bicarbonate therapy should be guided by blood gas measurement indicating a marked base deficit. The usual dose of sodium bicarbonate is 1 mEq per kilogram initially, with repeat doses being 0.5 mEq per kilogram no more often than every 10 minutes. Increases in arterial and tissue carbon dioxide may be reduced if the bicarbonate is given by slow infusion rather than by rapid intravenous bolus.

Atropine

Atropine sulfate enhances sinus node automaticity and atrioventricular conduction by its vagolytic effects. It is used during cardiac arrest associated with an electrocardiographic pattern of asystole or slow idioventricular rhythm. However, heightened parasympathetic tone probably contributes little to these rhythms during cardiac arrest in adults. The predominate cause of asystole and electromechanical dissociation (EMD) is severe myocardial ischemia, and the most important treatment is improvement of coronary perfusion and myocardial oxygenation. The first priority should be effective chest compressions and epinephrine to improve coronary perfusion pressure. Since the use of atropine has minimal adverse effects and asystole/EMD is associated with a dismal prognosis, atropine is recommended as a second-line drug in refractory arrest with these rhythms. The usual dose is 1 mg, which is repeated

with in 5 minutes if the rhythm persists. A dose of 2 mg is fully vagolytic in most adults.

Calcium Salts

Because calcium increases myocardial contractility and enhances ventricular automaticity under normal physiologic circumstances, it has been used for years as treatment for asystole and EMD. In recent years, however, dangerously high calcium levels following CPR have been reported in humans. Retrospective studies and prospective clinical trials of calcium and placebo in out-of-hospital cardiac arrest with asystole and EMD have shown no improvement in resuscitation or survival. Therefore, calcium is currently recommended only if the arrest is contributed to or precipitated by calcium channel blocker overdose, severe hypocalcemia, or severe hyperkalemia. If calcium is used, the chloride salt, in a dose of 2 to 4 mg per kilogram, is preferred because it produces a higher and more consistent level of ionized calcium than other salts.

Calcium Channel Blockers

Diametrically opposed to calcium administration is the suggestion that calcium channel blockers should be given during CPR. Anoxia or ischemia results in a large shift of calcium into the cellular cytoplasm, and high intracellular calcium is associated with numerous adverse effects that might be counteracted by calcium channel blockers. Studies have focused on possible improved neurologic outcome when these drugs are given following cardiac arrest. Overall, there is no evidence of a beneficial effect. No studies have examined the effect of calcium channel blockers on the myocardium during or after cardiac arrest. Thus, there is currently no indication for the use of these drugs for the cardiac arrest victim.

Isoproterenol

Isoproterenol is contraindicated during cardiac arrest. It has been used during CPR when the electrocardiogram demonstrates a slow rhythm, especially idioventricular rhythm. However, the primary cause of this rhythm is myocardial ischemia. As a pure beta-adrenergic agonist, isoproterenol increases myocardial oxygen consumption while reducing aortic diastolic pressure and reducing coronary blood flow. Thus, it is counterproductive to myocardial resuscitation. The only possible use of the drug is after successful resuscitation to speed up temporarily a very slow perfusing rhythm while awaiting pacemaker placement. However, great care must be taken to ensure that it does not cause increased myocardial ischemia leading to recurrent arrest.

Assessing Adequacy of Circulation

Once life support measures are underway, there is an obvious need to assess whether CPR is producing myocardial and cerebral blood flow sufficient for viable resuscitation. The traditional method of palpating a pulse in a major artery is inaccurate. In experimental animals, an aortic diastolic pressure of more than 30 mm Hg and a coronary perfusion pressure (defined as aortic diastolic minus right atrial diastolic pressure) of more than 20 mm Hg correlate with myocardial blood flow adequate for restoration of spontaneous circulation. Recently, similar pressures have been found to be associated with successful resuscitation in humans. If an arterial line and central venous pressure are available during CPR, these pressures should be optimized by adjusting chest compression technique and/or administering additional epinephrine.

Although invasive pressure may be the ideal method of monitoring chest compressions, it is infrequently available during CPR. It has now been shown that end-tidal carbon dioxide monitoring is an excellent guide to the effectiveness of standard CPR. Carbon dioxide excretion during CPR with an endotracheal tube in place is flow dependent rather than ventilation dependent. Since alveolar dead space is large during low-flow conditions, end-tidal carbon dioxide is very low (frequently less than 10 mm Hg during CPR). If cardiac output increases, more alveoli are perfused and end-tidal carbon dioxide rises (usually 15 to 25 mm Hg during successful CPR). When spontaneous circulation resumes, the earliest sign is a sudden increase in end-tidal carbon dioxide to greater than 40 mm Hg. A recent study demonstrated that no patient with an end-tidal carbon dioxide less than 10 mm Hg during CPR could be successfully resuscitated. In the absence of invasive pressure monitoring, end-tidal carbon dioxide monitoring should be used to judge the effectiveness of CPR whenever possible. End-tidal carbon dioxide values are not useful for 3 to 5 minutes after sodium bicarbonate administration, since the carbon dioxide liberated when bicarbonate is given must be excreted through the lungs. Good perfusion pressures and end-tidal carbon dioxide values do not ensure the success of CPR. Damage to the myocardium from the underlying disease may preclude survival no matter how effective the CPR efforts. However, low perfusion pressures and/or end-tidal carbon dioxide values are associated with poor outcome even in patients who might be salvageable.

RESUSCITATION OF INFANTS AND CHILDREN

Although the differences in the approach to CPR for adults and that for infants and children may seem small, they are important to successful resuscitation. Respiratory arrest with hypoxia causing asystole or EMD as the primary mechanism for cardiac arrest is much more likely in the child than in the adult. For the purposes of CPR, an infant is defined as younger than 1 year of age and a child as 1 to 8 years of age. Children older than 8 years of age are treated as adults. Although the sequence of events for basic life support

is the same as for adults (see Table 1), several techniques differ. Because of the small facial features in the infant and small child, mouth-to-mouth ventilation is replaced by mouth-to-nose and mouth ventilation. The rate of ventilation is increased from 12 breaths per minute in the adult to 16 breaths per minute in the child and to 20 breaths per minute in the infant. Chest compressions in the infant are done with two fingers to a depth of 0.5 to 1 inch. In a child, compressions are performed with three fingers or the heel of one hand to a depth of 1 to 1.5 inches. The compression rate in the infant is 100 to 120 per minute, and in the child 80 to 100 per minute (same as for the adult). ACLS drug therapy indications are the same in infants and children as in adults and doses are similar relative to body size (see Table 2). All drugs can be given intraosseously in children younger than 3 years of age or intravenously. All but bicarbonate can be given via the endotracheal tube, although other routes are preferred. Difibrillation energy required for infants and children is higher than for adults. Initial energy should be 2 J per kilogram, and if defibrillation is unsuccessful, subsequent shocks should be at 4 J per kilogram. Paddles appropriate to the body size are used: 4.5 cm diameter for infants and small children, and 8 cm for adults and larger children.

POSTRESUSCITATION CARE

The major factors contributing to the high in-hospital mortality rate following successful resuscitation are progression of the primary disease and cerebral damage suffered as a result of the arrest. Active management during the postresuscitation period appears to mitigate postischemic brain damage and improve neurologic outcome without resulting in increased numbers of patients surviving in vegetative states. A patient who awakens within a few minutes of resuscitation may require only oxygen, monitoring, and observation. However, any patient who is comatose should receive mechanical ventilation for several hours, at least, maintaining the arterial oxygen partial pressure at greater than 100 mm Hg and the carbon dioxide partial pressure at 30 to 35 mm Hg. Restlessness, coughing, and seizure activity must be aggressively treated. Hemodynamic management is aimed at maintaining or improving cerebral blood flow. Increased intracranial pressure is uncommon after resuscitation from cardiac arrest and need not be an immediate concern. Blood volume should be maintained at normal or should be expanded slightly with nonblood solution, since moderate hemodilution to a hematocrit of 30 to 35 percent may be helpful. A brief 5-minute period of moderate hypertension (mean arterial pressure of 120 to 140 mm Hg) may help overcome the initial cerebral no-reflow. This frequently occurs without additional therapy because of the epinephrine given during CPR. Thereafter, blood pressure should be carefully controlled at a mean arterial pressure in the range of 90 to 110 mm Hg. Hyperglycemia during cerebral ischemia is thought to increase neurologic damage, although the effects during the postresuscitation period are unknown. It would seem prudent to keep blood glucose in the range of 100 to 250 mg per deciliter. These general supportive measures will help optimize neurologic outcome. No specific pharmacologic therapy has been shown to be of further benefit.

SUGGESTED READING

Proceedings of the 1985 National Conference on Standards and Guidelines for Cardiopulmonary Resuscitation and Emergency Cardiac Care. Circulation 1986; 74(suppl IV).
Standards and guidelines for cardiopulmonary resuscitation (CPR) and emergency cardiac care (ECC). JAMA 1986; 255:2905–2984.
Textbook of advanced cardiac life support. Dallas: American Heart Association, 1987.

DATA MANAGEMENT

AUTOMATED ANESTHESIA RECORDS

WILLIAM T. MERRITT, M.D.

There is a bit of anesthesia humor going around these days that suggests about 10 to 20 percent of anesthesiologists consider automated anesthesia records (AAR) as an essential part of the emerging role of the computer in the operating room, another 10 to 20 percent or so deride them as unwise and unnecessary, while the remainder hope they will retire before they are forced to use them! Such are the trials of new technology.

There are several pertinent questions about this technology. What must such a system do; what must it avoid? The primary function of the anesthesia record, as such, is to promote the recognition of trends through a visual representation that relates drug administration and surgical and anesthesia events to changes in vital signs. Data must be presented in a readily discernable format—a significant departure from records currently used (e.g., extensive columns or rows of digital data) will probably decrease acceptance. Electronic input from various monitors must be easily verifiable for accuracy and calibration purposes. The AAR screen will become the focus of our record-keeping attention, and "real-time" (or nearly so) vital signs must always be visible so that prompt recognition of change is possible. The frequency of data capture should preclude missing even transient events and should be adaptable for scholarly investigation in the proper setting. Such data resolution should shorten those periods of time for which no data are available (e.g., between the standard 5 minute recordings), thereby limiting assertions of uncertainty by plaintiff lawyers. Invasive monitoring lends itself well to automatic capture, but the majority of anesthetized patients require only noninvasive monitoring. Both must be handled equally well.

Diverse manufacturers provide innumerable pieces of monitoring equipment for use by the anesthesiologist. An AAR must be able to receive and process information from a variety of such devices, regardless of the type of output (e.g., analog or digital). Vital signs and functions that are not automatically processed, as well as descriptive annotations, will need to be entered easily through menu lists by keystroke, mouse-type selection, touch screen, or by voice activation; redundancy will be important. Such information must be readily available for review, if not constantly present on the screen.

General use operating room record-keeping computers must be "user friendly" in a most liberal sense. Many anesthesiologists may have little computer experience or may not be willing or able to devote the time to learn an overly complex system. Repeated and tedious forays into computer logic will not be accepted by many. Most of us will need to modify our information assimilation skills somewhat. Just as we have learned to accommodate a vast array of new monitors, we can learn to "cerebralize" data from an AAR. In addition, 24-hour telephone support must be provided and prompt service arrangements must be available, because these records represent *patient care documents!*

Cases must not get lost. Some systems will be run by "sneakernet,"—i.e., a runner will save the days' cases onto floppy disks for later entry into the departmental computer. The only practical long-term way to deal with this issue, however, is to use a networking system within one's operating rooms. Regardless of the method, there are strong financial and medicolegal reasons for not losing data. Fortunately, this has proved to be a very minor problem in hospitals where systems are currently in use.

Most discussions, positive or negative, eventually arrive at the subject of artifactual data, annotations, and corrections. Artifactual data are not much of a problem with a hand-kept record; it is screened out. Only important data make it through. AARs are at risk of recording a variety of artifactual information—the highs, lows, and straight lines constantly seen during the administration of anesthesia that are caused by electrical interference, line flushing, blood sampling, patient movement, monitor displacement, plugged sampling lines, and so forth. Some users will view these artifacts as the signature of a truly automated system. Most will want these events easily identifiable, preferably by software, and recognized as such; many will require that they be removed. The handling of artifact will be an evolving area of concern, and will probably be viewed as less important as experience is gained. Any good system also must readily perform user-customized, menu-type, explanatory "event" notes (e.g., breath sounds of good quality bilaterally), as well as permit notations by more conventional keystroke. A large degree of standardization is necessary, however, to permit database analysis. This brings up the subject of corrections. In the flow of anesthesia delivery, much annotation is done "after the fact"; this will be improved, but not eliminated, by an AAR. Not infrequently, an event that occurred earlier in a case is remembered, and a note inserted for the proper time. Some artifactual data may need to be amended (e.g., manual blood pressure to correct the reading from a damped arterial catheter or malfunctioning automated blood pressure device). Corrected information should appear in the record at the time of the event, to improve the quality of the trended information. The ability to correct or edit artifact, however, carries the responsibility of demonstrating that data, even that judged to be artifactual, is not being erased, and that it is available for review if necessary. Deletion of data may lead to the implication the record has been falsified. An audit trail, then, must track original information, corrections, editing, and the timing of such changes. Thus, evidence of decision-making and judgments is not lost.

Because the AAR is intended as the sole anesthesia record, it must be accepted as such. No hand-written "backup" records will be needed. Information must be saved (e.g., to a hard disk or network) frequently. If for some reason the individual AAR machine shuts down, the disk can be used to print the record to that point, and if necessary, a hand-written record can be kept for the remainder of that case.

Anesthesia departments vary widely in the numbers and complexity of cases performed; individuals will differ in their style of record keeping. Both institutional and individual customization should make the AAR more readily accepted; however, one must realize that database use will require considerable standardization.

Viewing an AAR keeper, however, solely in terms of a fancy operating room gizmo that spits out a neat anesthesia record falls far short of the mark. Such devices must ultimately become an integral component of an anesthesia data management system. Both improved efficiency of billing for anesthesia care and the clear potential (e.g., via bar codes) for a more accurate tracking of pharmaceuticals and expendables used are strong financial incentives for investments in this technology. Improved review of operating room utilization (start, stop, turnover, underposting, etc.) should permit more efficient scheduling, thus potentially improving revenues. The database derived from the AAR should assist both anesthesia and hospital administrators in the pursuit of quality assurance, peer review, and risk management activities and thus aid in the satisfaction of many JCAHO requirements. Verification of care should be enhanced, especially if "reminder windows" prompt the care provider to perform and/or document certain tasks (e.g., machine checkout, $ETCO_2$ presence at intubation, etc.). Such a system should be viewed favorably by mal-

practice insurers. For those departments with the desire to review large numbers of similar surgical/anesthetic cases or to study the patterns and pitfalls of anesthesia care, the AAR truly represents a major advance. The developer of any system must aggressively assist those interested in this capability.

To be truly part of a data management system, the AAR will need to participate fully in hospital-based patient information management systems currently in use or planned in many medical centers (i.e., laboratory data, radiology, ECG, catheterization reports, general medical/surgical and past anesthesia history). It will quickly become outdated if it does not. All of this information is potentially useful to the anesthesiologist.

AARs must of necessity participate in the development of "smart" monitoring. Eventually, rates of change of important physiologic parameters, drug combinations, drug dosage, and so forth will be followed by computers and, when necessary, warnings, doses, and suggestions, will be offered or available. The AAR screen becomes a logical site for the organization and coordination of such technology.

Actually, there is no reason that the use of AARs should not be sheer fun. Fun, that is, in the sense we all experienced during our residencies when we watched physiologic relationships unfold on cumbersome multichannel recorders, then, and even now, in use on complicated cases in many operating rooms. However, there are subtle, and not so subtle, events that occur in the most mundane of anesthetics that pique our interest, provide food for thought, and, if accurately recorded, afford the opportunity for animated discussions with both our anesthesia and surgical colleagues.

Black-box anesthesia is a term that can generate heated discussions, with views ranging from extremely positive to extremely negative. Those on the positive side believe AARs will allow closer patient care because less time will be used to physically generate a record, and believe that the document produced will be a superior representation of the care rendered. Those on the negative side, however, worry that very short-term undesirable events, or artifactual nonevents, will lead to recorded data susceptible to distorted interpretation by other health care providers or in a court of law. In addition, they believe that the use of computers in the anesthesia suite will be difficult to master. Polarized opinions aside, interest in this form of anesthesia record keeping recently resulted in the Committee on Standards for the New Jersey State Society of Anesthesiologists, in concert with the New Jersey Department of Health, to seriously consider, but later reject (for the immediate future), the pursuit of mandatory use of such devices.

Where is the middle ground? Unfortunately, there are little hard data to "prove" that an automated record leaves more time for patient care, or for that matter that the care is thereby improved. There are data suggesting that as many as 40 percent of manually generated anesthesia records contain significant errors and omissions. Other data document the considerable time spent recording data during complicated anesthetic delivery.

There are countless successfully litigated cases in which the deciding factor was a poorly documented anesthesia chart. Was good care poorly recorded, or was the poor documentation part of inadequate anesthesia care? Certainly a defense attorney will argue the former, the plaintiff's the latter. Since we as a group have not been able to consistently generate adequate anesthesia documents, should we not be open to technology that will work in that direction well before lawyers and insurers force it upon us? Unfortunately, an improved anesthesia record will not directly translate into an improvement in any care rendered, but it should permit better peer review and quality assurance endeavors, and in a roundabout way, ultimately improve the quality of anesthesia care. Recently, the quality of the AAR has resulted in two lawsuits being dropped before reaching a court of law.

Nearly 100 years have elapsed since the Codman/ Cushing anesthesia records of the 1890s ushered in an improved era of objectivity and accountability for the administration of anesthesia. In a similar sense, the advent of widespread use of AARs, predictable in the 1990s, represents a new horizon on anesthesia care.

SUGGESTED READING

Apple HP, Schneider AJ, Fadel J. Design and evaluation of a semiautomatic anesthesia record system. Med Instrum 1982; 16:69.

Edsall DW. Personal communication, ASA, 1990.

Eichorn JH, Edsall DW. Computerization of anesthesia information management. J Clin Monitor 1991; 7:71–82.

Gravenstein JS, de Vries A, Beneken JE. Sampling intervals for clinical monitoring of variables during anesthesia. J Clin Monitor 1989; 5:17–21.

Kennedy PJ, Feingold A, Wiener EL, et al. Analysis of tasks and human factors in anesthesia for coronary artery bypass. Anesth Analg 1976; 55:374.

Ream AK. Information management: What is it? How is it done? J Clin Monitor 1991; 7:75–77.

Smith NT. Perioperative anesthetic data—what to do with them? The role of the automated anesthesia record. IARS, 1991 Review Course Lectures, 65th Congress of the IARS.

Zollinger RM, Kruel JF, Schneider AJ. Man-made versus computer-generated anesthesia records. J Surg Res 1977; 22:419.

INDEX

Note: Page numbers followed by (f) indicate figures; page numbers followed by (t) indicate tables.

A

Abdominal aortic aneurysm, 139–144
  epidural anesthesia and, 412
Abdominal surgery, 305–317
  hepatic resection and, 308–310, 309f, 309t
  liver transplantation and, 311–317
  pheochromocytoma and, 314–317
  portal hypertension and ascites and, 305–308
  pulmonary function testing for, 12
Abdominal trauma, 392f, 392–396, 393f, 394t, 395t
Abuse, drug or alcohol
  abdominal trauma and, 395
  preoperative management and, 39
Accidental dural puncture, 407, 407t
Acetaminophen for chronic pain, 426, 426t
Acetylcholine
  diaphragmatic hernia and, 215
  eye and, 205
Acetylcholinesterase inhibitor, 495–496
Acid, epsilon-aminocaproic, 60
Acid-base balance, 495
Acid-base monitoring, 482t, 482–486, 485t
Acidosis
  aortic cross-clamping and, 143
  metabolic, liver transplantation and, 314
  postoperative, 483
  postoperative unresponsivenss and, 503
Acquired immunodeficiency syndrome, 74t, 74–78, 75t, 77t
  electroconvulsive therapy and, 183
  preoperative testing for, 19
Acromegaly, 163–164
ACTH
  adrenal insufficiency and, 73
  Cushing's disease and, 164–165
  pituitary tumor and, 163
Activated clotting time, 488–490, 489f
Adenoidectomy, 275–280
Adenoma, pituitary, 163
Adenosine, 201
Adenosine triphosphate, 201
Adrenal gland, pheochromocytoma of, 314–317
Adrenal insufficiency
  hypothyroidism and, 69
  preoperative medication for, 10
  steroid therapy and, 72–73
Adrenocorticosteroid hormone
  adrenal insufficiency and, 73
  Cushing's disease and, 164–165
  pituitary tumor and, 163
Advanced life support, 510, 511–514
Agonist, antagonist versus, 245
Agonist-antagonist opioid, chronic pain and, 427
AIDS, 74t, 74–78, 75t, 77t
  electroconvulsive therapy and, 183
  preoperative testing for, 19
Air bubble, cardiac surgery and, 135
Air embolism

head and neck cancer and, 259
  mediastinoscopy and, 291
Airway
  adenotonsillectomy and, 276, 280–281
  asthma and, 23–27
  burn injury and, 398
  cardiac arrest and, 5
  cardiopulmonary resuscitation and, 511
  cesarean delivery and, 359
  craniofacial reconstruction and, 262, 263–264
  head and neck cancer and, 257
  laryngotracheitis and, 235
  meconium staining and, 370–371
  myocardial contusion and, 391
  otolaryngologic procedures and, 251–282
  supraglottitis and, 233–235, 234t
  tracheal reconstruction and, 272–274, 274–275
Alcohol abuse
  abdominal trauma and, 395
  preoperative management and, 39
Alcohol block, 439
  celiac plexus and, 445
Alcoholic hepatitis, 41
Algorithm
  anemia and, 55, 56f
  cesarean section and, 365f
  jaundice and, 40f
Alkaline phosphatase, 40
Alkalosis
  postoperative, 483–484
  postoperative unresponsivenss and, 503
  respiratory, 142
Allen's test, 473
Allergic reaction
  neurologic disorder and, 175
  preoperative medication for, 10
Alpha-adrenergic agent, 9
Alpha-adrenergic blocking agent
  pheochromocytoma and, 315
  sympathetically maintained pain and, 424
Alveolar proteinosis, 294
Alveolar-arterial oxygen gradient, 216
Alveolus, lung hypoplasia and, 211
Ambulatory anesthesia
  for adults, 452–460, 463t, 464t
  for child, 461–464
Amide local anesthetic, 250
Aminophylline, 24, 25f
Amrinone
  aortic surgery and, 98
  ventricular septal defect and, 119
Amyotrophic lateral sclerosis, 65
Analgesia; see also Pain management
  burn injury and, 401
  in children, 242–250
    intrathecal and epidural, 248–249
    local anesthetics for, 249–250
    methadone, 248
    opioid receptors and, 244–246
    patient-controlled anesthesia and, 247–248

pharmacokinetics and, 246–247, 247t
  labor and, 340
  myocardial ischemia and, 37
  pneumonectomy and, 304
  preoperative, 7–8
Anemia, 53, 53t
  myocardial ischemia and, 36
  pregnancy and, 331
  renal disease and, 51
  renal transplantation and, 322
  sickle cell, 55
Aneurysm
  abdominal aortic, 139–144
    epidural anesthesia and, 412
  aortic, mediastinoscopy for, 291
  central nervous system, 158t, 158–162
  giant, 161–162, 176t
  thoracic aortic, 144–148
Angina pectoris
  outpatient anesthesia and, 456
  stellate ganglion block for, 441
Angiography
  coronary, 4
  neurologic disorder and, 176t, 179
Angiotensin-converting enzyme inhibitor, 31
Ankle nerve block, 198–199
Antacid
  aspiration prophylaxis and, 9
  pregnancy and, 334
Antagonist versus agonist, 245
Anterior percutaneous approach for celiac plexus block, 444–445
Anterior spinal cord syndrome, 379
Antibiotic
  necrotizing enterocolitis and, 229–230
  preoperative administration of, 10
  prolonged neuromuscular blockade and, 495
  unresponsiveness and, 502
Anticholinergic
  asthma and, 25
  preoperative administration of, 9–10
Anticholinergic eyedrops, 205
Anticoagulant
  epidural anesthesia and, 406
  native, 486–487
  ventricular septal defect and, 118
Anticonvulsant therapy
  chronic pain and, 429
  preeclampsia and, 350–351
Antidepressant
  chronic pain and, 428–429
  electroconvulsive therapy and, 183
Antihistamine, chronic pain and, 430
Antihypertensive agent
  central nervous system aneurysm and, 159
  outpatient anesthesia and, 456
  preeclampsia and, 351
  pregnancy-induced hypertension and, 340
Antimuscarinic agent, 252
Antithrombin III, 486
Anxiety
  coronary artery surgery and, 94